Nursing Care *of* Older Adults

Diagnoses, Outcomes, & Interventions

MERIDEAN L. MAAS
PhD, RN, FAAN
Professor and Chair, Adult and Gerontology
Senior Associate Director of Research
Director of Doctoral Studies
University of Iowa College of Nursing
Iowa City, Iowa

KATHLEEN C. BUCKWALTER
PhD, RN, FAAN
Professor
College of Nursing
Associate Provost for Health Sciences
University of Iowa
Iowa City, Iowa

LT. COL. MARY D. HARDY
PhD, RN
Assistant Chief, Nursing Education and Staff
Development
Landstuhl Regional Medical Center
Landstuhl, Germany

TONI TRIPP-REIMER
PhD, RN, FAAN
Professor, Associate Dean for Research
Director
Gerontological Nursing Interventions
Research Center
University of Iowa College of Nursing
Iowa City, Iowa

MARITA G. TITLER
PhD, RN, FAAN
Director, Nursing Research
Department of Nursing Services
University of Iowa Hospitals and Clinics
Iowa City, Iowa

JANET P. SPECHT
PhD, RN, FAAN
Assistant Professor
University of Iowa College of Nursing
Iowa City, Iowa

Mosby

A Harcourt Health Sciences Company

St. Louis   London   Philadelphia   Sydney   Toronto

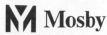
Mosby
A Harcourt Health Sciences Company

Vice President, Nursing Editorial Director: Sally Schrefer
Senior Editor: Michael S. Ledbetter
Senior Developmental Editor: Laurie K. Muench
Project Manager: John Rogers
Senior Production Editor: Mary Turner
Designer: Kathi Gosche
Cover Photograph: Steve "Stone" Taylor, Copyright ©2000.

FIRST EDITION

NOTICE

Pharmacology is an ever-changing field. Standard safety precautions must be followed, but as new research and clinical experience broaden our knowledge, changes in treatment and drug therapy may become necessary or appropriate. Readers are advised to check the most current product information provided by the manufacturer of each drug to be administered to verify the recommended dose, the method and duration of administration, and contraindications. It is the responsibility of the appropriately licensed health care provider, relying on experience and knowledge of the patient, to determine dosages and the best treatment for each individual patient. Neither the publisher nor the editor assumes any liability for any injury and/or damage to persons or property arising from this publication.

Mosby, Inc.

A Harcourt Health Sciences Company
11830 Westline Industrial Drive
St. Louis, Missouri 63146

Printed in the United States of America
Library of Congress Cataloging-in-Publication Data

Nursing care of older adults : diagnoses, outcomes & interventions / Meridean L. Maas
... [et al.].
   p. cm.
  Includes bibliographical references and index.
  ISBN 0-323-01259-0
    1. Geriatric nursing.   I. Maas, Meridean.

RC954 .N8825 2000
610.73'65—dc21
                                              00-045203

00 01 02 03 04 CL/MVY 9 8 7 6 5 4 3 2 1

CONTRIBUTORS

Jackie Akins, MA, RN, C
Nurse Clinician
Iowa Veterans Home
Marshalltown, Iowa

Jane M. Armer, PhD, RN, C
Associate Professor, Sinclair School of Nursing
Co-Director, Office of Research
University of Missouri—Columbia
Columbia, Missouri

Capt. Kathleen L. Atkins, RD, CNSD, LD
Consultant
USAR—United States Army
Columbus, Georgia

Mary Blegen, PhD, RN
Professor, School of Nursing
University of Colorado Health Science Center
Denver, Colorado

Karen S. Brasfield, RD
Certified Nutrition Support Dietitian
American Dietetic Association
Alexandria, Virginia

Veronica A. Brighton, MA, ARNP, CS
Lecturer
University of Iowa
Iowa City, Iowa

Donna Bunten, MA, RN, CNS
Staff Educator
VA Central Iowa Health Care System
Knoxville, Iowa

Cheryl Carter, RN, BSN, CIC
Nurse Epidemiologist
University of Iowa Hospitals and Clinics
Iowa City, Iowa

Patricia Clinton, PhD, RN, PNP
Clinical Assistant Professor, College of Nursing
University of Iowa
Iowa City, Iowa

Clare E. Collins, PhD, RN, FAAN
Professor, College of Nursing
Michigan State University
East Lansing, Michigan

Vickie S. Conn, PhD, RN
Potter Brinton Distinguished Professor
Director, Office of Research
Sinclair School of Nursing
University of Missouri—Columbia
Columbia, Missouri

Perle Slavik Cowen, PhD, RN
Associate Professor, College of Nursing
University of Iowa
Iowa City, Iowa

Kennith R. Culp, PhD, RN
Associate Professor, College of Nursing
University of Iowa
Iowa City, Iowa

Ruth E. Davidhizar, RN, DNS, CS, FAAN
Dean of Nursing
Bethel College
Mishawaka, Indiana

Linda Lindsey Davis, PhD, RN
Professor, School of Nursing
Senior Scientist, Center for Aging
University of Alabama at Birmingham
Birmingham, Alabama

Sheila A. Decker, MSN, RN, GNP
Instructor/Director of GNP Program, School of Nursing
Vanderbilt University
Nashville, Tennessee

Danielle N. DeVoss, MA
Doctoral Student, Humanities Department
Michigan Technological University
Houghton, Michigan

Cynthia M. Dougherty, PhD, RN, ARNP
Research Assistant Professor, Nurse Practitioner
School of Nursing
University of Washington
Seattle, Washington

Jan Drury, MA, RN
Administrator of Nursing
Iowa Veterans Home
Marshalltown, Iowa

Brenda Emick-Herring, MSN, RN, CRRN
Staff Development Specialist, Admission Liaison
Yamker Rehabilitation Center, Iowa Rehabilitation Network
Des Moines, Iowa

Carol J. Farran, DNSc, RN, FAAN
Professor, College of Nursing
Rush University College
Chicago, Illinois

Rita A. Frantz, PhD, RN, FAAN
Professor, College of Nursing
University of Iowa
Iowa City, Iowa

Col. Gwendolyn Fryer, MSN, RN
Chief, Army Nurse Branch, Headquarters
United States Army Recruiting Command
Fort Knox, Kentucky

Phyllis Gaspar, PhD, RN
Associate Professor
Winona State University
Winona, Minnesota

Linda A. Gerdner, PhD, RN
Post Doctoral Fellow/Instructor
Department of Psychiatry, Veteran's Administration
University of Arkansas for Medical Sciences
Little Rock, Arkansas

Joyce Newman Giger, EdD, RN, CS, FAAN
Professor of Graduate Studies, School of Nursing
University of Alabama at Birmingham
Birmingham, Alabama

Barbara A. Given, PhD, RN, FAAN
Professor of Nursing
Michigan State University
East Lansing, Michigan

Charles W. Given, PhD
Professor
Michigan State University
East Lansing, Michigan

Orpha J. Glick, PhD, RN
Associate Professor Emeritus, College of Nursing
University of Iowa
Iowa City, Iowa

Carla J. Groh, PhD, RN
Associate Professor
University of Detroit Mercy
Detroit, Michigan

Geri Richards Hall, PhD, ARNP, CS, FAAN
Associate Director for Outreach
University of Iowa Center on Aging
Iowa City, Iowa

Margo Halm, MA, RN, CCRN, CS
Advanced Practice Nurse
United Hospital
St. Paul, Minnesota

Pamela Harvey, DO, MHA, MA
Intern
U.S. Naval Hospital
San Diego, California

Karen S. Hayes, PhD, ARNP, CS
Assistant Professor
Wichita State University
Wichita, Kansas

Barbara J. Head, PhD, RN
Research Associate, Center for Nursing Classification
University of Iowa
Iowa City, Iowa

Keela A. Herr, PhD, RN
Associate Professor, College of Nursing
University of Iowa
Iowa City, Iowa

Barbara J. Holtzclaw, PhD, RN, FAAN
Associate Dean for Research/Director of Doctoral Studies/
  Hugh Roy Cullen Professor of Nursing, School of
  Nursing
University of Texas Health Science Center at San Antonio
San Antonio, Texas

Julie K. Hudson, MS, RD
Chief, Nutrition Care Division
Bassett Army Community Hospital
Fort Wainwright, Alaska

Todd N. Ingram, MA, RN
Lecturer, Clinical Nursing Specialist, College of Nursing
University of Iowa
Iowa City, Iowa

Ada Jacox, PhD, RN, FAAN
Associate Dean for Research, College of Nursing
Wayne State University
Detroit, Michigan

Rebecca A. Johnson, PhD, RN
Millsap Professor of Gerontological Nursing and Public
    Policy, Sinclair School of Nursing
University of Missouri—Columbia
Columbia, Missouri

Sharon L. Kozachik, MSN, RN
Project Manager
Family Care Studies, Walther Cancer Institute
Michigan State University
East Lansing, Michigan

Mary Kundrat, MA, RN
Nurse Researcher
VA Central Iowa Health Care System
Des Moines, Iowa

Priscilla LeMone, DSN, RN, FAAN
Associate Professor, Associate Dean—Undergraduate
    Program
Sinclair School of Nursing
University of Missouri—Columbia
Columbia, Missouri

Anne Lewis, MA, RN
Neuroscience Clinical Nurse Specialist
Genesis Medical Center
Davenport, Iowa

Susan Malan, MSN, RN, CRRN
Care Coordinator, Primary Care
Harry S. Truman Memorial Veterans Hospital
Columbia, Missouri

Maire B. McAnaw, MPT, PT
Senior Trauma Therapist
University of North Carolina Hospitals
Chapel Hill, North Carolina

Colette L. McKinney, BSN, RN
Officer in Charge, Primary Care Clinic
U.S. Army Nurse Corps
Fort Wainwright, Alaska

Audrey M. McLane, PhD, RN
Professor Emerita
Marquette University
Milwaukee, Wisconsin

Ruth E. McShane, PhD, RN
RN/BSN/MSN Program Coordinator, Clinical Assistant
    Professor, College of Nursing
Marquette University
Milwaukee, Wisconsin

Janet Mentes, PhD, MS, RNCS, GNP
Assistant Professor, School of Nursing
University of California at Los Angeles
Los Angeles, California

Paula Mobily, PhD, RN
Associate Professor, College of Nursing
University of Iowa
Iowa City, Iowa

Laurie Moore, MSN, RN, GNP
Nurse Practitioner, Extended Care Unit
Department of Veterans Affairs Medical Center
Decatur, Georgia

Sue A. Moorhead, PhD, RN
Associate Professor, College of Nursing
University of Iowa
Iowa City, Iowa

Mary Lynn Piven, MS, RN
Research Assistant, School of Nursing
University of North Carolina at Chapel Hill
Chapel Hill, North Carolina

Lori Popejoy, RN, MSN, CS, GCNS
Long-Term Care Research Nurse
University of Missouri—Columbia
Columbia, Missouri

Jean M. Pottinger, MA, RN, CIC
Nurse Epidemiologist
University of Iowa Hospitals and Clinics
Iowa City, Iowa

Marilyn J. Rantz, PhD, NHA
Professor, Sinclair School of Nursing
University of Missouri—Columbia
Columbia, Missouri

Carla Gene Rapp, PhD, RN
Postdoctoral Fellow, Department of Veterans Affairs,
    Health Services Research and Development; Instructor,
    Department of Psychiatry
University of Arkansas for Medical Sciences
Little Rock, Arkansas

Jean L. Reese, PhD, RN
Associate Professor Emerita
University of Iowa
Iowa City, Iowa

Chris Ressler, MSN, BA, FNP, GNP, ARNP-C
Nurse Practitioner
Mercy Family Clinic
Charles City, Iowa

Deborah Perry Schoenfelder, PhD, RN
Clinical Assistant Professor, College of Nursing
University of Iowa
Iowa City, Iowa

Joanne Sabol Stevenson, PhD, RN, FAAN
Professor, Associate Dean for Academic Affairs and
    Research, College of Nursing
Rutgers, The State University of New Jersey
Newark, New Jersey

Jacqueline M. Stolley, PhD, RN, CS
Professor
Trinity College of Nursing
Moline, Illinois

Elizabeth A. Swanson, PhD, RN
Associate Professor, College of Nursing
University of Iowa
Iowa City, Iowa

LuAnn Tandy, RN
Assistant Manager, Patient Access and Referral Services
University of Missouri Health Sciences Center
Columbia, Missouri

Karen R. Wadle, MA, RN
Chief, Education and Research Service
VA Central Iowa Health Care System
Knoxville, Iowa

Bonnie Wakefield, PhD, RN
Research Scientist, VA Medical Center
Clinical Assistant Professor, College of Nursing
University of Iowa
Iowa City, Iowa

James D. Waterman, MS, RN
Instructor, Department of Nursing
William Jewell College
Liberty, Missouri

Kay Weiler, JD, MA, RN
Associate Professor, College of Nursing
University of Iowa
Iowa City, Iowa

Elizabeth A. Weitzel, MA, RN
Parish Health Nurse
First Presbyterian Church
Marshalltown, Iowa

Ann L. Whall, PhD, RN, FAAN
Professor, Associate Director, School of Nursing
University of Michigan
Ann Arbor, Michigan

Gwen Whiting, MS, RN
Psychiatric Clinical Specialist
Mary's Place: Center for Health and Healing
Cary, Illinois

Lore K. Wright, PhD, RN, CS, FAAN
Professor, School of Nursing
Medical College of Georgia
Augusta, Georgia

Mary Zwygart-Stauffacher, PhD, RN, CS, GNP, GCNS
Associate Professor, School of Nursing
University of Minnesota
Minneapolis, Minnesota

REVIEWERS

Charlé C.F. Avery, MSN, RN, CS, ANP, GNP
Adult/Gerontologic Nurse Practitioner
Baylor Senior Health Center
Dallas, Texas

Tamara Espejo, RN, BS
Chief Nursing Officer
San Dimas Community Hospital
San Dimas, California

Stephanie D. Garrison, DSN
Associate Professor, College of Nursing
University of South Alabama
Mobile, Alabama

Joyce I. Harter, MSN, RN, CS, ANP, GNP
Adult/Gerontologic Nurse Practitioner
Baylor Senior Health Center
Dallas, Texas

Dorothy G. Herron, PhD, RN, CS
Assistant Professor, School of Nursing
University of Maryland
Baltimore, Maryland

Mary H. Housley, RN, CS, MS, GNP
Nurse Practitioner
Ho, Massa, Steyer, & Coskey
Burlingame, California

Barbara H. Kemerer, MSN, MBA
Assistant Professor, Department of Nursing
Shepherd College
Shepherdstown, West Virginia

Sharon Lambert, DNS, RN
Assistant Professor
McKendree College
Lebanon, Illinois

Laura Talbot, RN, CS, EdD, PhD
Program Director for Geriatric Nursing
Johns Hopkins University School of Nursing
Baltimore, Maryland

PREFACE

Since the First National Conference on the Classification of Nursing Diagnoses was held in St. Louis in 1973, interest in standardized languages to describe nursing phenomena among nurses in all practice settings and roles has steadily increased. The impact of the nursing diagnosis movement has reached every aspect of the profession. The North American Nursing Diagnosis Association (NANDA) maintains the NANDA Classification of Nursing Diagnoses (NANDA, 1999). More recently, the *Nursing Outcomes Classification (NOC)* and the *Nursing Interventions Classification (NIC)* were developed at The University of Iowa (Iowa Intervention Project, 2000; Iowa Outcomes Project, 2000). NANDA, NOC, and NIC are each comprehensive of all clinical specialties and care settings, and linkages among the classifications have been developed for clinical testing. The increasing use of standardized nursing languages, especially in nursing clinical information systems and practice, has stimulated research to describe the prevalence of diagnoses in specific populations, to validate and refine the classifications, to evaluate and sharpen diagnostic reasoning skills, and to test the outcomes of intervention strategies.

PURPOSE OF THE BOOK

This book is devoted to a discussion of nursing diagnoses, outcomes, and interventions for elderly persons. As such, the diagnoses selected for the volume are not exhaustive but represent a severely underdeveloped knowledge base. We have chosen diagnoses based on existing research of prevalence in the population and on our judgments as to the diagnoses that should be developed and shared with nurses (see Introduction).

Although most of the diagnoses included herein have been accepted for clinical testing by NANDA (NANDA, 1999), some are specific types of more general diagnoses; e.g., Risk for Poisoning: Drug Toxicity is viewed as a specific type of Risk for Poisoning. Other diagnoses that have not been approved by NANDA (e.g., Depression) are included because they are frequent and difficult-to-manage problems that nurses encounter among elders. Our intent is to expand the conceptual and operational development of the diagnoses, outcomes, and interventions; amplify discussion of their linkages to increase clinical usefulness; and promote further development and testing by nurse clinicians and researchers. Most of the labels and content of the diagnoses, outcomes, and interventions are consistent with those published by NANDA, NOC, and NIC

unless otherwise indicated. In a number of chapters diagnoses, outcomes, and interventions are compared with the published classifications with rationale provided for exceptions. In some chapters, however, it is left to the reader to determine whether or not the diagnoses, outcomes, and interventions are included in current classifications. Chapter authors were encouraged to critique existing standardized nomenclatures and to identify and develop new or revised diagnoses, outcomes, and interventions that were needed for the best and most useful practices in caring for elders.

ORGANIZATION

The book is organized in 11 parts, each representing one of Gordon's Functional Health Patterns (1994). Within each of the 11 parts, there is an overview and a brief chapter on normal aging. Most chapters within a part are organized as follows, although there are some exceptions. In most chapters outcomes are discussed before interventions. This is because in the natural sequence of clinical reasoning desired outcomes are identified before selection of interventions to achieve the outcomes. We allowed the authors some latitude in the organization of their chapters; however, overall there is substantial consistency of format.

I. Introduction and Presentation of the Nursing Diagnosis Concept
II. Significance to the Elder
III. Current Status of the Diagnosis: Assessment and Diagnosis
IV. Outcomes Sensitive to Nursing Intervention
V. Nursing Intervention Strategies
VI. Presentation of Case Study(s)
VII. Summary

In the Epilogue Jacox provides a discussion of salient issues regarding nursing diagnosis, the management of elders' care, and the emergence of standardized nursing languages. The implications she outlines for theory building, research, and clinical practice raise questions for debate and resolution.

PEDAGOGY

The aspects of normal aging that begin every Functional Health Pattern part are used to evaluate pathologic parameters for each diagnosis. It is important that readers realize, however, that elders are not a homogenous population, especially those over age 80. What was once thought of as "normal" to aging is now thought of as "usual" (Rowe & Kahn, 1987). Based on a synthesis of the literature, each of the 62 diagnosis chapters presents conceptual definitions and theoretical discussions of the diagnosis, the most relevant outcomes to assess the effectiveness of the interventions, and the nursing interventions selected to treat the diagnosis. Rationale are provided for the linkages of outcomes and interventions with each diagnosis. Diagnoses are presented using the problem label, the etiologies or related factors, and the defining characteristics or signs and symptoms, structural criteria developed by Gordon (1994). Likewise, NIC intervention labels are presented with definitions and specific activities to implement the interventions, and NOC outcome labels are given with definitions and the indicators that are needed to evaluate the status of each outcome. The use of NOC scales to measure the status of patient outcomes at selected intervals and the effectiveness of interventions is illustrated in a number of the chapters.

Significance of the diagnosis for the elderly population is discussed in terms of prevalence, consequences if not treated, predispositions or risk factors, and the importance for nurses to diagnose, treat, and measure outcomes in elders. The research base for the diagnosis, interventions, and outcomes and a critique of assessment tools also are presented, if available. Case studies are used to illustrate assessment data, diagnostic and treatment reasoning, and use of outcomes to assess the effects of interventions. Differential diagnosis is discussed for several problems experienced by elders and treated by nurses.

The majority of chapters highlight one intervention for each diagnosis and illustrate its use in case studies. Other relevant interventions are discussed briefly and may be cross-referenced to a more detailed discussion in another chapter. Readers are cautioned against interpreting diagnosis, intervention, and outcome linkages described in the chapters as "treatments of choice" in every case, because an adequate research base to predict "cause and effect" relationships is often lacking. Instead, nurses must use their judgment in choosing intervention strategies for the highly complex, rapidly changing, and often multicausal problems presented by elders. Further, although NOC outcome indicators have been evaluated for content validity, the indicators and measurement scales have not been validated with clinical data. It is for this reason that many chapters include summary sections with recommendations for future development and testing of the diagnosis, interventions, and outcomes, and their linkages.

THEORETICAL BASE

Although Gordon's Functional Health Patterns (1994), a middle range typology, are used to order and group the di-

agnoses and their linked outcomes and interventions, and the editors subscribe to the view that classifications of nursing diagnoses, interventions, and outcomes contain concepts representing factor isolating and factor relating levels of theory building, we did not otherwise explicitly adopt or attempt to force any particular nursing theory or model on the contributing authors. This fact may account for the varying approaches of some authors. We believe that the development of nursing diagnoses, outcomes, and interventions, along with their linkages, is more likely to be enriched and expanded by this eclectic approach, despite our awareness of NANDA, NOC, and NIC taxonomic structures. We opted to avoid the premature closure that a more explicit use of one particular taxonomy or theory might produce by encouraging authors to challenge and expand existing taxonomies. Again, authors were asked to critique existing diagnoses, outcomes, and interventions, to suggest modifications or alternative ideas, and to describe rationale for their alternatives.

CONTRIBUTORS

The authors were identified by the editors as doing research and/or having published in the area of the diagnosis. We also looked for contributors who could translate their research into the clinical reality of use to nurses in a variety of clinical settings. The editors are grateful to each of the contributing authors who raised important questions and provided their scholarship to make the book a reality. Perhaps we have benefited more than anyone from the challenge to ourselves and the authors to extend knowledge about nursing diagnoses, interventions, and outcomes that are responsive to the nursing care of elders.

ACKNOWLEDGMENTS

Many persons have contributed to the production of this book—some directly and others through support and encouragement of the editors over lifetimes and careers. Certainly, we are grateful to Linda Curran, who dedicated her time and skill to coordinating, editing, and processing the manuscript. We appreciate the contributors to the book *Nursing Diagnoses and Interventions for the Elderly* (1991). Without their contributions, this book also would not be possible. Our principal mentors, Ada Jacox, PhD, RN, FAAN, Myrtle Kitchell Aydelotte, PhD, RN, FAAN, and Joanne Stevenson, PhD, RN, FAAN, deserve acknowledgment. Finally, the book is dedicated to our parents, some deceased, who reared us to admire and value older persons and to see a project through to the end: Kenneth James and Miriam Jane Speas, Bill and Gertrude Coen, Arthur Hans Anderson and Helen Hart Anderson, Charles Robert Tripp and Harriett Jean Davis Tripp, Eugene Joseph Ball and Vlma Nadine Bowser Ball, Jean Moore Pringle and Anna Mae Struthers McCoy.

The aging aren't only the old: the aging are all of us.
  Alexandra Robbin
Of all the self-fulfilling prophecies in our culture, the assumption that aging means decline and poor health is probably the deadliest.
  Marilyn Ferguson
Age puzzles me. I thought it was a quiet time. My seventies were interesting and fairly serene, but my eighties are passionate. I grow more intense as I age.
  Florida Scott-Maxwell

We did not change as we grew older; we just became more clearly ourselves.
  Lynn Hall

Meridean L. Maas
Kathleen C. Buckwalter
Mary D. Hardy
Toni Tripp-Reimer
Marita G. Titler
Janet P. Specht

REFERENCES

Gordon, M. (1994). *Nursing diagnosis: Process and application* (3rd ed.). St. Louis, MO: Mosby.

Iowa Intervention Project. J. C. McCloskey & G. M. Bulechek (Eds.). (2000). *Nursing interventions classification (NIC)* (3rd ed.). St. Louis, MO: Mosby.

Iowa Outcomes Project. M. Johnson, M. Maas, & S. Moorhead (Eds.). (2000). *Nursing outcomes classification (NOC)* (2nd ed.). St. Louis, MO: Mosby.

Maas, M., Buckwalter, K. C., & Hardy, M. (Eds.) (1991). *Nursing diagnoses and interventions for the elderly.* Redwood City, CA: Addison-Wesley Nursing.

North American Nursing Diagnosis Association. (1999). *Nursing diagnoses: Definitions & classification 1999-2000.* Philadelphia: Author.

Rowe, J., & Kahn, R. (1987). Human aging: Usual and successful. *Science, 237,* 143-149.

INTRODUCTION: NURSING DIAGNOSES, NURSING-SENSITIVE OUTCOMES, AND NURSING INTERVENTIONS FOR ELDERS— EPIDEMIOLOGIC RATIONALE

Demographic trends have affected and will continue to affect both the future of long-term care services and the nurses who diagnose and treat responses to actual and potential illnesses in elders. Since 1900 the percentage of people in the United States age 65 and older has more than tripled (4.1% in 1900 to 12.8% in 1995), increasing nearly 11 times from 3.1 million to 33.5 million, representing about 1 in every 8 people in the United States. By 2030 there will be about 70 million older persons, more than twice their number in 1990, projected to be 20% of the total U.S. population. The older population itself also is getting older. In 1995 the 65-to-74 age-group (18.8 million) was 8 times larger than in 1900, but the 75- to 84-year-old group (11.1 million) was 14 times larger, and the 85-years-and-older group (3.6 million) was 29 times larger (U.S. Bureau of the Census, 1996).

At present, about 70% of the population can expect to live beyond age 65. Seventeen percent of these persons will survive to age 85, a percentage that will increase to over 50% according to projections for the year 2050. In 1995 persons reaching age 65 had an average life expectancy of an additional 17.4 years (18.9 years for females and 15.6 years for males); however, the majority of gain in life expectancy has been due to reduced death rates for children and young adults (U.S. Bureau of the Census, 1996).

The female population age 85 and older is expected to triple between 1980 and 2030. This segment of the population is more often single or widowed and thus at increased risk of needing long-term care assistance (Davis, 1986; U.S. Bureau of the Census, 1996). Minority populations are expected to represent 25% of elderly persons in 2030, up from 13% in 1990. Between 1990 and 2030, the white, non-Hispanic population 65 years and older is projected to increase by only 91% compared with 328% for older minorities, including Hispanics (570%) and non-Hispanic blacks (159%); American Indians, Eskimos, and Aleuts (294%); and Asians and Pacific Islanders (643%).

These elders may live within the community in a variety of settings ranging from high rises for elders to their own homes, or they may be institutionalized. Many, if not most, will be in a dependent role at least sometime during their remaining years, whether they are hospitalized, placed in a nursing home, or cared for at home by professionals and/or family caregivers.

Along with the rapid growth in the percentage of the population age 65 and older, there has been an even more dramatic increase in long-term care options. Accompanying a dramatic growth in home health care, more nursing homes are larger and offer more specialized nursing services (e.g., rehabilitation, subacute, dementia care), and there are a greater variety of housing and health care services along the long-term care continuum, such as Assisted Living. The number of nursing homes has decreased by 13% since 1985, but the number of beds has increased by 9%. The number of nursing home residents, however, was up only 4% between 1985 and 1995, despite an 18% increase in the age-65-and-older population. More than 35% of these nursing home residents were age 85 and older and predominantly white (88%) and female (72%) (National Center for Health Statistics [NCHS], 1995).

The aforementioned statistics suggest that the demand for cost-effective nursing care of elders will be enormous. This demand will make the development of nursing knowledge and practice applications around standardized nursing diagnoses, interventions, and outcomes that are sensitive to nursing imperative. Further, the development of knowledge to inform practice and influence policy makers will largely depend on the use of standardized nursing nomenclatures in clinical information systems. Inclusion of standardized nursing languages in clinical information systems will enable the construction and analysis of large local and national nursing databases, as well as the inclusion of nursing data in interdisciplinary data sets that can be used to assess the outcome effectiveness of all health care interventions (Iowa Outcomes Project, 2000; Maas, Johnson, & Moorhead, 1996).

Because of the deinstitutionalization movement, many elderly individuals were discharged from mental institutions and relocated in community long-term care facilities (Liptzin, 1986) or to communities. Some who were not relocated to community institutions and were unable to maintain "homes" because of a lack of support from community mental health systems account for the increase in homeless persons in the United States. In fact, today's nursing homes have been labeled modern-day "geropsychiatric ghettos," and many of the most challenging problems faced by nurses in these facilities are related to the emotional and behavioral disturbances and cognitive impairments of residents (Liptzin, 1986). It is estimated that 70% to 80% of nursing home residents have psychiatric problems (Dellasaga, 1991; Rovner, 1985; Roybal, 1984; Shea, Smyer, & Streit, 1994; Smith, Mitchell, & Buckwalter, 1995). Mental problems may influence whether an elderly person is able to manage at home or needs to enter a nursing home. Moreover, mental problems can develop after institutionalization. Therefore this book includes a number of relevant psychosocial nursing diagnoses, outcomes, and interventions that are responsive to nursing. Some examples of diagnoses are Chronic Confusion, Acute Confusion, Grieving, Depression, Body Image Disturbance, Fear, Anxiety, Powerlessness, Social Isolation, and Risk for Violence: Self-Directed or Directed at Others. Likewise, relevant psychosocial nursing interventions are discussed, such as Dementia Management, Counseling, Seclusion, Anxiety Reduction, and Grief Work Facilitation (Iowa Intervention Project, 2000), as are corresponding outcome states, including Anxiety Control, Information Processing, Mood Equilibrium, and Impulse Control (Iowa Outcomes Project, 2000). The elaboration of assessment, diagnosis, outcome measurement, and intervention strategies is intended to help prepare nurses to correct some of the inattention to psychosocial problems in elders. Attention to the signs, symptoms, and etiologies/related factors that distinguish psychosocial diagnoses is intended to help prevent misdiagnosis, enhance the appropriate selection of interventions, and focus measurement of progress on the most relevant outcomes.

Many elders also experience a number of chronic physical conditions that affect their functional health status and ability to perform activities of daily living (ADL). Because many elders have one or more chronic illnesses, responses to these illnesses combined with functional losses require nursing diagnosis and intervention if elders are to achieve optimal prevention, maintenance, and diagnosis-resolution outcomes.

The nursing diagnoses that are the most common functional responses to chronic illness also are reflected in the content of the book. Examples include Self-Care Deficit; Diversional Activity Deficit; Sexual Dysfunction; Impaired Physical Mobility; Activity Intolerance; Risk for Poisoning: Drug Toxicity; Bowel Incontinence; Impaired Skin Integrity; Impaired Verbal Communication; Risk for Injury: Falls;

and Altered Health Maintenance. The prevention and treatment of these problems are critical to the ability of elderly persons to be optimally independent in a variety of areas of daily living. Rehabilitation, encompassing prevention and optimization of healthy responses, is the appropriate approach, although it has not been a high-priority service for elders in our society (Brody, 1985). Nurses could do much to make rehabilitation a priority for elders, although concerted efforts to influence health policy makers to reimburse nurses to deliver these services will likely have to be successful before substantial gains are made. Nonetheless, it is important that knowledge about nursing diagnosis, intervention, and outcome effectiveness be further developed.

Research to validate nursing diagnoses among elderly and chronically ill persons has been limited. The work of Hoskins, McFarlane, Rubenfeld, Schreier, and Walsh (1986) on the validation of nursing diagnoses in the chronically ill is one of the first published studies that described nursing diagnoses among this population. Although no data on the frequency of the nursing diagnoses were reported by Hoskins et al. (1986) and the labels were somewhat different from those found in the North American Nursing Diagnosis Association (NANDA) taxonomy, most of the 51 nursing diagnoses found in their sample of community-dwelling chronically ill persons are represented in this book. Among those especially relevant to chronically ill persons are Sexual Dysfunction, Fear, Body Image Disturbance, Social Isolation, Anxiety, and Knowledge Deficit. A few prevalence studies of nursing diagnoses among elders and long-term care residents have been conducted by Hallal (1985); Leslie (1981); Rantz and colleagues (Rantz & Miller, 1987; Rantz, Miller, & Jacobs, 1985); and Hardy and associates (Hardy, Maas, & Akins, 1988). More recently, Daly and colleagues (Daly, Maas, & Buckwalter, 1995a, 1995b; Daly, Maas, McCloskey, & Bulechek, 1996) reported prevalence of nursing diagnoses and use of *Nursing Interventions Classification (NIC)* interventions (Iowa Intervention Project, 2000) in one long-term care setting.

Rantz and colleagues (Rantz, Vinz-Miller, & Matson, 1995) evaluated trends in nursing diagnoses of residents in a long-term care facility over a 10-year period. Similar to the most frequent diagnoses reported by Hallal (1985), Leslie (1981), and Hardy et al. (1988), they found Altered Nutrition: Less Than Body Requirements; Potential for Impaired Skin Integrity; Elimination Management Deficit; Decreased Cardiac Output; Impaired Physical Mobility; Self-Care Deficit; and Altered Thought Processes to be most frequent in both 1984 and 1993, although in 1993 Potential High Risk for Falls was added to the list of the most frequent diagnoses. Rantz et al. reported an increasing linear trend over the 10-year period for Altered Nutrition: Less Than Body Requirements; Potential for Fluid Volume Deficit; Fluid Volume Deficit; Elimination Management Deficit; Altered Peripheral Tissue Perfusion; Self-Care Deficit; and Depression. Decreasing linear trends were found for Potential for Infection; Potential for Trauma: Falls; Potential for Altered Nutrition: More Than Body Requirements; Potential for Impaired Skin Integrity;

Potential for Altered Neurological Status; Potential for Diversional Activity Deficit; Social Isolation; and Potential for Social Isolation. These results may reflect increases in the number and quality of activity programs and the heightened attention to therapeutic basic nursing care for problems such as skin, nutrition, and falls.

Several other important nursing diagnoses also emanate from the chronic physical illnesses that commonly affect the dependent elder (e.g., chronic obstructive pulmonary disease, cerebral vascular accident, pneumonia, heart disease, diabetes, cancer, arteriosclerosis), including Fluid Volume Deficit, Decreased Cardiac Output, Ineffective Breathing Pattern, Altered Tissue Perfusion, and Pain. Because nurses are the principal case managers of long-term health care, it is imperative that they are prepared to identify, intervene, and monitor the physiologic sequelae of common chronic illnesses. Prompt attention by nurses is essential for preventing acute exacerbation of the underlying pathology, for preventing unnecessary deterioration of the elderly person's physical condition, and for maintaining optimum mental and physical function.

Since the earlier published reports of the validation and prevalence of nursing diagnoses, the results of many studies reporting validation and prevalence have been published, many in the journal *Nursing Diagnosis*. The *Nursing Outcomes Classification (NOC)* (Iowa Outcomes Project, 2000) and *Nursing Interventions Classification (NIC)* (Iowa Intervention Project, 2000) research teams have evaluated the content validity of the standardized interventions and outcomes using expert nurse review. These teams also have conducted surveys of nurse experts in specialty practices regarding the use of NIC interventions and NOC outcomes; however, few clinical validation and use studies with patient populations have been reported. This is primarily due to the lengthy period required for inclusion of these languages in computerized clinical information systems and the slow development of the electronic patient record. Once NANDA, NOC, and NIC are included in clinical care planning and documentation systems, the databases needed for research will be available and an increase in nursing research to validate the phenomena and the linkages among diagnoses, interventions, and outcomes will markedly increase.

More than 25 diagnoses reported by at least one of the published prevalence studies are discussed in separate chapters of this book, including all of the diagnoses that were found to be among the 5 most prevalent in all of the studies. The editors added chapters to foster more detailed discussion of diagnoses that are specific types of more general nursing diagnoses and some that are characteristic of elderly persons in other settings, including discussions of health promoting behaviors, home maintenance management, and family caregiving. Finally, the editors, who have extensive knowledge and experience with nursing care of elders, have included diagnoses such as Depression; Activity Intolerance; Spiritual Distress; Altered Role Performance: Risk for Loss of Right of Self-Determination; and Altered Family Processes. These diagnoses are often poorly assessed and treated, and many are secondary to physical conditions and other losses that accompany aging.

Many NIC interventions and NOC outcomes also are described as they are relevant for each of the nursing diagnoses. Chapter authors were encouraged to illustrate the diagnoses and use of interventions and outcomes with case studies and to provide rationale for their use. The content of the book was designed to promote nurses' awareness of the occurrence of the diagnoses and to add to nurses' ability to recognize defining characteristics, make the appropriate diagnosis, select the pertinent outcomes to monitor and evaluate the elder's status, and prescribe the correct interventions. Finally, the content is intended to promote conceptual development and clinical validation of the diagnoses, interventions, and outcomes and to foster nursing effectiveness and efficacy research. Gordon's effort (1997) to validate nursing diagnoses among rehabilitation patients and to identify linkages among highly prevalent diagnoses and interventions and outcomes is an example of research that will hopefully be facilitated by the book. NOC outcomes are currently being tested for reliability and validity using clinical data (Iowa Outcomes Project, 2000).

Today's health care environment has been transformed into one that demands evidence-based practice and the use of quality indicators. Johnson and Maas (Iowa Outcomes Project, 2000) mention the growth of outcome and effectiveness research in nursing. Rather than intuition, this new paradigm stipulates the need for research evidence as the basis for practice. There also is an increase in the development of protocols and guidelines for use in a variety of practice settings, with registered nurses assuming the role of case manager or care coordinator, for which good, comprehensive assessment and care planning skills are essential. We included the use of standardized nursing diagnoses, interventions, and outcomes in the development of this book to assist nurses with assessment, diagnostic reasoning, and the evaluation of outcome effectiveness. Although the majority of nursing diagnoses, nursing-sensitive outcomes, and nursing interventions are those published by NANDA (1999), Iowa Outcomes Project (2000), and Iowa Intervention Project (2000), some included are not. Because no language classification is static, authors were encouraged to develop diagnoses, outcomes, and interventions for potential future inclusion in the classifications. The book will assist nurses to identify critical gaps and future research needs to support nursing practice and will illustrate why the use and documentation of nurses' decisions and actions using the standardized languages in computerized systems are essential for the development of evidence-based practice and to influence health policy decisions that benefit elders.

Meridean L. Maas
Kathleen C. Buckwalter
Mary D. Hardy
Toni Tripp-Reimer
Marita G. Titler
Janet P. Specht

REFERENCES

Brody, J. A. (1985). Rehabilitation and nursing homes. In E. L. Schneider (Ed.), *The teaching nursing home* (pp. 147-156). New York: Raven Press.

Daly, J. M., Maas, M., & Buckwalter, K. (1995a). Use of standardized nursing diagnoses (NANDA) and interventions (NIC) in long-term care. *Journal of Gerontological Nursing, 21*(8), 29-36.

Daly, J. M., Maas, M. L., & Buckwalter, K. C. (1995b). What nursing diagnoses do nurses use in long term care? *The Director, 3*(3), 115, 118-120, 123.

Daly, J., Maas, M., McCloskey, J., & Bulechek, G. (1996). A care planning tool that proves what we do. *RN, 59*(6), 26-29.

Davis, K. (1986). Paying the health bills of an aging population. In A. Pifer & I. Broute (Eds.), *Our aging society: Paradox and promise* (pp. 299-318). New York: W.W. Norton.

Dellasaga, C. (1991). Meeting the mental health needs of elderly clients. *Journal of Psychosocial Nursing, 29*(2), 10-14.

Gordon, M. (1997). Report of an RNF study to identify intervention-outcome links for highly prevalent nursing diagnoses. *Rehabilitation Nursing Research, 5*(4), 116-125.

Hallal, J. (1985). Nursing diagnosis: An essential step to quality care. *Journal of Gerontological Nursing, 11*(9), 35-38.

Hardy, M. A., Maas, M. L., & Akins, J. (1988). The prevalence of nursing diagnoses among elderly and long term care residents: A descriptive comparison. *Recent Advances in Nursing Science, 21,* 144-158.

Hoskins, L. M., McFarlane, E. A., Rubenfeld, M. G., Schreier, A. M., & Walsh, M. B. (1986). Nursing diagnosis in the chronically ill. In M. E. Harley (Ed.), *Clarification of nursing diagnosis: Proceedings of the sixth conference* (pp. 319-329). St. Louis, MO: Mosby.

Iowa Intervention Project. J. C. McCloskey & G. M. Bulechek (Eds.). (2000). *Nursing interventions classification (NIC)* (3rd ed.). St. Louis, MO: Mosby.

Iowa Outcomes Project. M. Johnson, M. Maas, & S. Moorhead (Eds.). (2000). *Nursing outcomes classification (NOC)* (2nd ed.). St. Louis, MO: Mosby.

Leslie, F. M. (1981). Nursing diagnosis: Use in long term care. *American Journal of Nursing, 81,* 1012-1014.

Liptzin, B. (1986). Major mental disorders/problems in nursing homes: Implications for research and public policy. In M. Harper (Ed.), *Mental illness in nursing homes: Agenda for research.* Washington, D.C.: U.S. Government Printing Office.

Maas, M., Johnson, M., & Moorhead, S. (1996). Conceptual and methodological issues and strategies in classifying nursing-sensitive patient outcomes. *IMAGE: Journal of Nursing Scholarship, 28*(4), 295-301.

National Center for Health Statistics. (1995). *1995 National nursing home survey. HHS News.* Washington, D.C.: National Center for Health Statistics, U.S. Department of Health and Human Services.

North American Nursing Diagnosis Association. (1999). *Nursing Diagnoses: Definitions & classification 1999-2000.* Philadelphia: Author.

Rantz, M., & Miller, T. (1987). How diagnoses are changing in long term care. *American Journal of Nursing, 87,* 360-361.

Rantz, M., Miller, T., & Jacobs, C. (1985). Nursing diagnosis in long term care. *American Journal of Nursing, 85,* 916-926.

Rantz, M., Vinz-Miller, T., & Matson, S. (1995). Nursing diagnoses in long-term care: A longitudinal perspective for strategic planning. *Nursing Diagnosis, 6*(2), 57-63.

Rovner, B. W. (1985). Mental illness among nursing home patients. *Hospital & Community Psychiatry, 36*(2), 119-128.

Roybal, E. R. (1984). Federal involvement in mental health care for the aged. *American Psychologist, 39*(2), 163-166.

Shea, D. G., Smyer, M. A., & Streit, A. (1994). Mental health services for nursing home residents. *The Journal of Mental Health Administration, 20*(3), 223-235.

Smith, M., Mitchell, S., & Buckwalter, K. C. (1995). Nurses helping nurses: The development of "internal specialists" in long term care. *Journal of Gerontological Nursing, 21*(3), 25-31.

U.S. Bureau of the Census. (1996). *Population projection of the United States by age, sex, race, and Hispanic origin: 1995-2050.* Washington, D.C.: U.S. Government Printing Office.

CONTENTS

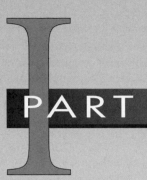

PART I

Health Perception–Health Management Pattern

OVERVIEW

Following Fryer's summary of normal changes in health perception and health management with aging, nursing diagnoses that focus on elders' problems with maintaining health are explored. The nursing diagnosis Altered Health Maintenance is particularly relevant for elders as they adjust both to the normal changes associated with aging and to personal and social expectations. This diagnosis, set forth by Glick and Ressler in Chapter 2, examines health behaviors and the individual's perceptions of health that influence those behaviors. Glick and Ressler distinguish Altered Health Maintenance from Self-Care Deficit and Impaired Home Maintenance Management but note the interrelationships among the three diagnoses. The elderly person's ability to maintain health independently is largely dependent on the ability to perform self-care and effectively maintain a home.

Falling is the most common accident, as well as the leading cause of accidental death, among elders. Most falls in elderly persons result either from changes that accompany the aging process or from disease entities. Chapter 3, by Stolley, Lewis, Moore, and Harvey, highlights other contributing factors that increase the risk of falling. Fall Prevention, Delirium Management, Environmental Management, Reality Orientation, Surveillance: Safety, Urinary Incontinence Care, and Home Maintenance Assistance are nursing interventions that are described to prevent falls. Safety Behavior: Personal, Safety Behavior: Home Physical Environment, Safety Behavior: Fall Prevention, Knowledge: Personal Safety, and Risk Control are patient outcomes that can be monitored to assess the effectiveness of interventions.

It is well known that elders are vulnerable for overprescription and overuse of medications, making the diagnosis Risk for Poisoning: Drug Toxicity an important area for nursing assessment, diagnosis, and intervention. In Chapter 4 Weitzel discusses the pharmacodynamics and pharmacokinetics among elderly persons, focusing on important variables in drug administration and polypharmacy. Weitzel developed a tool to monitor for digitalis toxicity that can serve as a prototype for identifying persons at risk for drug toxicity. Weitzel urges an interdisciplinary approach to the prevention of drug toxicity in elders, including drug holidays and careful monitoring of outcomes such as Knowledge: Medication, Risk Control: Drug Use, and Self-Care: Non-Parenteral Medication.

Infections are an increasing problem for institutionalized elders, with between 5% and 20% of patients residing in nursing homes manifesting one or more infections. Infections, especially those of the urinary tract and respiratory tract and decubitus ulcers, contribute to nursing home admissions and increased mortality. In Chapter 5, Risk for Infection, Carter and Pottinger enumerate a variety of predisposing factors to infection in elders. They propose interventions to maximize host resistance and to reduce the risk for common infections among institutionalized elders.

In Chapter 6 Head discusses Impaired Home Maintenance Management, underscoring the need for nurses to identify the signs of the problem, recommending interventions that can be used to assist elders with independent living, and describing outcomes that should be monitored to evaluate the effectiveness of the interventions. Similarly, Stevenson emphasizes the importance of optimizing Health Seeking Behaviors of elders in Chapter 7. Stevenson criticizes the nursing diagnosis approach for stressing illness rather than health and proposes that nurses will better serve elders if they give at least equal attention to interventions and outcomes that are health promoting.

Nonadherence with treatment, including medications, is a principal reason why elders' health is compromised. Zwygart-Stauffacher, in Chapter 8, explores Ineffective Management of Therapeutic Regimen, a problem that nurses are often in a position to treat with good outcomes. Likewise, nurses are often positioned to prevent and resolve Elder Mistreatment. In Chapter 9 Cowen describes the prevalence of elder mistreatment, outlines the signs and causes, and discusses how nurses can intervene to achieve desired outcomes.

CHAPTER 1

NORMAL CHANGES WITH AGING

Col. Gwendolyn Fryer

Nurses have an important role in assisting elderly clients to cope and choose health-protecting behaviors that will enhance their quality of life. When dealing with the elderly client, nurses will find themselves asking the question, "What is normal aging?" Some clients who "fit," by age alone, the category called "elder" will demonstrate compliance and adherence to health seeking behaviors. Others who fit the same age category will demonstrate an inability to cope with the changes of aging.

Aging and disease are not synonymous, and the effects of the aging process alone are not the primary contributors in terms of disability and disease. Pathologic changes combined with the normal changes of aging have the greatest impact on disability in elderly clients (Hart & Moore, 1992). As such, elderly persons may feel, look, and think no differently from how they did when they were younger. Nurses must evaluate older people carefully concerning their individual capabilities and needs when planning nursing care or helping them to meet their own needs for health maintenance. Their beliefs and behaviors about their health and their need to maintain it will not alter drastically as they transition to the later years of life.

Individuals who think that aging brings on uncontrollable consequences and changes in their health will be controlled by and eventually succumb to their thinking. A 1984 Longitudinal Study on Aging, in which 1391 persons older than age 70 were surveyed about their health status, lifestyle, and the principal cause of any illness, revealed that 45% of the respondents who had attributed their poor health to old age died 4 years later, compared with 30% of those who had blamed only the disease (Butler, 1992). As long as an elderly person is not afflicted with illnesses that are painful or impair functioning, aging is not noticeable until it has become advanced (Blazer, 1994).

HEALTH MAINTENANCE

The normal changes associated with the aging process have not changed and will be constant in all individuals approaching "old age." The perception that elderly people are at greater risk in terms of their ability to maintain a healthy state is both true and false. The degree to which an elderly person puts himself at risk is based on how well the elderly person adjusts to the normal conditions of both living and aging. In assessing an older person's belief

system or pattern pertaining to health in old age, nurses must determine what beliefs or perceptions were held as "most valuable" in younger years. Beliefs or perceptions of health and illness are intricately woven and developed in the "external life" that the elderly person has lived and perhaps continues to live. The social, psychologic, and economic life of the individual will affect how "normal" the health beliefs and perceptions of the elderly individual will be. The educational level, income potential, family and friendship bonds, status in society, personal philosophy, dietary habits, exercise routine, and self-indulgences like smoking and drinking will provide invaluable clues to how well the elderly person will maintain or manage health (Gallup, 1960). Elderly individuals who are highly educated, who have been economically "positioned" in both career and income, who have strong family ties, and who are held in high esteem within society are likely to value health over illness and seek a higher level of health maintenance.

A generalized approach to health care maintenance should include education related to current and future planning for the elderly individual and family members. Just as aging brings changes in physical stamina and mental acuity, financial, social, and economic changes develop as aging occurs. The most disciplined elderly persons who take pride in being "well adjusted" to old age may find themselves "buckling" under the pressures of increased medical expenses and decreased income. In addition, the elderly person should demonstrate general health care behaviors through increased understanding of good mental and physical health promotion, complying with medical and nursing prescriptions, and ensuring routine and timely follow-up care (Cheney, Diehm, & Seeley, 1992).

Awareness of the health risks is also an important factor in elderly individuals' ability to manage their health. Regardless of the decisions or choices elderly individuals may make based on their beliefs or perceptions, they are still potentially at greater risk than ever.

HEALTH PROMOTION AND DISEASE PREVENTION

Health promotion in the elderly patient focuses on preventing any decline in function while supporting abilities to remain independent. An important ingredient in preventive care for elders is ensuring optimal use of the health care resources available to them and the overall organization of health care institutions. A health maintenance program should be based on a clear understanding of the resources available for primary, secondary, and tertiary prevention.

When elderly patients are counseled about primary prevention, the nurse stresses the importance of exercise in preventing a wide range of health problems, including cardiovascular disease, falls, and depression. Walking is recommended to all persons who are physically able. The elder should be encouraged to maintain an activity level that is habitual and not unduly strenuous. Elderly clients who smoke should be told that they could increase their life expectancy, reduce their risk of heart disease, and improve the function of their lungs and circulation if they quit smoking. In addition, elderly clients should be warned of the negative impact of dietary excesses. They should be warned of the role excess dietary intake plays in disease development. Alcohol use is another area of concern in elders. Excessive alcohol use increases injuries, gastrointestinal illness, liver disease, and dementing disease (Williams, 1995).

Secondary prevention in the elder must focus on early detection and treatment of disease. Areas of priority for health promotion in the elder that nurses should emphasize include but are not limited to cancer screening, depression, falls, hypertension, infectious disease, misuse of medications, nutrition, oral health, osteoporosis, physical inactivity, sensory loss, and social isolation (Berg & Cassells, 1990).

Tertiary prevention of the elder usually begins when the elderly individual becomes symptomatic and enters the hospital milieu. Nursing personnel must ensure the completion of a comprehensive geriatric assessment to determine the current medical problems, sources of disability, and future care. This is especially important for identifying rapid changes in health status and determining future needs or living arrangements. The primary focus of tertiary care of the elder is rehabilitation. The primary goals should be to restore function and prevent future disability. The nurse must ensure that the elderly individual understands that preventive care can extend life and postpone the period of functional disability, increasing control over the quality of health in old age (Williams, 1995).

As a part of primary, secondary, or tertiary care of the elderly patient, nursing personnel must be aware that age-related changes in the immune system will predispose the elder to an increased likelihood of developing infections, tumors, and blood vessel and immune diseases. Because elderly clients are less able to produce antibodies, they will show less vigorous reactions to chemical substances normally used to detect infections, such as the skin test reactions for tuberculosis (Williams, 1995). Nurses must educate and encourage elderly clients to maintain an active immunization schedule, especially against viral influenza, pneumococcus, and tetanus. Tetanus antibodies may also wane in later life, leading to the development of tetanus. Cases of tetanus have occurred in elderly patients who have undergone bowel surgery or amputation of a limb. For this reason clients should ensure their tetanus toxoid boosters are current, especially before bowel surgery or surgery requiring amputation (William, 1989).

People who are older than 65 account for 25% of prescription drug use. This fact, coupled with the use of multiple medications (polypharmacy), places the elderly individual at increased risk of adverse drug reactions. The average elderly person uses five prescription medicines at any given time and fills 12 to 17 prescriptions each year. In addition, older adults use an average of 3½ over-the-counter medications. The cost of prescription medications used by older people is well over $10 billion a year (Williams, 1995). Increased use of medication leads to increased risk of adverse drug reactions. Nurses must educate elderly individuals about the development of unwanted symptoms, changes in blood or other tests being taken, and the possibility of death directly related to adverse drug reactions.

Elderly people must also be educated about the prevention of falls. Over 75% of falls occur at home. Tripping over objects or on stairs or steps is the most common cause. When assessing the elderly individual's potential for falls, the nurse must emphasize the need to eliminate environmental impediments through understanding the origin of the fall potential.

SUMMARY

Some people are convinced that "old age" is a period of decline and dissatisfaction. Although aging will bring about expected changes, these associated changes do not have to herald decline and dissatisfaction. There are pleasures, normal processes, and problems associated with aging. Older adults can approach age-related challenges with realism and develop increased knowledge about their health needs and about the resources that are available to help them manage their health.

REFERENCES

Berg, R., & Cassells, J. (1990). *The second fifty years: Promoting health and preventing disability.* Washington, DC: National Academy Press.

Blazer, D. G. (1994). *Intervention strategies for emotional problems in later life.* Northvale, NJ: Jason Aronson.

Butler, R. N. (1992). Attributing old age to poor health may lead to an earlier death (editorial). *Geriatrics, 47*(10), 16.

Cheney, W. J., Diehm, W. J., & Seeley, F. E. (1992). *The second fifty years: A reference for senior citizens.* New York: Paragon House.

Gallup, G. (1960). *The secrets of long life.* New York: Bernard Geis Associates, Random House.

Hart, B. G., & Moore, P. V. (1992). The aging workforce. *AAOHN Journal, 40*(1), 36-40.

William, R. (1989). *Clinical aspects of aging* (3rd ed.). Baltimore: Lippincott Williams & Wilkins.

Williams, M. E. (1995). *The American Geriatrics Society's complete guide to aging and health.* New York: Harmony Books, Crown.

CHAPTER 2

ALTERED HEALTH MAINTENANCE

Orpha J. Glick and Chris Ressler

The health of individuals and groups has been the focus of nursing practice throughout nursing history. Accordingly, education and counseling for disease prevention and health promotion have been a major component of nursing practice. More recently, federal public health initiatives such as *Healthy People 2000* (U.S. Public Health Service, 1990, 1996) and *The Guide to Clinical Preventive Services,* Second Edition (U.S. Preventive Services Task Force [USPSTF], 1996), have emphasized prevention of illness and disability and promoted self-responsibility in disease prevention and health promotion.

The focus of this chapter is the diagnosis and treatment of Altered Health Maintenance in elderly clients. Altered Health Maintenance is one of several diagnoses accepted for clinical testing at the 1982 (fifth) Conference of the North American Nursing Diagnosis Association (NANDA) (Kim, McFarland, & McLane, 1984). It is defined as the "inability to identify, manage and/or seek out help to maintain health" (NANDA, 1999, p. 94). This definition implies that maintaining and promoting health is the personal responsibility of the individual (as client); however, the actions of identifying, managing, and seeking out help for health maintenance and promotion can also be applied to the client as family, to the aggregate, or to a total community (Pender, 1996).

Conceptual meanings of health and distinctions among health promotion, disease prevention, and health maintenance have been a major focus of nursing literature for several decades (Brubaker, 1983; Kulbok & Baldwin, 1992; Moch, 1989; Newman, Sime, & Corcoran-Perry, 1991; Pender, 1987, 1996). Most authors have argued for broad "holistic" views of health that are consistent with the complexities of human existence and function. A broad view of health provides for individuals who experience a reduction in functional status or health secondary to aging-related biologic changes or to a specific disease process yet continue to carry out role functions, adapt to environmental changes, and achieve higher levels of health in other dimensions (McWilliams, Stewart, Brown, Desai, & Coderre, 1996). This is a particularly useful conception of health and health maintenance for older adults because many of them have chronic medical conditions (Van Nostrand, Furner, & Suzman, 1993; Young & Olson, 1991) and have experienced losses in their social network or material possessions (Mor-Barak, Scharlach, Birba, & Sokolov, 1992). A multidimen-

sional view of health is reflected in the writings of several authors who advocate health promotion for older adults (Frenn, 1994; Simmons, 1990). Spirduso (1995), for example, viewed health as the ability to live and function effectively in society and to exercise self-reliance and autonomy to the maximum extent feasible. Thus health is not necessarily total freedom from disease. Rather, a definition of health for older persons often includes successfully dealing with chronic illness to allow maximal functioning for that individual (McWilliams et al., 1996). This is also consistent with the notion that health behavior may be directed toward maintenance in one dimension and promotion in another.

Clearly, health is a highly personal concept and can be judged only in the context of the individual's personal and cultural or ethnic value system (Baldwin, 1996; Chen, 1996). Hill and Lindsey (1994) also emphasized the importance of considering the context of an individual's experience because each person creates unique meaning(s) from her life experience and makes choices based on those meanings. Further, the effects of aging-related changes on the body image of elderly adults and the effects of body image on health behavior in this population have not been studied. Although there are gaps in knowledge about health maintenance in older adults, health care professionals are challenged with distinguishing between "normal" aging and pathophysiology in their evaluation of health and health behavior in this population. Failure to accurately distinguish between normal aging and pathology may result in diagnosis and treatment of normal aging as disease. Conversely, pathology can be erroneously defined as normal aging and not receive appropriate intervention; for example, acute confusion and depression are two conditions that are frequently overlooked or misdiagnosed in this age-group (Mezey, Rauckhorst, & Stokes, 1993). Similarly, because sleep disturbances and the joint stiffness and discomfort accompanying osteoarthritis (Buchner, 1997; King, Oman, Brassington, Bliwise, & Haskell, 1997) are expected in late life, they are less likely to be actively treated.

Individual perceptions of what health is and personal descriptions of health status are partially formed by a person's environment and the individuals in it. This means that knowledge of sociocultural influences is important when assessing older adults' health perceptions and their behaviors. To respect cultural differences and to work within the framework and value structures of the elderly client, nurses must recognize their own attitudes and values, which may oppose the elder's perception. Knowledge of health conceptions and practices across population groups increases the ability to understand and predict other health-related variables such as health choices (Baldwin, 1996; Chen, 1996). Laffrey (1986) suggested that one's conception of health might be a more significant influence on health behavior than actual health status. She found, for example, that in a sample of healthy adults ($n = 95$), persons who held a more eudaemonistic health conception engaged in health behaviors to promote higher levels of health. On the other hand, persons whose health conception was more "clinical" engaged in behaviors primarily to prevent illness.

Societal and professional caregiver views of what constitutes preventive health care also affect expectations for services and self-care responsibility. For example, until recently, preventive and health promoting strategies were thought to have less application to older adults because there is a high prevalence of existing chronic disease (German et al., 1995). However, there is growing evidence that a number of chronic conditions can be prevented or delayed even after age 65 and that health care providers can assist older adults to maintain health and functional independence.

The core of health maintenance as a client initiative and responsibility is health behavior or health practices. Health behaviors are those activities initiated and performed by the person to preserve and enhance health and well-being (Pender, 1996). Simmons' (1980) definition of health behavior also included activities that promote recovery, maximize rehabilitation, and have the potential for improving the quality of a client's life: (1) nutrition; (2) sleep/rest; (3) physical activity; (4) personal hygiene; (5) substance misuse; (6) medical-dental supervision; (7) therapeutic regimen noncompliance (e.g., treatment, medication, diet); and (8) performance in technical procedures (Simmons, 1980). Several of these areas represent behaviors for health promotion, as well as for health maintenance. Pender (1987, 1996), however, has consistently distinguished behaviors that are undertaken to protect health (disease prevention) from behaviors that are designed to promote health. She has noted that health protection behavior is "directed towards decreasing the probability of experiencing health problems by active protection against pathological stressors or detection of health problems in the asymptomatic stage" (Pender, 1996, p. 34). Health promotion, on the other hand, is directed toward increasing the level of well-being and self-actualization (Pender, 1996, p. 34). In a review of health behavior literature, Kulbok and Baldwin (1992) also argued for emphasizing positive (promotion) rather than negative (prevention) language to characterize health promotion. These authors described a "subtle shift" in em-

phasis from prevention to promotion in the *Healthy People 2000* objectives in that health is being considered as a positive construct. Thus the meaning of health behavior is moving from a restricted view that is professionally driven and specific to disease prevention to an expanded view in which health is self-defined, nonorganized, and protective regardless of perceived wellness. This expanded view of health has increased the range of health behaviors beyond the medically (or other health care practitioners) recommended, self-care practices. Moreover, there has been professional and social movement toward individualized self-care with emphasis on beliefs, values, social support, personal resources, and individuals' rights to choose. Accordingly, in this chapter, health maintenance behavior is broadly defined as lifestyle choices and actions directed at early detection of health conditions, control of effects of chronic disease or its treatment, and actions that prevent accidental injury, preserve functional independence, and advance personal growth and resources.

Health behaviors are deeply integrated into an individual's lifestyle patterns. As previously noted, they are influenced by environmental constraints or resources and by personal and cultural beliefs and values. Assisting older adults to change health habits can enable them to postpone onset of chronic illness and remain active (Buchner, 1997; Spirduso, 1995). Improving health maintenance in older adults is likely to involve actual change in behaviors that are already well established. This is in contrast to the need to overcome resistance to social pressure that often operates in the young adult or adolescent. Chronic illness and multiple organ failure also can complicate health practices by decreasing physiologic reserves (Arking, 1991). In addition, the elder's own view of the future becomes very important to health practices, since self-actualizing behaviors require that the individual have the ability to perform the activity and be motivated to plan for the future based on the results of such practices. Elderly persons with the following positive developmental characteristics have participated in behaviors that support this aspect of their health status: (1) the desire to leave a legacy or to make contributions to the next generation; (2) positive interactions with the younger generation; (3) attachment to familiar objects, which provides continuity in day-to-day living; (4) a sense of immediacy related to the elder's opportunities to experience sensory and emotional stimuli on a daily basis; (5) a sense of life cycle reflective of introspection of previously held values and new understanding of philosophic matters; (6) creativity, curiosity, and surprise, which can be found in a zest for life; and (7) a sense of fulfillment in life to include the opportunity to review life, resolve conflicts, and be proud of personal achievements (Engle, 1984). Many of these characteristics were later verified in a phenomenological study of ways in which older adults with chronic illness engage in health promoting behaviors and thought patterns (McWilliams et al., 1996).

RELATED FACTORS/ETIOLOGIES

Problems with communication obviously decrease the older person's ability to maintain health independently. Similarly, a number of cognitive-perceptual and psychosocial factors affect health. NANDA (1999) has identified the following related factors (Box 2-1) as relevant to health maintenance behaviors: lack of ability to make deliberate and thoughtful judgments, perceptual/cognitive impairment (complete/partial lack of gross and/or fine motor skills), ineffective individual coping, ineffective family coping, dysfunctional grieving, unachieved developmental tasks, disabling spiritual distress, and lack of material resources (p. 95). Other related factors identified from the literature include loss of family or friends, abrupt changes in residence, acute or chronic illness or injury, lack of knowledge of positive or negative health behavior, low health value, inability to monitor self or environment, and insufficient motivation or self-efficacy (Tackenburg & Glick, 1991, pp. 6-17). Older persons often are more at risk because a number of these factors can accumulate and interact within their lives, ultimately influencing health status.

Researchers in several disciplines (e.g., sociology, public health, psychology, nursing) have attempted to identify factors that influence an individual to initiate and sustain health-related behavior for several decades. In 1980 Cummings, Becker, and Maile conducted a study of 14 conceptual models of health behavior developed by social scientists over a period of approximately 25 years. The purpose of their work was to lay the "groundwork" for a unified framework for explaining health action. Eight of eleven living authors of the health models participated in the study. Participants were asked to compare a set of 109 variables (obtained from a review of the 14 models of health behavior) and place them into categories on the basis of their similarities. The specific model from which the variables were drawn was not identified; however, the names and definitions of behaviors were given as they appeared in the literature describing the model. Analysis of study findings revealed the following six "clusters" of variables: (1) perception of illness and threat of disease; (2) knowledge of disease; (3) social network; (4) demographic variables; (5) access to health care; and (6) attitude toward health care. These investigators also observed subgroupings of behaviors within several of the categories. For example, the accessibility (to health care) variables aggregated into two distinct subgroups—those related to financial cost of care and

---

Box 2-1   **Defining Characteristics and Related Factors/Etiologies**
ALTERED HEALTH MAINTENANCE

Defining Characteristics
Demonstrated lack of knowledge regarding basic health practices
Demonstrated lack of adaptive behaviors to internal/external environmental changes
Reported or observed inability to take responsibility for meeting basic health practices in any or all functional pattern areas
History of lack of health seeking behavior
Expressed interest in improving health behaviors
Reported or observed lack of equipment, financial and/or other resources*
Reported or observed impairment of personal support systems*
Physical signs of ineffective symptom control (e.g., pedal edema, shortness of breath) that may indicate nonadherence to diet or medication prescription
Social withdrawal
Inattention to personal appearance
Inattention to home safety hazards
Misperceptions and engagement in behaviors that do not support health or that present hazards to health (e.g., skipping meals or unbalanced nutritional intake, smoking, excess use of alcohol or other controlled substances, lack of exercise)

Related Factors/Etiologies
Lack of, or significant alteration in, communication skills (written, verbal, and/or gestural)
Lack of ability to make deliberate and thoughtful judgments
Perceptual/cognitive impairment (complete/partial lack of gross and/or fine motor skills)
Ineffective individual coping
Dysfunctional grieving
Unachieved developmental tasks
Ineffective family coping
Disabling spiritual distress
Lack of material resources
Loss of relatives/friends
Abrupt change of residence
Acute or chronic illness/disability/injury
Lack of awareness of positive or negative health behaviors
Low health value
Inability to perform health behaviors
Inability to monitor self or environment

Data from Tackenburg, J., & Glick, O. (1991). Altered health maintenance. In M. Maas, K. Buckwalter, & M. Hardy (Eds.), *Nursing diagnoses and interventions for the elderly* (pp. 6-17). Redwood City, CA: Addison Wesley Longman.
*Suggest these items be deleted as defining characteristics because they are antecedent to Altered Health Maintenance and are included in the related factors.

those related to availability of services. The spatial arrangement of the major clusters in the Cummings et al. analysis is also of interest and suggests association between certain clusters of behaviors. For example, items pertaining to knowledge about the disease were situated in close proximity to items dealing with perception and evaluation of symptoms. Similarly, items related to individuals' attitudes toward health care and items on accessibility to health services suggest a relationship in which access factors are affected by one's evaluation of health care. Further, the proximity between demographic variables and access might be a function of social class. This analysis and summary of variables that influence health behavior illustrates the complexity of the diagnostic and treatment processes that surround health maintenance.

Lack of understanding and confusion from conflicting health messages also might explain why some older adults fail to participate in health protection services. For example, individuals might not understand the value of seeing their clinicians to stay well. Moreover, some individuals do not request preventive services, especially if they have no symptoms and must pay for the services. They often avoid clinicians' offices because of fear of finding a serious problem. These persons find it easy to defer the investment of time and money to avoid diseases or symptoms that are not imminent and benefits that are not immediate (Cimino, 1996). Thus insurance coverage can determine whether a patient is willing to undergo screening tests (Meyer, 1995). In contrast to individuals who avoid preventive health services, other persons present with a set of expectations and demand care based on incomplete information about the efficacy of a treatment (Jackson, Leininger, Harris, & Kaluzny, 1994). It can be difficult for consumers and health care providers when an organization, such as a specialty society, announces a new screening guideline for which there is insufficient evidence-based research. Clinicians need to be aware of controversial recommendations and be prepared to discuss them with clients who have read or heard about them (Meyer, 1995).

In addition to knowledge and cost issues, some older clients hesitate to take responsibility and want a more traditional provider-consumer arrangement in which the provider makes the decisions and assumes responsibility for management; however, intervention can assist them to actively participate in diagnostic and treatment decision making (Alto, 1995) and to take greater responsibility for their health. Some clients may also resist counseling about behavioral change because it may be unpleasant. Warner and Warner (1993) illustrated this view by noting, "Who wants to be lectured about a bad habit that you already know you should break, but that you find exceedingly difficult to alter?" (p. 42). The clinician can guide, but clients must take responsibility for their daily behavior, for accurate reporting of progress, and for initiating discussion of health-related problems (USPSTF, 1996). Health-

maintaining activities should go further than providing services to passive recipients. Instead, the potential of the clients to expedite their own health should be emphasized (Lindsey & Hartrick, 1996).

Insufficient provider knowledge and related attitudinal factors also can be reasons for failure to become engaged in disease prevention and health promotion. Many health care systems are oriented toward acute care and do not emphasize preventive care. Although many providers are motivated to give preventive care, treatment of the current illness takes precedence during an acute care visit, often leaving little time for preventive counseling and education (Jaen, Stange, & Nutting, 1994). Preventive care is often seen as an add-on or a service that could be performed at a more convenient time (Jackson et al., 1994). Stange, Fedirko, Zyzanski, and Jaen (1994) found that time-consuming counseling activities focusing on issues that may be uncomfortable to discuss were unlikely to be offered by the physicians they surveyed. Similarly, Morgan et al. (1996) studied a counseling intervention in a randomized, controlled trial designed to promote tobacco cessation in older smokers age 50 to 74. The 49 physicians who participated in the trial spent 3 to 10 minutes per patient implementing the counseling and did follow-up counseling during subsequent visits. Early in the trial 50% of the physicians believed that their patient's compliance with medical advice to quit smoking was unlikely. After results of the study showed that quit rates for participants in the intervention group were double those in the control group, 93% of the physicians expressed increased confidence in the benefits of counseling (Morgan et al., 1996). In addition to requiring time and seldom being rewarded financially, prevention often shows no immediate results. Alto (1995) noted that "the rewards from disease prevention and health promotion are more subtle and less tangible than the gratitude of a patient cured of pneumonia by an antibiotic" (p. 551).

Nurse practitioners, who have traditionally educated and counseled patients, might have more favorable attitudes toward prevention. Data from a national, government-sponsored survey of 17 of the *Healthy People 2000* objectives showed that nurse practitioners working in adult settings (including older adults) exceeded the targets related to reviewing clients' medications and assessing mobility and fall prevention. However, the data indicated that significant improvement was needed in the provision of adult immunization services, including tetanus-diphtheria boosters and pneumococcal and influenza vaccines (Lemley, O'Grady, Rauckhorst, Russell, & Small, 1994).

ASSESSMENT

Gordon (1982) suggested that assessment of health perception and health management be a part of the nursing history. The following interview questions are offered as examples of stimuli to assist clients to reflect on their health behavior:

1. How would you evaluate your current state of health?
2. What practices do you routinely perform that contribute to your health?
3. What do you do to manage common illnesses such as colds or the flu?
4. How would you describe your activity and sleep patterns for a typical day?
5. What kinds of things do you do to keep mentally healthy?
6. How would you describe your personal relationships with family? Friends?
7. Describe what interests, persons, or events give purpose and meaning to your life.
8. What changes in your health status would prompt you to see your doctor or other health care professional?

Although these questions are still relatively open-ended, they are specific to general health behaviors of adults in late life.

A tool designed to elicit a more comprehensive database for diagnosing Altered Health Maintenance was developed by Johnson-Saylor, Pohl, and Lowe-Wickson (1982). These clinical specialists developed an eight-item assessment form that directs some of its questions to the following goals: raising the patient's health consciousness, helping the patient identify health risks in terms of lifestyle and family history, and helping the patient identify strengths and resources. The self-administered assessment form is applicable to the health behaviors of older adults, although it might present some difficulties for the elder who has poor eyesight or motor difficulty and cannot fill out the form. Its strength is that it helps persons become aware of psychologic health issues and health maintaining strategies that are available within their lifestyle, thereby reinforcing a sense of control.

The Detroit assessment tool begins with a checklist of overall self-perception. Items from the Assessment of Life Condition Scale (ALCS) were selected for evaluation of strengths, resources, and stressors. Of particular importance to older adults are the items in this section that relate to role satisfaction and issues of control over environment, self, and lifestyle choices. This is especially important to institutionalized elderly adults, given the regimentation frequently seen in health care institutions and nurses' attitudes toward elderly adults (Alexy, 1985). Because institutional care tends to be directed toward outcomes for the majority, it is often difficult to honor individual needs. Disregard for individuality and adulthood can lead to depression and compromise positive health behaviors (Bahr, 1992; Taft, 1985). Taft suggested that resistance to the institution's mode of operation might leave the elder open to retribution from the staff and peers.

Another tool that could be used to determine health perceptions of older adults is the Health Self Determinism Index (HSDI). This 20-item Likert scale measures intrinsic motivation constructs that influence health behaviors (Deci, 1975). Subcategories in this instrument are self-determined health judgments, self-determined health behaviors, and perceived sense of competency in health matters. Cox (1985) demonstrated overall reliability for the items of this index, emphasizing the multidimensionality of motivation. The advantage of the tool is that it can identify to what extent motivation is a related factor in the incidence of health maintenance alteration. The HSDI is a tool that could refine motivational components after an assessment of health behaviors has been made. It does not address preventive or maintenance activities.

The Health Belief Model (HBM) has also been used as a basis for understanding and assessing health behavior (Rosenstock, 1974). After numerous revisions, the HBM instrument (Becker & Rosenstock, 1984) contains items that assess an individual's perceptions regarding (1) susceptibility to a specific disease, (2) association between severity of a health condition and health-related behaviors, (3) benefits of a health recommendation, and (4) effects of barriers (e.g., pain or cost) to the health-related behaviors. Like the HSDI, this model deals with motivation, a specific component of health behavior. The HBM is helpful when evaluating health practices of older adults because it addresses the realistic barriers experienced by many of them, such as cost, transportation, fatigue, and interpersonal relationships with health care providers. Because motivation is multidimensional (e.g., self-image, culture), the HBM does not recommend interventions based on assessment findings, but identifies motivational or perceptual issues that might help to individualize nursing interventions within a relevant lifestyle framework.

An assessment tool that addresses both aspects of health perception and health management was developed by the Department of Health and Human Services (1985). Items in this tool focus on general and specific preventive and health maintenance behaviors. The 56-item Likert scale is self-administered and includes assessment categories of interest to older adults (e.g., home safety, stress, dental care) that cannot be found in other instruments. It also assesses the elder's knowledge about specific health behaviors, for example, controlling high blood pressure and diet. Although quite long, the tool assesses environmental problems of the person who lives alone and many of the chronic health conditions to which older adults are predisposed.

NURSING DIAGNOSIS

Altered Health Maintenance is a diagnosis that is made when health or functional status is potentially or actually threatened by existing health behaviors. See Box 2-1 for the related factors and defining characteristics of Altered Health Maintenance as presented by NANDA (1999) with several additions obtained from the literature.

As shown, the concept of health maintenance is very broad and incorporates physical, psychosocial, and cultural behavioral domains. Because of this range, it is conceivable that the diagnosis could be made based on a problem in only one behavioral sphere or based on multiple problems from several domains. Peret and Stachowiak (1984) conceptualized health maintenance as a continuum ranging from complete dependence on a "second party" for health care needs (dysfunctional health maintenance) to a partial level of dependence to relative independence in health maintenance. These authors viewed health maintenance as a focus of nursing care when there are developmental disabilities or deficits in adaptive behavior or when there is an inability to communicate health care needs. It is unclear, however, to what extent knowledge, beliefs, values, and motivation enter into this conception of health maintenance. Moreover, viewing health maintenance as a functional dependence-independence continuum minimizes the self-actualizing dimensions of health for older adults who have severe physical limitations.

Because the scope of health maintenance is very broad, specifying the particular behavioral domain (e.g., eating patterns, medication use) as a subtitle of the diagnosis has been suggested as a useful way of delineating the specific behaviors to be targeted for intervention (Carpenito, 1987; Fehring & Frenn, 1986). Although specifying the behavioral domain might clarify the intervention target, it raises a question concerning the advantage of using a broad diagnosis rather than diagnoses that address the specific lifestyle pattern (e.g., Altered Nutrition: More Than Body Requirements). It is suggested that the concept of maintenance is applicable when individuals could benefit from acquiring new health promoting behaviors, as well as changing non–health supporting behavior (Prochaska, Norcross, & DiClemente, 1994). In addition, Altered Health Maintenance can be used for (1) an asymptomatic person who is at risk, (2) a person who has a chronic health condition but could attain a higher level of wellness, (3) a person having an acute problem but also having other areas of health at risk, or (4) someone who expresses a desire to change an unhealthy behavior pattern (Carpenito, 1987, 1997).

The defining characteristics of Altered Health Maintenance listed in the NANDA classification (1999) include a "demonstrated lack of knowledge regarding basic health practices" and/or "demonstrated lack of adaptive behaviors to internal/external environmental changes" (p. 94). (See Box 2-1.) The client might report (or the health care professional might observe) an inability to take responsibility for engaging in basic health practices. There might be a history of lack of health seeking behaviors, or the client might express an interest in improving health behaviors.

In addition to the defining characteristics listed in the NANDA classification (1999), the client might show persistent signs of physical or mental health disorders (e.g., shortness of breath, pedal edema, anxiety, dysphoria) that indicate self-management of recommended medical therapies is ineffective or incomplete either by choice or because of lack of awareness or knowledge. Clients also might self-report making changes in health care and medical (or nursing) recommendations or reveal misperceptions of self-care information or of their own symptoms and severity of their medical problem(s). Evidence of inattention to personal hygiene or to home safety hazards also signals an alteration in health maintenance. Finally, persistent engagement in lifestyle patterns that do not support health provide evidence of Altered Health Maintenance.

CASE STUDY

C. James is a 72-year-old man who lives alone. He is undergoing treatment for emphysema, including bronchodilators, antibiotics, fluid intake of at least 2000 ml, and low-flow oxygen at home. Mrs. James died 18 months ago from colon cancer. Since then, Mr. James's health has deteriorated, causing his daughters' concern. His ability to care for himself at home has decreased. Indeed, his records show that he has missed several clinic appointments or has not made them at the recommended intervals. Before his retirement, he was a department manager in a local industry. According to his daughters, Mrs. James managed all health care behaviors such as health care appointments, diet, and exercise. According to Mr. James, he did those things only "when I finally got tired of her nagging," although he "never did quit smoking," and "it gave her something to do."

Mr. James stated that his health is "good," that the doctors are trying to "make me older than I am," and that many of his friends "are worse off" than he because "they're in nursing homes." He disregards his daughters' reports of intermittent confusion and increased frequency of chest pain and dyspnea, saying, "those girls think everyone over 65 belongs in an old-age home."

Mr. James adheres to his health care program intermittently. He rarely goes out to socialize except for coffee once a month with a "few buddies." His level of physical activity is quite compromised, and the nurse notices that he becomes short of breath walking across the room. Further, he needs to support himself by holding on to furniture as he moves about. He reports sleeping poorly but "catnaps" during the day. Mr. James says he does not take his bronchodilators on a regular basis because "they taste so bad." His daughters report that he has had several colds within the last 6 months. They expressed fear that hospitalization will be required if his condition continues to deteriorate. Mr. James has lost 22 pounds the past year because he is "too tired to fix meals."

The assessment shows that Mr. James has many health care needs that are not being met because of Altered Health Maintenance related to role disturbance, nonsupportive health behavior choices, compromised physical health status (i.e., presence of chronic illness), a negative perception of health for older adults, loss of spouse, and negative perceptions of medical treatment. This diagnosis is manifested by the presence of cardiovascular and respiratory signs and symptoms, failure to assume health behaviors previously managed by his spouse, social withdrawal, and lack of knowledge regarding disease management and self-care.

NURSING-SENSITIVE OUTCOMES

In general, the aims of nursing intervention for Altered Health Maintenance are to facilitate (1) lifestyle changes, (2) acquisition of new health promoting thought patterns and behavior, and (3) self-care in managing chronic health conditions or risks. Several broad categories of patient outcomes in the *Nursing Outcomes Classification (NOC)* (Iowa Outcomes Project, 2000) are relevant to health maintenance: knowledge about conditions, risks, and self-care; beliefs, attitudes, and values (thought pattern, schema) regarding health and lifestyle issues; and health behavior that minimizes risk and supports or advances health. Table 2-1 lists nine of these outcomes with selected indicators that can be useful in assessing the effectiveness of nursing interventions. Note that the use of specific outcomes and/or indicators would depend on each client's situation. The indicators and corresponding scale would also be operationalized with markers, targets, and time intervals for assessing progress that are specific to the client.

Health Orientation

The outcome Health Orientation refers to the patient's "personal view of health and health behaviors as priorities" (Iowa Outcomes Project, 2000, p. 231). The five-point indicator scale reflects the strength of the perception and ranges from very weak (1) to very strong (5). The indicators target a range of perceptions (i.e., attitudes, beliefs, and values) about the importance of health, the relationship between lifestyle patterns and health, and the importance of self-responsibility in promoting and maintaining health.

Health Beliefs

The outcome Health Beliefs refers to "personal convictions that influence health behavior" (Iowa Outcomes Project, 2000, p. 226). The NOC includes five outcomes that address different sets of beliefs (e.g., perceived control, perceived resources) and like Health Orientation are scaled according to the strength of the belief or conviction. Although all of these outcomes are relevant to determining intervention effectiveness, only two (Health Beliefs and Health Beliefs: Perceived Ability to Perform) are included here.

The Health Belief outcome indicators incorporate ideas

from the HBM (Rosenstock, 1974) and health locus of control concepts (Wallston & Wallston, 1982). The indicators include perceived benefits of action, perceived threat from inaction, perceived importance of taking action, and perceived ability to perform action (Iowa Outcomes Project, 2000, p. 226).

Because considerable empirical evidence shows that self-efficacy is a major antecedent to engaging in health supporting behavior (Hurley & Shea, 1992; Strecher, DeVellis, Becker, & Rosenstock, 1986), the outcome Health Beliefs: Perceived Ability to Perform (Iowa Outcomes Project, 2000) can be an important intermediate outcome for health maintenance. The indicators for Health Beliefs: Perceived Ability to Perform also focus on perceptions regarding the complexity of health behavior, the amount of effort and time required to execute it, and the likelihood of maintaining the behavior over time. In addition to perceptions of difficulty, the amount of confidence that the client demonstrates (or verbalizes) in his ability to perform the targeted behavior is an important indicator of self-efficacy.

Knowledge Outcomes

See the two knowledge outcomes listed in Table 2-1, which focus on knowledge of health behaviors and knowledge of health resources. Again, depending on the client situation, other "knowledge" outcomes could be relevant (e.g., Knowledge: Disease Process). The reader is referred to the NOC (Iowa Outcomes Project, 2000). Knowledge: Health Behaviors is defined as the "extent of understanding conveyed about the promotion and protection of health" (Iowa Outcomes Project, 2000, p. 268). The scale ranges from none (1) to extensive (5) understanding. Indicators used to assess understanding reflect the client's ability to describe what constitutes "healthy" nutrition practices, benefits of exercise, effective stress management techniques, the negative health effects of substance use, and home or environmental safety hazards. Indicators for this outcome also include clients' descriptions of what age-specific health protection measures such as screening are needed.

Knowledge: Health Resources refers to understanding what health resources are available and how and when to access these resources as judged by the client's verbal description. This outcome also includes indicators specific to planning for follow-up care and to understanding of emergency measures. Again, the indicator scale ranges from none (1) to extensive (5) understanding (Iowa Outcomes Project, 2000, p. 271).

Health Behavior Outcomes

The behavioral (or health action) category of outcomes listed in Table 2-1 includes Health Seeking Behavior, Health Promoting Behavior, Risk Control, and Risk Detection. The Health Seeking Behavior outcome refers to the frequency (never demonstrated = 1, consistently demon-

NURSING DIAGNOSIS

ALTERED HEALTH MAINTENANCE

Defining Characteristics

Demonstrated lack of knowledge regarding basic health practices

Demonstrated lack of adaptive behaviors to internal/external environmental changes

Reported or observed inability to take responsibility for meeting basic health practices in any or all functional pattern areas

History of lack of health seeking behavior

Expressed interest in improving health behaviors

Reported or observed lack of equipment, financial and/or other resources

Reported or observed impairment of personal support systems

Physical signs of ineffective symptom control (e.g., pedal edema, shortness of breath) that may indicate nonadherence to diet or medication prescription

Social withdrawal

Inattention to personal appearance

Inattention to home safety hazards

Misperceptions and engagement in behaviors that do not support health or that present hazards to health (e.g., skipping meals or unbalanced nutritional intake, smoking, excess use of alcohol or other controlled substances, lack of exercise)

Related Factors/Etiologies

Lack of, or significant alteration in, communication skills (written, verbal, and/or gestural)

Lack of ability to make deliberate and thoughtful judgments

Perceptual/cognitive impairment (complete/partial lack of gross and/or fine motor skills)

Ineffective individual coping

Dysfunctional grieving

Unachieved developmental tasks

Ineffective family coping

Disabling spiritual distress

Lack of material resources

Nursing-Sensitive Outcomes

HEALTH ORIENTATION

Indicators

Focus on wellness

Focus on disease prevention and management

Focus on maintaining functional abilities

Focus on adjustment to life situations

Expectation that individual is responsible for choices

Perception that health behavior is relevant to self

Perception that health is a high priority in making lifestyle choices

Perception that health care provider expectations are congruent with one's cultural background

HEALTH BELIEFS

Indicators

Perceived importance of taking action

Perceived threat of inaction

Perceived benefits of action

Perceived internal control of action

Perceived control of health outcome

Perceived improvement in lifestyle from action

Perceived resources to perform action

Perceived absence of barriers to action

Perceived reduction of threat from action

RISK CONTROL

Indicators

Monitors environmental risk factors

Monitors personal behavior risk factors

Nursing Interventions

SELF-AWARENESS ENHANCEMENT

Activities

Encourage patient to recognize and discuss thoughts and feelings

Assist patient to identify the values that contribute to self-concept

Facilitate patient's identification of usual response patterns to various situations

Assist patient to be aware of negative self-statements

Assist patient to identify positive attributes of self

Assist patient to identify source of motivation

VALUES CLARIFICATION

Activities

Think through the ethical and legal aspects of free choice, given the particular situation, before beginning the intervention

Use appropriate questions to assist the patient in reflecting on the situation and what is important personally

Pose reflective, clarifying questions that give the patient something to think about

Encourage patient to make a list of what is important and not important in life and the time spent on each

Encourage patient to list values that guide behavior in various settings and types of situations

Use multiple sessions as directed by the specific situation

Avoid cross-examination questions

Create an accepting, nonjudgmental atmosphere

Continued

Nursing-Sensitive Outcomes	Nursing Interventions

RISK CONTROL—cont'd
Indicators—cont'd
Develops effective risk control strategies
Follows selected risk control strategies
Modifies lifestyle to reduce risk
Avoids exposure to health threats
Participates in screening for associated health problems
Participates in screening for identified risks
Recognizes changes in health status
Monitors health status changes

RISK DETECTION
Indicators
Recognizes signs and symptoms that indicate risks
Identifies potential health risks
Seeks validation of perceived risks
Performs self-examination at recommended intervals
Participates in screening at recommended intervals
Acquires knowledge of family history
Maintains updated knowledge of family history
Uses health care services congruent with needs

HEALTH SEEKING BEHAVIOR
Indicators
Asks questions when indicated
Completes health-related tasks
Performs self-screening when indicated
Contacts health care professionals when indicated
Describes strategies to eliminate unhealthy behavior
Seeks current health-related information
Adheres to self-developed strategies to maximize health
Performs prescribed health behavior when indicated

KNOWLEDGE: HEALTH BEHAVIORS
Indicators
Description of healthy nutritional practices
Description of benefits of activity and exercise
Description of effective sleep-wake patterns
Description of health effects of substance use (tobacco, alcohol, drugs)
Description of safe use of prescription drugs (and/or nonprescription)
Description of measures to reduce risk of accidental injury
Description of health promotion and protection services
Description of appropriate use of self-screening

VALUES CLARIFICATION—cont'd
Activities—cont'd
Help patient define alternatives and their advantages and disadvantages
Help patient to evaluate how values are in agreement with or conflict with those of family members/significant others

LEARNING READINESS ENHANCEMENT
Activities
Provide nonthreatening environment
Maximize the patient's hemodynamic status to facilitate brain oxygenation
Fulfill the patient's basic physiologic needs
Decrease the patient's level of fatigue, as appropriate
Control the patient's pain, as appropriate
Avoid use of medications that may alter the patient's perception
Monitor the patient's level of orientation/confusion
Maximize sensory input by use of eyeglasses, hearing aids, and so on, as appropriate
Encourage verbalization of feelings, perceptions, and concerns
Assist the patient to develop confidence in ability, as appropriate
Assist the patient to realize the severity of the illness, as appropriate
Assist the patient to realize ability to control the progression of the illness, as appropriate

TEACHING: INDIVIDUAL
Activities
Appraise the patient's current level of knowledge and understanding of content
Determine the patient's ability to learn specific information
Determine patient's motivation to learn specific information
Set mutual, realistic learning goals with the patient
Identify learning objectives necessary to reach goals
Determine the sequence for presenting the information
Select appropriate teaching methods/strategies
Adjust instruction to facilitate learning, as appropriate
Provide an environment conducive to learning

Nursing-Sensitive Outcomes	Nursing Interventions
	TEACHING: INDIVIDUAL—cont'd
	Activities—cont'd
	Evaluate the patient's achievement of stated objectives
	Correct information misinterpretations, as appropriate
	Include the family/significant other, as appropriate
	Include follow-up sessions or call-backs to assess comprehension and determine use of knowledge/skill
	Discuss ways that knowledge/skill can be used in everyday living
	Assist to develop a plan for integrating the knowledge acquired into everyday living
KNOWLEDGE: HEALTH RESOURCES	**HEALTH SYSTEM GUIDANCE**
Indicators	***Activities***
Description of resources that enhance health	Explain the immediate health care system, how it works, and what the patient/family can expect
Description of when to contact a health care professional	Instruct patient on what type of services to expect from each type of health care provider
Description of resources for emergency care	Inform patient of appropriate community resources and contact persons
Description of plan for follow-up care	Inform the patient the meaning of signing a consent form
Description of how to connect with needed services	Identify and facilitate communication among health care providers and patient/family, as appropriate
Description of emergency measures	Coordinate referrals to relevant health care providers, as appropriate
	Coordinate/schedule time needed by each service to deliver care
	Inform patient of the cost, time, alternatives, and risks involved in a specific test or procedure
	Give written instructions for purpose and location of health care activities, as appropriate
	Provide follow-up contact with patient, as appropriate
	Encourage the patient/family to ask questions about services and charges
	Assist individual to complete forms for assistance, such as housing and financial aid, as needed
HEALTH PROMOTING BEHAVIOR	**MUTUAL GOAL SETTING**
Indicators	***Activities***
Seeks balance among exercise, work, leisure, rest, nutrition	Determine patient's recognition of own problem
Performs health habits correctly	Encourage the patient to identify own strengths and abilities
Uses financial and physical resources to promote health	Assist the patient in identifying realistic, attainable goals
Uses social support to promote health	Assist the patient in breaking down complex goals into small, manageable steps
Uses effective stress reduction behaviors	Recognize the patient's value and belief system when establishing goals
Monitors personal behavior for risks	Avoid imposing personal values on patient during goal setting
Maintains satisfactory social relationships	Assist the patient in prioritizing (weighting) identified goals
HEALTH BELIEFS: PERCEIVED ABILITY TO PERFORM	Clarify with the patient roles of the health care provider and the patient respectively
Indicators	Assist the patient in developing a plan to meet the goals
Perception that health behavior is not too complex	Assist the patient in setting realistic time limits
Perception that health behavior requires reasonable effort	Review the scale (as developed with the patient) during review dates for assessment of progress
Perception that the frequency of health behavior is not excessive	Assist the patient in specifying the period of time in which each indicator will be measured
Perception of likelihood of performing health behavior over time	Explore with the patient methods of measuring progress toward goals
Confidence related to past experience with health behavior	
Confidence related to observation or anecdotal experiences of others	
Confidence in ability to perform health behavior	

strated = 5) with which actions are taken that promote optimal wellness, recovery, and rehabilitation (Iowa Outcomes Project, 2000, p. 233). The indicators include behaviors such as asking questions when indicated, completing health-related tasks, performing self-screening when indicated, describing strategies to eliminate unhealthy behavior, and performing prescribed health behavior when indicated (Iowa Outcomes Project, 2000, p. 233). A related outcome, Health Promoting Behavior, includes a wide range of "actions to sustain or increase wellness" (Iowa Outcomes Project, 2000, p. 232). The indicators for this outcome have the following foci: monitoring the environment and individual behavior for risks; seeking to achieve balance in practices such as exercise, sleep/rest, work, leisure, and nutrition; acquiring and maintaining social ties and relationships; and sociopolitical community action. Like the Health Seeking Behavior outcome, a frequency scale of 1 (never demonstrated) to 5 (consistently demonstrated) is used.

The Risk Control outcome refers to the extent to which the patient demonstrates "actions to eliminate or reduce actual, personal, and modifiable health threats" (Iowa Outcomes Project, 2000, p. 353). The indicators first focus on the client's acknowledging that she has the particular risk and then modifying and monitoring her lifestyle patterns to reduce the risk. Specific behavioral indicators include participating in screening, obtaining immunizations, using social support resources, recognizing changes in own health status, and developing risk control strategies. A related outcome, Risk Detection, is defined as "actions taken to identify personal health threats" (Iowa Outcomes Project, 2000, p. 369). The behavioral indicators include recognizing signs and symptoms that indicate risks, seeking validation of perceived risks, performing self-examinations at recommended intervals, acquiring knowledge of family history, and using resources to stay informed about potential risks.

CASE STUDY

As previously noted, Mr. James has several self-care needs that are not being met because he has elected to change the prescribed treatment for his chronic emphysema. Although he perceives his health as "good, even better than that of my friends in nursing homes," the professional health care team, as well as his family, is concerned about his deteriorating physical condition and the probability of hospitalization or institutionalization. Given the assessment findings, it has been determined that his negative health behaviors (Altered Health Maintenance) are related to role disturbance, knowledge deficit, a loss of control, and grieving over his wife's death.

Desired goals for Mr. James include the following:

1. Positive health perception beliefs regarding the benefits of taking action and the threats (consequences) of inaction

2. Perception of maintaining maximum control and resources to take action
3. Risk control, as evidenced by positive health behaviors and self-monitoring

To determine if nursing intervention for Mr. James is effective, the nursing staff would observe for health behavior outcome indicators including the following:

1. Taking medications as prescribed
2. Eating regular, nutritionally balanced meals
3. Increasing body weight to appropriate range
4. Reporting sleep patterns normal for him before the loss of his wife
5. Reporting less fatigue
6. Engaging in regular physical and social activities
7. Describing health resources and the effect of self–health regulating behaviors on health maintenance

Achieving these outcome benchmarks would indicate that Mr. James is changing his present health maintenance behaviors to more positive perceptions and activities. Although nurses should be positive regarding the potential for change in clients such as Mr. James, they should acknowledge that they may not wish to change all of the behaviors that are considered nonsupportive of health. Any intervention that helps to bring about more positive health perceptions can be considered successful because attitude is basic to engaging in health maintenance. Stuifbergen and Rogers (1997, p. 2) noted that the "concept of health promotion emphasizes self-care rather than expert care and promotes an active, independent attitude toward health care." It should also be clear that facilitating lifestyle integration of small changes or "one habit at a time" is more likely to be successful than overwhelming the client with a barrage of changes to be made (Prochaska, Norcross, & DiClemente, 1994).

NURSING INTERVENTIONS

The diagnosis of Altered Health Maintenance indicates a dysfunction in one or more components that contribute to health maintenance: physical, psychologic, social, or cultural. Thus a wide range of nursing interventions are appropriate.

Few interventions that influence Altered Health Maintenance in older adult populations have been examined from a research perspective. Many of the interventions for Altered Health Maintenance are based on the Transtheoretical Model of change (Prochaska, Norcross, & DiClemente, 1994), motivation theory, and learning theory with various educational principles. The generalizability of the Transtheoretical Model has been demonstrated with a wide range of health behaviors and client populations (Prochaska, Velicer, et al., 1994), thus providing a useful framework for nursing interventions. Although not a comprehensive list, the following interventions from the *Nursing Interventions Classification*

(NIC) (Iowa Intervention Project, 2000) are given as examples and are based on theoretical and/or clinical perspectives. See Table 2-1, which lists these interventions with selected activities and corresponding outcomes with indicators developed by the Iowa Outcomes Project (2000).

Self-Awareness Enhancement

Self-Awareness Enhancement can be used for persons who deny or are unaware of their need for change (precontemplation) or for those who have been thinking about unhealthy patterns but have not yet been able to make a change (contemplation) (Prochaska, Velicer, et al., 1994). Individuals with an alteration in health management might not perceive their problems clearly. Therefore a first step in facilitating behavior change is to increase their awareness of their situation. According to Damsteegt and Christoffersen (1982), self-awareness involves a process of self-evaluation in which a person compares his behavior with external standards or internal values. This comparison can lead to a negative self-evaluation that initially decreases self-esteem. It is hypothesized that this decrease in self-esteem leads to a behavior or attitude change to decrease the dissonance between behavior and salient standards.

The intervention Self-Awareness Enhancement is defined as "assisting a patient to explore and understand his/her thoughts, feelings, motivations, and behaviors" (Iowa Intervention Project, 2000, p. 574). The activities for Self-Awareness Enhancement focus on assisting a client to examine thought patterns regarding the self and her situation. This examination process includes expressing feelings of anxiety or fear and identifying her strengths and barriers to behavior change or acquisition of new health behavior. Self-Awareness Enhancement also includes assisting the client to evaluate lifestyle patterns and determine what is important in her life. One mechanism for assisting clients to evaluate what is important is to engage them in projecting images of "possible selves." Possible selves are images of who a person wants to be in the future. Research has shown that thinking about and projecting possible selves play a powerful role in motivating and regulating behavior and that generating detailed self-images as one is working toward a goal actually shapes and organizes the behavior as it is being enacted (Hooker & Kaus, 1992). Cross and Markus (1991) found that older adults' possible selves include more health-related images than those of younger adults. Thus assisting older adults to visualize themselves as becoming or remaining healthy or independent in the future might influence them to engage in behavior patterns that drive them toward that possible self.

Values Clarification

A "companion" intervention to Self-Awareness Enhancement that may be useful during the contemplation phase of health behavior change is Values Clarification. Values Clarification is a process of "assisting another to clarify his/her own values in order to facilitate effective decision-making" (Iowa Intervention Project, 2000, p. 693). Values are antecedents to beliefs, which, in turn, influence behavior; thus Values Clarification can be used as a basis for acquiring a new health behavior or changing a pattern that does not support or advance health. Activities for Values Clarification focus on using queries that stimulate reflection and evaluation of a client's own beliefs, attitudes, and values. A number of paper-pencil activities have also been suggested as tools to promote reflection (Pender, 1987) and to evaluate advantages and disadvantages of alternatives available to the individual. An important component of Values Clarification is for the client to consider consequences of a given behavior. In implementing this intervention, nurses must consider the ethical and legal aspects of free choice in a given situation before initiating the Values Clarification process.

Although not tested as a research protocol, the Values Clarification process has been used clinically to assist older adults to develop advanced directives for health care (M. Heffner, personal communication, February 1992). Nurses have likely included discrete activities that are listed in this intervention when assisting clients to make important health-related choices.

Learning Readiness Enhancement

Learning Readiness Enhancement includes actions that help in "improving the ability and willingness to receive information" (Iowa Intervention Project, 2000, p. 425). The focus of this intervention is to stabilize illness-related biomedical factors that can impede the learning process. For example, actions to maximize the hemodynamic state and fulfill basic physical or safety needs, as well as measures to control subjective states such as pain and fatigue, can decrease barriers to learning self-care. Activities for enhancing learning readiness are also directed toward minimizing use of pharmacologic agents that alter perception and toward maximizing sensory input. Finally, the intervention focuses on assisting the client to comprehend the severity of the illness or consequences of behavior choices and his ability to control progression of the illness or functional impairments.

Learning Readiness Enhancement is an intervention that could be used in the contemplation and/or planning stages of the Transtheoretical Model (Prochaska, Velicer, et al., 1994). It can also be used in clinical situations where it is necessary for the client to learn how to manage the symptoms and treatment of one or more disabling medical conditions. In this context the client could also be assisted to manage symptoms and redevelop confidence in the functional capacities of the body and the self.

Teaching: Individual

Teaching is a major component of health maintenance intervention. Teaching (often referred to as "patient teaching") is a process of planning, implementing, and evaluating instruction in a way that helps clients learn (Rakel, 1992). The current NIC (Iowa Intervention Project, 2000) includes two general patient teaching interventions. Teaching: Individual focuses on one-to-one (individual) teaching (Iowa Intervention Project, 2000, p. 643), whereas Teaching: Group focuses on group teaching (Iowa Intervention Project, 2000, pp. 641-642). In addition, there are 10 "content-specific" interventions (e.g., Teaching: Prescribed Activity/Exercise, Teaching: Prescribed Medication) (p. 648) that could be used according to the client's particular content learning needs. Only the Teaching: Individual intervention is described here for purposes of illustration.

The activities for this intervention begin with determining the client's existing level of knowledge and the motivation and ability to learn. It also includes assisting the client to identify resources for and barriers to learning and engaging in health maintenance. An understanding of the client's knowledge, perceptions, and readiness is then used to mutually establish realistic learning objectives and to project time lines for outcomes achievement. Again, emphasis is placed on identifying small, sequential steps toward a larger, more long-term goal. Using small, incremental goals is less overwhelming and less likely to arouse intense emotional responses that block decisions to act (Prochaska, Norcross, & DiClemente, 1994).

Attending to the learning environment is also critical to achieving desired learning outcomes. Diminished sensory function and slowed information processing capacity require minimal distractions, short sessions, and basic "how-to" information. Including significant others in the instruction facilitates reinforcement and clarification of information and assists in executing newly acquired behavior and thought patterns. Finally, follow-up sessions and/or "call-backs" can be used to reinforce achievement and to identify misperceptions and difficulties encountered in using the knowledge and skill in everyday life. Clearly, teaching goes beyond simple dissemination of information to include repeated discussions of ways the information can be integrated into everyday living patterns. This translation of health maintenance actions into everyday living goes a long way in facilitating acquisition of new behavior. Similarly, focusing on small, discrete actions that can be integrated on a regular (daily) basis (rather than focusing on what has to be given up) can assist persons to gradually change negative attitudes and perceptions regarding health maintenance. Basler (1995) has argued that health behavior change is a dynamic process that progresses through stages over time and that educational and counseling interventions be tailored to whatever stage the client is experiencing. This means that client contact is maintained over time.

Mutual Goal Setting

Mutual Goal Setting is an intervention that can be used in the planning stage of behavior change. Mutual Goal Setting is defined as "collaborating with patient to identify and prioritize care goals, then developing a plan for achieving those goals" (Iowa Intervention Project, 2000, p. 462).

Determining the patient's perceptions of the "problem(s)" is a first step in engaging him in the work of identifying goals and making a plan to move toward the goals. Specific activities include assisting the patient in breaking down complex goals into small, manageable steps and prioritizing activities used for goal achievement (Iowa Intervention Project, 2000, p. 462). It is also important to clarify with the patient what actions he will perform and what actions informal or formal caregivers will perform. Identifying with the patient what personal, environmental, and social resources are available and how these resources can contribute to self–health maintenance is another Mutual Goal Setting activity. In addition, setting time limits for goal achievement or "benchmarking" progress toward goal achievement is useful in structuring actions. Finally, Mutual Goal Setting intervention includes exploring with the patient methods of measuring progress toward goals (e.g., logs, diaries, progress charts) and coordinating periodic review dates for assessment of progress toward goals (Iowa Intervention Project, 2000, p. 462).

Mutual Goal Setting is an intervention based on educational theory that identifies the adult learner as a problem solver. In this approach active participation is preferred to passive response. Goal setting is intended to improve participation in health care over a period of time. Alexy (1985) found that goal setting was an effective intervention for selected behaviors and that totally managed provider goals made a significant change in risk-reduction health behaviors related to alcohol intake, seat belt use, and exercise. Collaboratively determined goals were effective for weight-reduction behaviors, exercise levels, and global measures of life expectancy. Because the control group also had increased exercise levels, Alexy speculated that media influence independent of the study contributed to increased exercise in all three groups. Overall, goal setting was found to be effective for developing risk-reduction behaviors.

Health System Guidance

Health System Guidance is "facilitating a patient's location and use of appropriate health services" (Iowa Intervention Project, 2000, p. 368). The activities focus on explaining the operations of the particular health care system(s) of interest. This information includes an explanation of services that can be expected, their cost and time requirements, and the alternatives and risks. The activities also include assisting clients to form questions for other health care providers, interpreting responses to these questions as needed, and assisting with required paperwork (e.g., health history, insurance forms, living wills). Because many diagnostic and treatment procedures require written informed consent, this intervention also includes explaining the meaning and process of providing informed consent. Finally, in addition to providing health service information verbally, it is also critical to provide written information for contacting or locating agencies or departments within agencies.

CASE STUDY

Although Mr. James was obviously a man of great control in his employment position, his spouse managed most of his personal activities at home. Attending to his health behaviors is new to his self-image, and he is having difficulty managing them in his wife's absence.

One of the first actions for the nurse is to determine Mr. James's level of knowledge and readiness to learn more about his condition and the recommended treatment. Counseling regarding his recent loss should also occur concurrently with knowledge assessment. This could include professional counseling or referral to a support group or individuals who have experienced a similar loss. Possible referrals to social services, to a psychologist, or to a mental health nurse are discussed. While recognizing his personal loss, the counseling and self-awareness enhancement might assist Mr. James to develop a more positive self-image and in turn achieve a sense of personal control as his role is reestablished. Establishing mutual goals with Mr. James also might be useful. The health care team, in collaboration with Mr. James, can prioritize goals so that they are acceptable to him yet will meet therapeutic goals for symptom control. One goal that the health care team shares with Mr. James is the desire to keep him independent in his home. Explaining how the health care regimen can help to accomplish this goal may cause the required treatments to become more meaningful to Mr. James. It is anticipated that working through the barriers to effective symptom management, such as the bad taste of medications, will enhance his ability to incorporate the treatment with a limited number of major changes in his daily lifestyle patterns.

Although correcting Mr. James's current physiologic status might be possible through hospitalization, failure in assisting him to change and integrate more positive perceptions and health behaviors would likely result in reversion to the same condition. Changing behaviors and attitudes takes time and can occur in small increments. Referral to other supportive services such as "Meals on Wheels" or home health care might be necessary, depending on the mutual goals established and Mr. James's preferences. Particular attention should be paid to Mr. James's ethnic and cultural values regarding health behavior.

One of the goals of the nurse and team is to increase Mr. James's awareness of feeling better physically. Although documentation in a log or diary is a common method for monitoring change, Mr. James might not be motivated enough to be complete in this activity. An alternative would be to monitor his progress through his activity levels in his home, which could then be used to give Mr. James an immediate reward for having the physical stamina to complete agreed on tasks or activities.

SUMMARY

The amount of research related to the motivational components of health maintenance behavior in older adults is limited, as are studies that relate the perceptions and developmental tasks of older adults to health maintenance behaviors. Thus the search for effective interventions for this diagnosis continues and becomes increasingly important as health care costs rise and the need for self-care in symptom management, health promotion, and disease prevention increases.

The interventions described here represent examples of interventions that can be used for Altered Health Maintenance. Most of them are broad and target health attitudes, perceptions, and behavior with the goal of facilitating attitude and behavior change. The NIC (Iowa Intervention Project, 2000) contains many other interventions that target specific health protection and health promotion behaviors, including Smoking Cessation Assistance, Exercise Promotion, Nutritional Counseling, Patient Contracting, Weight Management, Substance Use Prevention, Support System Enhancement, and Health Screening (see the Taxonomy of Nursing Interventions, pp. 90-103). The interventions with a more discrete content focus can be used in situations in which a client or caregiver targets a specific health area for change. The emphasis on general health perceptions, values, attitudes, and behavior in this chapter is intentional and is grounded in beliefs that self-care and self-responsibility are at the core of maintaining and promoting health and that individuals are capable of developing the knowledge, attitudes, and skills necessary for making and enacting healthful decisions (Simmons, 1990). Thus nurses have a responsibility to assist older adults to understand their health-related experiences and to enhance their abilities to make informed choices (Hill & Lindsey, 1994). Nursing responsibilities also include promoting the understanding that health behavior change involves lifestyle change. That is, the health behavior becomes a part of everyday life and not just a time-limited self-care program (Southard & Lombard, 1997). As Kulbok and Baldwin (1992) state, "health promotion is more than the adaptation of positive health habits or the avoidance of negative health behaviors" (p. 59). Health promotion involves a complicated web of knowledge, attitudes, and behavior related to health.

Although nursing has the commitment and capability to provide interventions for health maintenance and promotion, the issues of cost and payment for these services remain. In spite of the evidence for the role of lifestyle patterns in the genesis of disease and illness and the maintenance and promotion of health, third-party reimbursement for many clinical health promotion and preventive services is lacking, especially in the area of health behavior counseling. However, for patients 65 years of age and older, Medicare now covers mammography every 24 months, Papanicolaou tests every 3 years, influenza immunizations yearly, and pneumococcal immunizations at age 65.

Although the efficiency, safety, and cost of preventive services must be considered, society's primary goal must be to improve health status at a reasonable cost and not simply to contain cost (Thacker et al., 1994). It should not be assumed that prevention would necessarily save money. For example, in a randomized, controlled study involving 4195 Baltimore residents age 65 and over, individuals in the intervention group were offered free preventive visits (under waivers) to their physicians. Over a 2-year period the control group showed a 2% decline in general health over the group that was offered the intervention. The 2% difference in health might not seem significant at the individual level, but if the results are representative of the impact on the large number of Medicare recipients nationally, the difference becomes important. The researchers found that approximately two thirds of the intervention group members took advantage of the opportunity for at least one preventive visit to their primary care physician; there was little or no impact on charges under Medicare. They concluded that there appeared to be a modest health benefit with no negative cost impact (Burton et al., 1995). Results of this intervention indicated that adults over 65 years of age are interested in preventive services and can benefit from them and that such services can be cost-effective. The researchers concluded that adding preventive benefits to Medicare could improve the health of older people (German et al., 1995).

The value society places on preventive health care is reflected in the emphasis placed on cost-effectiveness. It is often stated that prevention will save money, either by decreasing medical costs or by increasing the number of productive work years. Older adults have not been included as part of this economic justification, even though many elderly individuals remain economically productive and some contribute to society in other ways such as engaging in volunteer activities. In the end our society will have to decide what resources we are willing to devote to health care for older individuals and what portion will be used for health promotion and prevention care (Klinkman, Zazove, Mehr, & Ruffin, 1992).

REFERENCES

Alexy, B. (1985). Goal setting and health risk reduction. *Nursing Research, 34*(5), 283-288.

Alto, W. A. (1995). Prevention in practice. *Primary Care, 22*(4), 543-553.

Arking, R. (1991). Modifying the aging process. In R. F. Young & E. A. Olson (Eds.), *Health, illness and disability in later life* (pp. 11-24). Thousand Oaks, CA: Sage.

Bahr, R. T., Sr. (1992). Personhood: A theory for gerontological nursing. *Holistic Nursing Practice, 7*(1), 1-6.

Baldwin, D. (1996). A model for describing low-income African-American women's participation in breast and cervical cancer early detection and screening. *Advances in Nursing Science, 19*(2), 27-42.

Basler, H. (1995). Patient education with reference to the process of behavioral change. *Patient Education and Counseling, 26,* 93-98.

Becker, M. H., & Rosenstock, I. M. (1984). Compliance with medical advice. In A. Steptoe & A. Matthews (Eds.), *Health care and human behavior.* San Diego, CA: Academic Press.

Brubaker, B. (1983). Health promotion: A linguistic analysis. *Advances in Nursing Science, 5*(3), 1-14.

Buchner, D. (1997). Physical activity and quality of life in older adults. *Journal of the American Medical Association, 277*(1), 64-66.

Burton, L. C., Steinwachs, D. M., German, P. S., Shapiro, S., Brant, L. J., Richards, T. M., & Clark, R. D. (1995). Preventive services for the elderly: Would coverage affect utilization and costs under Medicare? *American Journal of Public Health, 85*(3), 387-391.

Carpenito, L. (1987). *Nursing diagnosis: Application to clinical practice* (2nd ed.). Baltimore: Lippincott Williams & Wilkins.

Carpenito, L. (1997). *Nursing diagnosis: Application to clinical practice* (7th ed.). Baltimore: Lippincott Williams & Wilkins.

Chen, Y. (1996). Conformity with nature: A theory of Chinese American elders' health promotion and illness prevention processes. *Advances in Nursing Science, 19*(2), 17-26.

Cimino, J. A. (1996). Why can't we educate doctors to practice preventive medicine? *Preventive Medicine, 25*(1), 63-65.

Cox, C. (1985). The health self-determinism index. *Nursing Research, 34*(3), 177-182.

Cross, S., & Markus, H. (1991). Possible selves across the life span. *Human Development, 34,* 230-255.

Cummings, K. M., Becker, M. H., & Maile, M. C. (1980). Bringing the models together: An empirical approach to combining variables used to explain health actions. *Journal of Behavioral Medicine, 3*(2), 123-145.

Damsteegt, D. C., & Christoffersen, J. (1982). Objective self-awareness as a variable in the counseling process and outcome. *Journal of Counseling Psychology, 29*(4), 421-424.

Deci, E. (1975). *Intrinsic motivation.* New York: Plenum.

Department of Health and Human Services. (1985). *Health promotion and disease prevention survey.* Washington, DC: U.S. Government Printing Office.

Engle, V. F. (1984). Newman's conceptual framework and the measurement of older adults' health. *American Nursing Society, 3*(1), 24-33.

Fehring, R. J., & Frenn, M. (1986). Nursing diagnoses in a nurse-managed wellness resource center. In M. E. Hurley (Ed.), *Classification of nursing diagnoses: Proceedings of the Sixth National Conference.* St. Louis, MO: Mosby.

Frenn, M. (1994). Older adults' experience of health promotion: A guide for taxonomic development. In R. Carroll-Johnson & M. Paquette (Eds.), *Classification of nursing diagnoses: Proceedings of the Tenth National Conference* (pp. 242-249). Baltimore: Lippincott Williams & Wilkins.

German, P. S., Burton, L. C., Shapiro, S., Steinwachs, D. M., Tsuji, I., Paglia, M. J., & Damiano, A. M. (1995). Extended coverage for preventive services for the elderly: Response and results in a demonstration population. *American Journal of Public Health, 85*(3), 379-386.

Gordon, M. (1982). *Nursing diagnosis: Concepts and practices* (2nd ed.). Hightstown, NJ: McGraw-Hill.

Hill, M. D., & Lindsey, E. (1994). Health promotion: A viable curriculum framework for curriculum. *Nursing Outlook, 42*(4), 158-162.

Hooker, K., & Kaus, C. (1992). Possible selves and health behaviors in later life. *Journal of Aging and Health, 4*(3), 390-411.

Hurley, C. C., & Shea, C. A. (1992). Self-efficacy: Strategy for enhancing diabetic self-care. *The Diabetes Educator, 18*(2), 146-150.

Iowa Intervention Project. J. C. McCloskey & G. M. Bulechek (Eds.). (2000). *Nursing interventions classification (NIC)* (3rd ed.). St. Louis, MO: Mosby.

Iowa Outcomes Project. M. Johnson, M. Maas, & S. Moorhead (Eds.). (2000). *Nursing outcomes classification (NOC)* (2nd ed.). St. Louis, MO: Mosby.

Jackson, R. S., Leininger, L. S., Harris, R. P., & Kaluzny, A. D. (1994). Implementing continuous quality improvement in primary care: Implications for preventive services. *Journal of Ambulatory Care Management, 17*(3), 8-14.

Jaen, C. R., Stange, K. C., & Nutting, P. A. (1994). Competing demands of primary care: A model for the delivery of clinical preventive services. *Journal of Family Practice, 38*(2), 166-171.

Johnson-Saylor, M. T., Pohl, J., & Lowe-Wickson, B. (1982). An assessment form for determining patients' health status and coping responses. *Top Clinical Nursing, 6*(2), 20-27.

Kim, M. J., McFarland, G., & McLane, A. (Eds.). (1984). *Classification of nursing diagnoses: Proceedings of the Fifth National Conference.* St. Louis, MO: Mosby.

King, A. C., Oman, R. F., Brassington, G. S., Bliwise, D. L., & Haskell, W. L. (1997). Moderate-intensity exercise and self-rated quality of sleep in older adults. *Journal of the American Medical Association, 277*(1), 32-37.

Klinkman, M. S., Zazove, P., Mehr, D. R., & Ruffin, M. T. (1992). A criterion-based review of preventive health care in the elderly. Part 1: Theoretical framework and development of criteria. *Journal of Family Practice, 34*(2), 205-224.

Kulbok, P., & Baldwin, J. H. (1992). From preventive health behavior to health promotion: Advancing a positive construct of health. *Advances in Nursing Science, 14*(4), 50-64.

Laffrey, S. (1986). Development of a health conception scale. *Research Nursing Health, 9,* 107-113.

Lemley, K. B., O'Grady, E. T., Rauckhorst, L., Russell, D. D., & Small, N. (1994). Baseline data on the delivery of clinical preventive services provided by nurse practitioners. *Nurse Practitioner, 19*(5), 57-63.

Lindsey, E., & Hartrick, G. (1996). Health-promoting nursing practice: The demise of the nursing process. *Journal of Advanced Nursing, 23,* 106-112.

McWilliams, C., Stewart, M., Brown, J., Desai, K., & Coderre, P. (1996). Creating health in chronic illness. *Advances in Nursing Science, 18*(3), 1-15.

Meyer, D. L. (1995). Screening for disease, cost-effectiveness and guidelines. *Primary Care, 22*(4), 591-599.

Mezey, M. D., Rauckhorst, L., & Stokes, S. A. (1993). *Health assessment of the older individual.* New York: Springer.

Moch, S. D. (1989). Health within illness: Conceptual evaluation and practice possibilities. *Advances in Nursing Science, 11*(4), 23-31.

Mor-Barak, M., Scharlach, A., Birba, L., & Sokolov, J. (1992). Employment, social networks and health in retirement years. *International Journal of Aging and Human Development, 35*(2), 145-149.

Morgan, G. D., Noll, E. L., Orleans, C. T., Rimer, B. K., Amfoh, K., Phil, M., & Bonney, G. (1996). Reaching midlife and older smokers: Tailored interventions for routine medical care. *Preventive Medicine, 25*(3), 346-354.

Newman, M. A., Sime, A. M., & Corcoran-Perry, S. A. (1991). The focus of the discipline of nursing. *Advances in Nursing Science, 14*(1), 1-6.

North American Nursing Diagnosis Association. (1999). *Nursing diagnoses: Definitions & classification 1999-2000.* Philadelphia: Author.

Pender, N. (1987). *Health promotion in nursing practice* (2nd ed.). Norwalk, CT: Appleton & Lange.

Pender, N. (1996). *Health promotion in nursing practice* (3rd ed.). Norwalk, CT: Appleton & Lange.

Peret, K. K., & Stachowiak, B. (1984). Alteration in health maintenance: Conceptual base, etiology and defining characteristics. In M. J. Kim, G. McFarland, & A. McLane (Eds.), *Classification of nursing diagnoses: Proceedings of the Fifth National Conference* (pp. 364-370). St. Louis, MO: Mosby.

Prochaska, J., Norcross, J., & DiClemente, C. (1994). *Changing for good.* New York: Avon.

Prochaska, J. O., Velicer, W. F., Rossi, J., Goldstein, M. G., Marcus, B., Rakowski, W., Fiore, C., Harlow, L., Redding, C., Rosenbloom, D., & Rossi, S. (1994). Stages of change and decisional balance for 12 problem behaviors. *Health Psychology, 13*(1), 39-46.

Rakel, B. (1992). Interventions related to patient teaching. In G. Bulechek & J. McCloskey (Guest Eds.). *Nursing Clinics of North America, 27*(2), 397-405.

Rosenstock, I. M. (1974). Historical origins of the health belief model. In M. Becker (Ed.), *The health belief model and personal health behavior.* Thorofare, NJ: Slack.

Simmons, D. A. (1980). *A classification scheme for client problems in community health nursing* (DHHS Publication No. HRA 80-16). Washington, DC: U.S. Department of Health and Human Services.

Simmons, S. J. (1990). The health promoting self-care system model: Directions for nursing research and practice. *Journal of Advanced Nursing, 15,* 1162-1166.

Southard, D. R., & Lombard, D. (1997). Principles of health behavior change. In S. O. Roberts, R. A. Robergs & P. Hanson (Eds.), *Clinical exercise testing and prescription, theory and application* (pp. 263-280). Boca Raton, FL: CRC Press.

Spirduso, W. (1995). *Physical dimensions of aging.* Champaign, IL: Human Kinetics.

Stange, K. C., Fedirko, T., Zyzanski, S. J., & Jaen, C. R. (1994). How do family physicians prioritize delivery of multiple preventive services? *The Journal of Family Practice, 38*(3), 231-237.

Strecher, V. J., DeVellis, B., Becker, M. H., & Rosenstock, I. M. (1986). The role of self-efficacy in achieving health behavior change. *Health Education Quarterly, 13*(1), 73-91.

Stuifbergen, A. K., & Rogers, S. (1997). Health promotion: An essential component of rehabilitation for persons with chronic disabling conditions. *Advances in Nursing Science, 19*(4), 1-20.

Tackenburg, J., & Glick, O. (1991). Altered health maintenance. In M. Maas, K. Buckwalter, & M. Hardy (Eds.), *Nursing diagnoses and interventions for the elderly* (pp. 6-17). Redwood City, CA: Addison Wesley Longman.

Taft, L. B. (1985). Self-esteem in later life: A nursing perspective. *Advances in Nursing Science, 8,* 77-84.

Thacker, S. B., Koplan, J. P., Taylor, W. R., Hinman, A. R., Katz, M. F., & Roper, W. L. (1994). Assessing prevention effectiveness using data to drive program decisions. *Public Health Reports, 109*(2), 187-194.

U.S. Preventive Services Task Force. (1996). *The guide to clinical preventive services* (2nd ed.). Baltimore: Lippincott Williams & Wilkins.

U.S. Public Health Service. (1990). *Healthy people 2000: National health promotion and disease prevention objectives.* Washington, DC: U.S. Department of Health and Human Services.

U.S. Public Health Service. (1996). *Healthy people 2000: Midcourse review and 1995 revisions.* Washington, DC: U.S. Department of Health and Human Services.

Van Nostrand, J., Furner, S., & Suzman, R. (Eds.). (1993). Health data on older Americans in the United States. *Vital Health Statistics, 3,* 27.

Wallston, K. A., & Wallston, B. S. (1982). Who is responsible for your health? The construct of health locus of control. In G. Saunders & J. Suls (Eds.), *Social psychology of health and illness* (pp. 65-95). Hillsdale, NJ: Lawrence Earlbaum & Associates.

Warner, K. E., & Warner, P. A. (1993). Is an ounce of prevention worth a pound of cure? Disease prevention in health care reform. *Journal of Ambulatory Care Management, 16*(4), 38-49.

Young, R., & Olson, E. (1991). Overview of health and disease in later life. In R. F. Young & E. A. Olson (Eds.), *Health, illness and disability in later life* (p. 107). Thousand Oaks, CA: Sage.

CHAPTER 3

RISK FOR INJURY: FALLS

Jacqueline M. Stolley, Anne Lewis, Laurie Moore, and Pamela Harvey

Falls are a major health concern for the elderly, causing injury, impaired mobility, and death. Although 75% of falls do not result in serious injury, the risk of injury related to falls increases with age, particularly for persons over 75 years of age (Sattin, 1992). Falls in elderly persons can produce dependence and invalidism (Baker, 1996). Close to 5% of falls end in a fracture, most frequently of the hip, pelvis, humerus, or wrist (Nevitt, Cummings, Kidd, & Black, 1989; Sattin, 1992; Tinetti, Speechley, & Ginter, 1988). Older women are more likely to experience serious injury because of osteopenia (Vecht-Hart, Peters, & Collette, 1996). Hip fractures have the greatest impact of all fall-related injuries. An estimated 85% of persons who have suffered hip fractures with subsequent hospitalization and recovery experience prolonged periods of impaired mobility at 6 months following the injury (Marottoli, Berkman, & Cooney, 1992). Falls are the leading cause of injury-related mortality and rank as the sixth leading cause of death among the elderly (Runge, 1993; Sattin, 1992). Elders represent 12% of the population, yet 70% of deaths caused by falls occur in those over age 65 (Commodore, 1995).

In addition to physical injury related to falls, persons can experience psychologic effects such as fear of falling again, loss of confidence, increased dependency, and social isolation (Downton & Andrews, 1990; Tideiksaar, 1997; Tinetti & Powell, 1993). These persons are likely to become functionally dependent in walking, requiring the help of another person or assistive devices for locomotion. Loss of independence and immobility are related to temporary or permanent institutionalization in long-term care facilities.

The health care system bears a particularly large portion of the economic impact of falls and fractures (Miller, 1995). One fourth of hospital admissions of elderly individuals are related directly to falling, and the average length of acute stay for a faller is twice that of a nonfaller. Added to the immediate cost of falls and recovery is the cost of long-term care. Nearly half of the approximately 200,000 yearly hip fracture patients who are hospitalized for falling become institutionalized in long-term care (Dwyer, 1987; Meier, 1988; Tideiksaar, 1989; Tinetti, Liu, & Claus, 1993). Thus falls are an important health care issue for gerontologic nurses, both from a quality of life standpoint and for their economic impact.

RELATED FACTORS/ETIOLOGIES

The elderly are particularly vulnerable to serious injury as a consequence of falls. Osteoporosis causes bones to become fragile and predisposed to fractures (Nevitt, Cummings, & the Study of Osteoporotic Fractures Research Group, 1993; Vecht-Hart et al., 1996). Changes in baroreceptor reflexes can make the elderly prone to postural hypotension, causing episodes of light-headedness, loss of balance, and falls. An elderly person can be inhibited from "catching" herself when falling because of slowed reaction time associated with normal aging. Changes in visual fields, decreased dark adaptation, and diminished peripheral vision, depth perception acuity, and color perception can cause a misinterpretation of the environment and lead to tripping and falling. Gait and balance change with diminished functioning of the nervous, muscular, skeletal, sensory, circulatory, and respiratory systems. These changes alter the center of gravity, body sway, and balance, contributing to falls (Alexander, 1994; Chu et al., 1999; Hu & Woolacott, 1994; Maki, Holliday, & Topper, 1994; Tideiksaar, 1989). Changes in balance and proprioception make the elderly particularly vulnerable to changes in floor surfaces (e.g., glossy, slick floors or carpet). Finally, extreme age or disease can interfere with the function of protective reflexes and place the affected person at risk for falls (Lord, 1996).

RISK FACTORS

Specific risk factors for falling can be categorized as either intrinsic or extrinsic. Intrinsic risk factors are internal in nature and include patient variables such as age or disease. Extrinsic risk factors include things in the environment that can contribute to falls, such as poor lighting, clutter, slick floors, and poor footwear. Intrinsic and extrinsic factors related to the risk for falls are summarized in Box 3-1.

Intrinsic Factors

Intrinsic factors that contribute to the incidence of falling include the aging process (Craven & Bruno, 1986; Das & Kataria, 1985; Runge, 1993; Tideiksaar, 1989) and numerous disease conditions, including cardiac disease, cere-

Box 3-1	Intrinsic and Extrinsic Fall Risk Factors and Risk for Injury Defining Characteristics	
Intrinsic Fall Risk Factors	**Extrinsic Fall Risk Factors**	**Risk for Injury Defining Characteristics**
Older age	Environmental change	Presence of risk factors such as:
Medications	Mobility aids	Internal
• Cardiovascular	Floor surfaces	• Biochemical
• CNS depressants	• Slippery	• Regulatory function (sensory dysfunction)
• Laxatives	• High gloss	• Integrative dysfunction
Diseases	• Sloped	• Effector dysfunction
• Cardiovascular	High furniture	• Tissue hypoxia
• Cerebrovascular	• Beds	• Malnutrition
• Orthopedic	• Chairs	• Immune-autoimmune dysfunction
• Neurologic	Use of restraints	• Abnormal blood profile
Elimination		• Physical (broken skin, altered mobility)
• Incontinence (bowel or bladder)		• Developmental age
• Urgency		• Psychologic (affective orientation)
Sensory deficits		External
• Visual		• Biologic
• Hearing		• Chemical (pharmaceutic agents, alcohol, caffeine)
Communication deficits		• Nutrients
Altered mental status		• Physical (design, structure, and arrangement of community, building, and/or equipment)
• Confusion		• Mode of transport or transportation
• Agitation		• People or provider
• Depression		
• Anxiety		
History of falls		

brovascular disorders, and orthopedic and neurologic disorders (Innes, 1985; Kippenbrock & Soja, 1993). Patients with complex diagnoses, those with shorter lengths of acute care stay, and those who initiate early rehabilitation also are susceptible to falling (Baker, 1992). These data are important when considering the current health care climate of short acute hospital stays and critical pathways that can force elderly persons into physical rehabilitation for which they are not ready.

Another intrinsic factor that commonly has been associated with falls among the elderly is the individual's need for elimination. Many falls occur while elderly persons are on the way to, using, or returning from the bathroom (Hendrich, Nyhuis, Kippenbrock, & Soja, 1995; Innes, 1985; Kippenbrock & Soja, 1993). Falls associated with elimination can result from unfocused locomotion related to feelings of urgency or from a slip on incontinent body fluids on the floor. Furthermore, nighttime visits to the bathroom can be particularly perilous because of the diminished night vision that occurs as a normal part of aging.

Altered mental status also is related to the increased incidence of falls (Hendrich et al., 1995; Kippenbrock & Soja, 1993; Reinboth & Gyldenvand, 1982; Tideiksaar, 1989; Tinetti & Powell, 1993; Tinnetti et al., 1988). Studies have associated agitation, depression, and anxiety with the occurrence of falls (Hendrich et al., 1995; Tinetti & Powell, 1993; Vaughn, Young, Rice, & Stoner, 1993). A history of falls (Hendrich et al., 1995; Tinetti & Powell,

1993) might indicate illness in the elderly person (Kuehn & Sendelweck, 1995; Tinetti & Powell, 1993). Treating the underlying illness can result in a decreased number of repeat falls, providing a viable alternative to using restraints. Finally, vision, hearing, and communication losses have been implicated in the increased incidence of falling (Lawrence & Maher, 1992; Tideiksaar, 1989, 1997).

Extrinsic Factors

Extrinsic factors also contribute to falls. Early researchers found that falls commonly occur during the first week of hospitalization, suggesting that familiarity with surroundings might reduce accidents (Tack, Ulrich, & Kehr, 1987; Walshe & Rosen, 1979). However, in today's health care climate elders are more likely to experience shorter lengths of stay, encounter multiple transfers within the health care setting (e.g., subacute, skilled nursing facility), and have a significant degree of illness on discharge. Thus the elderly person can experience multiple environmental changes, resulting in less familiarity with the environment and an increased potential for falling. Interestingly, the first 24-hour postoperative period and the first 24 hours after treatment with intravenous lines have emerged as times when falling is more likely to occur (Hendrich et al., 1995). Thus the current health care environment, with its emphasis on technology for treating illness, might actually contribute to the iatrogenic consequence of falling.

Medications are external agents introduced to the elderly person and are considered by the North American Nursing Diagnosis Association (NANDA, 1999) to be external risk factors, although some experts consider them to be intrinsic factors because of their effects on internal biologic processes. Research has shown that medications affecting the cardiovascular and central nervous systems (Hendrich et al., 1995; Lawrence & Maher, 1992; Watson & Mayhew, 1994) increase the risk of falling, most likely because of the potential for orthostatic hypotension or for inducing altered mental status. Laxatives also have been implicated in the incidence of falling (Innes, 1985; Stolley, 1990).

Persons with impaired physical mobility are likely to use mobility aids such as wheelchairs, straight canes, quad canes, and walkers. An early study by Kalchthaler, Bascon, and Quintos (1978) revealed that older persons in wheelchairs had a greater number of falls than those using canes and walkers. Other studies report that patients who used assistive devices were more likely to fall than patients who did not (Berry, Fisher, & Lang, 1981; Lund & Sheafor, 1985). Foerster (1981), however, found that the use of assistive devices was not significantly related to the incidence or frequency of falls. The reason for this discrepancy between studies could be that patients who use assistive devices might suffer from more illnesses than patients who are not dependent on mobility aids. Generally studies implicate impaired mobility as a risk factor for falls and suggest that the use of mobility aids is an added risk, perhaps because of the health condition requiring a mobility aid or because of the aid itself. Ongoing research regarding the contribution of the use of mobility aids to the incidence of falling bears watching.

Other extrinsic factors that contribute to the risk of falling include elevated floor surfaces, bed heights that are either low or high, and the lack of grab bars in strategic locations, such as bathrooms and hallways (Tideiksaar, 1989, 1997). Tinetti, Liu, and Ginter (1992) found that persons who were restrained were more likely to suffer serious injuries than those with similar physical conditions who were not restrained. Furthermore, the extrinsic factor of restraint use contributes to muscle weakness and confusion, which are intrinsic risk factors for falls. These findings point to the importance of the recent trend toward restraint-free and restraint-appropriate environments.

ASSESSMENT

Assessment of a person's risk for falling entails determining whether the individual has relevant risk factors. The general risk factors associated with the NANDA diagnosis Risk for Injury are highlighted in Table 3-1. Internal risk factors are included in the following categories: biochemical; integrative dysfunction; effector dysfunction; physical: altered mobility; developmental age; and psychologic. External risk factors are included in the following categories: chemical/pharmaceutic agents; physical environment; and mode of transportation.

Several tools for fall risk identification have been reported in the literature (Morse, 1997; Morse, Morse, & Tylko, 1989; Perlin, 1992; Tinetti & Powell, 1993). The Risk Assessment for Falls II (RAFS II), developed by nurse investigators and tested in several settings (Ross, Watson, Gyldenvand, & Reinboth, 1991), is a 13-item assessment tool that predicts high risk for falling. The categories of indicators for risk of fall are (1) days since admission; (2) age; (3) date of last fall; (4) unsteadiness; (5) mental orientation; (6) agitation; (7) depression; (8) anxiety; (9) vision; (10) communication difficulties; (11) medications with cardiovascular and central nervous system effects; (12) chronic diseases; and (13) urinary problems. The RAFS II incorporates factors most frequently identified with falls and weights the magnitude of risk factors according to intensity.

The risk of falling increases dramatically with the number of risk factors. Tinetti et al. (1988) found that over a 1-year period fall risk rose from 8% for elderly persons with no risk factors identified to 32% for persons who had two risk factors and 78% for persons who had four or more risk factors. Morse, Tylko, and Dixon (1987) and Hogue, Studenski, and Duncan (1989) reported similar results.

The RAFS II was tested in several acute care (Gyldenvand, 1984) and extended care settings (Reinboth & Gyldenvand, 1982; Reinboth, 1985). The RAFS II showed an accuracy of 85% to 90% with fall prediction (Ross et al., 1991). However, because current health care trends lead to shorter lengths of stay, the RAFS II overpredicts falls in the acute care arena. Thus persons identified at high risk for falling will likely fall eventually, but probably not during an acute care stay.

Approximately 2.5 falls occur per 1000 patient days in acute settings, whereas nearly 420 falls occur per 1000 patient days in long-term care settings (Heslin et al., 1992). A risk assessment tool should be adaptable to several care settings. Heslin and colleagues developed a risk assessment tool that is adaptable across settings (acute, residential, and long-term care). Studies testing this tool revealed that falls in acute care were related to the patient's tendency to attempt to get out of bed unassisted. The following characteristics were identified as risk factors: age over 80, impaired mobility, generalized weakness, previous fall from a chair or wheelchair, and restraint use. Acute care patients who were predicted to have the greatest injury were those persons over age 80 and those individuals with mobility deficits. Interestingly, 54% of fallers were considered alert and 46% were confused.

In the long-term care setting characteristics of fallers included dependence in ambulating, wheelchair confinement, limited mobility, and presence of an internal medicine diagnosis or neurologic disorder. The combination of predictors that was most likely to result in injury was persons age 80 or over with a neurologic deficit who had fallen from a wheelchair or chair. In the residential setting fallers tended to be over age 80, have impaired gait, require total assistance for transfer, and have internal medicine and neurologic diagnoses. In this setting 24% of fallers ambulated without assistance. Risk factors that were most frequently associated with injury included a diagnosis in the internal medicine category, ambulation, mobility deficits, and use of restraints. Combined predictors that best identified fallers in all three settings were the use of a restrictive device, previous falls from chairs and wheelchairs, confusion, neurologic deficits, mobility deficits, and generalized weakness (Heslin et al., 1992).

Each risk factor found to predict falls was given a score reflecting its importance (Heslin et al., 1992). Three additional risk factors were added to the assessment form based on research results: (1) medications (sedatives, tranquilizers, narcotics, and general anesthesia) within 24 hours; (2) altered elimination (frequency, urgency, and nocturia); and (3) previous falls (Heslin et al., 1992).

The risk assessment tool developed by Heslin and colleagues (1992) was tested in an acute care hospital in the Midwestern United States (Stolley, Lewis, Moore, Hanrahan, & Carter, 1996). In a research utilization project 144 patients were assessed on an orthopedic nursing unit and a skilled nursing unit. Of these 144 patients, 21 fell. The risk factors of confusion, agitation, generalized weakness, and altered elimination were most predictive of falling. It might be possible for nurses to identify persons at risk for falling using these four risk factors, rather than a more comprehensive and time-consuming tool such as the RAFS II. Falls would not be overpredicted, and prevention strategies would target only those at risk for falling during the acute stay. However, nurses must be cautious in using this approach because the development of site-specific risk factors based on sound research methods is needed.

CASE STUDY

D. Murphy, age 82, was admitted to an acute care hospital from her home for pneumonia. The illness began as the flu but rapidly progressed to the point of requiring hospitalization. Mrs. Murphy's daughter, Ms. Wilson, was concerned because her mother sometimes seemed confused about the time of day and events. This confusion progressed with the emergence of difficulty in breathing and tachypnea. In addition to her pneumonia, Mrs. Murphy has a history of hypertension, for which she takes Cardizem ER, 120 mg bid. She is also on Lasix 40 mg bid for congestive heart failure (CHF).

Mrs. Murphy is a widow, but her daughter, who lives 2 miles away, is supportive and willing to assist with care. The patient is ordinarily alert and oriented and able to cook and to care for herself. Her mobility is somewhat impaired because of chronic arthritis affecting her hips, knees, and hands. Mrs. Murphy uses a cane for walking around her house but does not walk more than a few blocks without the assistance of another person. Her vision is impaired, and her daughter says that cataract surgery has been contemplated. In the meantime, Mrs. Murphy has arranged the furniture in her home so she can reach out to it for balance and support when ambulating. The lighting is sufficient to guide her ambulation, and she is careful to avoid clutter. This is especially important because Mrs. Murphy has urinary urgency and must get to the bathroom as quickly as possible to avoid being incontinent.

On admission to the hospital, it is obvious that Mrs. Murphy has respiratory distress, weakness, and intermittent confusion. Her daughter comments that Mrs. Murphy is even more confused since coming to the hospital. She already has experienced one episode of incontinence and was found trying to walk to the bathroom without assistance. An interdisciplinary care conference has been arranged to discuss the current plan of care and to begin to address potential discharge needs.

Mrs. Murphy exhibits several risk factors that contribute to the diagnosis Risk for Injury with a focus on falls. Internal or intrinsic factors that could increase the risk of injury include the following: regulatory function, physical factors (mobility), developmental age (physiologic), and psychologic factors (orientation). External or extrinsic factors that also might contribute to a risk for injury include chemical (medications) and physical (unfamiliarity with new environment). The patient is on several medications, has mental status changes, and is somewhat limited in her level of mobility. She also is in an environment with which she is unfamiliar, adding to the risk of injury from a fall.

NURSING DIAGNOSIS

NANDA defines Risk for Injury as "a state in which the individual is at risk of injury as a result of environmental conditions interacting with the individual's adaptive and defensive resources" (NANDA, 1999, p. 34).

Several NANDA diagnoses can be related to falls: Altered Thought Processes, developed in 1973; Risk for Injury, developed in 1978; Risk for Trauma, developed in 1980; and Impaired Environmental Interpretation Syndrome, Acute Confusion, and Chronic Confusion, developed in 1994. This chapter focuses on the nursing diagnosis Risk for Injury: Falls.

NURSING-SENSITIVE OUTCOMES

The optimal outcome in the nursing diagnosis Risk for Injury: Falls is absence of psychologic and physiologic injury. Thus as a cause of injury falls must be reduced to a minimum. Actual outcomes related to falls must be evaluated based on risk control efforts and the status of the individual and environmental safety factors that have been instituted in caring for the at-risk individual.

The *Nursing Outcomes Classification (NOC)* (Iowa Outcomes Project, 2000) provides several labels pertinent to the nursing diagnosis Risk for Injury: Falls. Risk Control is described as "actions to eliminate or reduce actual, personal, and modifiable health threats" (Iowa Outcomes Project, 2000, p. 353). The indicators of the outcome measure whether the patient demonstrates the actions: 1 = never demonstrated, 2 = rarely demonstrated, 3 = sometimes demonstrated, 4 = often demonstrated, and 5 = consistently demonstrated. Useful indicators of this outcome include the following: acknowledges risk, develops effective risk control strategies, monitors environmental risk factors, and follows selected risk control strategies. Other labels may apply to certain clients, and the reader is encouraged to review the entire label for thoroughness.

Knowledge: Personal Safety is the "extent of understanding conveyed about preventing unintentional injuries" (Iowa Outcomes Project, 2000, p. 281). This label is scaled as 1 = none, 2 = limited, 3 = moderate, 4 = substantial, and 5 = extensive. It is important to determine the client's and potential caregiver's level of knowledge regarding fall prevention strategies. This approach assists in determining the effectiveness of teaching interventions that are employed by nurses. Specific knowledge factors that might be useful under this label include description of measures to prevent falls, description of measures to reduce accidental injury, and description of home safety measures.

Several outcome labels address safety behavior of both the client and caregiver: Safety Behavior: Fall Prevention; Safety Behavior: Home Physical Environment; and Safety Behavior: Personal. Each of these labels contains indicators that measure the safety behaviors as 1 = not adequate, 2 = slightly adequate, 3 = moderately adequate, 4 = substantially adequate, or 5 = totally adequate.

Finally, two outcome labels address the safety status of the client. Safety Status: Physical Injury is defined as "severity of injuries from accidents and trauma," and Safety Status: Falls Occurrence is defined as the "number of falls in the past week." These outcome labels also can be included in an analysis of the effectiveness of a fall prevention program. Collaboration between the experts in nursing quality and risk management can prove very valuable in strengthening a fall prevention program that is based on sound interventions and measurable outcome data.

When evaluating a program of prevention, the incident report is the best source of data. When the patient or resident is assessed for risk, the risk score should be recorded in a central location in the patient's clinical record. When a fall occurs, the gerontologic nurse should investigate the incident and determine the variables involved, including determining if the patient or resident was at high risk and if the risk assessment and score were accurate. Evaluation also must be made regarding the appropriateness and individualization of prevention strategies.

Because a fall can be a symptom of a patient's or resident's deteriorating condition, the gerontologic nurse must assess for condition changes. The following are specific outcomes: (1) the number of falls decreases; (2) fewer injuries caused by falls are sustained; (3) individuals verbalize a reduced fear of falling; and (4) more patients or residents request assistance to ambulate and transfer.

CASE STUDY

Table 3-1 specifies NOC outcomes relevant to Mrs. Murphy. Outcomes were expected to be achieved gradually so that Mrs. Murphy reached level 4 or 5 in 10 days. These interventions and outcomes would be conveyed to her home care service to provide continuity and continued surveillance.

NURSING INTERVENTIONS

An enormous body of literature exists about nursing interventions for patient falls. However, much of it is in the form of suggestions rather than empirically validated strategies (Maciorowski et al., 1988; Uden, Ehnfors, & Sjostrom, 1999). Interventions include patient and family teaching, environmental management, and assessment of pharmacologic effects (Heslin et al., 1992; Innes, 1985; Isaacs, 1996; Miller, Morrison, Blair, Miller, & Morley, 1998).

Other discrete nursing actions in fall prevention include placement of the bed in low position, ensuring that the call light and other objects are within reach, providing adequate lighting, use of nonskid slippers, and urinary elimination management (Innes, 1985; Tideiksaar, 1996). Teaching patients and staff about environmental management for safety and fall prevention and about the dynamics of accidents also has been suggested. Instructions for patients include but are not limited to rising slowly and asking for assistance with toileting.

Environmental management for safety should include elimination of potential hazards such as clutter, unlocked bed or chair wheels, and spills. Confusion management for disoriented or agitated patients should be individually evaluated with regard to the proper use of side rails and other restraining devices. In essence, the interventions should be based on identified risk factors.

The *Nursing Interventions Classification (NIC)* (Iowa Intervention Project, 2000) has compiled a list of activities for the gerontologic nurse to consider when an elderly person is determined to be at risk for injury from falling. The intervention label Fall Prevention (see Table 3-1) is defined as "instituting special precautions with patient at risk for injury from falling" (Iowa Intervention Project, 2000, p. 326). Although this intervention label resulted

Suggested Nursing-Sensitive Outcomes and Nursing Interventions
Table 3-1   RISK FOR INJURY: FALLS

NURSING DIAGNOSIS
RISK FOR INJURY: FALLS
Risk Factors

Internal	External
Biochemical, regulatory function • Altered gas exchange due to impaired pulmonary function Physical • Arthritis resulting in mobility changes • Urinary urgency • Episode of incontinence • Impaired vision Development age • 82 years old Psychologic • Increased level of confusion • Attempting to get out of bed without assistance	Chemical • Medication use (diuretic, antihypertensive) Physical • Change in environment due to admission to hospital

Nursing-Sensitive Outcomes	Nursing Interventions
SAFETY BEHAVIOR: PERSONAL *Indicators* Balance of sleep and rest with activity Correct use of assistive devices	**FALL PREVENTION** *Activities* Monitor gait, balance, and fatigue level with ambulation Assist unsteady individual with ambulation Post signs to remind patient to call for help when getting out of bed, as appropriate Assist with toileting at frequent, scheduled intervals Provide nightlight at bedside
SAFETY BEHAVIOR: HOME PHYSICAL ENVIRONMENT *Indicators* Provision of lighting Provision of assistive devices in accessible location Arrangement of furniture to reduce risks	**DELIRIUM MANAGEMENT** *Activities* Initiate therapies to reduce or eliminate factors causing the delirium Encourage visitation by significant others, as appropriate Maintain a well-lit environment that reduces sharp contrasts and shadows Assist with needs related to nutrition, elimination, hydration, and personal hygiene Maintain a hazard-free environment
SAFETY BEHAVIOR: FALL PREVENTION *Indicators* Correct use of assistive devices Elimination of clutter, spills, glare from floors Adjustment of toilet height as needed Adjustment of chair height as needed Use of precautions when taking medications that increase risk for falls	**ENVIRONMENTAL MANAGEMENT** *Activities* Create a safe environment for the patient Identify the safety needs of patient, based on level of physical and cognitive function and past history of behavior Provide adaptive devices, as appropriate Place frequently used objects within reach

from a thorough review of the literature by nurse researchers, nursing activities must be individualized to fit the patient at risk. Other intervention labels to consider when developing a fall prevention plan include Delusion Management; Dementia Management; Environmental Management: Safety; Reality Orientation; and, most importantly, Surveillance: Safety.

Fall Prevention

Fall prevention programs have successfully reduced the number of falls by focusing on interventions that reduce or eliminate the incidence of falls once the risk for falling has been identified (Baker, 1996; Close et al., 1999; Heslin et al., 1992; Tack et al., 1987; Tideiksaar, 1996). Patients assessed as being at risk are identified by some method such as an

Table 3-1	Suggested Nursing-Sensitive Outcomes and Nursing Interventions—cont'd RISK FOR INJURY: FALLS—cont'd
Nursing-Sensitive Outcomes	**Nursing Interventions**
KNOWLEDGE: PERSONAL SAFETY *Indicators* Description of measures to prevent falls Description of measures to reduce risk of accidental injury **RISK CONTROL** *Indicators* Acknowledges risk Follows selected risk control strategies Uses health care services congruent with need (DC planning) Uses personal support systems to control risk **SAFETY STATUS: FALLS OCCURRENCE** *Indicators* Number of falls while walking Number of falls while sitting Number of falls from bed	**REALITY ORIENTATION** *Activities* Inform patient of person, place, and time, as needed Provide a consistent physical environment and daily routine Use environmental cues to stimulate memory, reorient, and promote appropriate behavior Provide for adequate rest/sleep/daytime naps **SURVEILLANCE: SAFETY** *Activities* Monitor patient for alterations in physical or cognitive function that might lead to unsafe behavior Provide appropriate level of supervision/surveillance to monitor patient and to allow for therapeutic actions, as needed Place patient in least restrictive environment that allows for necessary level of observation Communicate information about patient's risk to other nursing staff **URINARY INCONTINENCE CARE** *Activities* Monitor urinary elimination, including frequency, consistency, odor, volume, and color Modify clothing and environment to provide easy access to toilet Provide protective garments, as needed Schedule diuretic administration to have least impact on lifestyle **HOME MAINTENANCE ASSISTANCE** *Activities* Determine patient's home maintenance requirements Involve patient/family in deciding home maintenance requirements Provide information on how to make home environment safe and clean Order homemaker services, as appropriate

orange "dot" on their wrist bands, on the call light terminal at the nurses station, and/or on the spine of their chart.

A policy for assessing patients and implementing a fall prevention program (adapted from Heslin et al., 1992) can be found in Table 3-2. Heslin and colleagues (1992) found that this type of program led to a significant decrease in falls in all settings. In addition to the "spot the dot" program, interventions aimed at preventing falls in the acute care setting included instituting a benzodiazepine-free program and impaired mobility assessments.

Other long-term care interventions that contributed to a reduction in falls were restraint-free cushions and consultation on bed-to-chair transfers. Additionally, high-

Table 3-2	Guidelines for Completing Fall Risk Assessment and Scoring

RISK FACTOR ASSESSMENT

Risk Factor	Score
Age 65-79	0.5
Age ≥80	1
Confusion (unable to follow instruction to stay in bed)	2
Attempts to get out of bed/agitation	5
Previous fall related to patient condition	1
Impaired mobility, balance, or gait	1
Generalized weakness	1
Alterations in elimination (frequency, urgency, nocturia, incontinence, IV Lasix)	1
Medications within 24 hours (benzodiazepines, tranquilizers, narcotics, and anesthesia)	1
Immobile	−5
RISK ASSESSMENT TOTAL SCORE	

SCORING

Risk Assessment Total Score	Level of Risk
0.5-2	Level I
2.5-4	Level II
≥4.5	Level III

INTERVENTIONS BY RISK LEVEL

Risk Level	Intervention
Level I	Call bell in reach; bed in low position; side rails up; nonslip footwear
Level II	Spot the dot; assess and assist ambulation; elimination needs checked; nursing care plan; screen medications
Level III	Bed sensor

POLICY

1. A fall risk assessment will be completed on all newly admitted patients, excluding critical care, pediatrics, obstetrics, and psychiatry.
2. A flow sheet documenting fall risk assessment scores will be initiated for all Level II and Level III patients.

Adapted from Heslin, K., Towers, J., Leckie, C., Thornton-Lawrence, H., Perkin, K., Jacques, M., Mullin, J., & Wick, L. (1992). Managing falls: Identifying population-specific risk factors and prevention strategies. In S. G. Funk, E. M. Tornquist, M. T. Champagne, & R. A. Wiese (Eds.), *Key aspects of elder care: Managing falls, incontinence, and cognitive impairment* (pp. 70-88). New York: Springer.

tech transfer devices reduced the fall rate over 90%. Residential care interventions included rest stops, vigilance during dinner hour (falls related to postprandial hypotension), gait assessments, and muscle strengthening (Heslin et al., 1992). A combination of prevention strategies targeted both intrinsic and extrinsic risk factors, thus providing a safer internal and external environment for the older individual at risk for falling.

Staff education regarding fall prevention is imperative. It is important to educate not only the nursing staff involved, but also persons in other departments (e.g., housekeeping, maintenance, radiology, laboratory, dietary) who might come in contact with the patient. A highly effective strategy in preventing falls is to make all staff both aware that a particular patient is at risk for falling and responsible for reporting at-risk behavior to

the nursing staff. Persons identified at risk for falling should be reassessed periodically to determine continued risk. Assessment intervals depend on the severity of illness and the number of risk factors. During an acute illness, assessment every 24 to 48 hours might be indicated. However, with a stable patient 30-day assessment might be appropriate.

CASE STUDY

See Table 3-1 for specific nursing activities to address Mrs. Murphy's risk factors. The primary nurse educated the patient on using the call light and made sure that she had an uncluttered path to the bathroom. A discussion was held with the family regarding the use of one-to-one su-

Table 3-2	Guidelines for Completing Fall Risk Assessment and Scoring—cont'd

POLICY—cont'd

3. The flow sheet will be kept at the patient's bedside.

4. Fall risk reassessment and documentation on the flow sheet should be completed once per 12-hour tour for all Level II and Level III patients and maintained (for 3 days) for Level II patients who return to Level I.

5. For those patients scoring Level I on admission, reassessment is not required unless a significant change occurs in patient condition related to fall risk factors.

6. If in the nurse's judgment the patient does not require a bed sensor and the risk score is above 4.5, a note must be written in the core progress notes identifying the reasons for the decision; reassessment must be done every 12 hours.

7. All actual fall episodes must be documented on a fall report form.

PROCEDURE

1. Complete the fall risk assessment by marking the corresponding score in the appropriate column for the risk factors that apply to the patient. It may be necessary to collaborate with the registered nurse when completing the assessment. Consider the following:
   - Confusion: Inability to follow instructions, impaired short-term memory, impaired thought process (psychosis), and conditions that potentiate agitation, such as septicemia and hypoxia.
   - Attempts to get out of bed: Attempts to get out of bed related to factors such as agitation, alcohol, or poor pain control.
   - Previous fall related to risk factors: Note previous falls related to patient condition such as weakness, impaired mobility, or confusion. Do not include previous falls related to environmental factors such as faulty equipment.
   - Impaired mobility: Impaired gait (shuffling, small steps, slow pace, holding on to nurse, bed, walls, chairs, IV poles for support) and/or impaired balance (unsteady when standing or sitting).
   - Generalized weakness: Absence of two out of six ADL, unable to feed self, unable to turn self in bed yet is fully conscious, verbalizes is feeling weak, unable to sit on bed for 10 minutes without sliding off.
   - Alterations in elimination: Medications such as diuretics that may alter elimination patterns, including Lasix IV bolus and hs diuretics.
   - Immobile: Patient who is unable to initiate movement to get out of bed, patient who cannot attempt any self-movement. A score of −5 is assigned to prevent eligibility for a bed sensor.

2. Note whether patient has a Level I, Level II, or Level III level of risk.

3. Initiate a flow sheet to document level of risk for Level II and Level III patients.

4. Institute the interventions that correspond to the patient's level of risk.

5. Ensure that education is delivered to patient or family (or sitter) regarding fall prevention.

pervision if Mrs. Murphy's level of confusion increases. The possible use of a bed alarm also was discussed. The patient was placed on a toileting schedule of every 2 hours while awake following the administration of Lasix, and her fluids were limited in the evening hours. The importance of ensuring adequate hydration during daytime hours to prevent fluid volume deficit and subsequent problems was noted.

SUMMARY

Falls are a significant health problem for the elderly. It is important to identify risk factors and develop successful interventions to prevent falls and the devastating sequelae that may follow. The development of the nursing diagnosis Risk for Injury: Falls, based on risk factors and tested interventions, plays an important role in fall prevention and adds to the body of knowledge regarding falls in acute care settings. Successful implementation of the fall prevention program is anticipated to reduce morbidity and mortality rates and to improve the psychosocial well-being of those persons at risk for falling. A final anticipated benefit is a reduction in patient care costs for persons who are at risk for falling.

REFERENCES

Alexander, N. B. (1994). Postural control in older adults. *Journal of the American Geriatrics Society, 42,* 93-108.

Baker, D. I. (1996). Yale FICSIT: A strategy for reducing falls among older adults residing in the community. In C. Lafont, A. Baroni, M. Allard, R. Tideiksaar, B. J. Vellas, P. J. Garry, & J. L. Albarede (Eds.), *Falls, gait and balance disorders in the elderly* (pp. 5-11). New York: Springer.

Baker, L. (1992). Developing a safety plan that works for patients and nurses. *Rehabilitation Nursing, 17*(5), 264-266.

Berry, G., Fisher, R. H., & Lang, S. (1981). Detrimental incidents, including falls, in an elderly institutional population. *Journal of the American Geriatrics Society, 29*(7), 322-324.

Chu, L. W., Pei, C. K., Chiu, A., Liu, K., Chu, M. M., Wong, S., & Wong, A. (1999). Risk factors for falls in hospitalized older medical patients. *Journals of Gerontology. Series A, Biological Sciences & Medical Sciences, 54*(1), M38-M43.

Close, J., Ellis, M., Hooper, R., Glucksman, E., Jackson, S., & Swift, C. (1999). Prevention of falls in the elderly trial (PROFET): A randomised controlled trial. *Lancet, 353*(9147), 93-97.

Commodore, D. I. B. (1995). Falls in the elderly population: A look at incidence, risks, healthcare costs, and preventive strategies. *Rehabilitation Nursing, 20*(2), 84-90, 130.

Craven, R., & Bruno, P. (1986). Teach the elderly to prevent falls. *Journal of Gerontological Nursing, 12*(8), 27-33.

Das, S. K., & Kataria, M. S. (1985). Stability, movement and posture. In M. S. Kataria (Ed.), *Fits, faints and falls in old age* (pp. 11-13). Lancaster, England: MTP Press.

Downton, J. H., & Andrews, K. (1990). Postural disturbance and psychological symptoms amongst elderly people living at home. *International Journal of Geriatric Psychiatry, 5,* 93-98.

Dwyer, B. J. (1987). Putting the problem in perspective. *Focus on Geriatric Care and Rehabilitation, 1*(1), 1.

Foerster, J. (1981). A study of falls: The elderly nursing home resident. *Journal of the New York State Nurses' Association, 12,* 7-9.

Gyldenvand, T. (1984). *The construction and validation of the risk assessment for Fall Scale II (RAFS II).* Unpublished master's thesis, University of Iowa, Iowa City.

Hendrich, A., Nyhuis, A., Kippenbrock, T., & Soja, M. E. (1995). Hospital falls: Development of a predictive model for clinical practice. *Applied Nursing Research, 8*(3), 129-139.

Heslin, K., Towers, J., Leckie, C., Thornton-Lawrence, H., Perkin, K., Jacques, M., Mullin, J., & Wick, L. (1992). Managing falls: Identifying population-specific risk factors and prevention strategies. In S. G. Funk, E. M. Tornquist, M. T. Champagne, & R. A. Wiese (Eds.), *Key aspects of elder care: Managing falls, incontinence, and cognitive impairment* (pp. 70-88). New York: Springer.

Hogue, C. C., Studenski, S., & Duncan, P. (1989). Assessing mobility: The first step in preventing falls. In S. G. Funk, E. M. Tornquist, M. T. Champagne, L. A. Capp, & R. A. Wiese (Eds.), *Key aspects of recovery: Improving nutrition, rest and mobility* (pp. 275-280). New York: Springer.

Hu, M. H., & Woolacott, M. H. (1994). Multisensory training of standing balance in older adults: I. Postural stability and one-leg stance balance. *Journal of Gerontology: Medical Sciences, 49*(2), M52-M61.

Innes, E. (1985). Maintaining fall prevention. *Quality Review Bulletin, 11*(7), 217-221.

Iowa Intervention Project. J. C. McCloskey & G. M. Bulechek (Eds.). (2000). *Nursing interventions classification (NIC)* (3rd ed.). St. Louis, MO: Mosby.

Iowa Outcomes Project. M. Johnson, M. Maas, & S. Moorhead (Eds.). (2000). *Nursing outcomes classification (NOC)* (2nd ed.). St. Louis, MO: Mosby.

Isaacs, B. (1996). The prevention of falls in old people. In C. Lafont, A. Baroni, M. Allard, R. Tideiksaar, B. J. Vellas, P. J. Garry, J. L. Albarede (Eds.), *Falls, gait and balance disorders in the elderly* (pp. 5-10). New York: Springer.

Kalchthaler, T., Bascon, R. A., & Quintos, V. (1978). Falls in the institutionalized elderly. *Journal of the American Geriatrics Society, 26*(9), 424-428.

Kippenbrock, T., & Soja, M. (1993). Preventing falls in the elderly: Interviewing patients who have fallen. *Geriatric Nursing, 14*(4), 205-209.

Kuehn, A. F., & Sendelweck, S. (1995). Acute health status and its relationship to falls in the nursing home. *Journal of Gerontological Nursing, 21*(7), 41-49.

Lawrence, J. I., & Maher, P. L. (1992). An interdisciplinary falls consult team: A collaborative approach to patient falls. *Journal of Nursing Care, 6*(3), 21-29.

Lord, S. R. (1996). Instability and falls in elderly people. In C. Lafont, A. Baroni, M. Allard, R. Tideiksaar, B. J. Vellas, P. J. Garry, & J. L. Albarede (Eds.), *Falls, gait and balance disorders in the elderly* (pp. 125-139). New York: Springer.

Lund, C., & Sheafor, M. L. (1985). Is your patient about to fall? *Journal of Gerontological Nursing, 11*(4), 37-41.

Maciorowski, L. F., Munro, B. H., Dietrick-Gallagher, M., McNew, C. D., Sheppart-Hinkel, E., Wanich, C., & Ragan, P. (1988). A review of the patient fall literature. *Journal of Nursing Quality Assurance, 3*(1), 18-27.

Maki, B. E., Holliday, P. J., & Topper, A. K. (1994). A prospective study of postural balance and risk of falling in an ambulatory and independent elderly population. *Journal of Gerontology: Medical Science, 49*(2), M72-M84.

Marottoli, R. A., Berkman, L. F., & Cooney, L. M. (1992). Decline in physical function following hip fracture. *Journal of the American Geriatrics Society, 40,* 861-866.

Meier, D. E. (1988). Skeletal aging. In B. Kent & R. N. Butler (Eds.), *Human aging research: Concepts and techniques* (pp. 221-244). New York: Raven Press.

Miller, C. A. (1995). *Nursing care of older adults, theory and practice.* Philadelphia: Lippincott Williams & Wilkins.

Miller, D. K., Morrison, M. J., Blair, S. D., Miller, J. P., & Morley, J. E. (1998). Predilection for frailty remedial strategies among black and white seniors. *Southern Medical Journal, 91*(4), 375-380.

Morse, J. M. (1997). *Preventing patient falls.* Thousand Oaks, CA: Sage.

Morse, J. M., Morse, R. M., & Tylko, S. J. (1989). Development of a scale to identify the fall prone patient. *Canadian Journal of Aging, 8*(4), 366-377.

Morse, J. M., Tylko, S. J., & Dixon, H. (1987). Characteristics of the fall prone patient. *Gerontologist, 27*(4), 516-522.

Nevitt, M. C., Cummings, S. R., Kidd, S., & Black, D. (1989). Risk factors for recurrent nonsyncopal falls. *Journal of the American Medical Association, 261,* 2663-2668.

Nevitt, M. C., Cummings, S. R., & the Study of Osteoporotic Fractures Research Group. (1993). Type of fall and risk of hip and wrist fractures: The study of osteoporotic fractures. *Journal of the American Geriatrics Society, 41,* 1226-1234.

North American Nursing Diagnosis Association. (1999). *Nursing diagnoses: Definitions & classification 1999-2000.* Philadelphia: Author.

Perlin, E. (1992). Preventing falls in the elderly: A practice approach to a common problem. *Postgraduate Medicine, 9*(8), 241.

Reinboth, J., & Gyldenvand, T. (1982). *Pilot study of falls in an extended care setting.* Iowa City: University of Iowa.

Reinboth, J. L. V. (1985). *A study to investigate the interrater reliability of an assessment tool to assess risk for falling in elderly clients.* Unpublished master's thesis, University of Iowa, Iowa City.

Ross, J. E. R., Watson, C. A., Gyldenvand, T. A., & Reinboth, J. A. L. (1991). Potential for trauma: Falls. In M. Maas, K. C. Buckwalter, & M. Hardy (Eds.), *Nursing diagnosis and interventions for the elderly* (pp. 18-31). Redwood City, CA: Addison Wesley Longman.

Runge, J. (1993). The cost of injury. *Emergency Medical Clinics of North America, 11,* 241-253.

Sattin, R. W. (1992). Falls among older persons: A public health perspective. *Annual Review of Public Health, 13,* 489-508.

Stolley, J. M. (1990). *A secondary analysis of falls and medications in institutionalized persons with Alzheimer's disease.* Unpublished master's thesis, University of Iowa, Iowa City.

Stolley, J. M., Lewis, A., Moore, L., Hanrahan, B., & Carter, K. (1996). *Research utilization: Falls in acute care.* Unpublished manuscript. Davenport, IA.

Tack, K. A., Ulrich, B., & Kehr, C. (1987). Patient falls: Profile for prevention. *Journal of Neuroscience Nursing, 19*(2), 83-89.

Tideiksaar, R. (1989). *Falling in old age: Its prevention and treatment.* New York: Springer.

Tideiksaar, R. (1996). Reducing the risk of falls and injury in older persons: Contribution of a falls and immobility clinic. In C. Lafont, A. Baroni, M. Allard, R. Tideiksaar, B. J. Vellas, P. J. Garry, & J. L. Albarede (Eds.), *Falls, gait and balance disorders in the elderly* (pp. 163-182). New York: Springer.

Tideiksaar, R. (1997). *Old age: Prevention and management* (2nd ed., pp. 52-167). New York: Springer.

Tinetti, M., Liu, W., & Claus, E. (1993). Predictors and prognosis of inability to get up after falls among elderly persons. *Journal of the American Medical Association, 269*(1), 65-70.

Tinetti, M. E., Liu, W. L., & Ginter, S. (1992). Mechanical restraint use and fall-related injuries among residents of skilled nursing facilities. *Annals of Internal Medicine, 116*(5), 369-374.

Tinetti, M. E., & Powell, L. (1993). Fear of falling and low self-efficacy: A cause of dependence in elderly persons. *The Journals of Gerontology, 48,* (Special Issue), 35-38.

Tinetti, M. E., Speechley, M., & Ginter, S. (1988). Risk factors for falls among elderly persons living in the community. *New England Journal of Medicine, 319*(26), 1701-1707.

Uden, G., Ehnfors, M., & Sjostrom, K. (1999). Use of initial risk assessment and recording as the main nursing intervention in identifying risk of falls. *Journal of Advanced Nursing, 29*(1), 145-152.

Vaughn, K., Young, C. C., Rice, F., & Stoner, M. H. (1993). A retrospective study of patient falls in a psychiatric hospital. *Journal of Psychosocial Nursing and Mental Health Services, 31*(9), 37-42, 44-45.

Vecht-Hart, C. M., Peters, P. H. M., & Collette, H. J. A. (1996). Epidemiological risk factors for osteoporotic fractures. In C. Lafont, A. Baroni, M. Allard, R. Tideiksaar, B. J. Vellas, P. J. Garry, & J. L. Albarede (Eds.), *Falls, gait and balance disorders in the elderly* (pp. 91-100). New York: Springer.

Walshe, A., & Rosen, H. (1979). A study of patient falls from bed. *The Journal of Nursing Administration, 9,* 31-35.

Watson, M. E., & Mayhew, P. A. (1994). Identifying fall risk factors in preparation for reducing the use of restraints. *Medsurg Nursing, 3*(1), 25-28, 30, 35.

CHAPTER 4

RISK FOR POISONING: DRUG TOXICITY

Elizabeth A. Weitzel

Health care professionals and clients tend to think of drugs as the solution to certain health problems. However, drugs can have deleterious, as well as favorable, effects on the total body and can interact with other drugs and with foods. Drug toxicity occurs when the amount of a given drug in a person's body exceeds the amount necessary to bring about a desired therapeutic effect (therapeutic level) or when it has become a harmful agent in that person's body. Side effects are responses to the medication other than the intended therapeutic effect. If the side effects become harmful, they are called adverse effects and are part of the toxic response to the medication. A drug interaction occurs when a drug undergoes changes in pharmacokinetics in the presence of another drug. Drug interactions with other substances such as foods can result in subtherapeutic or toxic responses. Allergic reactions usually result when a drug acts as hapten, a low–molecular-weight substance that would not usually cause an allergic reaction and combines with an endogenous protein to form an antigenic complex and stimulate antibody formation. When the drug is reintroduced into the body, it can provoke a variety of allergic responses, ranging from skin rashes to exfoliative dermatitis, acute urticaria, or severe arthritis. Respiratory symptoms and anaphylactic shock are other allergic responses that can occur. Penicillin is a classic example of a drug that stimulates allergic response. Allergic response may be idiosyncratic in the aging person in terms of both what stimulates an allergic response and which precise symptoms are manifested (Klassen, 1980).

Medication can cause a cell to respond only to the extent that it is capable of responding, and the aging body has fewer functioning cells than the younger body. The effects of aging on pharmacokinetics (the fate of drugs in the body) and pharmacodynamics (the response of the body to a given drug) are important in identifying areas for drug monitoring. Health care professionals can use this information to maximize the effectiveness of drugs administered to elders. Unfortunately, health care professionals sometimes contribute to the problem of toxicity by having unrealistic expectations of what drugs will do for an individual.

One problematic expectation is that the right drug or drugs will improve all the health problems an older person is experiencing. This expectation is misleading for several reasons. Physiologically, cells can respond only to a certain level of maximum input. Aging diminishes most body cell populations and consequently decreases function. Also, many of the health problems for the aged are chronic and will not be cured even with extensive drug therapy. In some instances further cell deterioration leads to a narrowed therapeutic range. When the heart has become damaged, the upper limits of therapeutic levels of digoxin become lowered. Giving more digoxin will not make the heart function better but will lead to toxicity.

Another unrealistic belief is that all diagnosed problems of elders should be treated with medication. It often is advisable to treat with medication only one or two primary conditions causing the most problems and not attempt to administer medications for additional pathologies until the primary condition(s) is controlled. This helps to avoid the unfortunate situation of treating drug side effects with more drugs. Patients taking fewer than 5 drugs daily have a 4% incidence of adverse drug reactions, whereas the rate more than doubles to 10% when 6 to 10 drugs are taken (May, Stewart, & Leighton, 1977).

The belief that toxicity can be prevented by keeping blood levels within normal therapeutic levels is misleading. The complete clinical picture, including the functioning of the individual, must be evaluated to determine the appropriate level of medication, regardless of the "normalcy" of the blood level. Aronow (1996), for example, discusses the factors that can lead to "digitoxicity" despite normal digoxin levels, including reduced renal function, reduced skeletal mass, taking multiple drugs, lung disease, and a number of electrolyte and metabolic problems.

Finally, if social stress rather than physical illness is at the root of a problem an older person is experiencing, the solution to this problem might best lie in dealing with the social factors rather than in administering drugs (Davidson, 1978).

PREVALENCE

Elders are admitted to hospitals for drug-induced illnesses at a significantly higher rate than younger persons (Brady, 1978; Carnosos, Stewart, & Cluff, 1974; Grymonpre, Mitenko, Sitar, Aoki, & Montgomery, 1988). Lamy (1989) found that 30% of hospitalizations in elders were related to adverse drug reactions, many of which could be prevented. Thus potential for drug toxicity is an important area for nursing assessment, diagnosis, and management.

Furthermore, aging clients should expect the nurse to advocate in their behalf to prevent drug toxicity.

RELATED FACTORS/ETIOLOGIES

The risk factors that increase the probability that the aging person will develop a risk for drug toxicity include the effects of drugs in the aging body, the variables of drug administration, and the effects of polypharmacy.

Effects of Aging on Pharmacodynamics and Pharmacokinetics

Pharmacodynamics and pharmacokinetics are processes that determine how a given drug responds within the body. Both of these processes are somewhat altered within the aging body because of tissue loss and diminished organ function.

Pharmacodynamics refers to the responses of the body receptors to a given drug and the subsequent effects of that drug. The changes in body receptors caused by aging are particularly apparent with warfarin (Coumadin) and diazepam (Valium), which have increased effects even when serum drug concentrations are constant (Gromlin & Chapron, 1983; Lamy, 1980; Reidenberg, 1980). Altered sensitivity of central nervous system (CNS) receptors and beta-adrenergic receptors is a postulated but not proven explanation of this phenomenon.

Pharmacokinetics refers to the absorption, distribution, metabolism (biotransformation), and excretion of drugs in the body, all of which determine the amount of active components of a drug available to body tissues at a given time. Of the two processes, pharmacokinetics is probably the more important in producing the toxic effects of medication in the aging body.

Absorption of Drugs

Most oral medications are absorbed by passive diffusion, a process that is minimally altered with aging. Oral absorption can be altered in the following areas: (1) slowing in gastric emptying, especially when taking anticholinergics or antidepressants; (2) increased transit time through the bowel, which is influenced by altered dietary patterns and food intake and by changes in dentition; and (3) drug-drug or drug-food interactions such as those previously described, especially tetracycline with calcium-rich foods or medications (Lamy, 1982; Rock, 1985).

Absorption of parenteral medications is influenced by changes to the dermis and muscle mass and by changes in circulation, which generally slow absorption.

Distribution of Drugs

For drugs to be effective in the body they must be delivered to their sites of action. Distribution of a drug taken orally begins in the portal circulation, which takes the drug to the liver, where enzymes can change the chemistry of the drug or pass it on unchanged. From the liver, the drug enters the systemic circulation, where it can be in a free state or partially bound to blood proteins or tissues.

Muscle atrophy and other tissue decreases, along with a low-protein diet, contribute to protein loss among elders. When serum proteins decrease, drugs that are usually protein bound are found free in the serum in increased amounts. This increases the drug's effects on all the tissues with which it comes in contact, making both the therapeutic level and the toxic level occur at lower doses.

Another factor that increases the amount of free drug in the serum of the elderly person is the increased number of drugs taken. This enhances the chance of displacement by a drug that is more highly protein bound. In older persons, who are normally not as well hydrated as younger individuals, a decreased amount of body water further increases the concentration of drugs in the serum. Both of these factors are particularly problematic with drugs like aspirin, for which the therapeutic and toxic ranges are very close. The addition of a new drug that either displaces some of the bound aspirin or increases dehydration can be sufficient change to make the older person become aspirin toxic.

Distribution also is dependent on regional perfusion. Tissue perfusion and cardiac efficiency are often decreased in the elder relative to changes in blood vessels. There also is some empirical evidence that receptor systems and related tissue responses to drugs can be altered with aging (Tsujimoto, Hashimoto, & Hoffman, 1989). Thus a number of factors influence the distribution of drugs in the older person, with most of them contributing to the likelihood that drug toxicity will occur.

Metabolism or Biotransformation of Drugs

Metabolism is primarily a function of the liver and depends heavily on enzymes, which decrease with normal aging. Drugs such as cimetidine (Tagamet), chloramphenicol (Chloromycetin), and phenobarbital in high concentrations suppress enzymatic function. Hepatic blood flow decreases with aging, and some drugs are dependent on the amount of blood flowing through the liver for efficient metabolism.

Some metabolism also can occur in the intestinal wall during the process of absorption. Metabolism can inactivate a drug or change it into a form that continues to be active. Decreased liver function can increase the circulating active levels of a drug like propranolol (Inderal), which is dependent on enzymatic action to inactivate it. That same decreased liver function can decrease the active level of tricyclic antidepressants, since they are dependent on enzymatic action to change them into a more active form. Potempa and Folta (1992) document the influence of decreased activity and bed rest on metabolism, as well as on the distribution and excretion of drugs.

Excretion of Drugs

Excretion occurs primarily in the kidneys, with small amounts of drugs being excreted through saliva, sweat, lung exhalation, or lactation. Changes in renal function are more consistent and measurable than changes in hepatic function. The normal kidney loses 30% to 50% of its functioning between the ages of 35 and 70, and at the same time a considerable decrease in renal blood flow occurs. These changes cause decreased clearance of drugs. If the aging person also has hypertension, dehydration, urinary retention, diabetic nephropathy, pyelonephritis, atherosclerosis, or congestive heart failure, renal function can be compromised further (Lamy, 1982).

Loss of renal function is important to consider when a drug reaches the kidney in an active state. If the drug is not removed at the expected rate, the serum concentration rises. Each drug has an expected half-life ($t_{1/2}$), the amount of time it takes for half of the dosage given to be metabolized into an inactive form or to be excreted. When this does not happen in the expected amount of time, the half-life increases and, in effect, the dosage of the drug is increased. For example, digoxin, a commonly used drug among elders, reaches the kidney in an active state. Because the aging kidney might not excrete digoxin at the expected rate, it has an extended half-life. As a result, toxicity can occur when renal function is decreased and the dosage given is not decreased. Certain drugs may further decrease renal clearance. Lithium, commonly used in the treatment of bipolar disorders, can decrease renal function and thus reduce clearance of other drugs.

Variables in Drug Administration

Only 5% of persons 65 and older in the United States live in institutions. The remaining 95% live in the community, with most assuming responsibility for the medications they use. Medications are obtained from a variety of sources: physicians, dentists, and, in some states, nurse practitioners and physician assistants; over-the-counter (OTC) medications; and folk remedies. Elders living in the community consume about 50% of all OTC drugs sold in the United States, and 70% of these persons purchase and use OTC medications without consulting a health care professional (Berlinger & Spector, 1984; Gutman, 1977; Johnson & Moore, 1988). Two recent nursing studies documented the use of OTC medications in elders, one comparing urban and rural areas (Falvo, Holland, Brenner, & Benshoff, 1990; Moore & Johnson, 1993). Both found that elders rely on OTC medications to augment or in place of prescription medications.

Older persons, who constitute 12% of the population, purchase 30% of all medications prescribed in the United States, accounting for 30% to 40% of the health care dollar (Chrischilles et al., 1992; Lamy, 1989). They also spend three times more money on drugs than does the rest of the population. One study found the incidence of drug reactions to be about two and one-half times greater in persons over 60 than in those younger than 60, and some studies have found a steady age-related increase (Exton-Smith & Windsor, 1971; Stewart, 1987). Persons over age 85 contribute most to the growing number of older persons, which might mean a larger percent of the health care dollar expended on long-term care and more years of maintenance medications.

Adverse drug reactions requiring medical attention are more likely to occur to elderly persons living in the community than to institutionalized elders, since part of the role of the institution is to monitor for problems and seek early intervention (Lamy, 1982). Several studies have found drug-associated hospital admissions being more prevalent in elders (Bergman & Wilhelm, 1981; Grymonpre et al., 1988; Ives, Bents, & Gwythr, 1987).

Self-Administration

Self-administration of drugs by an elderly person presents considerable potential for error. Some studies have found omission of doses to be the most common error. Confusion, forgetfulness, or misreading the directions can lead to missed doses or to ingestion of more than the prescribed amount. Another very real factor for the elder is the cost of purchasing medication. An elderly individual might try to "make up" missed doses by taking several at once. Also, a dose might not be taken because the person wishes to avoid the side effects, feels the medication is too strong, or feels better and thinks the medication is no longer needed. Elderly persons can recognize the subtle symptoms of impending toxicity and adjust the dose, a behavior referred to as "intelligent" noncompliance (Vestal & Dawson, 1985).

Omission of doses usually does not lead to toxicity. However, omitting doses can change the balance among the drugs being taken and can lead to an exacerbation of illness. A physician who is unaware that an elderly person is omitting doses might increase the dosage or prescribe stronger medication, either of which could lead to toxicity.

An elderly institutionalized individual who omitted doses at home but functioned well with the actual amount ingested might be at risk when first institutionalized. When the staff begins to administer the medication as prescribed, the person can become toxic. Also, the stress of relocation can cause the newly admitted person to become toxic on a dose that was previously therapeutic (see Chapter 48). To avoid these problems, some long-term care facilities establish a "baseline" by removing most if not all of a client's medication on admission. The client is then carefully monitored to determine what medications are needed (Moss, 1978).

When the elderly person self-medicates with prescription drugs from a previous visit to the doctor, with someone else's prescriptions, with OTC medications, or with home remedies, drug interactions and toxicity are more likely. Alcohol consumption is also problematic. Alcohol itself can be toxic, and it can interact both with self-prescribed medications and with those prescribed by health care personnel (Forni, 1978).

The rate of medication errors in hospitals and long-term care facilities has been documented frequently (Hoffman, 1989; Moss, 1977). Although these errors certainly should be corrected, they rarely cause the client serious problems. Self-administration of medications by capable older persons in long-term care settings or in a hospital setting has not received frequent consideration. When monitored by the staff, this practice could have several benefits, including increased independence and self-esteem for the older person. In the hospital or long-term care facility, self-medication is good preparation for discharge and it allows the nurse to assess the accuracy of self-administration of medications. Perhaps the least important reason for implementing this practice is to decrease the amount of staff time required to administer medications.

Whether medications are self-administered by the older person or administered by a medication aide, LPN, or RN, it is the RN's responsibility to assess whether the client is receiving the medication as ordered, to know what actions are desired, and to document those that are not taking place. It also is the role of the RN to determine if side effects are occurring and to report these to the prescribing health care professional. At times it might be necessary for the RN to advocate for the aging client by pursuing changes in dosage or medications so that the client can function at an optimal level.

Effects of Polypharmacy

By definition, polypharmacy is the administration of several drugs to the same client, sometimes using more than one with similar effects. It is not unusual for an elderly person to have seven or more drugs prescribed for continuous maintenance therapy. If the elderly person develops an acute condition, the number of drugs often increases.

This becomes problematic, since pharmacologically it is difficult to know what chemicals are active within an elderly person who is taking several drugs at the same time. Drugs can interact with other drugs or cause body tissues to respond differently from expected.

CASE STUDY 1

V. Albert is a 75-year-old woman living in a nursing home. She had a seizure episode after a cerebrovascular accident a year ago and was started on phenytoin (Dilantin) 100 mg tid. She recently experienced nausea and high abdominal pain and ate poorly for 2 weeks. Following tests yes-

terday, her physician diagnosed a peptic ulcer. He prescribed cimetidine (Tagamet) 300 mg with meals and at bedtime and diazepam (Valium) 2 mg qid for 1 week to decrease Mrs. Albert's anxiety. The nurse, in reading a pocket drug reference, noted that phenytoin toxicity increases with decreased serum protein and also with the administration of either cimetidine or diazepam. The nurse also noted that Mrs. Albert's protein intake had been minimal for the past week. The nurse inferred that Mrs. Albert might have a lowered serum protein level and might be dehydrated. Dehydration would further concentrate the phenytoin in Mrs. Albert's blood.

The nurse suspected that Mrs. Albert was at increased risk for phenytoin toxicity related to concurrent administration of Tagamet and Valium, as well as to probable dehydration and lowered serum protein. After reading about the manifestations of phenytoin toxicity, the nurse noted that common signs and symptoms of phenytoin toxicity include CNS effects of ataxia, slurred speech, confusion, nystagmus, and diplopia and gastrointestinal (GI) effects of nausea and vomiting (Ford, 1986). The nurse planned to monitor Mrs. Albert for the common signs of toxicity and to promote increased fluid and protein intake to decrease Mrs. Albert's likelihood of developing toxicity. The nurse also planned to ask Mrs. Albert's physician to reconsider use of Tagamet and Valium.

ASSESSMENT

The precise signs and symptoms of drug toxicity are somewhat dependent on the drugs that are being taken. All body systems can show toxic effects (Box 4-1). Todd (1985) suggests that "in older adults, the first sign of adverse reaction is often a change in mental function" (p. 231). Confusion that develops after starting a medication or after a physical or psychologic stressor can be an early indicator of drug toxicity. Other CNS symptoms include gait changes, insomnia or drowsiness, visual changes, slurred speech, ototoxicity, seizures, tremors, irritability, and problems with temperature control. Anticholinergic effects of medications include dry mouth, constipation, blurred vision, urinary retention, headache, and restlessness. Preexisting pathology in the dependent elder can be exaggerated. For example, a man with benign prostatic hypertrophy who already has some urinary retention might experience increased retention caused by the adverse effects of medications.

Cardiovascular signs and symptoms include dysrhythmias, tachycardia, palpitations, hypotension, congestive heart failure, hypertension, and bone marrow depression resulting in leukopenia, thrombocytopenia, anemia, or agranulocytosis.

Hepatic changes can result in jaundice, clotting problems, and other symptoms of decreased liver function. GI signs and symptoms include anorexia, nausea, vomiting, diarrhea, GI bleeding, and pancreatitis.

General Defining Characteristics	
Box 4-1 DRUG TOXICITY	

Cardiovascular	Insomnia
Dysrhythmias	Drowsiness
Tachycardia	Blurred vision or other
Palpitations	visual changes
Hypotension	Slurred speech
Congestive heart failure	Ototoxicity
(CHF)	Seizures
Hypertension	Tremors
Bone marrow depression	Irritability
(leukopenia,	Problems with temperature
thrombocytopenia,	control
anemia, and	Anticholinergic effect
agranulocytosis)	
	Renal
Gastrointestinal	Electrolyte imbalances
Anorexia	Polyuria
Nausea and vomiting	Urinary retention
Diarrhea	Fluid retention
GI bleeding	
Pancreatitis	Liver
Metabolic problems	Jaundice
Lactic acidosis	Clotting problems
	Decreased liver function
Skin	
Rashes	Respiratory
Urticaria	Cough
Pruritis	Dyspnea
Photosensitivity	Asthmatic reactions
	Respiratory failure
Central Nervous	
System	
Confusion	
Gait changes	

Data from Barnhart, E. (1996). *Physician's desk reference.* Montvale, NJ: Medical Economics; United States Pharmacopeial Drug Information. (1996). USP DI Vol. I *Drug information for health care professionals.* Washington, DC: United States Pharmacopeial Convention.

Renal dysfunction from toxicity can result in electrolyte imbalances, polyuria, urinary retention, or fluid retention. Dyspnea, asthmatic reactions, and respiratory failure are respiratory signs and symptoms. Skin responses to toxicity include rashes, urticaria, pruritis, and photosensitivity.

The profile of the person most likely to develop drug toxicity is as follows: age greater than 75 years; small stature; female; history of allergic illness or adverse reaction; multiple chronic illnesses; kidney or liver dysfunction; more than five medications; taking "high-risk" drugs; and changes in overall condition, including mental status changes (Gambert, Grossberg, & Morley, 1994).

Because of the diversity of these defining characteristics, the nurse must suspect drug toxicity as the cause of developing confusion until another cause can be found, be aware of common toxic symptoms of drugs being used by the client, and always regard drugs as potential poisons.

General Drug History

Mullen and Granholm (1981) have developed a tool for gathering a comprehensive drug history, which could be used to identify potential for toxicity. This tool includes information on nonprescription and prescription drugs, as well as general information related to medications and the client's health problems.

Additional assessments also are warranted. Assessment of usual fluid and protein intake can help determine level of hydration and potential for hypoproteinemia. In addition, the use of alcoholic beverages should be singled out and explored more completely, since alcohol interacts with many drugs, particularly benzodiazepines (Valium, Dalmane) or theophylline. Chronic alcohol usage can change the action of many drugs that are metabolized in the liver. With these additions use of the tool should help identify what drugs the client is taking, what the client knows about them, future learning needs, and the potential for or current symptoms consistent with toxicity.

A Tool to Monitor for Digitalis Toxicity

Weitzel (1976) developed an instrument (Assessment Guide 4-1) to explore the effectiveness of both nursing observations and subjective changes reported by the older client in monitoring digitalis levels for the onset of toxic symptoms. This data collection tool was designed to be used as a follow-up to monthly nurse-administered cardiovascular clinics at the Iowa Veterans Home, a state-operated rehabilitation and long-term care agency serving about 700 residents. Following a pilot study, the tool was adopted for use in these clinics. The data collected by the tool have been instrumental in identifying monthly changes in individual residents. On several occasions its use has led to diagnosis of early digitalis toxicity and subsequent revision of medical orders.

This instrument also illustrates how nurses can develop tools for assessing signs and symptoms based on information in the literature for drugs that often cause toxicity in the elderly client. It gathers the data on one sheet so that signs and symptoms can be clustered and thereby give focus and direction to the monitoring activity.

CASE STUDY 2

J. Bean is an active 80-year-old man living with his wife in his own home. He developed complete urinary retention and general malaise. His family physician diagnosed a urinary tract infection and a heart dysrhythmia and pre-

Assessment Guide 4-1

POTENTIAL FOR DIGITALIS TOXICITY

Name _____ Date _____
Date started on digoxin _____ Dosage _____
Baseline: Creatinine _____ K _____ Apical rate _____ Rhythm _____
Current: Creatinine _____ K _____ Apical rate _____ Rhythm _____
Name of clinician _____
Evidence of: Resident Report Staff
Observation
Excessive fatigue _____
Headache that persists _____
Drowsiness _____
Confusion _____
Dizziness _____
Numbness or tingling _____
Blurred vision _____
Changes of color perception _____
Halo vision _____
Seeing frost on objects _____
Anorexia _____
Nausea _____
Vomiting _____
Diarrhea _____
Abdominal pain _____
Remarks: _____

scribed Bactrim and Procan SR. At his 2-week follow-up visit, his urine was free of infection and his dysrhythmia was converted to normal sinus rhythm. He was sent home and instructed to take half a Bactrim tablet each day and to continue the Procan SR. He was scheduled to return in 3 weeks to set a date for surgery for his benign prostatic hypertrophy. In a few days he awoke with joint pain, chills, and fever. He and his wife had been told "flu symptoms" were reason to contact the doctor immediately. Mrs. Bean called the doctor's office and talked with the RN, who recognized the symptoms as consistent with Procan toxicity.

The exact causes of Mr. Bean's developing a toxicity to Procan SR were not readily evident, but the onset of symptoms while taking the medication was sufficient reason to suspect toxicity. The nurse advised Mr. Bean to take no more Procan SR and said she would have the doctor call as soon as he was available. The doctor subsequently called, directing Mrs. Bean to discontinue the Procan SR but to continue the half tablet of Bactrim each day until Mr. Bean's return visit. On discontinuing the Procan SR, Mr. Bean's symptoms gradually disappeared. This case study demonstrates that although the nurse's role in actual drug toxicity is primarily dependent on the physician, the nurse can teach the patient and family about possible adverse effects for which to monitor and whom to call if adverse effects develop.

NURSING DIAGNOSIS

The diagnosis Risk for Poisoning: Drug Toxicity is not on the accepted North American Nursing Diagnosis Association (NANDA) list (Carroll-Johnson, 1992). It is subsumed under the diagnosis Risk for Poisoning (NANDA, 1999). However, the importance of the subdiagnosis to nurses who work with elders justifies developing it as a distinct diagnosis. NANDA defines Risk for Poisoning as "accentuated risk of accidental exposure to or ingestion of drugs or dangerous products in doses sufficient to cause poisoning" (NANDA, 1999, p. 36). Weitzel (1976) defines it as "the condition that exists when the amount of a given drug in a person's body exceeds the amount necessary to bring about therapeutic effect (therapeutic level), or it has become a harmful agent in that person's body, producing adverse effects." Box 4-2 lists the risk factors specified by NANDA (1999) and by Weitzel (1976).

NURSING-SENSITIVE OUTCOMES

The obvious desired outcome is prevention of drug toxicity or rapid recovery without sequelae if it should occur. Patient behaviors that might be a part of that outcome are Knowledge: Medication, defined as the "extent of under-

Box 4-2	Risk Factors RISK FOR POISONING

NANDA (1999)

Internal (Individual) Factors

Reduced vision

Verbalization of occupational setting without adequate
    safeguards

Lack of safety or drug education

Lack of proper precautions

Cognitive or emotional difficulties

Insufficient finances

External (Environmental) Factors

Large supplies of drugs in house

Medications stored in unlocked cabinets accessible to
    children or confused persons

Availability of illicit drugs potentially contaminated by
    poisonous additives

Flaking, peeling paint or plaster in presence of young
    children

Chemical contamination of food and water

Unprotected contact with heavy metals or chemical

Substances such as paint and lacquer in poorly ventilated
    areas or without effective protection

Presence of poisonous vegetation

Presence of atmospheric pollutants

Weitzel (1976)

Effects of drugs in the aging body

Variables of drug administration

Effects of polypharmacy

standing conveyed about the safe use of medication" (Iowa Outcomes Project, 2000, p. 279); Risk Control: Drug Use, which is the "actions to eliminate or reduce drug use that poses a threat to health" (p. 359); and Self-Care: Non-Parenteral Medication, which shows the "ability to administer oral and topical medications to meet therapeutic goals" (p. 386) (Box 4-3). Although Risk Control: Drug Use applies to habitual drug abuse, the outcome indicators are also appropriate for prevention of Drug Toxicity.

NURSING INTERVENTIONS

Nursing Interventions Classification (NIC) labels (Iowa Intervention Project, 2000) appropriate for Risk for Poisoning: Drug Toxicity include Medication Administration, Medication Management, and Teaching: Prescribed Medication (see Box 4-3). Medication Administration is defined as "preparing, giving, and evaluating the effectiveness of prescription and nonprescription drugs" (p. 434). Medication Management is "facilitation of safe and effective use of prescription and over-the-counter drugs," (p. 451), whereas Teaching: Prescribed Medication is "preparing a patient to safely take prescribed medications and monitor for their effects" (p. 650). The listed activities are general for use of

medications. Selected portions of the activities for these interventions have been amplified for this chapter.

Medication Management: An Interdisciplinary Approach

The very nature of drug administration makes prevention of toxicity an interdisciplinary function. The physician (or related health care professional) prescribes the drug for a specific function. The pharmacist dispenses the drug and applies knowledge of clinical pharmacy to the directions and counseling provided. At times the dietitian also can be involved, for example, if there are food interactions or the necessity for dietary adjustments. The RN takes responsibility for administration of the medication, whether giving it personally, supervising other health care personnel in giving it, or teaching the client and/or significant other how to give the medication. The nurse often is the first to help the client identify adverse effects as they develop, especially in a long-term care facility.

Elderly clients are best protected from toxic reactions when health care professionals work with them to teach, monitor, and promote those actions necessary to keep the drug from becoming toxic or to treat the toxicity promptly should it occur.

Clarifying Goals of Medication Administration

Davidson (1978) stated, "In geriatric medicine the aim of treatment is usually the amelioration of disease to the extent that the elderly person can return, in reasonable comfort, to his normal way of life. . . . or to a comfortable, dignified death" (p. 633). This statement implies that health care professionals need to keep the response of the older person as the prime measure of effective treatment. Individualization of care therefore becomes paramount when dealing with elderly clients.

Gerontologists agree on some basic tenets for prescribing medications for the aged (Davidson, 1978; Exton-Smith & Windsor, 1971; Rock, 1985; Tandberg, 1981). These are presented in Box 4-4. (See p. 44.)

Monitoring

The NIC interventions previously indicated list monitoring in at least 10 of the specified activities. Monitoring is usually the most effective intervention to prevent or minimize the effects of drug toxicity. Monitoring the client for therapeutic versus toxic response has been identified previously as an interdisciplinary function. The nurse's role is one of knowing what defining characteristics indicate toxicity, advocating for any appropriate laboratory tests, and presenting any evidence of toxic reaction to the physician for definitive treatment. If a toxic response is suspected and the physician is not readily available, the nurse is justi-

Box 4-3	Suggested Nursing-Sensitive Outcomes and Nursing Interventions **RISK FOR POISONING: DRUG TOXICITY**

Nursing Diagnosis
Risk for Poisoning: Drug Toxicity
Risk factors
Effects of drugs in the aging body
Variables of drug administration
Effects of polypharmacy
See Box 4-1 for defining characteristics for drug
   toxicity.

Nursing-Sensitive Outcomes
Medication Response
Indicators
Expected therapeutic effects present
Maintenance of therapeutic blood levels of medication

Knowledge: Medication
Indicators
Recognition of need to inform health care provider of all
   medications being taken
Statement of correct medication name
Description of appearance of medication
Description of actions of medication
Description of side effects of medications
Description of medication precautions
Description of use of memory aids
Description of potential adverse reactions when taking
   multiple drugs
Description of potential for interaction with other agents
Description of correct administration of medication
Description of self-monitoring techniques
Description of proper medication storage
Description of proper care of administration devices
Description of how to obtain required medication and
   supplies
Description of proper disposal of unused medications
Description of proper use of medication alert identification
Identification of needed laboratory tests

Risk Control: Drug Use
Indicators
Acknowledges risk for drug misuse
Monitors environment for factors encouraging drug
   misuse
Monitors personal drug use patterns
Develops effective drug use control strategies
Adjusts drug use control strategies as needed
Commits to drug use control strategies
Follows selected drug use control strategies
Participates in screening for associated health problems
Uses health care services congruent with needs
Uses personal support systems to control drug misuse
Uses support groups to control drug misuse
Uses community resources to control drug misuse
Monitor health status changes
Controls drug intake

Self-Care: Non-Parenteral Medication
Indicators
Identifies medication
States correct dose
Describes action of medication
Adjusts dose appropriately
Describes medication precautions
Describes side effects of medication
Uses memory aids
Performs self-monitoring activities
Uses monitoring equipment accurately
Maintains needed supplies
Administers medication correctly
Stores medication properly
Disposes of medication appropriately
Seeks needed laboratory tests

Nursing Interventions
Medication Administration
Activities
Develop agency policy and procedures for accurate and safe
   administration of medications
Develop and use an environment that maximizes safe and
   efficient administration of medications
Follow the five rights of medication administration
Verify the prescription or medication order before
   administering the drug
Prescribe and/or recommend medications, as appropriate,
   according to prescriptive authority
Monitor for possible medication allergies, interactions, and
   contraindications
Note patient's allergies before delivery of each medication and
   hold medications, as appropriate
Ensure that hypnotics, narcotics, and antibiotics are either
   discontinued or reordered on their renewal date
Note expiration date on medication container
Prepare medications using appropriate equipment and
   techniques for the drug administration modality
Restrict administration of medications not properly labeled
Dispose of unused or expired drugs, according to agency
   guidelines
Monitor vital signs and laboratory values before medication
   administration, as appropriate
Assist patient in taking medication
Give medication using appropriate technique and route
Use orders, agency policies, and procedures to guide
   appropriate method of medication administration
Instruct patient and family about expected actions and adverse
   effects of the medication
Monitor patient to determine need for PRN medications, as
   appropriate
Monitor patient for the therapeutic effect of the medication
Sign out narcotics and other restricted drugs, according to
   agency protocol

Continued

Box 4-3   Suggested Nursing-Sensitive Outcomes and Nursing Interventions—cont'd

RISK FOR POISONING: DRUG TOXICITY—cont'd

Nursing Interventions—cont'd

Medication Administration—cont'd

Activities—cont'd

Verify all questioned medication orders with the appropriate health care personnel

Document medication administration and patient responsiveness, according to agency guidelines

Medication Management

Activities

Determine what drugs are needed, and administer according to prescriptive authority and/or protocol

Determine patient's ability to self-medicate, as appropriate

Monitor effectiveness of the medication administration modality

Monitor patient for the therapeutic effect of the medication

Monitor for signs and symptoms of drug toxicity

Monitor for adverse effects of the drug

Review periodically with the patient and/or family types and amounts of medication taken

Facilitate changes in medication with physician, as appropriate

Determine factors that may preclude the patient from taking drugs as prescribed

Develop strategies with the patient to enhance compliance with prescribed medication regimen

Consult with other health care professionals to minimize the number and frequency of drugs needed for a therapeutic effect

Teach patient and/or family members the method of drug administration, as appropriate

Provide patient and family members with written and visual information to enhance self-administration of medications, as appropriate

Obtain physician order for patient self-medication, as appropriate

Establish a protocol for the storage, restocking, and monitoring of medications left at the bedside for self-medication purposes

Investigate possible financial resources for acquisition of prescribed drugs, as appropriate

Determine impact of medication use on patient's lifestyle

Provide alternatives for timing and modality of self-administered medications to minimize lifestyle effects

Assist the patient and family members in making necessary lifestyle adjustments associated with certain medications, as appropriate

Instruct patient when to seek medical attention

Identify types and amounts of over-the-counter drugs used

Provide information about the use of over-the-counter drugs and how they may influence the existing condition

Determine whether the patient is using culturally-based home health remedies and the possible effects of use of over-the-counter and prescribed medications

Provide patient with a list of resources to contact for further information about the medication regimen

Contact patient and family postdischarge, as appropriate, to answer questions and discuss concerns associated with the medication regimen

Institute measures to decrease risk of drug toxicity

Determine with prescribing health care professional if drug holidays are appropriate

Teaching: Prescribed Medication

Activities

Instruct the patient to recognize distinctive characteristics of the medication(s), as appropriate

Inform the patient of both the generic and brand names of each medication

---

fied in withholding a dose of the suspected drug until the physician can be apprised of both the client's reaction and any pertinent laboratory results.

Rock (1985) identified the following drugs as those most commonly monitored by laboratory tests in elders: digoxin (Lanoxin); gentamicin (Garamycin); propranolol (Inderal, Inderide); phenobarbital; diazepam (Valium); amitriptyline (Elavil, Endep, Etrafon, Limbitrol, Triavil); warfarin (Coumadin, Panwarfarin); theophylline; lidocaine; quinidine; and tolbutamide (Orinase). Sometimes monitoring will disclose subtherapeutic effects. At other times lab tests can report blood levels in the "therapeutic range" even though the individual has developed toxicity. Therefore monitoring must include not only the results of a given blood sample but also the clinical picture the person presents, including level of functioning. The cost of the lab test compared with the usefulness of the results also should be considered.

When blood levels are monitored, it is important to know if a "peak" or "trough" effect is being measured. Medical technologists or physicians are usually responsible for determining the timing, but they rely on the nurse to verify the time at which the prescribed dose has been given to the client. Accurate timing of drawing the sample is important. It is also important that the drug has been taken as prescribed for 24 to 72 hours before the test.

Practicing Client Advocacy

The role of client advocate involves the nurse and the physician in gathering and processing information about the older client's overall level of functioning. Even though the nurse does not usually prescribe medication, nursing input often helps identify a health problem, expected outcomes of treatment, and changes in function. The nurse also can influence the plan of treatment the physician will

---

Box 4-3 Suggested Nursing-Sensitive Outcomes and Nursing Interventions—cont'd

RISK FOR POISONING: DRUG TOXICITY—cont'd

Nursing Interventions—cont'd

Teaching: Prescribed Medication—cont'd

Activities—cont'd

Instruct the patient on the purpose and action of each medication

Instruct the patient on the dosage, route, and duration of each medication

Evaluate the patient's ability to self-administer medications

Instruct the patient to perform needed procedures before taking a medication (e.g., check pulse and glucose level), as appropriate

Inform the patient what to do if a dose of medication is missed

Instruct the patient on which criteria to use when deciding to alter the medication dosage/schedule, as appropriate

Inform the patient of consequences of not taking or abruptly discontinuing medication(s), as appropriate

Instruct the patient on specific precautions to observe when taking medication(s) (e.g., no driving or using power tools), as appropriate

Instruct the patient on possible adverse side effects of each medication

Instruct the patient on how to relieve and/or prevent certain side effects, as appropriate

Instruct the patient on appropriate actions to take if side effects occur

Instruct the patient on the signs and symptoms of over- or under-dosage

Inform the patient of possible drug/food interactions, as appropriate

Instruct the patient on how to properly store the medication(s)

Instruct the patient on the proper care of devices used for administration

Instruct patients on proper disposal of needles and syringes at home, as appropriate, and where to dispose of the sharps container in their community

Provide the patient with written information about the action, purpose, side effects, and so on, of medications

Assist the patient to develop a written medication schedule

Instruct the patient to carry documentation of prescribed medication regimen

Instruct the patient on how to fill prescription(s), as appropriate

Inform the patient of possible changes in appearance and/or dosage when filling generic medication prescription(s)

Warn the patient of the risks associated with taking expired medication

Caution the patient against giving prescribed medication to others

Determine the patient's ability to obtain required medications

Provide information on medication reimbursement, as appropriate

Provide information on cost savings programs/organizations to obtain medications and devices, as appropriate

Provide information on medication alert devices and how to obtain them

Reinforce information provided by other health care team members, as appropriate

Include the family/significant others, as appropriate

---

prescribe by clarifying treatment goals and by coordinating with the physician, pharmacist, medical technologist, dietitian, social worker, or other clinicians to keep the goals of the client and family members in focus.

If a client becomes toxic, the physician might decrease the drug dosage or stop the drug entirely, depending on the severity of the toxic reaction. After the drug has been withheld for at least the length of its half-life, it may be started again at a lower dosage. In some instances other medications will be given to reverse life-threatening toxic responses, such as antidysrhythmia drugs for the person with digitalis toxicity who is experiencing severe dysrhythmias.

Scheduling Drug Holidays

A drug holiday is a planned omission of a specific medication from the regimen of selected clients for 1 or more days each week (Keenan, Redshaw, Munson, & Mundt,

1983). Staff members of one 99-bed skilled nursing facility (SNF) (Keenan et al., 1983, p. 103) found the following benefits to drug holidays: increased alertness of residents; reduced medication use and consequently a reduction in medication costs; fewer restrictions in scheduling residents' activities on the drug holiday; and better use of professional nursing time and effort with use of drug holidays. The facility reduced consumption of medications by 9% and saved residents $4600 annually over a 2-year period by implementing drug holidays 1 day a week.

However, the use of drug holidays is a controversial intervention. Many early attempts were not successful because the plan was not individualized for each resident based on known responses to drugs for that person, serum drug levels, and so on. Some plans put more emphasis on decreasing the time staff spent administering medications rather than on the individual needs of the resident. Others scheduled the drug holidays for Saturdays or Sundays,

Box 4-4	Basic Tenets of Prescribing for the Aged

1. Diagnose the source of symptoms as clearly as possible.
2. Prescribe for the diagnosis that is primary at that time, not the symptoms.
3. Prescribe the shortest half-life possible and drug least likely to cause adverse effects.
4. Keep the regimen simple—three to four drugs if client is living at home.
5. Keep instructions simple, clear, and written so the older person can read them.
6. Consider stopping previously prescribed drugs if a new drug is needed.
7. Review the entire drug regimen on a regular basis.
8. Provide support for correct administration of medication for clients taking their own medications (e.g., a person coming into the home to monitor or assist with setting up the medications; use of memory devices, such as divided pill containers and egg cartons; and use of alarm clocks to help with timing).
9. Provide an accurate, effective, and efficient system of administration when someone other than the client is responsible for giving the medication.
10. Monitor blood levels when appropriate; compare with client's level of functioning.
11. Treat mental illness without prejudice to age; keep in mind that drugs can cause health problems, as well as cure or ameliorate them.

days when there are traditionally fewer staff members to monitor for and intervene in untoward effects of withholding medication.

Elderly clients often indicate some initial concerns over the withholding of medications, but most seem to accept drug holidays after adjusting to the change. Many residents have appeared more alert, and for some the omission of specific drugs 1 day a week has helped them to feel less dependent on the medications.

Professional nursing time can be structured to plan for the individual client, both in the process of establishing the drug holiday and by using time not spent in actual administration of medications. If ancillary staff are administering medication, time that had been spent dispensing medications can be used in planning other client-centered activities (Keenan et al., 1983).

Some physicians have questioned whether 24 hours is sufficient time to significantly decrease long-term drug accumulation in a patient's body stores. Some facilities have successfully implemented two drug holidays per week. This is still a short amount of time to effect a significant decrease in drugs that are stored in the body's fat supply; it can take weeks to deplete these body stores. It could be argued that individual clients might benefit physically from a simple reduction of the daily dose of drugs administered, although this does not take into consideration either the psychologic effects on a patient or staff time benefits. Perhaps both a decrease in the number of drugs

given and the implementation of drug holidays would be advisable in some situations.

The use of drug holidays is one intervention that can help prevent drug toxicity. Drug holidays are most effective if carefully planned for the individual client and appropriately administered to use the "free" time that occurs to benefit both the client and the staff.

CASE STUDY 3

G. Carr is a 72-year-old widow. She has diabetes, has had triple coronary bypass surgery, and has a hiatal hernia and diverticulitis. She is also hearing impaired and wears a hearing aid in her left ear. Mrs. Carr lives alone in her own home and administers her own medications.

Mrs. Carr recently sought nursing advice in establishing a schedule for taking her medications following hospitalization. She had exhibited signs of early digitalis toxicity—increased nausea, a dull, persistent headache, and circumoral tingling—and was hospitalized when her physician made the diagnosis. She was discharged from the hospital on Xanax 0.5 mg tid, Humulin 10 U q AM, Procardia 10 mg bid, Lasix 40 mg bid, Isordil 10 mg qid, Tagamet 300 mg ac and hs, Tonocard 40 mg bid, Lanoxin 0.125 mg q AM, Mylanta II 1 oz pc and hs, Surfak i bid, Valium 5 mg tid, and Rufen 400 mg ii with meals.

The nurse identified the following defining characteristics indicating potential for drug toxicity: (1) client confusion about what medications should be taken and when; (2) a medication schedule on the discharge sheet that had the client taking medication almost hourly from 6 AM to 10 PM; (3) omission of a potassium supplement, which the client had been taking in the hospital, and a low potassium level; and (4) client lack of knowledge about what symptoms to report to the physician. Outcomes identified were Knowledge: Medication; Risk Control: Drug Use; and Self-Care: Non-Parenteral Medication (Iowa Outcomes Project, 2000).

In consultation with the nurse, the physician confirmed that she wanted Mrs. Carr to take the medications as noted on the discharge summary, but that the timing could be altered. The physician also added a potassium supplement. Mrs. Carr's administration schedule was consolidated from 14 to 9 times daily. The nurse developed a chart for Mrs. Carr to follow, directing which medications to take at what times until her return appointment with the physician. However, Mrs. Carr's condition continued to deteriorate. The physician discontinued both the Tonocard and Xanax, and Mrs. Carr's condition began to improve slowly. Gradually some of her other medications were discontinued and dosages reduced on others. The nurse continued to advocate for Mrs. Carr.

This case study demonstrates monitoring, advocacy, attempts to clarify goals of therapy, and devices to assist the elder in taking medications (the chart). NIC labels Medication Management and Teaching: Prescribed Medication encompass the appropriate activities. It also demonstrates that patient advocacy can be an ongoing process.

SUMMARY

Risk for Poisoning: Drug Toxicity is a diagnosis that nurses should keep in mind as they work with aging clients. The defining characteristics are not always easily recognized. The nurse must be aware that any change in function might be related to medications the older person is taking and report these changes to the physician. The nurse might need to become the client's advocate and present information to the physician in such a way that medications are reviewed systematically, dosages are adjusted, or medications are discontinued. Decisions about medications should be based on knowledge of changes generally experienced by elders. The goal is to maintain an optimal level of function for the dependent elder by administering the smallest number of medications at the lowest dosage. In some situations drug holidays may be a way for institutions to decrease serum blood levels in selected residents and also to give more flexibility to residents and staff. With effective monitoring of the older client, the actuality of drug toxicity should be minimized, allowing the client to live a more healthy life.

REFERENCES

Aronow, W. S. (1996). Heart drug may be overused in the elderly. *Drug Topics, 13,* 64.

Barnhart, E. (1996). *Physician's desk reference.* Montvale, NJ: Medical Economics.

Bergman, V., & Wilhelm, B. E. (1981). Drug-related problems causing admission to medical clinic. *European Journal of Clinical Pharmacology, 20,* 193.

Berlinger, W. G., & Spector, R. (1984). Adverse drug reactions in the elderly. *Geriatrics, 39,* 45.

Brady, E. S. (1978). Drugs and the elderly. In R. Haynes (Ed.), *Drugs and the elderly* (Rev. ed., pp. 1-7). Los Angeles: University of Southern California Press.

Carnosos, G. J., Stewart, R. B., & Cluff, L. E. (1974). Drug induced illness leading to hospitalization. *Journal of the American Medical Association, 228,* 713-717.

Carroll-Johnson, R. M. (Ed.). (1992). *Classification of nursing diagnoses: Proceedings of the Tenth National Conference.* Philadelphia: Lippincott Williams & Wilkins.

Chrischilles, E. A., Foley, D. J., Wallace, R. B., Lemke, J. H., Semla, T. P., Hanlon, J. T., Glynn, R. J., Ostfeld, A. M., & Guralnik, J. M. (1992). Use of medications by persons 65 and over: Data from the established populations for epidemiologic studies of the elderly. *Journal of Gerontology, 47*(5), M137-M144.

Davidson, W. (1978). The hazards of drug treatment in old age. In J. C. Brockelhurst (Ed.), *Textbook of geriatric medicine* (pp. 632-637). New York: Churchill Livingstone.

Exton-Smith, A. N., & Windsor, A. C. M. (1971). Principles of drug treatment in old age. In I. Rossman (Ed.), *Clinical geriatrics* (pp. 369-375). Philadelphia: Lippincott Williams & Wilkins.

Falvo, D. R., Holland, B., Brenner, J., & Benshoff, J. J. (1990). Medication use practices in the ambulatory elderly. *Health Values, 14*(3), 10-16.

Ford, R. (Ed.). (1986). *Mediquick cards.* Springhouse, PA: Springhouse.

Forni, P. J. (1978). Alcohol and the elderly. In R. Haynes (Ed.), *Drugs and the elderly* (Rev. ed., pp. 75-83). Berkley, CA: University of Southern California Press.

Gambert, S. R., Grossberg, G. T., & Morley, J. E. (1994). How many drugs does your aged patient need? *Patient Care, 28*(6), 61-66, 69-72.

Gromlin, I. H., & Chapron, D. J. (1983). Rational drug therapy for the aged. *Comprehensive Therapeutics, 9,* 17.

Grymonpre, R., Mitenko, P. A., Sitar, D. S., Aoki, F. Y., & Montgomery, P. R. (1988). Drug-associated hospital admissions in older medical patients. *Journal of the American Geriatrics Society, 36,* 1092-1098.

Gutman, D. (1977). *A survey of drug taking behavior in the elderly.* Rockville, MD: National Institute on Drug Abuse.

Hoffman, R. P. (1989). *Drug death: A danger of hospitalization. An exposé of life threatening adverse drug reactions and medication errors in hospitals.* Springfield, IL: Charles C. Thomas.

Iowa Intervention Project. J. C. McCloskey & G. M. Bulechek (Eds.). (2000). *Nursing interventions classification (NIC)* (3rd ed.). St. Louis, MO: Mosby.

Iowa Outcomes Project. M. Johnson, M. Maas, & S. Moorhead (Eds.). (2000). *Nursing outcomes classification (NOC)* (2nd ed.). St. Louis, MO: Mosby.

Ives, T. J., Bents, E. J., & Gwythr, R. E. (1987). Drug related admissions to a family medicine inpatient service. *Archives of Internal Medicine, 147,* 1117.

Johnson, J. E., & Moore, J. F. (1988). Drug taking practices of rural elderly. *Applied Nursing Research, 1,* 128-131.

Keenan, R., Redshaw, A., Munson, J., & Mundt, W. (1983). The benefits of a drug holiday. *Geriatric Nursing, 4*(2), 103-104.

Klassen, C. D. (1980). Principles of toxicology. In L. Goodman & A. Gilman (Eds.), *The pharmacological basis of therapeutics* (pp. 1602-1614). New York: Macmillan.

Lamy, P. P. (1980). *Prescribing for the elderly.* Littleton, MA: PGS.

Lamy, P. P. (1982). Comparative pharmokinetic changes and drug therapy in an older population. *Journal of the American Geriatrics Society, 30*(Suppl.), 11-19.

Lamy, P. P. (1989). Pharmacotherapeutics in the elderly. *Morbidity and Mortality Journal, 39,* 144-148.

May, F. E., Stewart, R. B., & Leighton, E. C. (1977). Drug interactions and multiple drug administration. *Clinical Pharmaceutical Therapeutics, 22,* 322-328.

Moore, J. F., & Johnson, J. E. (1993). Over the counter drug use by the rural elderly. *Geriatric Nursing, 14,* 190-191.

Moss, B. B. (1978). Effective drug administration as viewed by a physician administrator. In R. Haynes (Ed.), *Drugs and the elderly* (pp. 29-34, Rev. ed.). Los Angeles: University of Southern California Press.

Moss, F. F. (1977). *Too old, too sick, too bad: Nursing homes in America.* Gaithersburg, MD: Aspen.

Mullen, E. M., & Granholm, M. (1981). Drugs and the elderly patient. *Journal of Gerontological Nursing, 7*(2), 108-113.

North American Nursing Diagnosis Association. (1999). *Nursing diagnoses: Definitions and classification 1999-2000.* Philadelphia: Author.

Potempa, K. M., & Folta, A. (1992). Drug use and effects in older adults in the United States. *International Journal of Nursing Studies, 29*(1), 17-26.

Reidenberg, M. M. (1980). Drugs in the elderly. *Bulletin of the New York Medical Society, 56,* 703.

Rock, R. C. (1985). Monitoring therapeutic drug levels in older patients. *Geriatrics, 40,* 75-86.

Stewart, R. R. (1987). Drug use and adverse reactions in the elderly: An epidemiologic perspective. In C. B. Lewis (Ed.), *Topics in geriatric rehabilitation and aging* (pp. 1-11). Rockville, MD: Aspen.

Tandberg, D. (1981). How to treat and prevent drug toxicity. *Geriatrics, 36,* 64-73.

Todd, B. (1985). Identifying drug toxicity. *Geriatric Nursing, 4,* 231-234.

Tsujimoto, G., Hashimoto, K., & Hoffman, B. B. (1989). Pharmacokinetic and pharmacodynamic principles of drug therapy in old age. Part 1. *International Journal of Clinical Pharmacology, Therapeutics and Toxicology, 27,* 13-26.

United States Pharmacopeial Drug Information. (1996). USP DI Vol. 1 *Drug information for health care professionals.* Washington, DC: United States Pharmacopeial Convention.

Vestal, R. E., & Dawson, G. W. (1985). Pharmacology and aging. In C. E. Finch & E. L. Schneider (Eds.), *Handbook of biology in aging* (2nd ed., pp. 744-819). New York: Van Nostrand Reinhold.

Weitzel, E. A. (1976). *Client report and nursing observations as early indications of digitalis intoxication.* Unpublished study.

CHAPTER 5

RISK FOR INFECTION

Cheryl Carter and Jean M. Pottinger

As persons age, normal, age-related changes in multiple body systems lead to a decreased ability to defend against infection. The number of organisms required to cause an infection is smaller for an older adult than for a young adult. Older persons do not always respond to infections in the same manner as a younger client. Symptoms can be decreased or masked or can mimic other diseases. Chronic illnesses, which are very common in older adults, constitute risk factors for infection. Even many of the medications prescribed for older adults increase the risk for infection. In a 2-year study of nosocomial infections in an acute care hospital, 64% of the infections occurred in patients over the age of 60, even though the over-60 age-group represented only 23% of the total number of hospitalized patients (Gross, Rapuano, Adringnolo, & Shaw, 1983). Risk for infection represents an ongoing concern for nurses who care for older adults.

RELATED FACTORS/ETIOLOGIES

Age-related changes occur in virtually every body system. These changes affect an individual's ability to resist infection. Moreover, underlying chronic diseases are themselves risk factors for infection. Kramarow and colleagues (1999) estimated that more than 79% of elderly persons have at least one chronic condition. Some chronic conditions commonly found in elders are chronic respiratory disease, heart disease, peripheral vascular disease, arthritis, diabetes, cancer, and dementia. Physicians frequently prescribe multiple medications to control these chronic diseases, but drugs such as antibiotics, antiinflammatory agents, and steroids themselves can impair the older person's ability to resist infection.

Changes in the Immune System

The human body is protected by the immune system in two ways. The humoral immune system is initiated by immunoglobulins that are produced when exposed to antigens. This response occurs during bacterial infections (Blaylock, 1993). The second type of immunity is cell-mediated immunity (CMI). In the presence of antigens CMI is activated in response to parasites, fungi, viruses, allergic reactions, and transplant rejection (Abrams, 1986; Paul, 1988).

The human immune system reaches optimum functioning capacity at about the time of puberty and then declines by 5% to 30% of its original capacity over a person's lifetime (Haddy, 1988). Certain functional immune parameters decline with age, although physiologic aging is far more important than chronologic age. There is general agreement that lymphocyte function decreases with age, but studies have been confusing because they were done on ill rather than healthy elderly persons.

The proportion of T-cells that can respond to new antigens decreases as involution of the thymus occurs with age, and as a result most T-cells in elders have already had contact with an antigen. This might explain why elderly persons respond to antigens they encountered in the past but not to new antigens (Terpenning & Bradley, 1991). Although changes in the immune system are associated with aging, older adults should not be considered immunocompromised in the same sense as the patient with AIDS.

A decrease in immune function can lead to the following changes:

- Skin turgor decreases; skin becomes more dry and less acidic, predisposing elders to skin breakdown.
- Estrogen level decreases, predisposing females to urinary tract infections (UTIs) or vaginitis.
- Cough reflex is reduced, ciliary action of the respiratory tract is limited, and dysphagia can occur, leading to possible aspiration or pneumonia.
- Incomplete bladder emptying, bladder muscle weakening, and prostatic disease may lead to UTI.
- Motility of the gastrointestinal (GI) system decreases, and acid production decreases; these changes predispose the elderly to gastroenteritis or diarrhea.
- Bacterial growth in the oral cavity increases because of decreased ability to perform oral hygiene. These bacteria can travel to the lungs during microaspiration events, which could lead to an increase in respiratory infections.

Malnutrition and dehydration play pivotal roles in immune function. Protein and calorie malnutrition is common in elders; it occurs in 40% to 80% of patients over age 70 (Plewa, 1990). Second to the immunodeficiency consistent with aging, malnutrition is the most common cause of immune system dysfunction in older individuals (Makris, 1996). Without adequate protein and other nutrients, older adults have a longer healing period for wounds and a lower resistance to fight off infection. Dehydration can lead to electrolyte imbalance and possible mental status changes. Other factors that can contribute to immune function impairment include medications, depression, immobility, isolation, alcohol abuse, and chronic medical conditions such as diabetes, cancer, and renal failure.

Changes in the Skin

Age-related changes in the skin begin at about age 30 and result in decreased protection and increased susceptibility to injury (Wiersema, 1995). Wiersema (1995) and Rusnak (1996) described the effects of aging on the skin. Skin cells have decreased cohesiveness and are replaced at a slower rate. Thus wound healing is delayed and the risk for infection is increased because the skin barrier remains broken for a longer period of time. The dermis and subcutaneous connective tissue become thinner, more fragile, and more prone to tear easily. Temperature regulation is affected as subcutaneous fat is lost. Consequently elderly persons become chilled or suffer from heatstroke more easily. The inflammatory and immune responses are decreased. Blood perfusion and the number of small blood vessels diminish. In addition, circulation to the extremities decreases. A decrease in sensory perception leads to increased risk of injury caused by things such as hot water and heating pads. The sebaceous glands secrete less sebum; hence the skin is more susceptible to cracking. Pruritus can result from the dry skin, causing the elder to scratch and break the skin. Atherosclerotic arterial disease and venous insufficiency can worsen normal aging factors.

The structural changes that occur in the skin increase the elder's risk for developing soft tissue infections and pressure ulcers. Pressure, shearing forces, friction, and moisture can cause skin injuries. Friction and moisture usually cause superficial skin breakdown and are most harmful when combined with excessive pressure. Prolonged or repeated pressure causes injury to muscle and subcutaneous tissue.

Immobility is the primary risk factor for developing a pressure ulcer. Related risk factors are urinary and fecal incontinence, diarrhea, dementia, malnutrition, anemia, spasticity, poor skin care, and diabetes (Allman, 1989). The pressure sore itself is a physical wound and not an infectious process. Wound infection, osteomyelitis, and sepsis are the infections associated with pressure sores.

Scabies is a skin infestation caused by the mite *Sarcoptes scabiei*. The mite is transferred by direct skin contact with infested persons (Rusnak, 1996). Caregivers who are infested transmit the mite and often do so before they develop symptoms. Scabies commonly occurs in dependent elders. Home care agencies have reported cases in their clients, and several nursing home outbreaks have been identified. The usual symptoms of scabies are pruritic linear lesions on the hands, fingers, wrists, arms, waist, and buttocks. Itching is more intense at night (Pien, 1996). In elderly persons, however, the presentation may be atypical and not easily recognized. The typical rash is not seen because of the diminished immune response, and itching is not intense because of decreased sensation. Therefore an infestation can become advanced before it is diagnosed (Rusnak, 1996).

Changes in the Respiratory System

The effects of aging on the respiratory system are subtle but progressive. Many older adults are not aware of these changes unless they have coexisting diseases such as chronic obstructive pulmonary disease (COPD), congestive heart failure (CHF), diabetes mellitus, or carcinoma. As the respiratory muscles lose tone and elasticity, the chest wall expands less, air flow and lung volume are reduced, and the maximum breath capacity declines (Johnson, 1995). The result is increased dead space in the lungs. Poor posture, partially caused by weakened muscles or osteoporosis, limits lung capacity (Rusnak, 1996). The lungs provide one-third less oxygen at age 80 than at age 20. Rales at the lung bases are common because of decreased respiratory function and are not necessarily caused by pneumonia (Johnson, 1995).

The activity of the ciliated epithelial cells in the upper respiratory tract decreases. The cough reflex is diminished, and the ability to cough and raise secretions is hampered. The cellular and humoral components of lung immunity decline, i.e., immunoglobulin A secretion is less efficient and the number of alveolar macrophages decreases. Consequently elders are less able to effectively kill organisms or clear them and particulates from the respiratory tract (Rusnak, 1996).

The normal flora in the throat changes, and the elder becomes colonized with more pathogenic gram-negative bacilli. This colonization is significant because bacterial pneumonia is usually preceded by microaspiration of oropharyngeal secretions (Esposito, 1991). Aspiration increases with esophageal disorders, altered level of consciousness, inactivity, physical dependency, cerebrovascular accidents, and dementia.

Lower respiratory tract infections are the fifth leading cause of death in elders, and pneumonia is the most common infectious disease necessitating hospitalization for elders (Bentley & Mylotte, 1991). *Streptococcus pneumoniae* is the most common cause of bacterial pneumonias occurring in community dwelling elderly persons (Advisory Committee on Immunization Practices, 1997). At least 500,000 cases of pneumococcal pneumonia occur each year in the United States, with 10% to 25% of adult persons also having concomitant bacteremia. Elders are at high risk for morbidity and mortality from serious pneumococcal infections. The death rate for elderly patients with pneumococcal bacteremia is 30% to 40%.

Influenza has caused major epidemics of respiratory infections in elders. During influenza seasons from 1972 to 1995, the influenza-associated mortality ranged from approximately 25 to more than 150 deaths per 100,000 persons age 65 or older. Greater than 90% of these deaths occurred among persons more than 65 years of age (Advisory Committee on Immunization Practices, 1999). Deaths are most frequently attributable to secondary bacterial pneumonia or to exacerbation of a preexisting chronic condition, such as COPD or CHF.

Changes in the Genitourinary System

The muscle of the bladder weakens with age; hence urine flow decreases as the strength of the bladder contractions diminishes. The volume of urine decreases with dehydration, resulting in the stasis of urine in the bladder. The urine pH is reduced. Obstruction of urinary flow occurs from neurogenic bladder, prostatic hypertrophy, and prolapse of the rectum, bladder, or uterus (Rusnak, 1996).

These physiologic changes allow microorganisms to multiply and cause UTIs. As many as 20% of elders are affected by UTI, and this percentage may increase to 25% to 50% among institutionalized elderly (Rusnak, 1996). Indwelling urinary catheters are the greatest risk factor for UTI. UTIs are the most frequent infections observed in hospitals and long-term care facilities, where as many as 30% of elderly patients have an indwelling urinary catheter in place (Smith & Rusnak, 1991). Most catheter-associated UTIs are caused by gram-negative bacteria that colonize the perineum and ascend up the urinary catheter.

Incontinence is the involuntary loss of urine so severe as to have social or hygienic consequences. An estimated 10 million adults in the United States are incontinent of urine, and the problem is greatest in the age-group over 65. Elderly individuals in the community comprise 9% to 30% of those with incontinence, hospitalized elders account for 19% to 35%, and 50% are elderly residents of long-term care facilities (Palmer & McCormick, 1991). Incontinence itself is not a risk factor for UTIs. Often, however, incontinence is managed by inserting an indwelling urinary catheter or applying an external catheter, which in turn places the elder at risk for a UTI. Incontinence also has implications for skin infections.

Changes in the Eyes

Many factors that protect the eye from infection and injury are absent or diminished in elders: sufficient tear production, the flushing action to remove debris from the eye, and the mechanical barrier of normal blinking. A common cause of conjunctivitis in elderly persons is *Staphylococcus spp.* Seborrhea can predispose the eye to chronic infection. In contrast to bacterial infections, the most common viral infection is adenovirus conjunctivitis. This type of conjunctivitis spreads rapidly by direct contact. Because a person has a red eye does not mean that it is conjunctivitis. Redness and irritation can be due to air pollution, lack of sleep, dry eyes, or other medical conditions such as an allergic reaction. Care must be taken to carefully differentiate between the two.

Infection of the lid margin, known as blepharitis, is common in elders and is usually associated with seborrhea of the eyebrows, skin of the nose, cheeks, and scalp. Secondary staphylococcus infections cause eye ulceration, chalazia, and abscesses. The elder may complain of itching, burning, scratching, tearing, and intolerance to smoke, light, and dust (Michaels, 1986).

Herpes simplex is the leading cause of corneal disease. The epidemiology is worldwide, and people seem to be the only natural reservoir. Attacks may be recurrent, so a history of prior eye or skin lesions is important. A number of triggers can be responsible: fever, sunburn, emotional stress, and topical steroids. Herpes zoster is a reactivation of the varicella zoster virus that causes chickenpox but has serious implications in elders.

Factors Related to Gastrointestinal Infection

The aging process affects nearly every part of the GI tract. Although aging alters GI function, many GI problems that older adults experience are more closely associated with their lifestyles (Joffrion & Leuszler, 1995). A decrease in the gastric pH occurs as one ages that might increase the susceptibility to pathogens.

Elders, especially those in long-term care facilities, frequently experience diarrhea. Mortality can occur if elders become dehydrated and symptoms go untreated. Diarrhea can be caused by tube feedings, medications, and viral and bacterial agents (Table 5-1). Most organisms that cause diarrhea are spread via the fecal and oral route or contaminated food and water.

Although noninfectious causes of diarrhea are common, infectious diarrhea must always be a consideration (Smith, 1987). Usually self-limiting, viral causes of diarrhea are common and antibiotic therapy is of no benefit (Smith, 1984). Rotavirus infections typically cause a mild form of diarrhea but may be more severe in elders. In nursing homes outbreaks have been reported with mortality rates ranging from 0% to 10%. Person-to-person spread is the main cause of viral outbreaks. The onset of gastroenteritis caused by a viral agent is usually very abrupt, 24 to 72 hours, and persists for 2 to 7 days. Symptoms associated with viral diarrhea may include fever, abdominal cramping, watery stools with or without blood, or mucous. Diarrhea caused by viral agents tend to occur in the winter.

Gastroenteritis caused by bacterial agents has a more insidious onset. The incubation period can last from 1 to 72 hours, with symptom duration persisting from less than 24 hours to weeks. Elders usually experience fever, loose bloody stools, or stools with occult blood. Leukocytosis can be present (Rusnak, 1996).

Table 5-1	Clinical Picture of Infections in the Elderly, Usual Pathogens Involved, and Diagnostic Tests	
Site	**Signs and Symptoms**	**Common Organisms**
Skin and soft tissue	Purulent drainage Pain, swelling, heat, induration, or erythema surrounding the lesion	*Staphylococcus spp.* *Streptococcus spp.* *Escherichia coli* *Proteus spp.* *Pseudomonas spp.* *Enterococcus spp.* *Bacteroides fragilis* *Clostridium perfringens*
Pneumonia	Shaking chills, fever, productive cough, pleuritic chest pain	*Streptococcus pneumoniae* *Haemophilus influenzae* *Staphylococcus aureus* *Moraxella catarrhalis*
Urinary tract	Dysuria, frequency, suprapubic or flank pain	*Escherichia coli* *Klebsiella spp.* *Proteus spp.* *Providencia spp.* *Pseudomonas spp.* *Serratia marcescens* *Enterococcus spp.*
Eye	Redness, drainage, itching, swelling	*Staphylococcus aureus* Adenovirus Herpes simplex Herpes zoster
Gastrointestinal	Diarrhea Vomiting	*Salmonella spp.* *C. perfringens* *E. coli* 0157:H7 *Shigella* *Staphylococcus aureus* *Giardia lamblia* *Entamoeba histolytica* *C. difficile*

Data from Rusnak, P. G. (1996). Long-term care. In R. N. Olmsted (Ed.), *APIC infection control and applied epidemiology: Principles and practice* (pp. 17-1 to 17-31). St. Louis, MO: Mosby.

Salmonellae are responsible for most of the large outbreaks of infectious diarrhea in long-term care facilities. Case fatality rates of 3% to 8% are typical (Smith & Rusnak, 1991). In one study of 25 nursing home outbreaks, the mean number of residents ill per outbreak was 22; 48 deaths occurred. These outbreaks were traced to such common vehicles as poultry, ungraded eggs, red meat, milk or other food products, or poor hygiene of the food workers. Attack rates for salmonella GI tract infections are higher in patients who are achlorhydric because of aging, previous surgery, or H_2-receptor antagonist (Markis, 1996). In a study by Gangarosa, Glass, Lew, and Boring (1992) of gastroenteritis in hospitalized patients, the case fatality ratio for gastroenteritis was .05% in infants and 3% in those 80 years and older.

Clostridium perfringens gastroenteritis can result from eating beef or poultry dishes that are cooked one day and inadequately cooled and stored before being served the next day. Antibiotic-associated colitis caused by a toxin of

C. difficile must be considered in cases of diarrhea occurring in long-term care facilities. *C. difficile* is a difficult pathogen for nursing staff to contend with. Patients can be asymptomatic carriers of the organism or develop antibiotic-associated diarrhea or pseudomembranous diarrhea. This organism is part of the normal flora of the GI tract but under certain situations can become pathogenically acquired from the environment via the hands of health care workers. Any patient who develops diarrhea within 10 weeks of receiving antibiotics should be screened for *C. difficile* (Keogh, 1993). Most often the use of cephalosporins, extended-spectrum penicillins, and clindamycin is responsible. These agents decrease the normal flora and allow overgrowth of *C. difficile*. Reports in the literature state that asymptomatic colonization may be seen in 2% of healthy adults and from 16% to 56% of hospitalized elderly adults. Persons with a *C. difficile* infection can present with foul-smelling, bloody diarrhea along with bloating, pain, and tenderness. Some patients may experience a prodrome of general malaise, drowsiness, and mental status changes before the onset of diarrhea such as with *C. difficile*. The natural course of *C. difficile* is usually self-limiting if the offending antibiotic is discontinued.

E. coli 0157:H7 has caused outbreaks of bloody diarrhea in long-term care facilities. Usually traced to a beef product, this organism should be kept in mind when cultures for common pathogens are negative (Smith & Rusnak, 1991).

The toxin produced by *Staphylococcus aureus* results from improperly stored food. Diarrhea caused by toxin producing organisms is usually sudden in onset. Typical symptoms for gastroenteritis caused by toxin producing organisms include nausea, vomiting, and profuse diarrhea (Rusnak, 1996).

Giardia is the most commonly isolated intestinal parasite in the United States and has been responsible for numerous community outbreaks. Ingestion of the cysts from contaminated water is the most common route of transmission. In long-term care facilities the mode of transmission is by direct person-to-person contact. In a Minnesota nursing home in 1986, an outbreak of *Giardia lamblia* that originated with an infected meal progressed by person-to-person spread and affected 35 residents and 38 employees. There was a child care center located within the facility, and it was evident that the children who often adopted "foster" grandparents served as the source for introducing the organism into the elderly community (White et al., 1989). *Giardia* can also be recovered from inanimate surfaces through indirect transmission. The incubation period is 7 to 14 days, and symptom duration is variable.

ASSESSMENT

Recognizing infections in elders can be difficult. The classic signs and symptoms and abnormal laboratory results of an infection are often absent; indeed, a nonspecific presentation is the norm (Blaylock, 1993). A change in functional status might be the only clue that an older adult has an infection. Functional status changes include the following: altered mental status, decreased appetite, increased confusion, increased dependence or disability, or unexplained increased heart or respiratory rates. The older person might fall or be incontinent of urine or feces. Another sign of infection in the elder might be an exacerbation of an underlying condition, such as uncontrolled diabetes or CHF. Dry mucous membranes often accompany infection because the older person becomes dehydrated.

Fever is absent in 20% to 30% of infectious episodes that occur in elders. Even if fever is present, it can be masked by medications the person is receiving for other conditions, e.g., aspirin, steroids, or antiinflammatory agents. Because the fever response is typically blunted in elders, a more specific definition of fever in this population is "persistent elevation of body temperature at least 2° F over baseline" (Norman & Yoshikawa, 1996).

See Table 5-1 for classic signs and symptoms of infections. The health care provider should look for these clinical symptoms when assessing the elderly patient. However, the provider should also be aware that these signs and symptoms may be absent or obscure. Pain with voiding may be absent in a UTI, and frequency may be difficult to detect if the person is incontinent. Even if the elderly person has pneumonia, cough may be absent because of the decreased cough reflex and sputum production. The silent presentation occurs most frequently with pneumonia. By the time the patient seeks health care assistance, the disease is in an advanced state and interventions are not successful (Fox, 1988). As many as 50% of elderly persons do not have leukocytosis when they have an infection. Some chronologically elderly patients are not immunologically old. In these patients infections appear as they do in younger patients.

NURSING DIAGNOSIS

Risk for Infection has been defined by the North American Nursing Diagnosis Association (NANDA) as "the state in which the individual is at increased risk for being invaded by pathogenic organisms" (NANDA, 1999, p. 11). It is important to distinguish between infection and colonization. Infection occurs when an organism invades and multiplies in the tissues of the host, resulting in cellular damage and producing an inflammatory response. Infections can be asymptomatic or can result in clinical signs and symptoms. Colonization is the presence of microorganisms that grow and multiply in or on a host but do not invade or damage tissue and do not produce clinical symptoms.

CASE STUDY 1

S. Jones is an 81-year-old woman who lives alone in her own home. She has arthritis, diabetes, hypertension, and CHF and controls her chronic conditions with diet and oral medications. Mrs. Jones is able to function at home but rarely leaves the house. A home health aide comes in to her home 2 mornings each week to bathe Mrs. Jones and do light housekeeping and laundry. An RN comes to the house once each month to assess Mrs. Jones. Mrs. Jones's children visit several times a week, bring her prepared meals, shop for her, and do errands for her.

Over the last year Mrs. Jones's appetite has been poor. She frequently prepared tea and toast for her meals during the day. One day she fell after her leg twisted while she was walking. She was admitted to the hospital and had a long leg cast placed for a fractured tibia and fibula.

The nurse assessed Mrs. Jones's risk for infection when she was admitted. Her temperature was 98° F. When the nurse examined Mrs. Jones's skin, she found no rash or open areas, but the nurse noted that Mrs. Jones's skin was very dry and the skin on her legs was flaky. Mrs. Jones's lungs were clear. Her urine was clear but very concentrated. Mrs. Jones was able to urinate without difficulty if she was helped to sit on the commode, but she was unable to urinate on the bedpan.

CASE STUDY 2

Sam Becker is a 70 year old with coronary artery disease, status post myocardial infarction, hypercholesterolemia, hypertension, and diabetes mellitus. He had a coronary artery bypass graft of two vessels and did well during the immediate postoperative period.

On the fourth postoperative day, the microbiology laboratory notified the nursing unit and the infection control team that Mr. Becker was growing vancomycin-resistant enterococcus (VRE) from a stool specimen that was submitted as part of a cluster investigation. The nursing unit was instructed by the infection control team to place the patient in contact precautions, which requires wearing gloves and gown and using antibacterial soap that contains 4% chlorhexidine or 60% isopropyl alcohol. The nurse manager followed the infection control guidelines by providing one-to-one nursing care for him to decrease the chance of transmitting VRE to newer postoperative patients. Mr. Becker was instructed in the basics of infection control: washing his hands to decrease the number of organisms, which in turn would decrease the chances of contaminating his vein harvest graft site and his surgical wound. Mr. Becker and his family had the following questions regarding care once he was released to home:

Can we catch this?
How long will I have this?
Is it safe for the grandchildren to be around?
What about cleaning the home?
Can I have visitors?
Should I use any special lotions or soaps?

NURSING-SENSITIVE OUTCOMES

The *Nursing Outcomes Classification (NOC)* (Iowa Outcomes Project, 2000) includes several nursing-sensitive outcomes that are appropriate for the diagnosis Risk for Infection. The primary outcomes include Infection Status, which is defined as the "presence and extent of infection" (Iowa Outcomes Project, 2000, p. 248); Knowledge: Health Behaviors, which is the "extent of understanding conveyed about the promotion and protection of health" (p. 268); and Risk Control, which shows "actions to eliminate or reduce actual, personal and modifiable health threats" (p. 353). Table 5-2 outlines the indicators for these outcomes and adds recommended outcomes and indicators that currently are not listed in NOC.

NURSING INTERVENTIONS

Nurses should take actions to compensate for the effects of aging and thereby reduce the risk of infection in the elderly patient. The *Nursing Interventions Classification (NIC)* (Iowa Intervention Project, 2000) includes several nursing interventions for Risk for Infection. Key NIC interventions are Infection Control, which is defined as "minimizing the acquisition and transmission of infectious agents" (Iowa Intervention Project, 2000, p. 398) and Infection Protection, which is the "prevention and early detection of infection in a patient at risk" (p. 401). Nursing activities that are appropriate for these and other nursing interventions are outlined in Table 5-2.

To reduce the incidence of infection in the elderly person, a thorough assessment and disease history is crucial. Oftentimes the smallest change in daily functioning is the first indication of a developing infection. Early clinical signs of a developing infection can include an elevated blood glucose, mild hypotension, or a slight increase in pulse and respiration. Nurses have the responsibility for continually assessing their patients for slight changes in functional status. Patient and family education on preventive measures and modes of transmission is essential.

To decrease the chance of a UTI, indwelling Foley catheters should be avoided if possible. If catheters are used, they should be secured to the leg. To reduce the number of organisms in the bladder, fluids should be offered and encouraged. Good hygiene when performing catheter care will decrease the potential for infection, as well.

Ensure equal weight distribution, especially for those who are immobile, to decrease risk for pressure sores. As mentioned earlier, immune function is affected by malnutrition, so enhancing the nutritional state of the patient is also of great importance. Infections in elders can have fatal outcomes if not addressed quickly. The best way to prevent the spread of organisms that cause infection is through the use of Standard Precautions and thorough hand washing.

One way to prevent infection in elders is to boost the immune system through immunization. The Centers for Disease Control and Prevention (CDC) recommends that persons age 65 and older receive influenza vaccine yearly. The CDC also recommends that persons age 65 and over receive a pneumococcal vaccine. A second dose of the vaccine should be given if they received the vaccine more than 5 years previously and were less than 65 at the time of the primary vaccine. One dose of the vaccine should be given to elderly persons with an unknown vaccine status. These immunizations are meant to lessen the severity of illness and complications should they occur. Table 5-3 is offered as a guide to immunizations for elders. The immune system also can be boosted through adequate nutritional intake and through the use of hormones or drugs.

Table 5-2	Suggested Nursing-Sensitive Outcomes and Nursing Interventions
	RISK FOR INFECTION

NURSING DIAGNOSIS

RISK FOR INFECTION

Defining Characteristics

Invasive procedures

Insufficient knowledge to avoid exposure to pathogens

Trauma

Tissue destruction and increased environmental exposure

Pharmaceutic agents

Malnutrition

Immunosuppression

Inadequate acquired immunity

Inadequate secondary defenses (decreased hemoglobin, leukopenia, suppressed inflammatory response)

Inadequate primary defenses (broken skin, traumatized tissue, decrease in ciliary action, stasis of body fluids, change in pH secretions, altered peristalsis), chronic disease

Nursing-Sensitive Outcomes	Nursing Interventions
TISSUE INTEGRITY: SKIN & MUCOUS MEMBRANES	**SKIN SURVEILLANCE**
Indicators	*Activities*
Skin intactness	Observe extremities for color, warmth, swelling, pulses, texture, edema, and ulcerations
Hydration IER*	Inspect skin and mucous membranes for redness, extreme warmth, or drainage
Color IER	Avoid daily bathing
Tissue temperature IER	Adjust hot water temperature to prevent scalding
Perspiration IER	Wear sunscreen and protective hat and clothing when outside
Tissue lesion free	Increase humidity in the environment to reduce drying of skin
	Ensure adequate fluid intake
	Minimize use of tape on the skin, and if tape must be used, ensure strength of adhesive is less than that of skin
	Avoid friction and shearing forces that can tear skin (Rusnak, 1996; Wiersema, 1995)
	SKIN CARE: TOPICAL TREATMENTS
	Activities
	Dress patient in nonrestrictive clothing
	Avoid use of rough-textured bed linens
	Keep bed linen clean, dry, wrinkle free
	Refrain from using alkaline soap on skin
	PRESSURE ULCER PREVENTION
	Activities
	Remove excess moisture on skin from perspiration, wound drainage, fecal or urinary incontinence
	Use established risk assessment tool to monitor risk factors (e.g., Braden scale)
	Keep skin clean, such as washing perineal area after each bowel movement
	Keep skin dry; use powder if necessary
	Apply lotion with little or no alcohol
	Facilitate frequent, small shifts of body weight
	Encourage appropriate exercise/mobility
	Ensure adequate nutrition
	Turn every 1-2 hours continuously
	Place on therapeutic mattress, cushion
	Inspect skin of all elders

*IER, In expected range.

Continued

Suggested Nursing-Sensitive Outcomes and Nursing Interventions—cont'd	
Table 5-2 RISK FOR INFECTION—cont'd	
Nursing-Sensitive Outcomes	**Nursing Interventions**

Nursing-Sensitive Outcomes	Nursing Interventions
	Have a high index of suspicion for scabies of all rashes Obtain skin scrapings to confirm diagnosis Treat all scabies infestations promptly Treat all contacts to stop transmission
PARASITE STATUS *Indicator* Skin clear of scabies	**ORAL HEALTH MAINTENANCE** *Activity* Apply lubricant to moisten lips and oral mucosa, as needed **ORAL HEALTH RESTORATION** *Activity* Discourage smoking
INFECTION STATUS *Indicators* Fever Chest x-ray infiltration	**INFECTION CONTROL** *Activities* Encourage deep breathing and coughing Instruct and assist to perform oral hygiene after eating and as often as needed Administer immunizations Encourage physical activity Change position frequently to prevent pooling of secretions Increase fluid intake to decrease viscosity of pulmonary secretions Use sedating drugs sparingly Prevent aspiration by elevating head of bed, positioning the physically dependent, alleviating abdominal distension
URINARY CONTINENCE *Indicators* Absence of urinary tract infections (<100,000 WBC) Fluid intake in expected range Predictable pattern to passage of urine Empties bladder completely Underclothing or bedding dry during night	**URINARY ELIMINATION MANAGEMENT** *Activities* Monitor urinary elimination including frequency, consistency, odor, volume, and color, as appropriate Teach patients signs and symptoms of urinary tract infection Avoid using indwelling catheters **URINARY CONTINENCE CARE** *Activities* Identify multifunctional causes of incontinence Instruct to drink a minimum of 1500 ml fluids a day Cleanse genital skin area at regular intervals Establish toileting interval based on voiding pattern Habit training, or toileting on a schedule frequent enough to prevent wetting, usually between 1 and 4 hours Use bellpad for cognitively impaired persons Assign nursing personnel to a group of persons to focus on toileting instead of changing wet clothing and mopping floors Monitor staff and reward appropriate behavior Use mechanical lift for frequent toileting of elders with impaired mobility (Palmer, 1991)
KNOWLEDGE: HEALTH BEHAVIORS *Indicator* Description of measures to prevent transmission of infectious disease	**INFECTION CONTROL** *Activities* Teach patient and family members how to avoid infections Teach patient and family about signs and symptoms of infection and when to report them to the health care provider

Suggested Nursing-Sensitive Outcomes and Nursing Interventions—cont'd	
Table 5-2 RISK FOR INFECTION—cont'd	
Nursing-Sensitive Outcomes	**Nursing Interventions**

SAFETY BEHAVIOR: PERSONAL
Indicator
Prevents or minimizes threats to eye or visual integrity

EYE CARE
Activities
Remove contact lenses as appropriate
Apply cool compresses to decrease irritation
Apply warm compresses to soften crust around the eye
Apply eye shield as appropriate
Patch the eyes as needed
Apply lubricating eyedrops
Apply lubricating ointment as appropriate
Monitor tear production

BOWEL ELIMINATION
Indicator
Diarrhea not present

DIARRHEA MANAGEMENT
Activities
Obtain stool for culture and sensitivity if diarrhea continues
Monitor for signs and symptoms of diarrhea
Monitor safe food preparation
Perform actions to rest the bowel
Identify factors that may cause or contribute to diarrhea
Place patient on contact precautions (gown if soiling likely and gloves for touching infected material)
Private room if hygiene poor
Perform scrupulous hand washing to prevent person-to-person transmission
Notify local health department if foodborne outbreak suspected
Replace normal colonic flora by the use of agents such as *Lactobacillus acidophilus*
Perform proper food handling to prevent foodborne infections

FLUID/ELECTROLYTE MANAGEMENT
Activities
Give fluids, as appropriate
Promote oral intake, as appropriate
Monitor for fluid loss

ELECTROLYTE MONITORING
Activities
Monitor for abnormal serum electrolytes, as available
Maintain intravenous solution containing electrolyte(s) at constant flow rate, as appropriate
Consult physician if signs and symptoms of fluid and/or electrolyte imbalance persist or worsen

RISK CONTROL
Indicators
Prevents or detects infection
Monitors environmental risk factors
Monitors personal behavior risk factors
Participates in screening for identified risks
Prevents resistant organism transmission

INFECTION PROTECTION
Activities
Monitor for systemic and localized signs and symptoms of infection
Monitor vulnerability to infection
Inspect skin and mucous membranes for redness, extreme warmth, or drainage
Inspect condition of any surgical incision/wound
Obtain cultures, as needed
Promote sufficient nutritional intake
Encourage fluid intake, as appropriate
Encourage rest
Monitor for change in energy level/malaise

Continued

Table 5-2	Suggested Nursing-Sensitive Outcomes and Nursing Interventions—cont'd RISK FOR INFECTION—cont'd	
Nursing-Sensitive Outcomes	**Nursing Interventions**
	Encourage increased mobility and exercise, as appropriate
	Administer immunizing agent, as appropriate
	Assess for fatigue, confusion, and behavioral changes
	Monitor for increase in blood glucose, hypotension, pulse, and respirations
	Elevate head of bed 30-45 degrees to prevent aspiration
	Perform pulmonary toileting as needed
	Obtain rectal or stool swabs as needed
	Obtain nares swab, as appropriate
	Skin lesions (infected or colonized) should be covered with dressings that contain drainage at all times (Rusnak, 1996)
	If outbreak occurs, group patients and nursing staff
	INFECTION CONTROL
	Activities
	Teach the patient and family about signs and symptoms of infection and when to report them to the health care provider
	Health care worker should use mask if performing procedures that generate aerosolization of organism
	INFECTION PROTECTION
	Activities
	Report suspected infections to infection control personnel
	Report positive cultures to infection control personnel
	Maintain isolation techniques, as appropriate
	Teach improved hand washing to health care personnel
	Instruct patient on hand washing technique
	Instruct visitors to wash hands on entering and leaving patient's room
	Use antimicrobial soap for hand washing
	Wash hands before and after each care activity
	Institute contact precautions
	Teach patient and family about signs and symptoms of infection and when to report them to the health care provider
	Teach patient and family members about how to avoid infections

OTHER ISSUES

HIV and AIDS

The older adult is often considered by society to be asexual and not an intravenous drug user (Scura & Whipple, 1995). Although frequency of sexual activity declines with age, a majority of persons over 60 remain sexually active.

It is estimated that 10% of the persons with acquired immunodeficiency syndrome (AIDS) in the United States are over the age of 50. The CDC HIV/AIDS Surveillance Report in 1995 reported 52,097 known cases of AIDS in the 50-years-of-age-and-older group (CDC, 1995). These numbers are probably underestimated because of lack of recognition of the disease in this group. The perception of the medical community and the lay public is that human immunodeficiency virus (HIV) is not a disease of older individuals (El-Sadr & Gettler, 1995; Stall & Catania, 1994). This belief is reflected in the numerous studies and projects that are focused on the younger person. In a seroprevalence study of 257 persons over the age of 60 who died in a New York hospital with no known history of HIV or AIDS, 5% of postmortem blood samples were found to have positive antibodies for HIV (El-Sadr & Gettler, 1995). Relative to younger AIDS patients, a higher proportion of elderly AIDS patients are female and Caucasian (Wallace, Paauw, & Spach, 1993). The United States has an estimated 1 million homosexual men over age 65 (McCormick & Wood, 1992).

HIV infection occurs because of transmission of the virus from an infected person through one of three routes: (1) sexual, (2) bloodborne, or (3) vertical from mother to child. The highest concentrations of the virus can be found in blood, semen, breast milk, female genital secretions, spinal fluid, and to a lesser extent saliva and tears.

Sexual contact with homosexual or bisexual men remains the chief mode of transmission for HIV. This is true for all age-groups except for the over-65 group, for

Table 5-3	Recommended Immunizations for the Elderly	
Vaccine	**Frequency**	**Comments**
Influenza	Immunize fall of each year if over age 65, has chronic cardiopulmonary system disorders, anyone who requires regular medical follow-up or required hospitalization during the preceding year because of chronic metabolic disease (including diabetes), renal dysfunction, immunocompromised, disorders of the cardiopulmonary system, residents of long-term care facilities	Highly recommended for persons with chronic illnesses and residents of long-term care facilities. Contraindicated in persons allergic to eggs.
Pneumococcal	Age 65 and over and anyone with chronic conditions that increase the risk of pneumococcal disease and its complications (heart disease, diabetes, renal failure, alcoholism, immunosuppression, persons with functional or anatomic asplenia): one dose	Consider revaccination every 6 years for adults at high risk for fatal pneumococcal disease or rapid decline in antibody levels (nephrotic syndrome, renal failure, organ transplantation).
Tetanus/diphtheria	Booster every 10 years	Persons with unknown or uncertain histories of receiving diphtheria or tetanus should be considered unvaccinated and should receive a full three-dose primary series of Td.

Data from Advisory Committee on Immunization Practices. (1989). Pneumococcal polysaccharide vaccine. *MMWR Morbidity and Mortality Weekly Report, 38,* 64-67, 73-76; Advisory Committee on Immunization Practices. (1997). Prevention of pneumococcal disease: recommendations of the Advisory Committee on Immunization Practices (ACIP). *MMWR Morbidity and Mortality Weekly Report, 46*(RR-8), 1-24; Advisory Committee on Immunization Practices. (1999). Prevention and control of influenza: recommendations of the Advisory Committee on Immunization Practices (ACIP). *MMWR Morbidity and Mortality Weekly Report, 48*(RR-4), 1-28.

which transfusion-acquired infection is the second leading cause of HIV transmission in persons over 50. Stall and Catania (1994) identified three major groups within the elderly population thought to be at risk for acquiring HIV infection: pre-1985 blood product recipients, spouses of those recipients, and persons who participate in unprotected anal or vaginal intercourse outside a monogamous relationship (Schuerman, 1994).

Heterosexual transmission should not be overlooked. A case was reported in which an 88-year-old woman contracted HIV from her husband (Schuerman, 1994). Wallace and colleagues (1993) pointed out that elderly women might be at a higher risk for acquiring HIV from an infected partner than elderly men are.

Perhaps the biggest problem with AIDS in elders is making the diagnosis. The presentation of AIDS in this age-group can often be misleading (Weiler, 1989). In one case reported in the literature an 89-year-old man presented with easy bruisability and was found to have a low platelet count. The patient was treated with steroids, and the platelet count returned to normal. Later he traveled outside the United States and developed diarrheal illness that forced him to seek medical attention. It was the country's policy for medical treatment to include HIV testing; the patient tested positive. The patient's history revealed a blood transfusion in 1983, with no other risk

factors (Weiler, 1989). In another case a 73-year-old bachelor was admitted for confusion and falls. He suffered a cardiac arrest and died a week later before any diagnosis was made. Later it was discovered that he was a homosexual and had tested positive for HIV several days before admission (Schuerman, 1994).

Elderly patients with HIV might deteriorate more rapidly than younger persons with HIV. Shorter survival time might be due to delayed diagnosis. The five most common opportunistic infections in older HIV infected patients are *Mycobacterium tuberculosis* (TB), *Mycobacterium avium* complex (MAC), *Pneumocystis carinii* pneumonia (PCP), herpes zoster, and cytomegalovirus (CMV) (Wallace et al., 1993).

Elderly patients often exhibit nonspecific symptoms that are not readily attributed to HIV infection. Fatigue, anorexia, weight loss, and dementia might not be looked on as symptoms of AIDS, since they occur in many of the chronic illnesses that plague older adults.

Among HIV infected individuals there is an 8% to 10% risk per year of developing active tuberculosis disease if previously infected. For the non–HIV infected there is a 10% risk over the lifetime. Extrapulmonary TB is seen frequently in the HIV infected adult.

MAC is a common complication in patients with advanced HIV infection. MAC causes disseminated disease in up to 40% of patients with HIV. In a study conducted by Chaisson, McCutchin, and Young (1993), MAC disease developed within 1 year in approximately 8% of patients with CD4 cell counts below 100/mm^3 at baseline but in virtually no patients with counts above this level. Patients typically present with slowly progressive constitutional symptoms, including fever, night sweats, fatigue, anemia, and weight loss. Abdominal pain and nausea can be linked to abdominal adenopathy.

PCP was the most common life-threatening opportunistic infection during the first decade of HIV. Now that highly successful prophylaxis is available, it is seen primarily in untreated or poorly controlled cases. Among patients who do not receive prophylaxis, approximately 80% subsequently develop PCP (Masur, 1992). Patients who develop PCP almost always have a CD4 count <200 cells/mm^3, and in most the CD4 count is <100 cells/mm^3 (Wallace et al., 1993). Patients typically have a progression of symptoms associated with PCP, such as fever, fatigue, and weight loss. A dry cough and dyspnea on exertion can be predominate and become persistent later in the process. A rapid progression of these symptoms can occur in older adults (Wallace et al., 1993). Cotrimoxazole is the drug of choice for primary prophylaxis and for lifelong maintenance therapy in patients who have recovered from PCP (Schneider, Borleffs, Stolk, Jaspers, & Hoepelman, 1999).

Among homosexual men those who are HIV positive develop herpes zoster 15 times more frequently than in age-matched HIV-negative controls (Wallace et al., 1993); thus elderly HIV positive patients should be expected to have a high occurrence of zoster (Wallace et al., 1993). Zoster is not a predictor of the development of AIDS. Elderly patients are more prone to reactivation of zoster, but in the HIV infected patient the healing time can be prolonged and recurrent outbreaks are more common. Dissemination of zoster, defined as 20 or more lesions outside a dermatome, may be pronounced in the HIV infected patient.

CMV most typically presents in the HIV positive person as CMV retinitis. CMV retinitis is a sign of systemic CMV infection and signifies profound immune compromise and poor prognosis for vision and survival. It is estimated that CMV retinitis occurs in 15% to 40% of patients with AIDS. It is frequently bilateral and if left untreated will often lead to blindness. Floaters and a decrease in the visual acuity, along with a decrease in peripheral vision, may occur.

AIDS in elders is now being called the "great imitator." It is often mistaken for other chronic illnesses. Most often AIDS presents in a form of dementia that is sometimes confused with Alzheimer's disease (Sabin, 1987). Many clinicians fail to recognize AIDS as a possibility. Neurologic dysfunction occurs in approximately 60% of patients with AIDS and may be the initial manifestation of HIV infection in elders (Wallace et al., 1993).

The following features of HIV related dementia help to distinguish it from Alzheimer's disease:

- AIDS dementia complex is a subcortical dementia characterized by decreased attention and concentration, apathy, social withdrawal (which may be mistaken for depression), and psychomotor retardation (Wallace et al., 1993).
- AIDS related dementia progresses more rapidly (over months) than Alzheimer's disease and is more often associated with peripheral neuropathies, myelopathies, and general physical complaints (mild headache, weight loss, fatigue).
- Unlike Alzheimer's, the cerebrospinal fluid often reveals mildly elevated protein levels (mean 0.62g/L), and approximately 25% of patients will have mononuclear pleocytosis (mean 3×10^6 cells/L).
- HIV associated cognitive abnormalities can improve with antiretroviral therapy, and thus HIV encephalopathy is a reversible (albeit, usually only transiently) cause of dementia (Schmitt et al., 1988).

Other common neurologic processes observed in HIV infected patients include cryptococcal meningitis, toxoplasmosis, and primary brain lymphoma (Ho, Bredesen, Vinters, & Daar, 1989).

Since the initiation of highly active antiretroviral therapy (HAART) for HIV infection, there has been a marked decrease in the incidence of opportunistic infections and an improvement in clinical outcomes for patients. Studies have shown that the routine use of HAART has resulted in declines in morbidity and mortality among HIV infected persons. Although treatment recommendations for the elderly are not any different from those for younger people, consideration must be given to chronic conditions and the medications used to treat them. Such treatments must be considered and weighed against the use of antiretrovirals or other HIV related medications that may be prescribed (Emlet, 1997).

Tuberculosis

TB causes significant morbidity and mortality in elders. In fact, the number of TB cases in the United States is highest for persons in the age-group 65 years and older (CDC, 1990). Persons in this age group were most likely infected 50 to 70 years ago. Their immune system was able to contain the organisms, but now as the function of their immune system declines and they develop chronic diseases, they are at high risk for active disease from reactivation of old infection (Dutt & Stead, 1992).

Persons residing in long-term care facilities are at increased risk of developing active TB. Hutton, Cauthen, and Bloch (1993) found that nursing home residents were 1.8 times more likely to develop active TB than elders living in the community. In addition to the risk of reactivation, the elder may be exposed to active TB from another resident in the facility. TB outbreaks have occurred in several nursing homes.

The best strategy for controlling the transmission of TB is to identify as soon as possible any person who might be infectious, place him on airborne precautions, and initiate effective antituberculosis therapy. Nurses should have a high level of suspicion for active TB in a patient with weight loss and respiratory symptoms; symptoms in this age-group can be very subtle.

Long-term care facilities should have active TB prevention programs because of the high potential their residents have for active disease. One essential component of the program is performing annual tuberculin skin tests (TSTs) for residents and personnel. However, TSTs alone do not prevent transmission. In addition, all persons who convert from a negative to a positive TST should be evaluated for the source of exposure and given prophylaxis. A careful investigation of exposed patients, staff, and visitors should be conducted (Nicolle & Garibaldi, 1995).

Resistant Organisms

Methicillin-Resistant *Staphylococcus Aureus* **(MRSA).** *Staphylococcus aureus* is a gram positive organism found on the skin and in the nares of most people. At any given time 20% to 40% of adults are nasal carriers of *Staphylococcus aureus,* and up to 70% of the population carry *Staphylococcus aureus* in their nose at some time during their lifetimes (Boyce et al., 1994). It is also the single most common agent causing postoperative wound infections. In addition, the elder host can acquire infections such as impetigo, abscesses, folliculitis, septic arthritis, or cellulitis.

Methicillin became available in the early 1960s for treating infections caused by β-lactamase-producing, penicillin-resistant *Staphylococcus aureus.* However, strains resistant to methicillin were soon identified in England and then Europe. It was not until the mid-1970s that MRSA became a significant problem in the United States (Mylotte, 1996). The prevalence of MRSA varies considerably from one locale to another and often varies widely among neighboring hospitals and nursing facilities (Boyce et al., 1994). MRSA is difficult to eradicate, and because elders transfer back and forth between acute care and nursing homes, they are at risk for becoming colonized or infected. Colonization can occur in the nares, respiratory tract, wounds, decubuti, urinary catheters, or other invasive devices. The risks for colonization among elders are many, including chronic underlying illnesses, frequent hospitalizations, long-term antibiotic use, surgical wounds, and exposure to other colonized or infected persons. One common fallacy that exists about MRSA is that it is more virulent than methicillin-sensitive *Staphylo-*

coccus aureus. MRSA is of special concern because it is often multi-drug resistant and because treatment options for infections are often limited.

MRSA is spread from person to person by direct contact. Mupirocin ointment placed in the nares twice a day for five days is a proven method for decolonization. MRSA is difficult to permanently eradicate, and relapses do occur. Treatment for infection is vancomycin intravenously.

Enterococcus. Enterococcus is part of the normal flora of the GI tract. In the past enterococcus was not considered a virulent organism, but over the last several years this organism has gained notoriety. The reason for this change is due to increasing antimicrobial drug resistance. The first reported case of vancomycin-resistant enterococcus (VRE) was reported in England in 1988 (Uttley, Collins, Naidoo, & George, 1988). In the United States the National Nosocomial Infection Surveillance (NNIS) system reported that the incidence of VRE increased from 0.3% of enterococcal isolates in 1989 to 10.4% in 1995 (Gaynes & Edwards, 1996). VRE spread occurs mainly by the hands and on objects that are frequently touched. VRE can live on environmental surfaces for a long period of time. Detection of VRE is accomplished through collection of a rectal swab or stool culture. VRE can cause bloodstream, urinary tract, and wound infections. Immunocompromised persons, including individuals who have had a transplant or received chemotherapy, and persons who have been on antibiotics for a long period of time are more prone to carry VRE. Other persons at risk include those who have spent long periods of time in an intensive care unit. Because this organism is resistant to multiple-antibiotics treatment, options are few if infection results. Currently there is no available therapy to attempt decolonization with VRE. Most patients with VRE will recolonize with normal flora on their own. This can take anywhere from 2 weeks to 1 year and will depend on the health state of the individual.

Long-term care facilities, fearing the spread of resistant microorganisms, sometimes question the infection status of persons being transferred from an acute care setting and want evidence of negative cultures before admitting a patient. Colonization or infection with a resistant organism is not grounds for denial to a long-term care facility. The use of standard precautions in conjunction with contact precautions and thorough hand washing with an antimicrobial soap is necessary to control the spread of resistant organisms. A private room, if available, is preferred for patients with resistant organisms. Cohorting patients with the same resistant organism is also an option. If neither of these options is available, cohorting with a non-colonized person would be another alternative. Care must be taken to ensure that the person is not at high risk for infection (e.g., patient on long-term ventilator care, urinary catheter, immunocompromised). Further information on prevention and control of resistant organisms can be found in the 1995 Hospital Infection Control Practices Advisory Committee recommendations for preventing the spread of vancomycin resistance (HICPAC, 1995) and in "Recommendations From a Minnesota Task Force for the Management of Persons With Methicillin-Resistant *Staphylococcus Aureus*" (Bennett, Thurn, Klicker, Williams, & Weiler, 1992).

Infection Control Programs in Long-Term Care Facilities

In addition to the physical effects of aging, living in an institution further increases the elder's susceptibility to infection. Long-term care facilities' unique characteristics increase the risk of cross infection. The nursing home has a dual role of providing medical care, as well as a place of residence and social activity. Semiclosed environments promote a higher risk of infection with group activities, common washing and dining facilities, and crowding. Personnel go from room to room and patient to patient in the course of patient care activities and may not have adequate time or resources for hand washing. Social activities result in more frequent patient interactions than in the acute hospital setting, thus providing extensive opportunities for direct contact between patients. Furthermore, the ambulatory resident may spread organisms in the environment through coughing, poor personal hygiene, or incontinence. Finally, patients are transferred to and from hospitals frequently, which provides opportunities for the exchange of multiple resistant organisms acquired in these facilities.

The epidemiology of nosocomial infections occurring in long-term care facilities has not been well studied. The available data suggest that these infections are a frequent source of morbidity and sometimes mortality for residents of long-term care facilities. Investigators have described numerous nursing home outbreaks of infections caused by influenza virus, MRSA, rotavirus, TB, *Streptococcus pyogenes*, enterohemorrhagic *Escherichia coli*, and *C. difficile*.

Infection control investigators have reported incidence and prevalence rates of nosocomial infections that range between 2.6 and 6.7 infections per 1000 resident days (Farber, Brennen, Puntereri, & Brody, 1984; Hoffman, Jenkins, & Putney, 1990; Jacobson & Strausbaugh, 1990; Vlahov, Tenney, Cervino, & Shamer, 1987). Nosocomial infection rates in long-term care facilities vary widely depending on the level of care required by the patient population and the adequacy of infection control practices in the institution. Currently, there is not an accurate method to stratify residents in long-term care facilities for their risk of acquiring an infection. In addition to facility and resident differences, investigators have used different methods, surveillance techniques, and definitions in their studies. Consequently, comparing rates between facilities is probably not valid.

Infection control programs, although relatively new, have been instituted in many long-term care facilities to reduce the potential for transmitting organisms in nursing homes. Nicolle and Garibaldi (1995) and Smith and Rusnak (1991) have published infection control recommendations for long-term care facilities. In addition, McGeer et al. (1991) published definitions of nosocomial infections specific for long-term care. If hospital guidelines are used, they should be modified to fit the long-term care environment. The effectiveness of infection control program activities is highly dependent on health care personnel's understanding the principles and goals of the program and making a commitment to follow established patient care practices that will reduce the potential for infection. Orientation and ongoing in services for all health care personnel are essential.

CASE STUDY 1

The nurse determined that Mrs. Jones's baseline temperature was 98° F. The nurse noted on the nursing care plan that a sustained temperature of 100° F would indicate presence of a fever. Mrs. Jones's temperature ranged from 98° F to 98.6° F during her hospitalization.

Since Mrs. Jones's skin was dry, the nurse scheduled her to be bathed twice a week. The nursing staff applied a moisturizing lotion daily and did perineal care daily and after each bowel movement. The nurses also taught Mrs. Jones to shift her weight frequently while she was awake. Mrs. Jones's skin remained intact with no reddened pressure areas.

Because Mrs. Jones had not eaten a balanced diet at home, the nurse requested a nutrition consult. The dietitian helped Mrs. Jones choose a nutritionally balanced diet. The nurse also encouraged Mrs. Jones to drink fluids throughout the day and administered a daily vitamin.

The nursing staff helped Mrs. Jones get out of bed to void, initially on the commode; by the third hospital day Mrs. Jones used her walker to ambulate to the bathroom. Mrs. Jones was able to urinate and did not require a urinary catheter.

To prevent a respiratory tract infection, the nursing staff had Mrs. Jones do mouth care twice a day, get up in the chair to eat and remain sitting for 30 minutes after meals, and increase the distance she walked with a walker each day. The physical activity helped Mrs. Jones sleep at night without sedation.

The nursing interventions were effective, and Mrs. Jones remained free of infection during her 5-day hospitalization.

CASE STUDY 2

The nurse caring for Mr. Becker consulted the infection control team for answers to the questions raised by Mr. Becker and his family. She explained to Mr. Becker and his family that he did not have an infection but was only colonized with VRE. The nurse emphasized the importance of following instructions carefully to avoid contamination and possible infection of his surgical sites.

The nurse also educated Mr. Becker and his family on the following issues:

- Enterococcus is part of the normal flora of the GI tract.
- VRE is spread mainly by the hands and objects that are frequently touched, such as doorknobs, tabletops, and other objects in the environment.
- VRE can cause bloodstream, urinary tract, and wound infections.
- Immunocompromised persons, including individuals who have had a transplant or received chemotherapy, and persons who have been on many antibiotics for a long period of time are more prone to acquire VRE. Also persons who have spent long periods of time in the intensive care unit area are at an increased risk.
- Because the organism is resistant to certain antibiotics, VRE can be difficult to treat if an infection occurs.
- While in the hospital, ambulating outside his room would be permissible if proper precautions were taken, such as washing his hands, gloving, and gowning to decrease the risk of transmission through inanimate objects.
- His family members were not at any increased risk for acquiring VRE.
- Once discharged from the hospital, it will be important for family members to wear gloves if any dressing changes have to be performed and to use antibacterial soap.

The nurse also explained that while he was in the hospital the housekeeping staff would frequently clean his room to decrease the organism load in the room. In the home environment linens and other laundry items could be washed in hot, soapy water. Mr. Becker was concerned about his grandchildren coming to visit. The nurse alleviated those fears by informing him that as long as his grandchildren or other visitors were not immunocompromised or had not had any recent major operations they could visit. He was also concerned about how long he would have the organism. The nurse closed by stating that no one knows for sure. Individuals can carry it for a short period of time or for a very long time. Currently there is no treatment for persons colonized with VRE. Mr. Becker and his family felt more at ease. He was discharged to home without any further complications.

SUMMARY

Aging does not happen suddenly, and, overall, age-related changes are relatively mild and benign. However, age-related changes contribute to a general loss of physiologic reserve that begins after age 30. It is also interesting to note that the average life span of individuals has increased during the time of recorded history, but the maximum life span has not. Prevention of infection in the older adult is to some degree a matter of continuing to ensure a healthy lifestyle. Regular exercise and diet, personal hygiene, and regular medical care are all important factors in preventing infection (Crossley & Peterson, 1996).

REFERENCES

Abrams, G. (1986). Response of the body to immunologic challenge. In S. Anderson & L. M. Wilson (Eds.), *Pathophysiology: Clinical concepts of disease processes* (pp. 54-70). Hightstown, NJ: McGraw-Hill.

Advisory Committee on Immunization Practices. (1989). Pneumococcal polysaccharide vaccine. *Morbidity and Mortality Weekly Report, 38,* 64-67, 73-76.

Advisory Committee on Immunization Practices. (1997). Prevention of pneumococcal disease: recommendations of the Advisory Committee on Immunization Practices (ACIP). *Morbidity and Mortality Weekly Report, 46*(RR-8), 1-24.

Advisory Committee on Immunization Practices. (1999). Prevention and control of influenza: recommendations of the Advisory Committee on Immunization Practices (ACIP). *Morbidity and Mortality Weekly Report, 48*(RR-4), 1-28.

Allman, R. M. (1989). Pressure ulcers among the elderly. *The New England Journal of Medicine, 320,* 850-853.

Bennett, M. E., Thurn, J. R., Klicker, R., Williams, C. O., & Weiler, M. (1992). Recommendations from a Minnesota task force for the management of persons with methicillin-resistant *Staphylococcus aureus*. *American Journal of Infection Control, 20*(1), 42-48.

Bentley, D. W., & Mylotte, J. M. (1991). Epidemiology of respiratory infections in the elderly. In M. S. Niederman (Ed.), *Respiratory infections in the elderly* (pp. 1-23). New York: Raven Press.

Blaylock, B. (1993). The aging immune system and common infections in elderly patients. *Journal of ET Nursing, 20,* 63-67.

Boyce, J. M., Jackson, M. M., Pugliese, G., Batt, M. D., Fleming, D., Garner, J. S., Hartstein, A. I., Kauffman, C. A., Simmons, M., Weinstein, R., O'Boyle-Williams, C., & the AHA Technical Panel on Infections Within Hospitals. (1994). Methicillin-resistant *Staphylococcus aureus* (MRSA): A briefing for acute care hospitals and nursing facilities. *Infection Control Hospital Epidemiology, 15,* 105-115.

Centers for Disease Control and Prevention (1990). Prevention and control of tuberculosis in facilities providing long-term care to the elderly: Recommendations of the Advisory Committee for Elimination of Tuberculosis. *Morbidity and Mortality Weekly Report, 39*(RR-10), 7-20.

Centers for Disease Control and Prevention. (1995). HIV/AIDS surveillance report. *Morbidity and Mortality Weekly Report, 7,* 15.

Chaisson, R., McCutchin, A., & Young, L. (1993). Managing *Mycobacterium avium* complex infection. *AIDS Clinical Care, 5,* 1-8.

Crossley, K. B., & Peterson, P. K. (1996). Infections in the elderly. *Clinical Infectious Disease, 22,* 209-215.

Dutt, A. K., & Stead, W. W. (1992). Tuberculosis. *Clinics in Geriatric Medicine, 8,* 761-775.

El-Sadr, W., & Gettler, J. (1995). Underrecognized human immunodeficiency virus infection in the elderly. *Archives in Internal Medicine, 155,* 184-186.

Emlet, C. A. (1997). HIV/AIDS in the elderly: A hidden population. *Home Care Provider, 2*(2), 69-75.

Esposito, A. L. (1991). Pulmonary host defenses in the elderly. In M. S. Niederman (Ed.), *Respiratory infections in the elderly* (pp. 25-44). New York: Raven Press.

Farber, B. F., Brennen, C., Puntereri, A. J., & Brody, J. P. (1984). A prospective study of nosocomial infections in a chronic care facility. *Journal of the American Geriatrics Society, 32,* 499-502.

Fox, R. (1988). Atypical presentation of geriatric infections. *Geriatrics, 43,* 58-59, 63-64, 68.

Gangarosa, R. E., Glass, R. I., Lew, J. F., & Boring, J. R. (1992). Hospitalization involving gastroenteritis in the United States, 1985: The special burden of the disease among the elderly. *American Journal of Epidemiology, 135,* 281-290.

Gaynes, R., & Edwards, J. (1996). The national nosocomial infection surveillance (NNIS) system. Nosocomial vancomycin resistant enterococci (VRE) in the United States, 1989-1995: The first 1000 isolates. In: The Sixth Annual Meeting of the Society for Healthcare Epidemiology of America; April 1996; Washington, DC. *Infection Control and Hospital Epidemiology;* 17P18 Abstract.

Gross, P. A., Rapuano, C., Adringnolo, A., & Shaw, B. (1983). Nosocomial infections: Decade-specific risk. *Infection Control, 4,* 145-147.

Haddy, R. I. (1988). Aging, infections, and the immune system. *Journal of Family Practice, 27,* 409-413.

Ho, D. D., Bredesen, D. E., Vinters, H. V., & Daar, E. S. (1989). The acquired immunodeficiency syndrome dementia complex. *Annual Review of Internal Medicine, 14,* 608-615.

Hoffman, N., Jenkins, R., & Putney, K. (1990). Nosocomial infection rates during a one-year period in a nursing home care unit of a Veterans Administration hospital. *American Journal of Infection Control, 18,* 55-63.

The Hospital Infection Control Practices Advisory Committee. (1995). Recommendations for preventing the spread of vancomycin resistance: Recommendations of the Hospital Infection Control Practices Advisory Committee. *American Journal of Infection Control, 23,* 87-94.

Hutton, M. D., Cauthen, G. M., & Bloch, A. B. (1993). Results of a 29-state survey of tuberculosis in nursing homes and correctional facilities. *Public Health Reports, 108,* 305-314.

Iowa Intervention Project. J. C. McCloskey & G. M. Bulechek (Eds.). (2000). *Nursing interventions classification (NIC)* (3rd ed.). St. Louis, MO: Mosby.

Iowa Outcomes Project. M. Johnson, M. Maas, & S. Moorhead (Eds.). (2000). *Nursing outcomes classification (NOC)* (2nd ed.). St. Louis, MO: Mosby.

Jacobson, C., & Strausbaugh, L. J. (1990). Incidence and impact of infection in a nursing home care unit. *American Journal of Infection Control, 18,* 151-159.

Joffrion, L. P., & Leuszler, L. B. (1995). The gastrointestinal system and its problems in the elderly, with nutritional considerations. In M. Stanley & P. G. Beare (Eds.), *Gerontological nursing* (pp. 241-254). Philadelphia: F.A. Davis.

Johnson, A. P. (1995). The pulmonary system and its problems in the elderly. In M. Stanley & P. G. Beare (Eds.), *Gerontological nursing* (pp. 201-209). Philadelphia: F.A. Davis.

Keogh, S. V. (1993). *Clostridium difficile*-associated diseases in the long term care facility (LTC): Recognition and management. *Infection Control in Long Term Care Facilities Newsletter, 4,* 2-3.

Kramarow, E., Lentzner, H., Rooks, R., Weeks, J., & Saydah, S. (1999). *Health and aging chartbook: Health, United States 1999.* Hyattsville, MD: National Center for Health Statistics.

Makris, A. T. (1996). Infections in the elderly. In R. N. Olmsted (Ed.), *APIC infection control and applied epidemiology: Principles and practice* (pp. 45-1 to 45-11). St. Louis, MO: Mosby.

Masur, H. (1992). Prevention and treatment of *Pneumocystis carinii* pneumonia. *New England Journal of Medicine, 327,* 1853-1860.

McCormick, W. C., & Wood, R. W. (1992). Clinical decisions in the care of elderly persons with AIDS. *Journal of the American Geriatrics Society, 40*(9), 917-921.

McGeer, A., Campbell, B., Emori, T. G., Hierholzer, W. J., Jackson, M. M., Nicolle, L. E., Peppler, C., Rivera, A., Schollenberger, D. G., Simor, A.E., Smith, P. W., & Wang, E. E. (1991). Definitions of infection for surveillance in long-term care facilities. *American Journal of Infection Control, 19,* 1-7.

Michaels, D. D. (1986). Ocular diseases in the aged. In A. A. Rosenbloom et al. (Eds.), *Vision and aging: General and clinical perspectives.* New York: Professional Press Books Fairchild.

Mylotte, J. M. (1996). *Staphylococcus* species. In R. N. Olmsted (Ed.), *APIC infection control and applied epidemiology: Principles and practice* (pp. 78-1 to 78-12). St. Louis, MO: Mosby.

Nicolle, L. E., & Garibaldi, R. A. (1995). Infection control in long-term-care facilities. *Infection Control and Hospital Epidemiology, 16,* 348-353.

Norman, D. C., & Yoshikawa, T. T. (1996). Fever in the elderly. *Infectious Disease Clinics of North America, 10,* 93-99.

North American Nursing Diagnosis Association. (1999). *Nursing diagnoses: Definitions & classification 1999-2000.* Philadelphia: Author.

Palmer, M. H., & McCormick, K. A. (1991). Alterations in elimination: Urinary incontinence. In E. M. Baines (Ed.), *Perspectives on gerontological nursing* (pp. 339-356). Thousand Oaks, CA: Sage.

Paul, W. (1988). The immune system: Introduction. In J. Wyngaarden & L. Smith (Eds.), *Textbook of medicine* (pp. 1932-1937). Philadelphia: W.B. Saunders.

Pien, F. D. (1996). Ectoparasites. In R. N. Olmsted (Ed.), *APIC infection control and applied epidemiology: Principles and practice* (pp. 55-1 to 55-6). St. Louis, MO: Mosby.

Plewa, M. C. (1990). Altered host response and special infections in the elderly. *Emergency Medicine Clinics in North America, 8,* 193-206.

Rusnak, P. G. (1996). Long-term care. In R. N. Olmsted (Ed.), *APIC infection control and applied epidemiology: Principles and practice* (pp. 17-1 to 17-31). St. Louis, MO: Mosby.

Sabin, T. D. (1987). AIDS: The new "great imitator." *Journal of the American Geriatrics Society, 35,* 467-468.

Schmitt, F. A., Bigley, J. W., McKinnis, R., Logue, P. E., Evans, R. W., & Drucker, J. L. (1988). Neuropsychological outcome of AZT treatment of patients with AIDS and ARC. *New England Journal of Medicine, 319,* 1573-1578.

Schneider, M. M., Borleffs, J. C., Stolk, R.P., Jaspers, C. A., & Hoepelman, A. I. (1999). Discontinuation of prophylaxis for Pneumocystis carinii pneumonia in HIV-1-infected patients treated with highly active antiretroviral therapy. *Lancet, 353*(9148), 201-203.

Schuerman, D. A. (1994). Clinical concerns: AIDS in the elderly. *Journal of Gerontological Nursing, 20,* 11-17.

Scura, K. W., & Whipple, B. (1995). HIV infection and AIDS in the elderly. In M. Stanley & P. G. Beare (Eds.), *Gerontological nursing* (pp. 338-346). Philadelphia: F.A. Davis.

Smith, P., & Rusnak, P. (1991). APIC guideline for infection prevention and control in the long-term care facility. *American Journal of Infection Control, 19,* 198-215.

Smith, P. W. (Ed.). (1984). *Infection control in long-term care facilities.* New York: John Wiley & Sons.

Smith, P. W. (1987). Nursing home-acquired infections. *Infection Control, 81,* 55-57, 62-66.

Stall, R., & Catania, J. (1994). AIDS risk behaviors among late middle-aged and elderly Americans. *Archives of Internal Medicine, 154,* 57-63.

Terpenning, M. S., & Bradley, S. F. (1991). Why aging leads to increased susceptibility to infection. *Geriatrics, 46,* 77-80.

Uttley, A. H., Collins, C. H., Naidoo, J., & George, R. C. (1988). Vancomycin-resistant enterococci. *Lancet, 1,* 57-58.

Vlahov, D., Tenney, J. H., Cervino, K. W., & Shamer, D. K. (1987). Routine surveillance for infections in nursing homes: Experience at two facilities. *American Journal of Infection Control, 15,* 47-53.

Wallace, J. I., Paauw, D. S., & Spach, D. H. (1993). HIV infection in older patients: When to suspect the unexpected. *Geriatrics, 48,* 61-70.

Weiler, P. G. (1989). Why AIDS is becoming a geriatric problem. *Geriatrics, 44,* 81-87.

White, K. E., Hedberg, C. W., Edmondson, L. M., Jones, D. B. W., Osterholm, M. T., & MacDonald, K. L. (1989). An outbreak of giardiasis in a nursing home with evidence for multiple modes of transmission. *Journal of Infectious Disease, 160,* 298-304.

Wiersema, L. A. (1995). The integumentary system and its problems in the elderly. In M. Stanley & P. G. Beare (Eds.), *Gerontological nursing* (pp. 148-160). Philadelphia: F.A. Davis.

CHAPTER 6

IMPAIRED HOME MAINTENANCE MANAGEMENT

Barbara J. Head

This chapter suggests how standardized nursing languages can be used to address the identification, treatment, and evaluation of nursing intervention effectiveness with problems of home maintenance management for elderly clients. The nursing diagnosis Impaired Home Maintenance Management was accepted for clinical testing at the 1978 conference of the North American Nursing Diagnosis Association, and the current NANDA taxonomy (NANDA, 1999) includes Impaired Home Maintenance Management as a problem within the human response pattern of moving. Gordon (1994) lists Impaired Home Maintenance Management as one of 24 diagnostic groupings in the functional health pattern of Activity-Exercise. Functional impairment, specifically impairment in the performance of Instrumental Activities of Daily Living (IADL), also is identified as a (causal) factor related to Impaired Home Maintenance Management.

Impaired Home Maintenance Management is defined by NANDA (1999) as the "inability to independently maintain a safe growth-promoting immediate environment" (p. 93). Defining characteristics are related primarily to the environmental status of the residence or home and include the following: (1) unwashed or unavailable cooking equipment, clothes, or linen; (2) accumulation of dirt, food wastes, or hygienic wastes; (3) overtaxed family members, e.g., exhausted, anxious; (4) repeated hygienic disorders, infestations, or infections; (5) household members expressing difficulty in maintaining their home in a comfortable fashion; (6) household requests for assistance with home maintenance; (7) household members describing outstanding debt or financial crises; (8) disorderly surroundings; (9) offensive odors; (10) inappropriate household temperature; (11) lack of necessary equipment or aids; and (12) presence of vermin or rodents (NANDA, 1999, p. 94). Factors identified by NANDA as related to this problem are as follows: (1) individual/family member disease or injury; (2) insufficient family organization or planning; (3) insufficient finances; (4) unfamiliarity with neighborhood resources; (5) impaired cognitive or emotional functioning; (6) lack of knowledge; (7) lack of role modeling; and (8) inadequate support system (p. 94).

PREVALENCE

An American Association of Retired Persons (AARP, 1990) survey reported that 7 million people age 65 or older and living in the community had difficulty performing one or more home management activities. National Health Interview Survey results for the population 65 and over also support the presence of difficulty with these activities and reveal at least some discrepancy between self-identified need and help received (Dawson, Hendershot, & Fulton, 1987). Heavy work around the house creates difficulty for between a quarter and two thirds of disabled elders at home (AARP, 1990; Agency on Aging, 1990) and is the most frequently reported home management problem. Other activities creating difficulty are shopping, doing light housework, doing yard work and home repairs, preparing meals, managing money, and using the telephone (Dawson et al., 1987; Hereford, Suther, & Seifert, 1990; Seifert & Suther, 1994). Personal security and emergency communications have been suggested as potential household maintenance areas requiring further study (Lawton, 1990). Many individuals fear that their disabilities related to home maintenance will launch a process that ends with their placement in a nursing home (Hereford et al., 1990).

Available studies also provide evidence that community health nurses use diagnoses pertinent to environmental and home maintenance issues. Two studies examining the use of nursing diagnoses in public health nursing agencies found Impaired Home Maintenance Management among the 10 most frequently used diagnoses (Lambert & Jones, 1989; Myers & Stull, 1989). Martin, Scheet, and Stegman (1993) reported that 1% of the nursing problems specified for more than 2400 clients fell within the environmental domain of the Omaha Problem Classification Scheme.

RISK FACTORS

Risk factors for Impaired Home Maintenance Management include disability, low income, and lack of adequate family support. Disability has been defined as a gap between a person's capability and the environment's demand (Verbrugge, 1990). Disability can be measured in terms of difficulty performing without help at least one Instrumental Activity of Daily Living (IADL) or one Activity of Daily Living (ADL). Disability increases with age (over half of those 85 and older report disability) and is higher among elders 65 and older who live alone (25.5%). The most vulnerable groups of people—those 75 years of age and older, those with incomes under $12,000 annually, and widowed persons—are the most likely to want to age in their current homes (AARP, 1990).

The most frequent source of help for older people in the community is the family (Osterkamp & Chapin, 1995). However, there is evidence that families have trouble meeting disabled members' needs. The ratio of working-age adult family members to disabled elders is decreasing, more women are taking jobs outside the home, and kinship structures are becoming more complex. All of these factors create difficulties for a family attempting to meet an elderly member's home maintenance management needs (Cantor, 1989; Fowles, 1991; Osterkamp & Chapin, 1995).

ASSESSMENT

Defining characteristics for Impaired Home Maintenance Management include family member perceptions, environmental characteristics, and family member states (Table 6-1). The Omaha System, developed by Martin and Scheet (1992), includes an environmental problem domain with labels pertinent to nursing assessment: (1) income (moneys from wages, interest, dividends, or other sources available to family for living and health care expenses); (2) sanitation (environmental conditions pertaining to or affecting health with reference to cleanliness, precautions against infection or disease, and promotion of health); (3) residence (place where individual or family lives); and (4) neighborhood or workplace safety (freedom from injury or loss as it relates to the community or place of employment) (Martin & Scheet, 1992). Using the Omaha System, a nurse specifies whether a problem pertains to an individual or involves the family as a whole. Comparison of the defining characteristics of the NANDA diagnosis Impaired Home Maintenance Management with the Omaha System problems of income and sanitation suggests that similar phenomena are involved. Both classifications include the elements of financial resources, environmental hygiene, environmental safety, infection status, and comfort.

NURSING DIAGNOSIS

The language used to identify client problems encountered in nursing practice is important to nurses and to nursing. If a problem or diagnostic concept is not named, accepted, and used consistently in nursing practice and research, the contribution of nursing to the resolution of the problem is difficult to evaluate. Impaired Home Mainte-

nance Management is a proposed standardized diagnostic label for which conceptual clarity has not been fully achieved.

As it has been accepted for testing by NANDA, Impaired Home Maintenance Management is a multifaceted diagnosis with numerous elements: (1) individual physical functional performance; (2) family functional performance; (3) environmental safety; (4) environmental hygiene; and (5) human growth and development. Neither diagnostic usefulness nor responsiveness of this complex diagnosis to nursing intervention has been adequately explored through research.

Nursing textbook authors consistently include NANDA concepts in their coverage of Impaired Home Maintenance Management but disagree about whether other concepts might be appropriate beyond the NANDA definition (Carpentino, 1995; McFarland & McFarlane, 1993; Sparks & Taylor, 1993; Thompson, McFarland, Hirsch, & Tucker, 1997). Is caregiver stress a defining characteristic? Is the diagnosis appropriate for impaired management of the overall home health care plan? Is the absence of structural adaptation of the home an aspect of the problem? Are adaptive devices and equipment elements of home maintenance management? When nurses are not certain of the answers to these questions, the diagnosis cannot be used in a standardized way.

Although use of the diagnosis Impaired Home Maintenance Management has not been widely reported, nurses use the term *home maintenance* or one of its variants to refer to other phenomena that interest nursing. One commonly used expression is "maintenance at home" in reference to the goal of a family, formal care provider, or other intervener to keep or "maintain" the client in the home setting. Many home care agencies purport that they allow the client to remain living in her own residence despite age or health-related difficulties. Although maintenance at home seems to be a clear, cost-efficient, and worthy aim of community nursing care, Sorgen (1986) found the concept difficult to measure as an outcome of home health care. Helberg (1993) used client dependency status for successful maintenance at home, measured at discharge from home care according to the following ratings: (1) independent (e.g., could manage alone even though family and friends were available); (2) assistance of family and/or friends required to maintain patient at home; (3) assistance of community resources required to maintain patient at home; (4) assistance of family members and community resources required to maintain patient at home; (5) institutionalized; and (6) deceased.

Marek (1989) suggested that home maintenance refers to a category of outcomes related to functioning of the family in the home environment of the client. She identified issues in this domain as family living patterns, environment, support, and roles and included caregiver strain as an important measure in the area. Marek's use appears consistent with the present NANDA diagnosis Impaired

Suggested Nursing-Sensitive Outcomes Table 6-1 IMPAIRED HOME MAINTENANCE MANAGEMENT	
Nursing Diagnosis	**Nursing-Sensitive Outcomes**
IMPAIRED HOME MAINTENANCE MANAGEMENT **Defining Characteristics** Unwashed or unavailable cooking equipment, clothes, or linen Accumulation of dirt, food wastes, or hygienic wastes Offensive odors Presence of vermin or rodents Disorderly surroundings Lack of necessary equipment or aids Presence of safety hazards (definition implies) Household members express difficulty in maintaining home in a comfortable fashion Household requests assistance with home maintenance	
	SELF-CARE: INSTRUMENTAL ACTIVITIES OF DAILY LIVING (IADL) **Indicators** Performs housework Does own laundry Shops for household needs Shops for groceries Shops for clothing Prepares meals Serves meals Uses telephone Handles written communication Opens containers Performs household repairs Does yard work Travels on public transportation Drives own car Manages medication **SAFETY BEHAVIOR: HOME PHYSICAL ENVIRONMENT** **SANITATION BEHAVIOR: HOME PHYSICAL ENVIRONMENT** **Indicators** Cleaning of dishes and utensils Cleaning of food surfaces General cleaning of home
Household members describe debts, financial crises	**SELF-CARE: INSTRUMENTAL ACTIVITIES OF DAILY LIVING (IADL)** **Indicators** Manages money Manages business affairs
Overtaxed family members (e.g., exhausted, anxious)	**COPING** **Indicators** Verbalizes sense of control Verbalizes acceptance of situation Modifies lifestyle as needed Uses available social supports Reports decrease in negative feelings Reports increase in psychologic comfort **ROLE PERFORMANCE** **Indicators** Description of behavioral changes with elderly dependents Reported strategies for role change(s) Reported comfort with role expectation
Repeated hygienic disorders, infestations, or infections	**INFECTION STATUS** **Indicators** Pain/tenderness Induration

Home Maintenance Management but raises the issue of whether the caregiver's condition or state is an aspect of this phenomenon. Whereas "overtaxed family members (e.g., exhausted, anxious)" is a major defining characteristic of the NANDA diagnosis Impaired Home Maintenance Management, Carpentino (1995) has suggested that caregiver strain be conceptualized not as a defining characteristic but rather as either an etiology or a separate coexisting problem. This is but one example of the uncertainty with which nursing views the diagnosis and its defining characteristics.

The inclusion of family member perceptions and states as defining characteristics of Impaired Home Maintenance Management suggests that the family is sometimes the unit of analysis for this diagnosis. Problems encountered in a community setting are frequently not amenable to resolution outside the context of the family or household. About 50% of the elderly in the community live alone, but the other half live in family-type situations. The perceptions of family members concerning their ability to manage the physical maintenance of their home are important in assessing family roles and relationships. For example, the physical environment might be spotless, although the single family member responsible for housecleaning, dishes, laundry, and other tasks experiences considerable stress, even to the point of harming her health. Unfortunately, the state of the art with respect to the development of a standardized, comprehensive nursing language and the measurement of nursing diagnoses and nursing-sensitive outcomes makes the analysis of family and environmental states imprecise. Based on current knowledge, the use of individual client–level diagnoses and outcomes might be most useful. Clear and precise descriptions of individual client problems and defining characteristics (signs and symptoms) are likely to best document problems and measurable outcomes influenced by nursing intervention. See Table 6-1, which illustrates the two levels of analysis of the diagnosis Impaired Home Maintenance Management (individual and environmental) and the difficulty of matching the diagnosis with individual-level *Nursing Outcomes Classification* (NOC) outcomes for use in practice and research.

The NANDA diagnosis Impaired Home Maintenance Management has been criticized for being too inclusive. However, the diagnosis also limits the potential scope of nursing concern with respect to ADL. The diagnosis includes only a few activities that are commonly identified as IADL, and these activities are not included elsewhere in the NANDA taxonomy. IADL, considered by many experts to be the activities needed for an individual to live in the home or the community, are use of the telephone, shopping, food preparation, housekeeping, laundry, public transportation, taking medications, and handling of finances (Lawton, 1972; Lawton & Brody, 1969).

Rinke (1988) suggests that the functional perspective is particularly useful in community health nursing because of its similar philosophic tradition emphasizing the teaching of clients to maintain and promote their own health. She stresses that, from a practical perspective, functional status categories are understood across health care disciplines and understandable to consumers. Helberg (1993) used a multidisciplinary tool—the Older American Resources Survey (Pfeiffer, 1975)—to evaluate home health care client functional status, including ADL and IADL scales. She found that both ADL and IADL were significantly related to the likelihood of a client's being independent at discharge and being able to avoid institutionalization. Expansion of the definition and defining characteristics for Impaired Home Maintenance Management would enable nursing to describe its practice in relation to multidisciplinary problems and to employ established measurement tools for research and clinical practice.

To summarize, the present NANDA diagnosis includes selected IADL and extends beyond individual perceptions and states to environmental conditions. In future revisions of NANDA consideration should be given to whether an individual-level nursing diagnosis such as "Impaired Instrumental Activities of Daily Living (IADL)," defined as the inability of a person to perform activities necessary to function in the person's home or community, might be a cleaner, more precise problem concept. A label such as this would build on the classic definition of IADL (Lawton & Brody, 1969) rather than create a new name for a familiar concept and would correspond with the similar NOC outcome. NANDA should also focus attention on whether the diagnosis reflects (1) the assistance an individual requires to accomplish instrumental activities or (2) the performance of the instrumental activity. Reuben (1995) suggests that traditional scales that focus on the amount of assistance needed are most useful for economic analysis. For nursing, a human enterprise, the performance of the instrumental activities might well be more salient.

NURSING-SENSITIVE OUTCOMES

Table 6-2 lists NOC outcomes and indicators appropriate for the three diagnostic components of Impaired Home Maintenance Management: impaired environmental sanitation, impaired home safety, and impaired comfort of family members. This table also illustrates how the impaired environmental sanitation component might require somewhat different outcomes for evaluating progress of individual patient IADL performance and for evaluating progress in obtaining supplemental assistance.

CASE STUDY

D. and I. Long, a couple age 75 and 76, live with their 22-year-old nephew in a run down, rented frame home located in an inner city neighborhood. Their street is

Table 6-2	Selected Problem Components and Related Outcomes IMPAIRED HOME MAINTENANCE MANAGEMENT	
Outcomes Related to Identified Client Performing IADL to Improve Sanitation		**Outcomes Related to Supplemental Help With IADL to Improve Sanitation**

PROBLEM COMPONENT: IMPAIRED ENVIRONMENTAL SANITATION

SELF-CARE: INSTRUMENTAL ACTIVITIES OF DAILY LIVING (IADL) Performs housework Does own laundry Shops for household needs	**KNOWLEDGE: HEALTH RESOURCES** Description of community resources available for assistance Description of how to connect with needed services
ROLE PERFORMANCE Reported strategies for role change(s) Reported comfort with role expectation Ability to meet role expectations	**ROLE PERFORMANCE** Description of behavioral changes with elderly dependents Reported strategies for role change(s) Reported comfort with role expectation Ability to meet role expectations **SOCIAL SUPPORT** Reports of labor provided by others Reports of persons who can help when needed Reports of willingness to call on others for help Reports of help offered by others
KNOWLEDGE: ENERGY CONSERVATION Description of conditions that increase energy expenditure Description of conditions that decrease energy expenditure Performance of methods to conserve energy Performance of proper body mechanics Performance of work simplification techniques	**KNOWLEDGE: ENERGY CONSERVATION** Description of conditions that increase energy expenditure Description of conditions that decrease energy expenditure Performance of methods to conserve energy Performance of proper body mechanics Performance of work simplification techniques
ENERGY CONSERVATION Balances activity and rest Recognizes energy limitations Uses energy conservation techniques Adapts lifestyle to energy level Maintains adequate nutrition Endurance level adequate for activity	**ENERGY CONSERVATION** Balances activity and rest Recognizes energy limitations Uses energy conservation techniques Adapts lifestyle to energy level Maintains adequate nutrition Endurance level adequate for activity

PROBLEM COMPONENT: IMPAIRED HOME SAFETY

KNOWLEDGE: PERSONAL SAFETY
Description of measures to prevent falls
Description of measures to reduce risk of accidental injury
Description of home safety measures
Description of emergency procedures
Description of age-specific safety risks
Description of personal high-risk behaviors

SAFETY BEHAVIOR: HOME PHYSICAL ENVIRONMENT
All indicators
Additional indicators:

- Cleaning of dishes and utensils
- Cleaning of food surfaces
- General cleaning of home environment

PROBLEM COMPONENT: IMPAIRED COMFORT OF FAMILY MEMBERS

COMFORT LEVEL
Expressed contentment with physical surroundings
Reported satisfaction with level of independence

heavily traveled, and the front door is separated from passing traffic by a narrow sidewalk. The three wobbly, stacked cinder blocks that serve as "stairs" leading up to the house end 12 inches below the porch floor. Hundreds of schoolboys attend the local Boys' Club across the street each afternoon.

Mrs. Long is a friendly woman, talkative and eager to please. She suffers from multiple physical problems, including insulin-dependent diabetes and impaired physical mobility. She moves slowly with a walker throughout the first floor of the house and spends most of her time on the living room couch watching TV and monitoring visitors who enter by the front door.

Mr. Long, a tall, frail-looking, serious man, has long-term problems with arthritis, hypertension, and depression. Until his retirement, forced by disability 20 years ago, Mr. Long worked as a wood craftsman for a local manufacturer. He is now inactive, walks with a shuffling gait, and sleeps most of each afternoon. If awake, he stares quietly out the front window while sitting on a straight-backed chair. Mrs. Long complains that he occasionally leaves her to go "down the street" and comes back intoxicated. She is concerned about his safety on these occasions.

Nate, Mrs. Long's nephew, has lived with the Longs since his discharge from the Army last year. Although in good physical health, he is often home during the day and has had trouble finding a job. He stays with the Longs for financial reasons and plans to rent his own apartment when he gets a job. Nate arranges medical appointments and taxi service and accompanies the Longs to their health care visits at a large outpatient medical clinic across town. He feels discouraged about his life and often spends afternoons drinking at the Long home with Mr. Long and his friends.

The furnishings in the home are sparse and dilapidated. Wallpaper is peeling and dirty, and the wooden floor is often covered with visible dirt. The home has running water but no laundry facilities. Dirty dishes are stacked in the kitchen for several days at a time, awaiting the attention of a family friend, C. Dole. Mr. Dole and Mrs. Long were hospitalized on the same floor 2 years ago. Recognizing her need for help, Mr. Dole contacted Mrs. Long after discharge and began riding the bus across town to help with household tasks. Mrs. Long expresses discomfort and embarrassment about the family's environment, especially the cockroaches on walls and other surfaces.

The family's income consists of Social Security disability, which must cover rent, food, treatment supplies, and other expenses. Mrs. Long handles the household finances. She gives Nate a small allowance because "a young man got to have a little for his pocket" and pays Mr. Dole's daily bus fare when she can. She pays the rent regularly, but the nutritional quality of the food is often questionable. Mrs. Long reuses insulin syringes to save money and often lacks alcohol and cotton to clean her skin. Large, golf ball–sized necrotic areas are present at insulin injection sites on Mrs. Long's abdomen and legs.

Mr. Dole is very concerned about what will happen to Mr. and Mrs. Long when he is unable to continue helping with housework. He is uncomfortable with his responsibility as the Longs' only resource. At 85 his health is better than that of his younger friends, but he expresses fatigue and wonders how long he can "hold out." At times he is unable to make the bus trip because of illness or other commitments. Household tasks are not completed in his absence, and he complains of feeling overwhelmed if he misses a day. He is critical of Nate, who gives little household help in exchange for the Longs' support. The Longs' health insurance is limited to Medicare, which covered homemaker services only briefly following Mrs. Long's hospitalization last year.

Impaired Home Maintenance Management is one of several diagnoses identified by the nurse. Defining characteristics include environmental conditions, the overtaxed condition of the family friend, and the family's strained budget and unmet medical supply needs. Lack of supplies resulting in the reuse of insulin syringes suggests the presence of a second major problem, Ineffective Management of Therapeutic Regimen, for Mrs. Long. Family members also have physical and emotional challenges, in addition to home maintenance issues.

The NOC (Iowa Outcomes Project, 2000) outcomes most useful for measuring nursing impact on the NANDA diagnosis Impaired Home Maintenance Management are Self-Care: Instrumental Activities of Daily Living (IADL); Safety Behavior: Home Physical Environment; Coping; Role Performance; and Infection Status (see Table 6-1).

The NOC (Iowa Outcomes Project, 2000) outcomes that are most relevant for estimating the impact of nursing intervention to resolve home sanitation and home safety concerns are Self-Care: Instrumental Activities of Daily Living (IADL), which is the "ability to perform activities needed to function in the home or community" (Iowa Outcomes Project, 2000, p. 385); Role Performance, defined as "congruence of an individual's role behavior with role expectations" (p. 370); Knowledge: Energy Conservation, which is the "extent of understanding conveyed about energy conservation techniques" (p. 264); Knowledge: Health Resources, which shows the "extent of understanding conveyed about health care resources" (p. 271); Social Support, which is the "perceived availability and actual provision of reliable assistance from other persons" (p. 406); Knowledge: Personal Safety, which is the "extent of understanding conveyed about preventing unintentional injuries" (p. 281); Safety Behavior: Home Physical Environment, which is defined as the "individual or caregiver actions to minimize environmental factors that might cause physical harm or injury in the home" (p. 373); and Comfort Level, which is the "extent of physical and psychologic ease" (p. 173) (see Table 6-2).

CASE STUDY

The Self-Care: Instrumental Activities of Daily Living (IADL) outcome includes indicators to address the major areas in which change is desired in the Longs' situation:

housework, laundry, medication management, household shopping, and money management. Indicators for these NOC outcomes allow for measurement of client progress using the scale: 1 = dependent, does not participate; 2 = requires assistive person & device; 3 = requires assistive person; 4 = independent with assistive device; and 5 = completely independent (Iowa Outcomes Project, 2000, p. 385). The indicators are specific self-care activities, such as performs housework, does own laundry, and manages medications.

The difficulty in using this scale to estimate Mr. and Mrs. Long's progress is that for them dependency is a given. They do what they are physically able to do but lack adequate assistance with household tasks. To make the outcome more useful for chronically disabled clients, the outcome and the scale would have to be modified. An individual-level outcome concept more useful for these clients than self-care would be IADL Performance, defined as "ability to perform, with or without assistance, activities needed to function in the community." Alternatively, a new outcome, IADL Performance: Assisted (the ability to perform with assistance the activities needed to function in the community) could be developed. The scale for this outcome concept might be changed to measure the frequency with which the performance outcome and indicators are achieved, e.g., 1 = never, 5 = consistently. An additional modification might involve defining the outcome as a family-level concept so that progress involv-

ing instrumental activities by any part of the family system would indicate client progress.

Appropriate timing of the outcome measurements for the Long family should also be carefully considered. The patterns contributing to the current problem did not develop overnight, and most solutions will be long range. Suggested timing for the measurement of home maintenance–related outcomes is sometime during the initial month of service (baseline) and every 3 months until either satisfactory status is achieved or further progress is judged unlikely and the problem is no longer an active nursing diagnosis.

NURSING INTERVENTIONS

As noted previously, the amenability of the diagnosis Impaired Home Maintenance Management to nursing intervention has not been studied. Suggested nursing interventions selected from the *Nursing Interventions Classification (NIC)* (Iowa Intervention Project, 2000) with related NOC outcomes appear in Table 6-3. Intervention selections are based on related factors for the current NANDA Impaired Home Maintenance Management diagnosis. Nursing intervention effectiveness studies are needed to guide clinical practice. This type of nursing research will

Table 6-3	Selected Interventions to Achieve Outcomes IMPAIRED HOME MAINTENANCE MANAGEMENT	
Outcomes	**Interventions**
Self-Care: Instrumental Activities of Daily Living (IADL)	Home Maintenance Assistance
	Anticipatory Guidance
	Teaching: Individual
Role Performance	Role Enhancement
	Family Involvement Promotion
	Family Mobilization
	Family Therapy
Knowledge: Energy Conservation	Teaching: Individual
	Teaching: Group
Energy Conservation	Teaching: Individual
	Teaching: Group
Knowledge: Health Resources	Referral
	Advocacy
	Insurance Negotiation
	Health Policy Monitoring
	Teaching: Individual
	Teaching: Group
	Referral
Social Support	Support System Enhancement
Knowledge: Personal Safety	Teaching: Individual
	Teaching: Group
Safety Behavior: Home Physical Environment	Teaching: Individual
	Teaching: Group
	Surveillance: Safety
Comfort Level	Interventions listed above

become less difficult and more meaningful when standardized languages are used to describe the phenomena of client problem, nursing intervention, and client outcome.

The most obvious NIC intervention for the NANDA diagnosis Impaired Home Maintenance Management is Home Maintenance Assistance, defined by NIC as "helping the patient/family to maintain the home as a clean, safe, pleasant place to live" (Iowa Intervention Project, 2000, p. 378). The intervention offers several suggestions concerning nursing activities with problems of home maintenance, but like the diagnosis it is complex.

Although the intervention Home Maintenance Assistance is quite general, it provides an overview of activities that can guide nurses to more discrete interventions and activities. Nursing activities for the standardized Home Maintenance Assistance intervention include (1) determining a patient's home maintenance requirements; (2) providing information on how to make a home environment safe and clean; (3) assisting with hygiene; (4) assisting with finances or referring for financial assistance; (5) advising family members about realistic expectations for their roles; and (6) identifying and assisting the family to obtain outside help, including use of its existing social support network (Iowa Intervention Project, 2000, p. 378). Specific areas in which the family might benefit from help to improve home maintenance are suggested, such as pest control, home repair, homemaker assistance, and respite care.

The NIC intervention Home Maintenance Assistance does not include nursing activities pertinent to homemaker service beyond "order homemaker services, as appropriate." Nurses working in many community settings may use the NIC interventions Delegation and Staff Supervision in working with homemaker staff. Homemaking may be provided as a supplemental service in the absence of family help or to provide responsible family members with a needed break. Homemakers often provide service under the nursing plan for rehabilitation or prevention of further client disability. The nurse ensures that homemaker help provides the specific assistance needed while not reducing valued independence for the older person.

When the nursing problem is related to impaired IADL functioning of an individual or family member, nursing interventions may focus on (1) assistance to the individual or family toward realistic planning to meet household responsibilities in anticipation of a member's disability with resultant role and responsibility change or (2) assistance when the home has already deteriorated and the family must adapt to new circumstances. Families with members who have compromised cognitive or emotional function might benefit from similar assistance. Nurse counseling and guidance in anticipation of a family member's disability—a situational crisis—is the NIC intervention Anticipatory Guidance. Although activities included in the intervention are mainly directed toward the "patient," family and significant others should be involved as appropriate.

When the older person lives with family, the nurse can help prepare either an individual client or a family for change.

Interventions appropriate when there has been insufficient family organization or planning for an elder's disability might involve family living near the older disabled member(s) or, as is becoming increasingly common, a family distant geographically. Possible nursing interventions include Family Mobilization, Role Enhancement, and Family Therapy. Each of these interventions is unique, although some are similar and some of the nursing activities may overlap. Family Mobilization is defined as the "utilization of family strengths to influence patient's health in a positive direction" (Iowa Intervention Project, 2000, p. 332). This intervention would be appropriate for families demonstrating good family relationships who are willing and able to become engaged in home maintenance assistance. Role Enhancement is "assisting a patient, significant other, and/or family to improve relationships by clarifying and supplementing specific role behaviors" (Iowa Intervention Project, 2000, p. 569). Difficulty in acceptance of an elderly parent's dependency and role changes might impede the assistance of adult children who have known their parents as vibrant, energetic, and independent people more likely to give help to others than to need help themselves. Nursing activities are aimed at facilitating more appropriate roles. For many years in public health nursing Family Mobilization and Role Enhancement were thought of as interventions in the broad category known as Health Teaching, Guidance, and Counseling and used in the Omaha System Intervention Scheme (Martin & Scheet, 1992). These interventions often are directed at the family as a unit rather than at the individual client.

Counseling is a more encompassing NIC intervention that refers to the "use of an interactive helping process focusing on the needs, problems, or feelings of the patient and significant others to enhance or support coping, problem-solving, and interpersonal relationships" (Iowa Intervention Project, 2000, p. 238). This intervention focuses primarily on assistance to the ill or disabled person ("patient") rather than on the family group. Family Therapy, an intervention most often associated with an advanced nursing practice role, is "assisting family members to move their family toward a more productive way of living" (Iowa Intervention Project, 2000, p. 339). This nursing intervention might be appropriate when family relationships are severely impaired, for example, when neglect of the older person has become an issue and requires extensive and in-depth reconstruction.

The problems of impaired home sanitation and safety are sometimes related to the individual's or family's lack of knowledge, unfamiliarity with existing resources, or lack of social support. Older people are commonly knowledgeable concerning basic home hygiene, although their sex-role preparation might result in lack of knowledge about specific tasks and techniques (Seifert & Suther, 1994).

The United States Consumer Products Safety Commission (1996) has targeted home safety as an area for education of older U.S. citizens based on high rates of accidents in the home. In the areas of home repair and yard upkeep, one home care agency identified lack of knowledge caused by role rigidity, for example, widows who did not know how to use a hammer or change storm windows, as a common reason for expressed home maintenance assistance needs (Seifert & Suther, 1994). For housecleaning and laundry widowers are often baffled by tasks assumed for decades by the female spouse. The intervention Teaching: Individual can be used to identify knowledge gaps and facilitate learning of household maintenance tasks.

When problems of home safety and sanitation are related to the client's or family's unfamiliarity with community resources, the most likely nursing intervention is Referral. The nurse provides information and assists the individual or family to make contact with a resource providing acceptable, affordable help. In these areas of home maintenance the nurse may find that resources are either not available or not financially accessible to meet client (individual, family, or community) needs. Health Policy Monitoring and a modification of Insurance Authorization, Insurance Negotiation, are appropriate interventions in this situation. Health Policy Monitoring involves nursing activities directed at resolving the shortage of affordable resources. Insurance Negotiation involves the nurse's acting as an advocate for the client to present a case to the client's insurer (or other potential payer) demonstrating the benefits and cost-effectiveness of home maintenance assistance coverage.

Insufficient finances are a related factor encountered regularly with long-term care of elderly clients at home. In some areas the Area Agency on Aging offers services or subsidization of services that provide help with home maintenance. State funds also might assist.

The lack of affordable home maintenance programs for community elders stimulated a project funded by the Robert Wood Johnson Foundation to explore how these programs could be organized efficiently (Hereford et al., 1990), and volunteer services have been developed in some locations (Osterkamp & Chapin, 1995). The cost of services in relation to what elders felt they could reasonably pay was an issue for this project, as was acceptability of assistance to elderly clients. The agency learned, for example, that because of trust and security concerns having a single person visit the home to complete multiple maintenance tasks—handyman, lawn care, and chore services—was more acceptable to elders than sending separate individuals (Seifert & Suther, 1994).

Homemaker service might be covered for a limited time based on a client's eligibility for Medicare home health care benefits. Social concerns about health care costs and related Medicare expenditures have hampered the expansion of coverage of home health and homemaker services.

In the absence of affordable formal service providers the nurse works to identify and help the client develop resources of informal support. As mentioned above, volunteer services are available in some areas. Occasionally the nurse is able to "broker" an innovative arrangement such as bartering of room and board in the older person's home in exchange for help with cleaning, laundry, or other services.

CASE STUDY

Mrs. Long and her husband were physically and emotionally unable to perform many IADL independently, and they lacked a satisfactory means of getting help. Mrs. Long's elderly friend was attempting to hold the household together, but his endurance was wavering. Mrs. Long was open to suggestions but had not pursued any options on her own.

The major concern identified by Mrs. Long was housecleaning. She wanted a clean home, but neither she nor Mr. Long was physically able to perform the tasks. Nate was physically able and did help with minor cleaning duties when Mrs. Long asked, but his skills were limited and the family culture and values did not support a young male's assuming responsibility for household work. He was often away from home and hoped to be employed soon.

Mrs. Long was able to prepare simple meals, although she could not stand long enough to do the dishes, and Nate did not mind grocery shopping if she gave him a list. He was reluctant to go to the laundromat but had a girlfriend who might be willing to help out.

The Longs had benefited from homemaker services from the local visiting nurse association following Mrs. Long's hospitalization the previous year, but Medicare covered this service for only a short time. Their Social Security disability income was high enough to disqualify them from the social service programs offering the long-term household assistance they needed.

Calls to explore other community resources determined that neither the county homemaker program nor the Area Agency on Aging was able to help. Paid housecleaning help was one alternative to overtaxing Mr. Dole, but Mrs. Long's assessment of the family finances was that there was absolutely no way to pay. The county health department environmental health unit's insect extermination service was available free of charge, but cockroach infestation would return unless the family could improve its household sanitation.

Meals on Wheels was available in the community and would deliver a noon meal and evening snack for Mr. and Mrs. Long. Mrs. Long resisted this alternative because it did not provide her nephew with meals. The nurse recognized that the Longs' problem would not be resolved through a simple telephone referral.

The nurse discussed with Mr. and Mrs. Long three options for their consideration: (1) reducing their financial support for Nate to allow them to purchase housecleaning; (2) negotiating with Nate to provide housecleaning in exchange for their support; and (3) contacting the Boys' Club to explore some type of an exchange

Table 6-4	The Long Family's Ratings Over Time on the Outcome IADL: Assisted			
	Baseline	3 Months	6 Months	1 Year
Indicators				
Housework	2	2	3	4
Laundry	2	3	3	4
Medication management	2	2	3	3
Money management	2	2	2	3

Scale: 1 = Never; 5 = Consistently.

between the Longs and one or two of the boys. The Longs did not find any of these suggestions acceptable because they did not want to confront Nate and were fearful of having young people they did not know in their home. Consequently the nurse arranged a time with Nate and Mr. Dole for a "family meeting" to discuss how to proceed. After several reschedulings because of Mr. Dole's or Nate's being unavailable, the family finally convened with the nurse as facilitator for a problem-solving session.

This family, although somewhat dysfunctional, had strengths on which the nurse could build. They had resources, and family members shared a common goal, that of Mr. and Mrs. Long's being able to live in their own home. The nurse acted as advocate for Mrs. Long to help her articulate to the family her concerns. The nursing interventions Role Enhancement and Family Mobilization were used to assist the family to articulate to one another their expectations and needs with regard to housecleaning and other activities. Nate had been aware of the old couple's inability to handle things as they had previously but was unaware that his aunt was dissatisfied with household cleanliness. He indicated a willingness to lend a hand in cleaning activities. Nate had been under the impression that Mrs. Long preferred Mr. Dole's help with daily activities because it offered her a chance for socialization. He was unaware of the difficulties Mr. Dole had expressed. He was receptive to becoming more involved in specific activities but asked Mrs. Long and Mr. Dole to be patient because he had a lot to learn. The family discussed activities that were most strenuous for Mr. Dole and planned for Nate to assume these first. Mr. Dole wanted to continue helping 2 or 3 times a week and offered to keep up with some of the less taxing household tasks. The nurse provided information to both men about techniques to conserve energy while accomplishing their daily tasks. Mr. and Mrs. Long were unable to adjust their activity levels but resolved to continue supporting young Nate until he was able to get a job. The nurse provided Anticipatory Guidance with regard to their need to have an alternative plan should Nate begin work. For the short term the present transportation and meal arrangements would remain.

A major nursing concern was Mrs. Long's lack of adequate supplies for insulin injection (sterile needles, alcohol, and cotton). Inadequate supplies were the result of (1) supporting three adults on a low, fixed income, (2) Mrs. Long's pattern of placing the needs of others before the needs of herself, and (3) inadequate understanding of her symptoms and the risks infection posed for her dia-

betes control. Ultimately the resolution of this problem would involve (1) Nate's employment and (2) an increase in Mrs. Long's understanding and behavior change using motivational strategies (she could not help others if she was hospitalized). Education and motivational work was begun while the nurse made arrangements using Insurance Negotiation with the Medicare fiscal intermediary to supplement Mrs. Long's syringe supply. The nurse also used Referral and Client Advocacy (non-NIC) strategies to encourage Nate's enrollment in a job-training program. Table 6-4 shows the family's ratings over time for the outcome IADL: Assisted.

SUMMARY

Impaired Home Maintenance Management, the inability to maintain a safe, growth-producing immediate environment, is a multifaceted diagnosis. Neither its diagnostic usefulness nor its responsiveness to nursing intervention has been adequately explored through research. The NANDA diagnosis has been criticized for being too inclusive, yet it includes only a few activities related to IADL. The inclusion of multiple concepts (physical environmental status, individual physical functional status, family functioning, comfort, and growth) in this single diagnosis creates methodological problems in researching its use. Despite these problems, the diagnosis remains in high use in public health nursing agencies. A family unit–level outcome would be a useful addition to the relevant NOC outcomes. The NIC intervention Home Maintenance Assistance also is complex yet offers several useful and appropriate suggestions concerning relevant nursing activities.

REFERENCES

Agency on Aging. (1990). *Interesting facts about older Americans.* Washington, DC: Author.

American Association of Retired Persons. (1990). *Understanding senior housing in the 1990s: An AARP survey of consumer preferences, concerns and needs* (D13899). Washington, DC: AARP Fulfillment.

Cantor, M. H. (1989). Social care: Family and community support systems. *ANNALS, AAPSS, 503,* 99-112.

Carpentino, L. J. (1995). Home maintenance management, impaired. In *Nursing diagnosis: Application to clinical practice* (pp. 471-478). Baltimore: Lippincott Williams & Wilkins.

Dawson, D., Hendershot, G., & Fulton, J. (1987). *Functional limitations of individuals age 65 years and over* (Advance data: Vital and health statistics No. 133). Washington, DC: U.S. Public Health Service.

Fowles, D. G. (1991). The numbers game: Pyramid power. *Aging, 362,* 58-59.

Gordon, M. (1994). *Nursing diagnosis: Process and application* (3rd ed.). St. Louis, MO: Mosby.

Helberg, J. L. (1993). Patients' status at home care discharge. *IMAGE: Journal of Nursing Scholarship, 25*(2), 93-99.

Hereford, R. W., Suther, M., & Seifert, M. (1990). Creating and building home maintenance program in a home health agency. *Caring, 9*(9), 64-66.

Iowa Intervention Project. J. C. McCloskey & G. M. Bulechek (Eds.). (2000). *Nursing interventions classification (NIC)* (3rd ed.). St. Louis, MO: Mosby.

Iowa Outcomes Project. M. Johnson, M. Maas, & S. Moorhead (Eds.). (2000). *Nursing outcomes classification (NOC)* (2nd ed.). St. Louis, MO: Mosby.

Lambert, M. A., & Jones, P. E. (1989). Nursing diagnoses recorded in nursing situations encountered in a department of public health. In R. M. Carroll-Johnson (Ed.), *Classification of nursing diagnosis* (pp. 234-238). Baltimore: Lippincott Williams & Wilkins.

Lawton, M. P. (1972). Assessing the competence of older people. In D. Kent, R. Kastenbaum, & S. Sherwood (Eds.), *Research, planning, and action for the elderly* (pp. 122-143). New York: Behavioral.

Lawton, M. P. (1990). Aging and performance of home tasks. *Human Factors, 32*(5), 527-536.

Lawton, M. P., & Brody, E. M. (1969). Assessment of older people: Self-maintaining and instrumental activities of daily living. *The Gerontologist, 9,* 179-186.

Marek, K. (1989). Classification of outcome measures in nursing care. In *Classification systems for describing nursing practice* (pp. 37-42). Kansas City, MO: American Nurses Association.

Martin, K. S., & Scheet, N. J. (1992). *The Omaha system: Applications for community health nursing.* Philadelphia: Harcourt Brace.

Martin, K. S., Scheet, N. J., & Stegman, M. R. (1993). Home health clients: Characteristics, outcomes of care, and nursing interventions. *American Journal of Public Health, 83*(12), 1730-1734.

McFarland, G. K., & McFarlane, E. A. (1993). Impaired home maintenance management. In *Nursing diagnosis and intervention: Planning for patient care* (3rd ed., pp. 308-317). St. Louis, MO: Mosby.

Myers, J. L., & Stull, M. K. (1989). The use of nursing diagnoses in community-based nursing agencies. In R. M. Carroll-Johnson (Ed.), *Classification of nursing diagnosis* (pp. 223-227). Baltimore: Lippincott Williams & Wilkins.

North American Nursing Diagnosis Association. (1999). *Nursing diagnoses: Definitions and classification 1999-2000.* Philadelphia: Author.

Osterkamp, L. B., & Chapin, R. K. (1995). Community-based volunteer home-repair and home-maintenance programs for elders: An effective service paradigm? *Journal of Gerontological Social Work, 24*(1/2), 55-75.

Pfeiffer, E. (1975). *Multidimensional functional assessment: The OARS methodology.* Durham, NC: Center for the Study of Aging and Human Development.

Reuben, D. B. (1995). What's wrong with ADLs? *Journal of the American Geriatrics Society, 43*(8), 936-937.

Rinke, L. T. (1988). *Outcome standards in home health: State of the art.* New York: National League for Nursing.

Seifert, S., & Suther, M. (1994). Breaking home care tradition with home repairs and other services. *Caring, 13*(6), 60-63.

Sorgen, L. M. (1986). The development of a home care quality assurance program in Alberta. *Home Health Care Services Quarterly, 7*(2), 13-28.

Sparks, S. M., & Taylor, C. M. (1993). Home maintenance management impairment related to impaired cognitive, emotional, or psychomotor functioning. In *Nursing diagnosis reference manual* (pp. 505-506). Springhouse, PA: Springhouse.

Thompson, J. M., McFarland, G. K., Hirsch, J. E., & Tucker, S. M. (1997). Impaired home maintenance management. In *Mosby's clinical nursing* (4th ed., pp. 1511-1515). St. Louis, MO: Mosby.

United States Consumer Products Safety Commission. (1996). *Safety for older consumer home safety checklist.* Washington, DC: U.S. Consumer Products Safety Commission.

Verbrugge, L. M. (1990). The iceberg of disability. In S. M. Stahl (Ed.), *The legacy of longevity.* Thousand Oaks, CA: Sage.

CHAPTER 7

HEALTH SEEKING BEHAVIORS

Joanne Sabol Stevenson

In the ancient world being healthy meant being (looking and behaving) whole and normal. Physical and mental normality was necessary for societal acceptance; the disabled were ostracized and lived apart. As education and affluence evolved in Western cultures, attitudes toward the ill and disabled became more positive and hopeful. During the last half of the twentieth century much attention was focused on mainstreaming people with physical and mental disabilities and chronic illnesses.

In recent decades a large body of evidence has been accumulated regarding the effects of lifestyle on health. McGinnis and Foege (1993) quantified the major non-genetic factors that contributed to all deaths in the United States during 1990. They found that by conservative definitions 50% of all (nongenetic) deaths could be attributed to harmful individual lifestyle factors (e.g., tobacco, sedentary lifestyle, poor diet, alcohol, stress, violence, high-risk sexual behavior) or environmental factors (e.g., toxic agents).

Blair and colleagues (1989) performed maximal stress tests and then followed 13,344 adult men and women for 8 years or 110,482 person-years. They found the following age-adjusted all-cause mortality differences between the least and most physically fit: the least fit men exhibited 64 deaths per 10,000 person-years compared with 18.6 deaths per 10,000 for the most fit men; the least fit women exhibited 39.5 deaths per 10,000 person-years compared with 8.5 deaths per 10,000 for the most fit women. Physical fitness was correlated with lower risk for all-cause and cause-specific mortality even when the subjects engaged in other nonhealthy behaviors such as smoking or had parental history of coronary heart disease (Blair et al., 1989). These and hundreds of other studies point to the importance of health promoting behaviors on longevity, functional independence, and high quality of life.

The terms *health, vigor, physical fitness, athletic prowess, nutritional soundness,* and *stress management* resonated primarily for young urban professionals during the 1980s, and orchestrating physical fitness programs was primarily the domain of exercise physiologists and allied specialists. Then in the 1990s the focus shifted toward higher levels of health achievement for all: for all age-groups, including

even the oldest old; for all physical ability levels, including the blind, the paralyzed, and many others; and for all intellectual levels, including the cognitively impaired. Sports such as basketball, swimming, distance running, golf, and even skiing were adapted to accommodate many age-groups and many persons with physical and cognitive disabilities. Olympic-style competition grew for many challenged groups whose members previously never dreamed of engaging in athletic or other physical and cognitive competitions.

Accordingly, the concepts of health, vigor, fitness, athletic prowess, nutrition, and stress management became applied to many age-groups and levels of ability, including the elderly, the disabled, and the chronically ill. These groups are the very ones who are in client-provider relationships with health care professionals, especially nurses, on a regular and long-term basis.

In the twenty-first century nearly every living person will qualify for some level of physical fitness work and other forms of health promotion. As more older adults, disabled of all ages, and chronically ill of all ages seek out opportunities to learn about and engage in health promoting lifestyles, the distinctions in professional training of health promoters will blur. Most notably, nurses and others will focus their health promoting interventions on persons within their service arena. That arena will be the greatly expanded health care system of the twenty-first century, most of the work of nurses will be in the community, and most of the clients will be older adults.

There are myriad definitions of health and of wellness. Some are old and out of fashion, some emanated from a narrow or mechanistic focus, and some focused only on the absence of disease. Broader and more holistic current definitions target different levels of society. There are definitions of health for the individual, the family, the community, the environment, and the society. The focus here will be primarily on the individual level, and the terms *health* and *wellness* will be used interchangeably.

Dunn's (1980) concept of higher level wellness embodied the idea of actualizing and maximizing the human potential through the pursuit of three subgoals: making progress toward a higher level of functioning, having an open-ended expanding goal to seek a fuller potential, and progressing toward a more integrated and mature human existence throughout the entire life course. Pender at-

The author wishes to acknowledge the contribution of Patricia Davis, whose able assistance in searching the literature and help with other tasks related to this chapter are greatly appreciated.

tempted to incorporate both Dunn's actualizing focus and Dubos's (1965) concept of health as maintaining stability through adaptation to the environment. According to Pender (1996) "health (or wellness) is the actualization of inherent and acquired human potential through goal-directed behavior, competent self-care, and satisfying relationships with others while adjustments are made as needed to maintain structural integrity and harmony with relevant environments" (p. 22). By modifying Pender's 1987 definition, one can define health promoting behaviors as those behaviors enacted by persons of any age and any level of ability to increase wellness and promote optimal well-being, self-actualization, and personal fulfillment (Pender, 1987).

In *Healthy People 2000*, the most relevant fact about health promotion is that only 22% of the United States' population over age 18 engage in such behaviors on a regular basis. This figure probably is even smaller for elders (United States Department of Health and Human Services [USDHHS], 1991). There are several reasons, but two important ones are lack of full understanding of the costs and benefits of health promotion and personal and environmental impediments to action even when in possession of full and accurate factual information about benefits.

Nurses of the twenty-first century will work in the community, as well as in more acute types of health care agencies. Regardless of work site, nurses will be expected to incorporate health promotion into the total package of nursing services provided to consumers. Clients, third party payers, and policy makers will expect health care practitioners to promote wellness because it is essential to the cost containment goals of a mature comprehensive managed care system. In a mature managed care system the objective is to focus resources toward facilitating people to "live long and die short." That is, the emphasis will be on maximizing functional independence for as long as possible and on minimizing both the length and severity of dependency as much as possible.

ASSESSMENT

According to Pender (1996) the components of a thorough health promotion assessment are functional health patterns, physical fitness evaluation, nutritional assessment, health risk appraisal, life stress review, spiritual health assessment, social support systems review, health belief review, and lifestyle assessment. This list is too lengthy for one session with elderly clients, so the components should be prioritized depending on the immediate goals of the client. In most instances clients want one or two of three things: (1) help with diet (weight loss or gain); (2) an exercise prescription; or (3) help with a crisis or stressful situation. The client's priority can help determine the staging of the assessment plan. Furthermore some aspects, such as physical fitness evaluation, require special training and accreditation. In the next several years

many more nurses will be trained in the various aspects of health promotion evaluation and program supervision through specialization at the graduate level.

The most basic step in assessing health seeking behaviors is to measure interest in or readiness to learn about and engage in health promotion. A number of investigators have used Pender's (1996) model of health promotion as the basis for building predictive models of the tendency to engage in health promoting activities (Duffy, 1993; Foster & Tamboli, 1992; Stuifbergen & Becker, 1994). Duffy (1993) found that the three determinants of a health promoting lifestyle in older persons, which accounted for 89% of the variance, were a positive belief about controllability of one's own health, higher self-esteem, and internal locus of control. For elderly persons the strongest predictors of engaging in a health promoting lifestyle were higher self-efficacy for health behaviors, a wellness-oriented definition of health, less need for mechanical assistance (e.g., walker), and being female (Stuifbergen & Becker, 1994).

Many investigators have used the Health Promoting Lifestyle Profile (Walker, Sechrist, & Pender, 1987) as their predictor instrument with moderately positive results. Other frequently used instruments have included the Health Locus of Control Scale (Wallston & Wallston, 1981), the Health Self-Determinism Index (Cox, Miller, & Mull, 1987), and the Health-Related Hardiness Scale (Pollock & Duffy, 1990). A new instrument that holds promise is the Perceived Health Competence Scale (Smith, Wallston, & Smith, 1995).

In general, between 20% and 30% of the variance in actually implementing health promoting behaviors is explained by these instruments, indicating that many other factors are at play (Palank, 1991). Knowledge about health promotion, motivation to engage in behaviors, barriers to engaging in behaviors, and resiliency in engaging in behaviors over time are but a few of many complex concepts for theorists, measurement problems for researchers, and challenges for practitioners in this field.

NURSING DIAGNOSIS

In 1988 the North American Nursing Diagnosis Association (NANDA) added "Health-Seeking Behaviors (Specify)" to the list of approved nursing diagnoses. The definition is "a state in which an individual in stable health is actively seeking ways to alter personal health habits and/or environment in order to move toward a higher level of health" (Carpenito, 1995, p. 463; NANDA, 1999, p. 83). Stable health is defined as "age appropriate illness prevention measures achieved, client reports good or excellent health, and signs and symptoms of disease, if present, are controlled" (Tripp & Stachowiak, 1989, p. 433). The defining characteristics include an expressed or observed desire to seek a higher level of wellness, expressed or observed desire for increased control of health practice, expressed concern about or observed attempts to alter the negative effects of current environmental conditions on health status, stated or observed unfamiliarity with wellness community resources, and demonstrated or observed lack of knowledge in health promotion behaviors (NANDA, 1999, p. 83). The *Nursing Interventions Classification (NIC)* system (Iowa Intervention Project, 2000) includes a list of nursing interventions to accompany the diagnosis Health Seeking Behaviors. Several of these interventions are pertinent to elders, including Health Education, Exercise Promotion, Nutrition Management, Self-Modification Assistance, Weight Management, and Spiritual Support (Iowa Intervention Project, 2000). The *Nursing Outcomes Classification (NOC)* group at the University of Iowa is developing a related set of nursing-sensitive outcomes. The relevant outcomes that have been developed include Balance, Perceived Ability to Perform a Given Health Behavior, Health Promoting Behavior, Knowledge: Health Behaviors, Well-Being, and Spiritual Well-Being (Iowa Outcomes Project, 2000).

Health Promotion and Nursing Diagnosis: A Mismatch of Concepts

In health promotion and wellness the focus is not on adjectives such as average, normal, adequate, effective, or adapted/adaptive but is on higher level and more ambitious adjectives such as optimizing, enriching, or actualizing. Such adjectives do not belong in the same classification system as problem or deficit identification, signs and symptoms, diagnosis, and treatments or interventions. The processes of nursing diagnosis and nursing intervention make very strange bedfellows with the processes of health promotion and wellness. By its nature an intervention means that some outside person or power is attempting to change the course of events because of a problem or undesirable situation. Health promotion is a joyful and positive process; it focuses on making the best ever better. Milz (1992) provided the warning to the medical community that health promotion is not a new medical treatment but is a social, ecologic, and holistic concept that is fundamentally different from medical care. Likewise, health promotion is not just another nursing treatment but constitutes a fundamentally different paradigm of care.

The concept of health promoting behaviors is antithetical not only to the basic concept of nursing diagnosis but also to all the literature that has attempted to discuss and promote the idea of positive nursing diagnoses. The concepts do not mix, and the processes do not mix. To talk about health promoting behaviors in a logical way, it is necessary to step out of the frame of nursing diagnosis. There are no signs and symptoms in the usual sense; there is no diagnosis to define within the standard NANDA protocol. The so-called diagnosis Health Seeking Behaviors is a mismatch with all the other nursing diagnoses; it is out of place. The related factors for Health Seeking Behaviors

listed by Carpenito (1995) include marriage, parenting, empty nest, and retirement. The situations in this list are not typical "nursing intervention" situations; this list reinforces the argument that "nursing diagnosis" is the wrong language to be using for this constellation of goals and activities.

Several authors have attempted to make the square peg of health or wellness fit into the round hole of nursing diagnosis (Allen, 1989; deSilva et al., 1987; Frenn, 1994; Stolte, 1986, 1994; Tripp & Stachowiak, 1989). Some of these authors attempted to focus on the diagnosis of strengths (Houldin, Salstein, & Ganley, 1987; Popkess-Vawter, 1984), but that is a conundrum because if the patient possesses these strengths, there is no necessity for a nurse to perform an act of professional service. Some of the authors focused on changing modifiers. This ends up with diagnoses such as sleep pattern, healthy; tissue perfusion, adequate; gas exchange, adequate; bowel elimination, regular; nutrition, adequate; or self-concept, healthy (Allen, 1989). Mere absence of a health problem is not equivalent to the pursuit of higher level wellness.

Frenn, Jacobs, Lee, Sanger, and Strong (1987) conducted a Delphi Survey to gain consensus on what they called "wellness and health promotion nursing diagnoses"; the resulting list is similar to Allen's (1989). Examples are sleep pattern, effective; stress management, effective; community resource use, effective; and so on in the same vein. Such diagnoses are out of sync with the essence of health promotion or wellness; they continue to be the stuff of a medical model with superficially altered modifiers. They sound more like positive outcomes of actions taken to solve the patients' problems than health promotion or wellness goals and activities in any primary or core sense.

Wellness and Health Promotion Practice: A Taxonomy of Its Own

During the ninth NANDA Conference in 1989 the Taxonomy Committee presented its early work on Taxonomy II (Fitzpatrick, 1991). A critical part of the conceptual development of Taxonomy II included the potential integration of "axes" in a fashion similar to their use in *Diagnostic and Statistical Manual of Mental Disorders*, Fourth Edition (DSM-IV). Hoskins (1991) and Warren (1991) explained that each diagnosis would be on one or more axes. Suggested axes included ages or stages of life, unit of analysis (individual, family, community), wellness, and illness. If wellness becomes an axis, it might partially address the conceptual dilemma. But it would create a new challenge, since many of the existing diagnoses would have to be rewritten to elaborate on their wellness dimension. Axes would not, however, solve the basic problem of mixing an illness-oriented model of diagnosis and intervention with the separate and distinct paradigm embodied by health promotion and wellness. The only good solution to dealing with a phenomenon as different from the illness model as health promotion would be to develop a separate classification system.

Although nursing may continue to work in isolation on developing a way to integrate health promotion within the existing NANDA or any other purely nursing classification system, other options would be more appropriate and useful to the consumer public. Since health promotion is by nature a multidisciplinary field, it is only fitting that representatives of the relevant disciplines and practitioners in that field develop its classification schema. Nursing is a major player but not the only player in that field. Currently the people who are most suitable to engage in classification development include behavioral health researchers (e.g., members of the Society of Behavioral Medicine), nurses, nutritionists, exercise physiologists, community and public health researchers, and several groups of nonmainstream practitioners, such as chiropractors, herbalists, massage therapists, acupuncturists, biofeedback experts, natural foods nutritionists, athletic coaches, personal trainers, and meditation trainers.

It is illogical to put energy into trying to make health promotion an add-on to the traditional system of diagnostic categories in nursing (or in medicine). It would be best to develop a separate classification system for health promotion—one that could be agreed on by the major players in health promotion and that would serve all the practitioners engaged in the practice of health promotion. If there were a separate classification schema for health promotion with its own set of strategies and measures of effect, the consumer public would find it easier to understand and ultimately would be better served. Such a system would provide clarity for a practice field (health promotion) that is currently very murky indeed. It would help to set norms and standards; it would help to decrease fraud and deception—both in products and services and in untrained and unscrupulous purveyors of useless or potentially harmful products and services.

Perhaps a more fitting language for a taxonomy of health promotion and wellness would include goals (rather than diagnoses), strategies with research-based activities by the client (rather than interventions by the caregiver), process measures, and intermediate outcomes (rather than discharge outcomes). This list may seem like trivial play on words, but it actually represents a substantive difference in orientation from a diagnosis-driven classification system to a wellness-oriented system.

NURSING-SENSITIVE OUTCOMES

In evaluating health seeking behaviors, two categories of outcomes are needed. First are measures of the processes of health promotion: whether the client is engaging the intervention, whether the "dosage" is adequate to fulfill his needs, and whether intermediate indicators are within the desired range. These process measures are very important for two reasons: beneficial outcomes cannot be achieved unless the behavior is implemented correctly and consistently over time, and proper dosage is critical to outcome measurement in health promoting behaviors. For example, it is self-deceiving to engage in exercise that is too slow, too low powered, too short, or too infrequent. Hence a process measure of exercise level would be the percent of heart rate reserve to be maintained during the exercise session. The desirable range of heart rate to be maintained is set as part of the exercise prescription. The client and/or the fitness supervisor monitors the exercise heart rate throughout the exercise sessions to make sure that the "dosage" of exercise is in the efficacious range. Analogous process measures exist for resistance training, diet, and other health promoting behaviors.

The second category of outcomes that should be specified is composed of measures of both short-term and long-term effects. Within the domain of effect requirements different levels are of interest. The results experienced by the individual client in each component of health promotion effort—e.g., aerobic exercise, resistance training, spiritual growth—is one level. The mean of the effects for the clients of the entire program at specified time intervals is another level of measurement. Finally, measurement of results from several programs, population groups, or communities is a third level of evaluation (Pruitt, 1992; Thompson, 1992). Each of these levels of evaluation is important, and each requires a different kind of expertise to develop and test the instrumentation. The totality of all that is to be developed is massive and complex. This fact adds another argument to the list of reasons that health promotion should be treated as a separate (multidisciplinary) service entity and not just one component of nursing diagnosis, intervention, and outcome.

Intermediate-effects outcome measures are focused on elements of time. Since health promotion is a lifelong endeavor, it is positively reinforcing to measure improvements or other changes in smaller segments of time. For example, the number of pounds or kilograms of weight lost or gained in 1 month and the time required to lose one half of the weight desired to be lost are examples of intermediate outcomes. From these measures trends can be drawn and progress (or lack of it) can be monitored. In this way it is possible to alter the strategy, the dosage, or both before too much time is lost engaging in a strategy that is not achieving the desired aims. At the individual level it is usually advisable to designate specific time lines for intermediate outcome measures. Intervals of 6 months, 1 year, or 2 years are often set as the designated outcome intervals to measure effects of individual health promotion efforts (Prochaska, Velicer, Rossi, Goldstein, & Marcus, 1994). Intervals of 4, 8, and 12 months are more often used with older adults.

Long-term outcome measures also are needed because health promotion is not episodic. Engaging in health promoting behaviors is not completed until death. Thus the provision of health promotion services is analogous to the provision of chronic illness care: there is no end but the final end. The ultimate evaluation of the effectiveness of health promotion strategies and programs is comparative morbidity and mortality data. In the area of morbidity functional independence (or the converse, functional dependence) statistics are used to determine the effectiveness of health promotion programming for populations. The expected outcomes are that the groups who engage in health promoting lifestyles will remain functionally independent and in control of their lives for longer periods of time compared with groups who do not participate. Population-level data send a very powerful message. One example is the decrease in lung cancer following the decrease in adult smoking during recent decades in the United States.

NURSING INTERVENTIONS

The gerontology literature is replete with health promotion experimental studies. This literature is dominated by findings that elders—even the oldest, most frail, and most sedentary—can and do benefit from health promotion interventions on their behalf. The cardinal principle behind working with the frail hypokinetic elder is that the more out of condition the person or group, the slower their progression and the longer the experimental program will take to produce measurable effects. This finding is a general principle of physical fitness practice with the elderly; patience and persistence are paramount.

A variety of strategies or activity groupings are subsumed under health promotion for elders: (1) a planned and supervised program of aerobic conditioning, resistance training, flexibility work, and gait or balance work; (2) nutritional management, including dietary modifications for under or over nutrition; (3) stress management, which can include any of several approaches or programs such as imagery, yoga, meditation, or biofeedback or an integrated exercise and antistress system such as tai chi; (4) spiritual growth, which often requires assistance from someone trained in spiritual guidance; and (5) maintenance or enhancement of interpersonal relationship skills, social support networks, and environmental safety strategies (Haber, 1994). Each of these components is a significant workload in its own right, and clients cannot focus on all these things or make all these changes at one time. The activities should be staged using the client's successes and readiness as the trigger points to add more components to the mix. Table 7-1 provides a matrix of goals, indicators for intermediate outcomes, and activities that are useful for providing health promotion services to the elder.

Exercise Promotion

Aerobic fitness is the most commonly studied health promoting intervention among elders. The overwhelming majority of studies over the past 30 years have shown positive results (Lowenthal, Kirschner, Carpace, Pollock, & Graves, 1994). Results consistently were positive among younger and community-dwelling elders with no health problems (Adams & de Vries, 1973; de Vries, 1970; Molloy, Beerschoten, Borrie, Crilly, & Cape, 1988; Stevenson & Topp, 1990; Topp & Stevenson, 1994), as well as among more frail and older subjects in a variety of settings (Fisher, Pendergast, & Calkins, 1991; Hall, DeBeck, Johnson, & Mackinnon, 1992; Jirovec, 1991; McMurdo & Rennie, 1993; Morey, Crowley, Robbins, Cowper, & Sullivan, 1994; Stevenson, 1988; Valentine-Garzon, Maynard, & Selznick, 1992). Stamford (1988) concluded after his exhaustive review of exercise studies that both elderly males and elderly females experienced positive training responses regardless of their previous training patterns or initial fitness statuses.

A number of investigators found secondary benefits, including significant improvements in several areas of cognition and short-term memory, following exercise interventions (Clarkson-Smith & Hartley, 1989; Lindenmuth & Moose, 1990; Molloy, Beerschoten, et al., 1988; Stevenson & Topp, 1990), whereas others reported little or no improvement (Molloy, Richardson, & Crilly, 1988; Perri & Templer, 1985).

Optimum physical functioning of the human body requires flexible joints, adequate muscle strength, and adequate bone strength. Buchner and Wagner (1992) confirmed that 25% of the variance in disability over several studies was explained by overall physical functioning status. Sedentary elderly men and women and even very hypokinetic elderly subjects can significantly increase their muscular strength (Fisher & Pendergast, 1994; Fisher, Pendergast, & Calkins, 1991; Nelson et al., 1994), balance (Sauvage et al., 1992), joint flexibility, bone density, and functional capacity (Fisher, Kame, Rouse, & Pendergast, 1994) through progressive training as long as the training is tailored to their initial capabilities, is strong and progressive enough, and lasts long enough.

A combination of aerobic exercise, strength training, balance training, and in one site tai chi was tested in the Frailty and Injuries: Cooperative Studies of Intervention Techniques (FICSIT) clinical trials. These activities assuaged frailty, increased independent mobility, and decreased fall proneness in several middle-old (70 to 85) and old-old (85 and older) samples (Buchner, 1993; Fiatarone et al., 1993; Fiatarone et al., 1994; Wolf, Kutner, Green, & McNeely, 1993; Wolf et al., 1996; Wolfson et al., 1993). A meta-analysis of seven FICSIT trials showed significant decreases in the 1.5 year (median) follow-up fall rates for community ($n = 2133$) and nursing home ($n = 295$) subjects (Province et al., 1995).

Nutrition Management

It is apparent from a wide array of studies that maintaining proper nutrition is complex but essential to the

Table 7-1	Interdisciplinary Health Promotion Goals, Indicators for Intermediate Client Outcomes, and Activities	
Goals	**Indicators**	**Activities**
Generate predictive profile of wellness status.	List of high-risk areas from history to address in health promotion program List of individual emphases and adaptations to fit into program List of social relationships and behaviors to be addressed	Interview, history, and physical exam. Include: Family history of ages Causes of disease and death Personal past and current health history Areas for special emphasis and adaptation of wellness plans Current family and social relationships Areas for improvement
Optimize aerobic fitness.	Weekly METS of effort expended Periodic fitness retesting (at 4, 8, 12 months) Increases in maximum stress test times	Fitness testing Aerobic exercise prescription Coaching/motivating Teaching and reinforcement
Improve strength in major muscle groups	Documentation of increased workload (capacity) at 4-, 8-, 12-month retests of strength in isolated muscles and muscle groups	Strength testing Program of resistance training with incremental increases Coaching and guidance Teaching and reinforcement
Improve flexibility in all joints	Documentation of increased flexibility (goniometry, dynamometry) at 4-, 8-, 12-month retests	Flexibility testing Program of flexibility and stretching exercises for large and small joints/muscles Coaching and guidance Teaching and reinforcement
Improve balance and gait.	Documentation of improved balance and gait rhythm, step height, and swing through at 4, 8, 12 months	Balance and gait testing Program of exercises and activities for gait and balance

optimum functioning of elders (Berry, 1994; Evans, 1992). Nutritional supplementation combined with exercise was efficacious in reducing frailty in the Boston FICSIT clinical trial (Fiatarone et al., 1994). The age-85-and-older experimental subjects gained more muscle strength, gait velocity, stair-climbing power, thigh-muscle mass, and self-initiated activity than the control subjects, who actually lost function.

Promotion of Well-Being

Few controlled experimental studies are extant on progressive relaxation or imagery for stress management in elder groups. However, interesting findings have emerged that suggest beneficial effects (Collison & Miller, 1987; Howell, 1994; Moody, Fraser, & Yarandi, 1993; Slivinske & Fitch, 1987). Intervention studies to promote subjective well-being of elders in order to promote health are few. The main forms of intervention were patient education programs (Hunter & Hall, 1989; Neuberger, Smith, Black, & Hassanein, 1993), self-help groups or provider-led

groups (Braden, 1993; Ruffing-Rahal, 1993, 1994), or both (Felker, 1988; Newman, 1993). Outcomes tended to be especially positive for those who engaged in long-term self-help groups. Peer groups over long time periods appear to work better than professionally led groups. However, professionals can facilitate the initial development of such groups.

Spiritual Support

Spiritual growth is another important component of health promotion. Koenig and colleagues (Koenig, George, & Siegler, 1988; Koenig, Kvale, & Ferrel, 1988) assessed the contributions of spirituality and religiosity to well-being (morale) independent of the confounding variables of health status, financial status, and social support. They found that higher spirituality scores correlated with greater overall morale and less agitation, loneliness, and dissatisfaction with life. There are few skeptics left who would deny the validity of the myriad studies indicating that old age does not have to be a time of physical depen-

Table 7-1	Interdisciplinary Health Promotion Goals, Indicators for Intermediate Client Outcomes, and Activities—cont'd	
Goals	**Indicators**	**Activities**
Optimize nutritional status	Pretest and periodic retesting of BMI, skin folds, BP, skin turgor, nails, hair, blood, urine, and stool Nutrition diaries at 4, 8, 12 months	Nutritional history Assessment of current likes, dislikes, allergies, chewing and swallowing capacities Comprehensive plan of food portions, fluids for meals and snacks Plan of vitamins, minerals, dietary supplements Guidance at the buffet over time Teaching and reinforcement
Enhance socioeconomic and spiritual health.	Annual objective and subjective retesting Reassessment by client of progress made, new goals, area for improvement in the coming year Unobtrusive measures and interviews about progress in social interactions and family relationships	Assessment of morale, stress, subjective well-being, spiritual fitness Planning of spiritual readings, group activities, individual activities, consultation with spiritual advisors or others
Address financial and legal issues.	Annual assessment of financial affairs and return on investments Completion of legal documents—will/trusts Completion of health self-determination documents and death arrangements	Assessment of financial and legal state of affairs Comprehensive plans for handling assets to maximize income Legal planning including will or trusts Assess status of health self-determination documents and death arrangements
Address hearing, dental, and eye health	Documentation of hearing status Documentation of dental health status Improvement in hearing or dental problem areas Maintaining vision at optimum level for the individual	Periodic hearing examination and address any problems Periodic teeth cleaning and dental examination Care of acute and chronic problems Periodic eye examination Eyeglasses (prescription) Changes of eye treatment as indicated

dence, depression, and cognitive incompetence. Rather, it can be a time of positive health and high quality of life. However, this does not occur for the majority without considerable effort devoted to a health promoting lifestyle. Furthermore, the vast majority of elders do not possess adequate knowledge and skills, nor do they have the inner motivation to develop, implement, and maintain a health promoting lifestyle without professional assistance and encouragement.

A Model for Promoting Healthy Lifestyle Changes

Nurses who will engage in health promotion work with elders will want to obtain specialized training in many of the specialized strategies, since none of them is simple and all of them have to be integrated into a smooth whole for maximum benefit. In addition, many components of the totality require consultation from experts. However,

nurses make excellent generalists with the capacity to pull the health promotion components into one integrated whole in concert with their clients. One of the most difficult steps in lifestyle change is the decision to take the first step. The theoretical model formulated by Prochaska and DiClemente (1984) is one of the more successful models in use today by practitioners involved in promoting health behavior change. The essence of the model is that there are stages of decision making that go into the final decision to make a health behavior change. The earlier stages are very critical to the process, and during these stages nurses play a major part in moving clients toward readiness for change.

The stages are precontemplation; contemplation; planning and preparation; action; and maintenance, continuation, and stabilization of the change. The stage of precontemplation is the stage when the client is not even thinking about making the behavior change; it is the point at which a nurse could do consciousness raising and start the thinking process that leads the client to contemplation. During contemplation nursing input is critical, since that is the time for providing factual information, motivational support, and positive reinforcement about the client's ability to make the change successfully. Social support from the nurse and significant others is equally important during the planning and preparation phase. During the action phase the expert advice of nurses and others is critical to make the actions efficient, safe, and healthful and to help the client avoid pitfalls and overcome problems encountered while adopting the new behavior. Finally, during the maintenance phase it is important to have support from knowledgeable and empathetic others who can provide positive reinforcement and relevant support services when the need arises. If one uses the example of exercise, it is important in the maintenance phase to help the client develop alternative routines to avoid boredom and to rotate muscle groups and types of exercises to keep the body from becoming overly adapted to the routine. Fitness experts refer to this rotation process as keeping the muscle groups confused and challenged, thus stimulating them to be constantly rebuilding and strengthening.

Prochaska and DiClemente (1984) do not have a separate stage for relapse; they seem to treat it as a return to one of the earlier stages, and the client then proceeds through the ensuing stages anew. In real life the relapsed client becomes depressed and feels like a failure. The nurse is in an important position to help the client focus on her former successes and make the effort to go through the change steps once again.

Health behavior change is a difficult and complex human endeavor. It rarely can be done alone, and this may be even more true for the current cohort of elderly persons. They lived through their childhood and adult life expecting to "retire" not only from their occupation but also from everything requiring large expenditures of effort and self-discipline. Converting many of them to self-responsibility for health is a major task. Convincing them that exercise is good for older persons (rather than dangerous or even foolhardy) is a monumental undertaking. It takes enormous patience, salesmanship, and creativity to convert the more reticent among this population. On the other hand, many elders are excited about health promotion and are eager to find someone who will advise and guide them through the process. Nurses will be expected to work successfully with elders of both polar persuasions, as well as those in-between.

CASE STUDY

N. Turner is an 82-year-old woman in generally good health. She recently sold her home of almost 50 years and used the proceeds to move to a Lifecare Retirement Community. The community signed a guarantee to provide whatever level of care she needs for life. Mrs. Turner in

turn paid an endowment and signed a contract that included a commitment to engage in a health promoting lifestyle and to work with the wellness staff to maintain functional abilities and independence to the best of her ability for her remaining lifetime. While making the decision to sell her house and move in to this particular lifecare community, Mrs. Turner progressed through the first two stages of the change model described earlier. So following the move, she was ready to initiate the planning stage with the wellness staff.

Previously she had kept active by raising a large family and then by maintaining a large house and garden after she was widowed. More recently she helped clean and maintain her church's physical plant. She has never engaged in exercise "without a purpose." Mrs. Turner settles into her apartment in the independent section of the community and begins a series of assessment interviews and planning sessions with the interdisciplinary wellness staff. A nurse with graduate training and certification in health promotion coordinates the team. The testing sessions are scheduled to avoid fatigue and consist of the areas shown in Table 7-1. Mrs. Turner is at or above average for her age on the fitness and strength measures, so goals are set to achieve higher levels of both over a series of months. Prescriptions are written for exercise, resistance training, and flexibility training. She has one-on-one sessions to get started and then joins the group sessions led by certified trainers.

Consistent with the matrix in Table 7-1, the dietary consultant assesses her past diet and helps her set up plans for choosing the three meals and snacks from the buffet of healthy choices. All foods in the community are prepared to maximize low-fat and high-fiber options in attractive "gourmet" preparations. Residents are taught about portion sizes, since undesirable weight gain can occur with even the healthiest foods if taken in large portions. Mrs. Turner also participates in the socioemotional testing and program planning. She sets goals for herself with staff guidance. She meets with a member of the clergy of her choice and makes decisions about whether to participate in group worship. She begins to consider her goals for higher levels of spiritual maturity.

During the following year she shows progress at the 4-, 8-, and 12-month reassessment sessions and participates in setting new goals for the following year. She is helped to understand that if an illness or any crisis causes a setback, she can begin again with appropriately reset goals and can continue to live a life of wellness within her personal areas of limitation.

Process measures over the first year, as shown in Table 7-1, include indicators of engaging in a fitness-promoting level of exercise and an adequate but safe level of resistance training. Examples would include exercise pulse rates and progressive changes in muscular strength and flexibility. Intermittent food diaries would provide data about nutrition goals, and some type of morale scale could be used to monitor mood and perceived quality of life. The minister consults with her about the spiritual progress and areas to focus on in the future.

Longer term outcome measures could be set at 1-year intervals. Comparisons through trend lines could be determined for each 12-month period, keeping in mind that as aging continues, maintenance of the status quo might be more reasonable than an expectation of continued improvement on the physical parameters. By engaging in such a comprehensive plan of health promoting behaviors, Mrs. Turner can look forward to living out the final stage of her life to the fullest. Through the subsequent 10 years that Mrs. Turner lives in the independent apartment, she continues to make progress in the socioemotional and spiritual areas of her life and relationships with family, neighbors, and staff. She embraces tai chi and yoga for their benefits in stress management and flexibility. Inherent in the plan developed for and by Mrs. Turner is staging so that she never feels overwhelmed or coerced but can participate in new behaviors at a reasonable and comfortable pace. At age 92 Mrs. Turner, her family, and the staff decide that movement to the assisted living building would be advantageous. Many of her goals and activities remain the same, and some can still be implemented in the independent area. However, her aerobic exercise, resistance training, and flexibility work are now done with the more frail residents using seated cycle ergometers or other adaptive devices. The other areas of development, such as her spiritual and socioemotional growth work, go on. Hence health promotion moves forward through creative planning and adjustments by the interdisciplinary staff in collaboration with Mrs. Turner for as long as she is willing and able. For Mrs. Turner, "health promotion isn't done 'til life's done."

SUMMARY

Health promotion does not fit into traditional classifications of nursing diagnoses or interventions. It is a unique field of its own, and nursing is but one of the practice disciplines that provide health promotion services. Health promotion services would serve humankind best if presented under the aegis of a separate classification schema, with its own set of strategies or activities and with a separate outcomes classification system. It is recommended that organized nursing provide the leadership to amass the relevant disciplines to develop this classification system. In the future this system could be even more important and advantageous to humankind than the current system of International Classification of Diseases, Injuries, and Causes of Death (ICD) codes, diagnostic criteria, and treatments focused on illness care. When managed care systems completely dominate the health care scene, the focus will be on maintaining all elderly persons in the lowest level of care for the maximum period of time. That means keeping them functioning independently in their own homes or apartments for as long as possible. To do this, health promotion among elders will achieve a critical level of importance and large segments of nursing time will be spent helping elders to engage in health promoting lifestyles.

Nurses in the twenty-first century working in a managed care environment will be expected to have the expertise to develop, implement, and evaluate programs to promote healthful lifestyles among their clients. Nursing practice with elders will increasingly become a balanced combination of chronic illness symptom management and health promotion programming for individuals, groups, and populations. But the fact that nurses are providers in both service domains (illness care and health promotion services) does not legitimize the unfortunate attempt to subsume health promotion within the nursing diagnosis classification schema. Health promotion is a distinct service entity; a parallel classification system should be developed to explicate it properly and thoroughly.

REFERENCES

Adams, G. M., & de Vries, H. A. (1973). Physiological effects of an exercise training regimen upon women aged 52-79. *Journal of Gerontology, 28,* 50-55.

Allen, C. J. (1989). Incorporating a wellness perspective for nursing diagnosis in practice. In R. M. Carroll-Johnson (Ed.), *Classification of nursing diagnoses: Proceedings of the eighth conference* (pp. 37-42). Baltimore: Lippincott Williams & Wilkins.

Berry, E. M. (1994). Chronic disease: How can nutrition moderate the effects? *Nutrition Reviews, 52* (8), S28-S30.

Blair, S. N., Kohl, H. W., III, Paffenbarger, R. S., Jr., Clark, D. G., Cooper, K. H., & Gibbons, L. W. (1989). Physical fitness and all-cause mortality: A prospective study of healthy men and women. *Journal of the American Medical Association, 262,* 2395-2401.

Braden, C. J. (1993). Promoting a learned self-help response to chronic illness. In S. G. Funk, E. M. Tornquist, M. T. Champagne, & R. A. Wiese (Eds.), *Key aspects of caring for the chronically ill: Hospital and home* (pp. 158-169). New York: Springer.

Buchner, D. M. (1993). The Seattle FICSIT/MOVEIT study: The effect of exercise on gait and balance in older adults. *Journal of the American Geriatrics Society, 41,* 321-325.

Buchner, D. M., & Wagner, E. H. (1992). Preventing frail health. *Clinics in Geriatric Medicine, 8,* 1-17.

Carpenito, L. J. (1995). *Nursing diagnosis* (6th ed.). Baltimore: Lippincott Williams & Wilkins.

Clarkson-Smith, L., & Hartley, A. A. (1989). Relationships between physical exercise and cognitive abilities in older adults. *Psychology and Aging, 4,* 183-189.

Collison, C., & Miller, S. (1987). Using images of the future in grief work. *IMAGE: Journal of Nursing Scholarship, 19*(1), 9-11.

Cox, C. L., Miller, E. H., & Mull, C. S. (1987). Motivation in health behavior: Measurement, antecedents, and correlates. *Advances in Nursing Science, 9*(4), 1-15.

deSilva, P., Dickson, G. L., Falconer, N., Frenn, M., Lee, H., Miller, K. M., & Strong, K. A. (1987). Toward a nursing diagnosis in wellness. In A. M. McLane (Ed.), *Classification of nursing diagnoses: Proceedings of the seventh conference* (p. 270). St. Louis, MO: Mosby.

deVries, H. A. (1970). Physiological effects of an exercise training regimen upon men aged 52-88. *Journal of Gerontology, 25,* 325-366.

Dubos, R. (1965). *Man adapting.* New Haven, CT: Yale University Press.

Duffy, M. E. (1993). Determinants of health-promoting lifestyles in older persons. *IMAGE: Journal of Nursing Scholarship, 25*(1), 23-28.

Dunn, H. L. (1980). *High-level wellness.* Thorofare, NJ: Slack.

Evans, W. J. (1992). Exercise, nutrition and aging. *75th annual meeting of the Federation of American Societies for Experimental Biology: Nutrition and Exercise* Boston: American Institute of Nutrition.

Felker, M. P. (1988). A recovery group for elderly alcoholics. *Geriatric Nursing, 9,* 110-113.

Fiatarone, M. A., O'Neill, E. F., Doyle, N., Clements, K. M., Roberts, S. B., Kehayias, J. J., Lipsitz, L. A., & Evans, W. J. (1993). The Boston FICSIT study: The effects of resistance training and nutritional supplementation on physical frailty in the oldest old. *Journal of the American Geriatrics Society, 41,* 333-337.

Fiatarone, M. A., O'Neill, E. F., Ryan, N. D., Clements, K. M., Solares, G. R., Nelson, M. E., Roberts, S. B., Kehayias, J. J., Lipsitz, L. A., & Evans, W. J. (1994). Exercise training and nutritional supplementation for physical frailty in very elderly people. *The New England Journal of Medicine, 330,* 1769-1775.

Fisher, N. M., Kame, V. D., Rouse, L., & Pendergast, D. R. (1994). Quantitative evaluation of a home exercise program on muscle and functional capacity of patients with osteoarthritis. *American Journal of Physical Medicine and Rehabilitation, 73,* 413-420.

Fisher, N. M., & Pendergast, D. R. (1994). Effects of a muscle exercise program on exercise capacity in subjects with osteoarthritis. *Archives of Physical Medicine and Rehabilitation, 75,* 792-797.

Fisher, N. M., Pendergast, D. R., & Calkins, E. (1991). Muscle rehabilitation in impaired elderly nursing home residents. *Archives of Physical Medicine and Rehabilitation, 72,* 181-185.

Fitzpatrick, J. J. (1991). Taxonomy II: Definitions and development. In R. M. Carroll-Johnson (Ed.), *Classification of nursing diagnoses: Proceedings of the ninth conference* (pp. 23-34). Baltimore: Lippincott Williams & Wilkins.

Foster, C., & Tamboli, H. P. (1992). Exercise prescription in the rehabilitation of patients following coronary artery bypass graft surgery and coronary angioplasty. In J. R. Shepard & H. S. Miller, Jr. (Eds.), *Exercise and the heart in health and disease* (pp. 283-298). Boca Raton, FL: Marcel Dekker.

Frenn, M. (1994). Older adults' experience of health promotion: A guide for taxonomic development. In R. M. Carroll-Johnson & M. Paquette (Eds.), *Classification of nursing diagnoses: Proceedings of the tenth conference* (pp. 242-245). Baltimore: Lippincott Williams & Wilkins.

Frenn, M. D., Jacobs, C. A., Lee, H.A., Sanger, M. T., & Strong, K. A. (1987). Delphi survey to gain consensus on wellness and health promotion nursing diagnoses. In A. M. McLane (Ed.), *Classification of nursing diagnoses: Proceedings of the seventh conference* (pp. 154-159). St. Louis, MO: Mosby.

Haber, D. (1994). *Health promotion and aging.* New York: Springer.

Hall, N., DeBeck, P., Johnson, P., & Mackinnon, R. (1992). Randomized trial of health promotion for frail elders. *Canadian Journal of Aging, 11,* 72-91.

Hoskins, L. M. (1991). What is the focus of taxonomy II? Nursing diagnosis axes. In R. M. Carroll-Johnson (Ed.), *Classification of nursing diagnoses: Proceedings of the ninth conference* (pp. 35-37). Baltimore: Lippincott Williams & Wilkins.

Houldin, A. D., Salstein, S. W., & Ganley, K. M. (1987). *Nursing diagnoses for wellness: Supporting strengths.* Baltimore: Lippincott Williams & Wilkins.

Howell, S. L. (1994). Natural/alternative health care practices used by women with chronic pain: Findings from a grounded theory research study. *Nurse Practitioner Forum, 5*(2), 98-105.

Hunter, S. M., & Hall, S. S. (1989). The effect of an educational support program on dyspnea and the emotional status of COPD clients. *Rehabilitation Nursing, 14,* 200-202.

Iowa Intervention Project. J. C. McCloskey & G. M. Bulechek (Eds.). (2000). *Nursing interventions classification (NIC)* (3rd ed.). St. Louis, MO: Mosby.

Iowa Outcomes Project. M. Johnson, M. Maas, & S. Moorhead (Eds.). (2000). *Nursing outcomes classification (NOC)* (2nd ed.). St. Louis, MO: Mosby.

Jirovec, M. M. (1991). The impact of daily exercise on the mobility, balance and urine control of cognitively impaired nursing home residents. *International Journal of Nursing Studies, 28,* 145-151.

Koenig, H. G., George, L. K., & Siegler, I. C. (1988). The use of religion and other emotion-regulating coping strategies among older adults. *The Gerontologist, 28,* 303-310.

Koenig, H. G., Kvale, J. N., & Ferrel, C. (1988). Religion and well-being in later life. *The Gerontologist, 28,* 18-28.

Lindenmuth, G. F., & Moose, B. (1990). Improving cognitive abilities of elderly Alzheimer's patients with intense exercise therapy. *The American Journal of Alzheimer's Care and Related Disorders & Research, 1,* 31-33.

Lowenthal, D. T., Kirschner, D. A., Carpace, N. T., Pollock, M., & Graves, J. (1994). Effects of exercise on age and disease. *Southern Medical Journal, 87*(5), S5-S12.

McGinnis, J. M., & Foege, W. H. (1993). Actual causes of death in the United States. *Journal of the American Medical Association, 270,* 2207-2212.

McMurdo, M. E., & Rennie, L. (1993). A controlled trial of exercise by residents of old people's homes. *Age and Ageing, 22,* 11-15.

Milz, H. (1992). "Healthy ill people": Social cynicism or new perspectives? In A. Kaplun (Ed.), *Health promotion and chronic illness: Discovering a new quality of health* (pp. 32-39). Copenhagen, Denmark: World Health Organization.

Molloy, D. W., Beerschoten, D. A., Borrie, M. J., Crilly, R. G., & Cape, R. D. T. (1988). Acute effects of exercise on neuropsychological function in elderly subjects. *Journal of the American Geriatrics Society, 36,* 29-33.

Molloy, D. W., Richardson, L. D., & Crilly, R. G. (1988). The effects of a three-month exercise program on neuropsychological function in elderly institutionalized women: A randomized controlled trial. *Age and Ageing, 17,* 303-310.

Moody, L. E., Fraser, M., & Yarandi, H. (1993). Effects of guided imagery in patients with chronic bronchitis and emphysema. *Clinical Nursing Research, 2,* 478-486.

Morey, M. C., Crowley, G. M., Robbins, M. S., Cowper, P. A., & Sullivan, R. J., Jr. (1994). The Gerofit program: A VA innovation. *Southern Medical Journal, 87*(5), S83-S87.

Nelson, M. E., Fiatarone, M. A., Morganti, C. M., Trice, I., Greenberg, R. A., & Evans, W. J. (1994). Effects of high-intensity strength training on multiple risk factors for osteoporotic fractures: A randomized controlled trial. *Journal of the American Medical Association, 272,* 1909-1914.

Neuberger, G. B., Smith, K. V., Black, S. O., & Hassanein, R. (1993). Promoting self-care in clients with arthritis. *Arthritis Care and Research, 6,* 141-148.

Newman, A. M. (1993). Effect of a self-help course on adaptation in people with arthritis. In S. G. Funk, E. M. Tornquist, M. T. Champagne, & R. A. Wiese (Eds.), *Key aspects of caring for the chronically ill: Hospital and home* (pp. 150-157). New York: Springer.

North American Nursing Diagnosis Association. (1999). *Nursing diagnosis: Definitions and classification 1999-2000.* Philadelphia: Author.

Palank, C. L. (1991). Determinants of health-promotive behavior: A review of current research. *Nursing Clinics of North America, 26,* 815-832.

Pender, N. J. (1987). Health and health promotion: Conceptual dilemmas. In M. E. Duffy & N. J. Pender (Eds.), *Conceptual issues in health promotion: Report of proceedings of a Wingspread Conference* (pp. 7-23). Indianapolis, IN: Sigma Theta Tau International Honor Society of Nursing.

Pender, N. J. (1996). *Health promotion in nursing practice* (3rd ed.). Norwalk, CT: Appleton & Lange.

Perri, S., & Templer, D. I. (1985). The effects of an aerobic exercise program on psychological variables in older adults. *International Journal of Aging and Human Development, 20,* 167-172.

Pollock, S. E., & Duffy, M. E. (1990). The health-related hardiness scale: Development and psychometric analysis. *Nursing Research, 39,* 218-222.

Popkess-Vawter, S. (1984). Strength-oriented nursing diagnosis. In M. J. Kim, G. K. McFarland, & A. M. McLane (Eds.), *Classification of nursing diagnoses: Proceedings of the fifth national conference* (pp. 433-440). St. Louis, MO: Mosby.

Prochaska, J. O., & DiClemente, C. C. (1984). *The transtheoretical approach: Crossing traditional boundaries of change.* Homeward, IL: Dow Jones-Irwin.

Prochaska, J. O., Velicer, W. F., Rossi, J. S., Goldstein, M. G., & Marcus, B. H. (1994). Stages of change and decisional balance for 12 problem behaviors. *Health Psychology, 13,* 39-46.

Province, M. A., Hadley, E. C., Hornbrook, M. C., Lipsitz, L. A., Miller, J. P., Mulrow, C. D., Ory, M. G., Sattin, R. W., Tinetti, M. E., & Wolf, S. L. (1995). The effects of exercise on falls in elderly patients: A preplanned meta-analysis of the FICSIT trials. *Journal of the American Medical Association, 273,* 1341-1347.

Pruitt, R. H. (1992). Effectiveness and cost efficiency of interventions in health promotion. *Journal of Advanced Nursing, 17,* 926-932.

Ruffing-Rahal, M. A. (1993). An ecological model of group well-being: Implications for health promotion with older women. *Health Care for Women International, 14,* 447-456.

Ruffing-Rahal, M. A. (1994). Evaluation of group health promotion with community dwelling older women. *Public Health Nursing, 11,* 38-48.

Sauvage, L. R., Myklebust, B. M., Crow-Pan, J., Novak, S., Millington, P., Hoffman, M. D., Hartz, A. J., & Rudman, D. (1992). A clinical trial of strengthening and aerobic exercise to improve gait and balance in elderly male nursing home residents. *Journal of Physical Medicine and Rehabilitation, 71,* 333-342.

Slivinske, L., & Fitch, V. (1987). The effect of control enhancing interventions on the well-being of elderly individuals living in retirement communities. *The Gerontologist, 27,* 176-181.

Smith, M. S., Wallston, K. H., & Smith, C. H. (1995). The development and validation of the Perceived Health Competence Scale. *Health Education Research, 10*(1), 51-64.

Stamford, B. A. (1988). Exercise and the elderly. In K. B. Pardolf (Ed.), *Exercise and Sports Sciences Reviews, 16,* 341-379.

Stevenson, J. S. (1988). *Effects of preventive exercise in frail elders.* (Final Rep. No. RF717732). Columbus, OH: The Ohio State University Research Foundation.

Stevenson, J. S., & Topp, R. (1990). Effects of moderate and low intensity long-term exercise by older adults. *Research in Nursing and Health, 13,* 209-218.

Stolte, K. (1986). A complementary view of nursing diagnosis. *Public Health Nursing, 3*(1), 23-28.

Stolte, K. (1994). Health oriented nursing diagnoses: Development and use. In R. M. Carroll-Johnson & M. Paquette (Eds.), *Classification of nursing diagnoses: Proceedings of the tenth conference* (pp. 143-148). Baltimore: Lippincott Williams & Wilkins.

Stuifbergen, A. K., & Becker, H. A. (1994). Predictors of health promoting lifestyles in persons with disabilities. *Research in Nursing and Health, 17,* 3-13.

Thompson, J. C. (1992). Program evaluation within a health promotion framework. *Canadian Journal of Public Health, 83*(S1), S67-S71.

Topp, R., & Stevenson, J. S. (1994). The effects of attendance and effort on outcomes among older adults in a long-term exercise program. *Research in Nursing and Health, 17,* 15-24.

Tripp, S., & Stachowiak, B. (1989). Nursing diagnosis: Health seeking behaviors (specify). In R. M. Carroll-Johnson (Ed.), *Classification of nursing diagnoses: Proceedings of the eighth conference* (pp. 433-436). Baltimore: Lippincott Williams & Wilkins.

United States Department of Health and Human Services. (1991). *Healthy people 2000: National health promotion and disease prevention objectives* (Pub. No. 91-50212). Washington, DC: U.S. Government Printing Office.

Valentine-Garzon, M. A., Maynard, M., & Selznick, S. Z. (1992). ROM dance program effects on frail elderly women in an adult day-care program. *Physical & Occupational Therapy in Geriatrics, 11,* 63-83.

Walker, S. N., Sechrist, K. R., & Pender, N. J. (1987). The health-promoting lifestyle profile: Development and psychometric characteristics. *Nursing Research, 36*(2), 76-81.

Wallston, B. S., & Wallston, K. A. (1981). Health locus of control scales. In H. M. Lefcourt (Ed.), *Research with the locus of control construct: Vol. I. Assessment methods* (pp. 189-243). New York: Academic Press.

Warren, J. J. (1991). Implications of introducing axes into a classification system. In R. M. Carroll-Johnson (Ed.), *Classification of nursing diagnoses: Proceedings of the ninth conference* (pp. 38-44). Baltimore: Lippincott Williams & Wilkins.

Wolf, S. L., Barnhart, H. X., Kutner, N. G., McNeely, E., Coogler, C., & Xu, T. (1996). Reducing frailty and falls in older persons: An investigation of Tai Chi and computerized balance training. *Journal of the American Geriatrics Society, 44,* 489-497.

Wolf, S. L., Kutner, N. G., Green, R. C., & McNeely, E. (1993). The Atlanta FICSIT study: Two exercise interventions to reduce frailty in elders. *Journal of the American Geriatrics Society, 41,* 329-332.

Wolfson, L., Whipple, R., Judge, J., Amerman, P., Derby, C., & King, M. (1993). Training balance and strength in the elderly to improve function. *Journal of the American Geriatrics Society, 41,* 341-343.

CHAPTER 8

INEFFECTIVE MANAGEMENT OF THERAPEUTIC REGIMEN

Mary Zwygart-Stauffacher

The diagnosis Ineffective Management of Therapeutic Regimen can be useful for nursing in almost all settings (Carpenito, 1995). Both individuals experiencing a variety of health problems and family members are challenged by complex treatment programs that require changes in lifestyle and function. These changes or adaptations are frequently instrumental in influencing the positive outcome of their care. Ineffective Management of Therapeutic Regimen describes those who are experiencing difficulty in achieving positive outcomes. Though certainly not exclusively used for older adults, it clearly is a diagnosis of great utility when working with elderly individuals.

The goal of nursing care is to provide client-focused care, which enables clients to effectively manage their therapeutic regimen to live the highest quality of life. The therapeutic nurse-client relationship is one in which the client and nurse are considered equal partners. Jointly these parties establish goals, negotiate strategies, and plan for care (Keeling, Utz, Shuster, & Boyle, 1993). With successful management of the therapeutic regimen, individuals are able to manage illness and promote their highest level of functioning.

RELATED FACTORS/ETIOLOGIES

Therapeutic regimens are sets of rules or habits of diet, exercise, and manner of living that are intended to improve health and treat or cure disease (Thorndike & Barnhart, 1979, as cited in Lunney, 1993). Chronic illness, impaired sensory function, social isolation, diminished self-care and self-care ability, environmental changes, and financial limitations make older adults vulnerable to Ineffective Management of Therapeutic Regimen (Carpenito, 1995; Ebersole & Hess, 1998; Lunney, 1993; North American Nursing Diagnosis Association [NANDA], 1999) (Box 8-1). These factors are magnified when taking into consideration the impact of past life experiences, personal health habits, and the need for potential life-modifying health regimens.

The complexity of the therapeutic regimen has substantial influence, especially for older persons who have sensori-perceptual, manual dexterity, or mobility deficits.

Because of multiple changes that are linked to aging, the number and types of cues previously used by an older adult might be inadequate to bring about implementation of the nursing plan of care. Emotional and psychologic stressors also affect an individual's ability to follow a designated regimen. The elderly are confronted with multiple losses and can be overwhelmed in their efforts to cope with them. Achieving health care goals may not always be possible, especially for older adults who need substantial guidance and assistance.

Knowledge deficit, not understanding either what was intended or the significance of not following through with the therapeutic regimen, is a frequently cited factor related to ineffective management of a therapeutic regimen. Issues also arise around decision making, the appropriateness of care, the consistency of that care with previous lifestyles, and patterns of health care. Individuals also can fail to perceive the seriousness of their illness or their susceptibility to negative outcomes from not participating in the regimen. Hays and DiMatteo (1981) asserted that the patient's failure to follow the prescribed treatment regimen is not solely the patient's or physician's fault; rather it is a by-product of their interaction. Certainly a nurse-patient relationship could result in a parallel interaction failure or in confusion about the intent and goal of the interaction.

The older adult can perceive barriers to self-care, financial limitations, or lack of social support. Feelings of powerlessness can develop when an elder feels unable to really change or perceives that change will not make a difference. For instance, older adults might question whether smoking cessation will really have an impact on their health or doubt that their attempt to quit smoking could be successful.

Finally, the complex health care system often makes it difficult for an individual to maneuver through a maze of providers. An individual can mistrust health care professionals and personnel within a very complex health care delivery system, especially when she has never known or had any relationship with a provider. Yet patients are expected to trust these providers and to believe that they should modify their lifestyle as recommended.

Related Factors/Etiologies
INEFFECTIVE MANAGEMENT OF THERAPEUTIC REGIMEN

Complexity of health care system
Complexity of therapeutic regimen
Decisional conflicts
Excessive demands made on individual or family
Family conflict
Family patterns of health care
Inadequate numbers and types of cues to activities
Knowledge deficits
Mistrust of regimen and/or health care personnel
Perceived seriousness
Perceived susceptibility

Additional Factors (Carpenito, 1995)
Ability to perform prescribed procedures
Cultural factors
History of disease
Learning abilities
Presence of sensory deficits
Stage of adaptation to disease

Data from Kim, M., McFarland, G., & McLane, A. (1997). *Pocket guide to nursing diagnoses.* (7th ed.). St. Louis: Mosby; North American Nursing Diagnosis Association. (1999). *Nursing diagnoses: Definitions & classification 1999-2000.* Philadelphia: Author.

ASSESSMENT

Assessment is multifaceted. Nurses need to identify that an individual has ineffectively managed his therapies and also understand the rationale behind why this may have occurred. Further, nurses should explore what is contributing to ineffective management of the health care regimen.

The nurse needs highly developed history-taking and observational skills and must be able to determine everyday patterns of what the elderly person is truly doing, not what has been recommended or prescribed. Elderly clients, in their wish to portray themselves as "good patients," might not always be as forthright as necessary. Nurses must be able to build trust so that elderly clients will feel free to share what is occurring and how they are managing their health.

Nursing assessment should include other factors that may be affecting the patient, including culture, economics, family influence, lack of recognition for the need for change, and positive self-efficacy (Bandura, 1982). The growing cultural diversity of the aging population during recent decades has increased the need for culturally competent care providers (Yeo, 1997). It is therefore imperative that nurses recognize the impact of culture on dimensions of health and health care delivery that can affect the interactions and outcomes of elder care. Awareness of culturally unique care includes, for example, lifestyle, living circumstances, intercultural dynamics, epidemiology of

disease, health beliefs, and complementary practices (Langer, 1999; Yee et al., 1995). Reviews of culturally appropriate assessment models and tools exist to guide the nurse in the appraisal of cultural influence regarding health care decisions and care delivery (Giger & Davidhizar, 1995; Tripp-Reimer, Brink, & Saunders, 1984).

The availability of monetary resources, together with the client's priorities related to budgeting those resources, is another important dimension of assessment. The elderly individual might sincerely wish to follow through with all suggested interventions yet because of limited resources must make difficult decisions regarding what is possible. For instance, an individual with limited income might have to decide whether to purchase her own medications or those of significant others. Clear associations have been established between elderly medication adherence, drug and dosage form, race, cost of medications, number of medications, insurance coverage, and prescriber client community (Balkrishnan, 1998). Individuals with limited resources might be unaware of additional sources of income such as Supplemental Security Income (SSI), or they might not wish to depend on family for economic assistance. Additionally, the impact of prescribed interventions on perceived quality of life is another important dimension to explore (Williams, 1998).

The elderly client might lack recognition of the need for behavioral change. The belief that health promotion and maintenance activities are not necessary or effective for elders is a common myth held by elders, as well as some health care providers.

Nurses also need to be cognizant of the elderly individual's decision-making capacities and competencies. For instance, has he and how did he achieve success in managing other health problems? What does the patient view as a successful outcome of care? Is the individual able to hear or see the health care instructions and then comprehend and remember the instructions? A significant aspect of health care is lack of knowledge and barriers to learning. Knowledge deficits are frequently cited in the literature as a significant contributing factor to ineffective therapeutic regimen.

Carpenito (1995, p. 571) recommended the following assessment questions as appropriate for ineffective management of health care regimen:

1. What is his present level of knowledge regarding the illness, including severity, prognosis, susceptibility to complications and ability to cure or control its progression, the knowledge and diagnostic studies, and preventative measures?
2. What is the pattern of adhering to the prescribed health behaviors? Complete, modified, or not adhering?
3. Does anything interfere with adherence to the prescribed health behaviors?
4. What are the learning needs perceived by the client and family?

NURSING DIAGNOSIS

In 1992 NANDA approved the nursing diagnosis Ineffective Management of Therapeutic Regimen. The approval of this diagnosis represented a shift from the previous diagnostic terminology of noncompliance. The literature is replete with discussions of how the terms *compliance* and *noncompliance* are value laden, how these terms focus on the subordinate position of the patient in relation to the health care professional, and how assessments of compliance are inconsistent between health care professionals and patients (Bakker, Kastermans, & Dassen, 1995; Goldberg, Cohen, & Rubin, 1998; Keeling, Utz, Shuster, & Boyle, 1993). In addition, use of the term *noncompliance* did not recognize either the clients' ability to make decisions or the complexity of lifestyle and life decisions associated with effectively managing and promoting their health. Compliance was viewed as a relationship in which power is used by superiors (nurses) to control or direct subordinates (patients) (Edel, 1985). As early as the mid 1980s, Edel suggested eliminating noncompliance as a nursing diagnosis and encouraged nurses to direct their interventions toward therapeutic alliances with patients.

A diagnosis that was reported by Lunney in 1982, Alterations in Management of Illness, provided the basis for the diagnosis Ineffective Management of Therapeutic Regimen (Lunney, 1993). Ineffective Management of Therapeutic Regimen has been defined as "a pattern of regulating and integrating into daily life a program for treatment of illness and the sequelae of illness that are unsatisfactory for meeting specific health goals" (Lunney, 1993; NANDA, 1999, p. 80).

The determination of Ineffective Management of Therapeutic Regimen should be a joint process. This duality, though, contributes to the substantial challenge of addressing this diagnosis. Bakker et al. (1995) stated, "It is this dual focus of the diagnosis that can make it difficult to use in practice. What happens when professionals and patients do not agree about the question of how effective the management of therapeutic regimen has been" (p. 165). When the worlds of the client and provider collide, care outcomes may not be achieved.

NANDA (1999) has identified the major defining characteristic for Ineffective Management of Therapeutic Regimen as choices of daily living that are ineffective for meeting the goals of a treatment or preventative program. These choices are demonstrated by the following (Kim, McFarland, & McLane, 1997; NANDA, 1999, p. 80):

- Acceleration of illness symptoms
- Verbalized desire to manage the treatment of illness and prevention of sequelae
- Verbalized difficulty with regulation or integration of one or more prescribed regimens of treatment of illness and its effects on prevention of complications
- Verbalized that did not take action to include treatment regimens in daily routines
- Verbalized that did not take action to reduce risk factors for progression of illness sequelae

The diagnosis Ineffective Management of Therapeutic Regimen was found reliable in a study conducted by Fujita and Dungan (1994), who used clinical protocols to investigate the utility of the diagnosis with patients experiencing congestive heart failure (CHF). This study is one of the extremely limited number of reports in the literature regarding the reliability, validity, and clinical utility of this diagnosis. It is therefore imperative that gerontologic nurses conduct further research.

CASE STUDY

R. Black is an 87-year-old male who is still living in the home that he and his wife had resided in since the 1940s. Mr. Black's wife died 2 years ago, and since that time he has had frequent visits to the clinic and hospital. He has recently been discharged from the hospital following an acute myocardial infarction (MI) with subsequent complications of CHF. He is on multiple medications, including diuretics, antidysrhythmics, and anticoagulation therapy. His daughter, a recently retired schoolteacher, lives approximately 200 miles from him; his son died from cardiac disease only 2 months ago.

The home health care nurse makes the initial visit to Mr. Black 3 days after his discharge from the local hospital. Reviewing the hospital forms, the nurse finds that on discharge Mr. Black had mild pedal edema and no shortness of breath (SOB); he had been instructed on his medications and a low sodium diet on the day of discharge. The discharge nurse had also documented that, though weak, he was not confused or disoriented and appeared to follow all directions.

At the time of the visit the home health care nurse observed that Mr. Black was experiencing difficulty breathing when he greeted her at the door. The nurse also noticed that he was wearing slippers. When questioned about why he was wearing slippers, Mr. Black replied that his shoes were quite tight that day. After asking to review his medications, the nurse noted that some of the medications were not present and there were an inappropriate number of pills in some of the bottles, with some bottles containing excess medications and some less than expected. A partially uneaten meal of commercially canned soup was on the table, and a can of salted peanuts sat next to Mr. Black's favorite chair.

On further questioning, the nurse found that Mr. Black did attempt to take his medications as had been prescribed, but he had confused the number of pills and was taking the wrong number of the "heart pill and fluid pills." In addition, he was unclear about when to take his "blood thinner" and had taken it in the morning versus the afternoon as suggested. He also stated that he understood he should "put his feet up and was doing so," but he was using a very low footstool next to his chair for his edematous extremities. Finally, Mr. Black could explain the need for a low-sodium diet with regard to cardiac function, but he did not realize that the soup he was eating contained substantial sodium. Therefore the nurse concluded that Mr. Black was exhibiting Ineffective Management of Therapeutic Regimen not caused by a conscious choice to disregard directions. Rather, it was related to insufficient knowledge and insight on how to manage a complex medication regimen in addition to significant dietary changes that had been suggested to him.

NURSING-SENSITIVE OUTCOMES

Several nursing-sensitive outcomes developed by the Iowa Outcomes Project address the effective management of therapeutic regimen (Iowa Outcomes Project, 2000). Nursing-sensitive outcomes that appropriately fit the diagnosis Ineffective Management of Therapeutic Regimen and research literature illustrating use of the outcome measures are shown in Box 8-2. These outcomes, along with others that are appropriate for the diagnosis, are defined as follows:

1. Acceptance: Health Status—reconciliation to health circumstances (p. 108)
2. Psychosocial Adjustment: Life Change—psychosocial adaptation of an individual to life change (p. 346)
3. Coping—actions to manage stressors that tax an individual's resources (p. 192)
4. Health Beliefs: Perceived Ability to Perform—personal conviction that one can carry out a given health behavior (p. 227)
5. Health Promoting Behavior—actions to sustain or increase wellness (p. 232)
6. Knowledge—related to the extent of understanding and skill needed to manage such things as disease process, energy conservation, health behaviors, medications, and treatment regimen to name a few (pp. 262, 264, 268, 279, 294).

Instruments have not been developed to measure these or other outcomes solely for this diagnosis; however, proxy measures such as a Medication Event Monitoring System have been used to evaluate the degree to which outcomes are met (Paes, Bakker, & Soe-Agnie, 1998).

A variety of goals could be established and agreed on by the patient and nurse to facilitate achievement of designated outcomes. These goals should be centered around promoting and enhancing the individual's ability to manage his health care appropriately and within what is reasonable for that person. These goals must be both age and culturally sensitive. How and why people choose or do not choose to participate in their health care is extraordi-

narily personal and should be clearly explicated so that elders can achieve the best outcomes.

Finally, the literature includes discussion of three factors that can affect the achievement of positive outcomes: self-efficacy, adherence, and empowerment. Self-efficacy refers to an individual's belief that one's actions are effective in achieving personal goals (Bandura, 1982; Chenitz, Stone, & Salisbury, 1991). Self-efficacy implies a sense of mastery over body, environment, and finances and infers a high degree of independence. One's perceptions of ability and control are major factors in self-efficacious behavior. Chenitz and colleagues (1991) cited the work of Smith et al. (1984), who found that individuals over the age of 60 had a lower desire to have control over their health than did younger adults. The work of Woodward and Wallston (1987) appeared to support this premise because those most vulnerable to illness were most likely to see themselves as less competent to make decisions related to health care. Older adults, who are frequently vulnerable to illness, would seem to be at high risk for having less perceived control. If Bandura's (1982) assertions are correct that a low level of perceived self-efficacy can be detrimental to effective coping, older persons might not seek needed help or might be only a passive participant in the treatment regimen. It is important to keep in mind that efficacy is generally viewed as situation specific and requires the care provider to reassess for each new behavior.

Adherence to a therapeutic regimen is a challenge for all individuals, though possibly most difficult for the chronically ill elder. Adherence is influenced by numerous issues, including the complexity of the regimen, the amount of change needed, the level of obstacles, dissatisfaction with the system, inconvenience of obtaining necessary care, and health beliefs (Ebersole & Hess, 1998). Belief in the efficacy of an action implies that the action will decrease the threat to health. The Health Belief Model (HBM) provides a framework from which to guide investigation on this topic. Redeker (1988) attempted to explain the response to preventative health behaviors. The major belief factors are what value the individual places on a particular outcome and the individual's estimate of the likelihood of a particular outcome associated with adherence to the regimen. The measurement of adherence has been controversial, with many believing that the only truly accurate way to measure adherence is by direct observation (Seley, 1993). Direct observation is a very costly and possibly invasive method when compared with self-reports of behavior.

The intent of empowerment is ". . . to enable people to increase their capacity to enhance their own health as they define it, both individually and collectively" (Fahlberg, Poulin, Girdana, & Dusek, 1991, p. 186). Applying empowerment to the nurse-client interaction creates greater trust, increased sense of self-worth, and better use of resources (Matteson, McConnell, & Linton, 1997).

Box 8-2   Suggested Nursing-Sensitive Outcomes and Nursing Interventions
INEFFECTIVE MANAGEMENT OF THERAPEUTIC REGIMEN

Nursing Diagnosis
Ineffective Management of Therapeutic Regimen
Defining characteristics
Acceleration of s/s of CHF (e.g., edema, SOB)
Verbalizes desire to manage care and also that he was feeling overwhelmed
Verbalizes difficulty following diet with his present health status
Demonstrates lack of knowledge of medication administration (i.e., inappropriate number of pills)
Attempts to follow regimen (i.e., did raise feet, but not appropriate height)
Recent losses and incomplete grieving

Nursing-Sensitive Outcomes
Knowledge: Treatment Regimen
Indicators
Description of rationale for treatment regimen
Verbalizes correct time of day and dosage of each medication
Selection of foods recommended in diet
Identifies foods that are high in Na and appropriate substitutes from personal likes

Health Beliefs: Perceived Ability to Perform
Indicator
Confidence in ability to perform health behavior

Acceptance: Health Status
Indicators
Modifies daily activities to facilitate cardiac status (e.g., raised feet)
Coping with health situation
Recognizes aspects of care with which he requires assistance

Coping
Indicators
Expresses sadness
Demonstrates decrease in depressive symptoms
Reports decrease in physical symptoms of stress
Participates in previous fulfilling activities (e.g., gardening)

Nursing Interventions
Teaching: Prescribed Medication
Activities
Instruct the patient on the dosage, route, and duration of each medication
Instruct the patient on the purpose and action of each medication

Mutual Goal Setting
Activities
Review the scale (as developed with the patient) during review dates for assessment of progress
Self-medication assistance with weekly medication setup

Nutrition Management
Activities
Assist patient in receiving help from appropriate community nutritional programs, as needed
Establish rest/activity schedule to decrease fatigue and provide raised feet

Home Maintenance Assistance
Activity
Obtain assistance with home care activities 2 times per week (e.g., homemaker services)

Active Listening
Activity
Use active listening

Emotional Support
Activities
Provide emotional support such as contact with lay minister and daughter at least 2 times per week
Encourage diversional activities such as gardening

Behavior Management
Activities
Reinforce appropriate behavior
Praise efforts of self-control

NURSING INTERVENTIONS

Three nursing priorities have been suggested by Doenges and Moorhouse (1997) when planning for effective interventions with persons who have Ineffective Management of Therapeutic Regimen:

1. Determining the reason for nonadherence
2. Assisting elderly persons in developing strategies that facilitate successful management
3. Health promotion

The more tailored and individualized the health promotion, the more likely it will be implemented. The work of Walter, Volkan, Sechrist, and Pender (1988) indicated that the elderly are a very heterogeneous group with multiple

health care needs. The nurse needs to facilitate the successful meshing of healthy lifestyle practice with the elder's lifestyle and health needs.

The *Nursing Interventions Classification (NIC)* (Iowa Intervention Project, 2000) provides a list of interventions that are appropriate for Ineffective Management of Therapeutic Regimen. When cross-referencing this list with core interventions as identified by the National Gerontological Nursing Association (p. 811), four interventions are identified: Active Listening, Behavior Management, Coping Enhancement, and Emotional Support. Other interventions (Box 8-3) that are consistent with the literature and useful in providing care would include Mutual Goal Setting, Patient Contracting, Self-Modification Assistance, and Teaching.

Definitions of these interventions are as follows:

Active Listening: "Attending closely to and attaching significance to a patient's verbal and nonverbal messages" (Iowa Intervention Project, 2000, p. 127)

Behavior Management: "Helping a patient manage negative behavior" (p. 160)

Coping Enhancement: "Assisting a patient to adapt to perceived stressors, changes, or threats that interfere with meeting life demands and roles" (p. 234)

Emotional Support: "Provision of reassurance, acceptance, and encouragement during times of stress" (p. 300)

Mutual Goal Setting: "Collaborating with patient to identify and prioritize care goals, then developing a plan for achieving those goals" (p. 462)

Patient Contracting: "Negotiating an agreement with a patient that reinforces a specific behavior change" (p. 494)

Self-Modification Assistance: "Reinforcement of self-directed change initiated by the patient to achieve personally important goals" (p. 581)

Teaching: Planning, implementation, and evaluation of a teaching program designed to address a patient's particular needs

Box 8-3	Suggested Nursing Interventions **INEFFECTIVE MANAGEMENT** **OF THERAPEUTIC REGIMEN**
Active Listening*	Family Support
Behavior Management*	Health System Guidance
Cognitive Restructuring	Mutual Goal Setting
Complex Relationship Building	Patient Contracting
	Risk Identification
Coping Enhancement*	Self-Modification Assistance
Counseling	Teaching: Disease Process
Crisis Intervention	Teaching: Procedure/
Culture Brokerage	Treatment
Emotional Support*	Telephone Consultation

*Interventions consistent with the National Gerontological Nursing Association Core Interventions.

CASE STUDY

The nurse was able to determine that Mr. Black sincerely wished to manage his health but was overwhelmed by the regimen. His feeling of being overwhelmed was compounded by his feelings of profound sadness over the death of his son and continued grieving for his wife. Simply managing daily household chores was overwhelming to him, and Mr. Black's lack of culinary skills made meal preparation nearly impossible.

For Mr. Black appropriate outcomes included that he be able to verbalize acceptance of his condition changes and recognize that his lifestyle required alteration. Improved affect and verbalizations of resolving grief would indicate progress in coping with his losses. Additionally, the ability to follow a daily medication regimen and knowledge of how to proceed if he were unable to manage the medications would be measurable outcome criteria. For Mr. Black it remained important, on an ongoing basis, to identify his abilities and reinforce these whenever possible.

Some examples of goals for Mr. Black were for him to thoroughly discuss and describe foods that are low and high in sodium (knowledge) and to be able to identify foods in his home that would be appropriate choices. Additionally, Mr. Black should be able to describe, or at least develop with the nurse, a mechanism for taking his medications appropriately. Other goals were for Mr. Black to verbalize a feeling of power over his situation, to determine what he wished to manage on his own, and to identify those aspects of care that he could not manage by himself.

All of the interventions listed by NIC would be reasonable to include in care planning for Mr. Black (see Box 8-3). With Mr. Black's permission, the nurse planned for a weekly medication setup. They also agreed that at each nursing visit they would discuss just one of his medications, reviewing the content of the previous discussion and written materials. In this way Mr. Black's knowledge would be enhanced without overwhelming him, allowing for self-pacing and achievement of a positive outcome.

Arrangements were also made for a low-sodium diet to be delivered by Meals on Wheels. This activity could, for a slightly increased cost, ensure two meals a day that would be consistent with the prescribed dietary plan. His daughter also planned to hire a home health aide to assist twice a week with house chores and shopping. Mr. Black expressed appreciation and tearfully stated, "I just didn't realize I could receive this kind of help. My wife and then my son managed all of these kinds of things in the past. I think that I will be all right now." Eventually Mr. Black demonstrated acceptance and belief that he could successfully manage his health care. Additionally, Mr. Black demonstrated coping skills when he contacted his minister for guidance and assistance. A lay minister from the church agreed to telephone and stop in at least twice a week.

Within a month there was a noted improvement. Both Mr. Black's physical status and his emotional status improved. He asked for further instruction regarding his medications and was hoping to be able to manage medication administration without assistance. He also thought he might be able to undertake a few more household tasks and wished to do some gardening, which he had not done since his wife's death.

SUMMARY

Managing one's health care is a complex process that requires the interest and involvement of the patient. Breakdowns in this process are common and expected. The role of the nurse is to enhance the ability of elders to successfully manage their health care. Although there is limited research on the utility of this recently approved diagnosis, it remains useful when working with older adults who need to make significant lifestyle changes.

REFERENCES

Balkrishnan, R. (1998). Predictors of medication adherence in the elderly. *Clinical Therapeutics, 20*(4), 764-771.

Bakker, R., Kastermans, M., & Dassen, T. (1995). An analysis of nursing diagnosis ineffective management of therapeutic regimen compared to noncompliance and Orem's self care deficit theory of nursing. *Nursing Diagnosis, 6*(4), 161-166.

Bandura, A. (1982). Self-efficacy mechanism in human agency. *American Psychology, 37*(3), 122-147.

Carpenito, L. (1995). *Nursing diagnosis: Application to clinical practice.* Baltimore: Lippincott Williams & Wilkins.

Chenitz, C., Stone, J., & Salisbury, S. (1991). *Clinical gerontological nursing: A guide to advanced practice.* Philadelphia: W.B. Saunders.

Doenges, M., & Moorhouse, M. (1997). *Nurse's pocket guide: Nursing diagnosis and interventions.* Philadelphia: F. A. Davis.

Ebersole, P., & Hess, P. (1998). *Toward healthy aging: Human needs and nursing response* (5th ed.). St. Louis, MO: Mosby.

Edel, M. (1985). Noncompliance: An appropriate nursing diagnosis? *Nursing Outlook, 33,* 183-185.

Fahlberg, L., Poulin, A., Girdana, D., & Dusek, D. (1991). Empowerment as an emerging approach in health education. *Journal of Health Education, 22*(3), 185-193.

Fujita, L., & Dungan, J. (1994). High risk for ineffective management of therapeutic regimen. A protocol study. *Rehabilitative Nursing, 19*(2), 75-79.

Giger, J., & Davidhizar, R. (1995). *Transcultural nursing: Assessment and intervention* (2nd ed.). St. Louis, MO: Mosby.

Goldberg, A., Cohen, G., & Rubin, A. (1998). Physician assessment of patient compliance with medical treatment. *Social Science Medicine, 47*(11), 1873-1876.

Hays, R., & DiMatteo, M. (1981). Patient compliance assessment. *Journal of Compliance Health Care, 2,* 37-53.

Iowa Intervention Project. J. C. McCloskey & G. M. Bulechek (Eds.). (2000). *Nursing interventions classification (NIC)* (3rd ed.). St. Louis, MO: Mosby.

Iowa Outcomes Project. M. Johnson, M. Maas, & S. Moorhead (Eds.). (2000). *Nursing outcomes classification (NOC)* (2nd ed.). St. Louis, MO: Mosby.

Keeling, A., Utz, S., Shuster, G., & Boyle, A. (1993). Noncompliance revisited: A disciplinary perspective of a nursing diagnosis. *Nursing Diagnosis, 4*(3), 91-98.

Kim, M., McFarland, G., & McLane, A. (1997). *Pocket guide to nursing diagnoses* (7th ed.). St. Louis, MO: Mosby.

Langer, N. (1999). Culturally competent professionals in therapeutic awareness enhance patient compliance. *Journal of Health Care for the Poor and Underserved, 10*(1), 19-26.

Lunney, M. (1993). Ineffective management of therapeutic regimen. In G. McFarland & E. McFarlane (Eds.), *Nursing diagnosis and interventions* (pp. 79-86). St. Louis, MO: Mosby.

Matteson, M., McConnell, E., & Linton, A. (1997). *Gerontological nursing concepts and practice.* Philadelphia: W.B. Saunders.

North American Nursing Diagnosis Association. (1992). *Nursing diagnosis: Definitions and classifications 1993-1994.* Philadelphia: Author.

North American Nursing Diagnosis Association. (1999). *Nursing diagnosis: Definitions and classifications 1999-2000.* Philadelphia: Author.

Paes, A., Bakker, A., & Soe-Agnie, C. (1998). Measurement of patient compliance. *Pharmacy World & Science, 20*(2), 73-77.

Redeker, N. (1988). Health beliefs and adherence in chronic illness. *IMAGE: Journal of Nursing Scholarship, 29*(1), 31.

Seley, J. (1993). Professional development. Is noncompliance a dirty word? *The Diabetes Educator, 19*(5), 386-391.

Tripp-Reimer, T., Brink, P., & Saunders, J. (1984). Cultural assessment: Content and process. *Nursing Outlook, 32*(2), 78-82.

Walter, S., Volkan, K., Sechrist, K., & Pender, N. (1988). Health promoting lifestyles of older adults, correlates and patterns. *Advanced Nursing, 11*(1), 76-90.

Williams, G. (1998). Assessing patient wellness: New perspectives on quality of life and compliance. *American Journal of Hypertension, 11,* 186S-191S.

Woodward, N., & Wallston, B. (1987). Age and health care beliefs, self efficacy as a mediator of low desire for control. *Psychology of Aging, 2*(1), 3-8.

Yee, B., Henderson, N., McCabe, M., Scott, V.J., Talamantes, M., & Yeo, G. (1995). Ethnogeriatrics white paper. In S. Klein (Ed.), *A national agenda for geriatric education: White papers* (Vol. 1, pp. 1-15). Rockville, MD: Bureau of Health Professionals, Public Health Services and U.S. Department of Health and Human Services.

Yeo, G. (1997). Ethnogeriatrics: Cross-cultural care of older adults. *Generations,* Winter, 72-77.

CHAPTER 9

ELDER MISTREATMENT

Perle Slavik Cowen

During the last 20 years elder mistreatment increasingly has been recognized as a serious and complex problem with multiple etiologies and manifestations. It has often been described as the last form of family violence to receive attention from practitioners and researchers (Phillips, 1988). Although a variety of terms have been used to describe this phenomenon, including *granny bashing, battered elder syndrome, maltreatment of the elder,* and *elder abuse* or *neglect* (Anetzberger, 1987; Block & Sinnott, 1979; Cornell, 1987; Gelles & Cornell, 1982; Haviland & O'Brian, 1989; Labrousse, 1988; O'Connor, 1988), the current recommended framework for organizing the subcategories of this phenomenon is elder mistreatment (Breckman & Alderman, 1988).

Despite increasing scholarly publications, health care professionals still lack knowledge regarding assessment, diagnosis, intervention, outcome, and reporting criteria of elder mistreatment (Haviland & O'Brian, 1989; Jones, Veenstra, Seamon, & Krohmer, 1997; Kleinschmidt, 1997; Krueger & Patterson, 1997; Tilden et al., 1994). Standardized nursing care classification systems including nursing diagnoses (North American Nursing Diagnosis Association [NANDA], 1999), *Nursing Interventions Classification (NIC)* (Iowa Intervention Project, 2000), and *Nursing Outcomes Classification (NOC)* (Iowa Outcomes Project, 2000) offer the potential for a more effective approach to the prevention and treatment of elder mistreatment. However, since these systems were developed independently, their categorizations, definitions, variables, criteria, and prioritization for concept development often differ. A more seamless linkage among these classification systems could provide guidance to both practitioners and researchers in addressing this multidimensional problem. Nursing classifications that are specific to the type of mistreatment, victim population, caregiver risks and inabilities, and preventive level (prevention versus protection) would offer the most guidance to both practitioners and researchers.

The federal definitions of elder abuse, neglect, and exploitation, which first appeared in 1987 in the amendments to the Older Americans Act, were intended to serve only as guidelines for identifying problems and not for enforcement purposes (National Center on Elder Abuse [NCEA], 1997). Statutes defining elder mistreatment for enforcement purposes exist in all 50 states; however, dif-

ferences exist in both their definition and whether they are categorized as elder mistreatment legislation or as part of a more broadly constructed adult protective services legislation (Hunzeker, 1990). The three basic categories of elder mistreatment are (1) domestic elder mistreatment, (2) institutional elder mistreatment, and (3) self-neglect or self-abuse (self-abuse is not addressed in this chapter). Generally, elder mistreatment is also addressed in terms of acts of commission (intentional infliction of harm) or acts of omission (harm occurring through neglect) by a caregiver. Although the definition of a caregiver may vary among states, a typical definition is "a related or nonrelated person who has the responsibility for the protection, care or custody of a dependent adult as a result of assuming the responsibility voluntarily, by contract, through employment, or by order of the court" (Iowa Department of Elder Affairs, 1992).

The literature describes eight types of elder mistreatment (Capezuti, Brush, & Lawson, 1997; Fulmer, 1991; Hirst & Miller, 1986; Quinn & Tomita, 1986; Sengstock & Hwalek, 1985): physical abuse and neglect, sexual abuse, psychologic abuse and neglect, financial or material exploitation, violation of personal rights, and self-neglect (Table 9-1). Individual cases can exhibit characteristics of multiple types of mistreatment, with degrees of severity ranging from mild to lethal. Physical abuse refers to intentional use of physical force that results in bodily harm, anguish, or pain. Physical abuse includes such acts of violence as striking (with or without an object), hitting, beating, pushing, shaking, slapping, kicking, pinching, burning, the inappropriate use of drugs or physical restraints, force-feeding, and any other kind of physical punishment. Research has indicated that mistreatment of an elder seldom occurs as an isolated incident, with physical abuse and neglect reccurring in up to 80% of cases (O'Malley, O'Malley, Everitt, & Sarson, 1984). Among 3153 emergency department visits where elder physical abuse or neglect was reported, only 1975 different patients were seen, with 63% representing repeat visits and 60.3% having presented within the previous 30 days (Fulmer, McMahon, Baer-Hines, & Forget, 1992).

Physical neglect is defined as the refusal or failure to provide for the basic necessities of life, including food, water, shelter, clothing, personal hygiene, medicine, comfort, and personal safety. However, this category is

Table 9-1	Types of Elder Mistreatment
Type	**Definition**
Physical abuse	Intentional acts by a caregiver resulting in bodily harm, anguish, or pain; acts that are typically at variance with the history given of them; unreasonable confinement, punishment, or assault; repeated patterns of physical punishment with short- or long-term effects
Physical neglect	Willful or negligent acts or omissions by a caregiver that deprive the elder of minimum food, shelter, clothing, supervision, physical or mental health care, or other care necessary to maintain life or health; failure to provide for a care need despite having the resources or being aware of available resources that could fulfill the need
Sexual abuse	Any form of involuntary sexual contact, including incest, rape, molestation, prostitution, or participation in sexual acts; acts that are typically perpetrated through threats of force, coercion, or misrepresentation
Psychologic abuse	Verbal assault by a caregiver that dehumanizes and causes mental anguish to the elder, including name calling, ridiculing, humiliating, threatening, or inducing fear of isolation or removal
Psychologic neglect	Failure of the caregiver to satisfy the emotional or psychologic needs of an elder, including isolating the elder or not providing social or cognitive stimulation
Financial or material exploitation	The act or process of using or taking the material goods of an elder for personal or pecuniary gain without consent or authority or through the use of undue influence; includes theft, mismanagement, or the blocking of access to her property and contracts
Violation of personal rights	Taking unlawful advantage of the legally guaranteed rights of the elder, including denied contracting, which prevents the elder from marriage, divorce, preparing a will, buying, selling, leasing, or lending; involuntary servitude, thus preventing the elder from leaving his residence, deciding where to live, or participating in activities such as voting or religious worship; unnecessary guardianship; or misuse of professional authority

laden with definitional issues related to its multiple underlying etiologies. Some researchers advocate the further subdividing of physical neglect into the categories of active neglect (purposeful withholding of necessities) and passive neglect (legitimate inability of the care provider to perform caregiving duties) based on the intent and capacities of the caregiver (Bristowe, 1989). Societal ambiguity underlies questions related to the nature and extent of family caregiver duties owed to the elder, since the term *neglect* implies a failure to fulfill an obligation (Lachs & Fulmer, 1993; Phillips, 1988). Conceptual and practical problems of this type have led some researchers to abandon traditional definitions and to conceptualize the problem as inadequate care of the elderly individual (Fulmer, 1987) or to propose that a caregiving paradigm be used to formulate intervention strategies (Phillips, 1988). However, these models can place the elder at risk by employing interventions that focus on counseling and education when legal interventions are more appropriate (Phillips, 1988). Self-neglect refers to the demonstrated inability to provide for one's own basic needs caused by physical and/or mental impairments or diminished capacity (Capezuti et al., 1997).

Sexual abuse refers to any form of nonconsensual sexual contact or sexual contact with an elder incapable of giving consent and includes rape, sodomy, coerced nudity, molestation, prostitution, and sexually explicit photography. Psychologic or emotional abuse is defined as the infliction of mental anguish through verbal acts, including name calling, ridicule, humiliation, intimidation, threats, or harassment. Psychologic neglect refers to nonverbal infliction of mental anguish through use of the "silent treatment" or social isolation. Financial or material exploitation is the illegal or improper use of an elder's funds, property, or assets without permission or through deception. Violation of personal rights is the unlawful obstruction of an elder's legal rights and includes such actions as impeding his right to engage in marriage, divorce, preparation of a will, buying or selling of his assets, or deciding where to live, as well as unnecessary establishment of guardianship or misuse of professional authority.

PREVALENCE

Elder mistreatment, like other forms of family violence, can be difficult to detect. Victims often do not complain because of their perceived dependency on the perpetrator or because of their fears of reprisal or embarrassment. In addition, cognitive impairments can affect the elder's memory or her ability to communicate, and age-related vulnerabilities can confound mistreatment symptoms in such areas as falls, dehydration, malnutrition, and drug toxicity (Haviland & O'Brian, 1989). The incidence of elder mistreatment has been estimated to range from 4% (Block & Sinnott, 1979) to 10% (Fulmer, 1992; Lau & Kosberg, 1979) of the aged population, affecting between 700,000 and 2.5 million elders each year (Fulmer et al., 1992; Iowa Department of Elder Affairs, 1992). The discrepancy in prevalence rates has been attributed to methodologic limitations, to extrapolation of small samples to the total elderly population of the United States (Pillemer & Suitor, 1988), and to lack of specificity in elder mistreatment definitions.

In the first large-scale study of mistreatment in community-dwelling elders, prevalence rates of 32/1000 were reported for all types of abuse. Physical violence emerged as the most widespread form, with a prevalence rate of 20/1000 (Pillemer & Finkelhor, 1988). However, in a study of hospital-based elders, referrals for neglect occurred at approximately five times the rate of referrals for physical abuse (Carr et al., 1986). Although spouse abuse has not received much attention, several studies suggest that it is a major component of elder mistreatment (Pillemer & Finkelhor, 1988; Wolf, 1986). In a national family violence study, researchers found husband-to-wife physical violence among 3.3% of married, elderly respondents and wife-to-husband violence among 4.2% (Straus & Gelles, 1986).

A statewide review of elder mistreatment reports found that financial exploitation was the most frequently reported abuse (49%), followed by emotional abuse (36%) and neglect (33%) (Neale, Hwalek, Goodrich, & Quinn, 1996). These findings were consistent with those of others who have noted that financial exploitation is a common type of elder mistreatment (Ogg & Bennett, 1992), particularly among those with dementia (Rowe, Davies, Baburaj, & Sinha, 1993). Nationwide, the reporting of elder mistreatment has increased steadily, with 241,000 reports filed in 1994. This figure represents a 106.6% increase from 1986 (NCEA, 1997). Of the non–self-mistreatment reports that were substantiated in 1994, 58.5% involved neglect, 15.7% involved physical abuse, and 12.3% involved financial or material exploitation. The victims' median age was 76.5 years, and the majority were female (62.1%). Of all the victims, 65.4% were white, 21.4% were black, 9.6% were Hispanic, and less than 1% were Native Americans, Asian Americans, or Pacific Islanders (NCEA, 1997).

RELATED FACTORS/ETIOLOGIES

As with other forms of family violence, theoretical perspectives on the causes and correlates of elder mistreatment are many and varied. The inability of single dimensional models to adequately address the known characteristics of elder mistreatment has resulted in the proposal of several multidimensional models that address specific types of elder mistreatment, such as neglect or spouse abuse (Delunas, 1990; Hamilton, 1989b; Karuza, Zevon, Gleason, Karuza, & Nash, 1990; Phillips, 1988; Pillemer & Suitor, 1988). Additionally, the caregiver stress model emphasizes the combination of resentment (generated by the elder's increased financial, physical, and/or emotional dependency) and ineffective caregiver coping (related to the increased responsibilities and lack of resources) (Cicirelli, 1983).

The ecologic model was adapted to address the many overlapping etiologies of the different types of elder mistreatment and to serve as a guide for the differing levels of preventive interventions (Figure 9-1). This model is based on the ecologic model of child maltreatment (Garbarino, 1977), which in turn is derived from the ecologic model of human development (Bronfenbrenner, 1977). The model is a paradigm for examining the complex interactions among elder victims' and caregivers' characteristics, intrafamilial and extrafamilial stressors, and the social and cultural systems. It also offers a framework for considering risk factors, available supports, and resources in relation to a topology of four levels (individual, familial, social, and cultural) (Howze & Kotch, 1987). Inadequately buffered risk factors within these levels can be translated into defining characteristics within nursing diagnoses, thereby providing guidance to both the activities of nursing interventions and the patient indicators of nursing outcomes. The model also provides guidance to diagnoses, interventions, and outcomes directed at the primary, secondary, and tertiary levels of elder mistreatment prevention.

RISK FACTORS

The importance of early identification and intervention lies in its potential for reducing or preventing the occurrence of elder mistreatment. Although the elder mistreatment literature has expanded significantly, a dearth of scientific studies remains. Most existing knowledge is based on small studies, nonrepresentative samples, clinical reports, and informal surveys (Jones, 1994; Jones et al., 1997). Those variables that have been associated with elder mistreatment can be classified into four separate domains: sociocultural factors, family factors, caregiver factors, and individual characteristics of the elder (Box 9-1). Stress arising from these domains can be situational, acute, or chronic in nature. To date, research has not indicated that there are any factors that are both present in all mistreating circumstances and absent in all nonmistreating circumstances. Thus there is no litmus test for elder mistreatment, but only related risk factors whose identification provides the opportunity for preventive measures to be directed at stressful environments or interpersonal relationships.

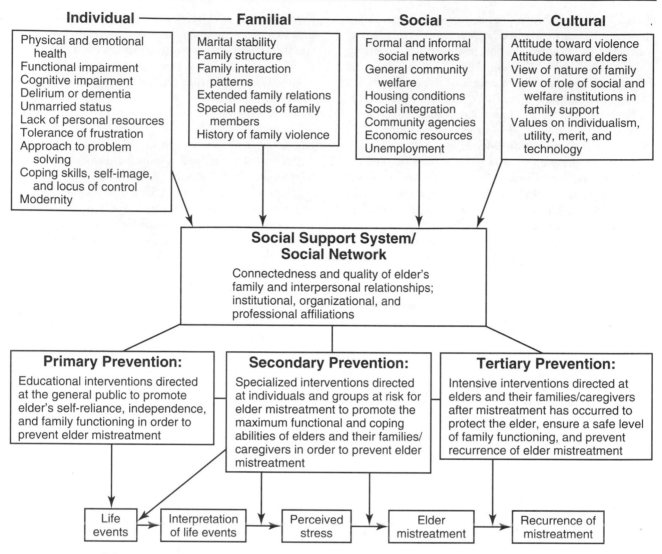

FIGURE **9-1**   The ecological model of elder mistreatment: Implications for prevention. (Adapted from Howze, D. C., & Kotch, J. B. [1984]. Disentangling life events, stress, and social support: Implications for primary prevention of child abuse and neglect. *Child Abuse and Neglect 8*[4], 401-409.)

Sociocultural Factors

Although elder mistreatment in the Western world tends to be regarded as a relatively recent phenomenon, research has demonstrated that the view of yesterday's family as a harmonious multigenerational unit that relied on mutual goodwill is largely a myth. Annuity contracts from preindustrial European agricultural settings contain references to the right of the elder to continue to sit at the family table or use the front door of the house, suggesting elders' distrust of their family's benevolence (Rosenmayr, 1979). In colonial America elders were forbidden entry into towns because it was feared they would increase the almshouses population, and poor widows were "warned-out" and forced to wander from town to town (Steinmetz, 1990). A 1772 New Jersey law required Justices of Peace to search arriving ships for old persons and other undesir-

ables and to send them away to prevent the growth of pauperism (Smith, 1980). In agrarian families parents with property often used economic coercion to control the family homestead and ensure the allegiance of their children in case they became disabled or unable to work (Steinmetz, 1990). Recent research has indicated that, although cultural variations exist that modify the nature of elder mistreatment, it remains a current threat for older adults in many progressively graying societies (Kosberg & Garcia, 1995). Ageism, sexism, poverty, unemployment, and disability have long been risk factors for elder mistreatment (Kosberg, 1988; Quinn & Tomita, 1986).

Modern medical technology has dramatically increased life expectancy, resulting in protracted periods of time during which elders are susceptible to physical and emotional disabilities and subsequently have greater depend-

---

Box 9-1

Risk Factors

ELDER MISTREATMENT

Sociocultural

Increased life expectancy with inadequate support for technologically dependent, chronically ill, or very elderly survivors

Lack of alternative support systems for independent living arrangements of frail elderly

Misguided societal values, attitudes, beliefs about violence, ageism, sexism, and disability

Unemployment; constrained financial resources

Substandard or questionable elder care facilities

Family

Competing demands on family members

History of family violence or intergenerational conflict

Immediate and extended family conflict

Inadequate or dysfunctional communication patterns among family members

Inadequate support systems

Overcrowded or stressful living conditions

Refusal to accept support services

Social or geographic isolation

Stressful life events

Unaware of available resources

Caregiver

Abuse or neglect in childhood, particularly by the elder

Competing role demands and responsibilities

Easily frustrated; intolerant; inflexible; impatient

External and interpersonal stress, including sudden situational stress; perception of caregiving as burden; caregiver burnout

Failure to understand the elder's mental or physical condition

Financial problems or dependency

Hypercritical personality

Immaturity; easily excitable

Impaired judgment caused by dementia, confusion, or substance abuse

Inexperience; inability or unwillingness to provide care

Lack of empathy; low self-esteem

Major mental disorders, including schizophrenia and bipolar affective disorder

Pattern of violent behavior, including intergenerational or domestic violence

Personal limitations, including restricted social life, lack of privacy, or lack of emotional support

Poor health; illness that exceeds ability to care for the elder

Presence of conditions associated with violent behavior, including diseases, exposure to toxins, and ingestion of psychoactive drugs

Unrealistic expectations of elder's cognitive or behavioral abilities

Elder

Adverse physiologic change or progressive impairment without assistive support

Emotional and behavioral patterns that irritate the caregiver, including threats of violence, verbal abuse, disruptive behavior, wandering, or passivity

Failure to report mistreatment or blame caregiver (excessive loyalty)

Female of advanced age (over 75); small stature

Financial dependency, limited economic resources, or property desired by caregiver

Frailty; functional impairment

History of abuse or neglect of the family or caregiver by the elder

Impaired cognitive ability caused by dementia, confusion, or substance abuse

Incontinence (fecal or urinary)

Major mental disorders, including schizophrenia and bipolar affective disorder

Pattern of violence or theft

Presence of conditions associated with violent behavior, including diseases, exposure to toxins, and ingestion of psychoactive drugs

Relinquishes financial management unnecessarily or transfers authority to others who usurp the elder's resources

Self-deprecation, low self-esteem, self-blame

Severely impaired health status

---

ency needs (Council on Scientific Affairs, 1987). In 1994 there were 33.2 million elderly people in the United States (age 65 or older), comprising one eighth of the country's population (United States Census Bureau, 1996). Among this group 18.7 million were 65 to 74, 11 million were 75 to 84, and 3.5 million were 85 or older. The "oldest old" (persons age 85 and over), the most rapidly growing segment, has increased by 274% since 1960, while the population of those 65 and over has doubled. The "oldest old" population is expected to reach a total of 7 million persons by 2020 (U.S. Census Bureau, 1996).

Although medical technology has produced mechanisms for extending the quantity of life, the frail elder might not experience the same general physical health that might have been experienced by previous old-age survivors (Steinmetz, 1990). The majority of elder mistreatment victims referred to social service agencies are dependent and frail and have multiple impairments; it has been proposed that dependency is a major factor in their mistreatment (Fulmer, 1989). Health care professionals have reported that recent cost-containment measures, implemented by hospitals in response to Medicare DRGs, have resulted in the vulnerable elders being discharged "quicker and sicker" and that such practices represent a form of institutional abuse (Baumhover, Beall, & Pieroni, 1990).

Current trends toward smaller family size and more blended families have resulted in fewer numbers of offspring who must share responsibility for elderly parents, parents-in-law, aunts, uncles, and relatives from current and previous marriages (Steinmetz, 1990). Although home visitation services and independent elderly housing can extend the frail elder's ability to remain self-sufficient, these services often are unavailable within rural or isolated areas. The alternative of relocating to a long-term care facility in an adjacent community may be rejected by frail elders and their family based on both their underestimation of the elders' care needs and their fear of mistreatment within "nursing homes."

Since the 1960s, patients' rights advocates have portrayed nursing homes as substandard environments in which the elderly are at serious risk of mistreatment (Pillemer, 1988). These reports are often based on anecdotal evidence or summary reports of state ombudsman programs (Monk, Kaye, & Litwin, 1984). However, a study that surveyed 577 staff (19% registered nurses, 20% practical nurses, 61% nursing aides) working in long-term care facilities reported that during the preceding year 36% had witnessed at least one incident of physical abuse and 81% had observed at least one psychologically abusive incident (Pillemer & Moore, 1989). Additionally, 10% of the respondents reported that they themselves had committed one or more physically abusive acts, and 40% reported they had committed at least one psychologically abusive act. The researchers reported that mistreatment appeared to be related not to the expected variables of institutional size or staff characteristics (demographic, educational, or experience levels), but instead to situational staff variables, including frequently thinking of quitting, beliefs that elder "patients are like children," high burnout, high patient conflict, and personal stress (Pillemer & Moore, 1989).

Family Factors

An estimated 80% of health care for the elderly is being provided by family members (Baines & Oglesby, 1992). It has been reported consistently that family caregivers are the primary perpetrators of elder mistreatment (Anetzberger, 1987; Baines & Oglesby, 1992; Brandl & Raymond, 1997; Council on Scientific Affairs, 1987; Fulmer & Cahill, 1984; Gelles & Cornell, 1982; Homer & Gilleard, 1990; Kosberg, 1988; Pillemer & Finkelhor, 1988, 1989; Tomita, 1982; Wolf, 1990). Researchers have reported that in 86% of mistreatment cases the abuser is a relative who lives with the elder approximately 75% of the time and who has cared for the elder an average of 9.5 years (O'Malley,

Everitt, & O'Malley, 1983). However, findings vary as to the nature of the perpetrator's relationship to the victim. Some studies have reported that the abuser is most likely the elder's adult child (Hirst & Miller, 1986; Mildenberger & Wessman, 1986). However, Pillemer and Finkelhor (1988) found that the perpetrator of mistreatment in 58% of the cases was a spouse, as compared with the 24% in which it was an adult child (Pillemer & Finkelhor, 1988). A recent nationwide study of state adult protective service agencies found that two thirds of the perpetrators of elder mistreatment were family members; of all reports, 36.7% of the perpetrators were adult children, 16.1% were other family members, and 13.8% were spouses (NCEA, 1997).

Families who do not have a network of relatives to assist with caregiving or who are unaware of or unwilling to access community resources place themselves in a precarious and isolated position. It has been reported that community resources are generally less available to elders who are cared for by their family than to the isolated individual in the community (Council on Scientific Affairs, 1987). Shorter hospital stays and early discharges of elderly patients often result in rushed, unplanned, and unrealistic placement decisions that fail to consider the elder's need for complex physical care, the family's lack of experience in providing such care, and the family's lack of preparedness for the long-term consequence of caring for a family member (Boland & Sims, 1996; Sims, Boland, & O'Neill, 1992). Additional factors that have been linked to elder mistreatment include lack of family support or competing demands on the family (Boland & Sims, 1996; Mildenberger & Wessman, 1986; Pillemer & Finkelhor, 1989; Steinmetz, 1990; Stephens & Zarit, 1989), isolation (Pillemer & Suitor, 1988), economic pressures (Lau & Kosberg, 1979), a history of family violence or conflict (Fulmer, 1989; Grafstrom, Nordberg, & Wimbald, 1992; Straus & Gelles, 1986), and being unaware of or ineligible for government or community assistance programs (Steinmetz, 1984).

Caregiver Factors

The unrelenting and constant demands of providing care may lead to caregiver stress and frustration, especially when the elder is mentally or physically impaired, when the caregiver is ill prepared for the task, or when needed resources are lacking (NCEA, 1997). However, caregiver stress may or may not lead to mistreatment. The likelihood of mistreatment is increased when the caregiver has personal impairments or when professional assistance is unavailable. Studies have indicated that elder-caregiver dependency is a bidirectional risk factor and that the continued dependency of the family caregiver on the elder for financial assistance, housing, or other necessities represents a major risk factor (Hwalek & Sengstock, 1986; Lachs & Fulmer, 1993; Pillemer, 1985; Wolf, 1986). Other identified caregiver risks include the following: a history of emotional illness and/or substance abuse (Pillemer & Finkelhor, 1989; Wolf, 1990); psychologic impairment, including senile dementia or confusion (Kosberg & Cail, 1986); a history of being mistreated as a child (Gelles & Cornell, 1982; Sengstock & Hwalek, 1985); a history of violent or antisocial behavior (Wolf, 1990); poor health or physical frailty (Lachs & Fulmer, 1993); unrealistic expectations and a lack of understanding of the elder's needs (Quinn & Tomita, 1986); a blaming, unsympathetic, hypercritical personality with a lack of empathy or concern for the elder (Sengstock & Hwalek, 1985); excessive stress; external pressures and role conflict (Hudson & Johnson, 1986; O'Malley et al., 1983); and being overwhelmed and stressed in the caregiver role (Lachs & Fulmer, 1993).

Violent behavior also has been associated with the following underlying health conditions in caregivers: (1) illnesses including hypoglycemia, seizure disorders, central nervous system vasculitis, hyperthyroidism, infections, cardiopulmonary insufficiency, dehydration with resulting electrolyte imbalances, severe pain, and brain lesions such as tumors, abscesses, and trauma-related conditions; (2) exposure to toxins including carbon monoxide, hydrocarbons, inorganic mercury, and boric acid; (3) ingestion, overdose, or withdrawal from psychoactive drugs including alcohol, benzodiazepines, amphetamines, phencyclidine (PCP), corticosteroids, digitalis, lidocaine, pentazocine, narcotic analgesics, and those with anticholinergic effects that can produce atropinism (atropine, scopolamine, anti-Parkinson drugs, neuroleptics, and tricyclic antidepressants); and (4) major mental disorders including schizophrenia and bipolar affective disorders (Barry, 1984).

Individual Factors

Characteristics that have been reported to place an elder at risk include advanced age (over 75 years old) (O'Malley et al., 1983), multiple health problems that decrease the elder's ability to function without assistance (Rounds, 1992), functional dependence (Council on Scientific Affairs, 1987; Lachs, Williams, O'Brien, Hurst, & Horwitz, 1997), incontinence (Lachs & Fulmer, 1993), cognitive loss or dementia (Coyne, Reichman, & Berbig, 1993; Fulmer, Street, & Carr, 1984; Lachs et al., 1997), substance abuse (Quinn & Tomita, 1986), stoicism or failure to blame the caregiver (Quinn & Tomita, 1986; Sengstock & Hwalek, 1985), financial dependency (Council on Scientific Affairs, 1987), relinquishment of financial management unnecessarily (Heisler & Tewksbury, 1991; Lachs & Pillemer, 1995), certain personality traits (Comijs, Jonker, van Tilburg, & Smit, 1999), and overly demanding behavior (Kosberg & Cail, 1986). Additionally, an elder's violent behavior toward her caregiver can result in defensive or retaliatory violent behavior on the part of the caregiver (Kleinschmidt, 1997; Pillemer & Suitor, 1992).

Although some studies have reported that mistreatment is associated with elder frailty or functional impairment, which presumably increases the caregiver's burden (Jones, Dougherty, & Schelble, 1988; Kosberg, 1988; Lachs et al., 1997), other studies have generally failed to find a direct relationship (Pillemer & Finkelhor, 1989; Pillemer & Suitor, 1992). However, researchers have noted that, at a minimum, greater impairment probably diminishes an elder's ability to defend herself or escape a mistreatment situation (Lachs & Pillemer, 1995).

ASSESSMENT

It has been suggested that all older adults be screened for elder mistreatment, even in the absence of symptoms (American Medical Association [AMA], 1992). Systematic assessment of the elder, her potential caregiver, and her family constellation before initial placement or caregiving arrangements offers the opportunity for primary prevention of elder mistreatment. Ongoing assessment allows emerging problems to be addressed before they escalate to a dangerous situation. However, the nurse's involvement with the elder and her family typically is initiated by her need for acute or health maintenance care services; the point of departure will most likely be the presenting problems or concerns of the elder.

In the acute care setting several aspects of the elder's presentation should alert the clinician to the possibility of mistreatment, including long delays between an injury and treatment (lacerations healing through secondary intention), unexplained, discrepant, or implausible explanations of illnesses or injuries, alleged self-inflicted injuries or claims that the elder is "accident prone," repeated emergency room visits or admissions caused by dehydration, noncompliance with medication or care prescriptions, and the arrival of unaccompanied cognitively impaired elders (Lachs & Fulmer, 1993). Initial contact in the community or home setting allows assessment of environmental clues such as inadequate hygiene or physical safety precautions, unused or grossly contaminated assistive equipment, inadequate provision for shelter, food, clothing, or care needs, and the absence of assisting behaviors on the part of the caregiver as observed or reported by neighbors or other relatives. In all settings observation of the interactions between the elder and the caregiver is important. Indicators of mistreatment include fearfulness, agitation, and overreticence on the part of the elder. Indicators displayed by the caregiver include repeated interruptions, attempts to discredit the elder, use of a harsh tone, demeaning statements, lack of concern or treating the elder as if she were invisible, hostile or negative nonverbal interactions, and insistence on providing the elder's history.

Accurate documentation in cases of suspected mistreatment is crucial and should include the following details: (1) verbatim information obtained from interviews of the elder, caregivers, alleged perpetrator, and witnesses; (2) the stated provocation for treatment or request for services; (3) health history, including any "accidental injuries"; (4) a detailed description of the physical examination, including the elder's functional, cognitive, nutritional, and hygiene status, precise descriptions and photographs of injuries or impaired skin integrity, including elder and caregiver explanations as to how and when they occurred; (5) observed behavior and interaction of the elder and his caregiver; and (6) an environmental assessment either during the initial interview or through follow-up. The tone of the discussion should be professional, nonjudgmental, and supportive.

Physical and behavioral indicators of elder mistreatment have been widely reported (Capezuti et al., 1997; Fulmer, 1989; Fulmer et al., 1984; Hamilton, 1989a; Haviland & O'Brian, 1989; Jones et al., 1988; Lachs & Fulmer, 1993; Lachs & Pillemer, 1995; NCEA, 1997; Pillemer & Finkelhor, 1989; Pillemer & Suitor, 1988; Quinn & Tomita, 1986; Sengstock & Hwalek, 1985; Wolf, 1990) and are summarized in Table 9-2. Although a single indicator does not necessarily prove that elder mistreatment is occurring, the repeated occurrence of an indicator, the presence of several indicators, or the appearance of serious injury should alert the nurse to the possibility of elder mistreatment. The physical indicators of elder mistreatment can be mild to severe. Dramatic cases of physical abuse or neglect are readily diagnosed by the experienced practitioner, but cases involving psychologic abuse or neglect can be more difficult to identify (Lachs & Pillemer, 1995). Behavioral indicators of abuse can exist alone or can accompany physical indicators. They can appear as subtle clues that something is amiss, or they can raise questions that leave one with the sense that "something is not right here."

The role of the informed inquisitor is absolutely fundamental to the assessment of elder mistreatment. The reporting of suspected elder mistreatment to state authorities enlists the assistance of the adult protective services, whose professional staff has expertise and resources in this area. Diagnosis, management, and prevention of elder mistreatment should never occur in isolation, but rather should involve a multidisciplinary team of well-coordinated professionals from nursing, medicine, social work, and many other disciplines (Jones et al., 1997; Lachs & Fulmer, 1993).

In addition to the reporting requirements of state mandatory reporting laws, the Joint Commission on Accreditation of Health Care Organizations (JCAHO) requires nurses working in emergency departments to make referrals for follow-up of elder mistreatment. JCAHO also requires all emergency departments to have written policies and procedures concerning mistreatment, a current list of referral agencies, and annual education for employees in mistreatment identification and interventions (JCAHO, 1995). All nurses who work with elders should have access to resources of this nature. A number of tools are available

to assist the practitioner with both assessment (Table 9-3) and intervention (Lachs & Fulmer, 1993; Lachs & Pillemer, 1995; Reis & Nahmiash, 1995, 1998).

A variety of factors that affect professional assessment of elder mistreatment have been identified. Researchers who examined factors that influence clinicians' assessment and management of family violence reported that elder abuse was not frequently suspected by any discipline, that 75% of professionals had not received any education on elder abuse, and that formal educational content in family violence significantly predicted the reporting of elder physical abuse. Among clinicians whose practice included elders, only 32% of nurses included reporting as an intervention they used (Tilden et al., 1994).

Clinicians also are affected in their judgment of elder mistreatment by the severity of the situation, the personalities of the elder and caregiver, and the degree of effort that the caregiver is perceived to expend (Phillips & Rempusheski, 1985). Additionally, the complex interaction between family or interpersonal dynamics and elder mistreatment laws may create additional ethical dilemmas for nurses involved in the care of elders (Capezuti et al., 1997). Educating health care professionals about elder mistreatment has been found to be effective in raising awareness and promoting active intervention (Hyman, Schillinger, & Lo, 1995; Tilden et al., 1994). Detection, assessment, and intervention could be further improved with formal and continuing education on pathophysiologic changes of aging, characteristics of elder mistreatment, advanced gerontologic physical assessment, and advanced therapeutic interview techniques (Jones et al., 1997; Krueger & Patterson, 1997).

CASE STUDY

S. Alberts, a 77-year-old woman, presents at the emergency department at 6 AM attended only by ambulance personnel who report that she was found wandering in a neighbor's yard. Although it is late fall with daytime temperatures averaging 50 degrees, she is dressed only in a torn, dirty, sleeveless dress and is without footwear. She appears very flushed, is encrusted with dirt and excrement, and smells foul. She appears delirious and is very combative, striking often at the staff or attempting to scratch them with her long, jagged fingernails. Her physical exam reveals that she is dehydrated and slightly malnourished (weight = 100 lbs, height = 5 ft). Her lab work confirms that she is dehydrated with resultant electrolyte imbalance. Her medical records document that she was treated 3 months ago for dehydration and although her hygiene was not as poor, it was noted as a problem. At that time she was prescribed a tricyclic antidepressant related to her flat affect, and in her son's report it was noted that she refused to eat or care for herself and that she cried all the time. Her records indicate that her only child, a son named Russ, lives with her and provides for her care. Mrs.

Table 9-2	Defining Characteristics ELDER MISTREATMENT	
Type of Mistreatment	**Physical Indicators**	**Behavioral Indicators**
Physical abuse	Bruises, chafing, excoriation on wrists or legs; other physical restraint marks (indicative of ropes or devices) Burns: cigarette, rope, chain, or immersion; scalding of the lips and mouth Dislocations and sprains inconsistent with victim's physical abilities or accompanied by fingertip pattern injuries Hematomas, contusions, welts, lacerations, scratches, punctures, or abrasions in various stages of healing on the face, lips, mouth, torso, back, buttocks, or arms (including defensive pattern on forearms) or clustered on the trunk Human bite marks Unusual pattern injuries (impression of a belt, hairbrush, fingertips) Fractures: simple or multiple (may be in various stages of healing) of the skull, nose, ribs, hips; fractures inconsistent with type of accident described or with victim's physical abilities Patches of missing hair or tender scalp Poisoning; drug toxicity or overdose	Prolonged interval between injury and professional treatment Injuries and trauma inconsistent with reported cause or unexplained injuries Illogical account of how injury occurred or information given reluctantly Vague health complaints Unexplained injuries or falls; frequent falls Depression, anxiety, nervousness, hostility Withdrawal, timidity, low self-esteem, passivity Unresponsiveness, stupor Confusion (confuses night and day) Death wishes or threats Overly anxious to please, overly compliant Shops around for physicians Reports erratic eating and sleeping patterns Speaks slowly with little feeling Appears humiliated and defeated Closely watches the caregiver, sits far away, or dodges as if expecting to be hit Elder's report of physical abuse Substance abuse
Physical neglect	Homelessness; inadequate shelter; inadequate environmental hygiene or physical safety precautions; inadequate protection from environmental hazards Poor hygiene; elder may be encrusted with dirt, food, and excrement; have foul odors; decayed teeth; overgrown fingernails or toenails; infestation of lice or other vermin; numerous insect bites Inadequate or inappropriate clothing or deprivation of footwear; hypothermia Perineal excoriation and skin breakdown caused by extended contact with urine and stool Restricted mobility or inadequate assistance with mobility or position changes as evidenced by skin breakdown, decubiti, or contractures Malnutrition or inadequate nutrition; dehydration, weight loss, anemia, physical evidence of inadequate or restricted foods being ingested; fecal impaction Deprivation or inadequate (damaged) aids to mobility and perception (canes, walkers, glasses, hearing aids, dentures) Untreated health problems Inadequate or inconsistent provision of medications or prescribed treatments Deprivation of social contacts	Substandard housing is common; housekeeping is practically nonexistent, and living areas may be littered with rotting food, garbage, and animal feces, with environmental hazards present and accessible. There is no routine for activities of daily living, accompanied by almost total emotional indifference to elder's well-being. Elder may sleep on mattress without sheets and often blankets; she is encrusted with dirt and has foul odors. Reports from home visitors of elders who are technology dependent that needed equipment is dirty, frequently contaminated, not used, or used infrequently Elder reports being left in an unsafe situation, abandoned, or driven out Prolonged interval between illness and medical treatment Repeated admissions caused by probable failure of health care surveillance Reports inability to obtain medications Failure to respond to warnings of obvious disease or injury Elder demonstrates listlessness, depression; low self-esteem, apathy Caregiver demonstrates emotional indifference to elder's well-being

Continued

Table 9-2	Defining Characteristics—cont'd ELDER MISTREATMENT—cont'd	
Type of Mistreatment	**Physical Indicators**	**Behavioral Indicators**
Sexual abuse	Reddened or traumatized genitals Vaginal or anal trauma or tenderness; recurrent urinary tract infections; sudden onset of poor sphincter tone; difficulty or pain with urination or defecation Acquired sexually transmitted diseases Contusions, scratches, or abrasions on extremities and trunk; increased muscular pain with movement Dramatic change in previously well-managed chronic illness	Reports sexual abuse Dramatic behavioral changes or undetermined etiology Depression, anxiety, nervousness Withdrawal; defensive posturing when approached Confusion Aggression against self, suicide ideation Erratic eating and sleeping patterns Appears humiliated and defeated; speaks slowly with little feeling Watches the caregiver closely or sits far away Substance abuse
Psychologic abuse or neglect	Victim may or may not exhibit sympathetic stimulation related to anxiety and fear, including cardiovascular excitation, restlessness, insomnia, hand tremors, extraneous movements (foot shuffling, hand and arm movements), facial tension, voice quivering, muscle tension, gastrointestinal irritability Dramatic change in previously well-managed chronic illness	Low self-esteem Depression, anxiety, listlessness Nervousness, restlessness Speaks slowly with little feeling or not at all Appears humiliated and defeated Eyes ask, "Can anyone help me?" Closely watches the caregiver and is overly cautious around the caregiver
Financial exploitation	Deprivation of personal possessions Evidence that the elder's personal assets (money, house, jewelry, car) are taken without consent or approval of the elder	Overly dependent; loyal to abuser Lacks knowledge of guardianships, powers of attorney, and other legal matters and resources Lacks knowledge of finances and economics Willingly turns over possessions to caregiver or gives into pressure to do so Caregiver's use of the elder's money for personal benefit Unexplained loss of Social Security or pension checks
Violation of personal rights	Victim may or may not exhibit sympathetic stimulation related to anxiety and fear, including cardiovascular excitation, restlessness, insomnia, hand tremors, extraneous movements (foot shuffling, hand and arm movements), facial tension, voice quivering, muscle tension, gastrointestinal irritability Dramatic change in previously well-managed chronic illness	Elder reports she is being prevented from marrying or divorcing Involuntary servitude: Elder reports or appears to be prevented from leaving residence, deciding where to live, or participating in activities such as religious worship or voting Unnecessary guardianship Misuse of professional authority

Alberts is given intravenous fluids, and additional blood is drawn to determine her serum imipramine level. Since she is suspected of atropinism related to her medication, she is given an injection of 1 mg of physostigmine salicylate. Her delirium symptoms are rapidly relieved following this injection, and her mental status continues to improve as she is rehydrated. She states that she does not know where her son is and that she does not remember leaving her home. Following consultation, the admitting nurse and physician file a phone report to the adult protective services.

The intake case worker is unable to contact Russ by phone, and 6 hours following Mrs. Alberts' admission she goes to Mrs. Alberts' previous listed address. The house is in an older neighborhood, and although the lot appears slightly run down, the external portion of the house appears in good condition. The front door is open, and following extended knocking and shouting into the house, Russ comes to the door. He appears to have just awakened, smells of alcohol, and is slightly staggering. He is surprised that his mother has been hospitalized and states that he thought she was in her bedroom. He admits the caseworker to look in his mother's room with him. The interior home is littered with rotting food, garbage, and animal feces from numerous cats. Russ states, "Yep,

Table 9-3	Elder Mistreatment Assessment Tools
Elder Mistreatment Assessment Tools	**References**
Barthel Self-Care Index	Granger, C. V., Albrecht, G. L., & Hamilton, B. B. (1979). Outcome of comprehensive medical rehabilitation: Measures of PULSES profile and BARTHEL INDEX. *Archives of Physical Medicine and Rehabilitation, 60,* 145-154.
BASE (Brief Abuse Screen for the Elderly)	IOA (Indicators of Abuse) & AID (Abuse Intervention Description). Reis, M., & Nahmiash, D. (1995). *When seniors are abused: A guide to intervention.* North York, Ontario: Captus Press.
Checklist for Families Considering Caretaking of Elders	Steinmetz, S. (1982). Family care of elders: Myths and realities. In Stinnet et al.: *Family Strengths, Vol. 5,* Lincoln, NE, University of Nebraska Press.
Elder Abuse Diagnosis and Intervention Model	Tomita, S. K. (1982). Detection and treatment of elderly abuse and neglect: A protocol for health care professionals. *Physical and Occupational Therapy in Geriatrics, 2,* 37-51.
Elder Assessment Instrument (EAI)	Fulmer, T. T., & Ashley, J. (1989). Clinical indicators of elder neglect. *Applied Nursing Research, 2*(4), 161-167.
The Elder Assessment Protocol (TEAP)	Fulmer, T. T., & Cahill, V. M. (1984). Assessing elder abuse: A study. *Journal of Gerontological Nursing, 10*(12), 16-20.
The Functional Assessment Inventory (FAI)	Pfeiffer, E. (1982). *Functional assessment inventory.* Tampa, FL: University of South Florida College of Medicine.
The Functional Assessment-Staging (FAST)	Reisberg, B. (1986). Dementia: A systematic approach to identifying reversible causes. *Geriatrics, 41*(4), 30-46.
Health Status Risk Assessment	Johnson, T. F. (1989). Greensboro, NC: University of North Carolina.
Health Status Within the Family, Attitudes Toward Aging, Living Arrangements, and Finances (HALF)	Ferguson, D., & Beck, C. (1983). H.A.L.F.—A tool to assess elder abuse within the family. *Geriatric Nursing, 4,* 301-304.
Older American Resource Scale—Multidimensional Functional Assessment Questionnaire (OARS-MFAQ)	Durham, NC: Duke University, 1978. In Fillenbaum, G., & Smyer, M. (1981). The development, validity and reliability of the OARS Multidimensional Functional Assessment Questionnaire. *Journal of Gerontology, 36,* 428-434.
PULSES (physical condition; upper limb functions; lower limb functions; sensory components; excretory functions; support factors)	Developed in 1957 by Moskowitz and McCann. In Calvani, M. S., & Douris, K. R. (1991). Functional assessment: A holistic approach to rehabilitation of the geriatric client. *Rehabilitation Nursing, 16*(6), 330-335.
Rapid Disability Rating Scale-2	Linn, M. W., & Linn, B. S. (1982). The rapid disability rating scale-2. *Journal of the American Geriatrics Society, 30*(6), 378-382.
Risk of Elder Abuse in the Home (REAH)	Hamilton, G. P. (1989). Using assessment to prevent elder abuse and neglect of the elderly: Assessment and intervention. *Orthopaedic Nursing, 8*(4), 11-19.

the crazy old bitch is gone again, I lock her in her room when I want some peace, but she crawls out the damn window." He also states that "the doctors gave her medicine because she wouldn't clean herself, work in the house, feed herself or me either. . . . Now she sneaks up on me and slaps or pinches me, so I lock her up at night so she won't take off and I can get some sleep." He cannot remember when he last locked her up but thought it was "about midnight when I went to bed." He states, "I put food out for her and tell her to clean herself up." He claims that he "can't deal with her crap, she's always been a mean old hag, but she's really starting to get on my nerves. . . . Hell, I moved back home to take care of her so she should be grateful and quit causing trouble." During the interview Russ states that he is 53 years old, that he never married, that his father died 7 months ago, and that he has been unemployed for "about 6 months," having worked at a local tire factory before being laid off. He moved in fol-

lowing his job loss and admits to having a "little drinking problem" and reports drinking a "half bottle of vodka and a six pack or so every day." He reports that his mother owns her home and they live on her Social Security and savings. He states that "she got insurance money when the old man died and I take care of things for her or she wouldn't spend a dime."

Within 24 hours Mrs. Alberts' condition is greatly improved and she is listed as stable. Mrs. Alberts tells her nurse that she wants to leave and go home. When the nurse discusses the need to plan for discharge and expresses concerns about Mrs. Alberts' returning to live with her son, Mrs. Alberts states, "He's a bum, always has been, but he's all I've got now that my husband is gone, and I'm going home." She states the nurse must "tell Russ that he can't lock me up at night anymore" and that she does not want any more of those "crazy pills."

NURSING DIAGNOSIS

Among nursing diagnoses elder mistreatment is addressed primarily through caregiver risks and/or inabilities such as Altered Family Processes, Altered Role Performance, Caregiver Role Strain, Risk for Caregiver Role Strain, Risk for Violence: Self-Directed or Directed at Others, and Ineffective Management of Therapeutic Regimen: Families. Although victim symptomatology can be addressed through a variety of physical and psychologic states that result from mistreatment (e.g., Altered Nutrition, Less Than Body Requirements; Pain; Anxiety; Fear), this is not a comprehensive or succinct method of clustering the defining characteristics related to the types of elder mistreatment. The only type of elder mistreatment that is specifically addressed is sexual abuse (Rape-Trauma Syndrome; Rape-Trauma Syndrome: Compound Reaction; and Rape-Trauma Syndrome: Silent Reaction); however, the defining characteristics are not population specific. Nursing diagnoses are available for primary preventive concepts (Potential for Enhanced Community Coping) and secondary and tertiary preventive concepts (Ineffective Management of Therapeutic Regimen: Community); however, they are not specific to the concept of mistreatment or to elderly populations.

Nursing diagnoses that incorporate the known risk factors and signs and symptoms of elder mistreatment are needed to provide guidance and direct linkages for primary, secondary, and tertiary preventive interventions and outcome indicators. Recommendations for the development or modification of elder mistreatment nursing classification labels and content are grouped under victim related (secondary and tertiary prevention), caregiver related (primary, secondary, and tertiary prevention), and community related (primary prevention) categories (Table 9-4). Improvement of both practice and research would greatly facilitate the identification of elder mistreatment within nursing minimum data sets, which could further assist local and state public health departments to benchmark progress toward patient and community health goals.

CASE STUDY

The following tentative nursing diagnoses were made for Mrs. Alberts:

1. Physical Neglect: Elder related to caregiver (son) omissions as evidenced by failure to provide minimum food, fluids, hygiene, clothing, and supervision despite having available financial resources.
2. Physical Self-Neglect: Elder related to undetermined etiology as evidenced by client's dehydration, malnutrition, poor hygiene, and inadequate clothing for weather conditions.

3. Potential Financial Abuse: Elder related to caregiver's control of client's adequate resources as evidenced by caregiver's statements and the demonstrated inadequate provision for client's basic needs, including minimum food, fluids, hygiene, clothing, and supervision.
4. Caregiver Role Strain related to son's inadequate care of mother as evidenced by failure to provide minimum food, fluids, hygiene, clothing, and supervision despite having available financial resources, substance abuse, and inadequate knowledge of caregiving skills.

The nurse also determined that the following additional data were needed:

1. Formal mental status testing with regard to competency. (Was admission delirium related to additional factors beyond drug reaction? R/O possible contribution of dehydration, early dementia, and depression.)
2. Consultation with hospital social worker and adult protective services. If the patient is determined or suspected to be incompetent (usually a result of dementia), adult protective services may petition the court for temporary or permanent guardianship (Capezuti et al., 1997).
3. Referral to multidisciplinary team for case assessment and management recommendations.

NURSING-SENSITIVE OUTCOMES

NOC is comprehensive in providing type-specific outcome indicators for the preventive and treatment concerns of both the elder and the caregiver (Iowa Outcomes Project, 2000). The addition of population-specific indicators would greatly increase their utility in addressing the differing issues of these groups. The patient and/or family members, in consultation with the nurse, usually select patient outcomes, since the outcomes must be important to the patient (Iowa Outcomes Project, 2000). However, the management of elder mistreatment often involves difficult ethical dilemmas in this regard. Among these is the maintenance of confidentiality in the nurse-patient relationship for patients who insist on remaining in a dangerous or abusive environment.

Mandatory reporting laws require the disclosure of suspected elder mistreatment despite the adult victim's wishes. This practice is based on the ethical principle of beneficence, which obligates the reporters to act in a way that will benefit the mistreated or at-risk elder (Capezuti et al., 1997). However, some researchers contend this is problematic, since adults of all ages have the right to accept or reject medical treatment or social services and to make decisions that can be viewed by others as wrong or eccentric (Capezuti et al., 1997). This contrasts with the situation for children, who under the law are unable to protect themselves or make decisions in their own best

Table 9-4	Linkage of Nursing Classification Systems for Elder Mistreatment	
Nursing Diagnoses	**Nursing-Sensitive Outcomes**	**Nursing Interventions**
ELDER VICTIM RELATED		
Physical Neglect: Elder*	Elder Neglect Recovery: Physical* Neglect Cessation*	Physical Neglect Protection: Elder* Abuse Protection: Elder*
Physical Self-Neglect: Elder*	Elder Self-Neglect Recovery* Risk for Violence: Self-Directed* Neglect Cessation*	Physical Self-Neglect Protection: Elder* Abuse Protection: Elder*
Physical Abuse: Elder*	Elder Abuse Recovery: Physical* Abuse Recovery: Physical*	Physical Abuse Protection: Elder* Abuse Protection: Elder*
Rape-Trauma Syndrome: Elder*	Elder Abuse Recovery: Sexual*	Sexual Abuse Protection: Elder*
Rape-Trauma Syndrome*	Abuse Recovery: Sexual*	Abuse Protection: Elder*
Emotional Abuse: Elder*	Elder Abuse Recovery: Emotional* Abuse Recovery: Emotional*	Emotional Abuse Protection: Elder* Abuse Protection: Elder*
Emotional Neglect: Elder*	Elder Neglect Recovery: Emotional* Abuse Recovery: Emotional*	Emotional Neglect Protection: Elder* Abuse Protection: Elder*
Financial Abuse: Elder*	Elder Abuse Recovery: Financial* Abuse Recovery: Financial*	Financial Abuse Protection: Elder* Abuse Protection: Elder*
Personal Rights: Impaired*	Elder Impaired Personal Rights Recovery* Abuse Protection*	Personal Rights Protection: Elder* Abuse Protection: Elder*
Risk for Elder Mistreatment*	Elder Mistreatment: Secondary Prevention* Abuse Protection*	Mistreatment Secondary Prevention: Elder* Abuse Protection: Elder*
CAREGIVER RELATED		
Caregiver Role Strain	Caregiver Stressors Caregiver Performance: Direct Care Caregiver Performance: Indirect Care Caregiver Emotional Health	Role Strain Protection: Family Caregiver*
Risk for Caregiver Role Strain Risk for Violence: Directed at Others	Caregiver Home Care Readiness Abusive Behavior Self-Control	Role Strain Prevention: Family Caregiver* Abusive Behavior Rehabilitation*
COMMUNITY RELATED		
Risk for Elder Mistreatment: Community* Potential for Enhanced Community Coping* Ineffective Management of Therapeutic Regimen: Community*	Elder Mistreatment Prevention: Primary* Abuse Protection: Elder*	Elder Mistreatment Primary Prevention*

*Recommended for development, changes, or further differentiation in existing NANDA, NOC, or NIC.

interests, including those involving medical treatment or social services (Capezuti et al., 1997). Recognition of these considerations, as well as those related to the significant developmental differences between these groups, lends support for the notion of population-based outcome indicators.

In practice this dilemma might involve a more personal quandary. Practitioners can damage the therapeutic nurse-patient relationship when they report mistreatment against the victim's emphatic wishes. Yet if they do not report, they violate their mandated reporting responsibil-

ity (Jones et al., 1988). More complications can arise if the victim chooses to protect the perpetrator through denial, withdrawal, or reversal of previous complaints. In these circumstances the clinician has an obligation to provide the minimum safety outcomes of explaining to the patient that she need not remain in a dangerous environment, providing information about safe alternatives, and reporting his suspicions to the adult protective services (Brandl & Raymond, 1997).

There are additional problems associated with establishing safe outcomes for mistreated elderly patients who are incompetent, and these problems are greatly compounded when the family caregiver is the perpetrator. The highest nursing-sensitive patient outcome priority is to ensure the safety of the mistreated elder while respecting the patient's autonomy. The answers to two critical questions dictate how to achieve this: (1) Does the patient accept or refuse intervention? and (2) Does she retain decision-making capacity? (Lachs & Pillemer, 1995). A useful algorithm, developed to guide the management of elder mistreatment cases (Lachs & Pillemer, 1995), has been adapted to provide guidance in establishing outcomes in situations involving the above problems (Figure 9-2).

The specific outcome indicators for each mistreated elder are tailored to address the etiology of the situation and to guide interventions directed at the patient's immediate needs, with promotion of optimum independence a primary goal. Outcomes indicators that address reme-

diation of environmental hazards and/or caregiver or patient behaviors can be initiated during this period in concert with adult protective services. The expertise and authority of this department are often helpful in sufficiently motivating the caregivers or family to address problems in a timely manner. A multidisciplinary approach also enables a more efficient method for evaluating goal achievement.

NURSING INTERVENTIONS

The NIC intervention Abuse Protection Support: Elder includes identifiers for all types of mistreatment, is restricted to a unique population, identifies caregiver risks and/or inabilities, and provides a variety of primary, secondary, and tertiary preventive activities (Iowa Intervention Project, 2000). The further delineation of interventions by mistreatment type could provide the opportunity

Text continued on p. 111.

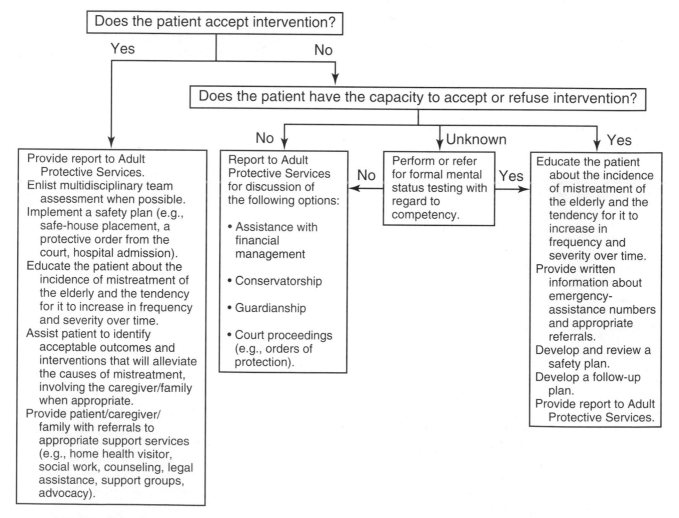

FIGURE **9-2**   Response to mistreatment of an elderly person. (Adapted from Lachs, M., & Pillemer, K. [1995]. Abuse and neglect of elderly persons. *The New England Journal of Medicine, 332*[7], 437-443. Copyright © 1995 Massachusetts Medical Society. All rights reserved.)

Table 9-5	Nursing Diagnoses, Outcomes, and Interventions for MRS. ALBERTS

Nursing Diagnoses	Nursing-Sensitive Outcomes	Nursing Interventions
PHYSICAL NEGLECT: ELDER *Defining Characteristics* Found wandering in neighbor's yard at 6 AM, disoriented, wearing sleeveless dress and no footwear in 40° temperature. Encrusted with dirt and excrement with generally very poor hygiene. Delirious and combative on admission, striking and scratching staff, found to be slightly malnourished, dehydrated with electrolyte imbalance and to have drug reaction (atropinism?) to imipramine. Stabilized with treatment. History of dehydration 3 months ago. Reported to be depressed, confused, and combative by son. APS data—Son reports being caregiver for 6 months, routinely locking patient in her bedroom at night to prevent wandering and violence toward him, was unaware his mother was missing 6 hrs after her admission. Son appears intoxicated and reports drinking approximately ½ bottle of vodka and 6 beers per day. House is littered with garbage, rotting food, and animal feces. Few indicators that son is providing direct assistance with ADL (see report). Patient wants to return home to live with son and states, "Tell Russ he can't lock me up anymore."	**ELDER NEGLECT RECOVERY: PHYSICAL** **NEGLECT CESSATION** *Indicators* Personal hygiene adequate Nutrition adequate Dresses appropriately for weather Supervision adequate Living environment clean Demonstrates interest in life Receives appropriate health care Behavior consistent w/social norms Adequate caregiver designated	**PHYSICAL NEGLECT PROTECTION: ELDER** *Activities* Determine whether elder demonstrates signs of neglect (see defining characteristics listed) Report suspected neglect to proper authorities Request multidisciplinary team and APS review to assess caregiver suitability and options Note patient relies on a single caregiver to provide extensive physical care and monitoring Assist patient/family to identify harmful care arrangements and identify mechanisms for addressing problem Discuss concerns about observations of at-risk indicators separately with patient and caregiver Determine caregiver's knowledge and ability to meet elder's needs and provide appropriate teaching Identify resources for elder/caregiver for functional support with ADL Promote maximum independence of elder and self-care through innovative teaching strategies Provide appropriate community resource information to elder/caregiver with details for accessing services Provide a public health nurse referral to ensure that home environment is monitored and patient continues to receive assistance Monitor for repeated visits to clinics, ER for inadequate supervision

Continued

Table 9-5	Nursing Diagnoses, Outcomes, and Interventions for MRS. ALBERTS—cont'd		

Table 9-5 Nursing Diagnoses, Outcomes, and Interventions for MRS. ALBERTS—cont'd

Nursing Diagnoses	Nursing-Sensitive Outcomes	Nursing Interventions
PHYSICAL SELF-NEGLECT: ELDER *Defining Characteristics* Found wandering in neighbor's yard at 6 AM, disoriented, wearing sleeveless dress and no footwear in 40° temperature. Encrusted with dirt and excrement with generally very poor hygiene. Delirious and combative on admission, striking and scratching staff, found to be slightly malnourished, dehydrated with electrolyte imbalance and to have drug reaction (atropinism?) to imipramine. Stabilized with treatment. History of dehydration 3 months ago. Reported to be depressed, confused, and combative by son. Husband died 7 months ago; periods of flat affect; lack of appetite and interest in self-care; confusion and violence reported by son. Etiology undetermined for history of confusion and violence.	**ELDER SELF-NEGLECT RECOVERY** **NEGLECT CESSATION** *Indicators* Personal hygiene adequate Nutrition adequate Dresses appropriately for weather Supervision adequate Living environment clean Demonstrates interest in life Receives appropriate health care Behavior consistent w/social norms Adequate caregiver designated Evidence of patient's competence for consent to treatment Evidence of court-ordered guardianship if indicated	**PHYSICAL SELF-NEGLECT PROTECTION: ELDER** **ABUSE PROTECTION: ELDER** *Activities* Determine whether elder demonstrates signs of neglect (see defining characteristics listed) Report suspected neglect to proper authorities Request multidisciplinary team and APS review to assess caregiver suitability and options Note patient relies on a single caregiver to provide extensive physical care and monitoring Assist patient/family to identify harmful care arrangements and identify mechanisms for addressing problem Discuss concerns about observations of at-risk indicators separately with patient and caregiver Determine caregiver's knowledge and ability to meet elder's needs and provide appropriate teaching Identify resources for elder/caregiver for functional support with ADL Promote maximum independence of elder and self-care through innovative teaching strategies Provide appropriate community resource information to elder/caregiver with details for accessing services Provide a public health nurse referral to ensure that home environment is monitored and patient continues to receive assistance Monitor for repeated visits to clinics, ER for inadequate supervision Determine if patient has the capacity to accept or refuse intervention; if unknown refer for formal mental status testing and APS with regard to competency
FINANCIAL ABUSE: ELDER *Defining Characteristics* Son reports that he takes care of money for mother. Son reports mother has adequate financial resources; demonstrated presence of unmet needs of mother. Found wandering in neighbor's yard at 6 AM, disoriented, wearing sleeveless dress and no footwear in 40° temperature. Encrusted with dirt and excrement with generally very poor hygiene.	**ELDER ABUSE RECOVERY: FINANCIAL** **ABUSE RECOVERY: FINANCIAL** *Indicators* Evidence of patient's competence to consent to treatment Evidence of court-ordered guardianship if indicated Protection of financial assets	**FINANCIAL ABUSE PROTECTION: ELDER** **ABUSE PROTECTION: ELDER** *Activities* Determine if patient has the capacity to accept or refuse intervention; if unknown refer for formal mental status testing and APS with regard to competency Determine whether patient demonstrates signs of exploitation including provision for basic needs when adequate resources are available

Caution patient to have Social Security or pension checks directly deposited, not to accept personal care in return for assets, and not to sign documents or make financial arrangements before seeking legal advice

Delirious and combative on admission, striking and scratching staff, found to be slightly malnourished, dehydrated with electrolyte imbalance and to have drug reaction (atropinism?) to imipramine. Stabilized with treatment.
History of dehydration 3 months ago.
Reported to be depressed, confused, and combative by son.
APS data—Son reports being caregiver for 6 months, routinely locking patient in her bedroom at night to prevent wandering and violence toward him, was unaware his mother was missing 6 hrs after her admission. Son appears intoxicated and reports drinking approximately ½ bottle of vodka and 6 beers per day. House is littered with garbage, rotting food, and animal feces. Few indicators that son is providing direct assistance with ADL (see report).

ROLE STRAIN PROTECTION: FAMILY CAREGIVER
ABUSE PROTECTION: ELDER

CAREGIVER STRESSORS
CAREGIVER PERFORMANCE:
DIRECT CARE
CAREGIVER PERFORMANCE:
INDIRECT CARE

Activities
Identify care arrangements that were made or continue under duress with only minimal consideration of the elder's care needs; caregiver's abilities; competing responsibilities, environmental accommodations, and quality of relationship between elder and caregiver
Identify situational stressors that may impede family coping
Assist caregivers to explore their feelings about care receiver and to identify factors that may contribute to mistreatment behaviors
Assist elders and their families in identifying inadequate or harmful care arrangements and help them to identify adaptive actions
Determine deviations from normal aging and note early signs and symptoms of compromised health through routine screening
Instruct on components of care plan, provide care teaching, and reinforce methods of monitoring changing care levels
Promote maximum independence and self-care of elder through innovative teaching strategies and the use of individualized pacing

Indicators
Reported stressors of caregiving; physical and psychologic limitations for caregiving; amount of care or oversight required
Assists with ADL; knowledge of treatment plan and disease process; monitoring of health status and behavior of care recipient; demonstration of competence in monitoring own caregiving skill level
Recognition of changes in health or behavior of care recipient; obtaining needed skills for care recipient's needs

CAREGIVER ROLE STRAIN

Defining Characteristics
Caregiver demonstrated inadequate care and supervision.
Patient found wandering in neighbor's yard at 6 AM, disoriented, wearing sleeveless dress and no footwear in 40° temperature. Encrusted with dirt and excrement with generally very poor hygiene.
Delirious and combative on admission, striking and scratching staff, found to be slightly malnourished, dehydrated with electrolyte imbalance and to have drug reaction (atropinism?) to imipramine. Stabilized with treatment.
History of dehydration 3 months ago.
Reported to be depressed, confused, and combative by son.
APS data—Son reports being caregiver for 6 months, routinely locking patient in her bedroom at night to prevent wandering and violence toward him, was unaware his mother was missing 6 hrs after her admission. Son appears intoxicated and reports drinking approximately ½ bottle of vodka and 6 beers per day. House is littered with garbage, rotting food, and animal feces. Few indicators that son is providing direct assistance with ADL (see report).
Patient wants to return home to live with son and states, "Tell Russ he can't lock me up anymore."

Continued

Table 9-5	Nursing Diagnoses, Outcomes, and Interventions for MRS. ALBERTS—cont'd	

Nursing Diagnoses	Nursing-Sensitive Outcomes	Nursing Interventions
CAREGIVER ROLE STRAIN—cont'd *Defining Characteristics—cont'd* Instability in care receiver's health and behavior. Inadequate coping as demonstrated by self-reported increased alcoholism problem. Situational stress—recent loss of father. Inexperience with caregiving. Lack of knowledge of caregiving activities. Inadequate use of community services. Caregiver isolation. Lack of respite and recreation for caregiver.		ROLE STRAIN PROTECTION: FAMILY CAREGIVER—cont'd ABUSE PROTECTION: ELDER—cont'd *Activities—cont'd* Provide environmental assessment and recommendations for adapting the home to promote physical self-reliance of elder Provide community resource information (e.g., residential respite, home health care, emergency care, transportation, substance abuse treatment, sliding-fee counseling services, Meals on Wheels) Help elders and their families identify coping strategies for stressful situations, including the difficult decision to discontinue home care Provide a public health nurse referral to ensure that the home environment is monitored and that appropriate care is provided

Nursing Outcomes Classification (NOC) 5-point Likert measurement scales:

Caregiver Stressors:	1 = Extensive; 2 = Substantial; 3 = Moderate; 4 = Limited; 5 = None.
Caregiver Performance: Direct Care:	1 = Not adequate; 2 = Slightly adequate; 3 = Moderately adequate; 4 = Substantially adequate; 5 = Totally adequate.
Caregiver Performance: Indirect Care:	1 = Not adequate; 2 = Slightly adequate; 3 = Moderately adequate; 4 = Substantially adequate; 5 = Totally adequate.

for more comprehensive type-specific interventions, as well as afford the clinician a more user-friendly format. Additionally, a category devoted to prevention of elder mistreatment could detail identification of high-risk factors before placement decisions and provide the nurse, elder, and family with an opportunity to more effectively review the potential consequences of their decisions (Kosberg, 1988).

The health care professional's role in comprehensive assessment and intervention in elder mistreatment has been well described (Arvanis et al., 1993; Capezuti et al., 1997; Capezuti & Diegler, 1996; Lachs & Pillemer, 1995; Nerenberg et al., 1990; Paris, Meier, Goldstien, Weiss, & Gein, 1995), and recently intervention models have been proposed (Reis & Nahmiash, 1995). Effective nursing interventions will include the following key steps: adequately identifying indicators of mistreatment; describing the nature of the mistreatment in a detailed and comprehensive manner; identifying necessary case management components as a key member or leader of a multidisciplinary team; promoting maximum independence and self-care of the elder through innovative teaching strategies; coordinating activities between acute and community settings to ensure continuity of care; providing direct care and serving as the elder's case manager; providing counseling to the elder, caregiver, and family to help them identify coping strategies for stressful situations; identifying social support resources available to the elder and his caregiver and assisting them in accessing needed services; determining the effectiveness of the elder and caregiver in their ability to meet the elder's safety and care needs; coordinating efforts with adult protective services to ensure the safety needs of the elder are met, to serve as an expert witness in cases involving legal intervention, and most importantly to provide guidance to the primary prevention of elder mistreatment.

CASE STUDY

In the case of Mrs. Alberts, the nurse was able to convince both Mrs. Alberts and her son that a more thorough diagnostic exam might provide cues to Mrs. Alberts' overall problems. Additionally, in discussion with team members the son was able to admit that he too had been having serious problems since the death of his father, who had been the "rock" of the family, including the escalation of his alcoholism problem. The outcomes selected for Mrs. Alberts are taken from the standardized nursing-sensitive outcomes developed by the Iowa Outcomes Project (Iowa Outcomes Project, 2000) (Table 9-5). Specific interventions for this case study also are listed in Table 9-4.

SUMMARY

Mistreatment is a harsh reality for many elders in the community and for many in institutions. Treatment is complicated by the multiple etiologies, types, and manifestations, process of diagnosis, time-intensive nature of interventions, resistance to their implementation, need for coordinated efforts with a host of other professionals, and the difficulty in evaluating efficacy of treatment. The lack of nursing diagnoses that address the signs and symptoms of the victim of elder mistreatment forms a major stumbling block to the linkage of the nursing classification systems. As the largest group of health care professionals providing care to elders and as the professionals most often serving as their advocate, nurses have a fundamental responsibility to provide leadership to primary, secondary, and tertiary prevention efforts.

REFERENCES

American Medical Association. (1992). *American Medical Association diagnostic and treatment guidelines on elder abuse and neglect.* Chicago: Author.

Anetzberger, G. J. (1987). *The etiology of elder abuse by adult offspring.* Springfield, IL: Charles C. Thomas.

Arvanis, S. C., Adelman, R. D., Breckman, R., Fulmer, T. T., Holder, E., Lachs, M., O'Brien, J. G., & Sanders, A. B. (1993). Diagnostic and treatment guidelines on elder abuse and neglect. *Archives of Family Medicine, 2,* 317-338.

Baines, E., & Oglesby, M. (1992). The elderly as caregivers of the elderly. *Holistic Nurse Practitioner, 7*(4), 61-69.

Barry, D. (1984). Pharmacotherapy in violent behavior. In S. Saunders, A. Anderson, C. Hart, & G. Rubenstein (Eds.), *Violent individuals and families: A handbook for practitioners* (pp. 226-242). Springfield, IL: Charles C. Thomas.

Baumhover, L. A., Beall, S. C., & Pieroni, R. E. (1990). Elder abuse: An overview of social and medical indicators. *Journal of Health and Human Resources Administration, 12*(4), 414-433.

Block, M. R., & Sinnott, J. D. E. (1979). *The battered elder syndrome: An exploratory study.* College Park, MD: University of Maryland Center on Aging.

Boland, D., & Sims, S. (1996). Family care giving at home as a solitary journey. *Image, 26*(1), 55-58.

Brandl, B., & Raymond, J. (1997). Unrecognized elder abuse victims. *Journal of Case Management, 6*(2), 62-68.

Breckman, R., & Alderman, R. (1988). *Strategies for helping victims of elder mistreatment.* Newbury Park, CA: Sage.

Bristowe, E. (1989). Family mediated abuse of noninstitutionalized frail elderly men and women living in British Columbia. *Journal of Elder Abuse and Neglect, 1*(1), 45-64.

Bronfenbrenner, U. (1977). Toward an experimental ecology of human development. *American Psychologist, 32,* 513-531.

Capezuti, E., Brush, B., & Lawson, W. (1997). Reporting elder mistreatment. *Journal of Gerontological Nursing, 23*(7), 24-32.

Capezuti, E., & Diegler, E. L. (1996). The role of the academic nurse and physician in the criminal prosecution of nursing home mistreatment. *Journal of Elder Abuse and Neglect, 8*(3), 47-58.

Carr, K., Dix, G., Fulmer, T., Kaulsh, B., Dravitz, L., Matlaw, J., Mayer, J., Minaher, K., Wetle, T., & Zarle, N. (1986). An elder abuse assessment team in acute hospital setting. *The Gerontologist, 35*, 115-118.

Cicirelli, V. (1983). Adult children's attachment and helping behavior to elderly parents: A path model. *Journal of Marriage and the Family, 45*, 815-825.

Comijs, H. C., Jonker, C., van Tilburg, W., & Smit, J. H. (1999). Hostility and coping capacity as risk factors of elder mistreatment. *Social Psychiatry & Psychiatric Epidemiology, 34*(1), 48-52.

Cornell, C. P. (1987). Elder abuse: The status of current knowledge. In R. J. Gelles (Ed.), *Family violence* (2nd ed., pp. 168-180). Newbury Park: Sage.

Council on Scientific Affairs. (1987). Elder abuse and neglect. *Journal of the American Medical Association, 257*, 966-971.

Coyne, A. C., Reichman, W. E., & Berbig, L. J. (1993). The relationship between dementia and elder abuse. *American Journal of Psychiatry, 150*, 643-646.

Delunas, L. R. (1990). Prevention of elder abuse: Betty Neuman health care systems. *Clinical Nurse Specialist, 4*(1), 115-118.

Fulmer, T. (1992). Clinical outlook: Elder mistreatment assessment as a part of everyday practice. *Journal of Gerontological Nursing, 18*(3), 42-45.

Fulmer, T., McMahon, D., Baer-Hines, M., & Forget, B. (1992). Abuse, neglect, abandonment, violence, and exploitation: An analysis of all elderly patients seen in one emergency department during a six-month period. *Journal of Emergency Nursing, 18*, 505-510.

Fulmer, T., Street, S., & Carr, K. (1984). Abuse of the elderly: Screening and detection. *Journal of Emergency Nursing, 18*, 505-510.

Fulmer, T. T. (1987). *Inadequate care of the elderly: A health care perspective on abuse and neglect.* New York: Springer.

Fulmer, T. T. (1989). Mistreatment of elders. Assessment, diagnosis, and intervention. *Nursing Clinics of North America, 24*(3), 707-716.

Fulmer, T. T. (1991). Elder mistreatment: Progress in community detection and intervention. *Family and Community Health, 14*(2), 26-34.

Fulmer, T. T., & Cahill, V. M. (1984). Assessing elder abuse: A study. *Journal of Gerontological Nursing, 10*(12), 16-20.

Garbarino, J. (1977). The human ecology of child maltreatment. *Journal of Marriage and the Family, 39*, 721-735.

Gelles, R. J., & Cornell, C. P. (1982). Elder abuse: The status of current knowledge. *Family Relations, 31* (July), 457-465.

Grafstrom, M., Nordberg, A., & Wimbald, B. (1992). Abuse is in the eye of the beholder: Reports by family members about abuse of demented persons in home care: A total population based study. *Scandinavian Journal of Social Medicine, 21*(4), 247-255.

Hamilton, G. P. (1989a). Risk of elder abuse in the home (REAH). *Orthopaedic Nursing, 8*(4), 11-19.

Hamilton, G. P. (1989b). Using a prevent elder abuse family systems approach. *Journal of Gerontological Nursing, 15*(3), 21-26.

Haviland, S., & O'Brian, J. (1989). Physical abuse and neglect of the elderly: Assessment and intervention. *Orthopaedic Nursing, 8*(4), 11-19.

Heisler, C. J., & Tewksbury, J. E. (1991). Fiduciary abuse of the elderly: A prosecutor's perspective. *Journal of Elder Abuse & Neglect, 3*, 23-40.

Hirst, S., & Miller, J. (1986). The abused elderly. *Journal of Psychosocial Nursing, 24*(10), 28-34.

Homer, A. C., & Gilleard, C. (1990). Abuse of elderly people by their carers. *British Medical Journal, 301*(6765), 1359-1362.

Howze, D. C., & Kotch, J. B. (1987). Disentangling life events, stress, and social support: Implications for primary prevention of child abuse and neglect. *Child Abuse and Neglect, 8*(4), 401-409.

Hudson, M. F., & Johnson, T. F. (1986). Elder neglect and abuse: A review of the literature (Monograph). *Annual Review of Nursing Research* (pp. 81-134).

Hunzeker, D. (1990). *State legislative response to crimes against the elderly.* Denver, CO: National Conference of State Legislatures.

Hwalek, M. A., & Sengstock, M. C. (1986). Assessing the probability of abuse of the elderly: Toward development of a clinical screening instrument. *Journal of Applied Gerontology, 5*, 153-173.

Hyman, A., Schillinger, D., & Lo, B. (1995). Laws mandating reporting of domestic violence: Do they promote patient well being? *Journal of the American Medical Association, 273*, 1781-1787.

Iowa Department of Elder Affairs. (1992). *Iowa Aging Information (Memo 92-72).*

Iowa Intervention Project. J. C. McCloskey & G. M. Bulechek (Eds.). (2000). *Nursing interventions classification (NIC)* (3rd ed.). St. Louis, MO: Mosby.

Iowa Outcomes Project. M. Johnson, M. Maas, & S. Moorhead (Eds.). (2000). *Nursing outcomes classification (NOC)* (2nd ed.). St. Louis, MO: Mosby.

Joint Commission on Accreditation of Health Care Organizations. (1995). *Accreditation manual for hospitals, Vol. I (Standards). Standards PEI.9 and PE6.2.* Chicago: Author.

Jones, J. (1994). Elder abuse and neglect: Responding to a national problem. *Annals of Emergency Medicine, 23*(4), 845-848.

Jones, J. S., Dougherty, J., & Schelble, D. (1988). Emergency department protocol for the diagnosis and evaluation of geriatric abuse. *Annals of Emergency Medicine, 17*, 1006-1012.

Jones, J. S., Veenstra, T. R., Seamon, J. P., & Krohmer, J. (1997). Elder mistreatment: National survey of emergency physicians. *Annals of Emergency Medicine, 30*(4), 473-479.

Karuza, J., Zevon, M. A., Gleason, T. A., Karuza, C. M., & Nash, L. (1990). Models of helping and coping, responsibility attribution, and well-being in community elderly and their helpers. *Psychology and Aging, 5*(2), 194-208.

Kleinschmidt, K. C. (1997). Elder abuse: A review. *Annals of Emergency Medicine, 30*(4), 463-472.

Kosberg, I., & Garcia, J. (Eds.). (1995). *Elder abuse: International and cross cultural perspectives.* Binghamton, NY: Haworth Press.

Kosberg, J., & Cail, R. (1986). The cost of care index: A case management tool for screening informal care providers. *The Gerontologist, 26*, 273-278.

Kosberg, J. I. (1988). Preventing elder abuse: Identification of high risk factors prior to placement decisions. *The Gerontologist, 28*(1), 43-50.

Krueger, P., & Patterson, C. (1997). Detecting and managing elder abuse: Challenges in primary care. *Canadian Medical Association Journal, 157*(8), 1095-1100.

Labrousse, W. (1988). Neglect of the elderly. *Florida Nurse, 36*(2), 5, 16.

Lachs, M., & Fulmer, T. (1993). Recognizing elder abuse and neglect. *Clinics in Geriatric Medicine, 9,* 665-681.

Lachs, M., & Pillemer, K. (1995). Abuse and neglect of elderly persons. *The New England Journal of Medicine, 332*(7), 437-443.

Lachs, M. S., Williams, C., O'Brien, S., Hurst, L., & Horwitz, R. (1997). Risk factors for reported elder abuse and neglect: A nine year observational cohort study. *The Gerontologist, 37*(4), 469-474.

Lau, E., & Kosberg, J. (1979). Abuse of the elderly by informal care providers. *Aging, 12,* 10-15.

Mildenberger, C., & Wessman, H. (1986). Abuse and neglect of elderly persons by family members. *Physical Therapy, 66*(4), 537-539.

Monk, A., Kaye, L., & Litwin, H. (1984). *Resolving grievances in the nursing home: A study of the ombudsman program.* New York: Columbia University Press.

National Center on Elder Abuse. (1997). *Elder abuse in domestic settings* (Elder Abuse Information Series #1). Washington, DC: Author.

Neale, A., Hwalek, M., Goodrich, C., & Quinn, K. (1996). The Illinois elder abuse system: Program description and administrative findings. *The Gerontologist, 36*(4), 502-511.

Nerenberg, L., Hanna, S., Harshbarger, S., McKnight, R., McLaughlin, C., & Parkins, S. (1990). Linking systems and community services: The interdisciplinary team approach. *Journal of Elder Abuse & Neglect, 2,* 101-135.

North American Nursing Diagnosis Association. (1999). *Nursing diagnoses: Definitions & classification 1999-2000.* Philadelphia: Author.

O'Connor, F. (1988). "Granny-bashing": Abuse of the elderly. In N. Hutchings (Ed.), *The violent family: Victimization of women, children, and elders* (pp. 104-114). New York: Human Sciences Press.

Ogg, J., & Bennett, G. (1992). Elder abuse in Britain. *British Medical Journal, 305,* 998-999.

O'Malley, T., Everitt, D., & O'Malley, H. (1983). Identifying and preventing family mediated abuse and neglect of elderly persons. *Annals of Internal Medicine, 98,* 998-1005.

O'Malley, T. A., O'Malley, H. C., Everitt, D. E., & Sarson, D. (1984). Categories of family-mediated abuse and neglect of elderly persons. *Journal of American Geriatrics, 32*(5), 362-369.

Paris, B. E. C., Meier, D. E., Goldstien, T., Weiss, M., & Gein, E. D. (1995). How to recognize warning signs and intervene. *Geriatrics, 50*(4), 47-52.

Phillips, L. R. (1988). The fit of elder abuse with the family violence paradigm, and the implications of a paradigm shift for clinical practice. *Public Health Nursing, 5*(4), 222-229.

Phillips, L. R., & Rempusheski, V. F. (1985). A decision-making model for diagnosing and intervening in elder abuse and neglect. *Nursing Research, 34*(3), 134-139.

Pillemer, K. (1985). The dangers of dependency: New findings on domestic violence against the elderly. *Social Problems, 33,* 146-158.

Pillemer, K. (1988). Maltreatment of patients in nursing homes: Overview and research agenda. *Journal of Health and Social Behavior, 29*(3), 227-238.

Pillemer, K., & Finkelhor, D. (1988). The prevalence of elder abuse: A random sample survey. *The Gerontologist, 28*(1), 51-57.

Pillemer, K., & Finkelhor, D. (1989). Causes of elder abuse: Caregiver stress versus problem relatives. *American Journal of Orthopsychiatry, 59*(2), 179-187.

Pillemer, K., & Moore, D. W. (1989). Abuse of patients in nursing homes. Findings from a survey of staff. *The Gerontologist, 29*(3), 314-320.

Pillemer, K., & Suitor, J. J. (1988). Elder abuse. In V. B. Van Hasselt, R. L. Morrison, A. S. Bellack, & M. Hersen (Eds.), *Handbook of family violence* (pp. 247-270). New York: Plenum Press.

Pillemer, K., & Suitor, J. J. (1992). Violence and violent feelings: What causes them among family caregivers? *Journal of Gerontology, 47,* 165-172.

Quinn, M. J., & Tomita, S. K. (1986). *Elder abuse and neglect: Causes, diagnosis and intervention strategies.* New York: Springer.

Reis, M., & Nahmiash, D. (1995). When seniors are abused: An intervention model. *The Gerontologist, 35*(5), 666-671.

Reis, M., & Nahmiash, D. (1998). Validation of the indicators of abuse screen. *The Gerontologist, 38*(4), 471-480.

Rosenmayr, L. (Ed.). (1979). *Socio-cultural change in the relation of the family to its older members: Towards an integration of historical, sociological and psychiatric perspectives* (Vol. 2). Paris: International Center of Social Gerontology.

Rounds, L. (1992). Elder abuse and neglect: A relationship to health characteristics. *Journal of the American Academy of Nurse Practitioners, 4*(2), 47-52.

Rowe, J., Davies, K., Baburaj, V., & Sinha, R. (1993). F.A.D.E.A.W.A.Y: The financial affairs of dementing elders and who is the attorney. *Journal of Elder Abuse & Neglect, 5*(2), 73-79.

Sengstock, M., & Hwalek, M. (1985). *Comprehensive index of elder abuse* (2nd ed.). Detroit, MI: SPEC Associates.

Sims, S. L., Boland, D. L., & O'Neill, C. (1992). Decision making in home health care. *Western Journal of Nursing Research, 14,* 186-200.

Smith, D. B. (1980). *Inside the great house: Planter family life in the 18th century Chesapeake society.* Ithaca, NY: Cornell University Press.

Steinmetz, S. K. (1984). Family violence toward elders. In S. Saunders, A. M. Anderson, C. A. Hart, & G. M. Rubenstein (Eds.), *Violent individuals and families: A handbook for practitioners* (pp. 137-163). Springfield, IL: Charles C. Thomas.

Steinmetz, S. K. (1990). Elder abuse by adult offspring: The relationship of actual vs. perceived dependency. *Journal of Health and Human Resources Administration, 12*(4), 434-463.

Stephens, M. A. P., & Zarit, S. H. (1989). Symposium: Family caregiving to dependent older adults: Stress, appraisal, and coping. *Psychology and Aging, 4*(4), 387-388.

Straus, M., & Gelles, R. (1986). Societal change and change in family violence from 1975 to 1985 as revealed by two national surveys. *Journal of Marriage and the Family, 48,* 1-15.

Tilden, V. P., Schmidt, T. A., Limandri, B. J., Chiodo, G. T., Garland, M. J., & Loveless, P. A. (1994). Factors that influence clinical assessment and management of family violence. *American Journal of Public Health, 84,* 628-633.

Tomita, S. K. (1982). Detection and treatment of elderly abuse and neglect: A protocol for health care professionals, *Physical and Occupational Therapy in Geriatrics, 2,* 37-51.

United States Census Bureau. (1996). *65+ in the United States* (P23-190). Washington, DC: Author.

Wolf, R. (1986). *Major findings from three model projects on elder abuse.* Dover, MA: Auburn House.

Wolf, R. S. (1990). Elder abuse: Scope, characteristics, and treatment. *Nurse Practitioner Forum, 1*(2), 102-108.

PART II

Nutritional-Metabolic Pattern

OVERVIEW

Nutrition is a concern for aging individuals at every stage of life; however, the needs of well and frail elders differ. In Chapter 10 dietitians Atkins, Brasfield, and Hudson discuss normal changes in nutritional-metabolic patterns, differentiating the nutritional requirements for these two types of elders. The authors point out common barriers to good nutrition and recommend health care provider interventions.

Pressure ulcers pose a major threat to elders, especially to those who are immobilized with chronic health problems. At present the accepted North American Nursing Diagnosis Association (NANDA) diagnoses Impaired Skin Integrity and Impaired Tissue Integrity do not have specific measurable signs and symptoms. As Frantz notes in Chapter 11, Impaired Skin Integrity: Pressure Ulcer, pressure ulcers can create life-threatening complications. In addition, financial costs for the health system and personal costs are great. Frantz explores the combination of pressure and time as the primary etiology in the development of pressure ulcers. She presents and critiques an assessment tool for grading pressure ulcers that is most useful to nurses in long-term care settings, describes interventions designed to promote circulation to ischemic tissue and healing of ulcers, and specifies the nursing-sensitive outcomes and indicators to be monitored to determine healing of these wounds.

In Chapter 12 Hardy addresses another significant diagnosis for elders, Impaired Skin Integrity: Dry Skin, which at present is not among the accepted NANDA diagnoses. Although dry skin is a common problem among elderly persons, the author notes that little systematic research has been done to identify etiologies or to test the efficacy of nursing interventions. Hardy reports her own research to test interventions related to this diagnosis using a psychometrically sound assessment and evaluation tool.

Nutritional problems account for one third to one half of all health problems in elders, and many independently living elders demonstrate nutritional deficiencies. In Chapter 13, Altered Nutrition: Less Than Body Requirements, Wakefield discusses risks of malnutrition, illnesses that interfere with nutrition, and psychosocial and economic factors that may influence nutritional intake. The role of the nurse in assessment of nutritional status and diet history is emphasized. Wakefield also offers a critical look at the NANDA diagnosis and suggests nursing-sensitive outcomes and interventions.

In Chapter 14, Impaired Swallowing, Tandy and Malan take the complex process of swallowing and identify each stage of the swallow by specific signs and symptoms. In so doing, the authors expand the broader NANDA conceptualization and advance nursing care planning for specific aspects of dysphagia in elderly clients.

Oral complications and poor oral hygiene are often problems that accompany aging, particularly among elders who have chronic illnesses and functional losses. In Chapter 15 Reese illuminates the diagnosis Altered Oral Mucous Membrane and sets forth plans for oral monitoring and oral hygienic care. Nursing-sensitive outcomes are suggested in relation to the diagnosis and recommended interventions.

In Chapter 16 Reese suggests modifications for the NANDA diagnostic label Fluid Volume Deficit according to tonicity, or the effect of the extracellular fluid on cellular volume. She discusses defining characteristics of the dehydration diagnosis, emphasizing the most common causes among elders. Nursing interventions and nursing-sensitive outcomes are evaluated and specified for each diagnostic type. Reese asserts that rehydration is the common nursing goal to treat all fluid deficits. She emphasizes that independent nursing interventions focus on prevention and notes assessment tools to detect fluid deficits and to test the effectiveness of preventive strategies.

A final metabolic problem common in advanced age is the increased risk of alterations in core body temperature. In Chapter 17 Holtzclaw clarifies the NANDA diagnosis Risk for Altered Body Temperature in the context of aging and elaborates on both hyperthermia and hypothermia risks. Holtzclaw proposes revisions in the NANDA diagnosis based on links with standardized nursing interventions and nursing-sensitive outcomes.

CHAPTER 10

NORMAL CHANGES WITH AGING

Capt. Kathleen L. Atkins, Karen S. Brasfield, and Julie K. Hudson

"Successful" aging occurs when the best possible adjustment to aging is achieved. "Usual" aging occurs among the population that succumbs to the effects of smoking, poor eating habits, and inactivity. Approaches to health promotion and wellness differ between the well elderly and the frail elderly. The frail elderly population continues to grow, and the number of people older than age 85 requiring long-term care is predicted to increase to 2.5 million by the year 2020 (Shoaf & Bishirjian, 1995). Although nutrition is significant at every stage in life, nutritional concerns differ between the successfully aging population and the frail elderly (Gray-Donald, 1995).

Older, healthy adults should enjoy a variety of foods but often require fewer calories secondary to decreases in activity, muscle mass, and basal metabolism. Healthy eating habits and regular exercise are key approaches for the well population. In contrast, meeting calorie and protein needs becomes the challenge for the frail elderly. With aging, regaining lost body cell mass becomes more difficult, making weight maintenance an important nutritional goal (Gray-Donald, 1995). Frequently the elderly do not eat a well-balanced diet because of social isolation, dental problems, depression, medications that affect food intake, poverty, and decreased physical ability to buy foods or prepare meals. A long-term decrease in calories puts the elderly at increased risk for specific vitamin and mineral deficiencies. A body mass index (BMI), kilograms/meters squared, below 24 is often indicative of compromised nutritional status in adults older than age 65. The lowest mortality rates have been found among men with BMIs between 23 and 30 and among women with BMIs between 22 and 30 (Coulston, Craig, & Voss, 1996).

Good nutrition can affect many aspects of the elder's life, including self-esteem, social structure, physical well-being, quality of life, and survival. Consequently, regular assessment of nutritional status is indicated. Tools such as the Nutrition Screening Initiative (Callagher-Allred, 1993) can be used to do standardized identification of older adults at nutritional risk. Nurses, dietitians, and other health care professionals also can undertake interventions to improve, correct, and even prevent problems leading to malnutrition and dehydration.

CHANGES RELATED TO AGING

A decline of bone mineral and matrix begins in early adult life. The severity of bone loss is individual and not totally understood. Changes in physical activity, the reproductive endocrine system, and calcium metabolism are thought to be the primary factors contributing to a decline in bone density. Postmenopausal women and men over age 60 experience a rapid decline in bone mass ranging from .6% to 6.0% loss per year (Kelley, 1992). Vitamin D intake decreases secondary to a decrease in exposure to sunlight and a decreased enzymatic production of vitamin D metabolites by the kidney and liver. Decreased vitamin D, in turn, has a profound effect on calcium use. The current recommended intake of calcium for postmenopausal women is 1000 to 1500 mg per day. These needs can be met through increased consumption of dairy products, green leafy vegetables, and supplementation.

Thinning of the skin, shortening of muscle fibers, and reduction of lean body mass give many elders the appearance of being frail and toneless. Anorexia, acute illness, and socioeconomic factors can result in a decrease in protein and energy intake. It is estimated that approximately 15% of the elderly suffer from protein energy malnutrition (PEM) and approximately 25% of the elderly individuals admitted to hospitals are malnourished (Powers & Folk, 1992). Malnutrition in the elderly is correlated with multiple hospital admissions, decubiti, and an increase in mortality and morbidity. Covinsky et al. (1999) found that malnutrition affected not only greater mortality, but delayed functional recovery and higher rates of nursing home use. In fact, it is considered a protective factor for the elder to weigh 10% above his ideal body weight (Powers & Folk, 1992). PEM can be difficult to identify because although lean body mass declines, fat does not and will sometimes mask the appearance of malnutrition. The consumption of a nutrient-dense diet with adequate protein will help prevent PEM and associated complications. Protein recommendations for the elder are currently being revised. It is thought that 1 gram of protein per kilogram of weight will help to maintain and prevent loss of visceral and skeletal mass (Campbell, Crin, Dallal, Young, & Evans, 1994).

Energy requirements for the elderly decline, but vitamin and mineral requirements remain stable or increase. This decrease in energy requirements should not impair nutritional status as long as nutritional value or density of the foods consumed is not sacrificed. However, meeting vitamin and mineral requirements with decreased caloric intake often is difficult.

One of the most remarkable changes with aging is the frequent development of atrophic gastritis and the inability to secrete gastric acid (Saltzman & Russell, 1998). *Helicobacter pylori* recently has been identified to cause this condition, which can lead to decreased absorption of nutrients and a decreased intake caused by irritation. Lactose intolerance, which seems to increase with age, can add to decreased intake of high protein foods such as milk and cheese.

Digestion of food begins in the mouth. Persons who have ill-fitting dentures, sores, or lesions in their mouth, loose teeth, or periodontal disease can find it difficult to consume adequate amounts of calories and nutrients. Often these individuals gravitate to eating soft foods, which have a tendency to be higher in fat and simple sugars and lower in protein.

Swallowing transports the food from the mouth to the stomach. Dysphagia is common in the elderly, and proper identification is necessary. Gastroesophageal reflux is also a complaint, causing individuals to experience heartburn after consuming a meal or within 2 to 3 hours of eating. Dietary restriction of certain foods may help with the symptoms. With both of these conditions it is necessary to treat the underlying condition while ensuring that adequate nutrition is maintained either by dietary modification or nutritional support. An age-related decrease in acid production by the stomach and a higher pH of gastric mucosa can result in an impaired absorption of iron, folate, calcium, and vitamins K and B_{12}.

Constipation, a common complaint among the elderly, also can alter nutritional status. First, a search for an underlying physiologic diagnosis should be made. Second, medications, dehydration, and lack of fiber in the diet should be examined. Third, the individual should be taught that normal bowel defecation ranges from 2 times per day to 3 times per week. Simple education may be helpful. The addition of dietary supplemental fiber is often included to help treat constipation; however, sugar-containing supplements may alter control in the individual with diabetes. Hydration, prescribed at the following rate, promotes good bowel function: 25 ml per kilogram of body weight or approximately 1 ml of water for each calorie consumed (Gottschlich, Matarese, & Shronts, 1993). For example, a 150-lb female would require approximately 1705 ml of water. Consumption of caffeinated beverages is not included in this amount because of their diuretic properties.

CHALLENGES TO NUTRITION

Assessing the physical capabilities of the elderly helps to evaluate their ability to eat a balanced diet. Many elders are confined to wheelchairs or walkers, have arthritis, or have other physical barriers to preparing meals. With poor vision, transportation is often limited. Shopping for groceries and meal preparation become restricted. Inability to self-feed decreases the quantity and quality of oral intake. In the elderly person with decreasing mental status, such as with Alzheimer's disease, memory loss, hyperactivity, depression, anorexia, and polypharmacy create further challenges to good nutrition. Altered cognition and psychiatric conditions can increase the risk of malnutrition in the elderly individual and should be investigated.

Changes in living conditions can have adverse effects on the elder's nutritional status. Coping with the loss of a mate, moving, social isolation, and loss of control is difficult at any age. The motivation to care for oneself is often lacking when an elderly person is faced with these and other challenges. Convenience items are often seen as simple alternatives in this segment of the elderly population but can cause an increase in fat and sodium consumption.

Anorexia and changes in taste perception, especially among smokers, are common in the elder. Poor fitting or lack of dentures can lead to decreased intake. Nutrient-dense food selections are essential to good nutrition for the elderly. Nutritional needs can be met by increased intake of dairy products, eggs, ground meat, and well-cooked chicken and fish. Canned juices or easy-to-chew fruit and cooked vegetables should be included in the diet. When self-feeding is not possible, the caregiver feeding the patient is crucial to adequate intake and nutrition. Frequent, small feedings of nutrient-dense foods are often required to achieve weight maintenance or gain. Nutritional supplements are an option if calorie and protein needs cannot be met through diet alone. However, nutritional supplements are not recommended for the healthy elder meeting his estimated needs through a regular diet.

Another potential challenge to good nutrition is living with a fixed income. Studies focusing on dietary intake indicate that low-income, black, and Hispanic elderly populations are at increased nutritional risk (Neyman, Zidenberg-Cherr, & McDonald, 1996). Elderly people with higher incomes generally have more nutritious diets. The elderly living in inner cities are often forced to pay higher prices because of their location and lack of transportation. As funds available for food decrease, fat consumption often increases secondary to price, convenience, and lack of nutrition education. Consumption of fresh fruits, vegetables, and meats often decreases, whereas consumption of convenience foods high in calories from carbohydrates and fat often increases. Targeting the elderly population with health and nutrition promotion messages geared to the special needs of this group is essential if this challenge is to be met.

Many elderly people are eligible for community-based nutrition programs. Title III-C of the Older Americans Act of 1965 provides for nutrition programs for persons age 60 and over. More than 50% of the elderly living at home do not meet recommended energy or protein intakes (Payette, Gray-Donald, & Cyr, 1995). Congregate meal programs provide food and socialization for many elderly people. A recent study by Neyman et al. (1996) showed that the mean dietary intake data and biochemical indices of nutritional status did not vary significantly between congregate-site meal program participants and nonparticipants. However, 28% of participants and 23% of nonparticipants were identified as having poor diets, eating less than 66% of the Recommended Daily Allowance (RDA) for at least three nutrients.

Meal delivery programs are another option available to many elderly people who are unable to leave their homes. In comparison with the congregate-site meal participants, 70% of the elderly population receiving home-delivered meals were identified as having poor diets (Neyman et al., 1996). The homebound elder may be put on waiting lists for home-delivered meal programs because of insufficient funds, thereby increasing her risk for malnutrition and related complications. The individual elder, a family member, or a health care provider can request home-delivered meal services. Many elderly people depend on these meals to provide their most nutrient-dense meal of the day. However, data indicate that these programs may not be nutritionally adequate. Gray-Donald (1995) reported that 36% of Meals on Wheels clients were at high risk for PEM. Coulston et al. (1996) reported that of 230 participants age 60 to 90 enrolled in a Meals on Wheels program, 74% were considered at risk for poor nutritional status using anthropometric, dietary, and lab indicators; 98% were deemed at risk using The Nutrition Screening Initiative's "Determine Your Nutritional Health" tool. The population identified at risk for poor nutritional status requires intervention to avoid the consequences associated with malnutrition (Coulston et al., 1996). Consult with your facility's registered dietitian or social worker for information on programs available in your community.

Good eating habits enhance health and longevity at all ages, contributing to prevention and delaying onset of many chronic diseases such as hypertension, diabetes, heart disease, and possibly some cancers. Weight reduction when BMIs are greater than 30, sodium restriction, regular aerobic exercise tailored to the elderly patient's ability, and avoidance of alcohol are important to the treatment of these diseases. Dietary education and follow-up geared toward the individual contributes greatly to the successful management of many chronic diseases and when adhered to will often decrease the need for polypharmacy.

MEDICATION AND NUTRITIONAL STATUS

Medication use, especially long-term medication use, and polypharmacy can affect nutritional status through decreasing appetite, decreasing nutrient intake, and decreasing nutrient absorption. Residents of nursing homes receive an average of eight different medications per day (Varma, 1994). Therefore awareness of potential food/nutrient-drug interactions that can affect medical nutrition therapy in the elderly population is critical for health care providers.

The most commonly used drugs in the elderly population include antihypertensives, vitamins, cardiovascular medications, and analgesics. Over-the-counter drug use of aspirin can contribute to iron-deficiency anemia. Laxative abuse leads to sodium and potassium depletion and to diarrhea. Antacids can inactivate thiamin and decrease folic acid and iron by increasing gastric pH (Worthington-Roberts, 1988).

Prescription drugs affect nutritional status as well. Many impair taste and cause dry mouth, nausea, malabsorption of nutrients, and abnormal nutrient metabolism. Vitamin K interferes with the effectiveness of warfarin sodium (Coumadin). Protein intake is regulated in persons taking the anti-Parkinson drug levodopa. Chemotherapy and radiation therapy cause many side effects affecting nutritional intake. Common drug-induced deficiencies include those of the B vitamins, vitamins C, D, and K, phosphate, potassium, calcium, magnesium, and zinc. According to Neyman et al. (1996), marginal zinc status has been suggested as responsible for changes in taste and smell acuity, delayed wound healing, and declining immune function sometimes observed in the elder. Dietary intervention is beneficial in avoiding complications associated with many food/nutrient-drug interactions and medication side effects. The full diet and drug history of the elderly patient is needed before undertaking dietary and supplement interventions and before changing medications to avoid drug-induced malnutrition (Varma, 1994).

An estimated 3 million people over the age of 65 in the United States abuse alcohol (Krach, 1998). Alcohol intake decreases serum potassium levels, increases zinc excretion, interferes with thiamin absorption, and can cause malabsorption of vitamin B_{12} and folate. It is difficult to diagnose a thiamin deficiency because symptoms such as heart disease, memory loss, and decreased sensation in the lower body are common in aging. Current and past alcohol use should be considered when assessing nutritional status in the elderly patient (Schlenker, 1984).

SUMMARY

Geriatric nutrition involves many complicated issues. As more people approach, pass, and live well beyond the age of 65, health care professionals must provide health promotion and care in the area of nutrition. Many resources are available to the health care provider caring for geriatric patients. The Nutrition Screening Initiative (Callagher-Allred, 1993) can be used as an assessment tool to identify older adults at nutritional risk. Interventions can be undertaken by nurses, dietitians, and other health care professionals to prevent problems leading to malnutrition and dehydration and, when appropriate, to help the elderly population improve and even correct nutritional problems. By addressing nutrition in a comprehensive manner, health care teams can assist the elderly in attaining improved self-esteem, social structure, physical well-being, quality of life, and survival.

REFERENCES

Callagher-Allred, C. R. (1993). *Implementing nutrition screening and intervention strategies.* Washington, DC: Nutrition Screening Initiative.

Campbell, W. W., Crin, M. C., Dallal, G. E., Young, V. R., & Evans, W. J. (1994). Increased protein requirements in elderly people: New data and retrospective reassessments. *American Journal of Clinical Nutrition, 13,* 277-284.

Coulston, A. M., Craig, L., & Voss, A. C. (1996). Meals-on-wheels applicants are a population at risk for poor nutritional status. *Journal of the American Dietetic Association, 96*(6), 570-573.

Covinsky, K. E., Martin, G. E., Beyth, R. J., Justice, A. C., Sehgal, A. R., & Landefeld, C. S. (1999). The relationship between clinical assessments of nutritional status and adverse outcomes in older hospitalized medical patients. *Journal of the American Geriatrics Society, 47*(5), 532-538.

Gottschlich, M. M., Matarese, L. E., & Shronts, E. P. (Eds.). (1993). *Nutrition support dietetics core curriculum.* Bodischebaugh, MA: American Society for Parenteral and Enteral Nutrition.

Gray-Donald, K. (1995). The frail elderly: Meeting the nutritional challenges. *Journal of the American Dietetic Association, 95*(5), 538-540.

Kelley, W. N. (Ed.). (1992). *Essentials of internal medicine.* Baltimore: Lippincott Williams & Wilkins.

Krach, P. (1998). Myths & facts. *Nursing 98, 28*(2), 25.

Neyman, M. R., Zidenberg-Cherr, S., & McDonald, R. B. (1996). Effect of participation in congregate-site meal programs on nutritional status of the healthy elderly. *Journal of the American Dietetic Association, 96*(5), 475-483.

Payette, H., Gray-Donald, K., Cyr, R. & Boutier, V. (1995). Predictors of dietary intake in a functionally dependent elderly population in the community. *American Journal of Public Health, 85*(5), 677-683.

Powers, J. S., & Folk, M. C. (1992). Nutritional concerns in the elderly. *Southern Medical Journal, 85*(11), 1107-1112.

Saltzman, J. R., & Russell, R. M. (1998). The aging gut. Nutritional issues. *Gastroenterology Clinics of North America, 27*(2), 309-324.

Schlenker, E. D. (1984). *Nutrition in aging.* St. Louis, MO: Mosby.

Shoaf, L. R., & Bishirjian, K. O. (1995). Standards of practice for gerontological nutritionists. A mandate for action. *Journal of the American Dietetic Association, 95*(12), 1433-1438.

Varma, R. N. (1994). Risk for drug-induced malnutrition is unchecked in elderly patients in nursing homes. *Journal of the American Dietetic Association, 94*(2), 192-194.

Worthington-Roberts, B. S. (1988). *Nutrition throughout the life cycle.* St. Louis, MO: Mosby.

CHAPTER 11

IMPAIRED SKIN INTEGRITY: PRESSURE ULCER

Rita A. Frantz

Despite advances in health care that extend life and improve functional status, pressure ulcers continue to be a frequent accompaniment of chronic illness in the elder. Pressure ulcers are generally defined as localized areas of cellular necrosis that occur over bony prominences exposed to pressure for a sufficient period of time to cause tissue ischemia. The National Pressure Ulcer Advisory Panel (NPUAP, 1989), an independent, nonprofit organization formed in 1987 and dedicated to education and research to prevent and treat pressure ulcers, has defined a pressure ulcer as a localized area of tissue necrosis that develops when soft tissue is compressed between a bony prominence and an external surface for a prolonged period of time. The Agency for Health Care Policy and Research (AHCPR) guideline (Clinical Practice Guideline Panel, 1992) defined pressure ulcer as "any lesion caused by unrelieved pressure resulting in damage of underlying tissue." Although these definitions dilute the complex processes involved in pressure ulcer development, they describe the basic nature of the problem. Normal tissue metabolism is dependent on a constant supply of nutrients and removal of waste products. Exposure of tissues to prolonged pressure in excess of capillary pressure inhibits circulation and limits normal exchange of metabolic substrates and waste products. If an inadequate level of circulation persists, cellular metabolism is disrupted and cell death ultimately occurs.

The financial and human costs of pressure ulcers are enormous. Pressure ulcers create the potential for life-threatening complications. Osteomyelitis and sepsis are ever-present threats for the patient with a pressure ulcer. Osteomyelitis has been reported to occur in 26% of patients with pressure ulcers, whereas bacteremia occurred at a rate of 3.5 episodes per 10,000 hospital discharges (Allman, 1989). The combination of bacteremia and pressure ulcers has been associated with a mortality rate of 50% among hospitalized patients (Bryan, Dew, & Reynolds, 1983). Recent figures on the cost of treating pressure ulcers reveal that the occurrence of complications is a major factor contributing to the overall cost of treatment. The mean cost of treating 45 ulcers that occurred over a 1-year period in a long-term care facility was $2731 per ulcer. When hospital treatment was excluded, the mean cost of treatment was $489 per ulcer (Xakellis & Frantz, 1996). On a national level the cost in treatment and hospital stays is estimated to be as high as $6 billion a year for ulcers that develop in hospital patients alone (Vasconez, Schneider, & Jurkiewicz, 1977). In the elder and institutionalized populations, pressure ulcers are estimated to encumber the health care system with an additional $1 billion in expenditures and 2.2 million Medicare hospital days (Staas & Cioschi, 1991). Preliminary evidence has suggested that an intensive program of prevention that significantly reduces pressure ulcer incidence is more cost-effective than treating ulcers that develop when routine prevention is absent (Xakellis, Frantz, Lewis, & Harvey, 1998). Clearly, in the absence of prevention the costs of incident ulcers are highest for patients who must endure financial hardship, pain, and disability directly attributable to pressure ulcers.

PREVALENCE

Although methodological limitations have made it difficult to assess accurately the magnitude of the pressure ulcer problem in the elder, epidemiologic studies suggest there is cause for concern. The prevalence of pressure ulcers, determined from cross-sectional counts of existing cases at a specific point in time, has been reported from 3% to 18% for hospitalized patients (Allman, Laprade, et al., 1986; Hawthorne, Jefferson, & Paduano, 1989; Maklebust, 1987; Meehan, 1990; Shannon & Skorga, 1989). Estimated prevalence rates of 11% to 24% are commonly reported in long-term care facilities (Brandeis, Berlowitz, Hossain, & Morris, 1995; Brandeis, Morris, Nash, & Lipsitz, 1989, 1990; Langemo et al., 1989; Pinchcofsky-Devin & Kaminski, 1986; Reed, 1981; Spector, Kapp, Tucker, & Sternberg, 1988; Weiler, Franzi, & Kecskes, 1990; Young, 1989). Isolated studies have found much lower prevalence, such as the 3% rate reported among elderly residents in one state-owned long-term care facility (Frantz, Bergquist, & Specht, 1994). The prevalence of pressure ulcers in community-based adults ranges from 6% to 33% (Bergquist & Frantz, 1999; Clark, Barbanel, Jordan, & Nicol, 1978; Fuhrer, Garber, Rintala, Clearman, & Hart, 1993; Hanson, Langemo, Olson, Hunter, & Burd, 1996).

Reports of pressure ulcer incidence, defined as the number or percent of "at risk" individuals who develop a pressure ulcer within a given time period, must be viewed within the historical context of prevention measures being introduced into routine management of this population. Before the introduction of turning as a routine preventive intervention, Norton, McLaren, and Exton-Smith (1962) found that 24% of patients developed a pressure ulcer following admission to a geriatric hospital. Subsequent studies of pressure ulcer incidence in the general hospital population have reported rates ranging from 1% to 29% (Allman, Laprade, et al., 1986; Andersen & Kvorning, 1982; Clark & Kahdom, 1988; Ek, 1987; Gerson, 1975; Gosnell, Johannsen, & Ayres, 1992; Olson, Langemo, Burd, Hanson, Hunter, & Cathcart-Silberberg, 1996). The reported incidence among hospitalized or nursing home elderly and orthopedic patients has been higher, with estimates ranging from 8.5% to 42% (Allman, Goode, Patrick, Burst, & Bartolucci, 1995; Bergstrom, Braden, Kemp, Champagne, & Ruby, 1996; Brandeis et al., 1990; Ek, 1987; Gosnell, 1973; Jensen & Juncker, 1987; Roberts & Goldstone, 1979; Versluysen, 1986). The intensity of the problem is even greater in intensive care units, as indicated by a 33% incidence rate (Bergstrom, Demuth, & Braden, 1987). Estimated incidence rates among less severely ill, community-based adults range from 2.2% to 28% (Bergquist & Frantz, 1999; Guralnik, Harris, White, & Cornoni-Huntley, 1988; Ramundo, 1995; Rodriquez & Garber, 1994). The wide range of incidence found in these studies is thought to arise from the highly variable nature of the case mix and staffing in the study settings (Brandeis et al., 1989, 1990; Langemo et al., 1991; Powell, 1989). Despite this variability, it is noteworthy that patients destined to develop pressure ulcers have been found to do so largely in the first 2 weeks after admission to a nursing home (Bergstrom & Braden, 1992).

Although pressure ulcers are a common occurrence in the institutionalized elder, recent studies suggest that their occurrence is not an inevitable consequence of aging-related functional decline. There is growing evidence that incidence can be reduced in the institutionalized elder with an active program of prevention. Xakellis, Frantz, and Lewis (1995) reported an incidence rate of 6.2 cases per 100 subject-years in a long-term care setting where aggressive prevention measures were being provided. Similarly, the incidence rate decreased from 23% to 5% when an intensive protocol for pressure ulcer prevention was instituted in a long-term care facility that previously had no systematic prevention program (Xakellis et al., 1998).

RELATED FACTORS/ETIOLOGIES

Although the occurrence of pressure ulcers is not limited to the geriatric population, biophysiologic changes associated with the aging process increase the risk of soft tissue injury in the elder. As a consequence of aging, the elastin content of the soft tissue decreases, thereby limiting the weight-bearing capability of these structures. The body's

mechanical load is shifted to the interstitial fluid and cells. Mechanical pressure squeezes the interstitial fluid out of the region, allowing cells to come in contact with each other. Having lost the cushioning protection of the interstitial fluid, cell membranes may rupture if the external pressure is high. Once pressure is removed, interstitial fluid pressure may be sufficiently low to cause capillary bursting in the area affected by the external pressure. When such damage occurs, the lymphatic system is unable to clear the area of toxic intracellular debris. The cells in the area are poisoned, and a large area of necrosis will develop (Krouskop, 1983).

Advancing age is accompanied by cellular changes that influence healing of pressure ulcers. There is a decrease in the density of collagen, fewer fibroblasts are present, there is fragmentation of elastin fibers, and the number of mast cells diminishes with age (van de Kerkhoff, van Bergen, Spruijt, & Kuiper, 1994). Despite these physiologic changes, in the absence of concomitant diseases the rate of healing in the elder is only slightly slower or within the normal range and it is predominantly reepithelialization that is delayed (Holt et al., 1992; Olerud et al., 1995; van de Kerkhoff et al., 1994).

In addition to the biophysiologic changes associated with aging, other factors that contribute to delay pressure ulcer healing occur with greater frequency in the elder. Chronic illnesses that lead to insufficient oxygenation and perfusion often contribute to impaired healing. Inadequate molecular oxygen results in slowed deposition of oxygen. As tissue oxygen levels fall below 40 mm Hg, fibroblast proliferation decreases and collagen synthesis is adversely affected. However, collagen lysis continues creating a condition where wounds may break down in response to the hypoxic environment (Hunt, 1988). Inadequate tissue oxygen levels also reduce tissue resistance to infection, since lack of sufficient oxygen inhibits phagocytic activity of neutrophils and macrophages and compromises the bacterial killing activity of leukocytes (Hunt, 1988). Protein-calorie malnutrition, defined as a weight loss of 20% of the body weight, is associated with impaired pressure ulcer healing. This nutritional deficit slows the gain of tensile strength during the healing process, thus increasing the potential for reoccurrence of the pressure ulcer (Daly, Vars, & Dudrick, 1972; Goodson & Hunt, 1988; Irvin, 1978). Altered immune competency that accompanies aging compromises pressure ulcer healing by delaying or totally disrupting the inflammatory response. The effects of immunocompromise can be compounded in elderly persons who are also taking nonsteroidal antiinflammatory agents to treat other chronic conditions. Abnormal glucose metabolism and ensuing hyperglycemia, which occur with greater frequency in older adults, increase the risk of impaired healing.

Although multiple factors are cited as variables in pressure ulcer development, most authorities agree that the primary etiologic factor is pressure (Husain, 1953; Kenedi, Cowden, & Scales, 1976; Kosiak, 1959; Lindan, Greenway,

& Piazza, 1965; Reuler & Cooney, 1981; Scales, 1976). Defined as the perpendicular load or force exerted on a given area, the predominant effects of pressure on human tissue occur in the capillary bed (Bennett & Lee, 1985; DeLisa & Mikulic, 1985). The rate of blood flow through tissue capillaries is related to perfusion pressure (Burton & Yamada, 1951). The classic study by Landis (1930) established that when transmural pressure is reduced, blood flow decreases rapidly and total cessation of capillary flow occurs at transmural pressures between 20 and 40 mm Hg. This level is considered the critical closing pressure and can be produced by increasing externally applied pressure or by decreasing intravascular hydrostatic pressure. Nichol, Girling, Jerrard, Claxton, and Burton (1951) demonstrated that capillary flow is unstable at low perfusion pressures and that low levels of positive pressure result in either cessation or temporary reversal of flow. This is particularly significant for functionally impaired older adults, who are commonly in a low fluid volume state.

An additional consideration in the etiology of pressure ulcers is the duration of the pressure. Animal studies have determined that an inverse relationship exists between the amount of time and the amount of pressure needed to produce pathologic changes in tissue (Kosiak, 1959; Parish, Witkowski, & Crissey, 1983). Application of 60 to 70 mm Hg of pressure has been shown to produce pathologic changes in muscle tissue within 1 to 2 hours (Kosiak, Kubicek, Olson, Danz, & Kottke, 1958). Higher pressures can be tolerated for the same or longer periods if pressure is relieved intermittently for as little as 3 to 5 minutes. Husain (1953) noted that low pressure applied for long periods caused more tissue destruction than high pressure maintained for brief periods. He further determined that the degree of injury associated with tissue compression increases when a certain threshold is exceeded. This threshold is the product of pressure multiplied by time. Below a certain pressure-time threshold, release of the compression allows blood to flow back into the tissue, flooding the ischemic cells with nutrients and oxygen and producing a bright red flush called reactive hyperemia. This localized vasodilatation has been shown to be a normal compensatory response to temporary ischemia (Lewis & Grant, 1925; Scales, 1976). However, when the pressure-time threshold is exceeded, ischemic injury will continue even with relief of the compression. The region develops interstitial edema, the blood vessels and lymphatic circulation become obstructed, and cellular destruction occurs. More recently, Salcido, Donofrio, and Fisher (1994) have suggested the role of free radicals in pressure ulcer formation. Anesthetized rats exposed to five 6-hour sessions of controlled pressure applied to the skin over the trochanter developed ulceration initially in the muscle layer. Recurrent pressure resulted in increasingly severe damage to the vascular system and parenchyma consistent with an ischemia/reperfusion insult initiated through a free radical mechanism.

Human tissue can tolerate a relatively high level of pressure as long as the stress or load is uniformly distributed over the whole body (Scales, 1976). However, when pressure is localized, as little as one pound per square inch is sufficient to cause tissue destruction, mechanical damage, and blockage of blood vessels (Chow & Odell, 1978). Local pressure of greater than one and one-half pounds per square inch, or approximately 80 mm Hg, applied over a long period has been documented to cause skin necrosis (Trumble, 1930). Such excesses of pressure have been shown to occur when the body is being supported by a relatively small proportion of the total body surface area. Pressure measurements taken in the supine, prone, and side-lying positions produce readings in excess of the mean capillary pressure at the sacrum, heels, spine, hip, knees, costal margins, and occiput (Kosiak, 1959; Lindan, Greenway, & Piazza, 1965). Movement from a supine to a sitting position increases the pressure over the ischial tuberosities from approximately 70 mm Hg to 300 mm Hg (Kosiak et al., 1958).

The close proximity of the bony prominence to the body surface results in the body's weight being supported by these small surfaces. The combination of pressure and time on bony prominence in excess of the critical pressure-time threshold is the primary etiology of pressure ulcers.

Other factors have been implicated in the etiology of pressure ulcers, although their role in producing tissue ischemia is less clear. Several authors have cited shearing force as a causative agent in pressure ulcer formation (Berecek, 1975; Brown, Boosinger, Black, & Gasper, 1981; Reichel, 1958). Sacral ulcers have been associated with elevation of the head of the bed and the accentuation of pressure on the posterior sacral tissues. As the patient's bony pelvic structure slides downward in bed, the sacral skin surface adheres by friction to the bed linen. The deeper fascia moves downward with the bone while the superficial fascia remains connected to the dermis. This results in stretching and distortion of the vessels that supply the skin from the underlying fascia and muscle. It is thought that if this state is allowed to persist for a sufficient period of time, a pressure ulcer will result (Reichel, 1958). Empirical studies of shearing force have been limited. Dinsdale (1974) showed that a combination of friction and pressure produced lesions in the epidermis of swine. Bennett and Lee (1985) reported that in the presence of a high level of shear, vascular occlusion occurred with half the amount of pressure needed in the absence of shear.

Friction is another frequently cited factor in the development of pressure ulcers. Although not generally viewed as a primary factor in the etiology of pressure ulcers, the force of skin rubbing against another surface strips away the protective stratum corneum and decreases the fibrinolytic reactions in the dermis. Having lost this protective layer, the skin that is subjected to pressure is at greater risk for necrosis. Loss of the stratum corneum is also accompanied by transepidermal water loss, which collects on the body surface. This causes the coefficient friction to rise, increasing the adherence of the skin to its supporting surface (Lowthian, 1976). When combined with shearing force, the skin-adhering effects of friction tend to intensify the disruption of underlying fascia and blood supply.

Pressure, shearing force, and friction all have been identified in the literature as factors that cause pressure ulcers. However, close scrutiny of the pathologic events that lead to the ischemic injury suggests that the primary etiology is a combination of pressure and time on a bony prominence in excess of a critical pressure-time threshold. The presence of shearing force and friction can intervene and accentuate the effects of pressure, further limiting available circulation to tissues. Similarly, other factors can limit the pressure-time threshold by compromising the usual vitality of the tissue and rendering it more susceptible to ischemic injury. Chronic illness and the accompanying physical weakness and immobility commonly associated with functional impairment can limit the individual's ability to respond to stimuli arising from compressed tissue. Nutritional deficiencies reduce the subcutaneous tissue and muscle bulk, decreasing the mechanical padding between the skin and underlying bone. Hypoproteinemia predisposes the individual to edema formation, which decreases the elasticity, resiliency, and vitality of the skin and slows the rate of oxygen diffusion from the capillaries to the cells. Deficiencies of ascorbic acid, which commonly occur in elderly individuals, have been shown to accentuate the intensity and rate of tissue destruction that accompanies prolonged compression (Husain, 1953). Incontinence leads to a marked rise in static friction between the surface of the bed linen and the skin, intensifying the destruction of superficial tissue layers and increasing the potential for infection. Any condition that leads to nutritional deficiencies, impaired perfusion, or infection can compromise the usual vitality of tissue, limit the pressure-time threshold, and render tissue more susceptible to ischemic injury.

ASSESSMENT

Several systems have been proposed for assessing and categorizing pressure ulcers using level of tissue injury as an organizing framework. However, a great deal of disparity exists among the proposed approaches. The number of categories or grades of tissue injury varies from three to six. Some systems use illustrations or visual representations to distinguish characteristics of the various levels of injury, whereas others rely on narrative descriptions. Until recently the classic classification system used for pressure ulcer assessment was the one developed by Shea (1975). It described four levels of tissue injury numerically labeled Grade I through Grade IV, with Grade I consisting of a superficial breakdown limited to the epidermis and subsequent grades defined by increased depth of tissue loss. Recognizing that Shea's grading system did not capture the changes observed on skin exposed to pressure in excess

of the critical pressure-time threshold, experts in skin care proposed an alternative staging system, which has become the current standard (National Pressure Ulcer Advisory Panel, 1989). The stages of tissue injury are defined in this system as follows:

Stage I: Nonblanchable erythema of intact skin, the heralding lesion of skin ulceration
Stage II: Partial thickness skin loss involving epidermis and/or dermis
Stage III: Full thickness skin loss involving damage or necrosis of subcutaneous tissue that may extend down to, but not through, underlying fascia
Stage IV: Full thickness skin loss with extensive destruction, tissue necrosis, or damage to muscle, bone, or supporting structures

Although this classification system provides a simple, easy-to-use method of quantifying level of tissue destruction, it is not without controversy. The validity of the Stage I pressure ulcer continues to be debated among experts in skin care. The lack of external soft tissue destruction, the difficulty accurately assessing a Stage I pressure ulcer in persons with darkly pigmented skin, and the reversibility of the phenomenon with relief of pressure are argued by some experts as justification for revising the definition of Stage I pressure ulcer.

It is this author's position that the phenomenon currently being defined as a Stage I pressure ulcer should be relabeled to distinguish it from pressure induced tissue ischemia resulting in observable tissue destruction. *Taber's Cyclopedic Medical Dictionary* (Thomas, 1985) defined ulcer as "an open sore or lesion of the skin or mucous membrane accompanied by sloughing of inflamed necrotic tissue" (p. 1791). Since the skin remains intact in a Stage I pressure ulcer, it is incongruent to refer to this phenomenon as an ulcer. Furthermore, the pathologic events that lead to irreversible cell injury are distinctly different from those that occur with reversible damage. Severe injury causes derangement in energy and substrate metabolism involving altered high-energy phosphate metabolism and a progressive reduction in cellular content of adenosine triphosphate (Buja, Eigenbrodt, & Eigenbrodt, 1993). The progression from reversible to irreversible injury is related to the deterioration of these processes. During ischemic cell death, pyknosis (thickening and condensing) of nuclear chromatin, intracellular swelling of organelles (endoplasmic reticulum, mitochondria, lysosomes, and other vesicles), subsurface cell blebbing, and general cell edema are associated with potentially reversible injury (Buja et al., 1993). Characteristics associated with irreversible injury include advanced changes in the nuclear chromatin, mitochondria lesions (amphorous matrix densities, linear densities, and in certain conditions, electrodense calcium phosphate deposits), and physical defects in the plasma membrane and organellar membranes (Buja et al., 1993).

Since a Stage I pressure ulcer will resolve with relief of pressure and restoration of tissue perfusion, it is pathologically different from tissue that has experienced irreversible injury and died. Tissue that has experienced irreversible injury must undergo repair and regeneration to restore functional integrity. Allman and colleagues (1995) demonstrated that nonblanchable erythema is a risk factor for development of a Stage II or greater pressure ulcer. An alternative approach to classifying what is currently defined as a Stage I pressure ulcer would be to include it with the label Risk for Impaired Skin Integrity. Identifying it as a risk would serve as a trigger for implementation of preventive interventions to reverse the pressure causing ischemia and restore functional tissue integrity. Stage II, III, and IV pressure ulcers could be reclassified as partial thickness pressure ulcer and full thickness pressure ulcer. Such a classification system would simplify the diagnosis of pressure ulcer while providing sufficient definition of the type of tissue injury to guide nursing interventions and outcomes.

NURSING DIAGNOSIS

Although pressure ulcers have posed a long-standing problem, only recently has nursing attempted to define the problem and its etiologies and signs and symptoms. Although there is general recognition that ulcerated lesions are areas of soft tissue necrosis resulting from pressure-induced ischemia, the terminology used to define them remains inconsistent. Historically, the terms *decubitus ulcer* and *bedsore* were widely used to describe the lesions, since they were observed to occur most frequently in individuals who were confined to bed. Arising from the Latin word *decumbere,* which means "to lie down," the term *decubitus ulcer* implies that the lesion is caused solely by prolonged recumbence. More recent clinical observations have confirmed that the ulcer can occur in any position exposed to excessive, unrelieved pressure. The term *pressure ulcer* or *pressure sore* evolved to reflect more accurately the etiology of the ulceration rather than a specific body position. In an effort to establish consistent terminology, the National Pressure Ulcer Advisory Panel Consensus Development Conference (NPUAP, 1989) determined that the term *pressure ulcer* be used universally. This label was reaffirmed by the AHCPR Guideline Panel (Clinical Practice Guideline Panel, 1992) in its clinical practice guideline on prediction and prevention of pressure ulcers.

The North American Nursing Diagnosis Association's efforts (NANDA, 1999) to place the phenomenon of pressure ulcers within the accepted taxonomy of nursing diagnoses have produced confusing, ambiguous results. Taxonomy I contained two diagnoses that relate to the phenomenon: Impaired Skin Integrity and Impaired Tissue Integrity (Carroll-Johnson, 1989). Table 11-1 compares the etiologies (related factors) and signs and symptoms (defining characteristics) specified by NANDA with those described in this chapter.

Table 11-1	Comparison of Related Factors/Etiologies and Defining Characteristics for Three Nursing Diagnoses Related to Pressure Ulcers	
Nursing Diagnoses	**Related Factors/ Etiologies**	**Defining Characteristics**
Impaired Skin Integrity	*External (environmental):* hyperthermia or hypothermia; chemical substance; mechanical factors (shearing forces, pressure, restraint); radiation; physical immobilization; humidity *Internal (somatic):* medication; altered nutritional state (obesity, emaciation); altered metabolic state; altered circulation; altered sensation; altered pigmentation; skeletal prominence; developmental factors; immunology deficit; alterations in turgor (change in elasticity)	Disruption of skin surface Destruction of skin layers Invasion of body structure
Impaired Tissue Integrity	Altered circulation; nutritional deficit/excess; knowledge deficit; impaired physical mobility; irritants; chemical (including body excretions, secretions, medications); thermal (temperature extremes); mechanical (pressure, shear, friction); radiation (including therapeutic radiation)	Damaged or destroyed tissue (cornea, mucous membrane, integumentary, or subcutaneous)
Impaired Skin Integrity: Pressure Ulcer	Pressure × Time; shearing force; friction	Partial thickness Full thickness

The definitions for the NANDA diagnoses lack specificity in delineating the phenomenon of pressure ulcer. Both Impaired Skin Integrity and Impaired Tissue Integrity are defined as disruptions in the skin or integument. The defining characteristics are identified broadly as disruptions or destruction of skin tissue. Specific, measurable signs and symptoms have not been delineated, although preliminary work has attempted to operationalize the diagnosis Impaired Skin Integrity. Cattaneo and Lackey (1987) analyzed open-ended responses given by 42 enterostomal therapy nurses to the statement, "When I see the nursing diagnosis, impaired skin integrity, to me it means . . ." Following validation by a panel of nurse experts, 28 terms or phrases were identified that define Impaired Skin Integrity. Although this listing provides more specific descriptors of the diagnosis than the NANDA taxonomy, their terms are not conceptually distinct, with signs and symptoms, antecedents, and assessment factors collectively represented. The lack of a narrowly focused diagnosis with a specific underlying etiology further contributes to this state of conceptual confusion.

Confusion could be eased by formulating a nursing diagnosis specifically directed at pressure ulcers and identified by the label Pressure Ulcer. It would be conceptually congruent with the well-established etiology of pressure over a bony prominence in excess of a critical pressure-time threshold, and the label would be consistent with the terminology recommended by other expert panels in skin and wound care. Furthermore, the documented pathologic events that occur in the presence of this etiology give rise to a cluster of observable, measurable changes in the skin and underlying tissue. The pattern of these changes would define the signs and symptoms of the diagnosis as Partial Thickness Pressure Ulcer, which is skin loss involving epidermis and/or dermis, and Full Thickness Pressure Ulcer, which is loss involving damage or necrosis of subcutaneous tissue that may extend down to or through underlying fascia and involve muscle, bone, or supporting structures.

CASE STUDY

M. Owen is an 82-year-old female with left-sided hemiplegia secondary to a right-sided cerebral vascular accident (CVA). She is unresponsive to verbal and painful stimuli. Since her CVA she has been confined to bed and has been unable to reposition herself. During the acute phase of her CVA she was positioned supine for extended periods of time and her heels were constantly in contact with the surface of the bed.

At the time of discharge to a long-term care facility, Mrs. Owen had an open wound over the left heel that extended through the dermis and subcutaneous tissue, exposing the deep fascia. Adherent necrotic tissue covered the floor of the wound, and the sides were diffusely covered with granulation tissue. Wound edges were dis-

tinct and attached to the wound base. The periwound tissue was pale pink and without evidence of edema, induration, or erythema and blanched with digital pressure. Two small, irregular areas of ecchymosis were visible superior and lateral to the wound edges. A moderate amount of thin purulent exudate was draining from the wound. Digitized tracings of the wound edges revealed a circumference of 12.6 cm and a surface area of 7.2 cm^2.

The diagnosis Impaired Skin Integrity: Pressure Ulcer was inferred from the clinical data. The hospital report of being confined to bed and unable to reposition and spending extended periods of time supine with the heels constantly in contact with the bed established the etiology of pressure. Further delineation of the diagnosis was made from examination of the signs and symptoms. The full thickness tissue loss extending to the deep fascia and the presence of necrotic tissue confirmed that this individual had a Stage IV pressure ulcer on her left heel.

NURSING-SENSITIVE OUTCOMES

Since a pressure ulcer is injured tissue, the obvious outcome desired is repair and regeneration of new tissue. The body responds to tissue injury by an ongoing sequential reparative process characterized by three phases: inflammation, proliferation, and remodeling. The ultimate outcome of this process is wound closure. Along the trajectory to wound closure, intermediate markers of progress can be identified. These intermediate outcomes are linked to the cellular events that characterize each of the phases of wound healing.

The inflammatory phase of healing is characterized by a cascade of cellular events that are initiated in response to tissue injury. The cellular and vascular disruption that accompanies injury exposes blood to collagen, which activates coagulation factors and causes platelet aggregation and clot formation (Clark, 1988). The platelets also release several growth factors that attract other cells and chemical substances needed for repair. Tissue injury and activation of clotting factors stimulate the release of vasoactive substances such as histamine, which cause the surrounding vessels to dilate and become more permeable. Vasocongestion and leakage of serous fluid ensue, causing the wound to appear erythematous, edematous, and warm with varying amounts of exudate. Chemoattractants produced by the platelets, activated clotting factors, and fibrin breakdown products attract leukocytes into the wound bed (Clark, 1988). Polymorphonuclear leukocytes initially migrate into the interstitial space and begin to digest and transport devitalized organic matter from the wound. After 24 hours leukocytes recede and monocytes enter the wound. Monocytes are rapidly converted to macrophages. They are responsible for debriding the wound, regulating fibroplasia, and degrading collagen in the wound healing process. Additionally, the macrophage orchestrates subsequent events in healing by release of angiogenic factor (which stimulates formation of new blood vessels to feed the growing new tissue) and by deposition of a growth factor (which stimulates fibroblast production and promotes collagen synthesis in the proliferative phase of wound healing). The primary function of the inflammatory phase of healing is to initiate the wound healing cascade, to remove debris, and to prepare the wound for regeneration of new tissue (Goodson & Hunt, 1980; Hotter, 1982). Clinically, local erythema, edema, exudate, and tenderness of the injured tissue characterize this phase.

The proliferative phase of wound healing overlaps the inflammatory phase and serves to deposit connective tissue and collagen cross-linking. Fibroblasts multiply and actively synthesize collagen, the essential protein of connective tissue. Collagen provides the matrix that fills the wound and gives it strength. During collagen production, capillaries form as budlike structures from nearby vessels, creating a granular appearance on the wound surface termed *granulation tissue*. As the wound matures and the synthesis of collagen decreases, the new vascular channels recede. The wound is transformed from capillary-dense, highly cellular tissue to a relatively avascular, cell-free scar composed of dense collagen bundles (Goodson & Hunt, 1980; Hotter, 1982). During the proliferative phase, full thickness wounds that are healing by secondary intention undergo wound contraction mediated by special contractile cells called myofibroblasts. This process reduces the volume of the open wound so that less granulation tissue is needed to fill the defect and there is less surface area for epithelial cells to cover. The final component of the proliferative phase is epithelialization, which creates a protective epithelial covering over the wound surface. Epithelial cells are inherently attracted to contact cells of their own type and will migrate from the wound edges across the wound until contact inhibition occurs. In wounds with minimal tissue loss, such as partial thickness wounds, epithelial migration occurs concurrently with collagen synthesis. In full thickness wounds epithelialization is delayed until a bed of granulation tissue is established. Once the wound is covered by epithelial cells, weeping of body fluid and electrolytes ceases. Although this phase of healing normally is completed in approximately 15 to 16 days, the duration is prolonged in chronic wounds such as pressure ulcers that are healing by secondary intention.

Repeated degradation and resynthesis of collagen in the scar characterize the remodeling phase of healing. During this phase, which persists for years, the neovascularization of granulation tissue retracts and the scar fades from a deep red to a silvery white as the granulation buds retract. The scar decreases in bulk and gains tensile strength, achieving a maximum of 80% of normal tissue strength.

The orderly, sequential process of regeneration and repair leading to wound closure suggests that outcomes can be represented by a series of intermediate outcomes culminating in wound closure. As a pressure ulcer moves from inflammation into the proliferative phase of healing, erythema, induration, and edema diminish and the wound bed clears of necrotic tissue. During the proliferative phase, granulation increasingly fills the open wound bed. Epithelial cells begin to migrate across the wound surface from the edges. Exudate decreases as the wound is increasingly covered with epithelium. As epithelial coverage is completed, the wound can be considered closed. However, the new epithelial tissue is fragile and easily wiped off with slight trauma. Therefore some experts would suggest that a more desirable outcome of healing is epithelialization capable of sustaining functional integrity during activities of daily living (Lazarus et al., 1994). This more functional outcome occurs during the remodeling phase, when the scar flattens out, becomes smoother in appearance, and gains in tensile strength. The color fades from deep red to silvery white as the granulation buds retract. At this point the injured tissue has been restored to the maximum level of function achievable through normal repair processes.

Nursing Outcomes Classification (NOC), developed by the Iowa Outcomes Project (2000), describes only one outcome pertinent to pressure ulcers, Wound Healing: Secondary Intention, defined as "the extent to which cells and tissues in an open wound have regenerated" (p. 446). This outcome specifies 18 indicators of healing in addition to size assessed by wound area and depth. Each indicator is quantified from none to complete using a 5-point Likert-type scale. In its current form NOC provides a starting point for delineating outcomes for assessing the responsiveness of nursing interventions implemented to treat pressure ulcers. However, given the sequential nature of wound healing and the prolonged time that may elapse before the ultimate endpoint of wound closure is achieved, intermediate measures of progress are essential. This is especially true in settings populated by older adults, who often experience delayed healing (Eaglstein, 1986; Grove, 1982). The quarterly assessments mandated by federal long-term care regulations further reinforce the need for intermediate outcomes that can be used as benchmarks of progress leading to the primary outcome of wound closure. The ability to quantify NOC outcome indicators offers the potential to develop such markers of progress. Further testing of the NOC outcome is needed to validate which indicators most accurately represent healing and to determine the usual pattern of change in these indicators in a healing wound.

A number of individual parameters have been used to measure progression of a wound toward closure. However, no single measurement has been satisfactory to describe healing, resulting in the combination of several variables into an index tool (Rodeheaver & Stotts, 1995). In an effort to quantify multiple indices and arrive at a score of overall wound status, Bates-Jensen (1995) developed the Pressure Sore Status Tool (PSST). The 15-item instrument assesses location, shape, necrotic tissue amount, exudate type, exudate amount, surrounding skin color, peripheral tissue edema, peripheral tissue induration, granulation tissue, and epithelialization using a modified Likert scale. Location and shape are assessed but not scored. The individual items are summed, and the total score indicates overall wound status. Total scores range from 13 to 65. The tool allows for sequential monitoring of individual characteristics, as well as the total wound. Multiple scores over time provide an indication of deterioration or progression of the wound toward closure. Studies to establish reliability and validity of the tool are in progress. A panel of twenty experts established content validity, and the measure was refined by a nine-member panel of expert judges. Partial concurrent validity was determined by comparing the stage of the ulcer with the depth subscale. The correlation coefficient was $r = 0.91$ (Bates-Jensen & McNees, 1995). To date, predictive validity has not been established. Intrarater reliability was determined for each item using the kappa coefficient. Following a training program on the tool, the kappa values for enterostomal therapy nurses using the tool were 0.75 or greater for all items except exudate amount and exudate type for one rater and exudate type and skin color for a second rater (Bates-Jensen, Vredevoe, & Brecht, 1992). Interrater reliability, computed by using the Pearson product moment correlation coefficient, was assessed to be 0.78 for practitioners (Bates-Jensen & McNees, 1995) and 0.91 for enterstomal therapy nurses (Bates-Jensen et al., 1992). For individual items the kappa was 0.75 or greater following a training program on the tool. These values illustrate that training is essential to achieve desirable reliability and validity using the PSST. From a clinical perspective, the tool is relatively long and contains detailed information, some of which may be unnecessary or redundant. However, it does provide a comprehensive assessment of multiple attributes of a wound that inform clinicians about changing wound status and guide decision making related to treatment.

The indicators identified for the NOC outcome Wound Healing: Secondary Intention contain the elements of the PSST instrument but classify them into more discrete levels of measurement. For example, the PSST identifies exudate type as one assessment parameter and lists various forms of exudate from which the one that best describes the wound can be selected. NOC lists each potential type of exudate as a unique indicator (Table 11-2) and quantifies it on a Likert-type scale from none to complete. The relative merits of one outcome measuring system over the other remain to be clarified through additional empirical testing.

The Sessing Scale for assessing pressure ulcer healing was created as a simple, easy-to-use observational instrument that measures granulation tissue, infection, drainage, necrosis, and eschar on a 7-point scale (Ferrell, Arinian, & Sessing, 1995). The scale is scored by calculating the change in numeric values over successive wound assessments. Positive scores indicate ulcer improvement, and negative scores indicate deterioration. Correlational validity was assessed by comparing the Sessing Scale score to wound circumference measured by planimeter (Ferrell, Osterweil, & Christenson, 1993). Subsequently, circumference was transformed to diameter, using the square root of circumference to achieve a better fit of the data. The Sessing Scale was moderately correlated with wound diameter ($r = 0.35$) and the Shea stages ($r = 0.52$). Stepwise regression analysis identified the initial Sessing Scale score as highly predictive of the rate of ulcer healing (Ferrell, Keeler, Siu, Ahn, & Osterweil, 1995). The weighted kappas for interobserver and intraobserver reliability were 0.80 and 0.84 respectively. Some caution must be exercised in interpreting these results, since the variables used in this score each have several modifiers that require expertise to define. Furthermore, since only 54% of patients in the reported study were followed to complete closure, it is unclear how valid the tool is in benchmarking progress toward wound closure. It is not certain at this point whether the more detailed list of indicators contained in the NOC outcome will be more sensitive to change over time than the Sessing Scale. Further clinical testing of both methods of measuring healing outcomes is needed to determine the most valid and reliable approach to monitoring progress toward wound closure.

The Pressure Ulcer Scale for Healing (PUSH Tool) was developed by a task force of NPUAP to provide a method for monitoring the changing status of an ulcer. Its creation was prompted by the need for an alternative to downstaging that could be incorporated into the Minimum Data Set 2.0 (MDS). The scale consists of three parameters: surface area, exudate amount, and surface appearance (Thomas et al., 1997). Each parameter is scored, and the sum of the three yields a total wound status score. Observing the direction and magnitude of the score over time provides evidence of whether ulcer healing is occurring. The tool was developed from a database of 37 subjects with Stage III or Stage IV ulcers that were assessed weekly as part of a clinical trial. Using this existing data, principal component analysis was used to define those ulcer characteristics most associated with healing (Bartolucci & Thomas, 1997). Each variable was entered into the model, and the calculated amount of variance explaining the outcome was analyzed. Principal component analysis confirmed that surface area, exudate amount, and surface appearance provided the best model to explain the outcome of ulcer healing (Thomas et al., 1997). Predictive validity of the statistical model was evaluated in a separate database of 10 ulcers with similar outcome. Pairwise comparisons in mean surface area over time showed that the tool was sensitive to change in ulcer status over time. These findings suggest that the more detailed list of indicators contained in the NOC outcome could be pared down and still provide an acceptable level of sensitivity to change in ulcer status. Additional clinical evaluation of the PUSH

Table 11-2	Suggested Nursing-Sensitive Outcomes and Nursing Interventions IMPAIRED SKIN INTEGRITY: PRESSURE ULCER		
Nursing Diagnosis	**Nursing-Sensitive Outcome**	**Nursing Interventions**	
IMPAIRED SKIN INTEGRITY: PRESSURE ULCER *Defining Characteristics* Partial thickness pressure ulcer	WOUND HEALING: SECONDARY INTENTION *Indicators* Epithelialization Resolution of serous drainage Resolution of sanguineous drainage Resolution of serosanguineous drainage Resolution of surrounding skin erythema Resolution of periwound edema Resolution of abnormal surrounding skin Resolution of blistered skin Resolution of macerated skin Resolution of wound size Decreased area	PRESSURE ULCER CARE PRESSURE MANAGEMENT WOUND IRRIGATION TEACHING: INDIVIDUAL TEACHING: PROCEDURE/TREATMENT TEACHING: PSYCHOMOTOR SKILL NUTRITION MANAGEMENT NUTRITION THERAPY NUTRITIONAL COUNSELING	
Full thickness pressure ulcer	WOUND HEALING: SECONDARY INTENTION *Indicators* Granulation Epithelialization Resolution of sanguineous drainage Resolution of serosanguineous drainage Resolution of surrounding skin erythema Resolution of periwound edema Resolution of abnormal surrounding skin Resolution of blistered skin Odor Resolution of macerated skin Resolution of necrosis Resolution of sloughing Resolution of tunneling Resolution of undermining Resolution of sinus tract formation Resolution of wound Resolution of wound size Decreased area	PRESSURE ULCER CARE PRESSURE MANAGEMENT WOUND IRRIGATION TEACHING: INDIVIDUAL TEACHING: PROCEDURE/TREATMENT TEACHING: PSYCHOMOTOR SKILL NUTRITION MANAGEMENT NUTRITION THERAPY NUTRITIONAL COUNSELING	

Tool and NOC outcome indicators will be important in determining the most valid markers of changing wound status.

Although in the early stages of development, the PSST, the Sessing Scale, and the PUSH Tool offer alternative methods to systematically assess healing, and in so doing, provide outcome measures of interventions to treat pressure ulcers. Further research is needed to design an outcomes evaluation tool that monitors the biologic progress of pressure ulcer healing using intermediate and primary measures that are valid, reliable, and sensitive to change over time.

NURSING INTERVENTIONS

Nursing interventions for treatment of pressure ulcers are those activities directed toward supporting the normal biologic events of wound healing and preventing further injury to the tissue. The AHCPR Clinical Practice Guideline Treating Pressure Ulcers (Bergstrom et al., 1994) provides a comprehensive description of interventions for managing pressure ulcers. Compiled by a 15-member multidisciplinary panel of experts on pressure ulcers and wound healing, the guidelines are based on an extensive analysis of the research literature supplemented as needed by expert opinion. It is beyond the scope of this chapter to discuss all of the nursing and medical treatments for pressure ulcers. This chapter will focus on those interventions performed primarily by nurses. Interventions available to nurses that support the normal biologic events of wound healing include activities to remove necrotic tissue and debris, provide a moist wound environment, control bacterial levels in the wound, and supply essential substrates for cell regeneration and repair.

Debridement and Cleansing

The presence of nonviable tissue in the wound provides a culture medium for the growth of bacteria (Dhingra, Schauerhamer, & Wangensteen, 1976). Sapico et al. (1986) showed that both aerobes and anaerobes were present in large numbers only when necrotic tissue was present. When necrotic tissue was cleared from wounds, anaerobic organisms virtually disappeared and the number of aerobic organisms decreased dramatically. Robson and Heggers (1969) demonstrated that high levels of bacteria in pressure ulcers result in delayed healing. It follows that bacterial burden of chronic wounds will be reduced and healing enhanced by removal of necrotic tissue.

Four methods of debridement are available for removal of adherent nonviable tissue: sharp, mechanical, chemical, and autolytic. Conservative sharp debridement involves using a scalpel or scissors to remove macroscopically visible necrotic tissue from the wound surface. This is the most rapid and efficient method of debridement. Many state nurse practice laws define requirements for performance of this procedure within the scope of nursing practice (Fowler, 1992). Mechanical debridement uses wet-to-dry gauze dressings to physically remove dead tissue. Chemical debridement with enzyme agents targets specific types of necrotic tissue, such as protein, fibrin, and collagen. Selection of the enzyme is based on the type of necrotic tissue in the wound. Necrotic fibrins and proteins tend to develop more superficially in the wound bed than devitalized collagen. Enzymes affect a specific type of necrotic tissue and are generally classified into one of three groups: proteolytics, fibrinolytics, and collagenases (Feedar, 1994). Although capable of more selective debridement than mechanical methods, enzymes are expensive and relatively slow in breaking down necrotic tissue in the wound. Autolytic debridement uses the body's own enzymes to digest devitalized tissue. Application of a moisture-retentive dressing allows endogenous enzymes in the wound fluid to liquefy necrotic tissue selectively. The macrophages and neutrophils that are naturally present in wound fluid digest and make soluble necrotic tissue while maintaining the integrity of viable tissue. This method is the most highly selective debridement method, but it is also slow, which limits the range of wound conditions where it can be used effectively.

Although removal of necrotic tissue is considered essential for healing to progress, research on debridement is sparse. Chemical debridement is the only method that has established efficacy through randomized trials. These studies have reported the debriding efficacy of collagenase when compared with a placebo and have demonstrated that collagenase can make undenatured collagen soluble and facilitate debridement of necrotic tissue (Boxer, Gottesman, Bernstein, & Mandl, 1969; Lee & Ambrus, 1975; Varma, Bugatch, & German, 1973). To better optimize outcomes from debridement, additional research is needed to determine what debridement method is most effective for given patient and wound characteristics.

The presence of nonadherent foreign material such as exudate and metabolic wastes can slow the progression of cellular events in wound healing. Interventions to cleanse the wound bed of inflammatory material will facilitate optimal healing. Wound cleansing requires selection of a cleansing solution and a mechanical method of delivering the agent to the wound bed. Although multiple wound cleansers are available commercially, the most common and cost-effective wound cleansing solution is isotonic saline (Bergstrom et al., 1994). Recent studies have established that many wound cleansers are cytotoxic to white blood cells and therefore should be avoided in treating open wounds (Burkey, 1993; Foresman, Payne, Becker, Lewis, & Rodeheaver, 1993). The mechanical method used to deliver the solution should provide sufficient force to release the debris from the wound surface without causing trauma. Irrigation pressures in excess of 15 pounds per square inch (psi) have been shown to cause wound trauma and drive bacteria into the tissue (Bhaskar, Cutright, Hunsuck, & Gross, 1971; Wheeler, Rodeheaver, Thacker, Edgerton, & Edlich, 1976). Devices that deliver fluid streams of 4 to 15 psi will facilitate removal of debris from wounds without causing tissue trauma (Rodeheaver, Pettry, Thacker, Edgerton, & Edlich, 1975; Stevenson, Thacker, Rodeheaver, Bacchetta, & Edgerton, 1976).

Provision of a Moist Wound Environment

It is well established that a moist wound environment promotes reepithelialization and healing. Exposing a wound to air for prolonged periods allows the surface to dry and form a scab. Epidermal cells must tunnel under the dry crusts or scabs to reach a moist layer of tissue in order to migrate across the wound bed. Conversely, when the surface of the wound is kept constantly moist, epidermal cells are able to migrate more efficiently and closure of the wound with an epithelial covering occurs more rapidly (Winter & Scales, 1963).

Numerous dressing materials support a moist wound healing environment. In addition to maintaining a moist wound bed, dressings perform a number of functions that support healing under various circumstances, including debridement, absorption of exudate, filling of dead space, insulation, and protection from trauma and infection. There are hundreds of different wound dressings available to choose from, making it beyond the scope of this chapter to discuss all of them. No single dressing can provide an optimum environment for all wounds. However, it is noteworthy that randomized trials comparing one type of moist wound healing dressing with another consistently showed no differences in pressure ulcer healing outcomes (Alm et al., 1989; Colwell, Foreman, & Trotter, 1992; Neill, Conforti, Kedas, & Burris, 1989; Oleske, Smith, White, Pottage, & Donavan, 1986; Xakellis & Chrischilles, 1992). Selection of the appropriate dressing is dictated by characteristics of the wound bed, the functions provided by various dressings, and the desired intermediate outcome to be achieved along the trajectory to wound closure. As the wound moves through the phases of wound healing, the dressings should be modified to meet the changing environment of the wound bed.

Controlling Bacterial Levels

Quantitative bacteriologic studies involving patients with pressure ulcers have concluded that there is a direct correlation between the level of bacteria in a wound and healing (Bendy et al., 1964). Bacteria are active cells that consume nutrients and produce toxic products. For optimum wound healing to occur, these bacteria have to be controlled and their numbers have to be reduced to low levels. Heavy bacterial overgrowth or compromised host defenses can produce colony counts that are not compatible with wound healing. Pressure ulcers producing tissue biopsy cultures of less than 10^5 bacteria per gram of tissue have been shown to heal when treated with pressure relief and local wound management. In contrast, ulcers with greater than 10^5 bacteria fail to heal normally (Robson & Heggers, 1969). Bendy and colleagues (1964), using a quantitative swab technique, showed that significant healing of pressure ulcers occurred only when bacterial counts were less than 10^6 bacteria per milliliter. Although controversy exists over the appropriate technique for monitoring bacterial levels in wounds, the belief prevails that assessment for wound infection is essential. According to the Centers for Disease Control and Prevention, a pressure ulcer is infected when two of the following clinical findings are present: redness, tenderness, or swelling of wound edges *and* organisms are isolated from either a needle aspirate, tissue biopsy, or blood culture (Garner, Jarvis, Emori, Horan, & Hughes, 1988). Routine swab cultures are of no value in determining the presence of an infection, since they detect only the surface contaminants and not the level of bacteria present in the wound tissue.

To minimize bacterial growth in wounds, effective cleansing and debridement are indicated to remove the debris that supports organism growth and delays wound healing. Antiseptics should not be used to control the level of bacteria within the tissue. They are reactive chemicals that have been demonstrated to be toxic to all cells in the wound tissue (Lineaweaver et al., 1985). Systemic antibiotics are indicated for controlling bacterial levels only in the presence of bacteremia, sepsis, advancing cellulitis, or osteomyelitis and are not required for signs of local infec-

tion (Chow, Galpin, & Guze, 1977; Lewis et al., 1988). Topical antibiotics may be initiated as an intervention when the ulcer continues to produce exudate and fails to progress toward closure following sustained debridement and cleansing to remove nonviable tissue (Bendy et al., 1964; Kucan, Robson, Heggers, & Ko, 1981).

Provide Essential Substrates

Essential substrates for healing include protein, calories, vitamins, and minerals. Proteins in the form of amino acids are needed for angiogenesis, fibroblast activity, collagen synthesis, and scar formation. Sufficient carbohydrates and fats must be provided to prevent use of amino acids for energy expenditure. Vitamins A, B complex, and C support epithelialization and collagen synthesis, maintain the integrity of newly formed scar tissue, and increase resistance to infection. Zinc increases immunity and collagen synthesis, and iron is an important component of hemoglobin needed to transport oxygen to healing tissue. Although the role of specific substrates in wound healing has been well established, research to establish the prescriptive requirements needed to promote healing is incomplete. However, it is generally agreed that nutritional support sufficient to place the patient in a positive nitrogen balance (approximately 30 to 35 calories/kg/day and 1.25 to 1.50 grams of protein/kg/day) is a reasonable initial level of intervention (Chernoff, Milton, & Lipschitz, 1991; Kaminski, 1976). Since the majority of elderly nursing home patients have been shown to be vitamin and mineral deficient, it is advisable to provide a multiple vitamin with minerals supplement when deficiencies are suspected (Bergstrom & Braden, 1992; Pinchcofsky-Devin & Kaminski, 1986).

Prevention of Further Injury

Along with interventions to promote the normal biologic events of wound healing, support of the repair process necessitates that pressure on the ulcer be eliminated. Without attention to removing the etiology, all other interventions to support healing are futile. If possible, the patient with a pressure ulcer should be positioned to avoid any external force on the ulcer. When the ulcer is located in the sacral area, the patient should refrain from sitting until the wound has healed. A variety of support surfaces (mattress, beds) are marketed to relieve pressure over bony prominences. Although these surfaces have been shown to provide an environment in which pressure ulcers improve, there is not compelling evidence that one support surface consistently performs better than all others under all circumstances (Allman, Walker, et al., 1986; Conine, Daechsel, & Lau, 1990; Ferrell et al., 1993; Jackson, Chagares, Nee, & Freeman, 1988; Munro, Brown, & Heitman, 1989; Strauss, Gong, Gary, Kalsbeek, & Spear, 1991; Warner, 1992). Until more prescriptive research data are available, selection of a support surface should be guided by consideration of the clinical condition of the patient, the characteristics of the care setting, and the characteristics of the support surface.

The *Nursing Interventions Classification (NIC)* identifies Pressure Ulcer Care as an intervention to facilitate healing in pressure ulcers (Iowa Intervention Project, 2000). A second intervention, Wound Care, is defined as "prevention of wound complications and promotion of wound healing" (p. 706). The two interventions are categorized within the domain identified as Physiological: Complex, under the class labeled Skin/Wound Management. Although the label Pressure Ulcer Care appears to be the most appropriate intervention for nursing management of pressure ulcers, the definition for the Wound Care intervention suggests that it could also be used in caring for pressure ulcers. However, many of the activities listed for the Wound Care intervention appear more consistent with an acute wound condition rather than a chronic wound condition. Refinement of these definitions would increase clinicians' accuracy in selecting the most appropriate intervention for management of pressure ulcers.

Seventeen activities are listed under Pressure Ulcer Care. The level of specificity of the activities varies greatly. Some activities are general, which allows for individualization to specific patients. Others are quite specific, such as the use of a 19-gauge needle and 35-cc syringe to clean deep ulcers. The rationale for these varying levels of specificity remains to be clarified. There is no organizing framework for the activities and no linkages of these activities to the physiologic events that occur during the wound healing process. Certain of the activities identified, such as measure and describe characteristics of the ulcer at regular intervals, are assessments related to measurement of outcomes and are not activities to facilitate healing. The NIC intervention Pressure Ulcer Care represents a worthy initial effort to identify nursing activities appropriate to the treatment of pressure ulcers. Further expansion, refinement, and testing of the intervention are needed to develop a taxonomy that delineates specific foci for nursing activities and suggests a logical scientific rationale for their application. Ultimately, nursing interventions should be linked to diagnoses and outcomes.

CASE STUDY

Having confirmed the diagnosis of a Stage IV pressure ulcer, nursing interventions for Mrs. Owen were selected to reduce or eliminate pressure and to promote the normal biologic events of healing as the ulcer progressed through the phases of wound healing to closure. The presence of moderate exudate and necrotic tissue in the base of the ulcer indicated that an active inflammatory response was occurring in the wound. Since necrotic tissue tends to harbor bacteria and impede progression of healing, conservative sharp debridement was performed to quickly remove a majority of the nonviable tissue in the wound. Moist saline gauze dressings were used to maintain a moist environment on the wound surface. The dressings were changed 4 times a day initially; the frequency was reduced to 3 times a day as the exudate decreased. To ensure that the wound bed was kept continuously moist, the gauze in direct contact with the wound was remoistened between dressing changes. The wound was cleansed with isotonic saline at each dressing change using a 19-gauge angiocath and 35-cc syringe. The left lower extremity was fitted with a protective boot that suspended the heel so that pressure was totally eliminated. Mrs. Owen was maintained on tube feedings of Ensure and given a daily multiple vitamin with minerals supplement.

Outcomes were monitored weekly, including wound circumference and surface area measured by digitized tracings, the proportion of wound surface covered with necrotic tissue and granulation tissue, the proportion of original wound covered with new epithelial tissue, and the amount and type of exudate. The outcomes as they evolved until wound closure are presented in Table 11-3.

Table 11-3	Mrs. Owen's Outcomes With Pressure Ulcer Treatment						
Week	Circumference (cm)	Surface Area (cm^2)	Necrotic Tissue (%)	Granulation Tissue (%)	Epithelial Tissue (%)	Exudate Amount	Exudate Type
Start	12.6	7.2	50	50	0	Moderate	Purulent
1	12.6	7.2	25	75	0	Moderate	Purulent
2	12.6	7.2	0	100	0	Small	Serous
3	10.8	6.0	0	100	10	Small	Serous
4	9.9	4.4	0	100	10	Small	Serous
5	8.8	3.8	0	100	25	Small	Serous
6	8.3	3.1	0	100	25	Small	Serous
7	5.4	1.7	0	100	50	Small	Serous
8	3.6	0.5	0	100	75	Scant	Serous
9	1.2	0.2	0	100	90	Scant	Serous
10	0	0	0	0	100	0	0

SUMMARY

Although pressure ulcers are a frequently encountered problem in the elderly population, their diagnosis and treatment remain poorly defined. Multiple labels are used to delineate the problem, and treatments lack data to substantiate efficacy. Assessment measures to document the level of tissue injury remain controversial. Tools for monitoring outcomes of interventions are in their infancy, and numerous questions regarding valid indicators of pressure ulcer healing must be resolved. Efforts will have to be directed toward organizing the body of knowledge related to pressure ulcers so that it articulates with the physiologic events that underlie tissue injury and repair. Such an organization of knowledge would clearly define meaningful diagnostic labels based on measurable signs and symptoms and conceptually congruent etiologies. From this foundation nursing intervention labels could be defined and outcome measures described.

REFERENCES

Allman, R. M. (1989). Epidemiology of pressure sores in different populations. *Decubitus, 2*(2), 30-33.

Allman, R. M., Goode, P. S., Patrick, J. M., Burst, N., & Bartolucci, A. A. (1995). Pressure ulcer risk factors among hospitalized patients with activity limitation. *Journal of the American Medical Association, 273,* 865-870.

Allman, R. M., Laprade, C. A., Noel, L. B., Walker, J. M., Moorer, C. A., Dear, M. R., & Smith, C. R. (1986). Pressure sores among hospitalized patients. *Annals of Internal Medicine, 105*(3), 337-342.

Allman, R. M., Walker, J. M., Hart, M. K., Laprade, C. A., Noel, L. B., & Smith, C. R. (1986). Air-fluidized beds or conventional therapy for pressure sores: A randomized trial. *Annals of Internal Medicine, 107*(5), 641-648.

Alm, A., Hornmark, A. M., Fall, P. A., Linder, L., Bergstrand, B., Ehrnebo, M., Madsen, S. M., & Setterberg, G. (1989). Care of pressure sores: A controlled study of the use of a hydrocolloid dressing compared with a wet saline gauze compress. *Acta Derm Venereol (Stockholm), 149*(Suppl.), 1-10.

Andersen, K. E., & Kvorning, S. A. (1982). Medical aspects of the decubitus ulcer. *International Journal of Dermatology, 21*(5), 265-270.

Bartolucci, A. A., & Thomas, D. R. (1997). Using principal component analysis to describe wound status. *Advances in Wound Care: The Journal for Prevention and Healing, 10*(5), 93-95.

Bates-Jensen, B. M. (1995). Indices to include in wound healing assessment. *Advances in Wound Care, 8*(4), 25-33.

Bates-Jensen, B. M., & McNees, P. (1995). Toward an intelligent wound assessment system. *Ostomy/Wound Management, 41*(Suppl. 7A), 80S-86S.

Bates-Jensen, B. M., Vredevoe, D. L., & Brecht, M. L. (1992). Validity and reliability of the pressure sore status tool. *Decubitus, 5*(6), 20-28.

Bendy, R. H., Jr., Nuccio, P. A., Wolfe, E., Collins, B., Tamburro, D., Glass, W., & Martin, C. M. (1964). Relationship of quantitative wound bacterial counts to healing of decubiti: Effect of topical gentamicin. *Antimicrobial Agents and Chemotherapy, 4,* 147-155.

Bennett, L., & Lee, B. K. (1985). Pressure versus shear in pressure sore causation. In B. Y. Lee (Ed.), *Chronic ulcers of the skin* (pp. 39-56). Hightstown, NJ: McGraw-Hill.

Berecek, K. H. (1975). Etiology of decubitus ulcers. *Nursing Clinics of North America, 10*(1), 157-170.

Bergquist, S., & Frantz, R. (1999). Pressure ulcers in community-based older adults receiving home health care. *Advances in Wound Care, 12*(7), 339-351.

Bergstrom, N., Allman, R. M., Alvarez, O. M., Bennett, M. A., Carlson, C. E., Frantz, R. A., Garber, S. L., Jackson, B. S., Kaminski, M. V., Jr., Kemp, M. G., Kroskop, T. A., Lewis, V. L., Jr., Maklebust, J., Margolis, D. J., Marvel, E. M., Reger, S. I., Rodeheaver, G. T., Salcido, R., Xakellis, G. C., & Yarkony, G. M. (1994). *Treatment of pressure ulcers.* Clinical Practice Guideline, Number 15. AHCPR Publication No. 95-0652. Rockville, MD: Agency for Health Care Policy and Research, Public Health Service, U.S. Department of Health and Human Services.

Bergstrom, N., & Braden, B. (1992). A prospective study of pressure sore risk among institutionalized elderly. *Journal of the American Geriatrics Society, 40,* 747-758.

Bergstrom, N., Braden, B., Kemp, M., Champagne, M., & Ruby, E. (1996). Multi-site study of incidence of pressure ulcers and the relationship between risk level, demographic characteristics, diagnoses and prescription of preventive interventions. *Journal of the American Geriatrics Society, 44*(1), 22-30.

Bergstrom, N., Demuth, P. J., & Braden, B. J. (1987). A clinical trial of the Braden Scale for Predicting Pressure Sore Risk. *Nursing Clinics of North America, 22,* 417-428.

Bhaskar, S. N., Cutright, D. E., Hunsuck, E. E., & Gross, A. L. (1971). Pulsatile water jet devices in debridement of combat wounds. *Military Medicine, 264.*

Boxer, A. M., Gottesman, N., Bernstein, H., & Mandl, I. (1969). Debridement of dermal ulcers and decubiti with collagenase. *Geriatrics, 24*(7), 75-86.

Brandeis, G. H., Berlowitz, D. R., Hossain, M., & Morris, J. N. (1995). Pressure ulcers: The minimum data set and the resident assessment protocol. *Advances in Wound Care, 8*(6), 18-25.

Brandeis, G. H., Morris, J. N., Nash, D. J., & Lipsitz, L. A. (1989). Incidence and healing rates of pressure ulcers in the nursing home. *Decubitus, 2*(2), 60-62.

Brandeis, G. H., Morris, J. N., Nash, D. J., & Lipsitz, L. A. (1990). The epidemiology and natural history of pressure ulcers in elderly nursing home residents. *Journal of the American Medical Association, 264*(22), 2905-2909.

Brown, M. M., Boosinger, J., Black, J., Gasper, T. (1981). Nursing innovation for prevention of pressure ulcers in long-term care facilities. *The Journal of Plastic and Reconstructive Surgical Nursing, 5*(2), 51-55.

Bryan, C. S., Dew, C. E., & Reynolds, K. L. (1983). Bacteremia associated with decubitus ulcers. *Archives of Internal Medicine, 143,* 2093-2095.

Buja, L. M., Eigenbrodt, M. L., & Eigenbrodt, E. H. (1993). Apoptosis and necrosis: Basic types and mechanisms of cell death. *Archives of Pathology and Laboratory Medicine, 117,* 1208-1214.

Burkey, J. L. (1993). Differential methodology for the evaluation of skin and wound cleansers. *Wounds, 5*(6), 284-291.

Burton, A. C., & Yamada, S. (1951). Relation between blood pressure and flow in the human forearm. *Journal of Applied Physiology, 4,* 329-339.

Carroll-Johnson, R. (Ed.). (1989). *Classification of nursing diagnoses: Proceedings of the 8th conference.* Baltimore: Lippincott Williams & Wilkins.

Cattaneo, C. J., & Lackey, N. R. (1987). Impaired skin integrity. In A. M. McLane (Ed.), *Classification of nursing diagnoses: Proceedings of the seventh conference* (pp. 129-135). St. Louis, MO: Mosby.

Chernoff, R., Milton, K., & Lipschitz, D. (1991). The effect of a very high-protein liquid formula (Replete) on decubitus ulcer healing in long-term tube-fed institutionalized patients [Abstract]. *Journal of the American Dietetic Association, 90*(9), A-130.

Chow, A. W., Galpin, J. E., & Guze, L. B. (1977). Clindamycin for treatment of sepsis caused by decubitus ulcers. *Journal of Infectious Disease, 135*(Suppl.), S65-68.

Chow, W. W., & Odell, E. I. (1978). Deformations and stress in soft body tissues of a sitting person. *Biomedical Engineering, 100,* 79-82.

Clark, M., & Kahdom, H. M. (1988). The nursing prevention of pressure sores in hospitals and community patients. *Journal of Advances in Nursing, 13,* 365-373.

Clark, M. O., Barbanel, J. C., Jordan, M. M., & Nicol, S. M. (1978). Pressure sores. *Nursing Times, 74*(9), 363-366.

Clark, R. (1988). Overview and general considerations of wound repair. In R. Clark & P. Heneson (Eds.), *The molecular and cellular biology of wound repair.* New York: Plenum Press.

Clinical Practice Guideline Panel. (1992). *Clinical practice guideline: Pressure ulcers in adults: Prediction and prevention* (AHCPR Pub. No. 92-0047). Rockville, MD: Agency for Health Care Policy and Research, Public Health Service, U.S. Department of Health and Human Services.

Colwell, J. C., Foreman, M. D., & Trotter, J. P. (1992). A comparison of the efficacy and cost-effectiveness of two methods of managing pressure ulcers. *Decubitus, 6*(4), 28-36.

Conine, T. A., Daechsel, D., & Lau, M. S. (1990). The role of alternating air and Silicore overlays in preventing decubitus ulcers. *Journal of Rehabilitation Research, 13*(1), 57-65.

Daly, J. M., Vars, H. M., & Dudrick, S. J. (1972). Effects of protein depletion on strength of colonic anastomoses. *Surgical Gynecology and Obstetrics, 134,* 15-21.

DeLisa, J. A., & Mikulic, M. A. (1985). Pressure ulcers—what to do if prevention fails. *Postgraduate Medicine, 77*(6), 209-220.

Dhingra, U., Schauerhamer, R. R., & Wangensteen, O. W. (1976). Peripheral dissemination of bacteria in contaminated wounds; role of devitalized tissue: Evaluation of therapeutic measures. *Surgery, 80*(5), 535.

Dinsdale, S. M. (1974). Decubitus ulcers: Role of pressure and friction in causation. *Archives of Physical Medicine and Rehabilitation, 55,* 147-152.

Eaglstein, W. H. (1986). Wound healing and aging. *Dermatologic Clinics, 4*(3), 481-484.

Ek, A. C. (1987). Prediction of pressure sore development. *Scandinavian Journal of Caring Science, 1*(2), 77-84.

Feedar, J. A. (1994). Products that facilitate wound healing. *Topics in Geriatric Rehabilitation, 9*(4), 58-81.

Ferrell, B. A., Arinian, B. M., & Sessing, D. (1995). The Sessing scale for assessment of pressure ulcer healing. *Journal of the American Geriatrics Society, 43*(1), 37-40.

Ferrell, B. A., Keeler, E., Siu, A. L., Ahn, S. H., & Osterweil, D. (1995). Cost-effectiveness of low-air-loss beds for treatment of pressure ulcers. *Journal of Gerontology Series A: Biological Science & Medical Science, 50A*(3), M141-M146.

Ferrell, B. A., Osterweil, D., & Christenson, P. (1993). A randomized trial of low-air-loss beds for treatment of pressure ulcers. *Journal of the American Medical Association, 269*(4), 494-497.

Foresman, P. A., Payne, D. S., Becker, D., Lewis, D., & Rodeheaver, G. T. (1993). A relative toxicity index for wound cleansers. *Wounds, 5*(5), 226-231.

Fowler, E. (1992). Instrument/sharp debridement of nonviable tissue in wounds. *Ostomy/Wound Management, 38*(8), 26-33.

Frantz, R. A., Bergquist, S., & Specht, J. (1994). The cost of treating pressure ulcers following implementation of a research-based skin care protocol in a long-term care facility. *Advances in Wound Care, 8*(1), 36-45.

Fuhrer, M. J., Garber, S. L., Rintala, D. H., Clearman, R., & Hart, K. A. (1993). Pressure ulcers in community-resident persons with spinal cord injury: Prevalence and risk factors. *Archives of Physical Medicine and Rehabilitation, 74*(11), 1172-1177.

Garner, J. S., Jarvis, W. R., Emori, T. G., Horan, T. C., & Hughes, J. M. (1988). CDC definitions for nosocomial infections. *American Journal of Infection Control, 16*(3), 128-140.

Gerson, L. W. (1975). The incidence of pressure sores in active treatment hospitals. *International Journal of Nursing Studies, 12,* 201-204.

Goodson, W. H., & Hunt, T. K. (1980). Wound healing. In J. Kyle & J. D. Hardy (Eds.), *Scientific foundations of surgery.* Philadelphia: W. B. Saunders.

Goodson, W. H., & Hunt, T. K. (1988). Wound healing. In J. M. Kinney, K. N. Jeejeebhoy, G. L. Hill, & O. E. Owen (Eds.), *Nutrition and metabolism in patient care* (pp. 625-642). Philadelphia: W. B. Saunders.

Gosnell, D. J. (1973). An assessment tool to identify pressure sores. *Nursing Research, 22*(1), 55-59.

Gosnell, D. J., Johannsen, J., & Ayres, M. (1992). Pressure ulcer incidence and severity in a community hospital. *Decubitus, 5*(5), 56-62.

Grove, G. L. (1982). Age related differences in healing superficial skin wounds in humans. *Archives of Dermatological Research, 272,* 381-385.

Guralnik, J. M., Harris, T. B., White, L. R., & Cornoni-Huntley, J. C. (1988). Occurrence and predictors of pressure sores in the National Health and Nutrition Examination survey follow-up. *Journal of the American Geriatrics Society, 6*(9), 7-12.

Hanson, D. S., Langemo, D., Olson, B., Hunter, S., & Burd, C. (1996). Decreasing the prevalence of pressure ulcers using agency standards. *Home Healthcare Nurse, 14*(7), 525-531.

Hawthorne, M. H., Jefferson, J. W., & Paduano, K. J. (1989). The prevalence of dermal wounds. *Decubitus, 2*(3), 64.

Holt, D. R., Kirk, S. J., Regan, M. C., Hurson, M., Lindblael, W. J., & Barbul, A. (1992). Effect of age on wound healing in healthy human beings. *Surgery, 112*(2), 293-297.

Hotter, A. N. (1982). Physiologic aspects and clinical implications of wound healing. *Heart and Lung, 11*(6), 522-530.

Hunt, T. K. (1988). The physiology of wound healing. *Annals of Emergency Medicine, 17*(12), 2-10.

Husain, T. (1953). An experimental study of some pressure effects on tissues with reference to the bedsore problem. *Journal of Pathology and Bacteriology, 66,* 347-358.

Iowa Intervention Project. J. C. McCloskey & G. M. Bulechek (Eds.). (2000). *Nursing interventions classification (NIC)* (3rd ed.). St. Louis, MO: Mosby.

Iowa Outcomes Project. M. Johnson, M. Maas, & S. Moorhead (Eds.). (2000). *Nursing outcomes classification (NOC)* (2nd ed.). St. Louis, MO: Mosby.

Irvin, T. T. (1978). Effects of malnutrition on wound healing. *Surgical Gynecology and Obstetrics, 146,* 33-37.

Jackson, B. S., Chagares, R., Nee, N., & Freeman, K. (1988). The effects of a therapeutic bed on pressure ulcers: An experimental study. *Journal of Enterostomal Therapy, 15*(6), 220-226.

Jensen, T. T., & Juncker, T. (1987). Pressure sores common after hip operations. *Acta Orthopaedica Scandinavia, 58*(3), 209-211.

Kaminski, M. V., Jr. (1976). Enteral hyperalimentation. *Surgical Gynecology and Obstetrics, 143*(1), 12-16.

Kenedi, R. M., Cowden, J. M., & Scales, J. T. (Eds.). (1976). *Bedsore biomechanics.* London: University Park Press.

Kosiak, M. (1959). Etiology and pathology of ischemic ulcers. *Archives of Physical Medicine and Rehabilitation, 40*(2), 62-69.

Kosiak, M., Kubicek, W. G., Olson, M., Danz, J. N., & Kottke, F. J. (1958). Evaluation of pressure as a factor in the production of ischial ulcers. *Archives of Physical Medicine and Rehabilitation, 39,* 623-629.

Krouskop, T. A. (1983). A synthesis of factors that contribute to pressure sore formation. *Medical Hypotheses, 11,* 255-267.

Kucan, J. O., Robson, M. C., Heggers, J. P., & Ko, F. (1981). Comparison of silver sulfadiazine, povidone-iodine and physiologic saline in the treatment of chronic pressure ulcers. *Journal of the American Geriatrics Society, 29*(5), 232-235.

Landis, E. M. (1930). Micro-injection studies of capillary blood pressure in human skin. *Heart, 15,* 209.

Langemo, D. K., Olson, B., Hunter, S., Burd, C., Hansen, D., & Cathcart-Silberberg, T. (1989). Incidence of pressure sores in acute care, rehabilitation, extended care, home health, and hospice in one locale. *Decubitus, 2*(2), 42.

Langemo, D. K., Olson, B., Hunter, S., Hansen, D., Burd, C., & Cathcart-Silberberg, T. (1991). Incidence and prediction of pressure ulcers in five patient care settings. *Decubitus, 4*(3), 25-26, 28, 30 passim.

Lazarus, G. S., Cooper, D. M., Knighton, D. R., Margolis, D. J., Pecoraro, R. E., Rodeheaver, G., & Robson, M. C. (1994). Definitions and guidelines for assessment of wounds and evaluation of healing. *Archives of Dermatology, 130*(4), 489-493.

Lee, L. K., & Ambrus, J. L. (1975). Collagenase therapy for decubitus ulcers. *Geriatrics, 30*(5), 91-93, 97-98.

Lewis, T. Y., & Grant, R. T. (1925). Observations upon reactive hyperemia in man. *Heart, 12,* 73-120.

Lewis, V. L., Jr., Bailey, M. H., Pulawski, G., Kind, G., Bashioum, R. W., & Hendrix, R. W. (1988). The diagnosis of osteomyelitis in patients with pressure sores. *Plastic and Reconstructive Surgery, 81*(2), 229-232.

Lindan, O., Greenway, R. N., & Piazza, J. M. (1965). Pressure distribution on the surface of the human body. *Archives of Physical Medicine and Rehabilitation, 46,* 378-385.

Lineaweaver, W., Howard, R., Soucy, D., McMorris, S., Freeman, J., Crain, C., Robertson, J., & Romley, T. (1985). Topical antimicrobial toxicity. *Archives of Surgery, 120*(3), 267-270.

Lowthian, P. (1976). Underpads in the prevention of decubiti. In R. M. Kenedi, J. M. Cowden, & J. T. Scales (Eds.), *Bedsore biomechanics* (pp. 141-145). Proceedings of a seminar on tissue viability and clinical applications; 1975 August; Glasgow, Scotland. London: University Park Press.

Maklebust, J. (1987). Pressure ulcers: Etiology and prevention. *Nursing Clinics of North America, 22*(2), 359-377.

Meehan, J. (1990). Multisite pressure ulcer prevalence survey. *Decubitus, 3*(4), 14-17.

Munro, B. H., Brown, L., & Heitman, B. B. (1989). Pressure ulcers: One bed or another? *Geriatric Nursing, 10*(4), 190-192.

National Pressure Ulcer Advisory Panel. (1989). *Pressure ulcers: incidence, economics, risk assessment. Consensus development conference statement.* West Dundee, IL: S-N Publications.

Neill, K. M., Conforti, D., Kedas, A., & Burris, J. F. (1989). Pressure sore response to a new hydrocolloid dressing. *Wounds, 1*(3), 173-185.

Nichol, J., Girling, F., Jerrard, W., Claxton, B., & Burton, A. C. (1951). Fundamental instability of small blood vessels and critical closing pressures in vascular beds. *American Journal of Physiology, 164,* 330-344.

North American Nursing Diagnosis Association. (1999). *Nursing diagnoses: Definitions and classification 1999-2000.* Philadelphia: Author.

Norton, D., McLaren, R., & Exton-Smith, A. N. (1962). *An investigation of geriatric nursing problems in hospital.* Edinburgh: Churchill Livingstone.

Olerud, J. E., Odland, C. F., Burgess, E. M., Wyss, C. R., Fisher, L. D., & Matsen, F. A., III. (1995). A model for the study of wounds in normal and elderly adults and patients with peripheral vascular disease or diabetes mellitus. *Journal of Surgical Research, 59*(3), 349-360.

Oleske, D. M., Smith, X. P., White, P., Pottage, J., & Donavan, M. I. (1986). A randomized clinical trial of two dressing methods for the treatment of low-grade pressure ulcers. *Journal of Enterostomal Therapy, 13*(3), 90-98.

Olson, B., Langemo, D., Burd, C., Hanson, D., Hunter, S., & Cathcart-Silberberg, T. (1996). Pressure ulcer incidence in an acute care setting. *Journal of Wound, Ostomy & Continence Nursing, 23*(1), 15-25.

Parish, L. C., Witkowski, J. A., & Crissey, J. T. (1983). *The decubitus ulcer.* New York: Masson.

Pinchcofsky-Devin, G. D., & Kaminski, M. V., Jr. (1986). Correlation of pressure sores and nutritional status. *Journal of the American Geriatrics Society, 34,* 435-440.

Powell, J. W. (1989). Increasing acuity of nursing home patients and the prevalence of pressure ulcers: A ten year comparison. *Decubitus, 2*(2), 56-58.

Ramundo, J. M. (1995). Reliability and validity of the Braden Scale in the home care setting. *Journal of Wound, Ostomy & Continence Nursing, 22*(3), 128-134.

Reed, J. W. (1981). Pressure ulcers in the elderly: Prevention and treatment utilizing a team approach. *Maryland State Medical Journal, 30,* 45-50.

Reichel, S. M. (1958). Shearing forces as a factor in decubitus ulcers in paraplegics. *Journal of the American Medical Association, 166*(7), 762-763.

Reuler, J. B., & Cooney, T. G. (1981). The pressure sore: Pathophysiology and principles of management. *Annals of Internal Medicine, 94,* 661-666.

Roberts, B. V., & Goldstone, L. A. (1979). A survey of pressure sores in the over sixties on two orthopedic wards. *International Journal of Nursing Studies, 16,* 355-364.

Robson, M. C., & Heggers, J. P. (1969). Bacterial quantification of open wounds. *Military Medicine, 134*(1), 19-24.

Rodeheaver, G. T., Pettry, D., Thacker, J. G., Edgerton, M. T., & Edlich, R. F. (1975). Wound cleansing by high pressure irrigation. *Surgical Gynecology and Obstetrics, 141*(3), 357-362.

Rodeheaver, G. T., & Stotts, N. A. (1995). Methods for assessing change in pressure ulcer status. *Advances in Wound Care, 8*(4), 34-36.

Rodriquez, G. P., & Garber, S. L. (1994). Prospective study of pressure ulcer risk in spinal cord injury patients. *Paraplegia, 32*(3), 150-158.

Salcido, R., Donofrio, J., & Fisher, S. (1994). Histopathology of pressure ulcers as a result of sequential computer-controlled pressure sessions in a fuzzy rat model. *Advances in Wound Care, 7*(5), 23-40.

Sapico, F. L., Ginunas, V. J., Thornhill-Joynes, M., Canawati, H. N., Capen, D. A., Klein, N. E., Khawam, S., & Montgomerie, J. Z. (1986). Quantitative microbiology of pressure sores in different stages of healing. *Diagnostic Microbiology and Infectious Disease, 5,* 31-38.

Scales, J. T. (1976). Pressure on the patient. In R. M. Kenedi, J. M. Cowden, & J. T. Scales (Eds.), *Bedsore biomechanics* (pp. 11-17). London: University Park Press.

Shannon, M. L., & Skorga, P. (1989). Pressure ulcer prevalence in two general hospitals. *Decubitus, 2*(4), 38-43.

Shea, J. D. (1975). Pressure sores classification and management. *Clinical Orthopaedics and Related Research, 112,* 89-100.

Spector, W. D., Kapp, M. C., Tucker, R. J., & Sternberg, J. (1988). Factors associated with presence of decubitus ulcers at admission to nursing homes. *The Gerontologist, 28*(6), 830-834.

Staas, W. E., Jr., & Cioschi, H. M. (1991). Pressure sores: A multifaceted approach to prevention and treatment. *Western Journal of Medicine, 154,* 539.

Stevenson, T. R., Thacker, J. G., Rodeheaver, G. T., Bacchetta, C., & Edgerton, M. T. (1976). Cleansing the traumatic wound by high pressure syringe irrigation. *Journal of the American College of Emergency Physicians, 5*(1), 17-21.

Strauss, M. J., Gong, J., Gary, B. D., Kalsbeek, W. D., & Spear, S. (1991). The cost of home air-fluidized therapy for pressure sores: A randomized controlled trial. *Journal of Family Practice, 33*(1), 52-59.

Thomas, C. L. (Ed.). (1985). *Taber's cyclopedic medical dictionary.* Philadelphia: F. A. Davis.

Thomas, D. R., Rodeheaver, G., Bartolucci, A., Frantz, R., Sussman, C., Ferrell, B., Cuddigan, J., Stotts, N., Maklebust, J. (1997). Pressure ulcer scale for healing: Derivation and validation of the PUSH tool. *Advances in Wound Care: The Journal for Prevention and Healing, 10*(5), 96-101.

Trumble, H. C. (1930). The skin tolerance for pressure and pressure sores. *Medical Journal of Australia, 2,* 724.

van de Kerkhoff, P. C. M., van Bergen, B., Spruijt, K., & Kuiper, J. P. (1994). Age-related changes in wound healing. *Clinical and Experimental Dermatology, 19,* 369-374.

Varma, A. O., Bugatch, E., & German, F. M. (1973). Debridement of dermal ulcers with collagenase. *Surgical Gynecology and Obstetrics, 136*(2), 281-282.

Vasconez, L. O., Schneider, W. J., & Jurkiewicz, M. J. (1977). Pressure sores. *Current Problems in Surgery, 14*(4), 1-62.

Versluysen, M. (1986). How elderly patients with femoral fractures develop pressure sores in hospital. *British Medical Journal (Clinical Research Edition), 292,* 1311-1313.

Warner, D. J. (1992). A clinical comparison of two pressure-reducing surfaces in the management of pressure ulcers. *Decubitus, 5*(3), 52-55, 58-60, 62-64.

Weiler, P. G., Franzi, C., & Kecskes, D. (1990). Pressure sores in nursing home patients. *Aging, 2*(3), 267-275.

Wheeler, C. B., Rodeheaver, G. T., Thacker, J. G., Edgerton, M. T., & Edlich, R. F. (1976). Side-effects of high pressure irrigation. *Surgical Gynecology & Obstetrics, 143*(5), 775-778.

Winter, G. D., & Scales, J. T. (1963). Effect of air drying and dressings on the surface of a wound. *Nature, 197,* 91-92.

Xakellis, G. C., & Chrischilles, E. A. (1992). Hydrocolloid versus saline gauze dressings in treating pressure ulcers: A cost-effectiveness analysis. *Archives of Physical Medicine and Rehabilitation, 73*(5), 463-469.

Xakellis, G. C., & Frantz, R. A. (1996). The cost of healing pressure ulcers across multiple health care settings. *Advances in Wound Care, 9*(6), 18-22.

Xakellis, G. C., Frantz, R. A., & Lewis, A. (1995). Cost of pressure ulcer prevention in long-term care. *Journal of the American Geriatrics Society, 43,* 496-501.

Xakellis, G. C., Frantz, R. A., Lewis, A., & Harvey, P. (1998). Cost-effectiveness of implementing an intensive pressure ulcer prevention protocol in long-term care. *Advances in Wound Care: The Journal for Prevention and Healing, 11*(1), 22-29.

Young, L. (1989). Pressure ulcer prevalence and associated patient characteristics in one long-term care facility. *Decubitus, 2*(2), 52.

CHAPTER 12

IMPAIRED SKIN INTEGRITY: DRY SKIN

Lt. Col. Mary D. Hardy

Care of the integument has been within the defined scope of nursing practice since Nightingale (1946). Nightingale defined skin care as "personal cleanliness," suggesting that the ideal bath incorporates soap, rubbing, and a large quantity of soft water that the skin will absorb. Assessment and treatment of the patients' skin has traditionally centered around cleanliness, the condition of the skin being a sign of overall health. More recently nursing assessment has included a systematic measure of the condition of the skin and scalp, of which dryness is one factor (Lueckenotte, 1998). As problems associated with aging have gained more attention in the literature, nursing interventions for dry skin among elderly individuals have been addressed (Frantz & Gardner, 1994; Gilchrest, 1986; Hardy, 1990b) and tested (Hardy, 1992; Hardy, 1996).

PREVALENCE

Dry skin is a problem for 59% to 85% of elderly individuals (Beauregard & Gilchrest, 1987; Eliopoulos, 1988; Frantz & Kinney, 1986; Tindall & Smith, 1963). Up to 85% of pruritus in aging is associated with dry skin (Herman & Gilchrest, 1989).

RELATED FACTORS/ETIOLOGIES

As skin ages, it becomes less efficient at holding moisture and less pliable (Downing et al., 1987). Dry skin results primarily from a lack of water, not from a lack of skin oils.

RISK FACTORS

A variety of factors can increase the risk of dry skin in the elderly. External risk factors can include excessive exposure to sun, soaps, radiation, lack of humidity, and the winter season. Internal risk factors can include medications, dehydration, stress, and disease processes such as diabetes, liver disease, hyperthyroidism, hypothyroidism, and malignancies.

ASSESSMENT

Dry skin is considered to occur primarily on the extremities, although the trunk and face can be affected (Arndt, 1983; Parent, 1985). Extensive work exists on history and assessment of the integument (Delancy & North, 1983; Hannigan, 1978; Hogstel, 1983; Malkiewicz, 1981; Pearson & Kotthof, 1979; Urosevich, 1981). However, the research base for measurement of dry skin is limited to two extant instruments: the Black and Gaspar Foot Assessment Tool (BGFAT) and the Skin Condition Data Form (SCDF). The BGFAT measures skin condition on a scale of 1 (oily) to 7 (very dry) for dorsal and plantar surfaces of the feet. Brown, Boosinger, Black, Gaspar, and Sather (1982) used the BGFAT to evaluate the effectiveness of an intervention for treating elderly individuals with dry feet. The findings of the study indicated significant ($p < .01$) improvement in the condition of dry skin.

The SCDF includes questions pertaining to practices and etiologic factors and measures skin conditions, including redness, scaling, fissuring, rash, excoriation, greasy appearance, and thickening. The SCDF was used by Frantz and Kinney (1986) with 76 subjects over the age of 65 to analyze the relationship between sebum content and dry skin. One check was made each time a sign occurred on any of the 11 areas of the body rated, making the range of possible scores from 0 to 77. Hardy (1990a) reported the content validity and reliability of a modified SCDF as part of a pilot study. Content validity was judged by a panel of experts. Interrater reliability, using percents agreement between raters, was 87%, 63%, and 68%, respectively, on history, current skin practices, and observed dryness. Hardy tested an intervention to treat dry skin in a sample of 143 elderly subjects, using the SCDF with a modified scoring scheme to measure dryness on 22 areas of the body. For the skin dryness observation items, raters assigned a value of 1 (absent), 2 (mild), or 3 (severe) for observed redness, flaking, scaling, and cracking. The author reported an interrater reliability of 94% for 18 subjects using a method suggested by Polit and Hungler (1987), but they cautioned that the result might be an overestimate.

NURSING DIAGNOSIS

The diagnoses Impaired Skin Integrity: Actual and Impaired Skin Integrity: Potential were accepted for testing by the North American Nursing Diagnosis Association (NANDA) in 1975 (NANDA, 1989). Although the NANDA Taxonomy I (1989) continued to use the 1975 nomenclature, the terminology recently was altered to

"Impaired Skin Integrity" and "Risk for Impaired Skin Integrity" (NANDA, 1999). Impaired Skin Integrity is defined as "a state in which the individual has altered epidermis and/or dermis" (NANDA, 1999, p. 43). NANDA (1999) lists the defining characteristics as "disruption of skin surface (epidermis); destruction of skin layers (dermis); and invasion of body structures." Related factors for Impaired Skin Integrity include those that are external or environmental and those that are internal or somatic. The subdiagnosis Impaired Skin Integrity: Dry Skin is not on the list of diagnoses accepted for testing by NANDA. However, comparison of the etiologies and signs and symptoms described in the literature on dry skin with those listed with the Impaired Skin Integrity label make it clear that Dry Skin is an appropriate "specification" of Impaired Skin Integrity. Table 12-1 illustrates this comparison, showing that there are multiple similarities among the defining characteristics and etiologies for the diagnoses. It is reasonable to expect that the defining characteristics and etiologies for Impaired Skin Integrity: Dry Skin would be more specific than those for Impaired Skin Integrity, since the former is a further specified diagnosis of the latter.

CASE STUDY

H. Biggs is a 74-year-old woman living independently at home except for support from a niece for buying groceries and doing heavy housework. Mrs. Biggs remains active with volunteer work at the local community hospital once a month and has a small garden in the summer. Otherwise, she has little physical activity outside her usual light housekeeping, meal preparation, and a daily afternoon swing on the back-porch glider. She arrived at the family practice clinic with a large overnight bag full of lotions, creams, soaps, and oils she had purchased to treat dry skin and itching. She wanted to show the doctor and the nurse all the things that she "wasted money on because they had not worked."

Mrs. Biggs complained that for many years and especially in the winter she had suffered from severe itching, primarily on her lower legs and back. Inspection revealed mild scaling on her lateral upper arms. Severe flaking was observed on the dorsal surface of her feet, on the posterior and lateral surfaces of her lower arms, on the anterior and lateral surfaces of her lower legs, and on her back. Mild cracking was present on her elbows and heels. Otherwise, her skin was supple, without raised surfaces or destruction. As shown in Table 12-2, the SCDF scoring for Mrs. Biggs was 103 at the time of screening.

Mrs. Biggs lives in the Midwest and is aware that her dry skin is more intense in the winter when the furnace is on. Although she tried hard to take in adequate fluids, she was not able to drink 6 to 8 glasses of water daily. "I get too full; I don't have that much room in my stomach anymore." Moreover, Mrs. Biggs took 12.5 mg of hydrochlorothiazide for mild right-sided congestive heart failure and justified not drinking more because "I just have to go to the bathroom more, with this water pill that I take." As she had done since she was a child on the farm, Mrs. Biggs tub bathed once a week with "a mild soap." She had tried multiple oils, lotions, and other things over the past several years to alleviate the itching and dryness. She had no assistive devices on her tub for entering and exiting it, so each bath was a somewhat difficult process.

NURSING-SENSITIVE OUTCOMES

The literature reports few studies helpful in labeling outcomes of effective intervention for dry skin. Spoor (1958) reported "successful therapeutic affect" and "personal acceptance" in 10 of 12 subjects after using water-dispersible bath oil. Weiner et al. (1983) reported "limited success" in the treatment of dry skin with a topical moisturizing and lubricating lotion. Brown et al. (1982) reported significant ($p < .01$) "improvement in the skin condition" of the feet in subjects enrolled for 2 weeks in an intervention designed to reduce dryness of the feet. Hardy (1990a) reported significant reductions in "total skin dryness," "redness" ($F = 3.55$, $p = .031$), "scaling" ($F = 2.86$, $p = .007$), and "flaking" ($F = 3.44$, $p = .001$) in a pilot study of a bathing intervention. A larger study reported by Hardy (1996) further tested a treatment for dry skin, analyzing the effects of frequency (low, moderate, and high) and mode (shower versus tub bath) of bathing on dryness. Scaling, flaking, and redness again were significantly reduced over the 18-week study for subjects bathing or showering 5 or more times weekly ($p = .000$). Subjects who showered rather than tub bathed had a greater drop in flaking scores during the intervention ($p = .010$). High-frequency showers demonstrated significantly reduced scores on scaling ($p = .018$). No statistically significant reduction in cracking was found in either the 1990 or 1996 Hardy study, thus bringing into question the validity of the symptom, the validity or reliability of the symptom measurement, or the validity of the intervention for treating the symptom.

Skin changes can take up to 2 weeks to be manifested in elderly individuals (Fenske, 1982). Therefore it is not surprising that the effects of Hardy's (1996) intervention to treat dry skin did not clearly present until 2 weeks after the start of the treatment and continued to be observed 2 weeks after the treatment was terminated.

Three outcomes included in the *Nursing Outcomes Classification (NOC)* (Iowa Outcomes Project, 2000) are useful in evaluating effective treatment for Impaired Skin Integrity: Dry Skin. Specifically, the outcomes Comfort Level and Symptom Control with the following selected indicators are appropriate:

Comfort Level—Extent of physical and psychologic ease (p. 173)

Table 12-1	Comparison of Impaired Skin Integrity Label With That of Impaired Skin Integrity: Dry Skin
Nursing Diagnoses	
IMPAIRED SKIN INTEGRITY	**IMPAIRED SKIN INTEGRITY: DRY SKIN**
Defining Characteristics	
Disruption of skin surface (epidermis)	Raised skin edges (scaling)
Destruction of skin layers (dermis)	Destruction of skin layers (flaking and chapping)
Invasion of body structures	Redness
	Pruritus
Related Factors/Etiologies	
External (environmental)	
Hyperthermia or hypothermia	Excessive exposure to sun
Chemical substance	Soap
Mechanical factors	Radiation
Radiation	Lack of humidity
Physical immobilization	Too frequent bathing
Humidity	Winter season
Medication	
Internal (somatic)	
Altered nutritional state	Medication
Altered metabolic state	Dehydration
Altered circulation	Stress
Altered sensation	Disease process (diabetes, liver disease, hyperthyroid,
Altered pigmentation	hypothyroid, malignancy)
Developmental factors	
Skeletal prominence	Maturation related to aging
Immunologic deficit	Smoking
Alterations in turgor (elasticity)	

Nursing-Sensitive Outcomes	Nursing Intervention
COMFORT LEVEL	**BATHING**
Indicator	*Activities*
Reported satisfaction with symptom control	Use superfatted soap for cleaning
SYMPTOM CONTROL	Use water temperature of 90-105°
Indicators	Immerse in a tub up to chest or shower for 10 minutes
Recognizes symptom onset	Pat the skin dry with a cotton towel
Recognizes symptom persistence	Use linen that has been thoroughly rinsed
Recognizes symptom variation	Apply mineral oil over all body parts
Uses preventive measures	Wear cotton clothing
Uses relief measures	Assist with chair shower, tub bath, bedside bath, standing
TISSUE INTEGRITY: SKIN & MUCOUS MEMBRANES	shower, or sitz bath as appropriate or desired
Indicators	Wash hair, as needed and desired
Color in expected range	Assist with perineal care, as needed
Skin intactness	Administer foot soaks, as needed
	Shave patient, as indicated
	Offer hand wash after toileting/before meals
	Apply drying powders to deep skin folds
	Monitor skin condition while bathing
	Monitor functional ability while bathing

Table 12-2	Skin Condition Data Form for Mrs. Biggs on Preintervention Visit			
Enter a number in each box: 1 = Absent, 2 = Mild, 3 = Severe.				
Body Site	**Redness**	**Scaling**	**Cracking**	**Flaking**
Face	1	1	1	1
Neck	1	1	1	1
Upper arms				
• Anterior	1	1	1	1
• Posterior	1	1	2	1
• Lateral	1	2	1	1
Forearms				
• Anterior	1	1	1	1
• Posterior	1	1	1	3
• Lateral	1	1	1	3
Hands—dorsal	1	1	1	1
Trunk				
• Anterior	1	1	1	1
• Posterior	1	1	1	3
• Lateral	1	1	1	1
Thighs				
• Anterior	1	1	1	1
• Posterior	1	1	1	1
• Lateral	1	1	1	1
Lower legs				
• Anterior	1	1	1	3
• Posterior	1	1	1	1
• Lateral	1	1	1	3
Feet				
• Dorsal	1	1	1	3
• Plantar	1	1	1	1
• Heels	1	1	2	1
• Between toes	1	1	1	1
TOTALS	22	23	24	34

TOTAL SCORE = 103

• Reported satisfaction with symptom control (no itching)

Symptom Control—Personal actions to minimize perceived adverse changes in physical or emotional functioning (p. 419)

• Recognizes symptom onset
• Recognizes symptom persistence
• Recognizes symptom variation
• Uses preventive measures
• Uses relief measures
• Reports controlling symptoms

Additionally, although the outcome Tissue Integrity: Skin & Mucous Membranes is appropriate, indicators must be further specified as follows to be consistent with dry skin measurement and to make this outcome useful in evaluating effectiveness of treatment for dry skin:

Tissue Integrity: Skin & Mucous Membranes—Structural intactness and normal physiologic function of skin and mucous membranes (p. 427)

• Color in expected range (no redness)
• Skin intactness (no flaking)
• Skin intactness (no scaling)

Specifically, itching as a *symptom* will be decreased or eliminated, and feelings of ease and comfort will be increased. Flaking, scaling, and redness brought on by dryness are abnormal structural features of skin that will be reduced or eliminated with therapeutic treatment of dry skin.

These three outcomes (see Table 12-1) are consistent with the literature on effective treatment of dry skin. Unfortunately, no instruments have been sufficiently validated to accurately measure indicators of efficacy in dry skin treatment. The SCDF and a modified version of the SCDF, which measures structural intactness, have been used in three small studies, one study of etiology (Frantz & Kinney, 1986) and two studies of intervention (Hardy, 1990a, 1996). Since cracking was not reduced significantly in either Hardy study, it is recommended that cracking not be used as an outcome. However, reduction in flaking, scaling, and redness should be considered for use. Based on a delayed response to a patch test of up to 2 weeks in elderly individuals (Fenske, 1982), outcomes of treatment for dry skin are ideally measured every 2 weeks. Unfortunately, no empirical findings are available on the effect of dry skin treatment on itching as a symptom or physical and emotional barrier to a feeling of ease.

NURSING INTERVENTIONS

Aging skin is dry, not because it lacks skin oils, but because it becomes less efficient at holding moisture and less pliable (Downing et al., 1987). Water absorbed by the skin through bathing will hydrate the skin but will rapidly be lost to the atmosphere. Therefore current therapy for dry skin emphasizes maintenance of a controlled humidity and the use of occlusive emollients to prevent moisture loss from the skin (Arndt, 1983; Fitzsimmons, 1983; Hogstel, 1983; Parent, 1985; Shellchock, 1994)—Gilchrest (1986) suggests, "the greasier, the better."

Bathing is listed as one of the interventions in the *Nursing Interventions Classification (NIC)* (3rd ed.) (Iowa Intervention Project, 2000, p. 157) and is defined as "cleaning of the body for the purposes of relaxation, cleanliness, and healing." Clearly the intervention Bathing, when defined in this way, is aimed not only at cleaning and comforting but also at healing. It is therefore appropriate for the treatment of dry skin. However, bathing as an intervention for treating dry skin could be made more useful if either of the following changes would be adopted: (1) the activities within the current intervention Bathing were expanded to include those used in *healing* dry skin or (2) "Bathing: Dry Skin Treatment" were added as an intervention and defined as "cleaning of the body for the purposes of healing dry skin" and the definition of Bathing were revised to read "cleaning of the body for the purposes of cleanliness and comfort."

There is no research base and little agreement on brands of soap, frequency of bathing, shower versus tub, occlusive agents, or desired environmental humidity. Although there is agreement that water should be tepid, that rough clothing should be avoided (Arndt, 1983; Shelley & Shelley, 1982), that vigorous drying should be avoided (Parent, 1985), and that laundry should be treated without starch or antistatic drying agents, there is little research base supporting any of these multiple treatment choices (Boisits, 1986; Cornell, 1986; Epstein, 1983; Fenske, 1982; Fitzsimmons, 1983; Gaul & Underwood, 1951; Hogstel, 1983; Parent, 1985; Pearson & Kotthof, 1979; Porth & Kapke, 1983; Walther & Harber, 1984; Weiner et al., 1983). A recent article by Hardy (1996) synthesized the literature on the issues and research associated with dry skin bathing intervention.

Soaps

Beauregard and Gilchrest (1987) reported that among 68 independent living elderly individuals 90% used conventional soap that can make skin dry after the early and middle stages of life (Shelley & Shelley, 1982). "Mild," nonirritating soaps have decreased detergent content but also decreased cleansing ability. Superfatted soaps, on the other hand, provide an excess of emollient material, which results in a thick film of oil being deposited on the skin surface (Dotz & Berman, 1984). The consensus is that nonperfumed, superfatted soaps that do not contain hexachlorophene are most effective in treating dry skin in elderly individuals. Specific brands meeting these criteria include Basis, Dove, Tone, Caress (Arndt, 1983; Hardy, 1996; Walther & Harber, 1984), Neutrogena, and Emulave (Porth & Kapke, 1983). Dove has been reported as being tested in a laboratory study and found to be less "irritating" than other soaps (Frosch & Kligman, 1979).

Frequency of Bathing

There is little consensus in the literature about the frequency of bathing. Recommendations for elderly individuals vary from a partial bath daily and a complete bath 2 to 3 times per week (Hogstel, 1983) to one short, cool shower per week for any older individual suffering from itching caused by dry skin (Shelley & Shelley, 1982). Epstein (1983) suggests, however, that unless bathing more than once a day, there is no reason for those with dry skin to cut down on bathing. This suggestion is consistent with the theory that one element of effective treatment for dry skin is superhydration. However, older individuals may favor less frequent bathing (Arndt, 1983; Beauregard & Gilchrest, 1987; Hardy, 1996; Hogstel, 1983; Shelley & Shelley, 1982; Walther & Harber, 1984). Whether this is due to available bathroom facilities, physical limitations, tradition, or simple preference has not been ascertained.

Mode of Bathing

Walther and Harber (1984) suggest a bed-bath or partial bath for treatment of dry skin. This suggestion has not been tested, however, and is intuitively contradictory to the theory that water absorption must be maximized in dry skin treatment. Although Pearson and Kotthof (1979) suggest a soaking or submerging for 10 to 15 minutes and Spoor (1958) and Brown et al. (1982) reported successful treatment with soaking baths, total immersion may not always be practical. Hardy (1996) reported no statistically significant difference, except in reducing flaking, among 143 subjects age 55 to 102 who either bathed or showered during a 6-week bathing intervention. This finding is consistent with the statement made by Epstein (1983) that showering was as effective as bathing in treating dry skin.

In a study of 68 noninstitutionalized subjects age 50 to 91, subjects younger than 78 used both the tub and the shower frequently, whereas subjects age 80 years and older often related exclusive use of either tub (38%) or shower

(21%) (Hardy, 1990a). Hardy (1996) reported that among 143 subjects age 55 to 102 enrolled in a study to treat dry skin, more subjects showered ($n = 81$) than bathed ($n = 59$). No research reports the rationale used by elderly individuals or by nurses in making bathing mode treatment choices. Safety, time, mobility, physical support to enter or exit the tub, and the medical regimen are often major considerations. The clinical feasibility and outcomes of nursing intervention must be considered. For instance, Lindell and Olsson (1990) found that 89% of 28 institutionalized elderly women, compared with 20% of 35 living at home, complained of vaginal pruritus; the authors attributed these findings to the fact that the institutionalized women were bathed in bed and had inadequate rinsing of soap, whereas the women at home showered.

Emollient

An oil base is consistently suggested as the primary agent of choice following a bath, while skin is still wet and water will be trapped (Arndt, 1983; Dotz & Berman, 1984; Shelley & Shelley, 1982). Occlusive agents lubricate the skin surface and make the skin feel smoother and less dry. This improves the greasy feeling and, once the water has been trapped, the oily film remaining on the skin is generally sufficient to retard transepidermal water loss. Keratin softening agents, such as urea, lactic acid, and allantoin, may be added to dry skin products to soften the skin and improve its appearance. However, they do not affect the water content of the skin and should be used in conjunction with occluding agents. Among the emollient agents recommended in the literature are bath oil, vegetable oil, Keri, Nivea, Aquaphor, Eucerin, mineral oil, petrolatum, and lanolin (Arndt, 1983; Cornell, 1986; Dotz & Berman, 1984; Epstein, 1985; Hardy, 1996; Parent, 1985; Pearson & Kotthof, 1979; Porth & Kapke, 1983). Some debate exists about each of these products: bath oil because it may be hazardous; petrolatum because of the greasy feeling; lanolin because it is more expensive and may sensitize skin; mineral oil because it may act as a drying agent; and vegetable oil because it may leave an odor.

Research is limited to a very few studies. Weiner et al. (1983) used Dermo-Pedic Foot Lotion, a lotion containing "ethoxylated" lanolin in an aqueous base and allantoin. A study by Spoor (1958) used a water-dispersible bath oil. Studies by Brown et al. (1982) and Hardy (1996) suggest that mineral oil is the emollient of choice because of its cost, availability, and ability to hold water. However, a clinical trial of occlusive agents at a relative humidity of 20% resulted in a 98% reduction in moisture loss with petrolatum, an 83% reduction with lanolin, and a 31% reduction with mineral oil (Boisits, 1986). If the aesthetics of petrolatum are acceptable to a client, this may be the most appropriate choice. However, petrolatum as an emollient in the treatment of dry skin requires further study to be recommended.

Water Temperature

The consensus is that water that is 90° to 105° F be used for bathing (Arndt, 1983; Dotz & Berman, 1984; Fitzsimmons, 1983; Hogstel, 1983; Pearson & Kotthof, 1979; Porth & Kapke, 1983). Hardy (1996) reported use of a large water thermometer by subjects at home to easily measure the temperature of bath water. Institutions often have regulatory requirements for maintenance of safe temperatures for bath water, usually between 90° and 105° F.

Humidity

Dry skin is common at humidities of less than 30% and uncommon at humidities over 60% (Gaul & Underwood, 1951; Hogstel, 1983). Hardy (1996) reported that subjects living in environments of 40% humidity or greater responded more favorably to a bathing treatment designed to reduce skin dryness. Room temperature should be kept as low as is comfortable because the dry heat associated with winter contributes to further drying (Arndt, 1983). Humidifiers or pans of water on radiators should be used (Arndt, 1983; Walther & Harber, 1984) to increase ambient humidity. A hygrometer, used for measuring environmental humidity, is easily accessible and used.

The following activities for the treatment of dry skin should be added to those presently comprising the activities for the intervention Bathing:

1. Use superfatted soap for cleansing
2. Use water temperature of 90° to 105° F
3. Immerse in a tub up to chest while pouring water over body parts or shower with continuous spray over all body parts for 10 minutes
4. Pat the skin dry with a cotton towel rather than rubbing
5. Apply mineral oil over all body parts
6. Use linen that has been thoroughly rinsed of detergent and without antistatic agents
7. Wear cotton clothing

The currently listed activities of "bathe in water of a comfortable temperature" and "apply lubricating ointment and cream to dry skin areas" can be removed because they are further specified in the activities listed above. All of the other activities currently listed with the intervention Bathing (see Table 12-1) are appropriate for bathing for purposes of healing dry skin, as well as providing cleanliness and comfort.

CASE STUDY

The case manager who saw Mrs. Biggs at the family practice clinic collected the first baseline data (see Table 12-2). The case manager explained the etiologies, signs and symptoms, and interventions for dry skin so that Mrs. Biggs would understand the scope of the problem and see that it required more than adding lotion to dry skin. They mutually agreed that it would be appropriate for Mrs. Biggs to use a bathing intervention targeted at decreasing her dry skin for a period of 6 weeks, during which time she agreed not to use any of the other items in her bag. To facilitate this intervention, an assistive device would be installed to her tub. Mrs. Biggs agreed to fill a 1.5-qt container daily with fresh water and sip from a glass all day long, thus avoiding the necessity to drink an entire glass of water at a time. She would place pans of water on her radiators during the winter when she was most plagued by dry skin. In the summer she would wear a large-brimmed hat to work in the garden and sit on her porch.

The case manager explained to Mrs. Biggs that it would take at least 6 weeks to evaluate the effectiveness of the new bathing practice because the normal cell moves from the basilar level to the epidermis in about 26 days and can take twice as long in the elderly individual. Mrs. Biggs could use her lotions and other things she had purchased while the clinic's home health nurse collected baseline data 2 more times over a 6-week period before introducing a change in Mrs. Biggs' bathing routine. This was to allow adequate time to measure Mrs. Biggs' skin condition over time and provide adequate data with which to compare outcomes following intervention. Skin condition was observed every 2 weeks. Total scores on the SCDF at 2 weeks and 4 weeks following the first meeting with Mrs. Biggs were 106 and 100, respectively. She continued to complain of moderate to severe itching on her lower legs and back. At 6 weeks the case manager had Mrs. Biggs bring in her Dove soap and mineral oil so that they could discuss the precise intervention. The nurse gave Mrs. Biggs written instructions and a large laboratory thermometer that she could read to regulate the temperature of her bath water. Mrs. Biggs started tub bathing 3 times weekly using Dove soap, regulating her water temperature to between 90° and 105° F, applying mineral oil, and drying only excess water before application of the mineral oil. Her niece timed her visits with Mrs. Biggs so that she could apply the mineral oil to her back as often as possible. Mrs. Biggs was seen by the home health nurse for 2 weeks following the start of the bathing treatment. Her SCDF score of 100 was discouraging to Mrs. Biggs because it was the same as 2 weeks ago, before she changed her bathing routine. The home health nurse explained that changes due to treatment or toxins can take up to 2 weeks to be manifested in the elderly individual (Fenske, 1982) and she had been using the treatment for only 2 weeks. At 4 weeks after starting the new bathing routine, her SCDF score was 95 and the itching on her legs was much less, but the itching on her back continued to be severe when her niece was not able to apply her oil.

At week 6 following the start of the intervention, the case manager inspected Mrs. Biggs' skin and obtained a score of 90. The flaking on her lower legs and lower arms continued to be mild, the itching on her legs was absent, and the itching on her back was mild. At week 8, however, both her dryness and her itching were completely absent. Her skin was structurally intact and appeared supple, without flaking or cracking. Mrs. Biggs understood that she needed to continue this bathing treatment in order to maintain the positive outcomes she had obtained during the past 8 weeks. She gave away all of her lotions.

SUMMARY

Dry skin not only causes primary discomforts such as itching, redness, scaling, cracking, and flaking but can also add to risk for pressure sores (United States Public Health Service [USPHS], 1992) and secondary complications. Nurses must diagnose and treat the primary effects of dry skin, the associated disturbances to skin integrity and self-concept, and the secondary effects such as infection and increased anxiety that can further complicate the diagnosis and treatment of dry skin. Humidity, fluid intake, soaps, emollients, water temperature, bathing frequency, and mode of bathing are variables that can be incorporated independently by nurses in bathing practices and through counseling about self-care practices by clients. Clearly the healing outcomes of bathing are within the scope and accountability of the nurse.

REFERENCES

Arndt, K. A. (1983). *Manual of dermatologic therapeutics.* Boston: Little, Brown and Company.

Beauregard, S., & Gilchrest, B. (1987). A survey of skin problems and skin care regimens in the elderly. *Archives of Dermatology, 123,* 1638-1643.

Boisits, E. K. (1986). The evaluation of moisturizing products. *Cosmetics and Toiletries, May,* 31-39.

Brown, M., Boosinger, J., Black, J., Gaspar, R., & Sather, L. (1982). Nursing innovation for dry skin care of the feet in the elderly. *Journal of Gerontological Nursing, 8*(7), 393-395.

Cornell, R. C. (1986). Aging and the skin. *Geriatric Medicine, 5*(1), 26-33.

Delancy, V., & North, C. (1983). Skin assessment. *Topics in Clinical Nursing, 4,* 5-10.

Dotz, W., & Berman, B. (1984). Aids that preserve hydration and mitigate its loss. *Consultant, August,* 46-62.

Downing, D. T., Stewart, M. E., Wertz, P. W., Colton, S. W., Abraham, W., & Strauss, J. S. (1987). Skin lipids: An update. *Journal of Investigative Dermatology, 88,* 2s-6s.

Eliopoulos, C. (1988). *Gerontological nursing* (2nd ed.). Philadelphia: Lippincott Williams & Wilkins.

Epstein, E. (1983). *Common skin disorders* (2nd ed.). Oradell, NJ: Medical Economics Books.

Fenske, N. A. (1982). Problems of aging skin. *Consultant, January,* 287-300.

Fitzsimmons, V. M. (1983). The aging integument: A sensitive and complex system. *Topics in Clinical Nursing, 4*(6), 32-38.

Frantz, R. A., & Gardner, S. (1994). Clinical concerns: Management of dry skin. *Journal of Gerontological Nursing, 20*(9), 15-18, 45.

Frantz, R. A., & Kinney, C. N. (1986). Variables associated with skin dryness in the elderly. *Nursing Research, 35*(2), 98-100.

Frosch, P. J., & Kligman, A. M. (1979). The soap chamber test: The irritancy of soaps. *Journal of the American Academy of Dermatology, 1,* 35-41.

Gaul, L. E., & Underwood, G. B. (1951). Relation of dew point and barometric pressure to chapping of normal skin. *The Journal of Investigative Dermatology, 19,* 9-19.

Gilchrest, B. A. (1986). Skin diseases in the elderly. In E. Calkins, P. Davis, & A. B. Fords (Eds.), *The practice of geriatrics* (pp. 488-498). Philadelphia: W. B. Saunders.

Hannigan, L. (1978). Nursing assessment of the integumentary system. *Occupational Health Nursing, 10*(January), 19-22.

Hardy, M. (1990a). A pilot study of the diagnosis and treatment of impaired skin integrity. *Nursing Diagnosis, 1*(2), 57-63.

Hardy, M. (1990b). Impaired skin integrity: Dry skin. In M. Maas, K. Buckwalter, & M. Hardy (Eds.), *Nursing diagnoses and interventions for the elderly* (pp. 86-96). Reading, MA: Addison Wesley Longman.

Hardy, M. (1992). Dry skin care. In G. M. Bulechek & J. C. McCloskey (Eds.), *Nursing interventions: Essential nursing treatments* (pp. 34-47). Philadelphia: W. B. Saunders.

Hardy, M. (1996). What can you do about your patient's dry skin? *Journal of Gerontological Nursing, 22*(5), 10-18.

Herman, L., & Gilchrest, B. (1989). Pruritus in the elderly. *Geriatric Medicine Today, 8*(2), 23-44.

Hogstel, M. O. (1983). Skin care for the aged. *Journal of Gerontological Nursing, 9*(8), 431-437.

Iowa Intervention Project. J. C. McCloskey & G. M. Bulecheck (Eds.). (2000). *Nursing interventions classification (NIC)* (3rd ed.). St. Louis, MO: Mosby.

Iowa Outcomes Project. M. Johnson, M. Maas, & S. Moorhead (Eds.). (2000). *Nursing outcomes classification (NOC)* (2nd ed.). St. Louis, MO: Mosby.

Lindell, M., & Olsson, H. (1990). Personal hygiene in external genitalia of health and hospitalized elderly women. *Health Care for Women International, 11,* 151-158.

Lueckenotte, A. G. (1998). *Pocket guide to gerontologic assessment* (3rd ed.). St. Louis, MO: Mosby.

Malkiewicz, J. (1981). The integumentary system. *RN, 44*(December), 55-60.

Nightingale, F. (1946). *Notes on nursing. Facsimile of first edition, 1859.* Philadelphia: Stern and Company.

North American Nursing Diagnosis Association. (1989). *Nursing diagnoses: Definitions & classification.* Philadelphia: Author.

North American Nursing Diagnosis Association. (1999). *Nursing diagnoses: Definitions & classification 1999-2000.* Philadelphia: Author.

Parent, L. (1985). Therapy of skin problems in the elderly. *U.S. Pharmacist, 10*(4), 48-54.

Pearson, L. J., & Kotthof, M. K. (1979). *Geriatric clinical protocols.* Philadelphia: Lippincott Williams & Wilkins.

Polit, D., & Hungler, B. (1987). *Nursing research: Principles and methods.* Philadelphia: Lippincott Williams & Wilkins.

Porth, C., & Kapke, K. (1983). Aging and the skin. *Geriatric Nursing, 4*(3), 159-162.

Shellchock, L. (1994). Dry skin: Softening winter's effects. *Healthline,* November, 6-7.

Shelley, W., & Shelley, E. (1982). The ten major problems of aging skin. *Geriatrics, 37*(9), 107-113.

Spoor, H. J. (1958). Measurement and maintenance of natural skin oil. *New York State Journal of Medicine,* (October), 3292-3299.

Tindall, J., & Smith, J. (1963). Skin lesions of the aged. *Journal of the American Medical Association, 186,* 1039-1042.

United States Public Health Service. (1992). *Clinical practice guideline (Number 3): Pressure ulcers in adults: Prediction and prevention* (AHCPR Publication No. 92-0047). Rockville, MD: AHCPR.

Urosevich, P. R. (Ed.). (1981). *Nursing photobook.* Horsham, PA: Nursing 81 Books, Intermed Communications.

Walther, E. M., & Harber, L. C. (1984). Expected skin complaints of the geriatric patient. *Geriatrics, 39*(12), 67-80.

Weiner, E. M., Beiser, S., Giudice, R., Kanat, E., Kaplan, E., Kauth, B., & Stone, D. (1983). Treating the dry skin syndrome. *Journal of the American Podiatry Association, 63*(11), 571-581.

CHAPTER 13

ALTERED NUTRITION: LESS THAN BODY REQUIREMENTS

Bonnie Wakefield

The science of nutrition relates health, well-being, and disease to ingestion, absorption, and use of food and nutrients (Ebersole & Hess, 1998; Karkeck & Worthington-Roberts, 1993). The ability to obtain and maintain proper nutrition depends on multiple influencing factors. Good-quality food and nutrients must be available and obtainable for ingestion in appropriate types and amounts. The individual must be able and willing to eat. Finally, food must be absorbed to maintain body structure and function. The elder can have problems at one or more of these stages.

The most recent National Health and Nutrition Examination Survey (NHANES III) included persons over age 74 for the first time in the survey's history (Marwick, 1997). Findings from NHANES III for the elderly include the following:

- Median daily caloric intake was below recommended levels.
- Fat intake exceeded the recommended allowance of 30% of calories.
- Cholesterol intake was below recommended levels.
- Consumption of folate and vitamin B_{12} was higher than recommended, but calcium consumption was lower than recommended.
- Nutrient intake declines as age increases.

Malnutrition is a preventable and correctable cause of mortality in elders (Sullivan, Walls, & Bopp, 1995), and is associated with a number of adverse health outcomes (Covinsky, Martin, Beyth, Justice, Sehgal, & Landefeld, 1999), including altered immune response (Buzina-Suboticanec et al., 1998; Mazari, & Lesourd, 1998) cognitive impairment (Incalzi et al., 1996; Ortega et al., 1997), and decreased quality of life.

RISK FACTORS

A risk factor is a characteristic or occurrence that increases the likelihood of an outcome. Because of the heterogeneity of the elderly population, chronologic age is of less value in determining risk factors for altered nutrition than are functional groupings (White, 1994). When determining

important risk factors for altered nutrition, White (1994) suggests the following groupings: independent community-dwelling elders, dependent community-dwelling elders, and institutionalized elders. One additional category that could be included is acute hospitalized elders, who have unique needs in terms of risk factors and interventions. An alternative risk classification might be based on the interventions required: well elders who currently are not at risk but who might require nutritional counseling and educational preventive interventions; at-risk elders currently not nutritionally compromised but who have a potential for alteration in nutrition and who might require nutritional assessment and monitoring interventions; and elders with alterations in nutrition, who require nutrition therapy. Related factors are defined by the North American Nursing Diagnosis Association (NANDA) as an "inability to ingest or digest food or absorb nutrients due to biological, psychological, or economic factors" (NANDA, 1999, p. 10). More specifically, risk factors that have been identified in the literature for Altered Nutrition, Less Than Body Requirements, include illness, medications, alcohol use, oral health problems, functional limitations (including physical, cognitive, and social function), and financial limitations (Marwick, 1997).

Illness

In addition to normal changes associated with aging that can interfere with nutrition, the elderly population has an increased frequency of chronic illnesses. Recommended treatments for chronic illnesses can limit food types and palatability. Some examples are diabetes (decreased carbohydrate intake), chronic heart failure (decreased sodium intake), renal failure (decreased potassium, sodium, and protein intake), and hepatic disease (decreased protein intake).

Medications

Nutritional problems related to medication use result from misuse of prescribed drugs, inappropriate prescriptions, polypharmacy, and food-drug or alcohol-drug interactions (White, 1994). Medications can influence the ingestion or absorption of nutrients in several ways. Medications prescribed for chronic illnesses can be involved in drug-nutrient interactions and can induce nutritional deficiencies. Drug-nutrient interactions include (1) depression of drug absorption, (2) increases in drug absorption, and (3) nutrient depletion as an adverse drug reaction. Nutritional evaluation therefore is essential for any elderly patient receiving one or more drugs that could interact with nutrient intake or absorption. Ham (1994) recommends the "plastic bag test," in which a relative or the patient brings in every medication in the house. This will provide a good baseline to assess medications that might be causing anorexia or food-drug interactions.

Alcohol Use and Abuse

Alcoholism or alcohol abuse is accompanied by poor nutritional status. Estimates indicate that 3 million people over the age of 65 in the United States abuse alcohol (Krach, 1998). In older persons with new-onset alcoholism, loneliness and depression are contributing factors (White, 1994). Drinking creates nutritional problems when the elderly person substitutes drinking for eating nourishing food. Alcohol consumption increases nutrient requirements in the elder as a result of the increased metabolic effects of alcohol (White, 1994). Abuse of alcohol also is related to a number of vitamin deficiencies (Klein & Iber, 1991). Alcohol abuse can be hidden and difficult to assess. Questionnaires such as CAGE (Mayfield, McLeod, & Hall, 1974) can help identify problem drinking. Family education also might be needed because family members sometimes obtain alcohol for the elder.

Oral Health Problems

Poor dentition caused by lack of teeth or ill-fitting dentures can make chewing difficult. Even in elderly persons with adequate dentition, masticatory mandibular movements with chewing are not the same (Nagao, 1992). Almost half of people over age 75 in the United States and close to one third of those between the ages of 65 and 74 lack all of their teeth; this is compared with only 12% of 45 to 54 year olds (Dwyer, 1994).

Functional Limitations

Physical Function. Regardless of setting, losses of function can make an elderly individual dependent on others for meals or limit the choice of foods. One study found a relationship between body mass indexes (discussed in a subsequent section of this chapter) and risk for functional impairment. Greater extremes of body mass index (either high or low) are associated with greater risk for functional impairment (Galanos, Pieper, Cornoni-Huntley, Bales, & Fillenbaum, 1994), although the direc-

tion of the relationship is unclear. The decision of when and what to eat might be made for dependent elders, thus decreasing their control and choices.

Failing motor abilities and eyesight also can make meal preparation impossible. In one recent study 4% of those 60 to 69 years old were unable either to prepare their own meals or to walk around the room; among 80 year olds 23% were unable to prepare their own meals and 17% were unable to walk (Marwick, 1997). The number of people who own and are able to drive a car declines with each year over 65 years of age, and public transportation may be unavailable. The majority of grocery stores are now accessible only by car because neighborhood grocery stores are disappearing. Although convenience stores may be available, their prices are extremely high and the selection of fresh fruits, vegetables, and meats is limited.

Sensory impairment can create a situation of social isolation. Visual and hearing losses are fairly common in older adults. Hearing and vision loss, when combined with gradual declines in taste and smell, can result in diminished food intake and subsequent malnutrition. Both detection and recognition thresholds for taste and smell are elevated with aging, i.e., more intense taste and odor are required for the elderly person to detect and recognize the taste or odor. To compound this, a myriad of disease states and medications commonly used by the elderly affect the sense of smell and taste, including hypertension, cancer, chronic renal failure, diabetes mellitus, diuretics, antiinflammatory agents, vasodilators, sympathomimetics, and hypoglycemic agents (Schiffman, 1994).

Cognitive Function. Cognitive impairment can compromise nutrition in many ways, including inability to obtain and prepare food, poor judgment about food selections, or just not eating. In particular, people with dementia are at risk for poor nutrition because they have difficulty making decisions and adapting to new environments (e.g., when institutionalized). Depression also is associated with decreased food intake, which relates to the elder's ability to organize, choose, and take in enough nutrients (Ham, 1994). Conversely, nutritional deficits can cause or contribute to cognitive problems. Elders with low levels of vitamins B_{12} and C, folate, and riboflavin have been shown to score poorer on tests of memory and nonverbal abstract thinking (Goodwin, Goodwin, & Garry, 1983).

Social Function. Living alone is a significant risk factor for poor nutritional status. Older adults living alone do not make poorer food choices; rather they tend to consume fewer calories (Davis, Randall, Forthofer, Lee, & Margen, 1985). There can be a change in roles and increased loneliness because of the loss of a spouse or companion. Rolls' (1994) study found that young men and women ate up to 50% more when dining with friends;

however, eating with strangers did not increase food intake. The investigator concluded that use of socialization to improve food intake might depend on the type of social interaction. The use of socialization, in particular the effect of different types of socialization while eating, should be tested with older individuals.

The 1990 census in the United States found that about 25% of people over age 60 live alone (Himes, Hogan, & Eggebeen, 1996), a statistic that tends to be related to poor nutritional status. Munro (1985) found that men from 65 to 69 years of age averaged 9.3 years of independent living followed by 3.8 years of dependence. Women of the same age-group have 10.6 years of independent living but a lengthy 8.9 years of dependent living. Living alone can influence cooking and eating behaviors. Because mealtimes are a social activity, as well as an eating activity, the elderly who are alone may lack motivation to cook and eat.

Financial Problems

There is a consistent relationship between low income and poor nutritional intake. Low-income elderly often must choose among food, utilities, medications and medical care, and housing as to how to spend limited resources (White, 1994). The relationship between low income and poor nutritional status is explained by a lack of variety of food, inadequate intake of specific food groups or vitamins and minerals, overconsumption of fat and cholesterol, and inadequate intake of calories (White, 1994).

An estimated 20% of the elderly have limits imposed on nutritional intake by poverty. Total income decreases by one half for retirees, and many elderly live on fixed incomes that do not keep up with inflation. The elderly pay, on the average, 50% more for food because they buy food in smaller quantities, eat in restaurants, and purchase convenience foods. They may also be forced to buy poorer quality food. All of these factors place them at risk for inferior dietary intake.

Governmental and community-assisted programs, food stamps, Meals on Wheels, congregate meals, and shopping assistance are available in various communities. Even when available, however, they are not always used. Poor housing necessitated by low income can lack adequate food storage and preparation areas. Health care also can be affected by low income, especially dental care, resulting in loss of teeth, inability to obtain dentures, and lack of maintenance of dentures. If the elderly person cannot chew effectively, the diet is more likely to be inadequate in protein and fresh fruits and vegetables.

ASSESSMENT

A large multidisciplinary effort called the Nutrition Screening Initiative (1992) was undertaken by the American Academy of Family Physicians, The American Dietetic Association, and the National Council on the Aging, Inc.,

in partnership with over 25 national health, aging, and medical organizations. The purpose of the initiative, funded by Ross Products, Abbott Laboratories, was to unite the efforts of nutrition, medical, and geriatric experts in advocating for nutrition screening and intervention as a routine component of health care for the elderly (White, 1996). Major and minor indicators of poor nutritional status in the elderly have been identified by the initiative and are compared in Box 13-1 with those proposed by NANDA.

Some of the usual changes with aging, e.g., loss of lean muscle mass, skin dryness, and hair loss, can be confused with signs of malnutrition; this makes assessment of malnutrition challenging. The most common form of malnutrition in the elder is protein-calorie malnutrition (PCM) (Ham, 1994). PCM involves inadequate intake of both calories and protein and results from intake of a high-carbohydrate, low-protein diet. Findings in PCM include weight loss, pallor, dry, flaky skin, and loss of muscle mass. A decrease in serum albumin can occur with prolonged PCM (Ebersole & Hess, 1998). PCM increases hospital stay and can increase mortality. When PCM is present, the body's defense mechanisms are interrupted.

Nutritional assessment should be an integral component of health care for the elderly. Assessment of nutritional status can be complicated by changes that occur normally with aging and by the lack of standards for interpretation of measurements. Assessment includes clinical measures, dietary intake and energy status, anthropometrics, and biochemical measures.

Clinical Measures

Clinical measures include history, interview, and assessment of clinical signs, as well as the presence of the etiologies discussed earlier. The history and interview includes collecting information on attitude and interest in life, activities of daily living, a diet history including any problems with food intake and digestion, bowel and urinary habits, and a detailed medication history. A physical assessment should focus on signs indicative of nutritional deficiencies. Evidence of cheilosis (inflammation of the lips) and/or angular stomatitis can result from vitamin B deficiency. Mouth dryness can signal dehydration, as can variation in skin turgor. Evidence of a lack of subcutaneous fat and loose skin is a sign of weight loss. Bruising and poorly healing wounds may indicate undernutrition. Edema is a sign of hypoproteinemia (Ham, 1994). Persons should be examined for sore gums, decayed teeth, ill-fitting dentures, dysphagia, and poor oral hygiene, which can interfere with intake. Other problems that can affect intake, such as difficult breathing in patients with chronic respiratory disease, also should be considered. A chronically undereating person experiences early satiety (Ham, 1994), which can further reduce intake and exacerbate existing undernutrition.

Box 13-1	Major and Minor Indicators of Poor Nutritional Status in the Elderly

Altered Nutrition: Less Than Body Requirements

Defining characteristics

Loss of weight with adequate food intake

Body weight 20% or more under ideal

Reported inadequate food intake less than RDA

Weakness of muscles required for swallowing or mastication

Reported or evidence of lack of food

Aversion to eating

Reported altered taste sensation

Satiety immediately after ingesting food

Abdominal pain with or without pathology

Sore, inflamed buccal cavity

Capillary fragility

Abdominal cramping

Diarrhea and/or steatorrhea

Hyperactive bowel sounds

Lack of interest in food

Perceived inability to ingest food

Pale conjunctival and mucous membranes

Poor muscle tone

Excessive loss of hair

Lack of information, misinformation

Misconceptions

Nutrition Screening Initiative Indicators (Nutrition Screening Initiative, 1992)

Major indicators

Weight loss

Underweight or overweight

Low serum albumin

Change in functional status

Inappropriate food intake

Midarm muscle circumference <10th percentile

Triceps skinfold <10th percentile or >95th percentile

Obesity

Nutrition related disorders:

- Osteoporosis
- Osteomalacia
- Folate deficiency
- B_{12} deficiency

Minor indicators

Alcoholism

Cognitive impairment

Chronic renal insufficiency

Multiple concurrent medications

Malabsorption syndromes

Anorexia, nausea, dysphagia

Change in bowel habit

Fatigue, apathy, memory loss

Poor oral or dental status, dehydration

Poorly healing wounds

Loss of subcutaneous fat and/or muscle mass

Fluid retention

Reduced iron, ascorbic acid, zinc

Nutrient Intake

Nutritional requirements differ according to the age and health status of the elderly person. Requirements for the healthy elderly are similar to those for young or middle-age adults. Acutely ill elders have increased requirements caused by the stress of illness. Chronically ill elders typically have lower intake but increased need for specific nutrients (Guigoz, Vellas, & Garry, 1994). These differences have not been addressed in the established standards. The nutritional requirements for a 51 year old are probably different from those of a 95 year old. There is a consensus that, because of changes in metabolic rate and activity, caloric intake should be reduced as one ages by 5% per decade from age 55 to 75, with a further reduction of 7% beyond age 75 (Karkeck & Worthington-Roberts, 1993; Kart, Mestress, & Mestress, 1978). Caloric ranges for elderly men are from 2000 to 2800 calories and for elderly women from 1200 to 2200.

The National Research Council (1989) publishes the Recommended Dietary Allowances. The Recommended Dietary Allowances state the minimum levels of intake of essential nutrients needed to adequately meet the known nutritional needs of healthy individuals. The most recent version of the Recommended Dietary Allowances has somewhat more specific information for the elderly than has been provided in the past. For adults over age 50 with light to moderate activity, 2300 kilocalories are recommended for men and 1900 kilocalories are recommended for women. A normal variation of 20% is acceptable, as is true for younger adults. Requirements for persons beyond age 75 are said to be likely to be less because of reduced body size, resting energy expenditure, and activity.

There is no evidence that the need for nutrients decreases with age (Kart et al., 1978). However, recent evidence suggests that actual nutrient intake does decline with aging (Marwick, 1997). This suggests that, as one ages, food must be of better quality to fulfill nutrient needs. A recent study in malnourished hospitalized patients demonstrated success in increasing nutrient intake while maintaining normal portion sizes by using energy-enriched food (Olin et al., 1996).

Establishment of standard daily requirements obviously does not ensure that these requirements will be followed. Inappropriate or inadequate food intake and failure to consume the established Recommended Dietary Allowances of nutrients occur for many reasons, including cultural, ethnic, or religious preferences that result in restrictive food patterns, excessively restrictive dietary modifications related to chronic illness, mistaken health beliefs, poverty, lack of help with shopping, and eating alone. Dietary variety also declines as age increases (Rolls, 1994). Fruits, vegetables, breads, and cereal are the foods least likely to be consumed by people of *all ages* in the United States. The foods most commonly consumed by *older* people in the United States include white bread, coffee, whole milk, sugar, potatoes, tea, orange juice, eggs, butter, and bacon, although recently the elderly have been shifting to a lower-fat diet (Briley, 1994).

Measures of Healing, Immunity, and Strength

Nutritional requirements change in the presence of illness, injury, or surgery. Undernutrition can be reflected in delayed healing, reduced immunity, and loss of strength. Failure of a wound to heal, particularly in the absence of diabetes or circulatory disorders, should signal the need for evaluating nutritional status.

Malnutrition is known to affect immune function. Skin testing with common antigens has been used as a part of overall assessment, but cannot in and of itself diagnose malnutrition (Charney, 1995). Total lymphocyte count is a marker of immune function and nutritional risk, but like skin testing, should be part of a broader assessment protocol (Charney, 1995).

Structural and metabolic changes in skeletal muscle have been found with calorie and protein restriction, resulting in decreased muscle strength and mass (Ham, 1994). Several studies have found hand grip strength to be a more sensitive predictor of postoperative morbidity and mortality than usual assessment parameters such as weight loss, arm circumference, or albumin (Charney, 1995). A simple test of muscle strength and mobility is the Get up and Go test (Mathias, Nayak, & Issacs, 1986; Tinetti, Williams, & Mayewski, 1986). This test consists of asking the person to stand up from a chair, walk forward without assistance, turn around, bend and pick something up from the floor, return to the chair, rotate, and sit down. She should then be assessed for a sense of instability or dizziness.

Anthropometric Measurements

The most commonly used measures include height, weight, triceps skinfold, and mid-upper arm circumference measurements. Height should be measured as actual height, not an estimate given by the patient. Loss of height can indicate osteoporosis, in part a nutritional disorder. In persons with kyphosis or flexion contractures of the leg, formulas are available for calculating stature from knee height (Roe, 1990). Actual weight should be measured. However, a change in the fit of clothes can indicate weight

loss in the absence of measured weight (Ham, 1994). Weight change is a common sign of malnutrition, and a history of weight loss can be an important indicator of malnutrition in the elder. An unintended weight loss of 10 lb or more is regarded as significant (Ham, 1994). The more recent and severe the involuntary weight change, the greater the likelihood that the elder is at risk (White, 1994). Dehydration can complicate assessment of nutritional outcomes also, as weight loss or gain may reflect fluid status changes, i.e., edema and dehydration.

Several height-weight indices are available, including the Body Mass Index (BMI) (weight in kilograms/squared height in meters) and waist-to-hip ratio. A low BMI is an indicator of poor nutritional status. For individuals age 65 and older desirable BMI ranges from 24 to 29. Less than 24 is a significant sign of poor nutrition, and greater than 27 is a major risk factor for obesity (Ham, 1994). However, waist-to-hip ratio may be a more sensitive predictor of mortality in women. Women with the highest risk of mortality had low BMI but high waist-to-hip ratios. This pattern was similar for both smokers and nonsmokers (Folsom et al., 1993).

According to Chernoff, Mitchell, and Lipschitz (1984), several known changes in stature and body composition in the elderly can be attributed to the aging process itself. These changes are similar to those observed in malnutrition at any age. Because of this, it can be difficult to interpret abnormal values observed in the elderly person. Anthropometric body measurements are frequently part of the nutritional assessment. These include triceps skinfold and arm circumference, which indicate measurements of fat and protein stores. Standards for these measurements are set for young adults. When standards are available for the elderly, these measurements might improve the prediction of malnutrition in older persons. Because the elderly exhibit both a marked reduction in lean muscle mass and changes in the percentage of fat stores, these measurements might not be the best predictors of malnutrition; however, further study is needed. The Nutrition Screening Initiative recommended triceps skinfold as a measure of subcutaneous fat and mid-arm circumference as a measure of muscle mass (Ham, 1994). These are simple standardized measures requiring a triceps caliper and flexible tape measure.

Laboratory Values and Biochemical Measures

Laboratory measurements that frequently are used in nutritional assessment include serum albumin, total iron-binding capacity, serum transferrin, lymphocyte count, and 24-hour urinary creatinine. Serum transferrin is a poor predictor of malnutrition in the elderly, since older individuals have a reduced transferrin level that may be related to higher tissue iron stores and not malnutrition. Anemias and abnormalities in lymphocyte count are not uncommon in the well-nourished elder, making these variables poor predictors by themselves. Urinary creatinine is influenced by renal and liver dysfunction, which is common in the elderly. Serum albumin is only minimally altered by aging, and therefore hypoalbuminemia may be the best predictor of malnutrition in older persons (Chernoff et al., 1984; Ham, 1994; Mitchell & Lipschitz, 1982; Seltzer et al., 1979), particularly when interpreted in combination with clinical signs and weight changes.

Nutritional Assessment Tools

The goal of nutritional assessment is to assist in identification of problems so that a plan to improve and maintain nutritional status can be developed. Various parameters have been suggested for assessment. Most commonly included areas are a diet history, anthropometric measurements, laboratory values and immunologic assessments, and clinical presentation. Three pertinent assessment tools were found and are reviewed here.

Wolinsky et al. (1990) developed the Nutritional Risk Index (NRI) to screen for persons at risk of developing nutritional disabilities. The NRI includes 16 questions selected to tap five dimensions of nutritional risk: mechanics of food intake, prescribed dietary restrictions, morbid conditions affecting food intake, discomfort associated with food intake, and significant changes in dietary habits. The NRI was designed to be brief, easily scored, and suitable for telephone administration. The psychometric properties of the NRI have been tested in large groups (more than 1200) of community-dwelling elders in St. Louis and Houston, as well as with older outpatients from the St. Louis Veterans Affairs Medical Center. The developers suggest that the NRI is useful as a screening device to identify elderly individuals who are nutritionally at risk and who need more detailed standard clinical and laboratory nutritional assessment.

The Mini-Nutritional Assessment (MNA) (Guigoz et al., 1994) was developed to be included as part of functional geriatric assessment, since nutritional assessment is often absent from such assessments. Scoring from the MNA categorizes the elderly person as having one of the following: (1) normal or adequate nutrition, (2) borderline or being at risk for malnutrition, or (3) undernutrition. The MNA is a brief assessment that can be performed in 20 minutes or less and includes anthropometric measurements and questions on lifestyle, medication, mobility, food intake, autonomy of feeding, and self-perception of health. If needed (and available in the setting), biologic measures such as albumin and lymphocyte count can be included in the scoring. The MNA has been validated in more than 700 elderly people in France and the United States, and both French and English language versions are available. Tested groups included a range of individuals from the very frail to the healthy

elderly. The MNA includes 18 items covering both risk factors (e.g., more than three prescription drugs per day) and defining characteristics (e.g., weight loss and mid-arm circumference measure) of malnutrition.

Finally, a three-level assessment scheme was developed by the Nutrition Screening Initiative. The three levels are the DETERMINE screen, a risk self-assessment to be filled out by individuals, and Level One and Two screens, which are completed by a health care professional. The DETERMINE screen is an easy-to-use checklist highlighting nine risk factors for poor nutritional status. The overall score can cue the patient, caregiver, or health care professional to limitations in nutritional status. The Level One screen, designed to be used by health care professionals, aims to identify candidates for preventive interventions, such as home meal delivery or nutrition education (Grindel & Costello, 1996). The Level Two screen gathers detailed diagnostic information, such as changes in body weight and laboratory data, and usually takes place in a hospital, nursing home, outpatient clinic, or physician's office.

NURSING DIAGNOSIS

Altered Nutrition: Less Than Body Requirements is defined as "the state in which an individual is experiencing an intake of nutrients insufficient to meet metabolic needs" (NANDA, 1999, p. 9). The etiologies and defining characteristics associated with the diagnosis that are currently accepted for clinical testing by NANDA are listed in Box 13-2 (NANDA, 1999). Despite the prevalence and significance of this diagnosis for all age-groups, there are only two published studies related to this diagnosis. In the first study 101 nurses who were members of a nutritional support society were surveyed (Murphy, 1989). The nurses were asked to review a list of 18 etiologies and 32 defining characteristics for the diagnosis. Of these, the nurses rated eight etiologies and only two defining characteristics as being "quite" or "very" characteristic of the diagnosis (Box 13-3). These nurses listed six of the NANDA defining characteristics as not relevant. These six are misconceptions, lack of information/misinformation, pale conjunctiva and mucous membranes, capillary fragility, abdominal cramping, and lack of interest in food.

In the second study the etiologies and defining characteristics were validated in a group of 50 cancer patients from two medical centers (Chiang, Ku, & Lo, 1994). Eight items were selected as critical etiologies, and 14 defining characteristics were verified. These are compared with the findings of Murphy (1989) (see Box 13-3). The second study validated etiologies and defining characteristics with patients. However, since some of these factors might be unique to cancer patients, the study should be replicated using other patient groups.

| Box 13-2 | Suggested Nursing-Sensitive Outcome and Nursing Intervention
ALTERED NUTRITION: LESS THAN BODY REQUIREMENTS |

Nursing Diagnosis
Altered Nutrition: Less Than Body Requirements
Defining characteristics
Loss of weight with adequate food intake
Body weight 20% or more under ideal
Reported inadequate food intake less than Recommended
    Dietary Allowance
Weakness of muscles required for swallowing or mastication
Reported or evidence of lack of food
Aversion to eating
Reported altered taste sensation
Satiety immediately after ingesting food
Abdominal pain with or without pathology
Sore, inflamed buccal cavity
Capillary fragility
Abdominal cramping
Diarrhea and/or steatorrhea
Hyperactive bowel sounds
Lack of interest in food
Perceived inability to ingest food
Pale conjunctival and mucous membranes
Poor muscle tone
Excessive loss of hair
Lack of information, misinformation
Misconceptions
Related factors/etiologies
Inability to ingest or digest food or absorb nutrients due to
    biologic, psychologic, or economic factors

Nursing-Sensitive Outcome
Nutritional Status
Indicators
Nutrient intake
Food and fluid intake
Energy
Body mass
Weight
Biochemical measures
NOTE: Several of the indicators for the outcome Nutritional
    Status type of nutrients needed to meet are outcomes with
    more specific indicators (Nutritional Status: Body Mass;
    Nutritional Status: Nutrient Intake; Weight Control)

Nursing Intervention
Nutrition Therapy
Activities
Monitor food/fluid ingested and calculate daily caloric intake, as
    appropriate

Monitor appropriateness of diet orders to meet daily
    nutritional needs, as appropriate
Determine—in collaboration with dietitian, as appropriate—
    number of calories and nutrition requirements
Determine food preferences with consideration of cultural and
    religious preferences
Determine need for nasogastric tube feedings
Select malts, shakes, and ice cream to supplement nutrition
Encourage patient to select semisoft food if lack of saliva
    hinders swallowing
Encourage intake of high-calcium foods, as appropriate
Encourage intake of foods and fluids high in potassium, as
    appropriate
Ensure that diet includes foods high in fiber content to prevent
    constipation
Provide patient with high-protein, high-calorie, nutritious
    finger foods and drinks that can be readily consumed, as
    appropriate
Assist patient to select soft, bland, and nonacidic foods, as
    appropriate
Administer enteral feedings, as appropriate
Discontinue use of tube feedings, as oral intake is tolerated
Administer hyperalimentation fluids, as appropriate
Ensure availability of progressive therapeutic diet
Provide needed nourishment within limits of prescribed diet
Encourage bringing home-cooked food to the institution, as
    appropriate
Suggest trial elimination of foods containing lactose, as
    appropriate
Offer herbs and spices as an alternative to salt
Structure the environment to create a pleasant and relaxing
    atmosphere
Present food in an attractive, pleasing manner, giving
    consideration to color, texture, and variety
Provide oral care before meals, as needed
Assist patient to a sitting position before eating or feeding
Teach patient and family about prescribed diet
Refer for diet teaching and planning, as needed
Give patient and family written examples of prescribed diet

| Box 13-3 | Comparison of Related Factors/Defining Characteristics and Etiologies ALTERED NUTRITION: LESS THAN BODY REQUIREMENTS |

Defining Characteristics

Murphy (1989)
20% or greater under ideal body weight
Low serum albumin

Chiang, Ku, & Lo (1994)
Upper arm circumference too small
Fatigue
Reported inadequate food intake
Triceps skinfold too thin
Loss of body weight
Muscle wasting
Apathy
Slow reaction
Dry skin

Depression
Hemoglobin less than normal
Less than ideal body weight
Restlessness
Sleep disturbance

Related Factors/Etiologies

Murphy (1989)
Inability to ingest or digest food because of
    biologic factors
Hypermetabolic/catabolic states
Absorptive disorders
Inability to ingest or digest food or absorb
    nutrients because of psychologic factors

Nausea and vomiting
Anorexia
Dysphagia
Starvation

Chiang, Ku, & Lo (1994)
Anorexia
Taste or smell alteration
Decrease in salivary secretion
Emotional disturbance
Pain
Difficult to swallow
Nausea or vomiting
Feeling of not being well rested

CASE STUDY

C. Wright, a 71-year-old white female, was admitted to a local care facility following discharge from an acute care hospital. She was 5'3" tall and weighed 105 lb after a weight loss of 7 lb during the recent hospitalization. She was able to walk short distances without assistance but had right side arm and leg weakness and spent most of the day sitting in a chair. She had poor muscle tone. Mrs. Wright wore full dentures. On admission her serum albumin was 3.2 g/dl and her hemoglobin was 10 g. (Normal albumin is >3.5 g/dl, and normal hemoglobin for females ranges from 11 to 15 [Roe, 1990]). Her intake was less than 1000 calories each day. On physical examination the nurse noted a broken area of skin over the coccyx.

Mrs. Wright verbalized that she had "little appetite," that she does not "really need to eat much," and that she feels "weak." She also stated that she had lost 20 lb over the past year. From the history and interview the nurse determined that Mrs. Wright had had a left hemispheric cerebrovascular accident (CVA) complicated with pneumonia before admission to the care facility. She had been widowed for 2 years and had lived alone since her husband's death. One son and daughter visited occasionally.

since her husband's death, no longer felt the need or desire to cook complete meals, and missed the company of her husband at mealtimes. Without her husband to accompany her, she had decreased the amount of time she spent on social activities. Because of this diminished activity level, she felt that she needed to eat less to avoid weight gain.

NURSING-SENSITIVE OUTCOMES

Once the diagnosis Altered Nutrition: Less Than Body Requirements is determined, outcomes are selected to measure progress and the impact of interventions. Appropriate NOC outcomes in the current classification include the following: Nutritional Status; Nutritional Status: Biochemical Measures; Nutritional Status: Body Mass; Nutritional Status: Energy; Nutritional Status: Food & Fluid Intake; Nutritional Status: Nutrient Intake; Oral Health; Self-Care: Eating; and Knowledge: Diet (Iowa Outcomes Project, 2000). Selection of the appropriate outcome, and indicators within each outcome, depends on the individual needs and characteristics of the patient being treated. The NOC outcome labels and indicators are inclusive and comprehensive.

Ongoing, systematic assessment and evaluation are necessary to determine response to interventions. The goals of nursing interventions are to increase amounts of nutrients ingested, to improve the quality of nutrients ingested, to achieve adequate nutrition based on identified needs, and to promote client understanding of nutritional needs.

From this data the nurse made the following nursing diagnosis: Altered Nutrition: Less Than Body Requirements, related to social isolation, anorexia, emotional stress, and inability to prepare and procure food as evidenced by poor appetite, weight loss, hypoalbuminemia, and poor muscle tone.

Mrs. Wright was at risk because of poor nutritional status. Her weight loss and skinfold measurements demonstrated a lack of muscle and fat reserve. Her skin was broken down over her coccyx, and her condition was complicated by pneumonia. She had not been cooking much

NURSING INTERVENTIONS

Plans for ensuring adequate nutrient intake must be individualized according to the identified needs of the individual and the specific outcomes chosen. There is a range of NIC interventions for Altered Nutrition: Less Than Body Requirements, depending on the stage of malnutrition the patient is experiencing, including Teaching: Prescribed Diet, Nutritional Counseling, Nutrition Management, Nutritional Monitoring, and Nutrition Therapy. Other related interventions include Referral, Socialization Enhancement, Oral Health Maintenance, Oral Health Promotion, and Oral Health Restoration.

The risk level of the patient guides determination of which NIC label to use. Developers of the NIC taxonomy might want to reconsider activities within labels using this consideration. In most cases more than one NIC intervention will be appropriate.

Referral

Referral is the "arrangement for services by another care provider or agency" and is an appropriate NIC intervention for nutritionally at-risk or compromised elders (Iowa Intervention Project, 2000, p. 551). Referrals may be made to occupational therapy or physical therapy to evaluate the need for special utensils or exercises to improve the patient's ability and desire to eat. The ability to chew and swallow properly is essential to begin the process of ingestion. Elders experiencing oral health problems, which can interfere with nutrition, might need to be referred to a dentist, although the NIC interventions Oral Health Maintenance, Oral Health Promotion, or Oral Health Restoration might be appropriate. (A detailed discussion of these interventions is beyond the scope of this chapter.) Problems with dentition, fitting and use of dentures, and muscle difficulties in swallowing can influence ingestion and must be corrected so that the patient is able to eat. Those individuals who are edentulous or who have ill-fitting dentures may limit the type of food selected and eaten. Inability to chew could severely decrease the amount of protein intake (Hogstel & Robinson, 1989). The speech therapist can assist with difficulties with dysphagia.

For elders unable to buy or prepare adequate diet because of poverty, referrals can be made for financial assistance programs for nutrition, such as the Food Stamp Program, congregate or home-delivered meals, or local food banks. For elders with functional limitations, referrals for case management services, in-home health aides or homemaker and chore services, and adult day care might be appropriate.

Socialization Enhancement

Improving the setting and socialization at mealtime can improve nutrient intake. Making meal settings aesthetic and pleasant can improve an individual's will to eat (Ham, 1994; Irwin, 1987). Making mealtime a time of sharing and pleasant interchange can also improve the will to eat. Mealtime is traditionally the time for family sharing and socializing. Once families are gone, other socialization should be provided to return meaning to the mealtime. Even the socialization provided by the individual delivering the Meals on Wheels might provide positive socialization experiences for the elder at home. Congregate nutrition programs, adult day care services, and active senior citizen centers also can provide socialization for isolated elders.

Nutrition Education

Although the nurse can have a direct impact on nutritional status, a team approach to treating nutritional status is optimal and a collaborative effort between the nurse and the dietitian is necessary. Dugdale, Chandler, and Baghurst (1979) found that physicians and nurses generally know more about the theoretical basis of nutrition than the practical aspects. For patient education to be as beneficial as possible, the nurse must combine the theoretical knowledge of nutrition with practical, individual application. Principles of adult learning are used to design the educational intervention.

Efforts should be directed to assist the individual to substitute favorable eating habits for poor eating habits. Education also should encompass activity and exercise to improve appetite. Patients must have input into mutually agreed on goals. Knowing the type of food that is important to the patient is valuable, particularly in ethnic populations. Food likes and dislikes are important to identify in order to prepare food that the elderly person will actually eat at mealtime and to identify the need for supplemental nutrition. Family members also must be involved in the education process. Their attitudes and beliefs can influence the patient's response to teaching. Informed family members can be a useful source of supplemental nutrition.

Nutrition Therapy

Nutrition Therapy is the "administration of food and fluids to support metabolic processes of a patient who is malnourished or at high risk for becoming malnourished" (Iowa Intervention Project, 2000, p. 475). Nutrition Therapy is intended for individuals who cannot meet their nutritional needs by eating a nutritionally balanced diet normally. As seen in Box 13-2, this intervention appropriately includes monitoring and teaching activities, as well as encouraging or providing adequate nutrients. Nutrition Therapy can occur at several levels, including (1) modification of nutrient content and density, (2) modification in consistency and use of nutritional supplements, (3) enteral feeding, and (4) parenteral feeding (Nutrition Screening Initiative, 1992).

Several approaches can be taken to modify the nutrient content and density of foods: encouraging substitution of nutrient-dense foods such as broccoli, sweet potatoes, and enriched whole wheat bread for less nutrient-dense foods such as green beans, white potatoes, or white bread; trying six small meals per day rather than two or three larger meals; or adding vitamin and mineral supplements. Food consistency can be modified by using soft, pureed, or liquid diets. It is important to determine the particular chewing or swallowing difficulty when deciding how to alter the consistency of foods. Commercially available supplements also can be used for individuals with chewing and swallowing difficulties.

When feasible, oral intake is the preferred method of feeding. However, if oral intake proves inadequate, enteral feeding might be necessary. Enteral feeding solutions are nutritionally complete, and unlike parenteral feeding, enteral feeding promotes maintenance of the structural and functional integrity of the small intestine. Enteral feeding is a method used to provide supplemental nutritional support when persons are unable to chew and ingest food for adequate nutritional food and fluid intake. Nasogastric tubes or surgically placed gastrostomy or jejunostomy tubes can deliver enteral feedings. Cataldi-Betcher, Seltzer, Slocum, and Jones (1983) found three types of complications in those patients receiving enteral feedings: 6.2% experienced gastrointestinal complications, including diarrhea and inadequate gastric emptying, 3.5% experienced mechanical complications, and 2% experienced metabolic complications, including fluid and electrolyte imbalance (Seltzer, Slocum, Cataldi-Betcher, Seltzer, & Goldberger, 1984). When enteral feedings are used, the patient needs to be evaluated for tolerance to the feedings and nutritional benefit.

Table 13-1 Nursing Outcomes and Selected Indicators for MRS. WRIGHT

Nursing-Sensitive Outcomes	Selected Indicators	Rationale
NUTRITIONAL STATUS: NUTRIENT INTAKE	Caloric intake	Current intake of 1000 calories significantly lower than Recommended Dietary Allowance
	Protein intake	Serum albumin depressed, poor muscle tone, and potential pressure sore development
	Iron intake	Low hemoglobin
NUTRITIONAL STATUS: BIOCHEMICAL MEASURES	Serum albumin	Subnormal serum albumin, indicating chronic undernutrition
	Hemoglobin	Low normal hemoglobin
NUTRITIONAL STATUS: BODY MASS	Weight	Weight loss in the past year of 20 lb, including both chronic and recent loss
	Body mass index	BMI below normal range
NUTRITIONAL STATUS: ENERGY	Stamina	History of CVA, muscle weakness, diminished activity level, feelings of weakness
	Hand grip strength	
KNOWLEDGE: DIET	Describes recommended diet	Self-reported anorexia and need to eat less because of diminished activity level
	Explains rationale for recommended diet	
	Describes advantages of following recommended diet	Social isolation related to bereavement and living alone
	Develops strategies to change dietary habits	

Nursing Outcomes Classification (NOC) 5-point Likert Measurement Scales:

Nutritional Status: Nutrient Intake	1 = Not adequate; 2 = Slightly adequate; 3 = Moderately adequate; 4 = Substantially adequate; 5 = Totally adequate.
Nutritional Status: Biochemical Measures	1 = Extreme deviation from expected range; 2 = Substantial deviation from expected range; 3 = Moderate deviation from expected range; 4 = Mild deviation from expected range; 5 = No deviation from expected range.
Nutritional Status: Body Mass	1 = Extreme deviation from expected range; 2 = Substantial deviation from expected range; 3 = Moderate deviation from expected range; 4 = Mild deviation from expected range; 5 = No deviation from expected range.
Nutritional Status: Energy	1 = Extremely compromised; 2 = Substantially compromised; 3 = Moderately compromised; 4 = Mildly compromised; 5 = Not compromised.
Knowledge: Diet	1 = None; 2 = Limited; 3 = Moderate; 4 = Substantial; 5 = Extensive.

In some circumstances parenteral nutrition is necessary. Total parenteral nutrition can be used in the extremely malnourished individual when other methods are not appropriate (Starker et al., 1985).

CASE STUDY

The following outcomes were selected for Mrs. Wright: Nutritional Status: Nutrient Intake; Nutritional Status: Energy; Nutritional Status: Body Mass; Nutritional Status: Biochemical Measures; and Knowledge: Diet. Only selected indicators were chosen for each outcome. These are identified in Table 13-1. Nutritional Status was not selected as an outcome because it is very broad and the indicators are identified as other nutritional status outcomes. Nutritional Status: Food & Fluid Intake was not selected because it describes methods of intake. Oral Health was not selected because Mrs. Wright did not have evidence of signs of oral health problems, even though she had dentures. Self Care: Eating was not selected because Mrs. Wright was physically able to feed herself.

Collaboration between the nurse and the dietitian resulted in a nutritional plan for Mrs. Wright. Nutritional education was provided to Mrs. Wright and to her son and daughter. Improved nutritional intake was linked with increasing social contacts for Mrs. Wright. She was encouraged to eat with two of the other residents who she liked. Because Mrs. Wright enjoyed breakfast, increased amounts of food were provided at that meal. To improve both her appetite and her social contacts, Mrs. Wright was referred to an activity therapist for a plan of recreational activities. A referral also was made to physical therapy to determine if deficits related to the CVA had affected her ability to eat. Supplemental feeding was not indicated because Mrs. Wright was not extremely malnourished, was responsive to educational strategies, and was able to eat independently without difficulty. Within a few months Mrs. Wright had improved. Mobility and some swallowing difficulties detected by the physical therapist were being treated. She enjoyed her daily recreational activities. At times she would still become somewhat depressed over the loss of her husband; however, these periods were brief. She was eating a good breakfast and smaller meals for lunch and dinner, with occasional between-meal snacks. Mrs. Wright could also verbalize an understanding of the importance of good nutrition and its relationship to her physical and mental health status. A 10-lb weight gain was noted, along with improved muscle tone.

SUMMARY

Although a large body of literature is available related to the assessment of malnutrition, age-specific standards for nutritional requirements still should be identified. Relatively little work has been accomplished on the nursing diagnostic label. Hence, it is not known whether the approved defining characteristics and related factors are valid. The related factors approved by NANDA are vague, and the inclusion of risk factors within the defining characteristics, e.g., evidence of lack of food and lack of information, further cloud a clear characterization of the label. Based on the review of literature and work by the Nutrition Screening Initiative, the following indicators are recommended as defining characteristics: indicators of poor oral health, such as mouth dryness and sore gums; skin dryness; lack of subcutaneous fat; poor wound healing; early satiety or lack of interest in food; intake less than Recommended Dietary Allowances (although this could qualify as a related factor); diminished muscle strength and mass; BMI less than 24; recent weight loss greater than 10 lb; abnormal triceps skinfold and mid-arm circumference measures; and hypoalbuminemia. Risk factors include illness, medications, alcohol use, oral health problems, functional limitations, and financial problems. Nurses also need to be knowledgeable about normal aging changes so that signs associated with malnutrition can be differentiated and not assumed to be a part of "getting old." In this way, undernutrition can be recognized early and appropriate treatment can be instituted.

REFERENCES

Briley, M. E. (1994). Food preferences of the elderly. *Nutrition Reviews, 52*(8), S21-S23.

Buzina-Suboticanec, K., Buzina, R., Stavljenic, A., Farley, T., Haller, J., Bergman-Markovic, B., & Gorajscan, M. (1998). Ageing, nutritional status and immune response. *International Journal for Vitamin & Nutrition Research, 68*(2), 133-141.

Cataldi-Betcher, E., Seltzer, M., Slocum, B., & Jones, K. (1983). Complications occurring during enteral nutrition support: A prospective study. *Journal of Parenteral and Enteral Nutrition, 7*, 546-552.

Charney, P. (1995). Nutrition assessment in the 1990s: Where are we now? *Nutrition in Clinical Practice, 10*, 131-139.

Chernoff, R., Mitchell, C. O., & Lipschitz, D. A. (1984). Assessment of the nutritional status of the geriatric patient. *Geriatric Medicine Today, 3*, 129-141.

Chiang, L., Ku, N., & Lo, C. (1994). Clinical validation of the etiologies and defining characteristics of altered nutrition: Less than body requirements in patients with cancer. In R. M. Carroll-Johnson & M. Paquette (Eds.), *Classification of nursing diagnosis: Proceedings of the tenth conference* (pp. 188-193). Baltimore: Lippincott Williams & Wilkins.

Covinsky, K., Martin, G., Beyth, R., Justice, A., Sehgal, A., & Landefeld, S. (1999). The relationship between clinical assessments of nutritional status and adverse outcomes in older hospitalized medical patients. *Journal of the American Geriatrics Society, 47*(5), 532-538.

Davis, M. A., Randall, E., Forthofer, R. N., Lee, E. S., & Margen, S. (1985). Living arrangements and dietary patterns of older adults in the United States. *Journal of Gerontology, 40*(4), 434-442.

Dugdale, A. E., Chandler, D., & Baghurst, K. (1979). Knowledge and belief in nutrition. *American Journal of Clinical Nutrition, 32,* 441-448.

Dwyer, J. (1994). Nutritional problems of elderly minorities. *Nutrition Reviews, 52*(8), S24-S27.

Ebersole, P., & Hess, P. (1998). *Toward healthy aging: Human needs and nursing response.* (5th ed.) St. Louis, MO: Mosby.

Folsom, A., Kaye, S., Sellers, T., Hong, C., Cerhan, J., Patter, J., & Prineas, R. (1993). Body fat distribution and 5-year risk of death in older women. *Journal of the American Medical Association, 269,* 483-487.

Galanos, A. N., Pieper, C. F., Cornoni-Huntley, J. C., Bales, C. W., & Fillenbaum, G. G. (1994). Nutrition and function: Is there a relationship between body mass index and the functional capabilities of community-dwelling elderly? *Journal of the American Geriatrics Society, 42,* 368-373.

Goodwin, J. S., Goodwin, J. M., & Garry, P. J. (1983). Association between nutritional status and cognitive functioning in a healthy elderly person. *Journal of the American Medical Society, 249,* 2917.

Grindel, C., & Costello, M. (1996). Nutrition screening: An essential assessment parameter. *MEDSURG Nursing, 5*(3), 145-154.

Guigoz, Y., Vellas, B., & Garry, P. (1994). Mini nutritional assessment: A practical assessment tool for grading the nutritional state of elderly patients. *Facts and Research in Gerontology, 2,* 15-59.

Ham, R. J. (1994). The signs and symptoms of poor nutritional status. *Primary Care, 21*(1), 33-54.

Himes, C., Hogan, D., & Eggebeen, D. (1996). Living arrangements of minority elders. *Journals of Gerontology, 51*(1), S42-S48.

Hogstel, M. O., & Robinson, N. B. (1989). Feeding the frail elderly. *Journal of Gerontological Nursing, 15*(4), 16-20.

Incalzi, R., Gemma, A., Capparella, O., Cipriani, L., Landi, F., & Carbonin, P. (1996). Energy intake and in-hospital starvation. *Archives of Internal Medicine, 156*(4), 425-429.

Iowa Intervention Project. J. C. McCloskey & G. M. Bulechek (Eds.). (2000). *Nursing interventions classification (NIC)* (3rd ed.). St. Louis, MO: Mosby.

Iowa Outcomes Project. M. Johnson, M. Maas, & S. Moorhead (Eds.). (2000). *Nursing outcomes classification (NOC)* (2nd ed.). St. Louis, MO: Mosby.

Irwin, M. (1987). Encourage oral intake—yes, but how? *American Journal of Nursing, 87,* 100, 106.

Karkeck, J., & Worthington-Roberts, B. (1993). Nutrition. In D. L. Carnaveli & M. Patrick (Eds.), *Nursing management for the elderly* (3rd ed., pp. 208-238). Baltimore: Lippincott Williams & Wilkins.

Kart, G. S., Mestress, E. S., & Mestress, J. F. (1978). *Aging and health: Biologic and social perspectives.* Reading, MA: Addison Wesley Longman.

Klein, S., & Iber, F. (1991). Alcoholism and associated malnutrition in the elderly. *Nutrition, 7,* 75.

Krach, P. (1998). Myths & facts. *Nursing 98, 28*(2), 25.

Marwick, C. (1997). NHANES III health data relevant for aging nation. *Journal of the American Medical Association, 277,* 100-102.

Mathias, S., Nayak, U. S., & Issacs, B. (1986). Balance in elderly patients: The "Get up and Go" test. *Archives of Physical Medicine and Rehabilitation, 67,* 387-389.

Mayfield, D., McLeod, G., & Hall, P. (1974). The CAGE questionnaire: Validation of a new alcoholism instrument. *American Journal of Psychiatry, 131*(10), 1121-1123.

Mazari, L, & Lesourd, B. (1998). Nutritional influences on immune response in healthy aged persons. *Mechanisms of Ageing and Development, 104*(1), 25-40.

Mitchell, C. O., & Lipschitz, D. A. (1982). The effects of age and sex on the routinely used measurements to assess the nutritional status of hospitalized patients. *American Journal of Clinical Nutrition, 36,* 340-349.

Munro, H. N. (1985). Nutrient needs and nutritional status in relation to aging. *Drug-Nutrient Interactions, 4,* 55-74.

Murphy, L. (1989). Establishing and clarifying the etiologies and characteristics of the nursing diagnosis alteration in nutrition: Less than body requirements. In R. M. Carroll-Johnson (Ed.), *Classification of nursing diagnosis: Proceedings of the eighth conference* (pp. 341-344). Baltimore: Lippincott Williams & Wilkins.

Nagao, M. (1992). The effects of aging on mastication. *Nutrition Reviews, 50*(12), 434-437.

National Research Council. (1989). *Recommended dietary allowances* (10th ed.). Washington, DC: National Academy Press.

North American Nursing Diagnosis Association. (1999). *Nursing diagnoses: Definitions and classification 1999-2000.* Philadelphia: Author.

Nutrition Screening Initiative. (1992). *Nutrition intervention manual for professionals caring for older Americans.* Washington, DC: Author.

Olin, A. O., Osterberg, P., Hadell, K., Armyr, I., Jerstrom, S., & Ljungqvist, O. (1996). Energy-enriched hospital food to improve energy intake in elderly patients. *Journal of Parenteral and Enteral Nutrition, 20*(2), 93-97.

Ortega, R., Requejo, A., Andres, P., Lopez-Sobaler, A., Quintas, M., Redondo, M., Navia, B., & Rivas, T. (1997). Dietary intake and cognitive function in a group of elderly people. *American Journal of Clinical Nutrition, 66,* 803-809.

Roe, D. A. (1990). Geriatric nutrition. *Clinics in Geriatric Medicine, 6*(2), 319-334.

Rolls, B. J. (1994). Appetite and satiety in the elderly. *Nutrition Reviews, 52*(8), S9-S10.

Schiffman, S. (1994). Changes in taste and smell: Drug interactions and food preferences. *Nutrition Reviews, 52*(8), S11-S14.

Seltzer, M. H., Bastidas, J., Cooper, D., Engler, P., Slocum, B., & Fletcher, H. (1979). Instant nutritional assessment. *Journal of Parenteral and Enteral Nutrition, 3,* 157-159.

Seltzer, M. H., Slocum, B., Cataldi-Betcher, E., Seltzer, D., & Goldberger, D. (1984). Specialized nutrition support: Patterns of care. *Journal of Parenteral and Enteral Nutrition, 8*(5), 506-510.

Starker, P. M., LaSala, P., Forse, A., Askanazi, J., Elwyn, D., & Kinney, J. (1985). Response to total parenteral nutrition in the extremely malnourished patient. *Journal of Parenteral and Enteral Nutrition, 9,* 300-302.

Sullivan, D. H., Walls, R. C., & Bopp, M. M. (1995). Protein-energy under-nutrition and the risk of mortality within one year of hospital discharge: A follow-up study. *Journal of the American Geriatrics Society, 43,* 507-512.

Tinetti, M., Williams, T. F., & Mayewski, R. (1986). Fall risk index for elderly patients based on number of chronic disabilities. *American Journal of Medicine, 80,* 429.

White, J. V. (1994). Risk factors for poor nutritional status. *Primary Care, 21*(1), 19-31.

White, J. V. (1996). The Nutrition Screening Initiative: A 5-year perspective. *Nutrition in Clinical Practice, 11,* 89-93.

Wolinsky, F., Coe, R., McIntosh, A., Kubena, K., Prendergast, J., Chavez, M., Miller, D., Romeis, J., & Landmann, W. (1990). Progress in the development of a nutritional risk index. *Journal of Nutrition, 120,* 1549-1553.

CHAPTER 14

IMPAIRED SWALLOWING

LuAnn Tandy and Susan Malan

Impaired swallowing, or dysphasia, is a discomfort or a difficulty in swallowing. If not managed appropriately, impaired swallowing can lead to serious consequences, such as aspiration pneumonia, fluid and electrolyte imbalances, and undernutrition. Because eating is a significant part of normal daily life, it is difficult for patients to accept that something so satisfying can be life-threatening.

The long-term outcome of dysphagia management is to return the patient to normal functioning. With the geriatric population, however, this goal is not always realistic because of their multiple and chronic medical and nursing problems. A diagnosis of swallowing impairment can include cognitive, as well as physical, impairment, making patient education difficult. Therefore it is important that families are included in the plan of care so that they understand the importance of the treatment plan and risk control.

The nursing diagnosis Impaired Swallowing, approved and defined by the North American Nursing Diagnosis Association as "abnormal functioning of the swallowing mechanism associated with deficits in oral, pharyngeal, or esophageal structure or function" (NANDA, 1999, p. 98), is broad and encompasses all stages of swallowing (Box 14-1). This chapter proposes separate diagnoses for each stage of swallowing and describes signs and symptoms that are specific to each stage. This separation by stage assists with planning nursing care for the swallowing impaired elderly patient.

Swallowing is a complex process that involves the oral cavity, pharynx, larynx, and esophagus (Cherney & O'Neill, 1986; Ergun & Miskovitz, 1992; Hargrove, 1980; Maloof, 1985). These anatomic structures are illustrated in Figure 14-1. Swallowing occurs in four phases (Figure 14-2). A normal swallow takes 7 to 9 seconds: 1 to 2 seconds for the oral stage, 1 second for the pharyngeal stage, and 5 to 6 seconds for the esophageal stage (Hanak, 1992). Table 14-1 presents the function of cranial nerves during the various stages of swallowing.

The anticipatory phase of swallowing occurs before any food reaches the mouth. It is during this stage that decisions are made concerning the quantity, the type of food, the setting, and the rate at which food is eaten (Cherney & O'Neill, 1986).

During the oral preparatory stage a quantity of food is placed in the oral cavity and the lips close. The tongue ma-

nipulates and controls the food's location. The soft palate and uvula close off the nasopharynx to prevent reflux.

In the oral stage the bolus or mass of food passes the anterior fossa arches and the swallow reflex is triggered. The tongue moves the food posteriorly in an anterior-to-posterior rolling action. This stage of the swallow is under voluntary control.

The pharyngeal stage is the most essential stage, involving further movement of the bolus and protection of the airway. The triggering of the swallow reflex induces a number of physiologic activities simultaneously. The tongue prevents food from reentering the oral cavity; this is accomplished by closure of the velopharyngeal valve through elevation and contraction of the soft palate. The superior pharyngeal constrictor muscle, which narrows the upper pharynx, facilitates this action. Pharyngeal peristalsis is initiated, causing the downward squeeze of the bolus through the pharynx to the cricopharyngeal sphincter (Cherney & O'Neill, 1986; Hargrove, 1980; Maloof, 1985). At the same time, the larynx is elevated and brought forward by the suprahyoid and thyrohyoid muscles. This is observed as "bobbing of the Adam's Apple" (Dobie, 1978). The cricopharyngeal muscle then relaxes, allowing the material to pass from the pharynx into the esophagus, and respiration resumes. This aspect of the swallowing process is involuntary and reflexive and takes about 1 second (Broniatowski et al., 1999).

The last stage of swallowing is the esophageal stage. This stage starts with the lowering of the larynx; the primary peristaltic wave propels the bolus to the lower esophageal sphincter, causing the contraction of the cricopharyngeal muscle to guard against reflux. If the first peristaltic wave does not complete the task, successive stronger waves will move the bolus into the stomach (Hanak, 1992). Esophageal dysphagia is a common disorder in the elderly.

Several types of dysphagia have been described in the literature, including dysphagia mechanica, pseudobulbar dysphagia, dysphagia paralytica, and functional dysphagia (Kadas, 1983; Martin, Holt, & Hicks, 1985). Patients with dysphagia mechanica experience difficulty swallowing because of loss of sensory guidance of the structures needed to complete the process; this usually occurs with brain damage or pathology. Dysphagia mechanica is easily recognized by physical alteration of the swallowing mech-

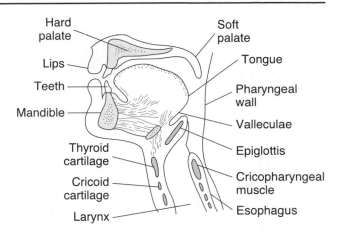

Box 14-1	Impaired Swallowing (NANDA, 1999)

Defining Characteristics
Major
Observed evidence of difficulty in swallowing (e.g., stasis of food in oral cavity, coughing/choking)

Minor
Evidence of aspiration

Related Factors/Etiologies
Neuromuscular impairment (e.g., decreased or absent gag reflex, decreased strength or excursion of muscles involved in mastication, perceptual impairment, facial paralysis); mechanical obstruction (e.g., edema, tracheostomy tube, tumor); fatigue; limited awareness; reddened, irritated oropharyngeal cavity

Pharynx	Larynx	Oral Cavity
Uvula	Single cartilages:	Lips
Epiglottis	Thyroid	Teeth
Valleculae	Cricoid	Hard palate
Tonsils	Epiglottis	Soft palate
Pharyngeal	Paired cartilages:	Cheeks
constrictor	Arytenoid	Floor of mouth
muscles	Corniculate	Tongue
	Cuneiform	Fossal arches
		Mandible

FIGURE **14-1**   Anatomy and physiology of swallowing.

anism, usually affecting the oral stage (Kadas, 1983; Martin et al., 1985).

Pseudobulbar dysphagia usually occurs because of upper motor neuron damage, especially to the right hemisphere. A patient with pseudobulbar dysphagia can lose the cortical controls of swallowing and cognitive control over the swallowing process. This condition usually affects the oral and pharyngeal stages (Kadas, 1983; Martin et al., 1985).

The elder with dysphagia paralytica has paralysis caused by disease or trauma. This patient usually has lesions in the lower motor neuron system that can result in muscle weakness and impairment of oral reflexes. Once again, the oral and pharyngeal stages of swallowing are affected, and the patient with this condition usually is dysarthric (Kadas, 1983; Martin et al., 1985). Functional dysphagia results from an emotional or behavioral disturbance that can cause spasms in the throat or distortion of messages from the cerebral cortex (Kadas, 1983).

Griffin and Tollison (1980) group dysphagias into three categories. Transfer dysphagia is caused by a disturbance in the process from the beginning of the swallow of the bolus from the oropharynx to the cervical esophagus. Transport dysphagia occurs when the bolus is interrupted during the esophageal stage by a lesion or disorder of the esophageal muscle. Delivery dysphagia results when the bolus has difficulty entering the stomach because of a lesion or abnormal functioning of the sphincter.

RELATED FACTORS/ETIOLOGIES

Impairment in the oral stage can occur both neurologically and mechanically. A neurologic problem in this stage will disrupt the grinding and shaping of food and the preparation of the bolus for the next stage. The close association of cranial nerves V, VII, IX, X, and XII, used in the oral stage, can produce certain generalizations. There may be decreased or reduced lip closure and reductions in oral

or facial sensation. A decrease in buccal tension can result in pocketing of food in the cheek. A reduction in mandibular movement can result in inadequately chewed food. Choking or coughing can be caused by decreased tongue movement that interferes with bolus formation. Another problem frequently encountered in the elderly is the loss or reduction of sensations, including taste, temperature, touch, and texture (Cherney & O'Neill, 1986; Dobie, 1978); these losses can interfere with swallowing. In general, patients who have had some type of oral surgery can have difficulty with mastication as well as formation and transportation of the bolus.

The greatest concern in managing swallowing impairment occurs during the pharyngeal stage. If there is impairment during this stage, problems can interrupt respiration and protection of the airway. The patient exhibits delayed or absent triggering of the swallowing reflex. This can be caused by food falling over the tongue into the vallecula, possibly causing aspiration. Decreased velar elevation can cause nasal regurgitation. Decreased closure of the glottis can also result in aspiration. Obstruction can occur at the cricopharyngeal muscle because of a decreased opening. When the bolus is liquid, it pools in the vallecular and pyriform sinuses (Cherney & O'Neill, 1986; Dobie, 1978). Another cause of problems during this phase is surgical resection of the pharyngeal and laryngeal areas for control of a

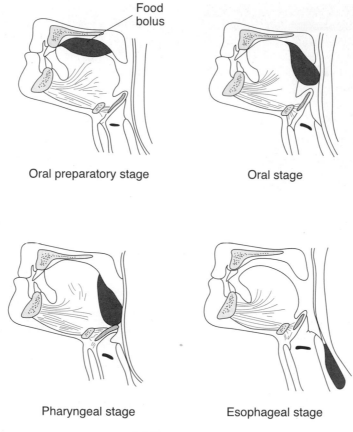

FIGURE **14-2**   Stages of swallowing.

malignancy while maintaining vocal and swallowing functions.

During the esophageal stage a disruption occurs in the transit of the bolus through the esophagus. These disruptions can be caused by obstruction, possibly because of tumors, esophageal reflux, pain caused by nonperistaltic contractions, and a diverticulum caused by dysfunction in the cricopharyngeal muscle (Cherney & O'Neill, 1986; Dobie, 1978).

ASSESSMENT

Impairment in uncompensated swallowing can take a number of forms because of the varied etiologies that can affect almost any stage of the swallowing process. In the anticipatory stage the elderly person might be afraid to swallow or might not find the food appealing. An aging patient might need either intense amounts of stimulation to maintain adequate alertness through mealtime or soft stimulation to avoid distraction at mealtime (Cherney & O'Neill, 1986).

Signs of oral stage impairments reflect involvement of cranial nerves V, VII, IX, X, or XII. Lip closure, oral or facial sensation, and buccal tension can be decreased. Food can be pocketed in the cheek or inadequately chewed. Loss or reduction of sensations, including taste, temperature, touch, and texture, can also occur (Cherney & O'Neill, 1986; Dobie, 1978). Reduction in mandibular and tongue movement may result in inadequately chewed food. Facial and

muscle weakness must be assessed along with tongue strength and coordination (Loustau & Lee, 1985).

Physical assessment of the swallowing, cough, and gag reflexes is important (Price & Dilorio, 1990b). A classic warning sign that a patient is choking is the protective cough. However, patients may not always cough, even if they are aspirating, because of decreased innervation to the mouth and esophagus. This silent aspiration can lead to aspiration pneumonia. A patient who aspirates over 10% of each bolus will probably develop aspiration pneumonia. The percentage of aspiration can be estimated by videofluoroscopy. A patient who aspirates may have a rapid heart rate and may suddenly turn gray. Gasping, choking, a hoarse voice, and gurgling sounds in the chest are other clinical indicators for which the nurse or caregiver should be observant (Groher, 1984). Chronic lung aspiration is indicated by increased temperature and adventitious lung sounds (Groher, 1984).

Mental status should also be evaluated throughout assessment and care (see Chapter 29). Poor short-term memory, distractibility, and inappropriate conversation can indicate perceptual impairments or impaired motor planning, which can interfere with the attention and planning needed for swallowing and eating (Groher, 1984). Impairment during the pharyngeal stage of the swallowing process can be evident through a "gurgling" voice or breathing, reduced or absent sensation to the pharynx, dysarthria, and a delayed or absent gag reflex.

Nerve	Activates	Stage
V (trigeminal)	Swallowing reflex Separates oral and nasal cavity Controls bolus movement Stimulates salivation and chewing Provides sensations to the face, teeth, gums, tongue *Impairment* Loss of sensation and inability to move mandible	Oral
VII (facial)	Provides sense of taste and control over muscles of face Swallowing reflex Separates oral and nasal cavity Controls movement of the bolus *Impairment* Increased salivation and pouching of food and inability to pucker lips	Oral
IX (glossopharyngeal)	Transmits sensation to soft palate, tonsils, pharynx Passage of air from nose to pharynx Influences sense of taste Influences production of saliva Moves food inside mouth *Impairment* Decreases taste sensations, salivation, and gag reflex	Oral, pharyngeal, and esophageal
X (vagus)	Sensation in palate, base of tongue, pharynx, larynx Moves food inside mouth Passage of air from nose to pharynx Passage of bolus to esophagus Passage of bolus to stomach *Impairment* Difficulty in swallowing, nasal regurgitation, decreased gag reflex	Oral, pharyngeal, and esophageal
XII (hypoglossal)	Controls the muscles of the tongue Moves food inside mouth Passage of bolus to the esophagus *Impairment* Inability to position food, pouching	Pharyngeal

Table 14-1   Cranial Nerves Involved in Swallowing Process

Assessment for swallowing impairment begins with a history of the current problem and type of neurologic damage. If the patient is unable to communicate, the nurse should obtain the history from the medical record and/or a family member. The patient should be questioned, if possible, to discover if she has experienced nasal regurgitation, hoarseness, or aspiration. The nurse should ask patients about the consistency of food they are able to handle. If liquids are more difficult, neurologic disease might be present; difficulty with solids is more indicative of a stricture or obstruction (Dobie, 1978). The nurse should also observe the elderly person eating during mealtime, assist the person with eating, and note how the elder handles and swallows a variety of foods and liquids.

Complaints of pain or comments such as "I feel like there's something stuck in my throat" warn the nurse that a patient is at risk for swallowing impairments. To determine the cause of discomfort an indirect laryngeal examination should be done by a credentialed practitioner. A probable finding would be food debris in the valleculas or pyriform sinuses, indicating that the swallowing mechanism has failed to clear the bolus from the pharynx into the esophagus. Since this debris could potentially be aspirated into the trachea, the bolus should be removed with suction.

Physical assessment can begin while taking the history. While conversing with the patient, abnormalities in speech pattern and tone should be noted. A hypernasal tone indicates a paralyzed palate and oropharynx; a hoarse voice results from partial paralysis of the tenth cranial nerve (Larsen, 1981).

It is important to assess the patient's saliva production. Saliva assists with bolus formation and prevents choking. Patients with a dry mouth can choke easily because the food cannot be formed into a bolus and may crumble in the mouth. Thick, ropy secretions also interfere with eating (Loustau & Lee, 1985). During the assessment interview, patients should be observed for drooling, poor lip closure, and facial muscle weakness. These symptoms indicate a possible problem with the oral stage of swallowing once the bolus is formed.

The nurse should observe for facial weakness by noting if the face is symmetric and test for muscle weakness by asking the elderly person to put the lips together. If a person cannot maintain closure, weakness is present (Loustau & Lee, 1985).

Tongue strength can be assessed laterally by asking the patient to press his tongue to the sides of the mouth against the assessor's hand. To check strength in the midline position, the patient should push his tongue against a tongue blade. Poor coordination or inability to use the tongue interferes with formation of the bolus in the oral stage (Loustau & Lee, 1985).

Physical assessment also includes checking the swallowing, cough, and gag reflexes (Loustau & Lee, 1985). To assess the swallowing reflex, the larynx is palpated by placing a finger on the thyroid cartilage when the patient swallows. The larynx should elevate, displacing the finger downward. Laryngeal elevation can also be evaluated by giving the patient a small sip of water or ice chips and observing swallowing. Patients who cough are exhibiting the cough reflex that protects the trachea from aspiration. If the patient does not cough, ask her to try to cough. The cough reflex can be evaluated by asking the patient to cough twice in rapid succession. Patients with intact voluntary cough reflexes are able to cough strongly and briskly. Because of the potential for aspiration, patients who cannot cough voluntarily should not be fed until further testing can be done.

The elderly patient who has experienced a recent unintentional weight loss or who exhibits signs of dehydration must be evaluated. This patient might fear choking and restrict dietary intake voluntarily. The nurse should also be aware of any indications of lung aspiration, such as increased temperature and adventitious lung sounds (Groher, 1984; Martin et al., 1981).

Throughout the interview and assessment the patient's mental status also should be noted (see Chapter 39). Poor short-term memory, distractibility, and inappropriate conversation should be assessed. Eating requires a great degree of attention and planning, and the patient who appears to have poor judgment, perceptual impairments, or motor planning is at risk for uncompensated swallowing impairment (Groher, 1984).

The Videofluoroscopic Swallowing Study (VFSS) is the gold standard for the academic and clinical analysis of swallowing physiology. The study is performed in the fluoroscopy room with a radiologist and speech pathologist present. The patient is given puree, liquid, and solid consistency barium in varied amounts. VFSS is a comprehensive test that assesses all phases of swallowing.

A new study, the Videoendoscopic Swallowing Study (VESS) complements the VFSS by addressing its weaknesses. The VESS is conducted by passing a fiberoptic na-

solaryngoscope through the nose to the nasopharynx to view the upper aerodigestive tract. The VESS provides a better assessment of neurologic status, including sensation and detailed anatomy (Bastian, 1998).

NURSING-SENSITIVE OUTCOMES

The most important *Nursing Outcomes Classification (NOC)* outcomes for the person with the diagnosis Impaired Swallowing or dysphagia are Nutritional Status, Risk Control, and Self-Care: Eating (Iowa Outcomes Project, 2000). Other related NOC outcomes include Concentration, Oral Health, Cognitive Ability, and Comfort Level.

To meet the NOC outcome Nutritional Status, a patient would need to have all indicators met at the mildly compromised level or not compromised. Adequate nutritional status also would be evidenced by normal skin turgor, stable weight, normal hemoglobin, hematocrit, and serum protein (Hanak, 1992) (Table 14-2).

Risk Control is met when the elder understands and accepts the fact that eating might be a risk. As discussed earlier, consistent demonstrations of strategies to prevent aspiration and choking are optimal to prevent aspiration (Hanak, 1992) (see Table 14-2). The Oral Health outcome is acceptable when the indicators are met at the mildly or not compromised level (see Table 14-2).

The NOC outcome Self-Care: Eating for a patient with difficulty in the oral-pharyngeal stage is met when the patient successfully takes food by mouth without aspirating. The elder may not be able to prepare the food but must be able to manipulate food orally, chew food, and swallow food with complete independence to reach the outcome Self-Care: Eating (Iowa Outcomes Project, 2000). The rest of the indicators (see Table 14-2) can be met by an assistive person and/or device. To achieve the outcome, the elder must be able to follow the correct swallowing sequence for safe oral intake (Hanak, 1992).

To meet the NOC outcome Concentration, a patient would need to demonstrate often or consistently the maintenance of attention and appropriate response to auditory, tactile, and olfactory cues. An elder who cannot achieve outcome indicators at this level is at risk for nutritional deficiency (see Table 14-2).

NURSING INTERVENTIONS

Several general strategies can be undertaken to improve swallowing. The elderly person must be in proper body alignment. The elder should be sitting upright with hips and knees at a 90-degree angle. The head should be flexed slightly forward to protect the airway. If a pillow is used to align the head, the pillow should be placed behind the patient's shoulders. Having the pillow behind the head places the patient in an incorrect position and may cause

Table 14-2	Suggested Nursing-Sensitive Outcomes and Nursing Interventions IMPAIRED SWALLOWING	
Nursing Diagnoses (Ter Maat & Tandy, 1991)	**Nursing-Sensitive Outcomes**	**Nursing Interventions**
IMPAIRED SWALLOWING: ANTICIPATORY STAGE *Defining Characteristics* Observed difficulty during or after swallowing Poor attention span/easily distracted Eats when fed Poor memory Confusion Sits down at meals, eats 3-4 bites	**RISK CONTROL** *Indicator* No aspiration **NUTRITIONAL STATUS** *Indicators* Nutrient intake Food and fluid intake Energy Body mass Weight stable Biochemical measures (hemoglobin, serum, protein, hematocrit) Skin turgor **CONCENTRATION** *Indicators* Maintains attention Responds appropriately to auditory cues Responds appropriately to olfactory cues	**POSITIONING** *Activities* Position in proper body alignment Elevate head of bed, as appropriate Position to flex head slightly forward Place chair and table at appropriate height **ENVIRONMENTAL MANAGEMENT** *Activities* Reduce environmental stimuli Provide safe environment (suction available) Provide calm, pleasant dining environment **NUTRITION MANAGEMENT** *Activities* Provide calm, unhurried assistance to eat Sit directly in front of person to feed Determine ability to meet nutritional needs Encourage appropriate nutrient intake **COGNITIVE STIMULATION** *Activities* Cue patient nonverbally to eat Provide group situation for mimicking others eating Reinforce or repeat information
IMPAIRED SWALLOWING: ORAL/PHARYNGEAL STAGE *Defining Characteristics* Observed difficulty during or after swallowing Drooling Poor lip closure Facial muscle weakness Poor tongue strength Inability to chew Reduction of oral sensation Reduced gag reflex Ineffective or absent cough Nasal regurgitation/aspiration Frequent pneumonia Recent weight loss Hoarse voice Gurgling breath sounds Generalized weakness/fatigues easily Chokes on liquids	**RISK CONTROL** *Indicators* Acknowledges risk Follows selected risk control strategies Monitors personal behavior risk factors No aspiration **SELF-CARE: EATING** *Indicators* Drinks from cup or glass Sips liquids Holds breath, tips chin Manipulates food in mouth Chews food Swallows food Raises chin, coughs twice to clear throat **ORAL HEALTH** *Indicators* Cleanliness of mouth, teeth, tongue Moisture of oral mucosa and tongue Breath odor	**SWALLOWING THERAPY** *Activities* Collaborate with other disciplines (OT, ST) Provide/monitor consistency of food/ liquid based on findings of swallowing study Instruct on emergency measures for choking Teach supraglottic swallowing technique **ASPIRATION PRECAUTIONS** *Activities* Monitor level of continuous cough reflex, gag reflex, swallowing ability Keep suction setup available Avoid liquids or use thickening agent (pudding, gelatin) **POSITIONING** *Activities* Position in proper body alignment Elevate head of bed, as appropriate

Continued

Table 14-2	Suggested Nursing-Sensitive Outcomes and Nursing Interventions—cont'd
	IMPAIRED SWALLOWING—cont'd

Nursing Diagnoses (Ter Maat & Tandy, 1991)	Nursing-Sensitive Outcomes	Nursing Interventions
	NUTRITIONAL STATUS *Indicators* Nutrient intake Food and fluid intake Energy Body mass Weight Biochemical measures (hemoglobin, serum protein, hematocrit) Skin turgor	Position to flex head slightly forward Place chair and table at appropriate height Keep upright 45-60 minutes after eating **NUTRITION MANAGEMENT** *Activities* Provide calm, unhurried assistance to eat Determine ability to meet nutritional needs Encourage appropriate nutrient intake **ORAL HEALTH MAINTENANCE** *Activities* Establish a mouth care routine Teach to clean food completely from mouth Suction constantly during oral hygiene Clean mouth with suction, cotton-tipped swab, or gauze
IMPAIRED SWALLOWING: ORAL STAGE *Defining Characteristics* Observed difficulty during or after swallowing Reduction of oral sensation Drooling Deviation of tongue Facial droop Inability to form bolus Inability to chew	**COGNITIVE ABILITY** *Indicators* Concentration Processes information **SELF-CARE: EATING** *Indicators* Drinks from cup or glass Places food in mouth Manipulates food in mouth Chews food Swallows food Completes a meal **NUTRITIONAL STATUS** *Indicators* Nutrient intake Food and fluid intake Weight Energy **ORAL HEALTH** *Indicator* Cleanliness of mouth	**COGNITIVE STIMULATION** *Activities* Use repetition to present new material Present information in small, concrete portions **SWALLOWING THERAPY** *Activities* Explain rationale of swallowing regimen to patient/family Assist patient to place food on back of mouth and on unaffected side Monitor patient's tongue movements while eating Monitor for sealing of lips during eating, drinking, and swallowing Instruct patient/caregiver how to check for pocketed food after meals Teach exercise for lips, facial muscle strength **NUTRITION MANAGEMENT** *Activities* Determine ability to meet nutritional needs

an abnormal reflex pattern (Groher, 1984; Loustau & Lee, 1985). If at all possible, elderly patients should not be fed in bed. If the elder cannot sit in a chair, the head of the bed should be raised as high as possible.

The nurse should remain unhurried and calm because the eating situation may be fearful for the elderly patient (Cole-Arvin, Notich, & Underrhill, 1994). Unless otherwise indicated, the nurse should sit or stand directly in front of the person while assisting with eating.

Prescribed dysphagia treatments usually are implemented for 3 to 4 months. By this time the patient should be able to take in sufficient calories orally. If im-

Table 14-2	Suggested Nursing-Sensitive Outcomes and Nursing Interventions—cont'd IMPAIRED SWALLOWING—cont'd	
Nursing Diagnoses (Ter Maat & Tandy, 1991)	**Nursing-Sensitive Outcomes**	**Nursing Interventions**
	RISK CONTROL *Indicators* Acknowledges risk Follows selected risk control strategies Monitors personal behavior risk factors No aspiration No tissue damage	Encourage appropriate (nutrient) intake Present ¼-⅓ tsp food until mouth opens Place food in center of tongue Vary temperature of food so aware of food in mouth Use assistive devices as needed **ORAL HEALTH MAINTENANCE** *Activities* Establish a mouth care routine after each meal Teach to clean food completely from mouth Clean mouth with suction, cotton-tipped swab or gauze **ASPIRATION PRECAUTIONS** *Activities* Monitor level of consciousness, cough reflex, gag reflex, and swallowing ability Keep suction setup available
IMPAIRED SWALLOWING: **ESOPHAGEAL STAGE** *Defining Characteristics* Observed difficulty during or after swallowing Heartburn Odorous breath Recent increase in dental problems Frequent eructation Heartburn worse at night	**COMFORT LEVEL** *Indicators* Reported satisfaction with symptom control Reports heartburn controlled Reports eructation controlled **ORAL HEALTH** *Indicators* Breath odor Cleanliness of tongue Tooth integrity **NUTRITIONAL STATUS** *Indicator* Nutrient intake	**SWALLOWING THERAPY** *Activities* Instruct to lie down after meals Instruct to eat smaller evening meals Instruct to drink carbonated beverage with meals **ORAL HEALTH MAINTENANCE** *Activities* Instruct/assist to perform oral hygiene after eating and as often as needed Encourage and assist patient to rinse mouth Arrange for dental checkups, as needed **NUTRITION MANAGEMENT** *Activity* Encourage increased intake of protein, iron, and vitamin C, as appropriate

provement does not occur within this time frame, the dysphagia treatment should be discontinued and an alternative method of nutrition considered. Treatment is deemed successful if aspiration is less than 10% of the bolus and the oral-pharyngeal stage is less than 5 seconds.

Various specific nursing interventions in the *Nursing Interventions Classification (NIC)* (Iowa Interventions Project, 2000) can be used to address Impaired Swallowing. However, the nurse must understand which part of the swallowing process is impaired in order to choose appropriate interventions. Therefore specific interventions are discussed in terms of particular swallowing stages and illustrated through case studies.

Interventions for Anticipatory Phase Impairments

Several factors can contribute to anticipatory phase impairments. To make feeding a success, the nurse must take into consideration the patient's mental status. A tired, confused, or lethargic patient does not create a successful feeding session. The session should be close to the patient's normal mealtime but not following a tiring trip for an x-ray examination or therapy. Eating takes concentration, and the elderly patient must be as alert and fresh as possible (Groher, 1984). The meal should be eaten in a pleasant environment away from excess stimulation (Cole-Arvin et al., 1994). When the patient first starts swallowing retraining, feeding should be done in a one-to-one situation close to suction equipment in case of choking. As the patient progresses and the nurse feels comfortable with his abilities, the elder may eat in a group situation. In some settings a speech pathologist may initiate the feeding process.

Memory impairment is a frequent problem. Group situations are helpful because they provide someone for the patient to mimic. An elderly patient placed across from someone who eats well will be cued nonverbally and will tend to eat in a more timely fashion. Furthermore, the group environment gives an air of normalcy to the eating situation, resembling a family situation.

CASE STUDY 1

H. Clark, a 69-year-old man with Alzheimer's disease, is evaluated for inability to eat. He sits down to eat a meal, eats three to four bites, and then sits without eating. Mr. Clark needs constant encouragement to eat; he is easily distracted by activities in the room or conversations with him. He eats only when fed by another person, has poor short-term memory, and is more confused toward evening. Table 14-3 summarizes this patient's signs and symptoms.

Impaired Swallowing: Anticipatory Stage was diagnosed, as evidenced by inability to complete a meal. Diagnoses related to other phases of swallowing were ruled out, as was the diagnosis Altered Nutrition: More Than Body Requirements. The nurse noted the need for the following additional data: neurologic assessment, including visual fields; weight history; current weight; mental status; orientation at mealtime; patient complaints of food sticking in throat; drooling; facial muscle weakness; and pocketing of food.

The following nursing-sensitive outcomes were specified for Mr. Clark:

Concentration: Ability to focus on a specific stimulus (Iowa Outcomes Project, 2000, p. 190).

Nutritional Status: Extent to which nutrients are available to meet metabolic needs (p. 319).

The following nursing interventions were undertaken in response to Mr. Clark's diagnosis:

Cognitive Stimulation: Promotion of awareness and comprehension of surrounding by utilization of planned stimuli (Iowa Intervention Project, 2000, p. 220).

Environmental Management: Manipulation of the patient's surroundings for therapeutic benefit (p. 305).

Nutrition Management: Assisting with or providing a balanced dietary intake of foods and fluids (p. 474).

Positioning: Deliberate placement of the patient or a body part to promote physiologic and/or psychologic well being (p. 514).

Interventions for Oral Phase Impairments

Many difficulties can occur in the oral stage. The elderly patient with oral and facial weakness has problems manipulating the bolus for swallowing. To strengthen the lips and facial muscles, the nurse can prescribe that the person practice the following exercises in front of a mirror (Groher, 1984):

1. Smile broadly with lips closed and open.
2. Frown tightly.
3. Alternate lip pursing and retraction.
4. Practice producing the letters *u, m, b, p,* and *w.*
5. Puff out cheeks with air and hold.
6. Purse lips and blow.
7. Suck hard on a frozen popsicle.
8. Hide tip of tongue under the top lip.

The nurse should also have the exercises rehearsed by any assisting staff or family caregivers to make sure the elderly person gets the appropriate assistance and actually does the exercises as prescribed.

To feed the elder with oral stage difficulties, ¼ to ⅓ teaspoon of food should be placed on a teaspoon and presented so the person can observe and smell. When the person's mouth opens, the spoon should be placed in the center of his tongue and the person should be allowed to remove the food with the lips. The pressure created by the spoon helps initiate mouth closure (Groher, 1984).

The pressure and placement of the spoon will help the elder keep the head lowered and in midline. Food should never be presented above mouth level, as this encourages raising of the head. After the elder has removed the food from the spoon, the nurse should withdraw the spoon with the same downward pressure and watch for the larynx to rise, indicating the elder has swallowed (Groher, 1984). It is important to make sure that the mouth is cleared from the first bite before serving the second bite and that food is not pocketed in the cheeks (Cole-Arin et al., 1994).

While the patient is eating, the nurse should observe for signs of hypersensitivity to hot or cold. Food temperature should be varied enough so that the elder is aware

Table 14-3	Nursing Diagnosis, Outcomes, and Interventions for MR. CLARK		
Nursing Diagnosis	**Nursing-Sensitive Outcomes**	**Nursing Interventions**
IMPAIRED SWALLOWING: ANTICIPATORY STAGE *Defining Characteristics* Poor short-term memory Easily distracted Sits at meal, eats 3-4 bites Confusion; more confused in evening Eats when fed	CONCENTRATION NUTRITIONAL STATUS	COGNITIVE STIMULATION ENVIRONMENTAL MANAGEMENT NUTRITION MANAGEMENT POSITIONING

that something is in her mouth, but not so extreme as to cause discomfort. The nurse should observe for signs of fatigue and discontinue feeding if the person becomes tired, so that lack of concentration on the eating task is prevented.

Assisting the patient who has problems moving a bolus posteriorly may require adaptive equipment such as a glossectomy spoon (Figure 14-3) or syringe. The glossectomy spoon is used to place the bolus at the back of the throat, where it may then be swallowed. The spoon has a plunger that pushes the food off the end of the spoon. Another useful item of equipment is a syringe with a tube attached that is the length of the distance from the lip to the uvula. A squeeze bottle used for drinking water at athletic events may also be used. The nurse can place pureed food in the bottle or syringe, then position the tube at the back of the throat. The bottle is squeezed so that the food is carefully deposited on the back of the tongue. Placement of the bolus on the back of the mouth prevents drooling and promotes swallowing. The nurse should assess which elderly persons are able to do this for themselves and teach those who cannot to do so if possible (Groher, 1984). After the feeding the nurse must check the mouth for retained food and provide mouth care. Effort should be made to assist the elder achieve at least moderately compromised cognitive ability.

CASE STUDY 2

A 78-year-old woman, L. Sutter, was admitted to the hospital with a right-sided cardiovascular accident (CVA). She had left facial droop, deviation of the tongue to the right, and reduction of oral sensation. She refused oral intake because of drooling and inability to chew and to form a bolus. Fluoroscopic evaluation determined that the patient was experiencing difficulty in the oral stage of swallowing. Table 14-4 summarizes this patient's signs and symptoms, NOC outcomes, and NIC interventions. Impaired Swallowing: Oral Phase Impairment was diagnosed, as evidenced by lack of tongue action to form bolus

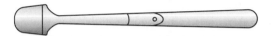

FIGURE **14-3**   Glossectomy spoon.

(NANDA, 1999, p. 99). Mrs. Sutter and her nurse agreed on the following nursing-sensitive outcomes:

Cognitive Ability: Ability to execute complex mental processes (Iowa Outcomes Project, 2000, p. 170).

Self-Care: Eating: Ability to prepare and ingest food (p. 382).

Nutritional Status: Extent to which nutrients are available to meet metabolic needs (p. 319).

Oral Health: Condition of the mouth, teeth, gums, and tongue (p. 325).

Risk Control: Actions to eliminate or reduce actual, personal, and modifiable health threats (p. 353).

The following nursing interventions were undertaken:

Cognitive Stimulation: Promotion of awareness and comprehension of surroundings by utilization of planned stimuli (Iowa Intervention Project, 2000, p. 220).

Swallowing Therapy: Facilitating swallowing and preventing complications of impaired swallowing (p. 638).

Nutrition Management: Assisting with or providing a balanced dietary intake of foods and fluids (p. 474).

Oral Health Maintenance: Maintenance and promotion of oral hygiene and dental health for the patient at risk for developing oral or dental lesions (p. 478).

Aspiration Precautions: Prevention or minimization of risk factors in the patient at risk for aspiration (p. 151).

Interventions for Pharyngeal Phase Impairments

Aspiration is the major problem in the pharyngeal phase. Many elderly patients aspirate without the nursing staff becoming aware of it. Dysphagia with aspiration is a fairly common occurrence after stroke. Approximately 40,000 deaths per year can be attributed to aspiration pneumonia after stroke (Lundy et al., 1999). Suction should be readily

Table 14-4	Nursing Diagnosis, Outcomes, and Interventions for MRS. SUTTER		
Nursing Diagnosis	**Nursing-Sensitive Outcomes**	**Nursing Interventions**
IMPAIRED SWALLOWING: ORAL STAGE *Defining Characteristics* Reduced oral sensation Drooling Inability to chew Inability to form bolus	COGNITIVE ABILITY SELF-CARE: EATING NUTRITIONAL STATUS ORAL HEALTH RISK CONTROL	COGNITIVE STIMULATION SWALLOWING THERAPY NUTRITION MANAGEMENT ORAL HEALTH MAINTENANCE ASPIRATION PRECAUTIONS

available if there is any question about the patient's ability to swallow.

As a rule, the nurse should not give thin liquids to the elderly patient who aspirates because transit time from lips to esophagus is too rapid and the liquid falls over the back of the tongue before the swallow is initiated. To thicken liquids a variety of techniques may be used. Adding gelatin to juice or adding powdered milk to milk products and creamed soups are two methods that are workable in almost any setting without additional cost. Baby cereal can also be added as an alternative thickening agent. Commercial thickeners are available, such as Thick It, Nutra Thick, Thick N Right, and Diamond Crystals Instant Food Thickener. The nurse should remember that milk products, unless baked into foods, should be avoided as a general rule because they produce mucus (Groher, 1984). Finally, straws are generally contraindicated for elderly patients with oral-pharyngeal problems because they cause the liquid to be propelled too quickly. Straws are also contraindicated for the impulsive stroke patient. Often there is weakness of the oral musculature. Lack of normal tongue control and coordination to form the liquids into a bolus makes liquids a much higher aspiration risk than soft food. Occupational therapy can often provide the patient with specially designed cups that enhance safe drinking. In the absence of occupational therapy a nose cup (Groher, 1984) can be created by cutting a semicircle one half the depth of the cup on one side. The patient drinks from the side of the cup that is intact, and the cut-out portion allows the patient to drink without tipping his head back (Figure 14-4).

To reduce the chance of aspiration the nurse can teach the patient to swallow supraglottically. This technique is simple. The patient is instructed to take a sip of fluids in the mouth, hold his breath, tip his chin to the chest, and swallow. Then the person is asked to raise the chin and cough twice to clear the throat. Tipping the head down closes off the larynx and trachea, thus preventing aspiration. Coughing clears the residue that may have accumulated around the opening to the trachea. The safest foods for an initial feeding are puddings or gelatin. These foods remain in a bolus and do not fall apart in the mouth. As

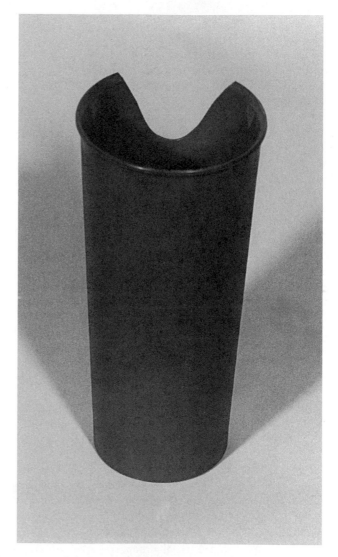

FIGURE **14-4**   Nose cup. (Courtesy Susan Malan and LuAnn Tandy.)

the patient makes progress, pureed foods and thickened liquids may be ingested.

Besides aspiration, the elder with dysphagia may experience oral-pharyngeal residue and stasis. Stasis occurs when food stays in the esophagus and pharynx, and residue occurs when food sticks to the side of the pharynx. The elderly patient with these problems clears the throat frequently and may feel as though something is stuck. The person can also experience a premature full feeling. The elder with stasis and residue is at risk for choking while eating but not when drinking.

The nurse can anticipate that the elderly patient who has been on pureed feedings for an extended period of time will become tired of the consistency and taste. If acceptable to the patient, these foods can be spiced up by adding ketchup, spaghetti sauce, or other spices. The nurse should avoid sticky foods, such as peanut butter, that can stay on the palate and cause choking or gagging. For the elder who cannot tolerate large meals, a six-feeding diet of smaller portions often works well.

After the meal the elder should be kept upright for at least 45 to 60 minutes to prevent reflux, decrease the risk of aspiration, and provide good oral care (Price & Dilorio, 1990a). The elder with a swallowing impairment is prone to dental problems because food pockets in the mouth. Since tongue movements are impaired, the patient is not able to sweep her mouth to remove food particles (Groher, 1984). It is sometimes effective to use a Yankaur suction tip and constant suction as the nurse provides or assists the elder with oral hygiene. Saliva and food particles can be suctioned out to avoid the risk of aspiration after oral care.

Family support is very important for the elder who is having feeding difficulties. Staff should encourage and instruct family members in the teaching and training process as much as possible (Groher, 1984).

CASE STUDY 3

D. Foster, an 82-year-old man, was evaluated for easy fatigability, generalized weakness, and a recent weight loss of 15 lb. His wife reported that while eating he experienced choking, predominantly with liquids, and nasal regurgitation. In the last 6 months he had been hospitalized for pneumonia 3 times. The physical examination revealed a reduced gag reflex and poor cough. Fluoroscopic examination revealed difficulty in the oral-pharyngeal stage of swallowing. Table 14-5 summarizes this patient's signs and symptoms.

Impaired Swallowing: Pharyngeal Phase was diagnosed, as evidenced by recent weight loss, generalized weakness, frequent choking on liquids, reduced gag reflex, poor cough, easy fatigability, nasal regurgitation, and frequent pneumonias (NANDA, 1999, p. 98). Mr. Foster agreed on the following nursing-sensitive outcomes:

Risk Control: Actions to eliminate or reduce actual, personal, and modifiable health threats (Iowa Outcomes Project, 2000, p. 353).

Self-Care: Eating: Ability to prepare and ingest food (p. 382).

Nutritional Status: Extent to which nutrients are available to meet metabolic needs (p. 319).

Oral Health: Condition of the mouth, teeth, gums, and tongue (p. 325).

The following nursing interventions were undertaken to help Mr. Foster reach the desired outcomes:

Aspiration Precautions: Prevention or minimization of risk factors in the patient at risk for aspiration (Iowa Intervention Project, 2000, p. 151).

Swallowing Therapy: Facilitating swallowing and preventing complications of impaired swallowing (p. 638).

Nutrition Management: Assisting with or providing a balanced dietary intake of foods and fluids (p. 474).

Positioning: Deliberative placement of the patient or a body part to promote physiologic and/or psychologic well-being (p. 514).

Oral Health Maintenance: Maintenance and promotion of oral hygiene and dental health for the patient at risk for developing oral or dental lesions (p. 478).

Interventions for Esophageal Phase Impairments

Esophageal reflux is a common problem in the elderly patient and is related to the esophageal stage of swallowing. Elders who have a gurgling voice, odorous breath, coated tongue, heartburn while eating, frequent eructations, and an increase in dental problems may have esophageal reflux. To improve the situation the nurse can instruct the elder not to lie down after a meal, since reflux is greater lying down. Instruction to eat a smaller evening meal and to drink 2 or 3 ounces of a carbonated cola beverage during meals also may be helpful. The carbon dioxide (CO_2) in the cola creates pressure in the lower esophageal sphincter, which holds the food in the stomach. In addition, eating a high-protein diet and elevating the head of the patient's bed 6 inches are recommended. Because the elderly person with esophageal reflux may also be prone to esophagitis, the nurse should be alert for this problem and make appropriate referrals to a physician or nurse practitioner for possible drug therapy.

CASE STUDY 4

P. Dirks, a 73-year-old man, had complaints of heartburn, frequent eructation, odorous breath, and a recent increase in dental problems. He did not complain of difficulty swallowing liquids or solids but stated that his heartburn was worse at night. Physical examination was normal for a man of his age. Diagnostic evaluation by radiology and speech pathology revealed esophageal reflux. Table 14-6 summarizes this patient's signs and symptoms, NOC outcomes, and NIC interventions.

Impaired Swallowing: Esophageal Phase (reflux as evidenced by pyrosis) was diagnosed. Mr. Dirks and

Table 14-5	Nursing Diagnosis, Outcomes, and Interventions for MR. FOSTER		
Nursing Diagnosis	**Nursing-Sensitive Outcomes**	**Nursing Interventions**
IMPAIRED SWALLOWING: ORAL-PHARYNGEAL STAGE *Defining Characteristics* Fatigues easily Generalized weakness Reduced gag reflex Recent weight loss Frequent pneumonias Chokes on liquids Nasal regurgitation Poor cough	RISK CONTROL SELF-CARE: EATING NUTRITIONAL STATUS ORAL HEALTH	SWALLOWING THERAPY ASPIRATION PRECAUTIONS NUTRITION MANAGEMENT POSITIONING ORAL HEALTH MAINTENANCE

Table 14-6	Nursing Diagnosis, Outcomes, and Interventions for MR. DIRKS		
Nursing Diagnosis	**Nursing-Sensitive Outcomes**	**Nursing Interventions**
IMPAIRED SWALLOWING: ESOPHAGEAL STAGE *Defining Characteristics* Heartburn Odorous breath Recent increase in dental caries Frequent eructation Heartburn is worse at night	COMFORT LEVEL ORAL HEALTH NUTRITIONAL STATUS	SWALLOWING THERAPY ORAL HEALTH MAINTENANCE NUTRITION MANAGEMENT

his nurse agreed on the following nursing-sensitive outcomes:

Comfort Level: Extent of physical and psychologic ease (Iowa Outcomes Project, 2000, p. 173).

Oral Health: Condition of the mouth, teeth, gums, and tongue (p. 325).

Nutritional Status: Extent to which nutrients are available to meet metabolic needs (p. 319).

Mr. Dirks and his care team agreed on the following nursing interventions:

Swallowing Therapy: Facilitating swallowing and preventing complications of impaired swallowing (Iowa Intervention Project, 2000, p. 638).

Oral Health Maintenance: Maintenance and promotion of oral hygiene and dental health for the patient at risk for developing oral or dental lesions (p. 478).

Nutrition Management: Assisting with or providing a balanced dietary intake of foods and liquids (p. 474).

SUMMARY

In geriatric populations swallowing remains a critical survival function. A good knowledge of head and neck anatomy and physiology and an understanding of the stages of swallowing are

essential for the nurse working with elders. Geriatric nurses have the opportunity to play an important role in dysphagia treatment both independently and as part of a swallowing retraining team. A swallowing retraining team (dysphagia team) consists of a nurse trained in dysphagia treatment, an occupational therapist, a dietitian, a speech pathologist, a physician, and a radiologist. Many of the interventions presented in this chapter are practical and can be used easily in any setting.

Nurses who engage in swallowing retraining need specific education and training. Knowledge and understanding of the anatomy and physiology of the mouth, neck, esophagus, and cranial nerves involved in the swallowing process is necessary to determine where the impairment is and how best to intervene with the elderly patient. The nurse on the team has direct responsibility for monitoring the elderly patient and reporting his status to the team. In some hospitals nurses serve as team leaders for the swallowing retraining team.

The nurse must be skilled with safety techniques, including CPR with blocked airway, suctioning, tracheostomy care, and use of resuscitation equipment. To provide swallowing rehabilitation the nursing staff must learn specific oral exercises and feeding and swallowing techniques. They also must be familiar with different dietary selections and what textures are available in the diets provided.

Eating and drinking have many meanings to the elderly person. The loss of pleasure of eating and drinking and the threat of choking cause older persons to feel anxious, depressed, and fearful. A successful retraining program will address these considerations, as well as procedural and educational components.

REFERENCES

Bastian, R. W. (1998). Contemporary diagnosis of the dysphagic patient. *Otolaryngologic Clinics of North America, 31*(3), 489-506.

Broniatowski, M., Sonies, B. C., Rubin, J. S., Bradshaw, C. R., Spiegel, J. R., Bastian, R. W., & Kelly, J. H. (1999). Current evaluation and treatment of patients with swallowing disorders. *Otolaryngology—Head & Neck Surgery, 120*(4), 464-473.

Cherney, L. R., & O'Neill, P. (1986). Swallowing disorders in the aged. *Topics in Geriatric Rehabilitation, 1,* 45-47.

Cole-Arvin, C., Notich, L., & Underrhill, A. (1994). Identifying and managing dysphagia. *Nursing, 24*(1), 48-49.

Dobie, R. (1978). Rehabilitation of swallowing disorders. *American Family Physician, 17,* 84-95.

Ergun, G. A., & Miskovitz, P. F. (1992). Aging and the esophagus: Common pathologic conditions and their effects upon swallowing in the geriatric population. *Dysphagia, 7,* 58-63.

Griffin, J., & Tollison, J. (1980). Dysphagia. *American Family Physician, 22*(5), 154-160.

Groher, M. (Ed.). (1984). *Dysphagia.* Newton, MA: Butterworth.

Hanak, M. (1992). Dysphagia management. In M. Hanak (Ed.), *Rehabilitation nursing for the neurological patient* (pp. 81-92). New York: Springer.

Hargrove, R. (1980). Feeding the severely disabled patient. *Journal of Neurosurgical Nursing, 12,* 102-107.

Horner, J., Massey, E., Riski, J., Lathrop, D., & Chase, K. (1988). Aspiration following stroke: Clinical correlates and outcomes. *Neurology, 38,* 1359-1362.

Iowa Intervention Project. J. C. McCloskey & G. M. Bulechek (Eds.). (2000). *Nursing interventions classification (NIC)* (3rd ed.). St. Louis, MO: Mosby.

Iowa Outcomes Project. M. Johnson, M. Maas, & S. Moorhead (Eds.). (2000). *Nursing outcomes classification (NOC)* (2nd ed.). St. Louis, MO: Mosby.

Kadas, N. (1983). The dysphagic patient: Everyday care really counts. *RN, 46,* 38-41.

Larsen, G. L. (1981). Chewing and swallowing. In N. Martin, N. Holt, & D. Hicks (Eds.), *Comprehensive rehabilitative nursing.* Hightstown, NJ: McGraw-Hill.

Linden, P., & Siebens, A. (1983). Dysphagia: Predicting laryngeal penetration. *Archives of Physical Medicine and Rehabilitation, 64,* 281-284.

Loustau, A., & Lee, K. A. (1985). Dealing with the dangers of dysphagia. *Nursing, 15*(2), 47-50.

Lundy, D. S., Smith, C., Colangelo, L., Sullivan, P. A., Logemann, J. A., Lazarus, C. L., Newman, L. A., Murry, T., Lombard, L., & Gaziano, J. (1999). Aspiration: Cause and implications. *Otolaryngology—Head & Neck Surgery, 120*(4), 474-478.

Maloof, M. (1985). Self feeding deficits. Application of rehabilitation concepts to nursing practice study guide. *Rehabilitation Nursing Institute,* 115-118.

Martin, N., Holt, N., & Hicks, D. (1985). *Comprehensive rehabilitation nursing.* Hightstown, NJ: McGraw-Hill.

North American Nursing Diagnosis Association (1999). *Nursing diagnoses: Definitions and classification 1999-2000.* Philadelphia: Author.

Price, M. E., & Dilorio, C. (1990a). Swallowing: A practice guide. *American Journal of Nursing, 7,* 42-46.

Price, M. E., & Dilorio, C. (1990b). Swallowing: An assessment guide. *American Journal of Nursing, 7,* 38-41.

Ter Maat, M., & Tandy, L. (1991). Impaired swallowing. In M. Maas, K. C. Buckwalter, & M. Hardy (Eds.), *Nursing diagnoses and interventions for the elderly* (pp. 106-116). Redwood City, CA: Addison-Wesley Nursing.

CHAPTER 15

ALTERED ORAL MUCOUS MEMBRANE

Jean L. Reese

During the last decade and a half toothlessness has declined considerably among elderly persons in the Western world (Haugen, 1992). The trend to retain natural teeth into old age has increased the use of dental services by the elder. The older adult requires costlier services that are replacement directed rather than preventive. Dental prepayment plans have increased in the last 2 decades, although few offer prepaid coverage after the insured reaches retirement age. Although older people in the United States control significant amounts of discretionary income, a sizable number of elderly individuals with low incomes will not be able to purchase dental care (Meskin & Mason, 1992). The economic burden and delivery of care problems seem to be greatest among the disabled and institutionalized. In long-term care facilities, it is the nurses' responsibility to meet the oral screening and care required by residents. Lack of knowledge and training, time constraints, and setting of priorities result in "daily oral hygiene care that is less than adequate" (Ettinger, 1992; Weeks & Fiske, 1994). Also of concern is the increased incidence of oral cavity cancer in the elderly. Although the low frequency of cancer at this site pales in comparison with rates for lung and colon cancer, early detection can reduce the need for major debilitating treatments. It is important to intervene with preventive actions for tooth destruction and soft tissue lesions in the elder, as well as to recognize when referral is necessary.

The oral cavity and its contents age in much the same way as other organ systems in the body. The oral status of the elder mirrors the effect of long-standing habits, such as the use of tobacco and alcohol, which are superimposed on changes resulting from aging itself (Axelsson, Paulander, & Linddhe, 1998).

Teeth (Dentition, Hard Tissue)

In the elderly individual the most common change in teeth is their numeric reduction. With tooth loss the corresponding alveolar bone shrinks significantly regardless of age, but bone loss is more extensive in the elder. Until recently, periodontal disease, which describes a group of diseases affecting the bone and soft tissues that support the teeth, was considered the main reason for the loss of teeth. However, the prevalence of untreated root caries and the secondary caries rate are high in the elder age-group and

appear to be important factors in tooth loss (Haugen, 1992). Root caries begin on the exposed cemental surfaces of the tooth root below the enamel margin (Figure 15-1). Exposure of the cemental surface to the oral environment occurs when the gingival margin has receded with the loss of periodontal attachment (Burt, 1992). On the average, over half of the institutionalized and close to one third of the independent dentate elders per year have coronal and root caries (MacEntree, Clark, & Glick, 1994).

Tooth enamel also undergoes changes with aging, including wearing down, darkening, and a tendency to develop longitudinal cracks. The age-related reduced water content of the enamel might explain the minor fractures (Haugen, 1992). The dentine of the tooth becomes more brittle, and the pulp chamber atrophies with age.

Oral Mucosa (Soft Tissue)

Studies of the oral epithelium lack consensus related to the structural change of cells caused by aging. Reports of the width, keratinization, rete pegs (projection of the epidermis into the dermis at the dermoepidermal junction), and mitotic activity of the epithelium vary from study to study. On the other hand, studies of connective tissue have demonstrated a consistent decrease in cellular elements, fibers, collagen synthesis, and acid mucopolysaccharides. These changes parallel those found in the skin with loss of cells, decreased vascular bed, and thickening of the bundles of collagen and elastin fibers (Haugen, 1992). The replacement of muscle fiber with loose, flabby connective tissue causes a loss of tissue resiliency and firmness of shape.

The sublingual varicose veins frequently observed in the elderly usually are without clinical importance. Fissure formation at the corners of the mouth (chronic angular cheilitis) may arise from the folding of the skin and reduction of circumoral muscle tone, allowing the escape of saliva.

The gingiva tissue can be maintained in the elderly with daily oral hygiene. Plaque accumulates constantly on the teeth. It is a clear, colorless, sticky film composed of broken-down food particles, bacteria, and saliva that must be removed every day. If it is not removed, it matures, causing redness, soreness, and bleeding of the gums. Calculus, or tartar, forms over the plaque, leaving a rough

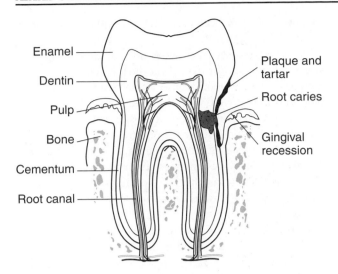

FIGURE **15-1**   Plaque formation, gingival recession, and root caries.

surface. If not removed, it will advance to gum and bone recession and ultimately result in periodontal disease.

Tongue

The number of taste receptors and the threshold for and discrimination of taste remain much the same with aging. An elderly person's complaint that she cannot enjoy flavorable foods might indicate problems with other sensory systems, particularly the olfactory, thermal, tactile, and textural sensors (Haugen, 1992). In addition, drugs, diseases, and tobacco use can reduce or alter the sensation of taste.

Salivary Glands

Saliva is critical for the well-being of the mouth. Saliva provides lubrication, protects the mucous membrane from dehydration and infection, and initiates digestion of the food bolus. Saliva contains antimicrobial elements that interfere with caries development, and it provides moisture for swallowing and speech functions. The production of saliva is controlled mainly by cholinergic innervation. Drugs such as atropine (an anticholinergic) are given specifically to control saliva flow during surgery.

Studies regarding the secretion of saliva show that elderly women have less saliva secretion than elderly men and tend to have more complaints of mouth dryness. However, as the elderly person ages, saliva secretion remains relatively constant (Osterberg, Birkhead, Johansson, & Svanborg, 1992). One study showed that the elderly had a less unstimulated saliva secretion rate than younger people but responded to sialogogues as well as younger people (Percival, Challacombe, & Marsh, 1994). A crude estimate of decreased saliva secretion leading to the complaint of "dry mouth" (xerostomia) in 611

elderly individuals was about 22.5%. Associated with the incidence of xerostomia among older adults were chronic medical conditions and reports of poor general health. Other problems involving eating, communication, and social interaction paralleled the reports of xerostomia (Locker, 1995). A variety of medications have been shown to significantly reduce saliva flow rate when medicated elders are compared with unmedicated elders (Narhi et al., 1992). Neither having hypertension nor having diabetes, per se, reduced salivation, but it was reduced in persons taking hydrochlorothiazide (Streckfus, Marcus, Welsh, Brown, & Cherry-Peppers, 1994; Streckfus, Wu, Ship, & Brown, 1994a, 1994b). Other classifications of drugs are closely associated with dry mouth, including sedatives, antipsychotics, antidepressants, and antihistamines.

Oral Cavity Lesions

Few studies have been conducted to determine the incidence of oral lesions in the elder. One study found a 23.1% rate for lesions in a sample of 629 noninstitutionalized, rural, and over–age 65 adults in Iowa. Denture-related lesions were found in 27% of the 382 subjects. The use of alcohol or tobacco increased the risk of denture-related lesions. No data were gathered regarding the rate of malignancy in these lesions (Hand & Whitehall, 1986).

Lesions of most concern are those suspected of being cancerous. Oral cavity lesions are not easily diagnosed because they appear variable and ill defined. Many lesions are benign and easily mistaken for a malignancy; conversely, an early malignant lesion can be mistaken for a benign lesion (Silverman, 1992). The oral cavity accounted for 3% of 1996 estimated new cancer cases in the United States, whereas the estimated death rate of oral cavity cancer was nearly 2% (Parker, Tong, Bolden, & Wingo, 1996). In a review of 844 oral cavity tumors, 65% were benign and 35% were malignant. The malignant tumors appeared more often between the fifth and seventh decade, were more frequently found in men than in women, and were located most often on the lip and tongue. Benign tumors occurred predominately in the gingiva and appeared between the third and sixth decades of life (Sortino & Milici, 1998).

Squamous cell carcinoma is the most frequent type of cancer of the oral cavity and occurs most often in older persons. Men have been more prone to oral cancers, although the ratio of incidence between men and women has narrowed to about 2 to 1. This change is thought to be related to the increase in smoking habits in women. The combination of alcohol consumption and smoking increases the incidence of oral cancers. Although the treatment combinations for oral cancer have improved, the survival rate after 5 years remains around 50%. Mortality is lowest in lip cancers and highest in cancers of the tongue.

ASSESSMENT

On entering a long-term care facility, each person should have a comprehensive oral examination, preferably performed by a dentist. Subsequent monitoring examinations can be performed by nurses or assistants who have had additional training.

Assessment of the oral cavity should include appraisal for loose teeth, missing fillings or missing parts of teeth, root tips, and caries. The amount of debris on the teeth indicates the elder's ability to clear food particles and the need for oral hygiene care. A person with hemiparesis might have food debris only on the affected side of the mouth. A change in food selection and/or chewing ability might indicate pain related to infectious processes or sores in the mouth. The lips, buccal membrane, gingiva, floor of the mouth, palate, tongue, and throat require inspection and palpation for lesions that indicate infection, irritation, or neoplasms (Figure 15-2). An example of an assessment

tool incorporating both hard and soft oral tissues appears in Assessment Guide 15-1.

A lesion that bleeds, grows rapidly, or causes paresthesia, dysphasia, and/or dysarthria must be considered malignant until proven otherwise. Other danger signals are a painful sore or irritation in the mouth that does not heal after 2 weeks and small areas of erosion (ulceration), erythema, and/or keratosis on the oral mucosa. A lump in the neck may indicate metastasis from a silent mouth lesion. An asymptomatic lesion does not rule out carcinoma. Slow-growing lesions that do not respond to standard treatment require further evaluation (Silverman, 1992).

The most common premalignant changes appear as areas of white lesions (leukoplakia). Lesions that are red (erythroplasia) or a combination of both red and white (erythroleukoplakia) carry a greater risk of developing into a carcinoma (Silverman, 1992). Leukoplakia is a white patch that cannot be wiped off and is not classified as any other disease. The cause is unknown. Size can vary from a minute circumscribed lesion to a large lesion with irregular and vague borders. Leukoplakia occurs most frequently at the lip commissure and buccal membrane. Location on the floor of the mouth or on the base of the tongue increases the probability of malignancy. Induration and rough texture also indicate malignancy. Risk factors for oral cavity carcinomas are sunlight, tobacco, alcohol, nutritional deficiency, infectious disease, and poor dentition (Beck & Watkins, 1992).

The most common candidal infection of the oral cavity is associated with upper dentures and is referred to as denture stomatitis. The mucosa is bright red, with the red color following the outline of the denture. Poor denture hygiene, broad-spectrum antibiotics, corticosteroids, xerostomia-causing drugs, vitamin A, and folate deficiencies are associated with candidal infection. Thrush, or acute candidiasis, appears as creamy, pearly white, or bluish white patches that are removable by gentle scraping (Beck & Watkins, 1992).

Gingival hyperplasia has been associated with the use of primidone, cyclosporine, and nifedipine, drugs used to treat diseases common in the elderly. The association of phenytoin with gingival hyperplasia is well known. Meticulous oral hygiene can control the secondary inflammation and excerbation of dental disease (Beck & Watkins, 1992).

NURSING DIAGNOSIS

The North American Nursing Diagnosis Association (NANDA) has defined Altered Oral Mucous Membrane as "Disruptions of the lips and soft tissue of the oral cavity." However, NANDA's diagnostic statement extends beyond the mucous membrane by including carious teeth in the defining characteristics (NANDA, 1999, p. 42). To increase consistency, it is proposed that the label for this area of nursing concern be broadened to include the teeth. The

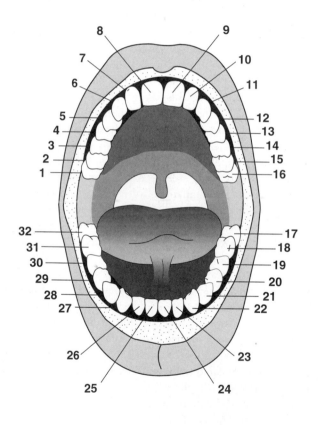

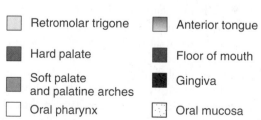

	Retromolar trigone		Anterior tongue
	Hard palate		Floor of mouth
	Soft palate and palatine arches		Gingiva
	Oral pharynx		Oral mucosa

FIGURE **15-2**   Structures of the oral cavity with numbering of the teeth.

Assessment Guide 15-1

ORAL MONITORING TOOL

Name _____ Room # _____

Care Ability		Upper Denture	Lower Denture
	Complete self-care	None	None
	Self-care with help	Full/partial	Full/partial
	Limited self-care	Does not wear	Does not wear
	No self-care	Wears at night	Wears at night
	Needs:	Labeled	Labeled
	Aids:	Broken/defects	Broken/defects
	Reminding	Food/debris	Food/debris
	Physical help	Check those that apply	

	Right	Left	Right	Left	U = Upper jaw
Missing teeth					L = Lower jaw
Loose teeth					
Large cavities					
Broken teeth					
Root tips					
Debris					
Root caries					
Gingivitis					Check if present

Location	Normal	Color of Lesion	Raised/ Swollen	Rough/ Smooth	Size of Lesion	Pain
Upper lip						
Lower lip						
Right cheek						

Continued

Assessment Guide 15-1—cont'd

ORAL MONITORING TOOL—cont'd

Name _____ Room # _____

Location	Normal	Color of Lesion	Raised/ Swollen	Rough/ Smooth	Size of Lesion	Pain
Left cheek						
Upper gums						
Lower gums						
Palate						
Tongue						
Floor mouth						
Throat						

Normal: Checkmark = Yes.

Color: red, white, red/white, blue, black, yellow.

Raised/swollen: Checkmark = Yes.

Rough/smooth: Record which it is.

Size: Use cm, or pinpoint, lacy, irregular: _____

Pain: Checkmark = Yes.   Evaluator _____ Date _____

label Altered Oral Tissues would include both the soft (mucous membrane) and hard (teeth) tissues of the mouth. The definition would then read "a state in which an individual experiences disruptions in the soft and hard tissues of the oral cavity." Box 15-1 includes NANDA's defining characteristics and related factors and suggested changes for this diagnosis.

NURSING-SENSITIVE OUTCOMES

The *Nursing Outcomes Classification (NOC)* outcome Oral Health is defined as the "condition of the mouth, teeth, gums, and tongue" (Iowa Outcomes Project, 2000, p. 325). Oral Health aims at measuring the cleanliness and integrity of the mucous membranes and teeth (Table 15-1). Again, the use of the term *oral health* is more encompassing than NANDA's term *mucous membrane*. None of the NOC indicators overlap, and each can be measured separately. The NOC outcome Oral Health does not include any indicator for pain. Inclusion of a pain indicator is critical because any oral mucosa interruption or decayed

tooth can cause pain. Determination of whether the outcome Oral Health is achieved requires reassessment of the same parameters evaluated during an initial nursing assessment. See Assessment Guide 15-1, which can be used to determine whether the outcome Oral Health is met. Reassessment activities are discussed as part of the nursing intervention Oral Monitoring.

NURSING INTERVENTIONS

The *Nursing Interventions Classification (NIC)* includes three interventions that are appropriate for a diagnosis of Altered Oral Tissues: Oral Health Maintenance, Oral Health Promotion, and Oral Health Restoration (Iowa Intervention Project, 2000). The activities listed for these three interventions often overlap. It is proposed here that nursing activities be reorganized into only two interventions. Monitoring activities can be grouped under an intervention labeled Oral Monitoring. Consolidation and grouping of oral monitoring activities provide easy access to oral assessment parameters regardless of whether the

Box 15-1	Related Factors/Etiologies and Defining Characteristics for Altered Oral Mucous Membrane and Suggested Changes With Altered Oral Tissues

Nursing Diagnosis
Altered Oral Mucous Membrane
Defining characteristics
Xerostomia
Vesicles, nodules, or papules
Oral pain/discomfort
Coated tongue
Stomatitis
Oral lesions or ulcers
Leukoplakia
Desquamation
Hyperemia
Edema
Halitosis

Related factors/etiologies
Decreased or no salivation:
• Radiation
• Dehydration
• Medications
No oral intake
Mouth breathing
Ineffective oral hygiene
• Cognitive deficits
• Motor deficits
Trauma:
Chemical
• Alcohol
• Smoking/chewing tobacco

Mechanical
• Ill-fitting dentures
• Braces
• Feeding/airway tubes
• Malocclusion
Surgical
• Lesion removal
• Tooth extraction
• Oral reconstruction
Malnutrition
Pathologic conditions:
• Infection
• Immunosuppression
• Malignancies

Nursing Diagnosis
Altered Oral Tissues
Defining characteristics
Orofacial pain
Edema
Difficulty chewing
Dried or ropy mucus
Xerostomia

Coated tongue
Halitosis
Leukoplakia
Erythroplakia
Erythroleukoplakia
Inflamed tissue mass
Ulcerated, indurated lesion
Gum recession
Inflamed, bleeding, edematous gums
Stomatitis
Glossitis
Hard tissue
Teeth sensitive to cold and/or heat
Broken teeth
Loose teeth
Root tips
Root caries
Carious teeth
Missing teeth
Toothache
Tooth debris

purpose is to promote, maintain, or restore oral health. The remaining nursing activities can be combined into a second intervention labeled Oral Hygiene Care (Box 15-2). Assimilation of these latter activities into one intervention will increase efficiency. Both NOC indicators and NIC activities for Oral Hygiene Care are combined in Table 15-1; nursing activities related to Oral Monitoring are not included.

Oral hygiene must be done daily to prevent gingivitis and bleeding of the gums. The level of interventions for oral care is based on the cognitive ability, neuromuscular ability, skeletal motion, visual adequacy, and motivation of the elderly person. Limited joint motion, which interferes with grasping a toothbrush, can be overcome by applying tin foil, a soft rubber ball, or a bicycle handle grip to the handle. Lengthening the toothbrush handle by attaching a rod can accommodate limited shoulder range of motion. The use of battery-driven toothbrushes provides friction without repetitive wrist movement. If a person has use of only one hand and wears dentures, suction cups attached to a brush in a sink filled with water provide a means for self-care. Often staff need only supply these aides for the motivated elderly person to use them.

Having the equipment for oral care organized in one place, such as in a cosmetic bag, a plastic box with a lid, or even a zippered plastic bag, increases the likelihood that oral care will be performed. Some persons who are physically able to brush their teeth will need only reminding, whereas others will need specific step-by-step directions to accomplish the task.

Persons who have bleeding gums need gum stimulation with a soft toothbrush to remove the tooth plaque that causes bleeding. Avoiding the bleeding areas only serves to make the gingivitis worse.

Chemical aids, such as fluoridated toothpaste, are the first choice for caries prophylaxis. Xylitol-flavored fluoride sucking tablets can stimulate salivary flow rate in persons with hyposalivation. The use of chlorhexidine in mouth rinses is helpful in reducing plaque formation, but it is not effective in preventing caries because of its short-lived effects on the level of mutans streptococci. Oral peroxidase mouth rinses are antimicrobial for lactobacilli, yeasts, and some viruses. The addition of hydrogen peroxide to toothpaste represents an attempt to increase antimicrobial action (Tenovuo & Soderling, 1992).

Increasing salivary flow is critical in maintaining oral health. Sugarless chewing gums and paraffin wax are stim-

Table 15-1   Suggested Nursing-Sensitive Outcomes and Nursing Interventions
ALTERED ORAL MUCOUS MEMBRANE

Nursing Diagnosis	Nursing-Sensitive Outcome	Nursing Interventions
ALTERED ORAL MUCOUS MEMBRANE *Related Factors/Etiologies* Lack of or decreased salivation; no oral intake; mouth breathing	**ORAL HEALTH** *Indicators* Painless chewing	**ORAL HEALTH MAINTENANCE** *Activity* Supply pureed diet **ORAL HEALTH RESTORATION** *Activity* Plan small, frequent meals, soft food, chilled
• Difficulty chewing		
• Dry mouth (xerostomia) • Coated tongue	Moisture of oral mucosa and tongue Cleanliness of tongue	**ORAL HEALTH MAINTENANCE** *Activities* Encourage and assist patient to rinse mouth Establish a mouth care routine Instruct patient to chew sugarless gum to increase saliva and cleanse teeth Use sialagogues Consult physician if dryness, irritation, or discomfort persists **ORAL HEALTH RESTORATION** *Activities* Avoid use of lemon-glycerin swabs Instruct to avoid commercial mouth rinses Increase liquids on food tray
• Dry, cracked lips	Moisture of oral mucosa and tongue	**ORAL HEALTH MAINTENANCE** *Activity* Apply lubricant to moisten lips and oral mucosa, as needed
• Halitosis	Breath odor	**ORAL HEALTH MAINTENANCE** *Activities* Facilitate toothbrushing and flossing at regular intervals Establish a mouth care routine **ORAL HEALTH RESTORATION** *Activity* Instruct to avoid commercial mouth rinses
Ineffective oral hygiene • Inflamed, bleeding, edematous gums	Gum integrity Cleanliness of gums	**ORAL HEALTH PROMOTION** *Activities* Promote regular dental checkups Massage gums **ORAL HEALTH MAINTENANCE** *Activity* Establish a mouth care routine **ORAL HEALTH RESTORATION** *Activities* Use soft toothbrush Instruct to avoid commercial mouth rinses

	Suggested Nursing-Sensitive Outcomes and Nursing Interventions—cont'd	
Table 15-1	ALTERED ORAL MUCOUS MEMBRANE—cont'd	
Nursing Diagnosis	**Nursing-Sensitive Outcome**	**Nursing Interventions**
• Tooth debris	Cleanliness of teeth	**ORAL HEALTH MAINTENANCE** *Activity* Facilitate toothbrushing and flossing at regular intervals
• Carious teeth	Tooth integrity	**ORAL HEALTH MAINTENANCE** *Activities* Refer to dentist Instruct to use fluoride toothpaste
• Toothache	Absence of pain	**ORAL HEALTH MAINTENANCE** *Activity* Refer to dentist
• Sensitive to cold/heat	Absence of pain	**ORAL HEALTH MAINTENANCE** *Activity* Supply warm foods
• Root caries	Tooth integrity	**ORAL HEALTH MAINTENANCE** *Activity* Refer to dentist
• Gum recession	Gum integrity Cleanliness of gums	**ORAL HEALTH PROMOTION** *Activity* Massage gums **ORAL HEALTH RESTORATION** *Activity* Use soft toothbrush
• Halitosis	Breath odor	**ORAL HEALTH MAINTENANCE** *Activity* Facilitate toothbrushing and flossing at regular intervals
• Dried or ropy mucus	Cleanliness of mouth	**ORAL HEALTH MAINTENANCE** *Activity* Encourage frequent mouth rising
Trauma		**ORAL HEALTH RESTORATION**
• Orofacial pain	Absence of pain	*Activities* Reinforce oral hygiene regimen with DC teaching Instruct to report signs of infection
• Broken teeth/jaw	Teeth integrity	**ORAL HEALTH RESTORATION** *Activities* Refer to dentist Consult physician/dentist for adjustment of wires
• Loose teeth	Teeth integrity	**ORAL HEALTH RESTORATION** *Activity* Refer to dentist
• Root tips	Teeth integrity	**ORAL HEALTH RESTORATION** *Activity* Refer to dentist
• Missing teeth	Fit of dentures Fit of dental appliance	**ORAL HEALTH RESTORATION** *Activity* Refer to dentist

Continued

	Suggested Nursing-Sensitive Outcomes and Nursing Interventions—cont'd	
Table 15-1	ALTERED ORAL MUCOUS MEMBRANE—cont'd	
Nursing Diagnosis	**Nursing-Sensitive Outcome**	**Nursing Interventions**
• Edema	Fit of dentures	**ORAL HEALTH RESTORATION** *Activity* Instruct to report signs of infection
• Difficulty chewing	Fit of dentures Fit of dental appliance	**ORAL HEALTH RESTORATION** *Activities* Supply liquid or pureed diet Refer to physician/dentist
Pathologic conditions/malnutrition		
• Difficulty chewing	Absence of pain	**ORAL HEALTH RESTORATION** *Activities* Assist selection of soft, bland, nonacidic foods Supply liquid or pureed diet
• Stomatitis/glossitis	Oral mucosa integrity Absence of pain Moisture of oral mucosa and tongue Color of mucosa membranes	**ORAL HEALTH RESTORATION** *Activities* Use Toothettes or disposable foam swabs Assist selection of soft, bland, nonacidic foods Remove dentures for severe stomatitis Increase mouth care to q2hrs & twice at night for stomatitis Apply topical anesthetics, pastes Consult physician for persistent stomatitis/glossitis
• Erythroplakia	Oral mucosa integrity Color of mucosa membranes	**ORAL HEALTH MAINTENANCE** *Activities* Refer to physician/dentist Discourage smoking and tobacco use
• Leukoplakia	Oral mucosa integrity Color of mucosa membranes	**ORAL HEALTH MAINTENANCE** *Activities* Refer to physician/dentist Discourage smoking and tobacco use
• Erythroleukoplakia	Oral mucosa integrity Color of mucosa membranes	**ORAL HEALTH MAINTENANCE** *Activities* Refer to physician/dentist Discourage smoking and tobacco use
• Inflamed tissue mass	Oral mucosa integrity Color of mucosa membranes	**ORAL HEALTH MAINTENANCE** *Activity* Refer to physician/dentist
• Ulcerated, indurated lesion	Oral mucosa integrity Color of mucosa membranes	**ORAL HEALTH MAINTENANCE** *Activities* Refer to physician/dentist Discourage smoking and tobacco use

ulants safe for teeth. If saliva-stimulating lozenges used several times a day are ineffective, then mucin-containing artificial salivas may help. However, water alone provides a therapeutic effect (Wiesenfeld, Stewart, & Mason, 1983). Lozenges containing citric acid are effective salivary stimulants, but they are also potential enamel demineralizers. Ending meals with cheese, peanuts, or uncooked vegeta-

bles and eating low-acid foods between meals can reduce acid production and plaque formation.

Oral care for persons who are demented requires adaptation to their usual response to stimulation. Not opening the mouth can occur because the verbal request is not understood. Stroking the cheek, touching the lips, or the opening of the caregiver's mouth can cue the person to

| Box 15-2 | Suggested Merging of the Maintenance, Promotion, and Restoration Activities for ORAL MONITORING AND ORAL HYGIENE CARE |

Oral Monitoring
Activities

Monitor oral mucosa on a regular basis

Monitor lips, tongue, moisture, color

Monitor teeth, color, shine, debris

Monitor every shift for dryness of oral mucosa

Monitor for glossitis, stomatitis

Identify the risk for stomatitis with drug therapy

Determine perception of taste, swallowing

Monitor for therapeutic effects of topical anesthetic

Oral Hygiene Care
Activities

Instruct in daily oral care routine

Establish a mouth care routine

Facilitate toothbrushing and flossing

Reinforce oral hygiene regimen with DC teaching

Promote, arrange regular dental checkups

Instruct to avoid commercial mouth rinses

Encourage frequent mouth rinsing

Encourage flossing with unwaxed floss with platelets >50,000

Instruct to chew sugarless gum to increase saliva

Instruct to report signs of infection

Discourage smoking and tobacco chewing

Remove, clean, and reinsert dentures

Remove dentures for severe stomatitis

Assist with oral care as needed

Apply lubricant to lips

Use soft toothbrush

Use Toothettes or disposable foam swabs

Massage gums

Avoid use of lemon glycerin swabs

Increase liquids on food tray

Increase mouth care to every 2 hrs & twice at night for stomatitis

Plan small, frequent meals, soft food, chilled

Assist selection of soft, bland, nonacidic foods

Apply topical anesthetics, pastes

Consult physician/dentist for adjustment of wires

Consult physician for persistent glossitis or stomatitis

Consult physician if dryness, irritation, or discomfort persists

---

what is wanted. The use of a padded tongue blade or a bite bar to hold the jaws apart to cleanse the tongue and medial aspects of the teeth might be necessary. Fingers should never be placed between the teeth of persons who are not reliable. Palpating the floor of the mouth or tongue for lesions is foregone in this situation.

Dentures must be removed during sleeping because saliva lubrication is at a diurnal low. Dentures must be labeled to identify those that are left in unusual places. Repair of cracked dentures or refitting of loose dentures requires professional expertise.

CASE STUDY

B. Jones, a 75-year-old Caucasian with Alzheimer's disease, had gradually exhibited increased irritability and pacing over a 1-week period. He stopped eating raw vegetables and meat but continued to eat mashed potatoes, cooked cereal, and rice. He lost 5 pounds. Unbeknownst to the nursing assistants, he was brushing his teeth on only one side of his mouth when reminded to do so. Betty, a nursing assistant who had recently completed an oral health care specialist program, became concerned about Mr. Jones. She assessed Mr. Jones's mouth and found a very reddened and swollen area on the gum surface of one of his upper molars and tooth debris on that side of his mouth. He reacted to pressure on the inflamed area and said, "That hurts!" The difficulty chewing, inflamed tissue mass, and orofacial pain were signs and symptoms for the diagnosis Altered Oral Tissues. She reported her findings to the nurse, who con-

sulted with a physician. Administration of an oral antibiotic was initiated immediately. In addition, the nursing intervention Oral Hygiene Care was highlighted in his care plan. Nursing assistants supervised Mr. Jones's oral hygiene, encouraging him to gently clean even the area that was inflamed. Daily Oral Monitoring was initiated to evaluate progress in healing. Within 2 weeks, the reddened area had receded, his agitated behaviors subsided, he reported that he no longer had pain, and he began eating raw vegetables again.

SUMMARY

Poor oral health can have deleterious effects on quality of life. Freedom from oral pain is highly valued by residents in long-term care facilities, by their relatives, and by their caregivers (Nordenram, Ronnberg, & Winbald, 1994). The ability to chew and enjoy food and have fresh breath and normal speech also are judged important. More frequent eating and esthetic problems are encountered in the elderly because of the associated greater tooth loss (Gift & Redford, 1992). Providing an elderly person with a freshly cleaned mouth can be one of the most important nursing activities.

REFERENCES

Axelsson, P., Paulander, J., & Linddhe, J. (1998). Relationship between smoking and dental status in 35-, 50-, 65-, and 75-year-old individuals. *Journal of Clinical Periodontology, 25*(4), 297-305.

Beck, J. D., & Watkins, C. (1992). Epidemiology of nondental oral disease in the elderly. *Clinics in Geriatric Medicine, 8*(3), 461-482.

Burt, B. A. (1992). Epidemiology of dental diseases in the elderly. *Clinics in Geriatric Medicine, 8*(3), 447-459.

Ettinger, R. L. (1992). Oral care for the homebound and institutionalized. *Clinics in Geriatric Medicine, 8*(3), 659-672.

Gift, H. C., & Redford, M. (1992). Oral health and the quality of life. *Clinics in Geriatric Medicine, 8*(3), 673-683.

Hand, J. S., & Whitehall, J. M. (1986). The prevalence of oral mucosal lesions in an elderly population. *Journal of the American Dental Association, 112,* 73-76.

Haugen, L. K. (1992). Biological and physiological changes in the aging individual. *International Dental Journal, 42*(5), 339-348.

Iowa Intervention Project. J. C. McCloskey & G. M. Bulechek (Eds.). (2000). *Nursing interventions classification (NIC)* (3rd ed.). St. Louis, MO: Mosby.

Iowa Outcomes Project. M. Johnson, M. Maas, & S. Moorhead (Eds.). (2000). *Nursing outcomes classification (NOC)* (2nd ed.). St. Louis, MO: Mosby.

MacEntree, M. I., Clark, D. C., & Glick, N. (1994). Predictors of caries in old age. *Gerodontology, 10,* 90-97.

Locker, D. (1995). Xerostomia in older adults: A longitudinal study. *Gerodontology, 12*(1), 18-25.

Meskin, L. H., & Mason, L. D. (1992). Problems in oral health care financing for the elderly. *Clinics in Geriatric Medicine, 8*(3), 685-692.

Narhi, T. O., Meurman, J. H., Ainamo, A., Nevalainen, J. M., Schmidt-Kaunisaho, K. G., Siukosaari, P., Valvanne, J., Erkinjuntti, T., Tilvis, R., Makila, E. (1992). Association between salivary flow rate and the use of systemic medication among 76-, 81-, and 86-year-old inhabitants in Helsinki, Finland. *Journal of Dental Research, 71*(12), 1875-1880.

Nordenram, G., Ronnberg, L., & Winblad, B. (1994). The perceived importance of appearance and oral function, comfort and health for severely demented persons rated by relatives, nursing staff and hospital dentists. *Gerodontology, 11*(1), 18-24.

North American Nursing Diagnosis Association. (1999). *Nursing diagnoses: Definitions and classification 1999-2000.* Philadelphia: Author.

Osterberg, T., Birkhead, D., Johansson, C., & Svanborg, A. (1992). Longitudinal study of stimulated whole saliva in an elderly population. *Scandinavian Journal of Dental Research, 100*(6), 340-345.

Parker, S. L., Tong, T., Bolden, S., & Wingo, P. A. (1996). Cancer statistics, 1996. *Ca-A Cancer Journal for Clinicians, 46*(1), 5-27.

Percival, R. S., Challacombe, S. J., & Marsh, P. D. (1994). Flow rates of resting whole and stimulated parotid saliva in relation to age and gender. *Journal of Dental Research, 73*(8), 1416-1420.

Silverman, S. (1992). Precancerous lesions and oral cancer in the elderly. *Clinics in Geriatric Medicine, 8*(3), 529-541.

Sortino, F., & Milici, A. (1998). Epidemiology of oral cavity tumors. *Minerva Stomatologica, 47*(5), 197-202.

Streckfus, C. F., Wu, A. J., Ship, J. A., & Brown, L. J. (1994a). Stimulated parotid salivary flow rates in normotensive, hypertensive, and hydrochlorothiazide-medicated. *Journal of Oral Pathology & Medicine, 23,* 280-283.

Streckfus, C. F., Wu, A. J., Ship, J. A., & Brown, L. J. (1994b). Comparison of stimulated parotid salivary gland flow rates in normotensive and hypertensive persons. *Oral Surgery, Oral Medicine, Oral Pathology, 77*(6), 615-619.

Streckfus, C. F., Marcus, S., Welsh, S., Brown, R. S., & Cherry-Peppers, G. (1994). Parotid function and composition of parotid saliva among elderly edentulous African-American diabetics. *Journal of Oral Pathology & Medicine, 23*(6), 277-279.

Tenovuo, J., & Soderling, E. (1992). Chemical aids in the prevention of dental diseases in the elderly. *International Dental Journal, 42*(5), 355-364.

Weeks, J. C., & Fiske, J. (1994). Oral care of people with disability: A qualitative exploration of the views of nursing staff. *Gerodontology, 11*(1), 13-17.

Wiesenfeld, D., Stewart, A. M., & Mason, D. K. (1983). A critical assessment of oral lubricants in patients with xerostomia. *British Dentistry Journal, 155,* 155-157.

CHAPTER 16

FLUID VOLUME DEFICIT— DEHYDRATION: ISOTONIC, HYPOTONIC, AND HYPERTONIC

Jean L. Reese

The term *dehydration* denotes a decrease in the amount of total body water. The decrease can involve water from both the extracellular (EC) and intracellular (IC) compartments or only from the EC compartment. The deficit can result from water loss, decreased water intake, or both. Fluid losses with varying serum sodium concentrations can have different causes and, although all require water for treatment, the composition of the rehydration fluids depends on the serum sodium concentration.

The effects of dehydration not only create morbidity problems for those affected but also have an economic impact. Dehydration was listed among other diagnoses for Medicare hospitalizations in 1991 at a rate of 236.2 per 10,000 elders' beneficiaries; it was the principal diagnosis at a rate of 49.7 per 10,000. Medicare reimbursed over $446 million for hospitalizations with dehydration as the principal diagnosis. Dehydration increased mortality when coupled with other diagnoses (Warren et al., 1991).

With normal aging the systems that control the volume and concentration of body fluids exhibit a reduction in reserve capacity and an inability to respond rapidly. These restrictions can create both fluid excess and fluid deficit problems for the elder. Under usual circumstances, maintenance of adequate fluid volume is not a problem of normal aging (de Castro, 1992), yet the Nationwide Food Consumption Surveys indicate that a portion of the population may be chronically mildly dehydrated (Kleiner, 1999).

Fluid Compartment Characteristics

The concept of fluid disbursement between the IC and EC compartments is basic to understanding the effects of fluid volume and concentration balances. Water flows through the cell wall passively, driven by the concentration gradient. The fluid surrounding the cells has to maintain osmotic equilibrium with the cellular fluid to prevent cellular volume changes. To maintain this osmotic equilibrium, water and/or solutes either move in and/or out of the cell with only a transient change in concentration in either compartment.

Tonicity refers to the effect that EC fluid has on cellular volume. EC solutes effect a change in cellular volume when they cannot cross the cell membrane and create an osmotic gradient, as is the case with excess EC glucose. Osmolality, on the other hand, reflects the concentration of water or solutes, which may or may not cause cellular volume change. Excess solutes that pass readily across the cell membrane do not create an osmotic gradient. Osmolality will be increased in both compartments, as with an elevated urea concentration, but will not result in hypertonicity or a movement of water between compartments (Sterns & Spital, 1990).

The EC compartment is divided into the interstitial space (the area between the cells) and the vascular space. The presence of red blood cells and the greater concentration of proteins differentiate the vascular fluid from the interstitial fluid. These two EC fluid compartments act essentially as a unit, with relatively unencumbered water and solute exchange occurring between them. In contrast, for water to flow into or out of cells the EC fluids must be either relatively hypotonic or relatively hypertonic to the IC fluids.

Sodium constitutes the major electrolyte contributing to the tonicity of the EC fluid compartment. Glucose and urea, if concentrated enough, can add significantly to the osmotic gradient. Sodium concentration is inextricably bound with fluid volume and must be considered in determining interventions. Aldosterone controls sodium reabsorption from the kidney tubules. Arginine vasopressin, also known as antidiuretic hormone (ADH), controls the reabsorption of water from the kidney tubules. Aldosterone determines the volume of body fluids, whereas ADH controls the concentration of body fluids.

Normal serum sodium ranges from 135 to 145 mEq/L, and serum osmolality, which closely follows serum sodium concentration, ranges from 280 to 295 mOsm/L. One study showed that healthy subjects ($n = 139$) had an age-related decrease of 1 mEq/L of sodium per decade from a mean of 141 +/− 4 mEq/L (Owen & Campbell, 1968). In contrast, an end range of normal osmolality (290 to 300 mOsm/kg) remained steady over a 6-month period, while the mean serum sodium level was at 143 mmole/L in 15 stable frail elderly men (Weinberg, Pals, McGlinchey-Berroth, & Minaker, 1994). Another study showed that 82% of elderly women registered serum osmolalities of more than 295 mOsm/Kg (O'Neill, Davies, & Wears, 1989). The range of urinary osmolality is usually 500 to

800 mOsm/L, which is about 1.5 to 3 times greater than the serum osmolality.

ASSESSMENT

Elders who initially come under a nurse's care should undergo a careful health history and physical assessment to establish a baseline level of functioning. Several initial and scheduled assessments (monitoring) are standard for people at risk for or having fluid imbalances, regardless of the type of imbalance. There is no substitute for accurate weights and accurate recording of intake and output. Measurement of vital signs, particularly blood pressure, and laboratory tests for blood and urine concentrations are common for any evaluation of fluid and/or electrolyte imbalances. The individual's degree of mental alertness, energy level, skin turgor, mucosal membrane moistness, and neurologic status provide valuable information as well.

Dehydration exhibits common characteristics regardless of tonicity. One of these is rapid weight loss, which directly reflects a decrease in fluid volume. Any weight loss greater than 500 g per day should be attributed to a loss of fluid volume. An exception to rapid weight loss as a symptom is "third spacing," in which fluid moves from the vascular compartment to other spaces, e.g., the pleural cavity, the abdominal cavity, or the interstitium. The trapped fluid maintains the body weight but is unavailable for blood circulation. Effective circulating blood volume (ECBV) may be decreased, showing volume depletion while weight remains the same or increases.

One of the most sensitive tests for detecting vascular volume depletion is the measurement of blood pressure with the patient in lying and standing positions. A fall of more than 15 mm Hg in systolic blood pressure and an increase of 15 beats per minute of the heart rate on standing suggests intravascular volume depletion (Briggs, Sawaya, & Schnermann, 1990). Hypotension can occur with isotonic, hypotonic (hyponatremic), and hypertonic (hypernatremic) dehydration. Hypotension develops later in the hypertonic dehydration sequence because the tonicity of the EC fluids draws water from the cells, thus maintaining vascular volume. When the EC volume losses continue, decreasing replacement from the cells, hypotension appears. The development of hypotension may also be delayed with hyponatremic dehydration if another substance, such as excess glucose, provides enough osmotic pull to maintain vascular volume. A common characteristic of vascular plasma loss is an increase in the hematocrit. Actually, as plasma volume decreases, both hematocrit and hemoglobin rise.

Urine output varies, depending on the reason for the volume depletion. If the cause for plasma volume depletion is active loss, such as from the gastrointestinal tract, and there is no kidney impairment, urine will be concentrated, urine volume will be small, and urine sodium concentration will be less than 10 mEq/L. Aldosterone saves sodium to boost the vascular volume. When water

and sodium conservation by the kidney is impaired, urine output may be dilute and in normal or large amounts, and urine sodium concentration will be more than 10 mEq/L.

NURSING DIAGNOSIS

The NANDA definition for Fluid Volume Deficit is "the state in which an individual experiences decreased in-

---

Box 16-1 | Defining Characteristics and Related Factors/Etiologies FLUID VOLUME DEFICIT AND RISK FOR FLUID VOLUME DEFICIT

1.4.1.2.2.1 Fluid Volume Deficit (1999)
Defining characteristics
Decreased urine output
Increased urine concentration
Sudden weight loss
Decreased venous filling

Other possible characteristics
Hypotension
Thirst
Increased pulse rate
Decreased skin turgor
Decreased pulse volume/pressure
Change in mental state
Increased body temperature
Dry skin
Dry mucous membranes
Increased body temperature
Weakness

Related factors/etiologies
Active fluid volume loss
Failure of regulatory mechanisms

1.4.1.2.2.2 Risk for Fluid Volume Deficit (1978)
Defining characteristics
Presence of risk factors such as:
- Extremes of age
- Extremes of weight
- Excessive losses through normal routes (e.g., diarrhea)
- Loss of fluid through abnormal routes (e.g., indwelling tubes)
- Deviations affecting access to or intake or absorption of fluids (e.g., physical immobility)
- Factors influencing fluids needs (e.g., hypermetabolic state)
- Knowledge deficiency related to fluid volume
- Medications (e.g., diuretics)

Related factors/etiologies
See risk factors.

Data from North American Nursing Diagnosis Association. (1999). *Nursing diagnoses: Definitions and classification 1999-2000* (p. 28). Philadelphia: Author.

travascular, interstitial, and/or intracellular fluid. This refers to dehydration, water loss alone without change in sodium" (NANDA, 1999, p. 28). Risk for Fluid Volume Deficit is "the state in which an individual is at risk of experiencing vascular, cellular, or intracellular dehydration" (NANDA, 1999, p. 28).

The present definitions by NANDA of Fluid Volume Deficit and Risk for Fluid Volume Deficit name three sites for dehydration to occur: vascular, cellular, and intracellular. The last two terms are redundant. A more accurate replacement for the term *cellular* would be *interstitial*. Replacing "fluid volume deficit" with "dehydration" is more efficient. It is a well-known, frequently used term and is readily understood. However, the term *dehydration* also has a narrow definition, namely, the presence of solute in excess of water in the body determined by an elevated serum sodium concentration (Alpern, Saxton, & Seldin, 1990).

The nursing diagnosis Fluid Volume Deficit is subdivided by two related factors: (1) failure of regulatory mechanisms and (2) active loss (NANDA, 1999). This division provides discernment in determining interventions (Box 16-1). Another needed discrimination is the concentration of the dehydration. Isotonic, hypertonic, and hypotonic dehydration require slightly different treatments (Box 16-2). The current NANDA categorization blurs a precise specification for interventions.

Box 16-2   Dehydration: Isotonic, Hypotonic, and Hypertonic

Dehydration: Isotonic
Related factors/etiologies
Hemorrhage
Burns
Vomiting
Diarrhea
Elevated environmental temperature—diaphoresis
Physical activity during hot weather
Third spacing of fluid
Gastrointestinal drainage
Diuretic therapy

Defining characteristics
Thirst
Orthostatic hypotension
Tachycardia
Decrease in venous filling
Weight loss (except in third spacing)
Weakness
Normal serum sodium level
Dry mouth
Decrease in skin turgor
Scant, concentrated urine
Elevated hematocrit, blood urea nitrogen (BUN)
Low urinary sodium

Dehydration: Hypotonic (Hyponatremic)
Related factors/etiologies
Same as Dehydration: Isotonic
Increased ADH production
Adrenal or pituitary insufficiency
Diuretic therapy
Excessive sweating
Salt-losing nephritis
Tube feedings with low sodium
Renal tubular acidosis
End-stage renal disease
Acute emotional distress

Defining characteristics
Weight loss
Supine tachycardia
Supine hypotension that worsens on rising
Poor skin turgor

Low serum sodium
Elevated hematocrit, BUN
Low volume, concentrated urine
Normal or low urinary sodium
Diminished vein filling
Dry mucous membranes
Anorexia, nausea, vomiting
Lethargy, weakness
Confusion, coma, convulsions
Paralysis, hypertonic reflexes
Decorticate posturing

Dehydration: Hypertonic (Hypernatremic)
Related factors/etiologies
Diabetes insipidus
Excess diuretic therapy
Hypercalcemia
Hypokalemia
Decreased fluid intake
Lack of thirst
Inability to obtain water
NPO for tests
Mental, physical incapacity
Loss of urine concentration
High-protein tube feedings without sufficient water

Defining characteristics
Rapid weight loss
Orthostatic hypotension
Thirst
Dry mucous membranes
Elevated serum sodium level
Decrease in pulse pressure
Increase in heart rate
Low-volume, concentrated urine
Fever, flushed, warm skin
Loss of sweating
Decrease in intensity of heart sounds
Decreased energy level
Decreased mental alertness
Personality changes
Hallucinations, manic behavior
Delirium, convulsions, coma

NURSING-SENSITIVE OUTCOMES

Nursing outcomes are based on changes in the signs and symptoms. Those signs and symptoms that indicated the problem fade as the problem recedes. When hemodynamic changes have occurred because of fluid loss, outcomes would include a rise in blood pressure, a decrease in pulse rate, and absence of dizziness on standing. With rehydration, urinary output should increase toward 40 mL/hr with lessening concentration and a BUN decrease. Quenching of thirst, moist mucous membranes, moist axilla, and restoration of energy level indicate a return to preillness level. During fluid replacement, attention must be directed to the patient's neurologic status. The level of alertness should increase and, hopefully, there will be a return to pre–volume deficit personality.

By judging the outcome with the initial signs and symptoms and interpreting its meaning, the nurse determines whether interventions should be continued, modified, or discontinued. Are the signs and symptoms lessening? Is the rate of change commensurate with expectations? Outcomes also serve as the basis for determining the types and frequencies of assessment or monitoring activities.

The *Nursing Outcomes Classification (NOC)* (Iowa Outcomes Project, 2000) includes two outcomes relevant to fluid volume deficits. Fluid Balance is defined as the "balance of water in the intracellular and extracellular compartments of the body" (p. 221), and Hydration is the "amount of water in the intracellular and extracellular compartments of the body" (p. 236). Unfortunately, the indicators for these two outcomes overlap widely. This overlap in indicators makes it difficult to choose which outcome is related to a given problem. It is not clear how to differentiate between the two definitions of these outcomes, "balance of water" versus "amount of water." It is recommended that these two outcomes be combined into one.

NURSING INTERVENTIONS

The *Nursing Interventions Classification (NIC)* categorized fluid and electrolyte monitoring and intervention activities into 20 sets (Iowa Intervention Project, 2000). Of these 20 interventions, 11 are related to fluid volume deficit as defined in this chapter. The activities specified for these interventions overlap widely, resulting in multiple intervention choices for one diagnosis. There is no conceptual grouping or patterning of activities within or between interventions, nor is there consistency with the specificity of the activities. The addition of the phrase "as appropriate" implies that the person using the classification already knows whether or not the activity will aid in the problem's resolution.

Monitoring activities, such as "Monitor weight," do not indicate the findings that are expected to occur and the findings that indicate a problem. It would be more informative to say "Monitor weight daily for sudden change." Statements such as "Monitor for fluid overload" (from the Fluid Resuscitation Intervention) are useful only if the user knows what the indicators are for "overload." In contrast, "Monitor for distended neck veins, crackles in the lung, peripheral edema, and weight gain" (from the Fluid Monitoring intervention) has the indicators incorporated.

The activities from NIC (Iowa Intervention Project, 2000) applicable to content in this chapter are Electrolyte Management, defined as "promotion of electrolyte balance and prevention of complications resulting from abnormal or undesired serum electrolyte levels" (p. 268); Electrolyte Management: Hypernatremia, which is the "promotion of sodium balance and prevention of complications resulting from serum sodium levels higher than desired" (p. 275); Electrolyte Management: Hyponatremia, which is the "promotion of sodium balance and prevention of complications resulting from serum sodium levels lower than desired" (p. 284); Electrolyte Monitoring, or the "collection and analysis of patient data to regulate electrolyte balance" (p. 288); Fluid Management, defined as the "promotion of fluid balance and prevention of complications resulting from abnormal or undesired fluid levels" (p. 348); Fluid and Electrolyte Management, which is the "regulation and prevention of complications from altered fluid and/or electrolyte levels" (p. 350); Fluid Monitoring, or the "collection and analysis of patient data to regulate fluid balance" (p. 352); Fluid Resuscitation, which is "administering prescribed intravenous fluids rapidly" (p. 353); Hypovolemia Management, or the "expansion of intravascular fluid volume in a patient who is volume depleted" (p. 390); Intravenous Insertion, defined as the "insertion of a needle into a peripheral vein for the purpose of administering fluids, blood, or medications" (p. 408); and Intravenous Therapy, the "administration and monitoring of intravenous fluids and medications" (p. 409).

To simplify the complexities present in the NIC, the following steps are recommended: (1) collapsing Electrolyte Monitoring and Fluid Monitoring into Fluid and Electrolyte Monitoring; (2) omitting Electrolyte Management, Fluid Management, Fluid and Electrolyte Management, and Fluid Resuscitation and moving some of their activities to other specific situations; (3) combining Intravenous Insertion and Intravenous Therapy; and (4) placing intervention activities into specific conditions. The effect of these changes would be to reduce the 11 interventions to the following five: Fluid and Electrolyte Monitoring (Table 16-1); Intravenous Therapy; Hypovolemia Management (Box 16-3); Electrolyte Management: Hypernatremia; and Electrolyte Management: Hyponatremia (Table 16-2).

Selection of nursing-sensitive outcomes and nursing interventions depends on the type of fluid volume deficit that is present. Consequently, specific etiologies, risk factors, signs and symptoms, outcomes, and interventions are discussed in the context of specific types of dehydration.

Table **16-1**	Assessment Parameters and Monitoring Activities for the Combined Intervention Fluid and Electrolyte Monitoring
Assessment Parameters	**Monitoring Activities**
Baseline history	Determine history of fluid intake and output
Risk factors	Identify risk factors for fluid and electrolyte imbalances
Weight	Monitor weight daily for changes
Intake/output	Compare intake and output
	Monitor for fluid losses: weight loss, thirst, dry mouth
	Monitor for fluid gains: weight gain, edema, lung crackles
	Include oral, IV, and enteral feeding amounts for intake
	Include urine, emesis, stools, tube, and drainage amounts for output
	Monitor the amount, color, and specific gravity of urine
	Monitor consistency of stools
Temperature	Monitor for high or low temperature
Blood pressure	Monitor blood pressure—lying and standing
	Monitor for dizziness on standing
	Monitor for venous filling in peripheral and neck veins
	Monitor invasive hemodynamic parameters
Pulse	Monitor pulse—lying and standing
	Monitor for cardiac dysrhythmias
	Monitor EKG tracings for changes related to abnormal serum potassium, calcium, and magnesium levels
Respirations	Monitor respiratory rate and note adventitious sounds
	Monitor saturated oxygen level
Gastrointestinal system	Monitor for constipation
	Monitor for nausea, vomiting, and diarrhea
Skin and mucous membranes	Monitor skin for dryness or sweating
	Monitor moistness of mucous membranes
Neuromuscular activity	Monitor for excitation, twitching, tetany, hyperreflexia, cramping, numbness, tingling, disorientation, seizures
	Monitor for muscle weakness, hyporeflexia, lethargy, altered mentation, coma
Energy level	Monitor for tiredness, lethargy, malaise
Laboratory tests	Monitor hemoglobin and hematocrit
	Monitor serum sodium, calcium, potassium, magnesium levels
	Monitor BUN/creatinine
	Monitor serum albumin
	Monitor serum osmolality
	Monitor urine osmolality
	Monitor urinary sodium

Dehydration: Isotonic

Losses of isotonic fluids decrease the volume of the EC fluid compartment but not the volume of the IC compartment. The vascular compartment, which constitutes about 7% of the body weight in the normal adult, is affected first. If the blood loss is rapid and large enough, shock develops from hypovolemia. If the loss is slow, as with gastrointestinal losses, the interstitium, which acts as a reservoir, will have time to move fluid to the vascular compartment. This movement of fluid moderates the effects of vascular volume loss. However, even a slow loss of 6 liters of isotonic fluid will produce shock (Pestana, 1985). A 2% reduction of body weight because of fluid loss causes thirst and oliguria; a 5% to 10% weight loss produces tachycardia and hypotension; and a 10% to 20% reduction can result in stupor and shock (Carroll & Oh, 1978).

Related Factors/Etiologies.   Vascular fluid losses of 1 to 2 liters, as in hemorrhage or burns, require immediate attention with packed red blood cells and isotonic fluids. A loss of 500 mL of blood by a healthy adult can cause short-lived lightheadedness. Vasoconstriction and movement of fluid from the interstitium prevent major changes in hemodynamics, as evidenced by the cardiovascular adjustment of blood donors. In an elderly person with the same amount of blood loss, arteriosclerosis may slow the arteriolar compensation and indicators of hypovolemia may appear.

Vomiting and diarrhea frequently cause isotonic EC fluid losses in the elder. Gastrointestinal infections can spread very easily among residents of a nursing home. Marrie, Lee, Faulkner, Ethier, and Young (1982), summarizing four studies of rotavirus-related diarrhea in geri-

Box **16-3**	Combining of Intravenous (IV) Insertion and Intravenous (IV) Therapy Interventions Into Intravenous (IV) Therapy; Combining of Fluid Resuscitation and Hypovolemia Management Into Hypovolemia Management

Intravenous (IV) Therapy

Verify order for IV therapy
Note bleeding risks of patient
Choose needle size based on purpose: #18 for transfusion
Instruct patient about procedure
Ask parents to hold and comfort child as necessary
Maintain standard precautions
Administer 1% lidocaine at insertion site by protocol
Start IV in opposite arm in patients with arteriovenous fistulas or shunts
Apply and maintain transparent dressing over insertion site
Prevent air from entering infusion line
Administer IV fluids at room temperature
Document time and placement of IV site
Monitor IV flow rate and site during infusion
Check IV patency before administering medications
Flush intravenous lines between administration of incompatible solutions
Maintain sterility of infusate and tubing
Replace IV cannula, tubing, and infusate according to protocol
Change dressings for central line according to protocol
Monitor site for infusion phlebitis and local infection
Change IV site if redness, swelling, warmth, and/or pain occurs
Record IV intake and urinary output
Compare intake and output
Monitor for fluid overload: restlessness, lung crackles, dependent peripheral edema
Monitor vital signs
Limit IV potassium chloride to 20 mEq/hr or 200 mEq/24 hrs

Hypovolemia Management

Initiate prescribed fluid challenge
Maintain patent IV access
Give extra oral fluids between meals
Provide frequent oral hygiene
Distribute oral fluid intake over 24 hours
Assist with ambulation
Instruct patient to avoid rapid lying to standing changes
Place patient in Trendelenburg if needed and not contraindicated
Control rate of isotonic solutions to prevent hypervolemia
Withhold vasodilators with low blood pressure
Administer isotonic solutions for EC rehydration
Administer hypotonic solutions for IC rehydration
Calculate fluid needs based on body surface and burn size
Maintain steady infusion flow rate
Obtain blood specimens for cross matching
Arrange availability of blood products for tranfusion
Administer blood products: packed red blood cells, platelets, fresh frozen plasma
Start protocol if blood reaction occurs
Institute autotransfusion of blood loss
Instruct patient/family about diuretic therapy
Instruct patient/family on means to avoid hypovolemia
Administer oxygen as needed
Collaborate with physician for administration of both crystalloids and colloids if needed
Combine crystalloid and colloid solutions for intravascular replacement

---

atric populations, reported that, of 395 persons at risk, 153 became ill and 4 died. Clearly, hypermotility of the bowel decreases absorption of intestinal fluids. Gastric suctioning represents another source of isotonic fluid loss.

Intestinal obstruction causes sequestering of fluids in the gut, reducing the effective circulating blood volume (ECBV) but not the body weight. Increased abdominal girth and discomfort with nausea and vomiting are indicators of fluid collecting in the gut. Fluid shifts to extravascular spaces, such as the peritoneal or pleural cavities, can lead to decreased ECBV as well.

Elevated environmental temperatures affect elders more than they affect younger people because of the elder's sluggish circulatory adaptive responses and reduced total body fluids. In addition, decreases in the concentrating ability of the kidney and in the sensation of thirst increase the risk for fluid loss and lack of fluid replacement in elders in hot weather. Hart et al. (1982) and Applegate et al. (1981) reported that economically depressed elders were more affected by heat waves than were elders with a higher economic status. Not having access to air-conditioned living quarters was cited as a factor in the

occurrence of heatstroke. Cooling measures and volume replacement constituted the basic treatment modalities.

Engaging in physical activity during hot weather raises added concern about dehydration and heatstroke in the elder. In a study by Irion, Wailgum, Stevens, Kendrick, and Paolone (1984), older men did not dissipate as much heat as younger men during exercise, apparently because of decreased skin blood flow associated with reduced cardiac output.

Signs and Symptoms. Orthostatic hypotension, tachycardia, weakness, a decrease in venous filling, dry mouth, and a decrease in skin turgor are typical signs and symptoms of an isotonic fluid deficit. Skin turgor in the elder, however, is extremely hard to assess. The skin of the healthy adult, after being pinched in a fold, returns to its original shape within 1 second, whereas in the well-hydrated elder the return may take 20 seconds. The time it takes for the return of the pinched fold of skin to its original position increases both with the severity of the fluid loss and with increasing age (Dorrington, 1981). Metheney (1996) suggested testing skin turgor over the

Table **16-2**	**Suggested Activities** **ELECTROLYTE MANAGEMENT: HYPERNATREMIA AND** **ELECTROLYTE MANAGEMENT: HYPONATREMIA**

Electrolyte Management: Hypernatremia	Electrolyte Management: Hyponatremia
Report decreased skin turgor, concentrated low urinary output (if water loss from route *other* than kidney), fever, dry mucous membranes, increased hematocrit and BUN (with plasma loss), weight loss, elevated serum sodium, lethargy, muscle irritability, seizures, coma	Report decreased serum sodium, decreased serum osmolality, lethargy, headache, confusion, increased intracranial pressure, anorexia, nausea, vomiting, muscular twitching, seizures, coma; if associated with hypovolemia: supine hypotension, tachycardia, weight loss
Obtain laboratory specimens	Obtain laboratory specimens
Maintain prescribed fluid infusion rates	Maintain prescribed fluid infusion rates
Maintain IV access	Maintain IV access
Contact physician for changes in fluid needs based on signs and symptoms	Contact physician for changes in fluid needs based on signs and symptoms
Adjust infusion rate based on patient's change in signs and symptoms and laboratory reports	Adjust infusion rate based on patient's change in signs and symptoms and laboratory reports
Assist with ambulation	Assist with ambulation
Instruct patient to avoid rapid lying to standing changes	Instruct patient to avoid rapid lying to standing changes
Place patient in Trendelenburg position if needed and not contraindicated	Place patient in Trendelenburg position if needed and not contraindicated
Administer prescribed diuretics with associated hypervolemia	Restrict free water in dilutional hyponatremia
Space extra fluids throughout day with associated hypovolemia	Provide for oral fluid intake (e.g., fluid preferences, easy access)
Administer 0.9% or 0.5% saline solution with associated hypovolemia	Administer 0.9% saline solution for sodium replacement
Provide free water with tube feedings	Control the rate of 3.0% and 5.0% saline administration closely for correction of acute hyponatremia per protocol
Provide fiber with tube feedings to reduce fluid loss with diarrhea	
Avoid administration of high sodium medications (e.g., Kayexalate, sodium bicarbonate)	Avoid administration of hypotonic infusions with hypervolemia
Maintain dietary sodium restrictions	Give saline infusion with correction for hyperglycemia
Provide frequent oral hygiene	Provide frequent oral hygiene
Institute seizure precautions with high serum sodium levels	Give enteral formulas that have sufficient sodium content
Instruct patient/family on use of salt substitutes	Irrigate gastric tubes with normal saline solution
Instruct patient/family on sodium diet restrictions	Institute seizure precautions with low serum sodium levels
Instruct patient/family on high sodium over-the-counter medications (e.g., selected antacids)	Supply food with sufficient sodium content
Instruct patient on prevention for dehydration (e.g., drinking extra fluids on hot days, drinking when not thirsty, avoiding caffeine)	Instruct patient/family on signs and symptoms of hyponatremia
Instruct patient/family on causes of dehydration	Instruct patient/family on causes for hyponatremia
	Instruct patient/family about diuretic therapy

sternum or forehead in older patients to obtain a more valid assessment. The presence of a dry axilla supports the diagnosis of hypovolemia with isotonic losses (McGee, Abernethy, & Simel, 1999).

Persons with isotonic fluid losses will exhibit normal sodium levels, since an equal ratio of sodium and water has been lost. A scanty, concentrated urine with low urinary sodium reflects the saving of water and sodium by the kidneys, provided the lack of tubule reabsorption is not the cause of the deficit. Blood urea nitrogen and creatinine levels are elevated. Hematocrit, which reflects the ratio of red blood cells to plasma, will rise in proportion to the plasma deficit. However, if the person is losing whole

blood, the hematocrit value remains the same until fluid from the interstitium moves into the plasma or crystalloid replacement occurs.

Nursing Interventions. Isotonic fluid losses are treated by replacement of the lost fluid with fluid of like tonicity. Oral fluids, given frequently in small amounts, can be sufficient to replace a small deficit. Severe deficits require intravenous fluid therapy so that immediate and controlled replacement occurs. For gastrointestinal losses the administration of intravenous fluids depends on the severity of the diarrhea and the presence of nausea and vomiting. Parceling fluids throughout the day is necessary to prevent gastric distention while replacing lost fluids. The often-suggested intervention of providing the elderly person with preferred fluids aims at increasing fluid intake. Fluids, such as Gatorade, milk, and weak beef broth, provide vital sodium, potassium, and calories. Treatment is also aimed at reducing bowel hypermotility and severity of the nausea and vomiting.

Eisenman (1986) suggested several preventive measures for physically active elders during hot weather: ex- ercise during cooler times of the day and in the shade; wear light, porous, and white clothing; drink 16 to 32 ounces of fluid a half hour before starting exercise; and continue drinking 6 to 8 ounces every 15 minutes during the physical activity regardless of absent thirst. Another caution is to avoid large meals during hot weather to reduce the metabolic production of heat. Box 16-4 shows the NANDA, NOC, and NIC linkages for isotonic dehydration.

Box 16-4 — Suggested Nursing-Sensitive Outcomes and Nursing Interventions
FLUID VOLUME DEFICIT: ISOTONIC DEHYDRATION

Nursing Diagnosis
Fluid Volume Deficit: Isotonic Dehydration
Defining characteristics
Decreased urine output
Increased urine concentration
Weakness
Sudden weight loss (except in third spacing)
Decreased venous filling
Increased body temperature
Decreased pulse volume/pressure
Change in mental state
Elevated hematocrit
Decreased skin/tongue turgor
Dry skin/mucous membranes
Thirst
Increased pulse rate
Decreased blood pressure
Output more than intake
Orthostatic hypotension
Tachycardia
Dry mouth
Dry axilla
Scant, concentrated urine
Elevated hematocrit/hemoglobin (except with blood loss)
Normal serum Na^+
Elevated BUN
Low urinary Na^+

Related factors/etiologies
(All etiologies except hemorrhage can produce the same defining characteristics in isotonic extracellular fluid losses.)
Active fluid volume loss
Failure of regulatory mechanisms
Burns
Physical activity during hot weather
Vomiting
Gastrointestinal drainage
Diarrhea
Diaphoresis
Third spacing of fluid
Diuretic therapy
Hemorrhage

Nursing-Sensitive Outcomes
Fluid Balance
Indicators
Orthostatic hypotension not present
Blood pressure in expected range
Pulmonary wedge pressure in expected range
Mean arterial pressure in expected range
Central venous pressure in expected range
24-hour intake and output balanced
Body weight stable
Abnormal thirst not present
Moist mucous membranes
Urine specific gravity within normal limits
Hematocrit within normal limits
Serum electrolytes within normal limits
BUN within normal limits
Heart rate within normal limits

Hydration
Indicators
Skin hydration
Moist mucous membranes
Peripheral edema not present
Ascites not present
Abnormal thirst not present
Fever not present
Urine output within normal limits
BP within normal limits
Hematocrit within normal limits
Perspiration ability

Nursing Interventions
Intravenous (IV) Therapy
Activities
Verify order for IV therapy
Instruct patient about procedure
Maintain strict aseptic technique
Examine the solution for type, amount, expiration date, character of the solution, and lack of damage to container
Select and prepare an IV infusion pump, as indicated
Spike container with appropriate tubing
Administer IV fluids at room temperature

Box 16-4 Suggested Nursing-Sensitive Outcomes and Nursing Interventions—cont'd
FLUID VOLUME DEFICIT: ISOTONIC DEHYDRATION—cont'd

Identify whether patient is taking medication that is incompatible with medication ordered

Administer IV medications, as prescribed, and monitor for results

Monitor IV flow rate and IV site during infusion

Monitor for fluid overload and physical reactions

Monitor for IV patency before administration of IV medication

Replace IV cannula, apparatus, and infusate every 48 hours, according to agency protocol

Maintain occlusive dressing

Perform IV site checks on a regular basis

Perform IV site care according to agency protocol

Monitor vital signs

Limit IV potassium to 20 mEq/hr or 200 mEq/24 hrs, as appropriate

Flush IV lines between administration of incompatible solutions

Record intake and output

Monitor for signs and symptoms associated with infusion phlebitis and local infection

Maintain universal precautions

Fluid/Electrolyte Management
Activities
Monitor for abnormal serum electrolyte levels, as available

Obtain laboratory specimens for monitoring of altered fluid or electrolyte levels

Weigh daily and monitor trends

Restrict free water intake in the presence of dilutional hyponatremia with serum Na level below 130 mEq per liter

Give fluids, as appropriate

Promote oral intake, as appropriate

Administer prescribed nasogastric replacement based on output, as appropriate

Administer fiber as prescribed for the tube-fed patient to reduce fluid and electrolyte loss through diarrhea

Minimize the number of ice chips consumed or amount of oral intake by patients with gastric tubes connected to suction

Irrigate nasogastric tubes with normal saline

Provide free water with tube feedings, as appropriate

Set an appropriate IV infusion (or blood transfusion) flow rate

Monitor laboratory results relevant to fluid balance

Monitor laboratory results relevant to fluid retention

Monitor hemodynamic status, including CVP, MAP, PAP, and PCWP levels, if available

Keep an accurate record of intake and output

Monitor for signs and symptoms of fluid retention

Institute fluid restriction, as appropriate

Monitor vital signs, as appropriate

Correct preoperative dehydration, as appropriate

Maintain IV solution containing electrolyte(s) at constant flow rate, as appropriate

Monitor patient's response to prescribed electrolyte therapy

Monitor for manifestations of electrolyte imbalance

Provide prescribed diet appropriate for specific fluid or electrolyte imbalance

Monitor for side effects of prescribed supplemental electrolytes

Assess patient's buccal membranes, sclera, and skin for indications of altered fluid and electrolyte balance

Consult physician if signs and symptoms of fluid and/or electrolyte imbalance persist or worsen

Administer prescribed supplemental electrolytes, as appropriate

Administer prescribed electrolyte binding/excreting resins, as appropriate

Institute measures to control excessive electrolyte loss, as appropriate

Institute measures to rest the bowel, if appropriate

Follow quick-acting glucose with long-acting carbohydrates and proteins for management of acute hypoglycemia, as appropriate

Prepare patient for dialysis, as appropriate

Monitor for fluid loss

Promote a positive body image and self-esteem, if concerns are expressed as a result of excessive fluid retention, if appropriate

Hypovolemia Management
Activities
Teach patient the rationale for use of diuretic therapy

Instruct patient and/or family on measures instituted to treat the hypervolemia

Arrange availability of blood products for transfusion

Administer blood products: packed red blood cells, platelets, fresh frozen plasma

Start protocol if blood reaction occurs

Institute autotransfusion of blood loss

Administer isotonic solutions for EC rehydration

Distribute oral fluid intake over 24 hours

Give extra oral fluids between meals

Assist with ambulation

Withhold vasodilators with low blood pressure

Instruct patient to avoid rapid lying to standing changes

Place patient in Trendelenburg position if needed and not contraindicated

Administer oxygen as needed

Collaborate with physician for administration of both crystalloids and colloids if needed

Calculate fluid needs based on body surface and burn size

Give extra oral fluids between meals

Administer isotonic solutions for EC rehydration

Initiate prescribed fluid challenge

Control rate of isotonic solutions to prevent hypervolemia

CASE STUDY 1

J. Thomas, a 76-year-old retired anthropologist, lived in a retirement village apartment. She called the village nurse and reported that she had had two large diarrheal stools during the night and was feeling somewhat tired; she had no nausea. The nurse called on her within the hour and discovered that Mrs. Thomas had returned the day before from an intercity tour. On this tour she drank water and ate at gourmet restaurants in various cities. She had no other health problems and took no medications except supplemental calcium.

Mrs. Thomas had abdominal cramping with the diarrheal stools and hyperactive bowel sounds, but no abdominal tenderness on palpation. Her temperature was normal, as were her other vital signs. She had drunk milk, weak tea, and broth totaling about "a quart and a half" in the early morning. She was "somewhat thirsty" but not hungry. She reported her urine as being "a darker yellow than usual." The nurse recognized that Mrs. Thomas was experiencing an isotonic fluid loss.

The nurse reinforced Mrs. Thomas's efforts for maintaining fluid volume, made certain that fluids were readily available, and verified that Mrs. Thomas understood that she should continue drinking small glasses (150 mL) of fluids at least every hour. When the nurse called Mrs. Thomas 3 hours later, she reported that she had had two more diarrheal stools. The nurse contacted the village physician, who wrote an order for Lomotil. Mrs. Thomas did not want to use the Lomotil prescription unless absolutely necessary. She decided to eat some cooked white rice, which was a standard treatment used by the people she studied in the Mediterranean area. She had a diarrheal stool 2 hours later and a small formed stool 3 hours later. The nurse called in the early evening for an update and advised Mrs. Thomas to continue taking fluids even though her diarrhea had lessened.

The physical and mental functioning of this elderly woman helped her to avoid a situation that could have become critical. She had not lost a lot of fluid before she requested help, and she had replaced the deficit with enough isotonic fluids to maintain vascular volume. In view of the age-related changes that reduced her compensatory range, continued monitoring was indicated.

Dehydration: Hypotonic (Hyponatremia)

The loss of sodium in excess of water from the body results in a hyponatremic fluid deficit. Pestana (1985) explains that there is no mechanism whereby hypertonic fluid can be lost from the body. Rather, hyponatremic deficits occur when an initial loss of isotonic fluid is partially replaced by hypotonic fluid. Specifically, the loss of isotonic fluid results in a contraction of the extracellular volume. The kidneys respond to this change in volume by reabsorbing more water than sodium. Retention of water, in turn, dilutes the EC fluid, creating hyponatremia or sodium dilution.

Related Factors/Etiologies. Sodium losses occur with diuretic therapy, vomiting, diarrhea, blood loss, adrenal insufficiency (Addison's disease), and renal salt-wasting diseases. These losses result in a decreased ECBV, which prompts renal salvage of water (Alpern et al., 1990). The lack of aldosterone caused by adrenal or pituitary insufficiency allows sodium loss by the renal tubules. Renal salt-wasting diseases include end-stage renal disease, salt-losing nephritis, and renal tubular acidosis (Lindeman, 1989). A decrease in renal concentrating capacity—meaning sodium and water is not reabsorbed by the renal tubules—leads to volume deficit with hyponatremia.

Another causative factor cited by Lindeman was severe metabolic alkalosis caused by vomiting, in which case the kidneys excrete sodium bicarbonate to adjust the pH. Miller, Morley, and Rubinstein (1995) reported in a 12-month review of 119 long-term care facility (LTCF) residents that 53% had been hyponatremic on at least one occasion. Eleven of the twelve residents receiving low sodium tube feedings were hyponatremic. Rudman, Racette, Rudman, Mattson, and Erve (1986), noting similar instances of hyponatremia, postulated that elders are less able to conserve sodium. Miller et al. (1995) found that 78% of the patients with hyponatremia had been given hypotonic fluids (oral water, 0.45% saline solution, or 5% glucose in water). The hyponatremia was associated with a wide variety of central nervous system (CNS) diseases, implicating abnormal antidiuretic hormone (ADH) secretion.

Booker (1984) cited three cases in which acute emotional stress was closely related to the onset of hyponatremic symptoms in previously healthy patients who were receiving diuretics. The stress-mediated release of ADH, which acts on the tubules to conserve water, was postulated as the factor that altered the electrolyte balance in these patients.

Excessive sweating can lead to hyponatremic volume depletion if replacement is with water only. These factors may have been responsible for the 81.2% increase in the death rate among geriatric admissions to two Great Britain hospitals during a summer heat wave, compared with the same time period the previous year when temperatures were typical (Fish, Bennett, & Millard, 1985).

Ayus, Krothapalli, and Arieff (1985) noted that hyponatremia resulted in less favorable outcomes among persons with alcoholism and/or severe malnourishment. A 53% difference in mortality occurred between alcoholic and nonalcoholic patients who had severe hyponatremia (serum sodium levels less than 120 mEq/L).

Signs and Symptoms. Fundamental hemodynamic signs of hypovolemic hyponatremia are supine tachycardia and hypotension that worsen on rising (Narins, Jones, Stom, Rudnick, & Bastl, 1982). Poor skin turgor also accompanies the depletion. BUN is elevated to a greater degree than is serum creatinine. If the kidneys are functioning normally, urine will have a low concentration of sodium but a high concentration of other waste products. However, renal disease and chronic partial urinary tract obstruction can cause excretion of isotonic urine with sodium. In these instances the increased urine volume and decreased concentration are actually the risks rather than the indicators for volume depletion.

Other signs and symptoms for hyponatremia include anorexia, nausea, intermittent or persistent vomiting, lethargy, weakness, confusion, grand mal seizures, coma with decorticate posture, bilateral rigidity, and extensor plantar reflexes. Neurologic symptoms, such as paralysis, can persist even after correction of low serum sodium levels. A serum sodium level of about 110 mEq/L or lower is associated with the central nervous system (CNS) signs (Ashouri, 1986). The gastrointestinal signs can occur when the serum sodium level is around 125 mEq/L.

Cerebral edema can result from hyponatremia. As the EC compartment becomes less concentrated than the IC compartment, water moves into the cells (Rymer & Fishman, 1973). Hyponatremia can mimic a stroke with neurologic signs of confusion, drowsiness, hypertonic reflexes, seizures, and coma (Booker & Crimmins, 1984).

Nursing Interventions. If hyponatremia is associated with neurologic symptoms, rapid correction with an intravenous hypertonic (3%) saline solution and a loop diuretic is warranted. The diuretic prevents vascular volume expansion in persons with a compromised cardiovascular system. Ayus et al. (1985) and Ashouri (1986) recommended treatment within 12 to 24 hours of the hyponatremic onset with hypertonic saline solution to a mild hyponatremic state of 125 to 130 mEq/L. Descriptions of patients' demise even with correction of the serum sodium level have been recorded (Arieff & Witte, 1979). Administration of this regimen requires meticulous control of the infusion rate. Inadvertent rapid administration of a hypertonic saline solution can cause death. The brain shrinks and pulls away from the cranial vault, causing rupture of cerebral vessels.

With less severe EC volume depletion, temporary withdrawal of diuretics and volume repletion with an isotonic solution or oral fluids are indicated. Replacement for mildly hyponatremic states with volume depletion can be in the form of salty liquids or foods. A sodium deficit disappeared in patients with low sodium tube feedings when sodium intake was elevated to 2 g per day (Miller et al., 1995). Avoiding the use of hypotonic fluids when increased water intake is required may prevent hyponatremia. Again, spacing and frequent small amounts should prevent gastric distention. Remember that nausea is a symptom of low serum sodium levels.

When diuretic therapy is initiated, awareness of the potential for hypovolemic hyponatremia is essential. Madias and Zelman (1982) suggested two ways to prevent volume depletion and hyponatremia with diuretic therapy: (1) a gradual increase in dosage accompanied by careful monitoring of weight and serum sodium levels and (2) the use of alternate-day administration, which allows adequate diuresis but prevents volume depletion. Also, persons who are prescribed low-sodium diets in conjunction with diuretics must be monitored even more closely for the development of hyponatremia and volume depletion. One nursing home discontinued low-salt diets because of their association with postural hypotension (Morley & Kraenzle, 1994).

Adrenal insufficiency is treated by means of hormonal replacement with adrenocorticotropic hormone (ACTH) and/or hydrocortisone along with a fluid intake that will replace both water and sodium losses. The amount and type of fluids for the fluid losses caused by intrinsic renal disease are adjusted individually. Box 16-5 shows the NANDA, NOC, and NIC linkages for hypotonic dehydration.

CASE STUDY 2

J. Hall, age 78 years, is a resident in a nursing home. He was admitted to the emergency room because of newly developed coma associated with diarrhea. At the nursing home he had received Isocal tube feedings (low sodium concentration of 23 mEq/L) diluted with water at a 1:1 ratio and given at a rate of 2500 mL per day because of dysphagia secondary to neuromuscular dysfunction. Hydrochlorothiazide 25 mg per day had been given for mild hypertension for several months. On admission to the hospital, Mr. Hall's serum sodium level was 112 mEq/L, his serum osmolality was 235 mOsm/kg, and his urine osmolality was 550 mOsm/kg.

Initial treatment was with 500 mL of 3% sodium chloride at a rate of 50 mL/hr. Mr. Hall began to respond to verbal stimulation within 3 hours. IV fluids were continued with 5% dextrose and 0.45 saline solution at 25 mL/hr. After 24 hours the serum sodium level rose to 130 mEq/L. By this time Mr. Hall was communicating with facial expressions and hand movements that equaled his preadmission level of performance. Fluid replacement continued until urinary output reached 40 mL/hr.

The associated factors leading to the low sodium levels included a decreased intake of sodium, an increased excretion of sodium, and water retrieval from the glomerular filtrate caused by an antidiuretic response to the volume depletion brought on by the diarrhea. Fluid losses by the bowel tend to be isotonic.

Rehydration and serum sodium adjustment demand frequent monitoring for level of mental alertness, focal neurologic signs, urinary output, vital signs, and breath sounds. Blood samples are needed to follow serum sodium level. Adventitious breath sounds are of concern because the administration of hypertonic saline solution can lead to hypervolemia, resulting in pulmonary edema. If pulmonary edema does occur, a potent diuretic, such as furosemide, is administered. It is not unheard of for persons who experience low serum sodium levels to develop neurologic deficits.

Nursing Diagnosis
Hypotonic Dehydration
Defining characteristics
Decreased urine output
Increased urine concentration
Weakness
Sudden weight loss (except in third spacing)
Decreased venous filling
Increased body temperature
Decreased pulse volume/pressure
Change in mental state
Elevated hematocrit
Decreased skin/tongue turgor
Dry skin/mucous membranes
Thirst
Increased pulse rate
Decreased blood pressure
Supine tachycardia
Supine hypotension that worsens on rising
Poor skin turgor
Low serum sodium
Elevated BUN
Elevated hematocrit
Normal or low urinary sodium
Low volume, concentrated urine
Anorexia, nausea, vomiting
Confusion, coma, convulsions
Paralysis, hyperreflexia
Decorticate posturing

Related factors/etiologies
(All etiologies except hemorrhage can produce the same
    defining characteristics in isotonic EC fluid losses.)
Active fluid volume loss
Failure of regulatory mechanisms
Burns
Physical activity during hot weather
Vomiting
Gastrointestinal drainage
Diarrhea
Diaphoresis
Third spacing of fluid
Diuretic therapy
Hemorrhage
Adrenal or pituitary insufficiency
Increased ADH production
End-stage renal disease
Excessive sweating
Salt-losing nephritis
Tube feedings with low sodium
Renal tubular acidosis
Acute emotional distress

Nursing-Sensitive Outcomes
Fluid Balance
Indicators
Orthostatic hypotension not present
Blood pressure in expected range
Pulmonary wedge pressure in expected range
Mean arterial pressure in expected range
Central venous pressure in expected range
24-hour intake and output balanced
Body weight stable
Abnormal thirst not present
Moist mucous membranes
Urine specific gravity within normal limits
Hematocrit within normal limits
Serum electrolytes within normal limits
Sunken eyes not present
Confusion not present
BUN within normal limits
Heart rate within normal limits

Hydration
Indicators
Skin hydration
Moist mucous membranes
Peripheral edema not present
Ascites not present
Abnormal thirst not present
Sunken eyes not present
Fever not present
Urine output within normal limits
Blood pressure within normal limits
Hematocrit within normal limits
Perspiration ability
Serum sodium within normal limits
Normal urinary sodium
Able to urinate

Nursing Interventions
Intravenous (IV) Therapy
Activities
Verify order for IV therapy
Instruct patient about procedure
Maintain strict aseptic technique
Examine the solution for type, amount, expiration date,
    character of the solution, and lack of damage to container
Select and prepare an IV infusion pump, as indicated
Spike container with appropriate tubing
Administer IV fluids at room temperature
Identify whether patient is taking medication that is
    incompatible with medication ordered
Administer IV medications, as prescribed, and monitor for
    results
Monitor IV flow rate and IV site during infusion

Box 16-5	Suggested Nursing-Sensitive Outcomes and Nursing Interventions—cont'd
	FLUID VOLUME DEFICIT: HYPOTONIC DEHYDRATION—cont'd

Monitor for fluid overload and physical reactions

Monitor for IV patency before administration of IV medication

Replace IV cannula, apparatus, and infusate every 48 hours, according to agency protocol

Maintain occlusive dressing

Perform IV site checks on a regular basis

Perform IV site care according to agency protocol

Monitor vital signs

Limit IV potassium to 20 mEq/hr or 200 mEq/24 hrs, as appropriate

Flush IV lines between administration of incompatible solutions

Record intake and output

Monitor for signs and symptoms associated with infusion phlebitis and local infection

Maintain universal precautions

Fluid/Electrolyte Management
Activities

Monitor for abnormal serum electrolyte levels, as available

Obtain laboratory specimens for monitoring of altered fluid or electrolyte levels

Weigh daily and monitor trends

Restrict free water intake in the presence of dilutional hyponatremia with serum Na level below 130 mEq per liter

Give fluids, as appropriate

Promote oral intake, as appropriate

Administer prescribed nasogastric replacement based on output, as appropriate

Administer fiber as prescribed for the tube-fed patient to reduce fluid and electrolyte loss through diarrhea

Minimize the number of ice chips consumed or amount of oral intake by patients with gastric tubes connected to suction

Irrigate nasogastric tubes with normal saline

Provide free water with tube feedings, as appropriate

Set an appropriate IV infusion (or blood transfusion) flow rate

Monitor laboratory results relevant to fluid balance

Monitor laboratory results relevant to fluid retention

Monitor hemodynamic status, including CVP, MAP, PAP, and PCWP levels, if available

Keep an accurate record of intake and output

Monitor for signs and symptoms of fluid retention

Institute fluid restriction, as appropriate

Monitor vital signs, as appropriate

Correct preoperative dehydration, as appropriate

Maintain IV solution containing electrolyte(s) at constant flow rate, as appropriate

Monitor patient's response to prescribed electrolyte therapy

Monitor for manifestations of electrolyte imbalance

Provide prescribed diet appropriate for specific fluid or electrolyte imbalance

Monitor for side effects of prescribed supplemental electrolytes

Assess patient's buccal membranes, sclera, and skin for indications of altered fluid and electrolyte balance

Consult physician if signs and symptoms of fluid and/or electrolyte imbalance persist or worsen

Administer prescribed supplemental electrolytes, as appropriate

Administer prescribed electrolyte binding/excreting resins, as appropriate

Institute measures to control excessive electrolyte loss, as appropriate

Institute measures to rest the bowel, if appropriate

Follow quick-acting glucose with long-acting carbohydrates and proteins for management of acute hypoglycemia, as appropriate

Prepare patient for dialysis, as appropriate

Monitor for fluid loss

Promote a positive body image and self-esteem, if concerns are expressed as a result of excessive fluid retention, if appropriate

Electrolyte Management: Hyponatremia
Activities

Teach patient the rationale for use of diuretic therapy

Instruct patient and/or family on measures instituted to treat the hypervolemia

Arrange availability of blood products for transfusion

Obtain lab specimens for analysis of altered sodium levels, as appropriate

Avoid excessive administration of hypotonic IV fluids, especially in the presence of syndrome of inappropriate anti-diuretic hormone (SIADH)

Institute seizure precautions

Encourage foods/fluids high in sodium, if appropriate

Administer hypertonic (3% to 5%) saline at 3 ml/kg/hr or per policy for rapid correction of hyponatremia, as appropriate

Assist with ambulation

Instruct patient/family on signs and symptoms of hyponatremia

Report decreased serum sodium, decreased serum osmolality, lethargy, headache, confusion, increased intracranial pressure, anorexia, nausea, vomiting, muscular twitching, seizures, and coma

If associated with hypovolemia: supine hypotension, tachycardia, and weight loss

Maintain prescribed fluid infusion rates

Maintain IV access

Contact physician for changes in fluid needs based on signs and symptoms

Adjust infusion rate based on patient's change in signs and symptoms and laboratory reports

Instruct patient to avoid rapid change from lying to standing

Provide for oral fluid intake

Restrict free water in dilutional hyponatremia

Administer 0.9% saline for sodium replacement

Give saline infusion with correction for hyperglycemia

Provide frequent oral hygiene

Irrigate gastric tubes with normal saline

Give enteral formulas that have sufficient sodium content

Mr. Hall's diarrhea subsided without specific medication. It was surmised that the diarrhea upset the fluid and sodium balance, since Mr. Hall had no weakness or nausea to indicate a low serum sodium level before the diarrheal episode. However, another formula was selected that had a similar osmolality to the Isocal, but a 10 mEq/L increase in sodium content. The agency transfer form to the nursing home contained information about hyponatremic states, as did a verbal report to the caregivers at the nursing home. Planned follow-up after Mr. Hall's return to the nursing home consisted of blood samples for serum sodium levels and recording of intake and output volumes.

Dehydration: Hypertonic (Hypernatremia)

A decrease in water intake or an increase in water loss relative to sodium loss leads to a reduction in total body water and an increase in sodium concentration. The kidneys must have a specific amount of water to remove solutes from the plasma. An increase in the solute load without a concomitant increase in water intake will result in the kidney's using body water to perform its functions.

Related Factors/Etiologies. The most common causes of hypernatremia in elders are mental incapacity and physical inability to obtain water even though thirst is present. Dehydration occurred 2 to 5 times more frequently in patients who had dementia as opposed to those who did not (Holstein, Chatellier, Piette, & Moulias, 1994). In more than half of study patients reported by Long, Marin, Bayer, Shetty, and Pathy (1991) the use of diuretics, depressed conscious level, and febrile illness were associated with hypernatremia. Another situation that limits water intake and can create volume depletion for the elderly person is the nothing-by-mouth (NPO) preparation for diagnostic tests. An increase in risk arises with the simultaneous cleansing of the bowel.

Lack of thirst can lead to decreased fluid volume. Miller, Krebs, Neal, and McIntrye (1982) reported that a group of six elderly patients whose mental status was considered normal and who lacked demonstrable hypothalamic or pituitary lesions had no sensation of thirst with hypertonicity. Phillips et al. (1984a) reported a decrease in thirst sensation in older men who experienced fluid volume depletion.

A tube-feeding formula has been mentioned previously as a possible cause for hyponatremia. In contrast, high protein formulas can produce hypernatremic fluid deficits with azotemia (Gault, Dixon, Doyle, & Cohen, 1968). Tube feedings with high osmolality require additional water supplementation because of the increased solute load presented to the kidneys. Advanced renal disease may contribute to the development of dehydration because the renal concentrating ability is lost, which increases the risk for hypernatremic fluid deficits when water replacement is inadequate.

Signs and Symptoms. Hypotension, which is a major indicator of isotonic and hypotonic dehydration, occurs later in the process of fluid losses with hypertonicity, because EC fluid volume is replenished by IC water. Urine volume may be low with maximal concentration. Conversely, if there is a high solute load being presented to the kidney, an increase in urine output will occur. If loss of body water continues, fever, flushing, loss of sweating, and dryness of mucous membranes occur with hemodynamic changes. Personality changes can progress to hallucinations, delirium, and manic behavior; ultimately, convulsions and coma develop.

Pals et al. (1995) found that institutional staff recognized decreased oral intake of residents and that subsequent laboratory evaluation revealed a high association with either increased BUN/creatinine or serum sodium concentration. Fevers, which may indicate a decrease in intake or loss of fluids, were most frequently found by the staff rather than by resident report. Cues, such as anorexia, myalgia, malaise, weakness, drowsiness, or coryza with fever, point to possible hypernatremic volume depletion (Pals et al., 1995).

Nursing Interventions. Interventions focus on providing water for intake. Hydrating residents at the first sign of impaired intake was the recommendation by Pals et al. (1995). Caregivers need to provide fluids between meals for dependent elders. For elderly persons with a decreased thirst sensation, ingestion of 2 quarts of water a day may be prescribed. Setting in the refrigerator the amount of water to be drunk in 1 day can serve as a reminder for the independent elder. High osmolar enteral tube feedings require extra water. Scheduling the elder early in the day for procedures that require her to be NPO after midnight can reduce the probability of a water deficit.

Weinberg et al. (1994) suggested a rehydration plan for institutionalized residents at risk for dehydration. All staff members would be alerted to medications that reduce free water and diseases that cause excess losses of fluids.

Increased water consumption is the usual treatment for volume depletion with hypernatremia. However, giving 5% dextrose in water IV for severe volume depletion can lead to cerebral edema because of the change in the osmotic gradient between the IC and EC compartments after metabolism of the dextrose. Phillips et al. (1984b) suggested that treatment with isotonic saline solution initially rather than water alone might avoid the risks of cerebral edema. Hughes-Davies (1984) suggested that fluid replacement with a salty soup might be safer than tap water for those able to swallow. What must occur is administration of more water than sodium while preventing a fluid shift to the IC compartment.

Pestana (1985) stated that the low side of volume replacement can be judged from the hourly urinary output, but cautioned that urinary output is less reliable as an indication of overhydration because pulmonary edema can occur before the kidneys react. Box 16-6 shows the NANDA, NOC, and NIC linkages for hypertonic dehydration.

Box 16-6

Suggested Nursing-Sensitive Outcomes and Nursing Interventions
FLUID VOLUME DEFICIT: HYPERTONIC DEHYDRATION

Nursing Diagnosis
Fluid Volume Deficit: Hypertonic Dehydration
Defining characteristics
Decreased venous filling
Decreased pulse volume/pressure
Change in mental state
Elevated hematocrit
Decreased skin/tongue turgor
Dry skin/mucous membranes
Thirst
Decreased intensity of heart sounds
Rapid weight loss
Tachycardia
Orthostatic hypotension
Elevated serum sodium
Elevated BUN
Low urinary sodium
Confusion
Delirium, convulsions, coma
Scant, concentrated urine
Fever
Tiredness/decreased energy level
Loss of sweating
Personality changes
Manic behavior

Related factors/etiologies
(All etiologies except hemorrhage can produce the same
    defining characteristics in isotonic EC fluid losses.)
Active fluid volume loss
Failure of regulatory mechanisms
Burns
Physical activity during hot weather
Vomiting
Gastrointestinal drainage
Diarrhea
Diaphoresis
Third spacing of fluid
Diuretic therapy
Hemorrhage
Diabetes insipidus
Excess diuretic therapy
Hypercalcemia
Hypokalemia
Decreased water intake
Lack of thirst
Inability to obtain water
Mental and/or physical incapacity
Loss of urine concentration
High protein feedings without sufficient water
Water loss more than solute loss

Nursing-Sensitive Outcomes
Fluid Balance
Indicators
Orthostatic hypotension not present
Blood pressure in expected range

Pulmonary wedge pressure in expected range
Mean arterial pressure in expected range
Central venous pressure in expected range
24-hour intake and output balanced
Body weight stable
Abnormal thirst not present
Moist mucous membranes
Urine specific gravity within normal limits
Hematocrit within normal limits
Serum electrolytes within normal limits
Sunken eyes not present
Confusion not present
BUN within normal limits
Heart rate in expected range

Hydration
Indicators
Skin hydration
Moist mucous membranes
Peripheral edema not present
Ascites not present
Abnormal thirst not present
Sunken eyes not present
Fever not present
Urine output within normal limits
Blood pressure within normal limits
Hematocrit within normal limits
Perspiration ability
Serum sodium within normal limits
Able to urinate

Nursing Interventions
Intravenous Therapy
Activities
Verify order for IV therapy
Instruct patient about procedure
Maintain strict aseptic technique
Examine the solution for type, amount, expiration date,
    character of the solution, and lack of damage to container
Select and prepare an IV infusion pump, as indicated
Spike container with appropriate tubing
Administer IV fluids at room temperature
Identify whether patient is taking medication that is
    incompatible with medication ordered
Administer IV medications, as prescribed, and monitor for
    results
Monitor IV flow rate and IV site during infusion
Monitor for fluid overload and physical reactions
Monitor for IV patency before administration of IV medication
Replace IV cannula, apparatus, and infusate every 48 hours,
    according to agency protocol
Maintain occlusive dressing
Perform IV site checks on a regular basis
Perform IV site care according to agency protocol
Monitor vital signs
Limit IV potassium to 20 mEq/hr or 200 mEq/24 hrs, as
    appropriate

Continued

Box 16-6

Suggested Nursing-Sensitive Outcomes and Nursing Interventions—cont'd
FLUID VOLUME DEFICIT: HYPERTONIC DEHYDRATION—cont'd

Flush IV lines between administration of incompatible solutions

Record intake and output

Monitor for signs and symptoms associated with infusion phlebitis and local infection

Maintain universal precautions

Fluid/Electrolyte Management
Activities

Monitor for abnormal serum electrolyte levels, as available

Obtain laboratory specimens for monitoring of altered fluid or electrolyte levels

Weigh daily and monitor trends

Restrict free water intake in the presence of dilutional hyponatremia with serum Na level below 130 mEq per liter

Give fluids, as appropriate

Promote oral intake, as appropriate

Administer prescribed nasogastric replacement based on output, as appropriate

Administer fiber as prescribed for the tube-fed patient to reduce fluid and electrolyte loss through diarrhea

Minimize the number of ice chips consumed or amount of oral intake by patients with gastric tubes connected to suction

Irrigate nasogastric tubes with normal saline

Provide free water with tube feedings, as appropriate

Set an appropriate IV infusion (or blood transfusion) flow rate

Monitor laboratory results relevant to fluid balance

Monitor laboratory results relevant to fluid retention

Monitor hemodynamic status, including CVP, MAP, PAP, and PCWP levels, if available

Keep an accurate record of intake and output

Monitor for signs and symptoms of fluid retention

Institute fluid restriction, as appropriate

Monitor vital signs, as appropriate

Correct preoperative dehydration, as appropriate

Maintain IV solution containing electrolyte(s) at constant flow rate, as appropriate

Monitor patient's response to prescribed electrolyte therapy

Monitor for manifestations of electrolyte imbalance

Provide prescribed diet appropriate for specific fluid or electrolyte imbalance

Monitor for side effects of prescribed supplemental electrolytes

Assess patient's buccal membranes, sclera, and skin for indications of altered fluid and electrolyte balance

Consult physician if signs and symptoms of fluid and/or electrolyte imbalance persist or worsen

Administer prescribed supplemental electrolytes, as appropriate

Administer prescribed electrolyte binding/excreting resins, as appropriate

Institute measures to control excessive electrolyte loss, as appropriate

Institute measures to rest the bowel, if appropriate

Follow quick-acting glucose with long-acting carbohydrates and proteins for management of acute hypoglycemia, as appropriate

Prepare patient for dialysis, as appropriate

Monitor for fluid loss

Promote a positive body image and self-esteem, if concerns are expressed as a result of excessive fluid retention, if appropriate

Electrolyte Management: Hypernatremia
Activities

Instruct patient on appropriate use of salt substitutes, as appropriate

Instruct patient/family about foods and over-the-counter medications that are high in sodium

Obtain lab specimens for analysis of altered sodium levels, as appropriate

Maintain IV access

Avoid administration/intake of high sodium medications

Provide frequent oral hygiene

Maintain sodium restrictions

Instruct patient/family on causes of dehydration

Instruct patient on prevention for dehydration (e.g., drinking extra fluids on hot days, drinking when not thirsty, avoiding caffeine)

Maintain prescribed fluid infusion rates

Assist with ambulation

Instruct patient to avoid rapid lying to standing changes

Report decreased skin turgor, concentrated low urinary output (if water loss from route other than kidney), fever, dry mucous membrane, increased hematocrit and BUN (with plasma loss), weight loss, elevated serum sodium level, lethargy, muscle irritability, seizures, coma

Administer 0.9% or 0.5% saline with associated hypovolemia

Administer hypotonic fluids with caution

Avoid administration of high-sodium medications (e.g., Kayexelate, $NaHCO_3$)

Space extra fluids throughout day with associated hypovolemia .

Provide free water with tube feedings

Provide fiber with tube feedings to reduce fluid loss with diarrhea

Adjust infusion rate based on patient's change in signs and symptoms and laboratory reports

Contact physician for changes in fluid needs based on signs and symptoms

Institute seizure precautions with high serum sodium levels

CASE STUDY 3

L. Gaines, an 81-year-old active woman, lived alone and maintained a garden. She generally worked in her garden in the mornings and continued doing so during a heat wave. She perspired but did not experience unusual thirst. She complained to her neighbors that she felt very tired and could not do her usual cleaning. Later that same day she called them because she became dizzy when she stood up. She was admitted to the hospital, where her blood pressure dropped from 142/88 mm Hg to 110/66 mm Hg on standing. She voided 100 ml of concentrated urine with a specific gravity of 1.026. She had not voided in 5 hours before admission. Her serum sodium level was 160 mEq/L, and her BUN was 58 mg/dL. She usually weighed 125 lb (56.8 kg), but on admission weighed just less than 119 lb (54 kg).

She was treated with 5% dextrose in water in 0.45% saline solution IV at 100 mL/hr for 24 hours. Oral intake of water and fruit juices totaled 750 mL the first 24 hours of admission. Her energy levels improved, as did the hypotension. Urine output increased to 950 mL, and serum sodium level dropped to 150 mEq/L in the first 24 hours of treatment. Oral intake increased to 2500 mL the second 24 hours. IV fluids were discontinued. Urine output rose to 1250 mL the second 24 hours of treatment. She was discharged after 3 days with home care instructions.

Decreased sensitivity to thirst and active loss of fluids through perspiration combined to reduce this elderly woman's fluid volume. Her history, along with such signs as hypotension, oliguria, weight loss, and elevated BUN, indicated fluid volume deficit. The elevated serum sodium level signaled hypernatremia.

Giving hypotonic saline solution rather than 5% dextrose in water reduced the likelihood of cerebral edema. The greater tonicity of the saline solution reduced the gradient for IC movement of water. Although the serum sodium level was elevated, the total body sodium level was probably decreased. In this instance, more water than sodium had been eliminated from the body. The rather cautious rate of IV fluid replacement was in consideration of the patient's age and the state of her cardiovascular system.

Oral administration of fluids was divided throughout the day, with increases being based on her tolerance for them. Improvement in the assessment parameters (blood pressure, pulse, urine output, serum sodium levels, and energy levels) validated the intervention strategies. Before going home, she received instructions on what to do during hot weather. She was shown how adequate fluid intake can be ensured by filling fluid containers in the morning from which she will drink during the day. In addition, she accepted a visiting nurse referral until increased fluid consumption became habitual.

SUMMARY

The treatment for dehydration beyond the mild level is often medically determined. Consequently, independent nursing interventions focus on prevention, that is, educating the elder about risk situations, modifying intake patterns, or altering the environment for those at risk. Research is needed to identify intake or eating regimens that prevent fluid imbalances and motivators that increase fluid intake. The classification systems available for linking nursing diagnosis, outcomes, and interventions in a logical manner related to fluid and electrolyte imbalances require refinement. Terms denoting fluid imbalances have been given different definitions in both medical and nursing literature. To interpret the current literature on fluid and electrolyte imbalances, one must understand the concepts of tonicity and osmolality, their effect on fluid movement between compartments, and the causes and results of these compartment changes. In other words, a conceptual understanding must be in place to use the nursing diagnosis, nursing outcomes, and nursing interventions.

REFERENCES

Alpern, R. J., Saxton, C. R., & Seldin, D. W. (1990). Clinical interpretation of laboratory values. In J. P. Kokko & R. L. Tannen (Eds.), *Fluids and electrolytes* (2nd ed., pp. 3-69). Philadelphia: W. B. Saunders.

Applegate, W. B., Runyan, J. W., Brasfield, L., Williams, M. L., Konigsberg, C., & Fouche, C. (1981). Analysis of the 1980 heat wave in Memphis. *Journal of the American Geriatrics Society, (July) 8*, 337-342.

Arieff, A. L., & Witte, J. M. (1979). Death or permanent neurological disability despite correction of protracted hyponatremia. (Abstract.) *Kidney International, 16*, 955.

Ashouri, O. S. (1986). Severe diuretic-induced hyponatremia in the elderly: A series of 8 patients. *Archives of Internal Medicine, 146*, 1355-1357.

Ayus, J. C., Krothapalli, R. K., & Arieff, A. I. (1985). Changing concepts in treatment of severe symptomatic hyponatremia: Rapid correction and possible relation to central pontine myelinolysis. *American Journal of Medicine, 78*, 897-901.

Booker, J. A. (1984). Severe symptomatic hyponatremia in elderly outpatients: The role of thiazide therapy and stress. *Journal of the American Geriatrics Society, 32*(2), 108-113.

Booker, J. A., & Crimmins, J. (1984). Hyponatremia or stroke? (Letter.) *Medical Journal of Australia, 140*(13), 799-800.

Briggs, S. P., Sawaya, B. E., & Schnermann, J. (1990). Disorders of salt balance. In J. P. Kokko & R. L. Tannen (Eds.), *Fluids and electrolytes* (2nd ed., pp. 70-138). Philadelphia: W. B. Saunders.

Carroll, H. J., & Oh, M. S. (1978). *Electrolyte and acid-base metabolism: Diagnosis and management.* Baltimore: Lippincott Williams & Wilkins.

de Castro, J. M. (1992). Age-related changes in natural spontaneous fluid ingestion and thirst in humans. *Journal of Gerontology, 47*(5), 321-330.

Dorrington, K. L. (1981). Skin turgor: Do we understand the clinical sign? *Lancet, 1*(8214), 264-266.

Eisenman, P. A. (1986). Hot weather, exercise, old age, and the kidneys. *Geriatrics, 41*, 108-114.

Fish, P. D., Bennett, G. C. J., & Millard, P. H. (1985). Heatwave morbidity and mortality in old age. *Age & Ageing, 14*, 243-245.

Gault, M. H., Dixon, M. E., Doyle, M., & Cohen, W. M. (1968). Hypernatremia, azotemia and dehydration due to high protein tube feeding. *Annals of Internal Medicine, 68,* 778-791.

Hart, G. R., Anderson, R. J., Crumpler, C. P., Shulkin, A., Reed, G., & Knochel, J. P. (1982). Epidemic classical heat stroke: Clinical characteristics and course of 28 patients. *Medicine, 61,* 189-197.

Holstein, J., Chatellier, G., Piette, F., & Moulias, R. (1994). Prevalence of associated diseases in different types of dementia among elderly institutionalized patients: Analysis of 3447 records. *Journal of the American Geriatrics Society, 42*(9), 972-977.

Hughes-Davies, T. H. (1984). Thirst in the elderly. (Letter). *New England Journal of Medicine, 312,* 247.

Iowa Intervention Project. J. C. McCloskey & G. M. Bulechek (Eds.). (2000). *Nursing interventions classification (NIC)* (3rd ed.). St. Louis, MO: Mosby.

Iowa Outcomes Project. M. Johnson, M. Maas, & S. Moorhead (Eds.). (2000). *Nursing outcomes classification (NOC)* (2nd ed.). St. Louis, MO: Mosby.

Irion, G., Wailgum, T. D., Stevens, C., Kendrick, Z. V., & Paolone, A. M. (1984). The effect of age on the hemodynamic responses to thermal stress during exercise. In V. J. Cristofalo, G. T. Baker, III, R. C. Adelman, & J. Roberts (Eds.), *Modern aging research* (vol. 6, pp. 187-195). New York: Alan R. Liss.

Kleiner, S. M. (1999). Water: An essential but overlooked nutrient. *Journal of the American Dietetic Association, 99*(2), 200-206.

Lindeman, R. D. (1989). Application of fluid and electrolyte balance principles to the older patient. In W. Reichel (Ed.), *Clinical aspects of aging* (3rd ed., pp. 248-263). Baltimore: Lippincott Williams & Wilkins.

Long, C. A., Marin, P., Bayer, A. J., Shetty, H. G., & Pathy, M. S. (1991). *Postgraduate Medical Journal, 67*(789), 643-645.

Madias, N. E., & Zelman, S. J. (1982). What are the metabolic complications of diuretic treatment? *Geriatrics, 37*(2), 93-96.

Marrie, T. J., Lee, S. H., Faulkner, R. S., Ethier, J., & Young, C. H. (1982). Rotavirus infection in a geriatric population. *Archives of Internal Medicine, 142,* 313-316.

McGee, S., Abernethy, W. B., & Simel, D. L. (1999). Is this patient hypovolemic? *Journal of the American Medical Association, 281*(11), 1022-1029.

Metheney, N. M. (1996). *Fluid and electrolyte balance: Nursing considerations* (3rd ed.). Baltimore: Lippincott Williams & Wilkins.

Miller, M., Morley, J. E., & Rubenstein, L. Z. (1995). Hyponatremia in a nursing home population. *Journal of the American Geriatrics Society, 43*(12), 1410-1413.

Miller, P. D., Krebs, R. A., Neal, B. J., & McIntyre, D. O. (1982). Hypodipsia in geriatric patients. *American Journal of Medicine, (Sept), 73,* 354-356.

Morley, J. E., & Kraenzle, D. (1994). Causes of weight loss in a community nursing home. *Journal of the American Geriatrics Society, 42*(6), 583-585.

Narins, R. G., Jones, E. R., Stom, M. C., Rudnick, M. R., & Bastl, C. P. (1982). Diagnostic strategies in disorders of fluid, electrolyte and acid-base homeostasis. *American Journal of Medicine, (March) 72,* 496-519.

North American Nursing Diagnosis Association. (1999). *Nursing diagnoses: Definitions and classification 1999-2000.* Philadelphia: Author.

O'Neill, P. A., Davies, I., & Wears, R. (1989). Elderly female patients in continuing care: Why are they hypersomolar? *Gerontology, 35,* 305-309.

Owen, J. A., & Campbell, D. G. (1968). A comparison of plasma electrolyte and urea values in healthy persons and in hospital patients. *Clinical Chim Acta, 22,* 611-618.

Pals, J. K., Weinberg, A. D., Beal, L. F., Levesque, P. G., Cunningham, T. J., & Minaker, K. L. (1995). Clinical triggers for detection of fever and dehydration: Implications for long-term care nursing. *Journal of Gerontological Nursing, 21*(4), 13-19.

Pestana, C. (1985). *Fluids and electrolytes in the surgical patient* (3rd ed.). Baltimore: Lippincott Williams & Wilkins.

Phillips, P. A., Rolls, B. J., Ledingham, J. G., Forsling, M. L. Morton, J. J., Crowe, M. J., & Wollmer, L. (1984a). Reduced thirst after water deprivation in healthy elderly men. *New England Journal of Medicine, 311,* 753-759.

Phillips, P. A., Rolls, B. J., Ledingham, J. G., Forsling, M. L. Morton, J. J., Crowe, M. J., & Wollmer, L. (1984b). Thirst in the elderly. (Letter). *New England Journal of Medicine, 312,* 247.

Rudman, D., Racette, D., Rudman, I. W., Mattson, D. E., & Erve, P. R. (1986). Hyponatremia in tube-fed elderly men. *Journal of Chronic Disease, 39*(2), 73-80.

Rymer, M. M., & Fishman, R. A. (1973). Protective adaptation of brain to water intoxication. *Archives of Neurology, 28,* 49-54.

Sterns, R. H., & Spital, A. (1990). Disorders of water balance. In J. P. Kokko & R. L. Tannen (Eds.), *Fluids and electrolytes* (2nd ed., pp. 139-194). Philadelphia: W. B. Saunders.

Warren, J. L., Bacon, W. E., Harris, T., McBean, A. M., Foley, D. J., & Phillips, C. (1991). The burden and outcomes associated with dehydration among U.S. elderly. *American Journal of Public Health, 84*(8), 1265-1269.

Weinberg, A. D., Pals, J. K., McGlinchey-Berroth, R., & Minaker, K. L. (1994). Indices of dehydration among frail nursing home patients: Highly variable but stable over time. *Journal of the American Geriatrics Society, 42*(10), 1070-1073.

CHAPTER 17

RISK FOR ALTERED BODY TEMPERATURE

Barbara J. Holtzclaw

Humans have the ability to maintain a relatively constant internal temperature despite wide variations in the environment. As *homeotherms,* or warm-blooded animals, humans have great adaptability to either adjust to or alter their environment. Alterations in body temperature are essentially problems of thermal balance, with physical factors, as well as physiologic abilities, affecting heat loss or heat gain. The dynamics of body temperature alterations must be clearly understood to plan effective care for any age-group. However, aging changes some of these dynamics significantly. Thermoregulatory ability changes throughout the life span as a function of maturation, metabolic rate, and relative health of circulatory and neurologic systems. A lower metabolic rate and a higher incidence of disease in advanced age increase the risk for alterations in core body temperature. Physical and behavioral incapacities also can contribute to thermal alterations in elders by limiting personal control of their environment. Consequently, the sequelae of thermoregulatory failure in the elderly can seriously affect patient outcomes.

This chapter is designed to clarify the nursing diagnosis Risk for Altered Body Temperature (NANDA, 1999) in the context of the aging (Gordon, 1994). Appropriate nursing interventions and outcomes are identified in the *Nursing Interventions Classification (NIC)* (Iowa Intervention Project, 2000) and the *Nursing Outcomes Classification (NOC)* (Iowa Outcomes Project, 2000). The diagnostic label Risk for Altered Body Temperature is reconsidered because its narrow focus on temperature leads to treatment of the temperature elevation itself rather than to treatment of the underlying dynamics that are causing the temperature alteration. An alternate diagnosis, Altered Thermal Balance, is proposed to link nursing interventions and outcomes to the underlying threats to heat gain or loss.

Body heat is produced continuously through life by expenditure of energy in cellular metabolic reactions and combustion of ingested foodstuff. Tissue friction resulting from circulating blood and muscle contraction produces additional heat. Basal cellular metabolism, the heat-producing "fire of life," declines with advanced age, leaving the older adult less able to generate heat. Metabolic rate falls to some extent by age 65, but by age 80 the reduction is significant (Reuler, 1984). Lower levels of available heat make it necessary for elders to expend energy during thermal emergencies. Unlike younger persons who stay warm during cold exposure by conserving or redistributing existing body heat, elders must either use musculoskeletal activity to generate heat or seek external sources of warmth. If physiologic or behavioral impairment interferes with heat replacement, the risk for hypothermia increases. Concern for heat loss is increasing in geriatric care; however, equal attention should be given to problems of overheating (Kolanowski & Gunter, 1983). Aging, illness, and drug therapy contribute to deficits in body water and vasomotor activity, so that the ability to dissipate body heat is impaired. The problem of overheating in warm climates increases when elders cannot afford air conditioning and live in neighborhoods where they feel unsafe to leave windows open. Fever creates another threat to thermal balance and often is manifested in a substantially different way among older persons (Norman, Grahn, & Yoshikawa, 1985).

Three conditions are common outcomes of altered thermal balance: hypothermia, hyperthermia, and fever. Each of these terms infers a deviation from normal body temperature, but one that is inadequately described by this measurement alone. In addition, these names do not define the causative factor. "Related factors" must be defined that attribute hypothermia or hyperthermia to failure of control mechanisms or overwhelming environmental factors. Likewise, fever requires further definition because it is not always attributable to infectious causes. Febrile activity is often caused by drugs, blood products, or substances that induce systemic host responses. Intervention can be more appropriate and specific when underlying related factors are identified. Even when the origin of fever remains unknown, there are predictable sequelae related to obligatory water and calorie expenditures that suggest reframing the diagnosis.

Hypothermia

The term *hypothermia* literally means "low heat." In most settings the term is used to describe a condition where deep body temperature falls below 35° C (95° F), with severity ranging from mild to profound. Hypothermia can occur in any person or situation where heat loss exceeds the body's ability to generate or conserve heat. The predisposition for hypothermia among older persons is great because the opportunity for heat loss frequently coexists with a decline in heat generation/conservation responses (Ballester & Harchelroad, 1999). Two situations tend to produce incidental hypothermia during cold weather: (1) a healthy individual is exposed for prolonged periods to severely cold environmental conditions or (2) a person with impaired thermoregulatory ability is exposed to room temperature without protection. An elderly person with some degree of thermoregulatory impairment may be at risk for both situations if he undergoes surgery, is injured in a fall or accident, or is lost or left unattended in a cool place. At brain temperatures below 20° C (68° F), thermoregulatory ability is suppressed and the person becomes *poikilothermic,* or lacking in thermoregulatory ability. Poikilothermia is potentially lethal, if untreated, as temperatures continue to fall below levels compatible with life. Every vital function is at risk when the hypothermic patient is unattended, but cardiac dysrhythmia and respiratory suppression represent the most immediate dangers.

Although the threats of fatal outcomes of hypothermia are well known, attention to the effects of cold stress on human immune functions is new. A generalized impairment of host defenses follows surgery in any person, but in the past this has been attributed primarily to anesthesia and tissue trauma (Cullen & van Belle, 1975). Low body temperature is known to suppress immune reactions in laboratory animals (Wang-Yang, Buttke, Miller, & Clem, 1990), yet has been largely ignored as a factor in postoperative immunosuppression. Hypothermia and infection were found to be significantly correlated in hospital admissions (Darowski, Najim, Weinberg, & Guz, 1991). Recent studies have suggested that maintaining thermal balance during surgery could lower postsurgical infections and shorten hospital stays (Kurz, Sessler, & Lenhardt, 1996). Surgical recovery in older patients is often complicated by infection. As evidence linking inadvertent cooling and altered immunity in elders continues to grow, it lends support to more aggressive interventions to maintain thermal balance during operative procedures. Meanwhile, there is sufficient rationale for doing so to prevent the cardiorespiratory and metabolic expenditures associated with rewarming after surgery.

When hypothermia is deliberately induced, such as during cardiac surgery, the therapeutic goal is not to maintain thermal balance. Instead, the focus is on minimizing the predictable sequelae and adverse responses. Hypothermic cardiopulmonary bypass is known to induce significant acute phase responses, often febrile in nature, after rewarming. Cell-mediated immunity is also depressed, even in younger patients (Roth, Golub, Cukingnan, Brazier, & Morton, 1981). With age-related reduction in immunocompetence, it is logical to expect that the elderly cardiac surgery patient will be at risk for infection even more than younger patients. Systemic rewarming by the bypass heat exchanger is usually not sufficient to completely restore heat to vasoconstricted regions and subcutaneous body tissue. Consequently, body temperatures often fall drastically when the patient is moved to the postsurgical care unit. Surveillance and external warming intervention must be intense to avoid temperature drift until thermal balance is restored.

Hyperthermia

Hyperthermia is the result of thermoregulatory dysfunction or failure of normal body cooling mechanisms. Injury to the hypothalamus, dehydration, or extremely high environmental heat can lead to hyperthermia. The older patient is particularly vulnerable to heatstroke, a condition that disturbs hypothalamic regulation activities. Inability to sweat and lose heat by vasodilation can quickly lead to death unless treated. As temperatures rise to levels above 40° C (104° F), the danger of irreversible damage to the brain increases. Persons who have a preexisting neurologic disorder, who use alcohol, and who take atropine-containing drugs might be even more susceptible. Hyperthermia requires active cooling and fluid replacement by caregivers. The more severe the condition, the less responsive the thermoregulatory responses will be. This relative poikilothermia, or reduced ability to control body temperature, creates another hazard during therapeutic cooling by increasing the danger of temperature "drift" downward. Accurate and frequent monitoring is imperative during these thermodynamic states.

Fever

Fever, also called hyperpyrexia, results when substances enter the body that provoke a systemic reaction termed the *acute phase response.* Fever-producing substances, or *pyrogens,* include infectious organisms, toxic drugs, chemical compounds, blood products, neoplastic cells, and foreign bodies. As a result of the release of cellular messengers called *cytokines,* endogenous pyrogens set off a chain of reactions within the body. Fever differs from hyperthermia in that thermoregulatory mechanisms remain intact and highly sensitive. Vasodilator and sweating mechanisms function normally but at a new higher set point level. Elevation of body temperature is but one part of the complex febrile response. An initial fall in neutrophil levels is followed in approximately an hour by a drastic neutrophilia. This sharp rise maximizes in 6 hours and lasts nearly 24 hours (Cooper, 1995). Other systemic reactions include release of lactoferrin, an iron binder, which may be responsible for the fall in plasma iron during fever. These reactions are in general immunostimulant, activating host reactions that kill microorganisms and deprive them of nutrients. However, certain cytokines, such as interleukin-1, tumor necrosis factor, and interferon-a, cause malaise, fatigue, and anorexia in the febrile patient.

Fever manifests three distinct stages in healthy younger persons: (1) the familiar *chill phase,* with febrile shivering and an uncomfortable sense of cold; shivering and vaso-constriction in this phase helps to generate and conserve heat to raise body temperature to the higher set point; (2) the *plateau phase,* which occurs when body temperature reaches the set point and no thermoregulatory responses are stimulated; and (3) the *defervescence phase,* which occurs when the pyrogen level subsides, the set point stabilizes to prefever levels, and febrile temperatures are sensed as uncomfortably hot. Here the patient typically sweats profusely, kicks off bedcovers, and complains of the heat.

Studies in humans and laboratory animals show an age-related impairment of the febrile response to interleukins and possibly other cytokines (Chassagne et al., 1996; Miller, Yoshikawa, & Norman, 1995). Febrile activity in elders can be blunted or even absent in the presence of serious infection. Even in the presence of bacteremia, elders have fewer febrile reactions, specifically, chills, sweating, and other symptoms, than do younger patients. Infectious processes can become dangerously severe before recognition and treatment. These findings point out the difficulty in using body temperature alone as an indicator of infection or the acute phase response in older patients. In a large population of elderly patients with fever, clinically identified bacteriuria was found to cause fewer than 10% of the episodes of significant fever (Orr et al., 1996). Rather than setting a particular temperature as a criterion for fever in elders, some authorities recommend using a 1° C (2° F) increase from the patient's baseline values (Norman & Yoshikawa, 1996). Although temperature levels may fail to indicate infectious processes in elders, other meaningful signs are induced by pyrogens: anorexia, fatigue, weight loss, and a fall in serum iron levels.

Although infectious fevers tend to be self-limiting among younger persons, the associated fluid loss and hypermetabolism make dehydration a risk in elders. In younger persons dehydration can destabilize the thermostatic set point and cause a fever. With advancing age the effects of dehydration are not as readily seen. Although fever contributes significantly to dehydration, an elevated body temperature is not a reliable predictor of dehydration in older patients. Thirst in the presence of dehydration also decreases with age, so caregivers must be attentive to clinical and laboratory indicators of fluid deficit (body weight, fluid intake, hemoconcentration, serum osmolality, sodium level, urine specific gravity). Changes in skin turgor and tissue resilience are difficult to see in elderly patients with declining subcutaneous tissue. Indicators found to correlate most closely with dehydration in elders admitted to an emergency room were tongue dryness and longitudinal furrowing, dry oral mucosa, upper body weakness, confusion, speech difficulty, and sunken eyes (Gross et al., 1992). Rapid changes in body weight are also sensitive indicators of body water loss or gain (approximately 1 lb = 1 pt of water). Physical examination and radiologic studies may be needed to determine if accumulated water is generally distributed normally.

For example, a dehydrated patient could have edema or "third space" accumulation of water in pleural or visceral spaces, large blisters, or an obstructed gut.

RELATED FACTORS/ETIOLOGIES OF ALTERED BODY TEMPERATURE

Thermal balance is defined as a dynamic state, a delicate equilibrium in which the rate of heat generated by the body is equivalent to the rate of heat lost to the environment. Because body temperature alterations are both the cause and the effect of problems with heat loss or heat gain, it is essential to rapidly identify related factors. In aging, physiologic changes tend to affect the generation, distribution, and conservation of heat. Physical changes in body density, water content, and insulation may contribute further to problems of heat exchange. Behavioral and environmental factors combine to threaten thermal balance when older persons are subjected to temperature extremes they cannot escape from or change.

Control Mechanisms

Thermoregulation is the regulation of heat gain and loss needed to keep the body at optimal levels for cellular function. In humans this is a relatively narrow range that is (1) warm enough to promote cellular chemical activity and neural transmission; (2) low enough to be safe for vulnerable tissues, such as the brain; and (3) efficient enough to operate with a minimum of energy expenditure. For most young adults, body temperature is maintained within 36.4° to 37.5° C (97.4° to 99.5° F) by an elaborate thermostatic control. Although several theories have been postulated and models tested, precise mechanisms for maintaining this range are not completely known. Currently, the most widely accepted explanation is that of the thermoregulatory set point. Control of body temperature is achieved by means of a complex feedback system: (1) sensory inputs that are sensitive to temperature change; (2) signal integration that centrally combines sensory inputs from throughout the body; (3) discrepancy detection that provides central thermostatic function; and (4) efferent outputs that initiate physiologic or behavioral heat-modifying responses. Even though central control mechanisms lack precise mapping, most experts agree that they are primarily located in the region of the anterior hypothalamus, preoptic area. Sensory inputs with the most dominant influence come from highly thermosensitive neurons of the skin, brain, and spinal cord. Thermal information is integrated, then relayed to the hypothalamus, where comparative functions take place. Sensed deviations from normal set point levels stimulate effector responses. Temperatures sensed above the set point initiate cooling responses of sweating and vasodilation. Deviations below set point levels stimulate the shivering center and sympathetic nervous system responses, including vasoconstriction. While compensatory physiologic responses involuntarily warm or cool the body, the person is inclined to take behavioral actions to keep warm or cool. Once the set point deviation is resolved, compensatory responses subside. There is evidence that thermoregulatory sensitivity declines with age, and both cooling and warming responses appear to be blunted (Kramer, Vandijk, & Rosin, 1989; Wongsurawat, Davis, & Morley, 1990). In addition, Fox, Woodward, and Exton-Smith (1973) found a general tendency among the majority of their subjects to "feel cool," whether or not body temperatures were lower. This suggests that inadequate responses to thermal stimuli may not only be physiologic, but perceptual and behavioral as well. Elderly patients have been found seriously compromised at both extremes of temperature, with poor perception of their body or environmental temperatures.

Ranges of Euthermia

Euthermia, the state of "normal" or usual body temperature, is not a single level, but rather a range of temperature that varies throughout the day. Whereas 37.5° C (99.5° F) reflects the state of euthermia for many people, other healthy individuals will range above or below this level. Large studies of elders report lower basal temperatures with advancing age (Fox et al., 1973). However, Wongsurawat et al. (1990) state that basal temperatures do not differ between young and old persons, but rather that low body temperatures in elders reflect susceptibility to transient heat losses. Whether vulnerability is caused by lower basal temperature or blunted response, the inability to defend against heat loss puts older patients at risk for hypothermia. Hormonal fluctuations throughout each 24-hour period cause diurnal temperature fluctuations of 0.2° to 0.3° C. Melatonin is responsible for approximately half of the nocturnal temperature decline in young adults. Levels of melatonin remain fairly stable in old age, but with aging this "hypothermic hormone" has weaker effects (Cagnacci, Soldani, & Yen, 1995). These changes have been implicated in some of the age-related disturbances in sleep and circadian rhythmicity in elders. This decline in thermal rhythmicity does not completely alter the fact that temperatures are at their nadir, or lowest point, during the night. There is still adequate evidence that elders sleep more comfortably with more stable core temperatures when additional insulation or warmth is provided during sleep (Holtzclaw et al., 1993).

Thermoregulatory Responses

Warming or cooling responses are proportional in intensity and energy expenditure to the sensed deviation or threat to thermal balance. Vasoconstriction may be transient during exposure to a draft and often causes little noticeable change in oxygen demand. If the sensed deviation persists despite vasomotor attempts to shunt blood to deeper, warmer tissues, shivering is stimulated. Shivering exacts a metabolic toll similar to bicycle riding or shoveling snow (Newstead, 1987). This aerobic activity can raise oxygen consumption 300% to 400% above resting levels in healthy younger subjects. The ability to shiver apparently diminishes as people age, yet they do appear to experience catecholamine release with exposure to cold (Wongsurawat et al., 1990). Sympathetic stimulation increases blood pressure and heart rate, leading to a rise in oxygen consumption and respiratory rate, although to a lesser degree than with shivering (Frank et al., 1995). The elderly person is often unable to effectively control heat loss by vasoconstriction and to generate sufficient heat by musculoskeletal kinetics (Collins, Easton, & Exton-Smith, 1981). For this reason, thermal and cardiovascular instabilities appear to be greater immediate threats than metabolic expenditure. These age-related vasomotor changes also make elders more vulnerable to the effects of heat than younger persons in extremely warm weather. With heat-induced vasodilation, elders cannot increase cardiac output sufficiently to compensate. This problem is particularly exacerbated by the use of antihypertensive drugs or alcohol. In extreme heat, age-related vascular rigidity makes it more difficult to increase cutaneous vasodilation, so heat loss is impaired (Minson, Wladkowki, Cardell, Paweldzyk, & Kenney, 1998). Sweating, the normal response that promotes evaporative heat loss, is diminished by age-related atrophy of the sweat glands (Wongsurawat et al., 1990) or by insufficient intake of oral fluid.

Behavioral Responses to Sensed Temperature Change

Appropriate behavioral responses to changes in environmental temperature include such actions as dressing for cool or warm weather, drinking warm or cool liquids, moving to a different location, or adjusting the room thermostat. These abilities require functional sensory and motor abilities. Alterations in both these dimensions are frequent after strokes or other neurologic insults but may also be a function of the aging process (Naver et al., 1995). The effects of aging on ability to sense temperature has been noted by several investigators, with thermal perception found to be decreased in elders (Natsume, Ogawa, Sugenoya, Ohnishi, & Imai, 1992). Actual reduction in thermal discrimination has been found in the skin, with greater thermal stimuli required to elicit a behavioral response (Taylor, Allsopp, & Parkes, 1995). At the same time, older persons tend to prefer warmer environmental temperatures in any season (Natsume et al., 1992).

RISK FACTORS

Underlying factors responsible for altered thermal balance are often amenable to nursing intervention, even if there are constitutional or pathologic conditions over which the

Box 17-1	Risk for Altered Body Temperature (Risk for Altered Thermal Balance): Ineffective Cooling Responses

Nursing Diagnosis
Risk for Altered Body Temperature (Risk for Altered Thermal Balance): Ineffective Cooling Responses

Risk factors
Age-related blunting of thermoregulatory sensory and cooling responses; neurologic impairment, such as paresis, paralysis, weakness, or sensory dysfunction; dehydration and decline of sudomotor (sweating) function; drugs that promote vasoconstriction; illness or trauma affecting temperature regulation; inappropriate clothing or shelter for environmental temperature

Defining characteristics
Hyperthermia
Absence of vasodilation and sweating, urinary output low; headache, nausea, intestinal cramping; cognitive dysfunction, dizziness, confusion, stupor; poor capillary filling

Heatstroke
History of heat exposure, high humidity; core temperatures >40° C, tachycardia, bounding pulse, hypotension, hot, dry skin

Heat Exhaustion
History of loss of sodium in heavy sweating; is exacerbated by diuretics; low serum sodium levels, high potassium levels

Nursing-Sensitive Outcomes
Safety Status: Physical Injury
Burns

Vital Signs: Body Temperature
Stabilized within normal range

Thermoregulation
Heat gain and loss

Fluid Balance
Gain, loss, and distribution

Risk Control
Surveillance to check environment and patient to avoid hyperthermia

Indicators
Stable body temperature within normal range; return of prevent cardiorespiratory signs, fluid volume, urinary output, thermoregulatory responses; electrolytes return to normal range; return of preevent cognitive status

Nursing Interventions
Temperature Regulation
Reducing body heat in hyperthermia; postevent, maintaining normal body temperature

Environmental Management: Safety
Avoiding overheating, overhumidification

Vital Signs Monitoring
Monitoring thermal status and thermal threats

Activities
Actively cool core body temperature with conductive cooling blankets to levels <40° C to avoid risk of neurologic damage; with loss of thermoregulatory control, must monitor temperature closely to avoid hypothermia; wrap extremities for protection, comfort, and to suppress warming responses; restore fluid balance to improve circulation to and heat loss from skin

caregiver has no control. The situation that puts the patient at risk for overheating or overcooling may be of neuroregulatory origin and beyond direct intervention. However, in many instances thermal balance can be restored and maintained by actively influencing heat exchange through therapeutic and environmental means. For example, risk for heat exhaustion and heatstroke can be related to dehydration and exposure to excessive heat. This condition can be coupled, at the same time, with the patient's inability to swallow or reach for a drink of water (Box 17-1). During surgery, inadvertent heat loss is usually related to the suppression of neuromuscular activity by drugs and low environmental temperatures (Boxes 17-2 and 17-3). In each of these situations the related factors of interest to nursing are those that can potentially be reversed or prevented. In fever the phase can dictate the diagnosis and management. During the chill phase, for example, the alteration in thermal balance is related to sensed heat loss, secondary to a higher thermoregulatory set point (Box 17-4). Appropriate interventions are to protect and keep extremities warm, while allowing excess heat to escape from the trunk and head. The interventions are not related to altered body temperature at all, but

rather to the underlying threat to thermal balance: factors that influence the exchange and generation of heat. If fever is related to fluid deficit, the threat to thermal balance may be "related to fluid volume deficit." Replacement of fluid is aimed at increasing circulatory perfusion to the skin and superficial tissues to dissipate heat.

ASSESSMENT

Accurate body temperature monitoring is the key activity for assessment. However, temperature monitoring simultaneously is a critical nursing intervention and a vital component of outcomes evaluation (see Boxes 17-1 through 17-4). Unfortunately, there is considerable variability in nursing skill and knowledge involving these measurements. Care units and families may use glass thermometers that cannot measure below 34.4° C (93.9° F). In some cases the individual taking the temperature may fail to shake the mercury column low enough to detect hypothermia. Preferably, electronic digital thermometers that measure at all possible human ranges should be used to assess thermal balance in older persons. Thermometers vary in their accuracy and ability to measure body tem-

---

Box 17-2   Risk for Altered Body Temperature (Risk for Altered Thermal Balance): Excessive Heat Loss

Nursing Diagnosis
Risk for Altered Body Temperature (Risk for Altered Thermal Balance): Excessive Heat Loss
Risk factors
Conditions such as injury, surgery, or unattended exposure in cold environments; although all humans are at risk, elders have lower metabolic heat generation and thermoregulatory defense against heat loss

Defining characteristics
History of cold exposure
Early signs
Thermal discomfort; core temperature $< 35°$ C; cutaneous vasoconstriction; "cold" diuresis; cool, mottled skin; increase in heart rate, blood pressure, respiratory rate; thermoregulatory shivering
Late signs
Thermoregulatory ability loss as temperature falls below $20°$ C; confusion, stupor, loss of consciousness; cardiac dysrhythmias; paradoxical sensation of warmth; cold, pale skin; exaggerated tendon reflex, hyperactivity; anuria

Nursing-Sensitive Outcomes
Thermoregulation
Thermal balance between heat gain and heat loss

Risk Control
Reduced likelihood of hypothermia by heightened patient awareness or caregiver surveillance; monitor system for gaining immediate assistance in event of fall or cold exposure

Indicators
Return of compensatory warming responses, which decline as temperature stabilizes; stable body temperature within normal range; stabilization of vital signs, cardiac function, urine output, tendon reflexes; skin color evenly distributed; return of preevent cognitive function; thermal comfort

Nursing Interventions
Hypothermia Treatment
Restoration of body heat postevent for induced or accidental hypothermia

Temperature Regulation
Conservation of existing body heat

Temperature Regulation: Intraoperative
Prevention of inadvertent hypothermia

Vital Signs Monitoring
Monitor thermal status

Environmental Management: Safety
Prevent overexposure to cold

Activities
Restorative
Transport to warm area; warmed convective air blankets, warmed oral and intravenous fluids, warmed humidified inhalation gases
Protective
Insulation with quilted or layered clothing/bedclothes, warmed humidified air; watch for falling core temperatures and drugs/substances that further lower warming or heat-conserving responses

---

perature, making investment in a reliable instrument important. Electronic devices should be calibrated regularly with unit-based calibration equipment or by the agency biomedical device department. For home use, reliable digital thermometers are recommended because they are easier for visually impaired persons to read and are less ambiguous for caregivers to interpret. Newer tympanic membrane (TM) thermometers can provide accurate, reliable information about "core" temperature, provided they are calibrated, of good quality, and used by trained caregivers. Unfortunately, several affordable TM thermometers commercially available to patients are not consistent or accurate in their measurement. TM measurement varies, depending on the angle at which the instrument is held and whether or not the infrared beam is reflected on the TM.

Caregivers are sometimes confused about which body temperature is meaningful. The site or method of measurement depends on which particular aspect of thermal balance is of concern. In cases of fever or hyperthermia the brain should be kept below $42°$ C ($107.6°$ F) to prevent irreversible damage to neurologic structures. Even though it is not presently possible to directly measure brain temperature, TM, pulmonary artery, and lower esophageal areas provide reasonably close estimates. Even though oral temperatures are usually $0.3°$ to $0.5°$ C lower than core temperatures, this measurement site can be used to monitor fever in conscious, alert persons. This is not the case when the patient cannot hold a thermometer securely under the tongue or keep the lips closed tightly in place. Significant variations in readings occur in mouth breathing, during coughing, or with poorly fitting dentures. Rectal temperature may closely approximate brain temperatures during fever, but it tends to be less reliable in conditions of thermal or hemodynamic instability. During shock and hypovolemic states the lower bowel and rectum are underperfused and thereby cooler. During rewarming from hypothermia, rectal temperature lags behind that of the core and brain. This limits usefulness of the rectal site for assessing brain temperature but makes this measurement an excellent one for measuring the speed and extent of rewarming.

Box 17-3	Risk for Altered Body Temperature (Risk for Altered Thermal Balance): Ineffective Warming Responses

Nursing Diagnosis
Risk for Altered Body Temperature (Risk for Altered Thermal Balance): Ineffective Warming Responses
Risk factors
Age-related blunting of thermoregulatory sensory and warming responses; neurologic or muscular impairment, such as paresis, paralysis, weakness, or sensory dysfunction; anesthesia or sedation, vasodilator drugs, alcohol intake

Defining characteristics
Range from diminished sensitivity to environmental temperature to heightened awareness but inability to "get warm"; falling core and skin temperatures; absent or attenuated shivering response; cognitive change: restlessness, confusion, stupor, loss of consciousness; cool, mottled skin; increase in heart rate, blood pressure, respiratory rate; thermoregulatory shivering; if untreated will progress to hypothermia (see Box 17-2).

Nursing-Sensitive Outcomes
Safety Behavior: Home Physical Environment
Safe thermal environment with patient awareness or caregiver surveillance

Vital Signs: Body Temperature
Stabilized within normal range

Thermoregulation
Thermal balance between heat gain and heat loss

Risk Control
Periodic check of factors that increase threat of hypothermia; accessible clothing/covering

Indicators
Thermoneutral environment with external control system; thermal comfort; stable body temperature within normal range; stabilization of vital signs, cardiac function, urine output, tendon reflexes; skin color evenly distributed; return of preevent cognitive function; thermal comfort

Nursing Interventions
Temperature Regulation
Maintaining normal body temperature

Temperature Regulation: Intraoperative
Protection (conservation) of existing body heat during surgery/anesthesia, procedures, transport

Environmental Management: Safety
Safe room warmth and humidity

Vital Signs Monitoring
Monitoring thermal status and thermal threats

Activities
Protective
Room thermometers and increased awareness of room temperatures in homes or institutions; humidifiers improve perceptions of warmth; precautions against drafts or body heat loss from radiation via windows; provide shawls, mittens, caps, earmuffs, thermal socks during sleep, as well as during outdoor exposure

Skin temperature is perhaps the most variable measurement of all, changing within seconds as circulation is shunted toward or away from the surface. Axillary temperature is, in effect, skin temperature of the axilla and can be expected to vary widely with circulatory state. Fever-induced vasodilation warms the skin so that axillary and skin temperatures correlate linearly to the temperature of internal organs. On the other hand, during cardiogenic shock, in hypovolemic states, or during aggressive cooling procedures, skin temperature is an unreliable indicator of internal thermal status.

NURSING DIAGNOSIS

The existing nursing diagnosis Risk for Altered Body Temperature, developed and defined by the North American Nursing Diagnosis Association (NANDA) as "the state in which an individual is at risk for failure to maintain body temperature within normal range" (NANDA, 1999, p. 11), was designed to state a clinical judgment about responses to actual or potential health problems related to thermoregulation (Gordon, 1994). By standard, NANDA requires that the diagnostic label be representative of a pattern of related cues. The modifying term *altered* means simply a change from baseline, but is without reference to the temperature site, extent of deviation, or direction of change. Adopted in 1986, the nursing diagnosis Risk for Altered Body Temperature lacks specificity or direction and is less developed than many other nursing diagnoses. A major drawback to the NANDA label is its present focus on body temperature. This tends to preoccupy caregivers with thermometer readings rather than with the dynamics of heat exchange. There already exists, in fever management, a misguided inclination to treat the temperature elevation rather than the underlying dynamics of the febrile response. Implied in the NANDA diagnosis is the notion that core or central temperature may have deviated from accepted norms. In reality the threats to thermal balance may exert considerable energy expenditure and discomfort to an individual before temperature levels deviate. The notion that there is just one important body temperature is also imprecise, and there is much confusion about what represents "core" temperature. Core could be interpreted to mean temperature from the rectum, brain, urinary bladder, or TM. Temperatures from these regions can differ significantly, particularly during conditions of hemodynamic or thermal instability. Likewise, the body has numerous different acceptable temperatures for various

Box 17-4	Risk for Altered Body Temperature (Risk for Altered Thermal Balance): Febrile Responses to Altered Set Point

Nursing Diagnosis
Risk for Altered Body Temperature (Risk for Altered Thermal Balance): Febrile Responses to Altered Set Point
Risk factors
Susceptibility to infection, exposure to pyrogenic substances (drugs, blood products); decreased fluid intake and dehydration, age-related blunting of diagnostic symptoms

Defining characteristics
Body temperatures increased over baseline (1° C or 2° F); chills, sweating, shivering are often blunted in elders; heart rate, respiratory rate, and systolic blood pressure may increase as oxygen and calories are expended; anorexia, fatigue, fall in serum iron may be present; headache and lassitude with higher fever

Nursing-Sensitive Outcomes
Thermoregulation
Thermal balance between heat gain and heat loss

Vital Signs: Body Temperature
During fever remains below 40° C

Risk Control
Surveillance to avoid threat of neural damage during fever

Indicators
During fever, temperature remains <40° C; thermal comfort ensured by diminished feelings of "chill"; fluid balance restored; cardiorespiratory function restored to preevent level; minimum of distress and shivering if cooling blanket is used; (NOTE: Nursing-sensitive outcomes indicate correction of febrile factors amenable to nursing care, not to recovery of underlying febrile infection)

Nursing Interventions
Fever Treatment Temperature Regulation
Reducing heat-generating febrile responses

Environmental Management: Safety
Avoiding drafts or chilling while allowing heat loss from body surface

Vital Signs Monitoring
Monitoring thermal status and thermal threats

Activities
Allow body heat to escape from trunk, but insulate hands/feet during chill phase; avoid drafts/chills during subsequent warm phases; offer and assist with fluid intake, warm or room temperature fluids to avoid chilling; if body temperatures rise above 40° C, actively cool with thermoconductive blankets to avoid risk of neural damage; loss of thermoregulatory control may follow, with cooling leading to hypothermia; monitor temperature closely; wrap extremities for protection, comfort, and to suppress warming responses; restore fluid balance to improve circulation to and heat loss from skin

---

anatomic regions. The more superficial and exposed the region, the more variable the temperature and the more likely it is to be influenced by environmental conditions. In most clinical situations it is the brain temperature that is of greatest concern. Physiologic and behavioral mechanisms are directed toward protecting the brain, a vital but vulnerable organ. However, temperatures of other regions are relevant to patient care because they reflect tissue perfusion and rewarming after hypothermic states.

An Alternative Diagnosis: Risk for Altered Thermal Balance

Temperature measurement remains an important part of assessing thermal balance, but other factors bear consideration. The nursing diagnosis is intended to state a clinical judgment about individual or group "responses to actual or potential health problems/life processes." In assessing human responses to thermal changes or to determining thermoregulatory responses to life events, clinical judgment must address the *altered process* rather than the *altered measurement outcome*. Altered Thermal Balance is proposed as an alternative diagnosis, with the contributory related factors flowing logically from actual or potential threats to the gain or loss of heat. The alteration in body temperature can be a clue, a warning, or a serious outcome. The temperature deviation might well be one of the critical signs that indicate the patient is at risk. The broader consideration of thermal balance, however, calls for attention to the underlying dynamics and raises several questions: (1) What is the threat or deficit? (What is the nursing diagnosis?); (2) What are the physical and physiologic contributory factors? (What is the threat or deficit related to?); (3) How is it manifested? (What are the signs and symptoms?); (4) Which of these factors are amenable to nursing interventions? (What interventions will improve the situation?); and finally (5) How can one tell the situation has improved? (What are the desired outcome indicators?). It is with this broader understanding that nursing interventions can be directed more appropriately toward alleviating these specific factors. See Boxes 17-1 through 17-4, which address four common situations in which elders encounter risk for alterations in thermal balance. The nursing diagnoses Risk for Altered Body Temperature (NANDA, 1999) and Altered Thermal Balance (proposed alternative) are both included for completeness. Conformity with national standards requires familiarity with the former, while understanding of the latter is crucial to reasoned action toward care. Related factors are included in the boxes with specific examples for high-risk situations.

CASE STUDY 1

K. Oliphant, age 80, was admitted by ambulance to the Emergency Department (ED) in a large urban city on a hot (38.3° C, or 101° F), humid (70%) day. City police broke through a barricaded door of his cramped basement apartment after a concerned telephone call from the corner grocery store owner. Mr. Oliphant failed to come in on schedule to cash his Social Security check, and attempts to deliver groceries ordered by phone the previous day were unsuccessful. Mr. Oliphant was found unconscious, unresponsive, and exhibiting symmetric decorticate posturing. The temperature in the apartment was 37.7° C (100° F), the electrical window cooling unit was not functional, and all windows were covered with thick plywood boards nailed to the window frames. The refrigerator held no food—only a nearly empty bottle of port wine. On admission to the ED, the following vital signs were obtained: pulse, 160; blood pressure, 90/70 mm Hg; respiration, 40; and rectal temperature, 41.1° C (106° F). Skin was dry and hot to the touch, respirations were labored, and mild seizure activity was noted. Medical records indicated that Mr. Oliphant had been taking diuretics and beta-blockers for chronic heart disease for the past 5 years.

Physician orders included intravenous fluids of half normal saline solution until laboratory tests could be completed. Urine was tested for myoglobinuria. Mr. Oliphant was intubated with an endotracheal tube, and 100% oxygen was administered by manual bagging. Arterial blood gas measurements were performed. Blood was also drawn for complete blood counts, platelets, prothrombin time/partial thromboplastin time (PT/PTT), fibrin split products and fibrinogen, electrolytes, blood urea nitrogen, creatinine, and glucose. Serum enzyme tests for hepatic and cardiac profiles were performed. Medical evaluation ruled out the competing possibilities of cardiac, endocrine, or infectious causes of disease. Nursing assessment of the neurologic impairment and abnormal posturing in the absence of cerebrovascular insult, combined with dehydration and absence of sweating, suggested hyperthermia. Mr. Oliphant was considered at high risk for altered thermal balance related to ineffective cooling responses because of the excessive thermal burden of high heat, humidity, and lack of air circulation. In addition, he had diminished capacity to dissipate body heat to the environment related to age, alcohol, and drug-related changes affecting circulation and hydration. Finally, poor intake of fluids decreased his ability to compensate for fluid loss, and hypovolemia prevented the distribution of heat to the body surface.

Tentative Diagnoses
1. Risk for Altered Thermal Balance: Ineffective Cooling Responses, as evidenced by history of heat exposure, high humidity, diuretic and alcohol use, and advanced age.
2. Risk for Altered Thermal Balance: Ineffective Cooling Responses as evidenced by core temperatures >40° C (104° F), cognitive dysfunction, stupor, tachycardia, low urinary output, and absence of vasodilation or sweating.

CASE STUDY 2

J. Fitz, age 78, is a lively woman who lives alone and is active on her church's altar committee. She has had few physical complaints in later life, except for her urinary bladder problems. For the past 5 years her urinary incontinence has grown increasingly worse, and when catheterized for residual urine on her last clinic visit, over 200 ml remained. The day she was admitted to the ED it had been unusual from the start. Her daughter had first become concerned because her mother had declined to attend church that morning, complaining of urinary urgency. By mid-afternoon Mrs. Fitz did not answer her telephone, so her daughter decided to bring a light supper over and check on her mother. She found Mrs. Fitz in bed, disoriented, picking at the sheet, and breathing with difficulty. Although she did not take her mother's temperature, Mrs. Fitz's skin felt warm to the touch. Mrs. Fitz's physician was called, and he ordered an ambulance. On admission, Mrs. Fitz's rectal temperature was 38.3° C (101° F). Symptoms included confusion, cough, dyspnea, and incontinence. Blood was drawn for a complete blood count (CBC), chemistry, and culture. A sterile catheterized urine specimen was obtained for complete urinalysis and urine culture; her urine was cloudy and foul smelling. Mrs. Fitz was poorly hydrated, with marked hemoconcentration. Further consultation with her daughter revealed that Mrs. Fitz believed that drinking liquids caused her bladder to "leak." She would therefore routinely restrict fluid intake when preparing to go out in public or to church. Intravenous infusions of half normal saline solution with potassium supplements and multivitamins were administered. Although her body temperature showed only a low-grade fever, her clinical picture was consistent with systemic infection. Chest films ruled out respiratory infection, but the blood cultures were positive for bacteremia. Urine microscopy revealed a bacterial colony count of greater than 1,000,000, with gross pyuria. Specific antimicrobial drugs are ordered after the blood and urine culture and sensitivity testing.

Tentative Diagnosis
Risk for Altered Thermal Balance: Febrile Responses to Altered Set Point secondary to urinary bladder stasis, susceptibility to uropathogens, and decreased fluid intake as evidenced by core temperatures >37.8° C (100° F), despite age-related blunting of febrile response.

CASE STUDY 3

L. Carter, age 84, was admitted to the ED on a cold 4.4° C (40° F) November Sunday. ED staff were concerned about *hypothermia* because of the weather. Vital signs revealed a rectal temperature of 31° C (87.8° F); a heart rate of 120 beats/minute that was irregular and had numerous premature ventricular beats; respirations that were 40/minute and labored; and a blood pressure of 160/100 mm Hg. Oxygen was administered by mask. Mrs. Carter was stuporous but hyperactive, showing exaggerated tendon reflexes. She was incontinent, and an indwelling urinary catheter was inserted to monitor diuresis. Urine output was 500 mL/hr. Serum enzyme tests for hepatic and cardiac profiles were negative. Cerebrovascular, endocrine, and infectious causes for her condition were ruled out.

Up to now Mrs. Carter had been in fairly good health except for failing eyesight and had no known cardiovascular problems. She had become more forgetful in the past year, however, and her son worried about her living alone at the old family home. Mrs. Carter had been found by her minister as he arrived at church to prepare for evening services. She was slumped over on an outside park bench. She had apparently been waiting, since the morning service ended at noon, for a ride home. Well-meaning church members usually provided her round-trip rides to church, but this Sunday had been different. The family who usually transported her was going out of town right after church and were unable to deliver her home. "Don't worry" insisted Mrs. Carter, who saw no difficulty in arranging for someone else to transport her home. Mrs. Carter apparently forgot her transportation needs once she arrived at church. The excitement of seeing friends, watching infant baptisms, and hearing a stirring sermon added to her distraction. Only after everyone filed out of the church and she stood on the church steps did she think about her ride; she could not remember what arrangements had been made. By this time she was alone on the steps and locked out of the building. She sat down to ponder, but grew colder and more confused. By the minister's estimation, she had been sitting on the cold concrete bench for 6 hours, exposed to light winds and wearing only a light coat. Medical evaluation eliminated cardiac or cerebrovascular events as the primary causes of Mrs. Carter's loss of consciousness. History and physical findings provided the basis for the following nursing diagnoses.

Tentative Diagnosis

Risk for Altered Thermal Balance: Severe Heat Loss and Ineffective Warming Responses (secondary to blunted thermoregulatory [physiologic and behavioral] responses of advanced age) evidenced by history of prolonged exposure to low environmental temperatures and low body temperature, core temperatures of < 32° C (89.6° F), cognitive dysfunction, stupor, elevated blood pressure, tachycardia, dysrhythmias, dyspnea, and high urinary output.

NURSING-SENSITIVE OUTCOMES

Management of patient care problems directed at maintaining thermal balance requires advanced assessment

skills to detect the need for and outcome of care. Ideally, one would expect outcomes that are sensitive to nursing care to reflect a correction of signs and symptoms identified in the nursing diagnosis (see Boxes 17-1 through 17-4). When the alteration is a "risk" rather than a reality, the outcomes may reflect safe, stabilized, and balanced conditions. Perhaps one of the most compelling reasons to change the diagnostic label from Altered Body Temperature to Altered Thermal Balance is to emphasize conditions that alter the generation and conservation of heat rather than the ultimate concentration of heat in a given region. If indeed the goal is to reduce the *risk* of altering thermal balance, nursing-sensitive outcomes will reflect changes in conditions that precede any measurable temperature alteration. Physiologic, behavioral, and environmental cues are often obvious to those who recognize their risks to thermal balance. Yet too often the clinical treatment of fever is based on a tradition of "bringing down" body temperature rather than on restoring fluids, preventing febrile shivering, or preventing thermal distress.

Declining basal body temperature is often symptomatic of age- or illness-related metabolic changes that are beyond nursing intervention. Therefore the goal for maintaining thermal balance is not to raise the patient's metabolic rate or existing body temperature. Instead, desired outcomes focus on making it unnecessary for the patient to expend additional energy to generate or conserve body heat. Nursing-sensitive outcomes to measure increased oxygen consumption include rising rates for respiration, pulse, and systolic blood pressure. If shivering and restless movement accompany chilling, oxygen consumption increases further. As thermal balance is achieved and the heat deficit is restored, these signs decrease.

Thermal comfort is an important outcome indicator. If the patient has complained of feeling cold, a nursing-sensitive outcome reflects relative success at achieving appropriate warmth by insulation, humidity, radiant heat, or convective heat. In a cognitively or neurologically impaired patient, nursing-sensitive outcomes must center on the pattern and stability of body temperature in light of ambient temperatures and heat replacement measures. Skin temperature yields minimal outcome information about thermal balance, except to assess the rate and extent of body rewarming after hypothermia. The rate of temperature rise and fall is as important as the level during cooling and rewarming, and gradual changes give objective nursing-sensitive indicators that interventions are responding appropriately. Rapid changes are indicators of thermal instability and can represent loss of thermoregulatory control. Temperature drifts below the level of hypothermia desired, "afterfall" when a cooling blanket is turned off, and "overshoot" of temperature above normal levels after rewarming indicate thermal instability. Patients with thermal instability are extremely vulnerable to all extraneous thermal influences. Nursing-sensitive outcomes are all aimed toward the successful maintenance of body temperature within safe thermal ranges, despite drastic and overwhelming heat loss. Assessment of these outcomes must be continuous and responsive to prevent permanent or hazardous sequelae.

Thermal stability is a nursing-sensitive outcome when interventions play a major role in returning thermoregulatory function (see Boxes 17-1 through 17-4). When thermal balance is altered because of excessive heat loss or heat gain, outcomes depend on the extent of the patient's impairment. In cases of heatstroke and heat exhaustion, there can be remarkable restoration of thermoregulatory ability when fluids are restored and body temperature is maintained at normothermia for several hours. Nursing-sensitive outcomes of thermal stability would be appropriate in this situation. Likewise, if a patient has been on a cooling blanket to treat fever, the slow rate and gradual lowering of temperature will contribute significantly toward reducing shivering and keeping temperatures stable. Because nursing intervention influences thermal stability during hypothermia, thermal stability remains an important outcome. However, if thermoregulatory failure is secondary to brain injury, endocrine failure, septic shock, or neuromuscular damage, nursing intervention is primarily focused on supportive maintenance of body temperature within safe ranges. Restoration of thermal stability, in this case, helps to define the patient's status but might not relate to the success of particular nursing interventions.

NURSING INTERVENTIONS

Interventions to Affect Heat Exchange

Physical laws governing the transfer or exchange of heat offer predictability in intervention. Physical interventions can directly influence this exchange by affecting the radiation, conduction, convection, and evaporation of heat. Heat is constantly in motion, passing by gradient from warmer molecules to cooler ones, until it is inevitably lost to the environment. Interventions can also indirectly influence heat exchange by actively stimulating physiologic warming or cooling responses. Physiologic responses influencing vascular blood flow work in concert with the physical properties of thermal exchange by directing heat toward or away from body surfaces.

Interventions Influencing Radiation.   Interventions can be designed to provide radiant heat or to protect the older person from its effects. In either case, it is helpful to consider this form of heat exchange broadly, beyond the use of heat lamps or radiant warmers. Heat passes as radiant energy through air or space from warm to cool objects. It is not necessary for the source of radiant heat to glow or to change the ambient temperature for heat to be radiated (Kleiber, 1961). Radiant waves, such as infrared and ultraviolet, can cause thermal injury to skin even when invisible to the eye. The potential for radiant heat

exchange requires constant surveillance by caregivers. The patient's skin radiates heat when it is uncovered. Exposure during bathing or surgical procedures allows heat to radiate easily from the body surface to the cooler environment. Patients sitting next to a closed window on a cool day risk heat loss by radiation through the glass to the cooler environment outside. By contrast, radiant heat from lamps and sunlight, even through a closed window, can warm exposed skin despite cool surroundings. Sunlight should be respected for the powerful radiant heat source it offers, that is, it provides warm and pleasant conditions for activities in day rooms, sun porches, and outdoors but requires vigilance to avoid overheating an immobilized elderly person sitting within its spectrum. In perioperative settings, heat lamps and radiant warmers require accurate controls and measurement of skin and ambient temperatures to prevent excessively warm conditions. It is safer practice, in any setting, to use radiant heat or heat lamps to warm surfaces, bedclothes, and equipment *before* they come in contact with the patient.

Interventions Influencing Conduction.   Transfer of heat by conduction is heavily influenced by the ability of one substance in contact with another to conduct heat away from another. Metals tend to be more rapid conductors than other substances, so when an older person is placed on a metal surface in cool conditions, the cooling effects are often drastic. Poor conductors, such as wool fabric, thermal knits, and goose down, are *insulators* that trap heat. When worn as clothing or used as bedclothes, they conserve existing body heat. Towels provide important insulation against burns when heating pads or hot water bottles are used. Precautions should be given to patients and caregivers about the potential dangers in using these devices. For example, patients should not place heating pads *under* their body. Insulation from protective covers on heating devices is lost when body pressure squeezes out trapped air.

Interventions Influencing Convection.   Heat is lost from the body by convection when air or liquid moves over its surface. Elders are at risk for convective heat loss from air conditioner vents, drafts, and breezes. Convective heat loss from wound irrigations, bladder irrigations, enemas, and shower baths can be reduced by warming solutions and environmental conditions. Heat gain by convection is achieved through convective air warming blankets, hot showers, and forced air heaters.

In warm weather, fans and air conditioners improve comfort and prevent overheating. Care must be taken, however, to avoid chilling and rapid evaporative loss. Fans should be used to circulate air and not be directed at the patient. Light coverings and clothing are likely to be more comfortable in summer to elders than bare extremities because they protect against abrupt convective and evaporative losses.

Moisture lost from wet skin or exposed mucous membranes constitutes a major source of evaporative heat loss for hospitalized patients during bathing, dressing changes, and surgical procedures. Use of bath blankets, rather than small towels, during a bed bath prevents evaporative loss from damp body surfaces. Replacement of wet clothing, especially with incontinent patients, removes a source of moisture that often contributes to evaporative, as well as conductive, heat loss.

Low humidity, high environmental temperature, and the presence of air currents all facilitate evaporative heat loss. In warm weather, heavy sweating evaporates more slowly and cools less effectively than a thin layer of moisture. Saturated skin should be blotted with a soft towel and sweaty clothing exchanged for dry, permeable garments. Alcohol should never be applied to skin to speed evaporation. Although a sense of cooling is perceptible with alcohol baths, this product is drying to skin and contains noxious vapors that can be harmful.

Combining Measures to Affect Heat Exchange in Perioperative Situations

The cool environmental conditions and patient exposure during surgical procedures are notorious for promoting inadvertent hypothermia. Efforts to conserve and replace heat in elders during and after surgery have been shown to be effective in both orthopedic and abdominal procedures (Carli, Emery, & Freemantle, 1989; Carli & Itiaba, 1985). Heat exchange interventions are combined to accomplish this by convective heat (warmed inhaled gases and intravenous fluids, warmed air-blowing blankets), conductive heat (bed and blanket warmers), radiant heat (thermal ceilings and warming lights), or insulation against heat loss (wrapping exposed body regions in warming blankets or warmed cotton padding, and covering patients with metallized plastic sheeting) (Tappen & Andre, 1996).

The greater the heat deficit, the less effective are single measures such as warmed intravenous fluids (Ellis-Stoll, Cantu, Englert, & Carlile, 1996) or warmed humidified gases (Tausk, Miller, & Roberts, 1976). In attempting to restore heat to persons after cardiac surgery with hypothermic bypass, the major restoration must be done by the heat exchanger in the bypass pump. This, however, is insufficient to completely maintain thermal balance, as large regions of underperfused tissue will not be warmed during this process. Administration of vasodilator drugs during recovery will enhance further heat loss. The time required for exchange and equilibration of heat throughout the body may take several hours beyond time on the bypass pump, extending long after the patient returns to the care unit. In older patients, whose rate of basal heat production is already reduced, environmental warmth is critical to the rewarming process. Measures that promote a slow, uniform warming of tissues are thought less likely to evoke shivering and adverse cardiovascular responses,

such as "rewarming shock" secondary to decreased systemic vascular resistance (Tappen & Andre, 1996). Acid-base disorders, common during rewarming, occur more frequently during rapid rewarming without adequate respiratory support. During this period, pH is lowered by metabolic byproducts from underperfused tissue, by lactic acid from shivering muscles, and by increased carbon dioxide production (Holtzclaw, 1986). Conversely, this stimulus can produce respiratory alkalosis.

Interventions Affecting Thermal Comfort

Many older individuals find warmer temperatures more comfortable for sleep. Two factors seem to be influential in promoting a warmer sensation: insulation of the head and extremities and the relative humidity (or sultriness) of the room. In clinical studies (Bedford, 1988), older patients who were provided with socks and a head covering had improved sleep and sensation of warmth, even though core temperatures were not significantly changed. Humidifying air with a steam vaporizer (Masse, 1988) improved comfort and slightly increased core and skin temperature in elderly patients. Insulative interventions include leg warmers, flannel sheets, quilted bed jackets, and sweaters. Loss of heat from the head causes significant distress for aging persons with little or no hair. Soft stockinet or knit caps should be provided that are loose enough to not compress the ears.

Sleep disruptions are common in older patients and, in part, might result from a decline in the pineal hormone melatonin. Levels of melatonin, along with thyrotropin, are in antiphase to that of temperature; that is, the body is cooler when melatonin levels are highest. Use of melatonin in pharmacologic doses is controversial, but some investigators believe it may hold clinical benefits for resynchronizing both sleep and body temperature in elders (Lushington, Pollard, Lack, Kennaway, & Dawson, 1997).

Providing Comfort and Preventing Sensory Responses

When younger persons experience the chill phase of fever, circulating pyrogens generally cause an elevation of thermostatic set point and a heightened sensitivity to cooling. Even while temperature rises to febrile levels, shivering and uncomfortable chills occur. Older persons vary in their response to pyrogens so that shivering and distressful chills may be absent, even with elevated levels of pyrogenic cytokines. Still others will complain bitterly of feeling cold but will not manifest shivering. In some cases where infection has not evoked a powerful febrile response, a drug or blood transfusion may do so. An effective treatment for febrile shivering and chills is extremity wraps, consisting of three layers of terry cloth toweling applied lengthwise and clipped or taped to form a seam. A light sheet is placed over the trunk. The wraps, which resemble "boots" or "mittens," protect hands and feet, the most thermosensitive regions of skin, while the less sensitive surface of the trunk loses heat to the environment (Holtzclaw, 1990).

In conditions of heatstroke and hyperthermia, it might be necessary to aggressively cool the older patient with a cooling blanket, ice packs, or cooling irrigations. These can be extremely distressful procedures to elders, despite age-related blunting of physiologic responses to cooling. When using cooling blankets, hands, feet, and bony prominences should be wrapped or padded to prevent possible "blanket burns" from pressure on poorly perfused skin surfaces. Use of the insulative towel wraps on extremities, described earlier, increases comfort and diminishes shivering during aggressive cooling (Abbey & Close, 1979). In this case the dominant heat-loss sensors of the hands and feet are protected, while heat is lost from the trunk to the conductive cooling blanket. Insulative extremity wraps are also useful when it is necessary to aggressively cool febrile patients by means of ice packs, electric fans, and tepid sponge baths. When hypothermia is induced by any means, surveillance must be intense to avoid uncontrollable temperature drift. Sedatives, which are often given during this period, can make the patient confused or unable to communicate. Temperature, level of consciousness, and all vital signs must be monitored continuously.

Interventions Affecting the Thermoregulatory Set Point

It might seem that one can do little to directly affect the neurologic control centers regulating thermoregulatory set point. However, nurses and caregivers do manage two care modalities that affect thermoregulatory set point: fluid intake and antipyretic drugs. Nurses frequently must decide if, when, how, and under what conditions this treatment takes place. The role of antipyretic drugs in fever management is primarily to reduce symptoms of malaise and headache. Aspirin and other nonsteroidal antiinflammatory agents are often effective in lowering the temperature during fever by blocking the production of and subsequent cytokine mediators from prostaglandins. Because prostaglandins play a role in forming the protective gastric mucous lining, prostaglandin-blocking drugs are irritating to gastric mucosa. They should be taken with food if possible. Absorption is facilitated by administering with a full glass of water. Acetaminophen (Tylenol) has less effect on prostaglandin but will mildly reduce fever. It is important to remember that a mild fever may hold host benefit effects. As long as thermoregulatory function remains intact, the goal of fever management is *not* to drive down the body temperature, but to maintain it within a safe range. Use of antipyretics and effective fluid replacement also is believed to improve thermoregulatory control by helping to resensitize hypothalamic set point control.

CASE STUDY 1

Measures were instituted to reduce Mr. Oliphant's body heat to prevent irreversible neurologic damage related to hyperthermia. Concurrently, he needed immediate oxygenation and fluid replacement. Intravenous infusions of normal saline solution were continued to promote heat loss, with careful assessment for circulatory tolerance. As hypovolemia was corrected, circulation to his skin improved. He was put on a mechanical ventilator until he became fully conscious. Then he was given 80% oxygen by nonrebreather mask at 8 L/minute. To lower body temperature by conductive transfer and to prevent heat generation, Mr. Oliphant's clothing was removed, his extremities were wrapped with terry cloth toweling, and a conductive cooling blanket was applied to his body trunk. Rectal and tympanic membrane temperatures were measured every 5 minutes to monitor heat loss. An indwelling urethral catheter was inserted, and urine output was monitored. When core temperatures reached 39° C (102° F), the blanket was turned off and removed and Mr. Oliphant was covered with a sheet. Body temperature was monitored at 10-minute intervals to be sure temperature did not "drift" to hypothermic levels. During active cooling, Mr. Oliphant began to regain consciousness and became frightened at his surroundings. He began to shiver and breathe more rapidly. Lorazepam 2 mg, was administered intravenously, which also would prevent heat generation by suppressing shivering, and the patient was given simple information about where he was and what happened. Mr. Oliphant was monitored in the ED for 4 hours, during which time his core temperature stabilized at 39° C (102° F). He was then transferred to the Medical Care Unit for thorough workup of his cardiac, renal, hepatic, and pulmonary function. During the 6 days of his recovery, Mr. Oliphant became more alert, with his cardiac and renal function returning to preadmission levels. Discharge planning included instructions to check the weather and temperature each day, to increase fluid intake, and to dress in cool, loose-fitting clothing during warm and humid weather. When outside, a large-brimmed hat for sun protection was recommended. Social services were contacted to seek replacement for Mr. Oliphant's broken air conditioner unit. They also worked with Mr. Oliphant's neighborhood contacts to check by telephone with him daily.

CASE STUDY 2

Mrs. Fitz's most immediate needs were rehydration and restoration of her blood volume to improve circulation to the skin and support normal heat exchange with the environment. Fluid restoration decreases serum osmolality, normalizing neuroendocrine responses and stabilizing hypothalamic centers. While Mrs. Fitz did not have a body temperature that posed a neurologic threat, an elevation to 38.3° C (101° F) in a woman of her age was interpreted as a serious febrile response. She began to shiver as she regained consciousness and required continuing oxygen support. The presence of thermoregulatory responses confirmed Mrs. Fitz's ability to thermoregulate. Oral and intravenous fluids were given with careful assessment of rising fluid volume. Supportive fluid and timing of urinary antimicrobials were essential to treatment of the underlying fever-producing infection. Because she was more susceptible to chilling in the febrile state, she was protected from drafts and *not* subjected to cooling measures. Antipyretic drugs, such as acetaminophen, were not appropriate to attempt to "bring down" such a mild febrile response. These drugs, however, could be useful for treating discomfort or headache accompanying a systemic infection. Mrs. Fitz was transferred to the Medical Care Unit for 5 days of follow-up care. She no longer required oxygen on the second day. Her body temperature was monitored every 4 hours, and she became afebrile after 24 hours of antimicrobial administration. Patient teaching included discussion, use of models, and illustrations appropriate to the patient's level of understanding. Key elements of prevention were (1) the importance of drinking liquids and keeping the "flow" through the bladder to prevent future urinary tract infections, and (2) the need to take heed of subtle symptoms or unusual feelings, such as urgency, as possible signs of urinary tract infection. She was discharged with a prescription renewal for the antimicrobial drug and urged to maintain her fluid intake at a minimum of 8 glasses of water per day. A referral was made to the urology clinic for evaluation of her incontinence and to the nurse practitioner who specializes in urinary bladder control training. Along with signing up Mrs. Fitz for training, the nurse gave her some immediate strategies for timing her voiding to accommodate her regular activities. Mrs. Fitz's daughter was engaged in supporting her mother's incontinence program and self-care by assisting her in checking the frequency, urgency, color, and odor of her urine.

CASE STUDY 3

Respiratory support and measures to stabilize cardiac rhythm were of utmost immediacy on Mrs. Carter's admission to the ED. These concerns initially took priority in care. Her rectal temperature of 31° C (87° F) raised concern for dysrhythmias. Below 28° C (82° F), the danger of atrial fibrillation and other dysrhythmias increases. Cardiac irritability makes cardiopulmonary resuscitation (CPR) undesirable, except in cardiac arrest or ventricular fibrillation, so drugs are used to maintain cardiac rhythm and acid/base balance. Oxygen support is maintained throughout the rewarming period to compensate for increased expenditure caused by shivering. Prolonged exposure to drastic environmental cooling could put Mrs. Carter at risk for temperature "drift" toward lower body temperatures, but rapid rewarming also was undesirable. She was covered with warmed bath blankets, and a radiant

heat lamp was used to maintain the warmth. Slow rewarming allowed restoration of body heat without promoting shivering. Intravenous fluids, warmed in the blood warmer, restored heat while expanding the circulatory volume. When Mrs. Carter regained consciousness and her vital signs had stabilized, her urinary output declined to a normal volume. With urinary output established and Mrs. Carter no longer at risk for cold diuresis, the indwelling catheter was removed. Body temperatures were measured every hour by TM thermometer until they stabilized at 37.5° C (99.5° F) for at least 3 hours. Concern for a rebound "overshoot" of temperature, or a febrile response indicating infection, made it important to monitor body temperature every 4 hours while she was hospitalized. Oxygen supplementation was discontinued on the second day. Intravenous infusions with vitamin supplements were continued for 3 days as Mrs. Carter's appetite and fluid intake gradually increased. Fortunately, Mrs. Carter did not develop pneumonia or infection related to her overexposure. A slight head cold was treated with antihistamines and decongestants. She remained in the hospital for 5 days before being discharged to her son's care. Predischarge teaching for Mrs. Carter and her son included precautions about hypothermia, the need for keeping up with weather predictions, and planning for a reliable transportation schedule for Mrs. Carter's outings. Her minister visits with the nurse on the unit and requested consultation for implementing a "weather awareness" program to better care for the community's elders during temperature extremes.

SUMMARY

Nurses have cared for fevers throughout the profession's history, yet understanding of the immunologic aspects and underlying dynamics of the febrile response is relatively recent. Still evolving is new knowledge about the effects of aging and illness on the responsivity and host benefits associated with fever. Information about the hazards and sequelae of hypothermia among elders can be attributed largely to better thermometers and observation during surgery. Electronic thermometers, capable of measuring low body temperature, have revealed a high incidence of hypothermia in institutionalized elders and those admitted to emergency facilities. Surveys of home-dwelling older persons raise consciousness that risk of hypothermia also poses a threat in the community. Assessment of underlying and contributory factors provides the targets for interventions in altered thermal balance. Monitoring body temperature is a key intervention for achieving and maintaining thermal balance. Other nursing interventions can influence heat exchange to promote thermal balance, improve thermal comfort, prevent chills and shivering, and decrease distress during aggressive treatment. Advances in the knowledge of thermoregulatory responses can improve the management of altered thermal balance in elders. Equally important will be the need to base future nursing care and innovation on evolving scientific information about thermoregulation and aging.

REFERENCES

Abbey, J. C., & Close, L. (1979). A study of control of shivering during hypothermia. *Communicating Nursing Research, 12,* 2-3.

Ballester, J. M., & Harchelroad, F. P. (1999). Hypothermia: An easy to miss, dangerous disorder in winter weather. *Geriatrics, 54*(2), 51-52, 55-57.

Bedford, N. K. (1988). *Thermal adaptation in elderly long-term care residents: The effect of thermal socks and caps on core temperature, thermal comfort and temperature perception.* Unpublished master's thesis, Vanderbilt University School of Nursing, Nashville, TN.

Cagnacci, A., Soldani, R., & Yen, S. S. (1995). Hypothermic effect of melatonin and nocturnal core body temperature decline are reduced in aged women. *Journal of Applied Physiology, 78,* 314-317.

Carli, F., Emery, P. W., & Freemantle, C. A. (1989). Effect of perioperative normothermia on postoperative protein metabolism in elderly patients undergoing hip arthroplasty. *British Journal of Anaesthesia, 63,* 276-282.

Carli, F., & Itiaba, K. (1985). Effect of heat conservation during and after major abdominal surgery on muscle protein breakdown in elderly patients. *British Journal of Anaesthesia, 58,* 502-507.

Chassagne, P., Perol, M. B., Doucet, J., Trivalle, C., Menard, J. F., Manchon, N. D., Moynot, Y., Humbert, G., Bourreille, J., & Bercoff, E. (1996). Is presentation of bacteremia in the elderly the same as in younger patients? *American Journal of Medicine, 100,* 65-70.

Collins, K. J., Easton, J. C., & Exton-Smith, A. N. (1981). Shivering thermogenesis and vasomotor responses with convective cooling in the elderly. *Journal of Physiology, 320,* 76P.

Cooper, K. E. (1995). *Fever and antipyresis: The role of the nervous system.* New York: Cambridge Press.

Cullen, B. F., & van Belle, G. (1975). Lymphocyte transformation and changes in leukocyte count: Effects of anesthesia and operation. *Anesthesiology, 43,* 563-569.

Darowski, A., Najim, Z., Weinberg, J. R., & Guz, A. (1991). Hypothermia and infection in elderly patients admitted to hospital. *Age and Ageing, 20,* 100-106.

Ellis-Stoll, C. C., Cantu, L. G., Englert, S. J., & Carlile, W. E. (1996). Effect of continuously warmed IV fluids on intraoperative hypothermia. *AORN Journal, 63,* 599-606.

Fox, R. H., Woodward, P. M., & Exton-Smith, A. N. (1973). Body temperatures in the elderly: A national study of physiological social and environmental conditions. *British Medical Journal, 1,* 200-206.

Frank, S. M., Fleisher, L. A., Olson, K. F., Gorman, R. B., Higgins, M. S., Breslow, M. J., Sitzmann, J. V., & Beattie, C. (1995). Multivariate determinants of early postoperative oxygen consumption in elderly patients: Effects of shivering, body temperature and gender. *Anesthesiology, 83,* 241-249.

Gordon, M. (1994). *Nursing diagnosis: Process and application* (3rd ed., pp. 108-109). St. Louis, MO: Mosby.

Gross, C. R., Lindquist, R. D., Woolley, A. C., Granieri, R., Allard, K., & Webster, B. (1992). Clinical indicators of dehydration severity in elderly patients. *Journal of Emergency Medicine, 10,* 267-274.

Holtzclaw, B. J. (1986). Postoperative shivering after cardiac surgery: A review. *Heart & Lung, 15,* 292-300.

Holtzclaw, B. J. (1990). Effects of extremity wraps to control drug induced shivering: A pilot study. *Nursing Research, 39,* 280-283.

Holtzclaw, B. J., Francis, R., Penzhover, F., Walker, B., Zembrzuski, C. D., & Robb, W. (1993). Keeping patients warm in bed. *Geriatric Nursing—American Journal of Care for the Aging, 14,* 180-181.

Iowa Intervention Project. J. C. McCloskey & G. M. Bulechek (Eds.). (2000). *Nursing interventions classification (NIC)* (3rd ed.). St. Louis, MO: Mosby.

Iowa Outcomes Project. M. Johnson, M. Maas, & S. Moorhead (Eds.) (2000). *Nursing outcomes classification (NOC)* (2nd ed.). St. Louis, MO: Mosby.

Kleiber, M. (1961). Temperature and heat. In *The fire of life: An introduction to animal energetics* (pp. 95-103). New York: John Wiley & Sons.

Kolanowski, A. M., & Gunter, L. M. (1983). Thermal stress and the aged. *Journal of Gerontological Nursing, 9,* 13-15.

Kramer, M. R., Vandijk, J., & Rosin, A. J. (1989). Mortality in elderly patients with thermoregulatory failure. *Archives of Internal Medicine, 149,* 1521-1522.

Kurz, A., Sessler, D. I., & Lenhardt, R. (1996). Perioperative normothermia to reduce the incidence of surgical-wound infection and shorten hospitalization. *New England Journal of Medicine, 334,* 1209-1215.

Lushington, D., Pollard, K., Lack, L., Kennaway, D. J., & Dawson, D. (1997). Daytime melatonin administration in elderly good and poor sleepers: Effects on core body temperature and sleep latency. *Sleep, 29*(12), 1135-1144.

Masse, H. (1988). *The effects of increasing ambient relative humidity on core temperature and the perception of warmth in sedentary elderly.* Unpublished master's thesis, Vanderbilt University School of Nursing, Nashville, TN.

Miller, D. J., Yoshikawa, T. T., & Norman, D. C. (1995). Effect of age on fever response to recombinant interleukin-6 in a murine model. *Journals of Gerontology. Series A, Biological Sciences & Medical Sciences, 50,* M276-279.

Minson, C. T., Wladkowski, S. L., Cardell, A. F., Paweldzyk, J. A., & Kenney, W. L. (1998). Age alters the cardiovascular response to direct passive heating. *Journal of Applied Physiology, 84*(4), 1323-1332.

Natsume, K., Ogawa, T., Sugenoya, J., Ohnishi, N., & Imai, K. (1992). Preferred ambient temperature for old and young men in summer and winter. *International Journal of Biometeorology, 36,* 1-4.

Naver, H., Blomstrand, C., Ekholm, S., Jensen, C., Karlsson, T., & Wallin, B. G. (1995). Autonomic and thermal sensory symptoms and dysfunction after stroke. *Stroke, 26,* 1379-1385.

Newstead, C. G. (1987). The relationship between ventilation and oxygen consumption in man is the same during both moderate exercise and shivering. *Journal of Physiology, 383,* 455-459.

Norman, D. C., Grahn, D., & Yoshikawa, T. T. (1985). Fever and aging. *Journal of the American Geriatrics Society, 33,* 859-863.

Norman, D. C., & Yoshikawa, T. T. (1996). Fever in the elderly. *Infectious Disease Clinics of North America, 10,* 93-99.

North American Nursing Diagnosis Association. (1999). *Nursing diagnosis: Definitions & classification 1999-2000.* Philadelphia: Author.

Orr, P. H., Nicolle, L. E., Duckworth, H., Brunka, J., Kennedy, J., Murray, D., & Harding, G. K. (1996). Febrile urinary infection in the institutionalized elderly. *American Journal of Medicine, 100,* 71-77.

Reuler, J. B. (1984). Hypothermia. In C. K. Cassel & J. R. Walsh (Eds.), *Geriatric medicine.* New York: Verlag.

Roth, J. A., Golub, S. H., Cukingnan, R. A., Brazier, J., & Morton, D. L. (1981). Cell mediated immunity is depressed following cardiopulmonary bypass. *Annals of Thoracic Surgery, 31,* 350-356.

Tappen, R. M., & Andre, S. P. (1996). Inadvertent hypothermia in elderly surgical patients. *AORN Journal, 63,* 639-644.

Tausk, H. C., Miller, R., & Roberts, R. B. (1976). Maintenance of body temperature by heated humidification. *Anesthesia & Analgesia, 55,* 719-723.

Taylor, N. A., Allsopp, N. K., & Parkes, D. G. (1995). Preferred room temperature of young vs. aged males: The influence of thermal sensation, thermal comfort and affect. *Journals of Gerontology Series A: Biological Sciences & Medical Sciences, 50*(4), M216-M221.

Wang-Yang, M. C., Buttke, T. M., Miller, N. W., & Clem, W. (1990). Temperature-mediated processes in immunity: Differential effects of low temperature on mouse T helper cell responses. *Cellular Immunology, 126,* 354-366.

Wongsurawat, N., Davis, B. B., & Morley, J. E. (1990). Thermoregulatory failure in the elderly. *Journal of the American Geriatrics Society, 38,* 899-906.

PART

III

Elimination Pattern

OVERVIEW

Problems with elimination consume a large proportion of nursing resources. They also affect the psychologic well-being, body image, and physical and social status of many older adults and are often related to the decision to institutionalize. McKinney overviews normal changes in elimination patterns with aging in Chapter 18. Changes in urinary and bowel elimination are presented with etiologic factors and practical suggestions to cope with problem patterns.

In Chapter 19 McLane and McShane consider the nursing diagnosis Constipation. They review the types of constipation and stress nursing interventions that develop health-related behaviors that contribute to healthy patterns of elimination. Numerous environmental and interactive variables related to this diagnosis are described, and data-based models of constipation are set forth, based in part on the authors' extensive research in this area. Nursing interventions directed toward the establishment of a comprehensive bowel management program are recommended, including development of a toileting routine, exercise, family instruction and problem-solving assistance, and development of an acceptable documentation process. Initial and long-term nursing-sensitive outcomes are identified and monitoring protocols suggested.

In Chapter 20, Diarrhea, Wadle discusses the diagnosis from the perspective of both acute and chronic diarrhea and the multiple etiologies. Tube-feeding interventions, as well as educational or teaching interventions, are highlighted to address this common and complex problem found among institutionalized elders.

In Chapter 21, Bowel Incontinence, Maas and Specht differentiate between normal defecation and bowel incontinence. The etiologies of this diagnosis are explicated, and the relationship to the problem of constipation is noted. Authors suggest key areas for assessment of bowel incontinence. Bowel training and environmental management are identified as important nursing interventions to treat this diagnosis.

In Chapter 22, Urinary Incontinence, Specht and Maas elaborate on the predisposing factors of this costly problem among institutionalized elders. They discuss the types of urinary incontinence found in this population, identify nursing-sensitive outcomes, and provide detailed advice on implementation of interventions for specific incontinence types. Specht and Maas discuss the bladder-filling incontinence diagnoses Urge Incontinence, Stress Incontinence, Reflex Urinary Incontinence, and Mixed Incontinence; the bladder-emptying incontinence diagnoses Overflow Incontinence and Total or Continuous Incontinence; and the incontinence diagnoses related to spurious factors, Functional Urinary Incontinence and Iatrogenic Incontinence. A guide for differential diagnosis is provided to assist nurses with differentiating specific types of incontinence.

CHAPTER 18

NORMAL CHANGES WITH AGING

Colette L. McKinney

Incontinence is one of the most common and distressing health care problems in elders and is expected to increase in incidence as the population of the United States continues to age. It can have a significant impact on health care costs, as well as on the individual's social status, physical health, and psychologic health. Complications include skin breakdown, urinary tract infections, social isolation, depression, and falls. Moreover, caregivers or families often use incontinence as a decisive factor in the institutionalization of elders.

URINARY SYSTEM

Urinary incontinence afflicts approximately 13 million people in the United States, 85% of whom are women (Shandra, 1998). Urinary incontinence cost society an estimated $26 million in 1995 for individuals 65 years of age and older (Wagner & Hu, 1995). Although urinary incontinence is not a concomitant of aging, several age-related factors contribute to its development. Bladder capacity and contractility decrease, and there is a general loss of muscle tone in the perineal floor, uterus, bladder, sphincter, and urethra. Residual urine volume has been noted to increase only slightly. The sensation of desire to void becomes more variable in elders, especially in those who receive medications that alter the micturition function or volume of urine. Although the etiology of detrusor overactivity is difficult to diagnose, it is a major contributing factor of urge incontinence in both sexes (Resnick, 1996). The development of stress incontinence (outlet incompetence) in women often results from relaxed pelvic muscles and atrophy of periurethral tissue due to estrogen deficiency, childbirth, and previous surgeries. Urinary incontinence in older men can be suggestive of benign prostatic hyperplasia (BPH), which affects 40% to 70% of men 65 years of age or older (Garraway & Kirby, 1994). An enlarged prostate gland can cause bladder outflow obstruction and lead to urinary retention and/or dribbling.

A disruption of the elder's lifestyle or environment can also result in urinary incontinence. During acute illness elders can experience hospitalization, immobility, inaccessible toilets, and delirium, each of which can contribute to incontinence. Elders sometimes refuse fluids to prevent episodes of incontinence, but in doing so actually put themselves at increased risk for dehydration.

The prevalence of urinary incontinence is higher in stroke survivors than in the general population (Burney, Senapati, Desai, Choudhary, & Badlani, 1996). Further research investigating the relationship of neurologic lesions involving micturition is needed, including the site versus the side and the role of apraxia or aphasia.

Functional changes of the aging kidney can leave the elder vulnerable to a variety of disease-related and drug-induced stresses; therefore careful evaluation of the elder's drug regimen should be taken into account. Structural changes include a loss of renal mass (primarily the renal cortex), a loss of nephrons, interstitial fibrosis, sclerotic glomeruli, and thickening of the glomerular and tubular basement membranes (Fillit & Rowe, 1992). Subsequently, a decline in renal blood flow leads to a decrease in glomerular filtration rate, although no rise in serum creatinine levels is observed. Structural changes can produce fluid and electrolyte abnormalities; the older kidney will have difficulty excreting hydrogen ions, leaving the elder in a state of metabolic acidosis. Renal changes in elders must be taken into account before initiating pharmacologic therapy, especially as more drugs with fewer side effects and more target efficacy are developed.

GASTROINTESTINAL SYSTEM

Although fecal incontinence is less common, it has been associated with 30% to 50% of elderly patients who exhibit frequent urinary incontinence. Fecal incontinence is noted to be higher in females secondary to postmenopausal connective tissue changes and to musculature weakness, nerve injury, and anal sphincter damage resulting from childbirth (Wald, 1994). Anorectal disorders usually follow childbirth, and symptoms increase with age. Hard stool (or scybalum) will irritate the rectum, leading to the production of mucus and fluid that leaks around the impaction. Problems with constipation, laxative use, or changes in cognitive status, such as delirium, can also contribute to fecal incontinence.

Although some structural changes lead to alterations in function, the gastrointestinal tract retains normal physiologic function during the aging process. Generalized muscle weakness of the pelvic floor, rectoanal incoordination, and slowing of the colonic transit time can interfere with normal defecation and induce constipation (Wald,

1994). In addition, diverticuli may develop in the lower colon with subsequent alteration in bowel habits, more often constipation than diarrhea. Hospitalization of the elder because of volume depletion, electrolyte imbalances, and malnutrition is often the result of diarrhea. Monitoring antimicrobial therapy and reducing the use of laxatives and diarrhea-causing medications will help to reduce the incidence of diarrhea.

Whether real or imagined, constipation is often reported among elders, especially those residing in institutions (Kinnunen, 1991). Decreased physical activity, lack of dietary fiber, and inadequate fluid intake all can slow the transit time of feces. Many hospitalized elders are faced with the discomfort of using a bedpan, which can lead to problems defecating. The longer the feces remain in the colon, the greater the amount of water reabsorbed back into the colon, further exacerbating the problem. Antihypertensives, analgesics, and antidepressants contribute to constipation through their anticholinergic effects.

MANAGING ALTERATIONS IN ELIMINATION

With proper evaluation and treatment the majority of patients with urinary incontinence can be helped. However, most patients do not volunteer information about urinary incontinence, and health care providers may be reluctant to ask. Nurses must ask specific questions about urinary incontinence, document their findings, initiate appropriate interventions, and see that management and evaluation occur. The first step in managing alterations in elimination is identification of all possible contributing factors. Careful assessment can help the nurse identify correctable causes and implement appropriate interventions. Assessment should include evaluation of bladder distention and enlarged prostate in males. An important fact to consider is that the elderly do not conserve water and are prone to fluid and electrolyte imbalances, especially when they are not eating and drinking appropriately. Indwelling catheters or incontinence undergarments should be used as a last resort because of the likely development of urinary tract infections and skin breakdown. Other therapeutic options include dietary modifications, pharmacologic agents, behavioral programs, and surgery. Pelvic floor muscle rehabilitation and bladder training are the two major types of behavioral modifications implemented; however, commitment is required from patients and nurses for these to be successful. Nurses should encourage fluids and see that fiber is regularly included in the diet in moderate amounts. If nocturia is troublesome, the amounts of fluids ingested in the evening can be limited. Regular toileting is important, since it provides a stimulus to evacuate the bowel and bladder. Some elders may need reminders to maintain a regular bathroom schedule. A bedside commode or urinal can help with patients who are weak, have immobility problems, or have increased frequency. Since less activity will result in reduced bowel function, a regular activity program can help initiate peristalsis. It is important to remember that improper positioning during toileting, restricted mobility including the use of restraints, and the inability to ask for or retrieve fluids all promote constipation and incontinence. Structured interventions geared toward the patient, education, frequent contact, and ongoing assessment are essential for optimal outcomes.

SUMMARY

Changes in elimination patterns create discomfort, embarrassment, and distress for millions of older adults. Yet elimination problems are not necessary sequelae to aging, nor are they always irreversible. The vital first step in helping older adults with elimination problems is to assess whether an elimination problem exists. A detailed assessment of elimination patterns and of factors that might contribute to problems serves as the foundation for intervention. Nurses can instruct older adults in dietary modifications, lifestyle changes, and toileting routines that might correct their elimination problems. Nurses can help individuals maintain commitment to behavioral interventions. When appropriate, nurses can also refer clients for medical evaluation. By actively assessing and addressing elimination problems, nurses have the potential to make lasting improvements in the lives of older adults.

REFERENCES

Burney, T. L., Senapati, M., Desai, S., Choudhary, S. T., & Badlani, G. H. (1996). Effects of cerebrovascular accident on micturition. *Urology Clinics of North America, 23*(3), 483-490.

Fillit, H., & Rowe, J. (1992). The aging kidney. In J. Brocklehurst, R. Tallis, & H. Fillit (Eds.), *Textbook of geriatric medicine and gerontology.* New York: Churchill Livingstone.

Garraway, W. M., & Kirby, R. S. (1994). Benign prostatic hyperplasia: Effects on quality of life and impact on treatment decisions. *Urology, 44*(5), 629-636.

Kinnunen, O. (1991). Study of constipation in a geriatric hospital, day hospital, old people's home and at home. *Aging, 3,* 161-170.

Resnick, N. M. (1996). Geriatric incontinence. *Urologic Clinics of North America, 23*(1), 55-74.

Shandra, K. C. (1998). Diagnosis and management of female urinary incontinence. *Hawaii Medical Journal, 57*(12), 746-748.

Wagner, T. H., & Hu, T. W. (1995). Economic cost of urinary incontinence in 1995. *Urology, 51*(3), 355-361.

Wald, A. (1994). Constipation and fecal incontinence in the elderly. *Seminars in Gastrointestinal Disease, 5,* 179-188.

CHAPTER 19

CONSTIPATION

Audrey M. McLane and Ruth E. McShane

An increase in the number of older adults and frail elders in the population has sparked a renewed interest in constipation as a phenomenon of concern. Individuals over age 85 represent the fastest growing segment of the aging population. Since the incidence of health problems usually increases with age, older persons are more subject to comorbidity, that is, they experience more than one health problem at any one time. In this context, constipation takes on new meaning in the daily life of the frail elder, and it can progress from a simple annoyance to a major health concern (Walsh, 1997; Wolfsen, Barker, & Mitteness, 1993).

There is no agreed upon definition of constipation in the clinical and research communities (Koch, Voderholzer, Klauser, & Muller-Lissner, 1997). Most definitions are symptom based, including the definition provided by the North American Nursing Diagnosis Association (NANDA, 1999). Probert, Emmett, Cripps, and Heaton (1994) studied a sample of 731 community-based women, using three definitions of constipation. They concluded that the term *constipation* is ambiguous and often misleading and that attempts to base a definition on symptoms are misguided. Their recommendation was to base epidemiologic studies about the prevalence of constipation on records of stool type and timing.

Patients who seek health care for constipation can present many challenges, including communication difficulties, problems in diagnosis, a history of mediocre therapy, uncorrectable conditions, or psychiatric problems that complicate management. A recent review by Stark (1999) describes both the challenges involved in managing constipation and management approaches that increase the likelihood of satisfactory outcomes.

PREVALENCE

Epidemiologic studies provide evidence that both self-reported and true clinical constipation increase with age despite the absence of physiologic changes in the lower bowel with normal aging. Prolonged transit through the sigmoid colon and rectum, especially in frail elders, is consistently reported (Harari, Gurwitz, & Minaker, 1993). Self-reported constipation and an increase in laxative use have been documented in both community-based and institutionalized older adults and frail elders (Campbell, Busby, & Horwath, 1993; Harari, Gurwitz, Avorn, Choodnovskiy, & Minaker, 1994; Petticrew, Watt, & Sheldon, 1997; Wolfsen et al., 1993).

Clinical evidence of constipation is not always found in individuals who self-report the problem. In one study only 62% met the study criteria for symptom-specific constipation. "Self-reporters" took almost twice as many laxatives, stool softeners, and enemas as subjects who did not self-identify the problem. At least one daily laxative, stool softener, or enema was taken by 50% of the subjects during the 1-month study period. More than half of laxative users ($n = 200$) took more than 60 doses a month (Harari et al., 1994).

RISK FACTORS

Factors placing persons at risk for developing constipation can be considered in the following categories: mental and emotional status, physical status, health beliefs and behaviors, environmental constraints, and economic status. Although the categories are not mutually exclusive, they do provide a heuristic device for thinking about a very complex problem and a framework for identifying additional factors unique to individuals or groups (Box 19-1).

Another way to view "at risk" is to look at groups of individuals who have a physiologic condition that increases the probability of constipation. For example, persons with diabetes mellitus can have a dysfunction of the autonomic nervous system resulting in loss of the gastrocolic reflex. Women, especially multiparas, can have sacral nerve root damage from obstetric trauma. Individuals with multiple sclerosis have clinical evidence of spinal cord disease that can cause constipation (Chia et al., 1995; Haines, 1995). However, identifying persons at risk in terms of mechanisms of injury or disease (many not reversible) tends to oversimplify the complexity of the phenomenon and provides only minimal guidance in the determination of expected outcomes and interventions. Risk factors are more powerful conceptual tools and play a major role in assessment, outcome specification, and the creation of unique interventions. Reducing risk by paying attention to all factors that place persons at risk is a more logical approach for preventing all types of constipation. Although it may not always be possible to eliminate the risk factors, e.g.,

Box 19-1	Proposed Categories of Risk Factors CONSTIPATION

Mental and Emotional
Altered thought processes
Impaired verbal communication
Affective state (depression)
Low intrinsic motivation
Altered awareness
Low/no social support

Physical Status
Self-care deficits
Weak pelvic floor muscles
Deterioration of innervation
Paradoxical contraction of the external anal sphincter
Altered mobility
Painful anorectal lesions
Constipating medications
Weak abdominal muscles
Ill-fitting dentures

Health Beliefs and Health Behaviors
Inadequate fluid intake
Minimal activity level

Failure to respond to gastrocolic reflex
No established toileting regimen
Diet: low in calories/quantity
Preference for low-fiber foods
Expectation of a daily bowel movement
Overuse of laxatives and enemas

Environmental Constraints
Unfamiliar surroundings
Limited access to toilet facilities
Change in daily routine
Poor lighting
Low decisional control
Hospitalization or relocation

Economic
Limited financial resources
Poor access to health services
Inadequate transportation

cancer patients receiving palliative care with large doses of constipating medication, prevention is more cost effective and more consistent with quality of life for elders (Bruera et al., 1994; Gattuso & Kamm, 1994). A more rigorous examination of research and clinical studies to confirm suspected risk factors has been recommended (Harari, Gurwitz, & Minaker, 1993).

ASSESSMENT

There are no validated and reliable assessment tools reported in the literature. Research-based and clinical reports usually include a definition of constipation, a bowel history guide, and a list of defining characteristics or signs and symptoms and contributing factors to serve as the basis for making an assessment. For example, a bowel history assessment guide was developed to screen homebound elders before their entrance into a study of a high-fiber pudding (Neal, 1995). Many individuals self-diagnose a problem with bowel elimination, which is then verified by a clinical assessment usually done by a nurse or physician. Minaker and Harari (1995) used two diagnostic algorithms and two management algorithms to present the case of an 85-year-old woman with constipation and elevated serum creatinine level. She was diagnosed as having both symptomatic and clinical constipation, two of three types defined by the investigators as clinically useful (Table 19-1). They listed the diseases and medications in Box 19-2 as the "causes" of slow transit constipation in the

elderly. With the exception of dehydration, immobility, and low-fiber and carbohydrate diet, none of these "causes" are easily impacted by nursing care.

The proposed categories of diagnostic indicators (McLane, McShane, & Sliefert, 1984), the model of factors contributing to constipation (McLane & McShane, 1991), and the identified risk factors could be used to design an assessment guide for use in practice and research that would reflect the complexity of the phenomenon and that would highlight those elements readily affected by nursing care.

Table 19-1	Types of Constipation With Definitions
Types	**Definitions**
Symptomatic constipation	Two or fewer bowel movements in a week; 25% involve straining
Clinical constipation	Fecal retention in the rectal ampulla on digital examination, excessive fecal retention in the colon on abdominal x-ray, or both
Subjective constipation	Self-reported constipation in the absence of clinical and symptomatic constipation

Data from Minaker, K. L., & Harari, D. (1995). Constipation in the elderly. *Hospital Practice, 30*(5), 67-70, 73-76.

<table>
<tr><td>Box 19-2</td><td>Causes of Slow Transit Constipation in the Elderly: Medications and Diseases/Conditions</td></tr>
</table>

Medications
Aluminum hydroxide antacids
Anticholinergics
Calcium channel blockers
Diuretics
Iron supplements
Narcotics

Diseases/Conditions
Colon cancer
Dehydration
Diabetes mellitus
Hypercalcemia/hypokalemia
Immobility
Low fiber and carbohydrate diet
Parkinson's disease
Stroke

CASE STUDY

T. Jackson is a 75-year-old widow who lives alone in a small brick house in a community of older adults. She cares for herself and her home with some assistance from a daughter and local contractors who take care of the yardwork. Mrs. Jackson is in moderately good health except for emphysema and chronic bronchitis that have resulted from a lifetime of smoking more than a pack of cigarettes a day. Sometimes she uses a cane to decrease right knee pain caused by degenerative osteoarthritis. She becomes fatigued easily and seldom leaves home except to go to church on Sunday and to do grocery shopping. Since her husband's death 2 years ago, she eats fewer fruits and vegetables, preferring a one-dish frozen meal such as lasagna or meatballs and spaghetti plus a large dish of ice cream. For breakfast, she eats a boiled egg, white toast, and coffee; for lunch she makes a sandwich of smoked sausage on rye bread. A home health care nurse visited Mrs. Jackson in response to her telephone request for a nurse to give her an enema for constipation.

In response to the nurse's questions, Mrs. Jackson reported the following signs and symptoms: no bowel movement for 4 days, no response to a suppository that had worked in the past, abdominal pain, and headache. During the preceding 2 weeks the stool in her bowel movements had been hard and difficult to pass. The nurse found a firm mass in the area of the descending colon on abdominal examination and impacted stool on rectal examination.

NURSING DIAGNOSIS

The North American Nursing Diagnosis Association (NANDA, 1999) has defined Constipation as "a decrease in a person's normal frequency of defecation accompanied by difficulty of incomplete passage of stool and/or passage of excessively hard, dry stool" (NANDA, 1999, p. 15). NANDA also has provided a definition of Perceived Constipation, namely "the state in which an individual makes a self-diagnosis of constipation and ensures a daily bowel movement through abuse of laxatives, enemas, and suppositories" (NANDA, 1999, p. 17). Defining characteristics and related factors for Constipation and Perceived Constipation are given in Table 19-2.

NURSING-SENSITIVE OUTCOMES

The initial outcome of treating an instance of constipation is to alleviate the acute problem immediately. Immediate relief from constipation is a priority and must be accomplished before a more comprehensive plan can be developed with an individual to achieve mutually agreed upon outcomes. Long-term outcomes include the following: to establish a regular pattern of bowel movements; to prevent future instances of constipation and/or impaction; to eliminate digital removal of feces; and to decrease use of a laxative, suppository, or enema to facilitate evacuation. Indicators that provide evidence of achieved outcomes rely on patient reports: modifies diet; increases physical activ-

Table 19-2	Defining Characteristics and Related Factors/Etiologies **CONSTIPATION AND PERCEIVED CONSTIPATION**		
	Defining Characteristics	**Related Factors/Etiologies**
Constipation	Decreased frequency; dry, hard, formed stool; palpable rectal mass; feeling of rectal fullness or pressure; straining with defecation	Functional; psychologic; pharmacologic; mechanical; physiologic
Perceived constipation	Major: Expectation of a daily bowel movement with the resulting overuse of laxatives, enemas, and suppositories; expected passage of stool at same time every day	Cultural/family health beliefs; faulty appraisal; impaired thought processes

ity; establishes a toileting routine without the use of suppositories, enemas, or oral laxatives; responds immediately to urge to defecate; passes stool easily; experiences sensation of complete passage of stool; has a soft formed stool every 2 to 3 days, using a suppository rarely (Kim, McFarland, & McLane, 1997; Iowa Outcomes Project, 2000).

Measuring outcome achievement is not a trivial process. Some research protocols specify the use of colon x-ray examinations and stool weights. Such indicators are impractical for routine use with older adults living in their own homes or some other community environment. Sharkey and Hanlon (1989) recommended use of a bowel elimination record to document the elements of a bowel management program. They suggested that the elimination record include the following items: date and time, description of bowel movement, medications including suppositories, and diet (p. 219). A list of descriptors with abbreviations was provided for each component of the program. Additional items unique to the individual could be added for a more complete record of outcomes achieved (McLane & McShane, 1992).

NURSING INTERVENTIONS

A comprehensive bowel management program for constipation includes the following components: diet modification; physical exercise; development and implementation of a toileting routine; pelvic floor exercises; instruction of patient/family with practice in problem-solving bowel elimination concerns; and development of an acceptable documentation process. Biofeedback-based behavior modification has been described for selected individuals with pelvic floor dysfunction, spasticity, and dyssynergia, a failure of muscle coordination in the pelvic floor, or paradoxically contracted external sphincters. Total or subtotal abdominal colectomy with anastomosis of the ileum to the colon has been reported as successful in treating intractable constipation. The drastic nature of the surgical approach should motivate health care workers to make a more serious commitment to implement interventions before constipation becomes intractable.

Diet

A diet high in fiber is consistently recommended to improve bowel function in older adults and frail elders. Fresh and dried fruits, raw and cooked vegetables, and whole grain breads are most often acceptable ways to add bulk to meals and between-meal snacks. Consuming bran in cereals, breads, and muffins may be rejected in favor of taking a high-fiber supplement. Bran has been reported to be more erratic than the refined fibers used in supplements, e.g., Metamucil. Raw bran can cause diarrhea and bloating and can bind calcium, iron, and fat-soluble vitamins, nutrients needed by older adults. Bran can bind with oral medications (e.g., cardiac glycosides, warfarin [Coumadin], and salicylates) and should be taken at a sep-

arate time. Bran adds more weight to the fecal contents, which helps to speed up its passage. A high-fiber supplement may cost less than a month's supply of bran. For some older adults on a fixed income, the cost advantage of the supplement will drive the decision in favor of the supplement (Gender, 1996; Minaker & Harari, 1995).

Nurses have developed some creative strategies to increase bulk in the diets of their patients. In one quality improvement study, patients hospitalized for vascular surgery were given high-fiber oatmeal raisin cookies and blueberry high-fiber muffins to prevent postoperative constipation and impaction. Constipation was reduced from 59% to 9%; impaction was eliminated; and requests for laxatives and enemas were reduced from 59% to 8% (Hall, Karstens, Rakel, Swanson, & Davidson, 1995). In another study, home health nurses used a "power pudding" for their patients over age 65 who reported periodic or chronic constipation. Nurses gave their patients varying amounts of the mixture (¼ to 1 cup) per day. The recipe was a mixture of applesauce, prunes and prune juice, wheat flakes, and whipped topping. The frequency of bowel movements, which was 0 to 3.5 per week before the intervention, increased to 3 to 6 per week. Half of the participants increased their fluid intake during the study, but the increase was not consistent. Fluid intake, age, and ambulatory status did not affect the results (Neal, 1995). In a related study of healthy volunteers, there was no difference whether 30 g of bran was taken with or without 600 ml of additional fluid (Klauser & Muller-Lissner, 1993).

Increasing fluid intake, especially water, is viewed as a logical adjunct to an increase in dietary fiber in the diets of older adults and frail elders, even though support from research is lacking. Fiber binds water in the form of a gel to prevent absorption from the large bowel, making fecal contents soft and bulky. Frail elderly who rely on walkers, canes, and personal assistance to ambulate frequently limit their fluid intake to decrease the number of trips to the bathroom. A special effort must be made to provide water, juices, and soups, a minimum of two liquids with each meal, and liquids between meals.

There is some evidence that number of meals and amount of caloric intake influence bowel elimination. In a small study of 36 community-dwelling outpatients over 60 years of age (18 constipated and 18 controls), constipated subjects reported consuming fewer meals per day compared with control subjects; constipated subjects also tended to consume fewer calories. Slow colonic transit was significantly related to low caloric intake, low fluid intake, higher protein in the diet, and psychologic symptoms (Towers et al., 1994). More studies are needed to determine whether increases in fluid intake are a necessary adjunct to increasing fiber in the diets of constipated older adults.

Physical Exercise

Conventional wisdom dictates an increase in physical activity as one component in a comprehensive bowel management program. Textbooks, clinical studies, and research reports describe the hazards of immobility and the almost inevitable constipation. Klauser and Muller-Lissner (1993) question the chain of reasoning that goes from immobility as a factor in causing constipation to an increase in physical activity as a treatment. An increase in physical activity is usually one element in many research protocols designed to test the effect of a comprehensive treatment program for constipation. Without component analysis, however, the outcomes achieved cannot be ascribed to any one element. Still, most expert nurses are quick to provide anecdotal evidence of the beneficial effect of physical activity on gastrointestinal motility.

Normally active older adults may not need to increase their physical activity to prevent or treat constipation, but fragile elders and persons with disabilities will benefit from planned increases in physical activity. Passive and active range of motion helps to maintain muscle tone in bedridden patients. A person with a disability can be taught self-care with a minimum of assistance. Wheelchair-bound individuals can learn to use the arms of the wheelchair to raise their bodies for a few moments to increase upper arm strength. Walking is the activity of choice for the frail elder. The type of activity and stepwise increases in physical activity must be dictated by the individual's overall health status, the environment in which the person lives, and the health and fitness of caregivers.

Development and Implementation of a Toileting Routine

Timing is a critical factor in establishing bowel regularity. The gastrocolic and duodenocolic reflexes are strongest when the stomach is empty and food is ingested. Breakfast is usually the meal that triggers the reflexes and produces mass movement of feces, forcing it into the rectum. Fatty acids delay reflex stimulation and must be excluded from the triggering meal. Some individuals respond to a cup of coffee or hot water and lemon before breakfast. Immediate response to the defecation reflex is a priority, since the reflex is weak and the rectum accommodates to the presence of feces. Some feces may move back into the sigmoid colon. Since the external and sphincter is under control of the conscious mind, it is possible to disrupt the normal mechanisms. Some individuals require digital stimulation to induce relaxation of the anal sphincter. Individuals who have been ignoring the defecation reflex may have to reestablish a consistent habit time by going to the toilet within 15 minutes of the triggering meal. Many older adults lead a very busy life and must be encouraged to provide a block of time to attend to their elimination needs (Gender, 1996; McLane & McShane, 1992).

Positioning is another critical element in establishing bowel regularity. Placing the knees higher than the hips in a squat position raises abdominal pressure and helps move the fecal mass into the rectum. Older adults using an elevated toilet seat can assume the proper position with the aid of a footstool, preferably one with a handle that is easy to move into place. A person with weak abdominal muscles can be helped by bending at the waist, using an abdominal binder, or massaging the abdomen beginning in the area of the right groin, moving upward and across the abdomen, and down to the left groin. Sitting on the toilet should be limited to 20 minutes. Persons using a bedside commode must be provided with privacy, since elimination is a very personal act. Once a pattern has been established, individuals need not try for a bowel movement every day if their pattern is every other day or every third day (Gender, 1996; McLane & McShane, 1992).

Pelvic Floor Exercises

Pelvic floor exercises are useful in the treatment of many bowel dysfunctions and urinary incontinence. They are frequently used as an adjunct to biofeedback in the treatment of pelvic floor disorders, e.g., pelvic floor dyssynergia. Pelvic floor exercises are repetitive contractions and relaxations of the puborectalis muscles and the anal sphincter. They must be performed 25 to 30 times, 3 times a day. Contractions must be maintained for 3 to 4 seconds and then repeated in a staccato fashion without tensing the muscles of the buttocks, legs, or abdomen. Sphincters tend to fatigue and then go into a refractory stage if contractions are maintained for more than 1 minute (Kim, McFarland, & McLane, 1997; McCormick & Burgio, 1984; McLane & McShane, 1992).

Instruction of Patient and Family

Instruction of the patient/family with practice in problem-solving bowel elimination concerns is an ongoing part of a bowel management program. All of the components of the program with the rationale for each must be shared with patient and family or caregiver. Outdated beliefs about the need for a daily bowel movement must be addressed. Patients and spouses or caregivers must be taught how to insert a suppository, perform digital stimulation, give an enema, or break up an impaction if an occurrence is likely. A review of factors placing someone at risk will help the patient and family recognize how risk can be decreased. Engaging the patient and family in problem-solving about managing an episode of diarrhea, incontinence, or constipation and deciding when to call the nurse or doctor will help relieve anxiety about the bowel management program.

Documentation

Documentation of each component of the bowel elimination program is essential. A comprehensive record includes the date and time, description of bowel movement, medications, suppositories, diet, physical exercise, pelvic floor exercises, assistance required, and problems encountered. Additional items could be added that are specific to the individual. Documentation provides a quick summary of the patient's daily and weekly progress. The records are extremely valuable when reporting to physicians or nurses and when requesting their assistance (McLane & McShane, 1992).

CASE STUDY

Mrs. Jackson's nurse made a diagnosis of Colonic Constipation. To provide immediate relief, the nurse instilled oil and followed it with two tap water enemas. In addition, she manually broke up the impacted stool to facilitate expulsion. After relieving the acute constipation, the next task for the nurse and Mrs. Jackson was to reach a mutual agreement about the outcome toward which new health practices would be directed. The outcome is followed by indicators, nursing interventions, and activities.

Nursing-Sensitive Outcome
Bowel Elimination
Indicators
- Elimination pattern IER*
- Ingests adequate fiber
- Ingests adequate fluids
- Stool soft and formed
- Exercise adequate
- Ease of stool passage
- Abuse of aids not present

Nursing Interventions
Bowel Management
Activities
- Monitor bowel movements
- Teach patient about specific foods that promote bowel regularity
- Instruct patient/family to monitor and record color, volume, frequency, and consistency of stools
- Instruct patient/family on foods that are high in fiber
- Instruct patient/family in proper use of and insertion of suppositories

Bowel Training
Activities
- Plan bowel program with patient and family
- Provide foods high in bulk and/or that have been identified as assistive by the patient
- Ensure adequate fluid intake
- Ensure adequate exercise
- Evaluate bowel status regularly
- Modify bowel interventions as needed

Nursing Intervention Activities and Rationales
Teach use of food diary to provide opportunity to analyze eating patterns with patient. Suggest gradual increase of high-fiber foods to add bulk to gastrointestinal contents, such as bran or high-fiber cereal, fresh fruit, and raw or cooked vegetables. Recommend that patient introduce high-fiber foods into the diet gradually to produce less cramping and flatus. Provide information about high-fiber supplements (e.g., Metamucil). Patient may need to use a supplement if she has difficulty tolerating high-fiber foods. Arrange joint meeting with patient and daughter to discuss elements of the program. Daughter's assistance might be required to shop more often for fresh fruits and vegetables.

Provide instruction about the importance of responding immediately to the urge to defecate, monitoring consistency of stool, and ease of passage of stool. (The rectum accommodates to the presence of feces, and water will continue to be absorbed, resulting in hard stool.) Collaborate with the patient to establish a toileting routine that does not rely on laxatives or suppositories. (Patient understanding of the role of stimulus behaviors, timing, and position on toilet will ensure success and compliance with the program.) Teach the correct time and way to insert bisacodyl (Dulcolax) suppository if constipation recurs. (Use of the suppository within 1 hour of the triggering meal will elicit the gastrocolic reflex if the suppository is in contact with the rectal wall. The suppository will not work if placed in the stool mass.)

Refer patient to physician or neighborhood clinic to obtain exercise prescription. (The patient's medical history and treatment will influence goal setting with respect to increase in physical activity.) Suggest walking outdoors with a companion to increase feelings of safety and to provide opportunity for increasing distance walked. For example, she might meet with neighbors to walk 15 minutes every morning and evening and gradually increase distance walked within exercise prescription. Suggest obtaining 3-point cane from church-run loan closet to increase feeling of stability and safety when walking. Teach and coach how to exercise abdominal muscles. Since mattress is firm, suggest doing abdominal exercises before getting up in the morning. (Developing the habit of exercising each morning will increase compliance.) Arrange to teach patient and daughter how to perform pelvic floor exercises. (Daughter will be able to coach patient and have a better opportunity to monitor her mother's physical condition.)

Collaborate with the patient to develop and implement a system for documenting the bowel movement, nutrient fiber, and exercise components of the bowel elimination program. (Keeping a record provides feedback to patients to monitor their own progress.) Review patient records, discuss progress, make suggestions, and answer questions. (Reviewing patient records conveys their importance to patient.)

IER, In expected range.

SUMMARY

Both self-reported and true clinical constipation increase with age. For many elderly persons, constipation poses a major health problem. Many of the nursing interventions included in the preceding care plan are not supported by scientific research. Many interventions are based on a nurse's understanding of normal physiology and a logical analysis of the risk factors that might have influenced the development or maintenance of the problem. Other nursing interventions fall into the category of "nursing wisdom," that is, interventions learned from working with expert nurses, interventions learned from colleagues at professional meetings, and interventions learned by systematically testing them in a case-by-case manner.

REFERENCES

Bruera, E., Suarez-Almazor, M., Velasco, A., Bertolino, M., MacDonald, S. M., & Hanson, J. (1994). The assessment of constipation in terminal cancer patients admitted to a palliative care unit: A retrospective review. *Journal of Pain & Symptom Management, 9*(8), 515-519.

Campbell, A. J., Busby, W. J., & Horwath, C. C. (1993). Factors associated with constipation in a community-based sample of people aged 70 years and over. *Journal of Epidemiology & Community Health, 47*(1), 23-26.

Chia, Y. W., Fowler, C. J., Kamm, M. A., Henry, M. M., Lemieux, M. C., & Swash, M. (1995). Prevalence of bowel dysfunction with multiple sclerosis and bladder dysfunction. *Journal of Neurology, 242*(2), 105-108.

Gattuso, J. M., & Kamm, M. A. (1994). Adverse effects of drugs used in the management of constipation and diarrhea. *Drug Safety, 10*(1), 47-65.

Gender, A. R. (1996). Bowel regulation and elimination. In S. P. Hoeman (Ed.), *Rehabilitation nursing: Process and application* (2nd ed., pp. 452-475). St. Louis, MO: Mosby.

Haines, S. T. (1995). Treating constipation in the patient with diabetes. *Diabetes Educator, 21*(3), 223-232.

Hall, G. R., Karstens, M., Rakel, B., Swanson, E., & Davidson, A. (1995). Managing constipation using a research-based protocol. *Medsurg Nursing, 4*(1), 11-20.

Harari, D., Gurwitz, J. H., & Minaker, K. L. (1993). Constipation in the elderly. *Journal of the American Geriatrics Society, 41*(10), 1130-1140.

Harari, D., Gurwitz, J. R., Avorn, J., Choodnovskiy, I., & Minaker, K. L. (1994). Constipation: Assessment and management in an institutionalized elderly population. *Journal of the American Geriatrics Society, 42*(9), 947-952.

Iowa Outcomes Project. M. Johnson, M. Maas, & S. Moorhead (Eds.). (2000). *Nursing outcomes classification (NOC)* (2nd ed.). St. Louis, MO: Mosby.

Kim, M. J., McFarland, G. K., & McLane, A. M. (1997). *Pocket guide to nursing diagnoses* (7th ed.). St. Louis, MO: Mosby.

Klauser, A. G., & Muller-Lissner, S. A. (1993). How effective is nonlaxative treatment of constipation? *Pharmacology, 47*(Suppl. 1), 256-260.

Koch, A., Voderholzer, W. A., Klauser, A. G., & Muller-Lissner, S. (1997). Symptoms in chronic constipation. *Diseases of the Colon & Rectum, 40*(8), 902-906.

McCormick, K. A., & Burgio, K. L. (1984). Incontinence: An update on nursing care measures. *Journal of Gerontological Nursing, 10*(10), 16-19, 22, 23.

McLane, A. M., & McShane, R. E. (1992). Bowel management. In G. M. Bulechek & J. C. McCloskey (Eds.), *Nursing interventions: Essential nursing treatments* (pp. 73-85). Philadelphia: W. B. Saunders.

McLane, A. M., & McShane, R. E. (1991). Constipation. In M. Maas, K. C. Buckwalter, & M. Hardy (Eds.), *Nursing diagnoses and interventions for the elderly* (pp. 147-158). Reading, MA: Addison Wesley Longman.

McLane, A. M., McShane, R. E., & Sliefert, M. (1984). Constipation: Conceptual categories of diagnostic indicators. In M. J. Kim, G. K. McFarland, & A. M. McLane (Eds.), *Classification of nursing diagnoses: Proceedings of the fifth conference* (pp. 174-179). St. Louis, MO: Mosby.

Minaker, K. L., & Harari, D. (1995). Constipation in the elderly. *Hospital Practice, 30*(5), 67-70, 73-76.

Neal, L. J. (1995). "Power pudding": Natural laxative therapy for the elderly who are homebound. *Home Healthcare Nurse, 13*(2), 66-70.

North American Nursing Diagnosis Association. (1999). *Nursing diagnoses: Definitions & classification 1999-2000.* Philadelphia: Author.

Petticrew, M., Watt, J., & Sheldon, T. (1997). Systematic review of the effectiveness of laxatives in the elderly. *Health Technology Assessment (South Hampton, NY), 1*(13), i-iv, 1-52.

Probert, C. S., Emmett, P. M., Cripps, H. A., & Heaton, K. W. (1994). Evidence for the ambiguity of the term constipation: The role of irritable bowel syndrome. *Gut, 35*(10), 1455-1458.

Stark, M. (1999). Challenging problems presenting as constipation. *American Journal of Gastroenterology, 94*(3), 567-574.

Sharkey, E. L., & Hanlon, D. (1989). Bowel elimination. In S. Dittmar (Ed.), *Process of rehabilitation* (pp. 196-226). St. Louis, MO: Mosby.

Towers, A. L., Burgio, K. L., Locher, J. L., Merkel, I. S., Safaeian, M., & Wald, A. (1994). Constipation in the elderly: Influence of dietary, psychological, and physiological factors. *Journal of the American Geriatrics Society, 42*(7), 701-706.

Walsh, M. B. (1997). The frail elderly population. In M. M. Burke & M. B. Walsh (Eds.), *Gerontologic nursing: Wholistic care of the older adult* (2nd ed.). St. Louis, MO: Mosby.

Wolfsen, C. R., Barker, J. C., & Mitteness, L. S. (1993). Constipation in the daily lives of frail elderly people. *Archives of Family Medicine, 2*(8), 853-858.

CHAPTER 20

DIARRHEA

Karen R. Wadle

Diarrhea is one manifestation of gastrointestinal (GI) disturbance. The word "diarrhea" originates from the Greek terms *dia* (through) and *rhein* (to flow) (Krejs & Fordtran, 1983, p. 257). Fine, Krejs, and Fordtran (1993) define diarrhea as an abnormal increase in stool liquidity (daily stool weight greater than 200 g) and stool frequency (greater than three per day); this definition is subject to variation among individuals. Bond (1982) defines diarrhea as the passage of over 200 g of stool per day (as compared with an average daily stool weight of 100 to 150 g per day), with a stool content of 70% to 90% water (compared with a normal stool content of 60% to 80% water). Sundaram (1993) emphasizes the importance of GI secretion as a contributing factor in diarrhea. The GI tract accommodates 9 liters of fluid each day, 2 liters from diet and 7 liters from secretions from the gut and pancreas. "All but 100 to 200 ml of this fluid must be absorbed . . . Diarrhea results when there is an imbalance between absorption and secretion in the intestine" (Sundaram, 1993, p. 353).

Sundaram (1993) defines acute diarrhea as 2 weeks or less in duration and chronic diarrhea as more than 3 weeks in duration. McLane and McShane (1993) define diarrhea as an acute problem lasting from 24 to 48 hours, or as a chronic problem lasting continuously or intermittently for several weeks. Ross (1993) found that elderly subjects' definitions of diarrhea could be grouped into five categories: (1) frequency of passing stools; (2) urgency to have a bowel movement; (3) consistency of the stool; (4) symptoms such as cramping or abdominal pain; and (5) other. Subjects' definitions tended to fall into multiple categories, with the most frequent definition (29% of subjects) involving consistency of stool. Twenty-three percent of elders viewed regular bowel habits as important for maintaining overall health.

In aging individuals, the GI system is subject to physiologic changes, as are other body systems. Decreases occur in motility, gastric juice secretion, free acid content, total acid production, and pepsin content. Salivary and pancreative digestive enzyme production also decreases. With aging, there is a decrease in the ability of the immune system to adapt to environmental stresses; thus, the elderly are more susceptible to infectious processes (Eglow & Burakoff, 1991; Schmucker & Daniels, 1986). Lifestyle changes brought about by physiologic, eco-nomic, and sociologic factors (e.g., nutritional habits and exercise patterns) also affect GI function in the aged. The three key processes of the GI tract are digestion, absorption, and metabolism (Broadwell, 1986). These factors all are subject to alterations from chronic illnesses, from the effects of the treatment of these illnesses, and from the decline of organ systems and their interdependent functioning.

Diarrhea is a complex phenomenon, with a variety of etiologies and related variations in characteristics. Consequently, defining characteristics will be described in the context of specific etiologies. Specific prevalence rates in the elderly also will be described in the context of specific etiologies.

RELATED FACTORS/ETIOLOGIES

It is useful to distinguish between large-stool and small-stool diarrhea. Table 20-1, based on Krejs and Fordtran (1983), lists several distinguishing characteristics. The etiologies and defining characteristics for acute and chronic diarrhea discussed later are listed in Table 20-2 and compared with those identified by the North American Nursing Diagnosis Association (NANDA) (Carroll-Johnson, 1989).

Acute Diarrhea

Etiologies for acute diarrhea include infection, drug reactions, alterations in diet, improper cooking of food, spoiled food, enteral feedings, heavy metal poisoning, fecal impaction, and treatment for other diseases (Dupont, 1997; Krejs & Fordtran, 1983; McLane & McShane, 1993; Sundaram, 1993).

Infection. Age-related changes in the mucosal surfaces, such as those of the respiratory and GI tracts, are associated with increased susceptibility to infectious diseases (Cooper, Shlaes, & Salata, 1994; Schmucker & Daniels, 1986; Stolley & Buckwalter, 1991). Institutionalization creates additional risks of infection for the elderly because of close proximity to other persons who may have infections.

Infectious diseases pose a greater threat to life in the elder than in younger patients (Vartian & Septimus, 1986).

Table 20-1	Differentiation of Defining Characteristics Commonly Associated With Small-Stool and Large-Stool Diarrhea	
	Small-Stool Diarrhea	**Large-Stool Diarrhea**
Location of underlying disorder or disease	Left colon and rectum	Small bowel or proximal colon
Stool qualities	Dark in color	Light in color
	Frequent small amounts	Large amounts
	Rarely foul-smelling	Foul smelling
	Flatus and mucus sometimes expelled without stool	Watery, soupy, or greasy
		Free of gross blood
	Stool, when passed, is mushy, mixed with visible mucus or blood	Contains undigested food particles
Pain location	When present, likely to be in hypogastrium, in left or right lower quadrant, or in sacral region	When present, likely to be periumbilical or in right lower quadrant
Pain quality	Gripping, aching, or with tenesmus (ineffective, painful straining at stool)	Intermittent, cramplike, accompanied by borborygmus (gurgling, splashing sound)

Data from Krejs, C., & Fordtran, J. (1983). Diarrhea. In M. H. Sleisenger & J. S. Fordtran (Eds.), *Gastrointestinal disease: Pathophysiology, diagnosis, management* (3rd ed.). Philadelphia: W. B. Saunders.

Statistics from the World Health Organization (1975) report a 400-fold increase in mortality associated with GI infections in the elder. Reduced motility and gastric acidity, which can accompany aging and result from either gastric surgery or the use of medication, can increase susceptibility to viral pathogens (e.g., rotavirus and Norwalk agent) (Sundaram, 1993) and to bacterial agents (e.g., *Shigella, Clostridium difficile, Salmonella, Campylobacter, Staphylococcus aureus, Clostridium botulism*) (Cunha, 1998; McFarland & Stamm, 1986; Sundaram, 1993; Vartian & Septimus, 1986). Bacterial endotoxins (e.g., clostridial and staphylococcal toxins) can be present in food that is improperly prepared or refrigerated or can be formed in the GI tract by organisms such as *Escherichia coli* (Bond, 1982). The elderly, particularly those living in rural areas where private and municipal water sources can become contaminated by infected animals, can become infected by intestinal parasites (e.g., protozoa *Giardia lamblia, Cryptosporidium*) or (less commonly in the United States) by *Entamoeba histolytic* (Bond, 1982; Sundaram, 1993). Infectious diarrhea can occur following travel, especially to a foreign country where bacterial contamination of water supplies is common. Diverticula are saccular outpouchings occurring through defects in the circular muscle layer of the colon (Burakoff, 1981). Fecal material becomes trapped within these diverticula, resulting in inflammation. Symptoms include lower quadrant abdominal pain, fever, and frequent episodes of diarrhea or diarrhea followed by severe constipation. Elders are especially prone to the development of diverticulitis, and the incidence increases with advancing age. It is estimated that as many as one half of adults over 70 years of age will have diverticular disease (Balson & Gibson, 1995; Burakoff, 1981; Vartian & Septimus, 1986).

Assessment factors specific to infection as an etiology in acute diarrhea differ depending on whether the organisms involve the small bowel or the colon. Small bowel infection usually produces "non-bloody, watery diarrhea and low-grade fever" (Vartian & Septimus, 1986, p. 55). Infection in the colon "can produce stools with blood, mucus and fecal leukocytes, usually in association with fever" (Vartian & Septimus, 1986, p. 56).

Drug Reactions.   Drugs can produce diarrhea as part of their intended effect, such as that produced by laxatives, or as a side effect other than the intended effect. Antibiotics frequently are accompanied by diarrhea because of alteration of normal flora or inflammation of intestinal mucosa. Antibiotics most often implicated in producing diarrhea are ampicillin, cephalosporin, clindamycin, lincomycin, neomycin, and tetracycline (Bond, 1982; Vogel, 1995). The prevalence of infections commonly treated with antibiotics (e.g., pneumonia, cholecystitis, and urinary tract infections) increases the magnitude of the problem of diarrhea in the elderly. An estimated 15% to 25% of the cases of antibiotic related diarrhea are caused by *Clostridium difficile*. Symptoms range from mild diarrhea to life threatening pseudomembranous colitis (Bartlett, 1990; Cartmill et al., 1994; Kelly, Pothoulakis, & LaMont, 1994; Vogel, 1995). Outbreaks of this infection pose a particular threat to institutionalized elders, since hospital or nursing home outbreaks can occur.

The prevalence of chronic illnesses in the elderly also increases their exposure to medications used to treat these conditions. A number of medications that commonly are prescribed for the elderly can cause diarrhea, including antacids, antibiotics, antihypertensives, cancer chemotherapeutic agents, colchicine, digitalis prepara-

Table 20-2 DIARRHEA
Related Factors/Etiologies and Defining Characteristics

NANDA (1999, p. 18)

Defining Characteristics

Abdominal pain
Cramping
Hyperactive bowel sounds
At least three loose liquid stools per day
Urgency

WADLE

Related Factors/Etiologies: Acute	Defining Characteristics
Infection	Small bowel; nonbloody; watery stools, low-grade fever; absence of fecal leukocytes; colon; bloody mucous stools with fecal leukocytes; fever
Drug reactions	Watery stools after medication ingestion, e.g., antibiotics, antihypertensives, digitalis preparations
Heavy metal poisoning (Krejs & Fordtran, 1983)	Watery stools of purging type with anorexia, abdominal pain, muscle cramps, and joint pain
Fecal impaction (Krejs & Fordtran, 1983)	Watery stools after a period of absence of bowel movement; digital identification of hard stool
Alteration in diet (McLane & McShane, 1993)	Change in diet pattern
	Increased fruit, vegetable, and lactose intake
	Tube feedings or formula
	Watery stools with cramping and flatulence

SPIRO (1993)

Related Factors/Etiologies: Chronic	Defining Characteristics
Lactase deficiency	Watery stools with gas and bloating
Laxative abuse	Severe, watery diarrhea, possible hypokalemia
Stress and anxiety	Watery stools, increased frequency
Inflammatory bowel disease, ulcerative colitis	Watery stools with abdominal cramps, rectal bleeding, fever, weakness
Irritable bowel syndrome	Alternating constipation and diarrhea, abdominal pain, psychologic factors, stressful life situations
Cancer of the colon	Reported change in bowel habits
Chemotherapeutic agents	Dependent upon agent
Radiation	Dependent upon site
Gastrointestinal surgery	Dependent upon site
Malabsorptive disorders, e.g., celiac sprue	Stools that are murky, frothy, and contain oil

tions, lactulose, potassium supplements, propranolol, and quinidine.

Obtaining a drug history is an important step in assessing the possibility of drug reaction as a cause of acute diarrhea. If the patient is unable to provide a reliable account of medications being taken, a record review or consultation with other health care professionals who have treated the patient is essential.

Diet Alterations. Dietary alterations among the elderly can be brought about by a number of factors, including economic problems, inability to shop for food fre-

quently, loss of teeth, and intolerance or inability to digest foods adequately. Ironically, changes in diet patterns can be brought about by institutionalization or dependence on mobile meal programs. In these situations, well-planned diets often are higher in fruit and vegetable products containing long-chain carbohydrates that are incompletely digested in the small intestine (Bond, 1982; Laurin, Brodeur, Bourdages, Vallee, & Lachapelle, 1994; McLane & McShane, 1993).

Economic factors can limit the elderly from purchasing expensive protein diet items and increase their consumption of carbohydrates or lactose-containing foods such as milk sugars. Lactose intolerance is associated with cramping, flatulence, and diarrhea (McLane & McShane, 1993). Tube feeding–associated diarrhea has been linked to milk-based formulas (Walike & Walike, 1973, 1977). Economic factors, as well as physical limitations, can inhibit the ability of the elderly to shop frequently for food items, limiting the types of foods they purchase and increasing the incidence of food spoilage caused by lengthy storage. Drug-food interactions can suppress or stimulate appetite, alter nutrient digestion and absorption, and alter the metabolism and excretion of nutrients (Roe, 1986).

The use of formula feedings in the elderly also can be associated with diarrhea. Suggested causes include the composition, osmolarity, and temperature of the feeding and the method of infusion (Taylor, 1982). Most formulas have been altered to be either low in lactose or lactose free, and some have been adjusted to be more compatible with the body's osmolarity requirements. Temperature of feedings and methods of infusion will be discussed in the section on nursing interventions. Assessment of diet habits, with particular attention to recent changes in eating patterns and foods ingested, is important in determining the effects of diet on elimination patterns.

Other Factors. Heavy metal poisoning can possibly cause acute diarrhea (Krejs & Fordtran, 1983). Because of their living conditions, elderly persons can be exposed to such things as lead content in old paint. The use of favorite old dishes or utensils with crazed or cracked finishes has been associated with heavy metal poisoning from lead content in pottery materials. Diarrhea of a purging type, along with anorexia, vomiting, abdominal pain, muscle cramps, and joint pain, is suggestive of heavy metal poisoning.

Fecal impaction is defined as a large, firm immovable mass of stool in the rectum or in some cases higher in the colon. Diarrhea is caused as liquid stool from the proximal colon is forced around the impaction (Krejs & Fordtran, 1983). This is a special risk factor for the elder because of dietary changes, decreased exercise patterns, and decreased GI function and circulation. The frequency of impaction is highest among institutionalized elders (Krejs & Fordtran, 1983). Assessment of fecal impaction is based on the presence of diarrhea after a period of absence of bowel movement and can be determined by digital examination of the lower bowel. X-ray examination is necessary to confirm fecal impaction high in the bowel.

Chronic Diarrhea

Sundaram (1993) identifies three categories of chronic diarrhea: (1) inflammatory diarrhea; (2) watery diarrhea without steatorrhea; and (3) steatorrhea. Inflammatory diarrhea is characterized by leukocytes and red blood cells in the stool, fever, abdominal pain, and often hypoproteinemia. Etiologies for chronic diarrhea include irritable bowel syndrome, lactase deficiency, cancer of the colon, inflammatory bowel disease, GI surgery, malabsorption disorders, laxative abuse, and alcohol use (McLane & McShane, 1993).

Irritable Bowel Syndrome. Irritable bowel syndrome is a motor disorder that is manifested by alternating constipation and diarrhea, abdominal pain, and the absence of detectable organic pathology. Psychologic factors and stressful life situations have been suggested as factors in the production of these symptoms (Schuster, 1983). The elder experiences many stressful life situations, such as retirement, loss of mate, chronic illness, and loss of independence, and can develop this syndrome as a response to these life losses. These factors should be assessed by interviewing the patient and family members familiar with significant life events.

Lactase Deficiency. Lactase deficiency and the resultant lactose intolerance are associated with diarrhea, gas, and bloating following the ingestion of milk, cheese, ice cream, or puddings and sauces made with milk or milk products (Alpers, 1983). Elders often include a high number of dairy items in their diet because they can be prepared quickly and they can be eaten comfortably by edentulous persons. In addition, dairy products often are more economically feasible to purchase than other foods. Lactase deficiency also can exaggerate symptoms of other intestinal disorders, such as irritable bowel syndrome or inflammatory bowel disease (Bond, 1982). A diet history can provide the nurse with useful assessment data. The incidence of lactose intolerance is highest among African-Americans, Native Americans, Mexican-Americans, and Jews (Englert & Guillory, 1986).

Colon Cancer. A change in bowel habits often is the earliest sign of cancer of the large bowel (Bond, 1982). Occult blood in stools or frank rectal bleeding, alternating diarrhea and constipation, increased gaseousness, and abdominal pain are presenting symptoms. Diets high in fat, protein, and beef and deficient in dietary fiber have been suggested as etiologic factors. Heredity also is a predisposing factor, as is inflammatory bowel disease. The malignancy itself, the agents used to treat the malignancy, and the immunocompromised state all can be implicated as causes of diarrhea (Ippoliti, 1998; Sundaram, 1993; Wadler et al., 1998). Risk for colorectal cancer rises sharply at age 50, doubling each decade after 40 years of age (Winawer & Sherlock, 1983).

Inflammatory Bowel Disease. Ulcerative colitis and Crohn's disease are the most common examples of inflammatory bowel disease. The diarrhea occurring in ulcerative colitis is accompanied by abdominal cramps, rectal bleeding, fever, and weakness (Bond, 1982). The cause is unknown, and although the disease often is diagnosed in younger persons, the incidence of onset in persons over age 50 is almost equal to the incidence of onset in younger persons. Treatment of inflammatory bowel disease is complicated by a high incidence of diabetes, arteriosclerosis, hypertension, emphysema, and diverticulosis in the elderly population (Cello, 1983). Crohn's disease also is of unknown etiology and, although a more common problem in younger persons, it is increasingly diagnosed in persons over 60 years of age (Foxworthy & Wilson, 1985). Symptoms of Crohn's disease are similar to those in ulcerative colitis, but rectal bleeding is less common. Perianal ulcerations, fistulas, and abscesses are associated with Crohn's disease.

Gastrointestinal Surgery. Surgery to treat ulcerative colitis, Crohn's disease, or tumors of the GI tract causes varying degrees of diarrhea and malabsorption, depending on the portion of the GI system removed. Gastric surgery increases the rate of entry of osmotically active carbohydrates through the small bowel, resulting in diarrhea. Major small bowel resections result in severe diarrhea and malabsorption (Bond, 1982) because of the decrease in surface area of the small bowel normally used to absorb fluid and nutrients into the bloodstream. As a result, the contents of the bowel contain a higher percentage of water as they pass through the GI system and are excreted. Record review, consultation with treating professionals, patient interview, and inspection for surgical scars are sources of assessment data for the nurse.

Malabsorption Disorders. Celiac sprue is a disease of malabsorption of nutrients associated with lesions of the small intestine and related to gluten intolerance. Gluten is a substance found in cereal grains. The first onset of symptoms often is in childhood, with a second onset in persons age 40 to 50 (Broadwell, 1986; Fine, Meyer, & Lee, 1997; Trier, 1983). The diarrhea of celiac sprue is related to increased volume and osmotic load introduced into the colon because it is malabsorbed by the small intestine and is aggravated by dietary fats and bile salts (Broadwell, 1986). Dietary habit assessment should include a review of specific foods associated with production of diarrhea. Stools of patients with malabsorption disorders are described as murky, frothy, and containing oil (Krejs & Fordtran, 1983).

Laxative Use. Laxative use and abuse can result from the elderly's concern for lessened frequency of bowel movements. A drug history taken by the nurse should include a review of laxative use.

Alcohol Use. Alcohol ingestion, an increasingly recognized problem in the elderly, is likely to cause malabsorption in the elderly patient (Roe, 1986). Other factors that link alcohol abuse to the production of diarrhea include exocrine pancreatic insufficiency, vitamin defi-

ciencies, hypermotility, inhibited jejunal water, and electrolyte absorption (Lipsitz et al., 1981; Martin, Justus, & Mathias, 1980). Patients' significant others should be interviewed to assess the use of alcohol as a factor contributing to diarrhea in the elder.

ASSESSMENT

Assessment Guide 20-1 presents an assessment tool developed for the nursing diagnosis of diarrhea.

NURSING DIAGNOSIS

"Diarrhea is the state in which an individual experiences a change in normal bowel habits characterized by the frequent passage of loose, fluid, unformed stools" (McLane & McShane, 1993, p. 1480). NANDA defines diarrhea as the "passage of loose, unformed stools" (NANDA, 1999, p. 18). Generally agreed on defining characteristics of the nursing diagnosis Diarrhea include the following: abdominal pain, cramping, increased stool frequency, hyperactive bowel sounds, at least 3 loose liquid stools per day, and urgency (McLane & McShane, 1993; NANDA, 1999, p. 18). Carpenito (1992) defined increased frequency of stools as meaning more than three stools per day.

CASE STUDY

T. Anderson, a 75-year-old man with multiinfarct dementia, has resided in a long-term care facility for 4 years as a result of increasing confusion and debilitation. He is unable to ambulate even with assistance and sits up in a chair for several short periods throughout the day and evening. Mr. Anderson is edentulous and recently was placed on nasogastric tube feedings because of his inability to swallow even soft foods without choking. He has aspirated food on two occasions and had to be treated for aspiration pneumonia. Mr. Anderson has been receiving a lactose-free, isotonic formula delivered by continuous drip infusion. Potassium chloride elixir was added to the formula. After 1 week on this feeding regimen, Mr. Anderson had watery stools four or five times for 2 days. Table 20-3 provides information about differential diagnosis and assessment.

NURSING-SENSITIVE OUTCOMES

The goals for nursing interventions are related to assessment of causative or contributing factors, assessment of fluid and electrolytes, and completion of health teaching as indicated (Carpenito, 1992). In addition, McLane and McShane (1993) include as outcomes symptom relief, taking medication correctly, understanding the mechanism of diarrhea, and ingesting adequate fluids and foods. The outcome Bowel Elimination is defined as the "ability

ASSESSMENT TOOL FOR NURSING DIAGNOSIS DIARRHEA

DEFINING CHARACTERISTICS	**Present**	**Absent**
Abdominal pain		
Cramping		
Stool frequency greater than 3/day		
Increased frequency of bowel sounds		
Loose, liquid stools		
Urgency		

RELATED FACTORS/ETIOLOGIES	**Present**	**Absent**
Infection:		
• Stool culture + for bacteria		
• Stool culture + for parasites		
Recent travel to foreign country		
Diverticular disease		
Small bowel infection signs		
Nonbloody, watery diarrhea		
Low-grade fever		
Absence of fecal leukocytes		
Colon infection signs		
Stools with blood, mucus		
Presence of fecal leukocytes		
Fever		

DRUG REACTIONS	**Present**	**Absent**
Drug regimen includes:		
• Antacids		
• Antibiotics		
• Antihypertensives		
• Chemotherapeutic agents		
• Colchicine		
• Digitalis preparations		
• Lactulose		
• Potassium supplements		
• Prepanolol		
• Quinidine		
• Other drugs known to cause diarrhea		

DIETARY ALTERATIONS	**Present**	**Absent**
Recent history of diet changes		
Increased fruit and vegetable intake		
Increased lactose-containing foods		
Tube-feeding formula instituted or changed		

Continued

Assessment Guide 20-1—cont'd

ASSESSMENT TOOL FOR NURSING DIAGNOSIS DIARRHEA—cont'd

FECAL IMPACTION   **Present**   **Absent**

Absence of bowel movements for several days prior to diarrhea onset

HISTORY OF CHRONIC BOWEL DISORDER   **Present**   **Absent**

Irritable bowel disorder
Lactase deficiency
Cancer of colon
Gastrointestinal surgery
Malabsorption disease
Laxative use
Alcohol abuse

Table 20-3	Diarrhea: Differential Diagnosis and Assessment for MR. ANDERSON	
Nursing Assessments	**Diagnoses Ruled Out**	**Additional Data Needed**
Watery stools, negative for blood 4-5 times/ day of 2 days' duration No history of chronic gastrointestinal disease	Diarrhea associated with chronic bowel diseases such as cancer, inflammatory bowel disease	Evidence of malabsorption
Lactose-free formula Negative stool culture and feeding/tubing cultures	Lactose intolerance Infectious disease	Additional cultures of feeding/ tubing to rule out contamination caused in administering
Absence of fever Normal WBC No recent change/significant life events Addition of potassium chloride nitrogen elixir to drug regimen	Irritable bowel syndrome	Serum albumin level Urine urea concentration Evidence of malnutrition (muscle wasting, skin and hair changes, edema)

---

of the gastrointestinal tract to form and evacuate stool effectively" (Iowa Outcomes Project, 2000, p. 127). The ultimate outcome goal is for the elder to experience as nearly normal an elimination pattern as possible: soft formed stool of normal volume and color. Additional desired outcomes include an intact defecation urge sensation, freedom from pain or cramping, and normal motility and bowel sounds. Table 20-4 relates the nursing diagnosis, outcomes, and interventions as described in the literature.

Additional outcomes formulated in the *Nursing Outcomes Classification (NOC)* (Iowa Outcomes Project, 2000) relate to specific causative factors (e.g., "fat within normal range in stool" or "free of blood . . . mucus in stool") (Iowa Outcomes Project, 2000). Refer to Table 20-2

for etiologies related to these symptoms. Similarly, additional nursing interventions identified by the Iowa Intervention Project (2000) would relate to specific causative factors (e.g., "obtain stool for culture and sensitivity" would relate to an infectious cause, whereas "suggest trial elimination of foods containing lactose" would relate to a suspected lactase deficiency). Such an intervention would be Diarrhea Management, which is defined as "management and alleviation of diarrhea" (Iowa Intervention Project, 2000, p. 256).

Monitoring of intake and output, of laboratory test results, and of skin, hair and muscle quality will provide ongoing evaluation of the patient's fluid, electrolyte, and nutritional status.

Table 20-4 **DIARRHEA**

Suggested Nursing-Sensitive Outcome and Nursing Intervention

Nursing Diagnosis	Nursing-Sensitive Outcome	Nursing Intervention
DIARRHEA *Defining Characteristics* At least three loose liquid stools per day	**BOWEL ELIMINATION** *Indicators* Stool soft and formed	**DIARRHEA MANAGEMENT** *Activities* Instruct patient/family members to record color, volume, frequency, and consistency of stools
Increased frequency of stools (more than three times diarrhea) Urgency	Elimination pattern in expected range Defecation urge sensation intact	Identify factors that may cause or contribute to per day diarrhea Consult physician if signs and symptoms of diarrhea persist
Cramping; abdominal pain	Ease of stool passage; painful cramps not present	Measure diarrhea/bowel output
Hyperactive bowel sounds	Normal bowel sounds present Intestinal motility in expected range	
Increased fluidity or volume of stools (Carpenito, 1992) Change in color of stools (McLane & McShane, 1993)	Stool amount normal for diet Stool soft and formed Stool color within normal limits	

NURSING INTERVENTIONS

Enteral Tube-Feeding Interventions

The major nursing intervention studies have focused on tube feedings. Anderson (1986) states that properly administered tube feedings do not cause diarrhea, but patients on tube feedings sometimes develop diarrhea from an underlying problem or from therapy. Malnutrition, osmolality, drug therapy, contaminated formula, and methods of administration can be associated with diarrhea in patients receiving tube feedings.

A research-based lactose-free tube-feeding protocol has been developed for clinical testing (Horsley, Crane, & Haller, 1981). The research suggests that diarrhea, as well as other symptoms of GI distress (e.g., nausea, belching, flatulence) for lactose-intolerant individuals, will be reduced if lactose is removed from tube-feeding formulas (Walike & Walike, 1973, 1977; Walike et al., 1975). Improved nutrition also is expected to result. In general, it is recommended that all persons with tube feedings be given lactose-free diets. Because of the special needs of elderly clients, lactose-free diets that also are low in sodium, residue, or protein should be available. Nurses, physicians, and dietitians need to be knowledgeable of the prevalence, the clinical significance, and the physiology of lactose intolerance among the elderly to implement and evaluate the protocol successfully.

Malnutrition, which can be a consequence of serious illness or of underfeeding, results in malabsorption of nutrients and diarrhea. The diarrhea, in turn, can worsen the malnutrition (Anderson, 1986). Malabsorption can be treated with a chemically defined or free amino acid formula to improve nutritional status (Konstantinides & Shronts, 1983). Slowing the rate of feeding to 20 to 30 ml/hr also can aid absorption of nutrients (Anderson, 1986).

Tube-feeding formulas frequently are diluted with water to "offset the diarrhea that the osmotic load of full-strength formula often is assumed to cause" (Anderson, 1986, p. 704). Anderson states that patients might be able to absorb undiluted, hyperosmotic loads unless malnutrition, poor visceral protein status, and depleted GI mucosa alter the osmotic gradient. Most formulas are isosmotic (approximately 300 mOsm/kg H_2O) and need not be diluted (Anderson, 1986). Malnourished patients with serum albumin levels below 3 g/dl can be given hyperosmotic solutions at half strength at a slow (25 ml/hr) rate (Anderson, 1986; Konstantinides & Shronts, 1983; Martyn-Nemeth & Fitzgerald, 1992).

Antibiotics or other drugs (e.g., potassium chloride) that change the osmolality of formula can be associated with diarrhea in tube-fed patients. Antacids, digitalis, and antidysrhythmic drugs also can cause diarrhea. Lactobacillus preparations can aid in combatting drug-induced diarrhea by slowing motility (Anderson, 1986; Konstantinides & Shronts, 1983).

Method of formula administration can be related to diarrhea in tube-fed patients. Replacing an intermittent or bolus feeding procedure with a continuous drip procedure, either by gravity flow or by mechanical feeding pump, is suggested to reduce the risks of GI side effects such as diarrhea. Taylor (1982), in a comparison of gravity flow and continuous infusion pump tube feeding in neurosurgical patients, found that diarrhea occurred in both methods of tube feeding. Another study of 80 patients found that use of an infusion pump controlled diarrhea in 10 of the patients who had serious GI disorders but was less successful in patients with poor gastric emptying or swallowing reflex impairment (Jones, Payne, & Silk, 1980).

The temperature of the formula has been suggested as a cause of diarrhea, with reference to the need to give the feeding at room temperature or to heat it to body temperature (Griggs & Hoppe, 1979). However, a study of gastric motility in monkeys found that the temperature of the formula affected gastric motility for only 6 minutes. The gastric motility rate then returned to fasting baseline rate (Williams & Walike, 1975). Heating formula can promote the growth of bacteria and, in itself, present a cause for diarrhea in debilitated patients (Bettice, 1971). Nursing interventions for infection control are recommended. Several studies of tube-feeding systems have found caregivers' hands to be the major source of contamination; these studies support the need for meticulous handwashing procedures (Iannini, Mumford, & Buckalew, 1983; Schreiner, Lemons, & Jansen, 1983; Schroeder, Fisher, & Paloucek, 1983). Additional measures to prevent contamination of tube-feeding systems include hanging a fresh feeding every 4 to 8 hours (never add new formula to formula that has been hanging) and changing feeding containers and tubing every day. Unnecessary handling or manipulation of the feeding system should be avoided (Konstantinides & Shronts, 1983).

The nurse can manage diarrhea associated with tube feedings by adjusting the type of tube feeding used, by monitoring the rate of infusion based on patient tolerance, and by preventing contamination of feedings by careful hand washing in preparing, administering, and monitoring the feeding (Carpenito, 1992; McLane & McShane, 1993). Because of the danger of greater dehydration, Anderson (1986) stresses that tube feedings should be continued while measures are instituted to treat the diarrhea, since stopping tube feedings poses an even greater danger from dehydration.

Teaching Interventions

Another area of suggested nursing interventions for Diarrhea involves patient teaching regarding prescribed medication use and side effects, medication management, prescribed diet, stress reduction, and aseptic techniques (Carpenito, 1992; McLane & McShane, 1993). Patient teaching can present a special challenge to the nurse working with the elderly. Alzheimer's disease or other organic brain disorders can limit the patient's ability to learn. The elder also might not have an available support

system wherein others can be taught to help the patient manage these aspects of life. Teaching should definitely be used as an intervention for elders who can profit from it. If teaching is not feasible, referral to appropriate support systems might be necessary.

Other Suggested Interventions

Monitoring food and fluid intake and replacement of lost fluids are other suggested nursing interventions (McLane & McShane, 1993). Carpenito (1992) suggests increasing oral intake to maintain urine specific gravity at normal levels (1.003 to 1.030) and encouraging fluids high in potassium and sodium. Intravenous replacement of fluid and electrolytes might be required. The nurse's role in diarrhea management, especially for cancer patients, is outlined by Hogan (1998). Nurses can monitor body weight, skin condition, and laboratory findings to assess nutrition, hydration, and electrolyte levels.

Perirectal skin can become excoriated because of the acidity and digestive enzyme content of diarrheal stools (Carpenito, 1992; McLane & McShane, 1993). Measures suggested in the literature to treat skin problems associated with diarrhea include thorough cleansing with mild soap and warm water following each diarrheal stool. Applying soothing ointment or spray and exposing the irritated skin to the air also are suggested (Englert & Guillory, 1986).

CASE STUDY

The nursing interventions instituted for Mr. Anderson included diluting the formula to half strength and slowing the rate of the continuous drip feeding to 25 ml/hr. An antidiarrheal agent was added to his drug regimen to slow gastric motility and aid in the absorption of nutrients in the feeding. The nurse did not mix any medications with the feeding. Rather, the feeding was stopped, the tubing was cleansed, and medications were given by feeding tube; the feeding was restarted in 30 minutes. Mr. Anderson's diarrhea subsided within 36 hours of these interventions, and he passed a small, soft, formed stool after 48 hours. The antidiarrheal agent was stopped.

Throughout the period of diarrhea Mr. Anderson's perirectal skin was cleansed with warm, soapy water, thoroughly rinsed with clean water, and allowed to air dry. Then the perirectal skin was lightly covered with a soothing, waterproof ointment to prevent further irritation and excoriation. Skin redness gradually lessened, and the area was healed with 3 days of the cessation of diarrhea. The addition of potassium chloride elixir had altered the osmolality of the feeding. Based on continuous monitoring of Mr. Anderson's laboratory findings, the potassium chloride elixir was stopped. The feeding was returned to full strength to deliver adequate calories to maintain adequate nutrition.

SUMMARY

The elderly are subject to physiologic changes of the GI system, which can be manifested as acute or chronic diarrhea. Most current interventions are based on an understanding of the physiology of the GI system. Nurses need to develop a comprehensive research base for nursing interventions used to manage acute and chronic diarrhea. Skin care methods, tube-feeding procedures, and the effectiveness of patient teaching all should be studied. Further studies on the effects of variables such as temperature, caffeine, tobacco products, and food substances on GI motility also are required. Finally, the feasibility of nursing interventions and their acceptability to the patient remain to be evaluated.

REFERENCES

Alpers, D. (1983). Dietary management and vitamin-mineral replacement therapy. In M. H. Sleisenger & J. S. Fordtran (Eds.), *Gastrointestinal disease: Pathophysiology, diagnosis, management* (3rd ed., pp. 1819-1831). Philadelphia: W. B. Saunders.

Anderson, B. J. (1986). Tube feeding: Is diarrhea inevitable? *American Journal of Nursing, 86*(6), 710F-710H.

Balson, R., & Gibson, P. R. (1995, February). Prescribing for the elderly: Lower gastrointestinal tract (2) Diarrhea and diverticular disease. *The Medicine Journal of Australia, 162,* 217-219.

Bartlett, J. G. (1990). Clostridium difficile: Clinical considerations. *Review of Infectious Diseases, 12*(Suppl. 2), 243-251.

Bettice, D. (1971). The case of vomiting of tube feedings by neurosurgical patients. *Journal of Neurosurgical Nurse, 3,* 93-111.

Bond, J. H. (1982, February). Office-based management of diarrhea. *Geriatrics, 37,* 52-64.

Broadwell, D. C. (1986). Gastrointestinal system. In J. M. Thompson, G. K. McFarland, J. E. Hirsch, S. M. Tucker, & A. C. Bowers (Eds.), *Clinical nursing* (pp. 1105-1279). St. Louis, MO: Mosby.

Burakoff, R. (1981, March). An updated look at diverticular disease. *Geriatrics, 36,* 83-91.

Carpenito, L. J. (1992). *Nursing diagnosis—Application to clinical practice* (pp. 190-194). Baltimore: Lippincott Williams & Wilkins.

Carroll-Johnson, R. (Ed.). (1989). *Classification of nursing diagnoses: Proceedings of the eighth conference.* Baltimore: Lippincott Williams & Wilkins.

Cartmill, T. D., Panigrahi, H., Worsley, M. A., McCann, D. C., Nice, C. N., & Keith, E. (1994). Management and control of a large outbreak of diarrhea due to clostridium difficile. *Journal of Hospital Infections, 27*(1), 1-15.

Cello, J. (1983). Ulcerative colitis. In M. H. Sleisenger & J. S. Fordtran (Eds.), *Gastrointestinal disease: Pathophysiology, diagnosis, management* (3rd ed., pp. 1122-1168). Philadelphia: W. B. Saunders.

Cooper, G. S., Shlaes, D. M., & Salata, R. A. (1994). Intraabdominal infection: Differences in presentation and outcomes between younger patients and the elderly. *Clinical Infectious Diseases, 19,* 146-148.

Cunha, B. A. (1998). Nosocomial diarrhea. *Critical Care Clinics, 14*(2), 329-338.

Dupont, H. L. (1997). Guidelines on acute infectious diarrhea in

adults. *American Journal of Gastroenterology, 92*(11), 1962-1975.

Eglow, R., & Burakoff, R. (1991, November 15). Acute diarrhea in the elderly patient. *Emergency Medicine, 23,* 19-34.

Englert, D. M., & Guillory, J. A. (1986). For want of lactase. *American Journal of Nursing, 86*(8), 902-906.

Fine, K. D., Krejs, G., & Fordtran, J. S. (1993). Diarrhea. In M. S. Sleisenger & J. S. Fordtran (Eds.), *Gastrointestinal disease: Pathophysiology, diagnosis, management* (5th ed., pp. 1043-1071). Philadelphia: W. B. Saunders.

Fine, K. D., Meyer, R. L., & Lee, E. L. (1997). The prevalence and causes of chronic diarrhea in patients with celiac sprue treated with a gluten-free diet. *Gastroenterology, 112,* 1830-1838.

Foxworthy, D. M., & Wilson, J. A. (1985). Crohn's disease in the elderly. Prolonged delay in diagnosis. *Journal of the American Geriatrics Society, 33,* 492-495.

Griggs, B. A., & Hoppe, M. C. (1979). Nasogastric tube feeding. *American Journal of Nursing, 79,* 481-485.

Hogan, C. M. (1998). The nurse's role in diarrhea management. *Oncology Nursing Forum, 25*(5), 879-886.

Horsley, J., Crane, J., & Haller, K. (1981). *Reducing diarrhea in tube-fed patients: CURN project.* New York: Grune & Stratton.

Iannini, P. B., Mumford, F., & Buckalew, F. (1983). *Microbial contamination of enteral liquid nutritional systems.* Proceedings of the Ross Laboratories Workshop on Contamination of Feeding Products During Clinical Use. Columbus, OH: Ross Laboratories.

Iowa Intervention Project. J. C. McCloskey & G. M. Bulechek (Eds.). (2000). *Nursing interventions classification (NIC)* (3rd ed.). St. Louis, MO: Mosby.

Iowa Outcomes Project. M. Johnson, M. Maas, & S. Moorhead (Eds.). (2000). *Nursing outcomes classification (NOC)* (2nd ed.). St. Louis, MO: Mosby.

Ippoliti, C. (1998). Antidiarrheal agents for the management of treatment-related diarrhea in cancer patients. *American Journal of Health System Pharmacy, 55*(15), 1573-1580.

Jones, B. J., Payne, S., & Silk, D. B. (1980). Indications for pump-assisted enteral feeding. *Lancet, 1*(8177), 1057-1058.

Kelly, C. P., Pothoulakis, C., & LaMont, J. T. (1994). Clostridium difficile colitis. *New England Journal of Medicine, 330,* 257-262.

Konstantinides, N. N., & Shronts, E. (1983). Tube feeding: Managing the basics. *American Journal of Nursing, 83*(9), 1312-1320.

Krejs, C., & Fordtran, J. (1983). Diarrhea. In M. H. Sleisenger & J. S. Fordtran (Eds.), *Gastrointestinal disease: Pathophysiology, diagnosis, management* (3rd ed., pp. 257-280). Philadelphia: W. B. Saunders.

Laurin, D., Brodeur, J. M., Bourdages, J., Vallee, R., & Lachapelle, D. (1994). Fiber intake in elderly individuals with poor masticatory performance. *Journal of Canadian Dental Association, 60*(5), 443-449.

Lipsitz, H. D., Porter, L. E., Schade, R. R., Gottlieg, G. P., Graham, T. O., & Van Thiel, D. H. (1981). Gastrointestinal and hepatic manifestations of chronic alcoholism. *Gastroenterology, 81,* 594-615.

Martin, J. L., Justus, P. G., & Mathias, J. R. (1980). Altered motility of the small intestine in response to ethanol (ETOH): An explanation for the diarrhea associated with the consumption of alcohol. *Gastroenterology, 78,* 1218.

Martyn-Nemeth, P., & Fitzgerald, K. (1992). Clinical considerations: Tube feeding in the elderly. *Journal of Gerontological Nursing, 18*, 30-36.

McFarland, L. V., & Stamm, W. E. (1986). Review of Clostridium difficile-associated diseases. *American Journal of Infection Control, 14*(3), 99-109.

McLane, A. M., & McShane, R. E. (1993). Bowel elimination, alteration in Diarrhea: Theory and etiology. In J. M. Thompson, G. K. McFarland, J. E. Hirsch, & S. M. Tucker (Eds.), *Clinical nursing* (pp. 1480-1481). St. Louis, MO: Mosby.

North American Nursing Diagnosis Association. (1999). *Nursing diagnoses: Definitions and classification 1999-2000.* Philadelphia: Author.

Roe, D. A. (1986, March). Drug-nutrient interactions in the elderly. *Geriatrics, 41*, 57-74.

Ross, D. G. (1993). Subjective data related to altered bowel elimination patterns among hospitalized elderly and middle-aged persons. *Orthopaedic Nursing, 12*(5), 25-32.

Schmucker, D. L., & Daniels, C. I. (1986). Aging, gastrointestinal infections and mucosal immunity. *Journal of the American Geriatrics Society, 34*, 377-384.

Schreiner, R. I., Lemons, J. A., & Jansen, R. D. (1983). *Microbial contamination of continuous-drip feedings in the newborn intensive care unit.* Proceedings of the Ross Laboratories Workshop on Contamination of Enteral Feeding Products During Clinical Use. Columbus, OH: Ross Laboratories.

Schroeder P., Fisher, D., & Paloucek, J. (1983). *A survey of factors leading to microbial contamination of enteral feeding solutions in a community hospital.* Proceedings of the Ross Laboratories Workshop on Contamination of Enteral Feeding Products During Clinical Use. Columbus, OH: Ross Laboratories.

Schuster, M. (1983). Irritable bowel syndrome. In M. H. Sleisenger & J. S. Fordtran (Eds.), *Gastrointestinal disease: Pathophysiology, diagnosis, management* (3rd ed., pp. 880-896). Philadelphia: W. B. Saunders.

Spiro, H. (Ed.) (1993). *Clinical gastroenterology* (4th ed). Hightstown, N. J.: McGraw-Hill.

Stolley, J. M., & Buckwalter, K. C. (1991). Nosocomial infections. *Journal of Gerontological Nursing, 17*(9), 30-34.

Sundaram, U. (1993). Small intestinal disorders: General considerations. In H. Spiro (Ed.), *Clinical gastroenterology* (4th ed., pp. 343-366). Hightstown, N. J.: McGraw-Hill.

Taylor, T. T. (1982). A comparison of two methods of nasogastric tube feedings. *Journal of Neurosurgical Nursing, 14*(1), 49-55.

Trier, J. (1983). Celiac sprue. In M. H. Sleisenger & J. S. Fordtran (Eds.), *Gastrointestinal disease pathophysiology, diagnosis, management* (3rd ed., pp. 1050-1069). Philadelphia: W. B. Saunders.

Vartian, C. V., & Septimus, E. J. (1986, February). Intra-abdominal infections in the elderly: Diagnosis and management. *Geriatrics, 41*, 51-56.

Vogel, L. C. (1995). Antibiotic-induced diarrhea. *Orthopaedic Nursing, 14*(2), 38-41.

Wadler, S., Benson, A. B., III, Engelking, C., Catalano, R., Field, M., Kornblau, S. M., Mitchell, E., Rubin, J., Trotta, P., & Vokes, E. (1998). Recommended guidelines for the treatment of chemotherapy-induced diarrhea. *Journal of Clinical Oncology, 16*(9), 3169-3178.

Walike, B., & Walike, J. (1973). Lactose content of tube feeding diets as a cause of diarrhea. *The Laryngoscope, 83*, 1109-1115.

Walike, B., & Walike, J. (1977). Relative lactose intolerance. *Journal of the American Medical Association, 238*, 948-951.

Walike, B. C., Padilla, G., Berstrom, N., Hanson, R. L., Kubo, W., Grant, M., & Wong, H. L. (1975). Patient problems related to tube feeding. In M. V. Bately (Ed.), *Communicating nursing research* (Vol 7, pp. 89-112). Boulder, CO: WICHE.

Williams, K. R., & Walike, B. C. (1975). Effect of the temperature of tube feeding on gastric motility in monkeys. *Nurse Research, 24*, 4-9.

Winawer, S., & Sherlock, P. (1983). Malignant neoplasms of the small and large intestine. In M. H. Sleisenger & J. S. Fordtran (Eds.), *Gastrointestinal disease: Pathophysiology, diagnosis, management* (3rd ed., pp. 1220-1249). Philadelphia: W. B. Saunders.

World Health Statistics Annual: I. (1975). *Vital statistics and cause of death.* Washington, DC: World Health Organization.

CHAPTER 21

BOWEL INCONTINENCE

Meridean L. Maas and Janet P. Specht

Bowel incontinence is a common problem for elderly persons, especially for those who are institutionalized or for those who suffer from chronic illnesses (Chassagne et al., 1999). The North American Nursing Diagnosis Association (NANDA) has defined bowel incontinence as "a state in which an individual experiences a change in normal bowel habits characterized by involuntary passage of stool" (NANDA, 1999). Whenever it occurs, bowel incontinence is degrading and embarrassing and creates distress for elders and for those who care for them. In addition to the inconvenience and psychologic distress it causes, bowel incontinence contributes to impaired skin integrity and urinary tract infections, especially among elderly women (Hogstel & Nelson, 1992).

Neural control of the bowel occurs through sympathetic and parasympathetic innervation. Sympathetic fibers at the level of thoracic vertebrae 11 and 12 (T11 and T12) and lumbar vertebrae 1 and 2 (L1 and L2) form the hypogastric nerve (adrenergic). The sympathetic system constricts sphincters and inhibits peristalsis. Parasympathetic fibers controlling the bowel, found in the vagus nerve and in fibers originating at sacral vertebrae 2, 3, and 4 (S2, S3, and S4), travel through the hypogastric plexus to form the plexus called the pelvic nerve (cholinergic). Normal defecation includes the action of two reflexes (King & Harke, 1994). The inferior myenteric plexus in the large colon joins with the hypogastric nerve to control the intrinsic reflex. The second reflex is in the sacral segments of the spinal cord (Figure 21-1). These reflexes are usually initiated after eating, especially after the first meal of the day, when a strong peristaltic wave pushes fecal matter into the rectum. The distention in the rectum stimulates a defecation reflex through the myenteric plexus to initiate further peristaltic waves from the descending colon toward the anus. The internal anal sphincter relaxes as the waves reach it, and if the external anal sphincter is also relaxed, defecation will occur. Voluntary control of evacuation is initiated by contracting the external sphincter, which reduces peristalsis and the urge to defecate. The external anal sphincter is innervated by the pudendal nerve, a voluntary motor nerve that originates in S2, S3, and S4.

Defecation is weak and ineffective unless aided by the spinal reflex. Stimulation to the rectum initiates signals through nerves to S2, S3, and S4 of the spinal cord, which in turn send impulses to intensify the peristaltic waves. A person with normal control is able to feel the desire to defecate when the stool enters and distends the rectum. The spinal reflex can be overridden by conscious inhibition from the anterior hypothalmic region of the brain, resulting in contraction of the external sphincter. The defecation reflex will die out in a few minutes if the person prevents defecation. The reflex may not return for several hours. The reflex may be reinitiated by taking a deep breath or bearing down (increasing intraabdominal pressure), but the reflex initiated in this way is not as effective as when it occurs naturally. Prolonged inhibition will result in progressive ineffectiveness of the defecation reflex.

Regular physical activity and exercise are important for maintaining normal bowel function. Physical activity assists with muscle tonicity needed for fecal expulsion and increases circulation to the digestive system, which assists with the development of feces that are more easily evacuated and promotes peristalsis. Anorectal continence refers to the ability to retain feces in order to evacuate at an appropriate time and place. Ordinarily the ability to control defecation is attained around 2 years of age.

Normal bowel function and continence depend on several factors (King & Harke, 1994; Wald, 1986). First, there must be normal delivery of feces to the rectum. Second, intact anal and rectal sensation is necessary. Third, the ability to contract the external anal sphincter and the puborectalis muscle to create the anorectal angle must be present, and the nervous system in general must be intact. Henry (1983) describes the preservation of an angle between the lower rectum and the upper canal, the anorectal angle, as the most important factor in preserving continence. Figure 21-2 illustrates the angle that is created by the pull of the puborectalis muscle away from the rectum. The fourth factor is the motivation and the cognitive ability to recognize rectal signals and make the appropriate decision to defecate or postpone defecation until a more appropriate time and place. The fifth factor is the ability of the rectum to accommodate the storage of feces. Hemorrhoids; inflammation due to colitis, infection, or irradiation; and surgical revisions are some of the causes of impaired reservoir capacity (Wald, 1986).

Loss of bowel continence by elderly persons is often a source of embarrassment, can deprive the person of social contacts, can affect self-esteem adversely, and creates un-

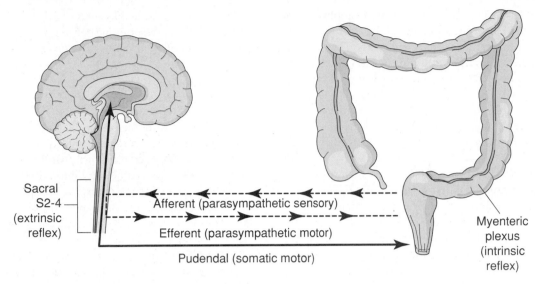

FIGURE **21-1**   Defecation reflex.

pleasant caregiving tasks for family or other attendants. Even if control of feces can be managed sufficiently to avoid socially disruptive occurrences, uncontrolled flatus can lead to altered lifestyle and limited social interactions. Furthermore, bowel incontinence can result in serious adverse consequences, such as impaired skin integrity and infection. Nurses who are sensitive to these consequences and who are equipped with the knowledge of bowel physiology and the ability to diagnose and treat bowel incontinence can positively affect the quality of life for many elderly persons.

Unfortunately, few articles in the nursing and medical literature have focused on bowel incontinence. More attention has been given to constipation and diarrhea, which often are associated with bowel incontinence (see Chapters 19 and 20). However, bowel incontinence can occur in the absence of these conditions. The focus on diarrhea and constipation alone limits comprehensive bowel management to achieve regularity and control of evacuation. The lack of development of this diagnosis is a reflection of the inattention to the problem of incontinence.

PREVALENCE

The incidence of Bowel Incontinence, often labeled fecal incontinence, is estimated to be from 10% to 23% among elderly persons in nursing homes (Chassagne et al., 1999; Tobin & Brocklehurst, 1986). The problem is less frequent among community dwelling elders but increases with age (Gordon et al., 1999). Along with urinary incontinence, fecal incontinence is a major problem experienced by institutionalized elderly persons (Chassagne et al., 1999; Tobin & Brocklehurst, 1986). Although it is a less frequent problem than urinary incontinence, bowel incontinence is more unpleasant for elderly persons and for caregivers. Fecal incontinence most frequently occurs with urinary incontinence among long-term institutionalized elders (Brockelhurst, 1985a; Nelson, Furner, & Jesudason, 1998).

RELATED FACTORS/ETIOLOGIES

There is a lack of documented information about age-related structure and function of the large intestine or

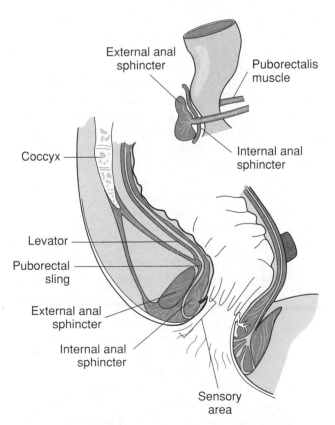

FIGURE **21-2**   Anorectal structural components.

changes in defecation. A slight decreased motility in the small intestine has been documented, but not enough to cause significant impairment of function. There are no documented changes in motility in the large intestine, although there is decreased mucus secretion and elasticity of the intestinal wall (Miller, 1990). Goldman (1979) reported that studies of stool specimens in elders showed little evidence of undigested nutrients. This is evidence that the digestive process is adequate in normal elderly persons.

Brocklehurst (1985b) discussed three major causes of bowel incontinence. The first is underlying disease of the colon, rectum, or anus, for example, diverticular disease, proctitis, cancer of the colon or rectum, hemorrhoids, prolapse, or colitis. Nurses should carefully observe and refer instances of fecal incontinence for further medical evaluation, since the underlying cause is often treatable, and more serious problems often can be prevented with prompt treatment.

Constipation of long standing, fecal impaction, is the second major cause of incontinence in the elder (Brocklehurst, 1985b; Kinnunen, 1991). Incontinence may take the form either of diarrhea around the impaction or of "smearing" from having the rectum full and not emptied. A study reported by Brocklehurst (1985b) found that a larger percentage of elderly persons with bowel incontinence had rectums with larger quantities of feces than did persons without incontinence. It is important for nurses to be aware that the stool found in the rectum of constipated individuals is not always hard and dry, but often can be soft and puttylike in consistency, even if transit time is as long as 7 days (Brocklehurst & Khan, 1969). This tends to negate the long-accepted belief that constipation can be eliminated simply by increasing fluids and fiber. Henry (1983) asserted that overdistention of the rectum by feces causes a continuous stimulation of the reflex, resulting in reduced internal and sphincter tone. If a client is constipated, nurses can monitor and intervene to prevent impactions (see Chapter 15).

The third major cause of bowel incontinence discussed by Brocklehurst (1985b) is a neurogenic change in the rectum similar to the hyperreflexia found in the bladders of elderly persons with urge urinary incontinence (see Chapter 22). In a study comparing the toleration of a distended balloon in the rectum between incontinent elderly men and elderly men without bowel incontinence, the incontinent men expelled the inflated balloon in response to rectal contractions that they were unable to inhibit (Brocklehurst, 1985b). On the other hand, the men who were not incontinent were able to retain the balloon by overriding the urge to defecate. Chassagne et al. (1999) documented five risk factors for the development of fecal incontinence in a sample of 1186 nursing home residents age 60 and older: a history of urinary incontinence, neurologic disease, poor mobility, severe cognitive decline, and age older than 70.

The most common etiologies of Bowel Incontinence in elders and the corresponding defining characteristics listed by NANDA (1999) and others are given in Table 21-1.

RISK FACTORS

Many elders have colon disorders. These disorders can result from a combination of factors such as diseases, dietary changes, environment, inadequate fluid intake, inadequate dietary fiber, improper positioning, and medication (Matteson, McConnell, & Linton, 1997; Wald, 1993).

The higher incidence of chronic illnesses and the functional losses with aging predispose the elder to increased problems with bowel continence. Elders not only are more apt to contract a disease that affects bowel function but also are more apt to have mobility and cognitive impairments that make them unable to maintain bowel control. For instance, an elderly woman who has had colitis for a number of years can anticipate frequent loose stools and plan trips to the toilet to avoid incontinence. If she becomes less mentally capable or less mobile, she will likely be incontinent. Bowel incontinence also is prevalent among elderly persons with diabetes mellitus, occurring in up to 20% of all persons with this disease (Wald, 1986). The probability of acquiring diabetes doubles each 10 years of a person's life, so elders are particularly predisposed to the illness (Blainey, 1986). More than 50% of elderly persons with diabetes have reduced rectal sensation, and many have rectosphincter abnormalities.

The main dietary changes that elders experience are a decrease in fiber intake and an increase in bulk. Because elders have an increased incidence of dentures, gum disease, and problems with swallowing, they often require foods that are easily chewed and swallowed. These foods are generally lower in fiber content. This is a problem because fiber intake is important for absorption of water in the bowel. Elders also are often prone to dehydration because of inability to obtain fluids, lack of knowledge of the importance of adequate fluid intake, and use of diuretics in the management of chronic illness. Thus the monitoring and provision of adequate fiber and fluid intake are important components of the nursing management of bowel programs for elders. Another dietary problem is lactose intolerance, which is frequently seen in the elder as a cause of diarrhea and may cause bowel irritation and incontinence. This problem is explained in more detail in Chapter 20.

Environmental factors often contribute to bowel incontinence for elders. Lack of privacy can be a major deterrent to maintaining regular bowel evacuation and can lead to impaction or "accidents," especially when the elderly person is institutionalized. Examples of other environmental impediments to regular defecation or to the ability to toilet are inadequate assistance for toileting; inaccessibility of the toilet because of stairs, distance, or other architectural barriers; and lack of knowledge of transfer

Text continued on p. 244

Table 21-1	Suggested Nursing-Sensitive Outcomes and Nursing Interventions BOWEL INCONTINENCE		
Nursing Diagnosis	**Nursing-Sensitive Outcomes**	**Nursing Interventions**

Nursing Diagnosis	Nursing-Sensitive Outcomes	Nursing Interventions

BOWEL INCONTINENCE	BOWEL CONTINENCE
	Indicators
	Predictable evacuation of stool
	Regular evacuation of stool q 3 days
	Free of incontinent episodes
	Ingests adequate amount of fluid
	Ingests adequate amount of fiber
	BOWEL ELIMINATION
	Indicator
	Exercises adequate amount
		BOWEL INCONTINENCE CARE
		Activities
		Determine goals of bowel management
		   program with patient/family
		Implement training program, as
		   appropriate
		BOWEL TRAINING
		Activities
		Ensure adequate fluid intake
		Ensure adequate exercise
		Provide foods high in bulk and/or that
		   have been identified as assistive by the
		   patient
		Evaluate bowel status regularly

Related Factor/Etiology
IMPAIRED COGNITION
Defining Characteristics
Low score on mental status measure
Unable to recognize, act on rectal
   fullness (urge)
Unable to find bathroom
Unable to recognize and name toilet
   articles
Normal rectal reservoir capacity
Normal rectal tightening with digital
   examination
Normal anal sphincter contraction
	SELF-ESTEEM
	Indicators
	Feelings about self-worth
	Free from feelings of embarrassment
	Fulfillment of personally significant roles
		DEMENTIA MANAGEMENT
		Activities
		Use symbols, other than written signs, to
		   assist patient to locate room,
		   bathroom, or other equipment
		Avoid unfamiliar situations, when
		   possible
		Give one simple direction at a time
		SELF-CARE ASSISTANCE: TOILETING
		Activities
		Provide assistive devices (handrails)
		Assist to toilet at specified intervals
		Provide privacy during elimination

Related Factors/Etiologies
GASTROINTESTINAL DISORDERS
Defining Characteristics
Colostomy
Fecal impaction
Diarrhea
Abnormally high abdominal pressure
Urgency
Inability to delay defecation
	BOWEL CONTINENCE
	Indicators
	Constipation not present
	Diarrhea not present
	Ingests adequate amount of fluid
	Ingests adequate amount of fiber
	Regular evacuation of stool q 3 days
	Free of incontinent episodes
	BOWEL ELIMINATION
	Indicators
	Exercises adequate amount
	Bloating not present
		BOWEL MANAGEMENT
		Activities
		Monitor for signs and symptoms of
		   diarrhea, constipation, and impaction
		Encourage decreased gas-forming food
		   intake, as appropriate
		Teach patient about specific foods that
		   are assistive in promoting bowel
		   regularity
		Evaluate medications for gastrointestinal
		   (GI) side effects
		Initiate bowel training program, as
		   appropriate
		BOWEL TRAINING
		Activity
		Ensure adequate exercise

Continued

Suggested Nursing-Sensitive Outcomes and Nursing Interventions—cont'd

Table 21-1   BOWEL INCONTINENCE—cont'd

Nursing Diagnosis	Nursing-Sensitive Outcomes	Nursing Interventions
Related Factor/Etiology Loss of rectal sphincter control *Defining Characteristics* Fecal smears in underclothing Constant dribbling of stool Inability to control passing flatulence	**BOWEL CONTINENCE** *Indicators* Sphincter tone adequate to control defecation Ingests adequate amount of fluid Ingests adequate amount of fiber Diarrhea not present **BOWEL ELIMINATION** *Indicator* Bloating not present	**BIOFEEDBACK** *Activities* Assist patient to learn to modify bodily responses to equipment cues Provide feedback of progress after each session **PELVIC MUSCLE EXERCISE** *Activities* Instruct patient to tighten, then relax the ring of muscle around urethra and anus, as if trying to prevent urination or bowel movement Write instructions and prescription for exercises **BOWEL MANAGEMENT** *Activities* Encourage decreased gas-forming food intake, as appropriate Monitor for signs and symptoms of diarrhea, constipation, and impaction Initiate bowel training program, as appropriate Teach patient about specific foods that are assistive in promoting bowel regularity Evaluate medications for GI side effects
Related Factor/Etiology Impaired reservoir capacity *Defining Characteristics* Idiopathic inflammatory disease Radiation proctitis Chronic rectal ischemia Frequent passage of loose stool	**BOWEL CONTINENCE** *Indicators* Ingests adequate amount of fluid Ingests adequate amount of fiber Free of incontinent episodes Diarrhea not present **BOWEL ELIMINATION** *Indicator* Bloating not present	**BOWEL TRAINING** *Activities* Ensure adequate exercise Ensure adequate fluid intake
Related Factors/Etiologies Environmental factors *Defining Characteristics* Unfamiliar setting Inconvenient toilet facilities Lack of privacy Physical restraint Lack of caregiver assistance	**BOWEL CONTINENCE** *Indicators* Reaches toilet facility independently before defecating Uses aids appropriately to achieve continence Manages bowel appliance independently Free of incontinent episodes **SELF-CARE: TOILETING** *Indicators* Gets to and from toilet Removes clothing Positions self on toilet or commode Gets up from toilet Adjusts clothing after toileting	**ENVIRONMENTAL MANAGEMENT** *Activities* Maintain accessible toilet facility Orient to setting **SELF-CARE ASSISTANCE: TOILETING** *Activities* Provide assistive devices (handrails) Assist to toilet at specified intervals Provide privacy during elimination

Table 21-1 BOWEL INCONTINENCE—cont'd
Suggested Nursing-Sensitive Outcomes and Nursing Interventions—cont'd

Nursing Diagnosis	Nursing-Sensitive Outcomes	Nursing Interventions
Related Factors/Etiologies Medications and treatments *Defining Characteristics* Laxative abuse Antibiotics Anticholinergic drugs Lactose Tube feedings Physical/chemical restraints Diuretics Antacids Narcotics Iron supplements	**BOWEL CONTINENCE** *Indicators* Constipation not present Diarrhea not present Ingests adequate amount of fluid Ingests adequate amount of fiber Regular evacuation of stool q 3 days Free of incontinent episodes **SELF-CARE: NON-PARENTERAL MEDICATIONS** *Indicators* Adjust dose and perform self-monitoring Describes side effects of medication **KNOWLEDGE: MEDICATION** *Indicators* Description of action of medication Description of correct administration of medication	**MEDICATION MANAGEMENT** *Activities* Monitor for adverse effects of the drug Teach patient and/or family members the expected action and side effects of the medication Review periodically with the patient and/or family types and amounts of medication taken **TEACHING: PRESCRIBED MEDICATION** *Activities* Instruct on criteria to use for altering medications Instruct on how to relieve/prevent side effects **BOWEL TRAINING** *Activities* Plan bowel program with patient and appropriate others Initiate consistent time for defecation Perform digital rectal dilatation, as necessary
Related Factors/Etiologies Neuromuscular disorders *Defining Characteristics* Upper motor nerve damage Damage to brain or spinal cord above T12 Unable to feel rectal fullness or urge Unable to control defecation reflex Frequent fecal impactions Digital stimulation is painful	**BOWEL CONTINENCE** *Indicators* Predictable evacuation of stool Regular evacuation of stool q 3 days Free of incontinent episodes Ingests adequate amount of fluid Ingests adequate amount of fiber	**BOWEL MANAGEMENT** *Activities* Teach patient about specific foods that are assistive in promoting bowel regularity Evaluate medications for GI side effects Give warm liquids after meals Monitor for diarrhea, constipation, and impaction Initiate a bowel training program, as appropriate
Related Factor/Etiology Lower motor neuron damage *Defining Characteristics* Damage to spinal cord T12 to L1 Fecal incontinence suddenly without warning Flaccid anal sphincter Absence of defecation reflex Constant dribbling of soft stool Inability to expel formed stool in rectum Belief that have to have 1 or more bowel movements (BMs) per day	**BOWEL CONTINENCE** *Indicators* Predictable evacuation of stool Regular evacuation of stool q 3 days Free of incontinent episodes Ingests adequate amount of fluid Ingests adequate amount of fiber **TISSUE INTEGRITY: SKIN & MUCOUS MEMBRANES** *Indicators* Skin intactness Color in expected range Tissue lesion free	**BOWEL MANAGEMENT** *Activities* Teach patient about specific foods that are assistive in promoting bowel regularity Monitor for diarrhea, constipation, and impaction Initiate bowel training program Instruct patient in foods high in fiber, as appropriate **BOWEL INCONTINENCE CARE** *Activity* Wash perianal area after toileting

Continued

Table 21-1	Suggested Nursing-Sensitive Outcomes and Nursing Interventions—cont'd BOWEL INCONTINENCE—cont'd		
Nursing Diagnosis	**Nursing-Sensitive Outcomes**		**Nursing Interventions**
Related Factor/Etiology Self-care deficit *Defining Characteristics* Impaired mobility Inability to reach toilet in timely manner Inability to get on and off toilet Inability to manage clothing Inability to complete toileting hygiene Inability to obtain appropriate foods/fluids Normal rectal reservoir capacity Normal rectal tightening with digital examination Normal anal sphincter contraction Decreased muscle strength Limited range of motion Impaired coordination	SELF-CARE: TOILETING *Indicators* Gets to and from toilet Removes clothing Positions self on toilet or commode Gets up from toilet Adjusts clothing after toileting Recognizes and responds to urge to have bowel movement BOWEL CONTINENCE *Indicator* Free of incontinent episodes MOBILITY LEVEL *Indicators* Ambulation: walking Transfer performance Joint movement		SELF-CARE ASSISTANCE: TOILETING *Activities* Provide assistive devices (handrails) Assist to toilet at specified intervals Provide privacy during elimination SELF-CARE ASSISTANCE *Activities* Monitor patient's ability for independent self-care Encourage independence, but assist if needed Establish a routine for self-care activities Teach skills to enable independent self-care EXERCISE PROMOTION *Activities* Assist patient to develop an appropriate exercise program Assist with exercise as needed Monitor patient's response to exercise program

techniques from wheelchair to toilet. The nurse should thoroughly assess environmental factors that might prevent the elderly person from maintaining continence. Because of the positive influence that activity and exercise have on regular bowel function, the nurse also should pay careful attention to the elderly person's ability to remain active in his environment. The advantages of activity and exercise for optimizing the elderly person's functional abilities are more fully discussed in Chapters 7 and 28.

Many elders take medications that adversely affect bowel function. Narcotics, barbiturates, propoxyphene hydrochloride, tranquilizers, and antacids can cause constipation. Iron can result in constipation or diarrhea, and magnesium-based antacids and digitalis preparations can cause diarrhea. A careful assessment of medications therefore is critical in addressing bowel incontinence. More information about the adverse effects of medications on elders can be found in Chapter 4.

ASSESSMENT

Assessment of bowel incontinence in elders involves the consideration of several contributing factors. Davis, Nagelhout, Hoban, and Barnard (1986) describe five types of bowel dysfunction: (1) uninhibited bowel dysfunction, which occurs when there is an upper motor neuron lesion above cervical vertebra 1 (C1); (2) reflex bowel dysfunction, caused by upper motor neuron damage between C1 and L1; (3) autonomic bowel dysfunction, which is due to lower motor neuron damage below L1; (4) sensory neuro-

genic bowel dysfunction, in which there is damage to the sensory component of the reflex arc (the message from bowel to spinal cord and back to bowel); and (5) motor neurogenic bowel dysfunction, in which there is damage to the motor component of the central nervous system or the reflex arc.

With uninhibited and reflex bowel incontinence the rectal reflex is intact but voluntary control of the reflex is absent. In autonomic bowel incontinence the reflex arc may be partially or completely damaged. Sensory bowel incontinence is distinguished by the individual having no awareness of stool in the rectum. In contrast, the elderly person with motor neurogenic bowel incontinence is aware of the stool in the rectum but cannot evacuate it. Assessment of anal sphincter tone can determine the presence of an intact reflex arc. Wald (1986) reported a poor correlation between digital evaluation of the internal rectal sphincter and objective tests in the laboratory. However, assessment for the presence of the reflex by sensing the internal rectal sphincter muscle tighten around a gloved finger inserted into the rectum is often recommended in general tests and provides some guidance for accurate diagnosis. An additional reason for digital rectal examination is to check for fecal impaction and other rectal abnormalities.

The evaluation for bowel incontinence should begin with a comprehensive history of the frequency, duration, and severity of the elderly client's bowel incontinence. Assessment should be alert for a perceived change that is associated with a change in health and/or function (McLane

ASSESSMENT TOOL FOR BOWEL INCONTINENCE

Name _____ Sex _____ Age _____

Previous Bowel Pattern

| Frequency: | Time: | Amount: | Consistency: |

Present Bowel History

| Frequency: | Time: | Amount: | Consistency: |

Impactions:

Methods Used to Initiate Defecation:

Recent Changes

| Color: | Bleeding: | Pain: | Other: |

Medical Diagnoses:

Relevant Bowel Disorders:

Rectal Examination

| Sphincter tone: | Fissure: | Fistula: | Hemorrhoids: |

Other:

Loss of Control

Partial/complete?

Patient's reaction:

Medications

Constipating drugs (opiates, antidiarrheals, iron supplements, aluminum antacids):

Laxatives:

Stool softeners:

Magnesium antacids:

Anticholinergics:

Others:

Physical Exercise/Activity

Abdomen

Scars/possible adhesions:	Hardness:
Bloating:	Ascites:
Muscle tone:	Masses:

Diet and Eating Habits

| Consistency: | Fiber: | Amount: | Schedule/Time: |
| Fluid intake: | Type: | Amount: | |

Laxative Use

| Frequency: | Type: | Amount: | History of use: |

Use of Enemas

| Frequency: | Type: | Amount: | History of use: |

Emotional/Mental Status

| Depression: | Anxiety: | Cognition: | Stressors: |

Coping Styles/Strategies:

Functional Abilities

Manual Dexterity in

- Removing clothing:
- Handling equipment:
- Toileting/hygiene:

Ambulation:

Transfer:

Neurologic Intactness:

Environmental/Iatrogenic Barriers:

Elder's Goals for Treatment

| Diagnoses: | Etiologies: |

& McShane, 1992). The pattern of incontinence should be carefully determined. The client interview should also elicit any symptoms that accompany the bowel incontinence, such as presence or absence of warning, time between sensation and defecation, amount of straining with defecation, and presence of constipation and diarrhea. Other items to assess include the following: presence of urinary incontinence; presence of diabetes; a history of anal, rectal, or spinal surgery; presence of cognitive deficits; and presence of other neurologic and bowel diseases. If the client is a woman, the number and character of vaginal deliveries should be noted. Finally, health management information such as fluid intake, dietary patterns and habits, usual activity and exercise, types and frequency of medications used, coping strategies, and the client's knowledge of bowel physiology and the process of defecation should be ascertained. For the assessment to result in an accurate diagnosis and effective treatment, environmental factors such as privacy and access to toilet and the functional ability of the elder for toileting must be determined (Assessment Guide 21-1).

CASE STUDY

G. Brown has lived at Get Rest nursing home for 6 months. He is 80 years old and married, but his spouse continues to live at home. Mr. Brown has been incontinent of both urine and feces since his admission to the nursing home. He is disoriented to time and place at all times. He has severe bilateral hearing loss and dense bilateral cataracts. He dislikes being touched and strikes out when he is touched. Mr. Brown receives a mechanical, soft, general diet with raw bran. He can feed himself about half of the time. Ordinarily he has a fluid intake of less than 1000 ml daily. He spends about 14 hours each day in bed and 10 hours each day in a wheelchair. He is able to walk about 5 feet with the assistance of two attendants. He suffered a hip fracture when he fell at home 3 years ago. The hip was pinned at the time of the fracture, and he has

never regained independent ambulation. He complains of pain when ambulation is attempted.

A rectal examination at the time of his admission to the nursing home revealed an enlarged prostate and poor sphincter tone. Mr. Brown has a history of laxative abuse. His wife reports that he has been incontinent of feces for approximately 1 year before admission. At present, if his bowels do not move daily, he develops a bowel obstruction. Consequently, he is on a vigorous bowel program of a daily Dulcolax suppository, followed by a Fleets enema if there are no results. In addition, he receives Lactulose and Senakot twice each day and Exlax prn. His abdominal muscles are flaccid, and he is unable to expel feces. He gives no indication of urge to defecate and wears disposable briefs at all times. Table 21-2 summarizes the significant signs and symptoms and lists the additional data needed for Mr. Brown's assessment.

NURSING DIAGNOSIS

NANDA has defined bowel incontinence as "a state in which an individual experiences a change in normal bowel habits characterized by involuntary passage of stool" (NANDA, 1999). See Table 21-1 for related factors/etiologies and defining characteristics that have been specified by NANDA.

NURSING-SENSITIVE OUTCOMES

The principal desired outcomes of interventions for bowel incontinence are to achieve a predictable pattern of defecation to avoid discomfort, embarrassment, and loss of self-esteem for the elderly person. Feelings of embarrassment and self-worth are important to preserve so that relationships with family and other sources of social support and opportunities for social interaction are not interrupted. Unpleasant odor and embarrassment that can accompany fecal incontinence can cause family, friends, and other social contacts to avoid the elderly person who is in-

Table 21-2	Bowel Incontinence: Differential Diagnosis for MR. BROWN		
Defining Characteristics	**Nursing Diagnoses Ruled Out**	**Additional Data Needed**	
No expression of urge to defecate Decreased rectal sphincter tone		Can identify rectal fullness? Rectal reservoir capacity?	
	IMPAIRED RESERVOIR CAPACITY **COGNITIVE IMPAIRMENT**	Stool in rectal vault?	
Unable to "bear down" to defecate Disoriented to time and place Soft, puttylike stools		Comprehensive mental status assessment Can name toilet articles and use appropriately? Complete evacuation? Presence of diarrhea?	
Poor food and fluid intake Minimal physical activity	**RECTAL SPHINCTER ABNORMALITY**	Tolerance for increased activity? Injury below T12?	
Frequent impactions	**CONSTIPATION**	Lower motor neuron damage?	

Table 21-3	Nursing Diagnoses, Outcomes, and Interventions for MR. BROWN		

Nursing Diagnoses	Nursing-Sensitive Outcomes	Nursing Interventions
BOWEL INCONTINENCE *Related Factors/Etiologies* Inability to delay defecation Disoriented to time and place Poor food and fluid intake Limited activity Frequent impactions Decreased rectal sphincter tone Unable to bear down to defecate Soft, puttylike stools	**BOWEL CONTINENCE** *Indicators* Free of incontinent episodes Predictable evacuation of stool Ingests adequate amount of fluid Ingests adequate amount of fiber Regular evacuation of stool q 3 days Constipation not present Diarrhea not present **BOWEL ELIMINATION** *Indicators* Exercises adequate amount Abuse of aids not present Passes stool without aids	**BOWEL TRAINING** *Activities* Initiate consistent time for defecation Administer suppository as appropriate Provide foods high in bulk Ensure adequate fluid intake Ensure adequate exercise Give warm liquids after meals Position to optimize bowel evacuation Teach family principles of bowel training **BOWEL MANAGEMENT** *Activities* Monitor bowel movements Monitor bowel sounds Monitor for signs and symptoms of diarrhea, constipation, and impaction **MEDICATION MANAGEMENT** *Activities* Monitor medications for adverse effects of the drug Review periodically types and amounts taken
IMPAIRED COGNITION *Related Factor/Etiology* Disoriented to time and place **LOSS OF RECTAL SPHINCTER CONTROL** *Related Factor/Etiology* Decreased rectal sphincter tone	**SELF-ESTEEM** *Indicators* Feelings about self-worth Free from feelings of embarrassment **TISSUE INTEGRITY: SKIN & MUCOUS MEMBRANES** *Indicators* Skin intactness Color in expected range	**ENVIRONMENTAL MANAGEMENT** *Activities* Provide adaptive devices as appropriate Orient to setting **SELF-CARE ASSISTANCE: TOILETING** *Activities* Assist patient to toilet at specified intervals Provide privacy during elimination Facilitate hygiene after elimination

Nursing Outcomes Classification (NOC) 5-point Likert measurement scales:

Bowel Continence:	1 = Never demonstrated; 2 = Rarely demonstrated; 3 = Sometimes demonstrated; 4 = Often demonstrated; 5 = Consistently demonstrated.
Bowel Elimination:	1 = Extremely compromised; 2 = Substantially compromised; 3 = Moderately compromised; 4 = Mildly compromised; 5 = Not compromised.
Self-Esteem:	1 = Never positive; 2 = Rarely positive; 3 = Sometimes positive; 4 = Often positive; 5 = Consistently positive.
Tissue Integrity: Skin & Mucous Membranes:	1 = Extremely compromised; 2 = Substantially compromised; 3 = Moderately compromised; 4 = Mildly compromised; 5 = Not compromised.

continent. The maintenance of skin integrity is another important outcome. The *Nursing Outcomes Classification (NOC)* (Iowa Outcomes Project, 2000) includes several outcomes that are appropriate for the diagnosis Bowel Incontinence: Bowel Continence, Bowel Elimination, Self-Esteem, and Tissue Integrity: Skin & Mucous Membranes (Table 21-3). Bowel Continence is defined as "control of passage of stool from the bowel" (Iowa Outcomes Project, 2000, p. 126). Bowel Elimination is the "ability of the gastrointestinal tract to form and evacuate stool effectively" (Iowa Outcomes Project, 2000, p. 127).

CASE STUDY

The following tentative nursing diagnosis was formulated for Mr. Brown: Bowel Incontinence related to upper motor neuron damage (sensory bowel incontinence) as evidenced by inability to feel rectal fullness, by inability to control defecation reflex, and by frequent impactions.

The following goals were developed with Mr. Brown, his wife, and his son: (1) Bowel Continence: Mr. Brown would demonstrate bowel continence 75% to nearly 100% of the time; (2) Bowel Elimination: Mr. Brown would demonstrate only mildly compromised bowel elimination; (3) Self-Esteem: Mr. Brown would report positive self-esteem 75% to nearly 100% of the time; and (4) Tissue Integrity: Mr. Brown would have uncompromised skin integrity. The nurse assessed and documented each of the outcomes and indicators at baseline and after 2, 4, and 8 weeks of intervention. Initial outcome assessments were recorded every 2 weeks for the first month, although the assessments were completed weekly. Weekly assessments of progress continued, but were again recorded at the end of the eighth week since Mr. Brown's progress was maintained and progressed to some extent. Thereafter weekly assessments continued and were recorded at least monthly.

NURSING INTERVENTIONS

Bowel incontinence is an important problem that nurses can treat. A recent study suggests that treatment of predisposing and associated conditions, such as tube feeding, impaction, and functional loss, is more important than anal sphincter corrective surgeries (Nelson, Furner, & Jesudason, 1998).

See Table 21-1 for NIC interventions (Iowa Interventions Project, 2000) for each of the etiologies of Bowel Incontinence associated with NOC outcomes. However, the interventions used to achieve the outcomes will differ depending on the specific etiology. Etiologies also can be mixed, so it is important to specify carefully all causes of Bowel Incontinence for the elderly individual. Because all of the interventions that could be used to treat the several etiologies of Bowel Incontinence cannot be discussed within the limitation of this chapter, we have focused on Bowel Training and Environmental Management, two interventions that are most often appropriate choices.

Bowel Training

Bowel Training is defined as "assisting the patient to train the bowel to evacuate at specific intervals" (Iowa Interventions Project, 2000, p. 190). The aim of Bowel Training is to train the bowel to evacuate at regular intervals and times planned with the elderly individual or family, resulting in a minimum of bowel accidents. Bowel training must be tailored to accommodate each elderly person's physiologic and psychosocial problems, the person's particular environment, and the individual's functional abilities. Habit training, control of diarrhea, digital and nondigital stimulation of the gastrocolic reflex, reduction of stool volume, and biofeedback are specific forms of bowel training that are used to treat bowel incontinence, depending on the etiology of the problem.

Before beginning any type of bowel training program the bowel must be empty. This can be accomplished by the use of enemas, suppositories, laxatives, or a combination of two or more. Brocklehurst (1985b) recommends cleansing of the bowel with phosphate enemas for 7 to 10 days before initiation of bowel training. He argues that this removes the etiology of constipation; however, most sources do not explicitly suggest such extreme cleansing (McLane & McShane, 1992). Bowel cleansing also can be used to control diarrhea when the elderly person is not constipated. This is especially effective when the source of diarrhea is an irritant that has been ingested and when there is intraintestinal infection. Cleansing can soothe inflammation and provide an opportunity for the bowel to heal and become less motile. However, nurses should prescribe enemas cautiously because of the risk of contributing to fluid and electrolyte imbalances. The elder can more easily experience fluid and electrolyte imbalance and become dehydrated, particularly if fluid intake is poor or restricted when enemas are given (Robinson & Demuth, 1985).

Ordinarily there are at least four components to Bowel Training. One component is appropriate diet and fluid. Fluid intake is usually recommended at 1500 to 2000 ml each 24 hours, excluding coffee, tea, and grapefruit juice because of their diuretic effects. Drinking a glass of warm or hot liquid before meals facilitates gastrocolic reflex. High-fiber foods are also important for nondigital stimulation of the gastrocolic reflex and for habit training because they prevent hard stools and promote peristalsis (McLane & McShane, 1986). Foods should be as fat free as possible to stimulate the gastrocolic reflex, since fats slow digestion and delay the reflex (Davis et al., 1986). When diarrhea is present but the elderly person is not constipated, the foods selected should be low in fiber. Any foods that produce a laxative effect, a great deal of gas, or an allergic reaction should be eliminated from the elder's diet. The reduction of stool volume is the form of bowel training that is needed when impaired reservoir capacity is the etiology of bowel incontinence. Reduction of stool volume is accomplished primarily through fiber restriction and the use of medications to increase transit time and absorption (Wald, 1986).

The second component of bowel training is increasing activity and exercise (McLane & McShane, 1992). Physical activity increases body circulation, including circulation to the bowel, and promotes digestion and peristalsis. The exercise program can include abdominal exercise to increase muscle strength for expulsion of feces. The most effective form of exercise in many cases will be getting the elderly person to do whatever is possible, given the individual's physical and cognitive functional abilities. Pelvic floor exercises, involving repetitive contraction and relaxation of the anal sphincter and the puborectalis muscles, can be used. The exercises should be done three times daily with 25 to 30 contractions held for approximately 3 seconds each (McCormick & Burgio, 1984). Electrostimulation also is used in some cases to train and strengthen muscles that assist with defecation and continence (King & Harke, 1994; McLeod, 1987) and is often used in combination with pelvic floor exercises. The electrical current stimulates the perineal muscles to contract. Although there are some reports of good results, success rates tend to be low because of a low level of patient acceptance (Brocklehurst, 1985a).

Timing is the third aspect of bowel training that is important to incorporate. A plan in which the elderly person defecates each day is usually the most successful. This involves establishing a regular time to sit on the toilet, usually 5 to 15 minutes, timed in such a way as to take advantage of the gastrocolic reflex. This reflex occurs in response to food intake and is strongest in the morning (Davis et al., 1986; Lewis, 1988). Combined with appropriate food and fluid intake and regular exercise, the consistency and regularity of the timing can lead to the formation of habit and can make other less natural measures to promote bowel movements unnecessary. Ouslander, Simmons, Schnelle, Uman, and Fingold (1996) found that the percent of continent bowel movements statistically significantly increased when a prompted voiding protocol was tested with elderly institutionalized persons, although the incidence of bowel incontinence did not decrease. This result suggests that regular toileting, in conjunction with more exercise and fluid intake, can decrease the number of episodes of bowel incontinence.

Finally, the fourth component of bowel programming includes laxatives, suppositories, massage of the anal sphincter, enemas, and antidiarrheals to promote regular, planned bowel evacuation. These approaches are most appropriate when bowel cleansing is required and when there is a spinal cord injury. With upper motor cord lesions, digital stimulation of the gastrocolic reflex is effective because the reflex arc is intact. Suppositories are helpful to use early on in initiating a bowel program. Suppositories stimulate the gastrocolic reflex similar to digital stimulation and relax the anal sphincter. Persons may progress from the use of suppositories to the use of only digital stimulation to trigger bowel evacuation (Sharkey & Hanlon, 1989). With lower motor cord lesions, enemas may be needed to evacuate the bowel. However, the nurse should attempt to establish regular evacuation by teaching the elder to bear down with abdominal muscles or to express manually by pushing on the lower abdomen if at all possible. The elderly person can be taught to massage the abdomen in the right groin in an upward direction and then down to the left, following the positions of the transverse large bowel, cecum, and rectum, to stimulate and hasten bowel action (Cannon, 1981). For controlling incontinence with diarrhea in persons who were not constipated, Imodium, up to 4 mg as often as four times a day, was found to be more effective than Lomotil.

Bowel training programs must be established and maintained for at least 10 to 15 days (Sharpless, 1982) and usually take from 6 to 8 weeks to produce a soft, formed stool within 1 hour of the designated time (Alterescu, 1986; Davis et al., 1986; Hanak, 1990). However, absence of defecation or frequent loose stools requires immediate attention. For this reason, the maintenance of a daily bowel record, which assesses food and fluid intake, laxative used, time and type of bowel evacuation, and the facility used, is important for evaluating the effectiveness of the intervention and identifying when there are problems.

Biofeedback as an adjunct to pelvic floor exercise for bowel training has been investigated at the National Institute on Aging, Laboratory of Behavioral Sciences (McCormick & Burgio, 1984). The biofeedback procedure for fecal incontinence gives the patient sensory feedback on anal sphincter activity (Wald, 1986). McCormick and Burgio (1984) reported that out of 13 older persons treated with biofeedback for fecal incontinence, "Four became continent and seven experienced more than 50% improvement" (p. 19). One patient in the McCormick and Burgio study was cognitively impaired and was not a candidate for biofeedback. This points out one disadvantage of biofeedback as an intervention to be used for the elderly who are incontinent of feces, since cognitive impairment is prevalent among institutionalized elders and is a frequent etiology. Bielefeldt, Enck, and Wienbeck (1990) suggest that emotional support by staff or behavioral modifications might be as important as the biofeedback for decreasing bowel incontinence among elders.

Environmental Management

Privacy, accessibility, comfort, functional positioning, and safety are the essential features of environmental structure that promote bowel continence. The elderly, especially if institutionalized, are often subjected to bowel elimination with minimal privacy. This can be particularly difficult for older persons who have been socialized to be modest. Most persons feel embarrassed when they must have bowel movements in the presence of another person. Thus lack of privacy can cause elders to avoid defecation, which can lead to constipation and incontinence. Nurses should carefully prescribe and monitor approaches that will ensure that the elderly person is able to defecate privately.

The nurse also should assess the elder's ability to ambulate to the bathroom, walking or in a wheelchair, as well as the person's ability to get to the bathroom in time to avoid an accident. If the elder is in a wheelchair, transfer ability must be evaluated and appropriate interventions prescribed to correct or compensate for any lack of ability. In addition, architectural barriers must be assessed, and care should be taken to remove or rearrange furniture and equipment that will obstruct the ambulant elderly person.

Assistive devices should be provided in bathrooms so that the elderly person has the needed support for safe transfer, clothing adjustment, and hygiene. Fecal evacuation is more apt to be successful if the elder feels safe and not in danger of falling. Prescriptions should incorporate the principles that peristaltic activity is greater when the person is in an upright position, as gravity assists the expulsion of feces. It is also important for the prescribed intervention to include instructions to staff to be responsive to the timing of defecation, impressing on staff the importance of consistency with the plan of care.

Table 21-4	Outcome and Indicator Ratings for MR. BROWN			
	Base	Week 2	Week 4	Week 8
BOWEL CONTINENCE	2	2	3	4
• Free of incontinence episodes	1	2	2	3
• Predictable evacuation of stool	1	2	4	4
• Ingests adequate amount of fluid	1	3	3	3
• Ingests adequate amount of food	2	3	4	4
• Regular evacuation of stool q 3 days	4	4	3	4
• Constipation not present	3	2	3	3
• Diarrhea not present	3	4	4	4
BOWEL ELIMINATION	1	2	2	3
• Exercises adequate amount	1	1	2	3
• Abuse of aids not present	1	3	4	4
• Passes stool without aids	1	2	2	2
SELF-ESTEEM	2	2	3	4
• Feeling about self-worth	3	3	4	4
• Free from feelings of embarrassment	2	2	3	4
TISSUE INTEGRITY: SKIN & MUCOUS MEMBRANES	3	3	4	4
• Skin intactness	5	5	5	5
• Color in expected range	2	2	4	4

Nursing Outcomes Classification (NOC) 5-point Likert measurement scales:

Bowel Continence: 1 = Never demonstrated; 2 = Rarely demonstrated; 3 = Sometimes demonstrated; 4 = Often demonstrated; 5 = Consistently demonstrated.

Bowel Elimination: 1 = Extremely compromised; 2 = Substantially compromised; 3 = Moderately compromised; 4 = Mildly compromised; 5 = Not compromised.

Self-Esteem: 1 = Never positive; 2 = Rarely positive; 3 = Sometimes positive; 4 = Often positive; 5 = Consistently positive.

Tissue Integrity: Skin and Mucous Membranes: 1 = Extremely compromised; 2 = Substantially compromised; 3 = Moderately compromised; 4 = Mildly compromised; 5 = Not compromised.

Finally, the nurse should provide emotional and social interventions (e.g., relaxation therapy, social support) if depression or anxiety is judged to be the etiology of incontinence. The need for all staff to be nonjudgmental when the elder requires assistance or when there is an incidence of incontinence is an essential, but often overlooked, aspect of the environment.

CASE STUDY

Specific activities for Mr. Brown's bowel training are included in his plan of care (see Table 21-3). Substantial progress with the outcome of regular bowel evacuation was not achieved until scheduled toileting had been initiated and maintained for 28 days. After implementation of the toileting schedule, which was prescribed after breakfast each day, Mr. Brown was continent except when his son visited each week and brought him chocolate bars. The nurse discussed with the son the importance of his father avoiding high-fat foods. The son then began to bring fresh fruit for Mr. Brown. Environmental structuring was prescribed specifically to provide privacy for toileting and to ensure that adaptive (grab bars, clock, hearing aid) devices were available for assistance because of his hearing and visual losses.

Table 21-4 presents a summary of Mr. Brown's progress with outcomes for the first 8 weeks of intervention as an example of how outcomes are assessed and documented at specified intervals. Although some of the staff complained about the difficulty of the toileting schedule, they were very pleased when Mr. Brown's "accidents" became infrequent, felt better about him, and agreed that the training and schedule were worth the effort. As mentioned previously, a bowel record is a useful tool for monitoring the effectiveness of the interventions for bowel incontinence. Mr. Brown had no skin impairment before the interventions for incontinence, and his skin integrity continued to be maintained. The outcome of avoiding embarrassment of Mr. Brown and his family was achieved by providing privacy and by achieving continence.

SUMMARY

Although much has been written about the prevalence and devastation of Bowel Incontinence, research has not validated the signs and symptoms of bowel incontinence and few studies have tested interventions for the diagnosis. Many discussions of the diagnosis and interventions are brief and lack sufficient detail to be optimally helpful to educators, clinicians, or researchers. The NANDA diagnosis Bowel Incontinence needs further development. Etiologies and the corresponding signs and symptoms must be expanded to be more useful for nursing education and clinical practice (Craft & Delaney, 1996). NIC and NOC offer many nursing interventions and outcomes that can be used to treat Bowel Incontinence. NIC lacks some clarity and inclusiveness of the Bowel Training and Bowel Management interventions. "Training" activities currently listed in the NIC Bowel Management intervention should be removed, and the

Bowel Training intervention should be revised to list only specific activities needed for bowel training. Also, activities for teaching self-care skills should be added to the NIC intervention Self-Care Assistance. There also are other NOC outcomes and indicators that nurses can find useful, depending on the patient's circumstances and Bowel Incontinence etiologies. "Free of incontinent episodes" should be added as an essential indicator for the outcome Bowel Continence, and "Free from feelings of embarrassment" should be added to the outcome Self-Esteem. It is hoped that further conceptual development of the diagnosis will stimulate and assist researchers, clinicians, and educators to study and use the diagnosis, outcomes, and interventions. These activities are essential for the further development and validation of the diagnosis, outcomes, and interventions and for improving the care provided to elderly persons.

REFERENCES

Alterescu, V. (1986). Theoretical foundations for an approach to fecal incontinence. *The Journal of Enterostoma Therapy, 13,* 44-48.

Bielefeldt, K., Enck, P., & Wienbeck, M. (1990). Diagnosis and treatment of fecal incontinence. *Digestive Diseases, 8,* 179-188.

Blainey, C. (1986). Diabetes mellitus. In D. Carnevali & M. Patrick (Eds.), *Nursing management for the elderly* (2nd ed., pp. 403-422). Baltimore: Lippincott Williams & Wilkins.

Brocklehurst, J. (1985a). *Textbook of geriatric medicine and gerontology* (3rd ed.). New York: Churchill Livingstone.

Brocklehurst, J. (1985b). The large bowel. In J. C. Brocklehurst (Ed.), *Textbook of geriatric medicine and gerontology* (3rd ed., pp. 534-556). New York: Churchill Livingstone.

Brocklehurst, J., & Khan, Y. (1969). A study of fecal stasis in old age and use of Dorbanex in its prevention. *Gerontology Clinics, 11,* 293-300.

Cannon, B. (1981). Bowel function. In N. Martin, N. B. Holt, & D. Hicks (Eds.), *Comprehensive rehabilitation nursing* (pp. 224-241). Hightstown, NJ: McGraw-Hill.

Chassagne, P., Landrin, I., Neveu, C., Czernichow, P., Bouaniche, M., Doucet, J., Denis, P., & Bercoff, E. (1999). Fecal incontinence in the institutionalized elderly: Incidence, risk factors, and prognosis. *American Journal of Medicine, 106*(2), 185-190.

Craft, M., & Delaney, C. (1996). *Revision and extension of the NANDA classification of nursing diagnoses* (Research Proposal to NINR). Iowa City: The University of Iowa College of Nursing.

Davis, A., Nagelhout, M. J., Hoban, M., & Barnard, B. (1986). Bowel management: A quality assurance approach to upgrading programs. *Journal of Gerontological Nursing, 12*(5), 13-17.

Goldman, R. (1979). Decline in organ function with aging. In I. Rossman (Ed.), *Clinical gerontology* (2nd ed., pp. 23-52). Baltimore: Lippincott Williams & Wilkins.

Gordon, D., Groutz, A., Goldman, G., Avni, A., Wolf, Y., Lessing, J. B., & David, M. P. (1999). Anal incontinence: Prevalence among female patients attending a urogynecologic clinic. *Neurourology & Urodynamics, 18*(3), 199-204.

Hanak, M. (1990). *Education guide for spinal cord injury nurses.* New York: American Association of Spinal Cord Injury Nurses.

Henry, M. (1983). Fecal incontinence. *Nursing Times, 79*(33), 61-62.

Hogstel, M., & Nelson, M. (1992). Anticipation and early detection can reduce bowel elimination complications. *Geriatric Nursing, 13*(1), 28-33.

Iowa Interventions Project. J. C. McCloskey & G. M. Bulechek (Eds.). (2000). *Nursing interventions classification (NIC)* (3rd ed.). St. Louis, MO: Mosby.

Iowa Outcomes Project. M. Johnson, M. Maas, & S. Moorhead (2000). *Nursing outcomes classification (NOC)* (2nd ed.). St. Louis, MO: Mosby.

King, B. D., & Harke, J. (1994). *Coping with bowel and bladder problems.* San Diego, CA: Singular Publishing Group.

Kinnunen, O. (1991). Study of constipation in a geriatric hospital, day hospital, old people's home, and at home. *Aging, 3,* 161-170.

Lewis, N. (1988). Nursing management of altered patterns of elimination. *Journal of Home Health Care Practice, 1,* 35-42.

Matteson, M., McConnell, E., & Linton, A. (1997). *Gerontological nursing: Concepts and practice* (2nd ed.). Philadelphia: W. B. Saunders.

McCormick, K., & Burgio, K. (1984). Incontinence: An update on nursing care measures. *Journal of Gerontological Nursing, 10*(10), 16-19, 22, 23.

McLane, A., & McShane, R. (1986). Elimination. In J. M. Thompson, G. K. McFarland, J. E. Hirsch, S. M. Tucker, & A. C. Bowers (Eds.), *Clinical nursing* (pp. 2059-2075). St. Louis, MO: Mosby.

McLane, A., & McShane, R. (1992). Bowel management. In G. Bulechek & J. McCloskey (Eds.), *Nursing interventions: Essential nursing treatments* (2nd ed., pp. 73-85). Philadelphia: W. B. Saunders.

McLeod, J. (1987). Management of anal incontinence by biofeedback. *Gastroenterology, 93,* 291-294.

Miller, C. (1990). *Nursing care of older adults: Theory & practice.* Glenview, IL: Scott Foresman.

Nelson, R., Furner, S., & Jesudason, V. (1998). Fecal incontinence in Wisconsin nursing homes: Prevalence and associations. *Diseases of the Colon & Rectum, 41*(10), 1226-1229.

North American Nursing Diagnosis Association. (1999). *Nursing diagnoses: Definitions and classification 1999-2000.* Philadelphia: Author.

Ouslander, J., Simmons, S., Schnelle, J., Uman, G., & Fingold, S. (1996). Effects of prompted voiding on fecal continence among nursing home residents. *Journal of the American Geriatrics Society, 44,* 424-428.

Robinson, S., & Demuth, P. (1985). Diagnostic studies for the aged: What are the dangers? *Journal of Gerontological Nursing, 11*(6), 7-12.

Sharkey, E., & Hanlon, D. (1989). Bowel elimination. In S. Dittmar (Ed.), *Process of rehabilitation nursing.* St. Louis, MO: Mosby.

Sharpless, J. (1982). *A problem oriented approach to stroke rehabilitation.* Springfield, IL: Charles C. Thomas.

Tobin, G. W., & Brocklehurst, J. C. (1986). Fecal incontinence in residential homes for the elderly: Prevalence, etiology and management. *Age & Ageing, 15,* 41-46.

Wald, A. (1986). Fecal incontinence: Effective nonsurgical treatments. *Postgraduate Medicine, 80*(3), 123-130.

Wald, A. (1993). Constipation in elderly patients: Pathogenesis and management. *Drugs & Aging, 3*(3), 220-231.

CHAPTER 22

URINARY INCONTINENCE: FUNCTIONAL, IATROGENIC, OVERFLOW, REFLEX, STRESS, TOTAL, AND URGE

Janet P. Specht and Meridean L. Maas

Urinary incontinence in the elderly population is a problem of considerable magnitude. Urinary incontinence is most simply defined as nonvoluntary voiding when the pressure in the bladder is greater than the resistance of the urethra. Urinary leakage that is objectively demonstrable and presents a social or hygienic problem is the definition accepted by the International Continence Society Committee on Standardization of Terminology (1990). The Agency for Health Care Policy and Research (AHCPR) Guideline defined urinary incontinence as "involuntary loss of urine which is sufficient enough to be a problem." Although these definitions oversimplify the complex processes that can occur with incontinence, they describe the essential nature of the problem for the person who experiences it. With normal urinary elimination the bladder stores urine that flows from the kidneys through the ureters into the bladder. As the bladder fills, it distends and sends a message along autonomic pathways to nerves in the spinal cord and cerebrum. Emptying of the bladder occurs when the parasympathetically innervated detrusor muscle relaxes concurrently with the bladder neck and urethral sphincters, which are innervated by sympathetic and somatic nerves. The distended detrusor muscle first gives the signal of a full bladder, which can be overridden with voluntary cortical control. Incontinence can result from the loss of voluntary control mechanisms, from deficits in neuromuscular function and urinary tract pathologies such as infection and obstruction, or from environmental and treatment-induced causes (Palmer, 1993).

Incontinence presents many secondary complications for the elderly person, including physiologic, social, psychologic, and economic effects. Physiologic effects include predisposition to impaired skin integrity, impaired skin hygiene, and a small hyperactive bladder. Social consequences are withdrawal from persons and activities, rejection by others, and the need to move to a nursing home. Urinary incontinence is one of the major reasons elderly persons are admitted to long-term care facilities (Fantl et al., 1996; Specht, 1986). The embarrassment and shame that the incontinent elder feels, combined with social rejec-

tion by others, often results in depression, self-neglect, low self-regard, and reclusion (Andrist & Maillet, 1992; Palmer, 1996). Urinary incontinence is a costly problem both for the incontinent person and for the health care system. Costs for equipment needed to manage the problem (e.g., adult briefs, laundry) and for institutionalization accrue to the individual. It has been estimated that the management of incontinence accounts for one third of the cost of nursing home care (Ouslander, 1981). Ouslander and Kane (1982) reported that $2000 to $4500 per year per person is spent in the United States to manage incontinent persons with disposable incontinence pads or catheters. Current estimates of the annual cost of incontinence management is $11.2 billion in the community and $5.2 billion in nursing homes (Hu, 1994). The management of incontinence in institutions is labor intensive and accounts for a large portion of the cost of care. It is estimated that expenditures for managing incontinence are second only to what is spent on food. The magnitude of the problem of urinary incontinence, particularly among elders, led to the formation of the Clinical Guideline Panel on Urinary Incontinence by the AHCPR and the subsequent publication of practice guidelines (McCormick, 1991).

PREVALENCE

According to the National Kidney and Urologic Diseases Advisory Board, approximately 13 million people in the United States are affected by urinary incontinence, with the highest incidence occurring among both noninstitutionalized and institutionalized elders. Although the incidence of incontinence in elders is known to be substantially higher than the 4% incidence identified in the general population, studies of prevalence vary widely in their findings. Available epidemiologic studies have several limitations: inconsistent definitions, biases in patient selection, methodologic differences that make comparisons impossible, and deficient documentation of relevant information in existing records (Kirschner-Hermanns, Scherr, Branch, Wetle, & Resnick, 1998; Mohide, 1986; Williams, 1983). Studies have documented that the incidence of incontinence in elders is from 14% to 40%, with twice as many women being affected as men. Yarnell and St. Leger (1979) reported that 11% to 17% of elderly persons living at home and 40% to 60% of elderly persons living in nursing homes in the United States were incontinent. Some claim that urinary incontinence plagues 15% to 30% of noninstitutionalized elders and at least half of the 1.5 million nursing home residents in the United States (Clinical Practice Guideline Panel, 1992; Diokno, Brock, Brown, & Herzog, 1986; Fantl et al., 1996; Resnick, Wetle, Scherr, Branch, & Taylor, 1986). Herzog, Diokno, Brown, Normolle, and Brock (1990) reported a prevalence of self-reported incontinence among noninstitutionalized older adults of 37.7% in females and 18.9% in males.

Incontinence is a regularly occurring problem, with about one third of persons afflicted reporting daily or weekly episodes of wetness (Burgio, Whitehead, & Engel, 1985). The seriousness of the problem for elders is underscored by the finding that elderly persons who are incontinent suffer the problem for an average of 9 years (Jeter & Wagner, 1990). It has been estimated that health care providers are aware of only half of the incontinent cases (Yarnell & St. Leger, 1979) because of patient reluctance to report this intimate and embarrassing problem to physicians or nurses and because of the absence of provider questioning about incontinence (Cohen et al., 1999). More than half of the people in the United States with urinary incontinence have had no evaluation or treatment (National Institutes of Health Consensus Development Conference on Urinary Incontinence in Adults, 1990).

Although incontinence is a common problem for elders and has major impact on the quality of their lives, incontinence is not an inevitable or irreversible consequence of aging. A number of interventions can be used to prevent or treat incontinence. There is growing evidence that treatment can reduce the incidence and cost of urinary incontinence in both institutionalized elders and elders living in their homes (Beheshti & Fonteyn, 1998; Ouslander, Palmer, Rovner, & German, 1993).

NURSING DIAGNOSIS

North American Nursing Diagnosis Association (NANDA, 1999) does not have a general definition for Urinary Incontinence. Rather, NANDA identifies five types of urinary incontinences: Stress Incontinence, Reflex Urinary Incontinence, Urge Incontinence, Functional Urinary Incontinence, and Total Incontinence. NANDA also includes Risk for Urinary Urge Incontinence as a diagnosis.

RELATED FACTORS/ETIOLOGIES

The risk of urinary incontinence increases with age. However, growing older itself does not cause incontinence. There is nothing involved with the normal aging process that makes incontinence inevitable. With normal aging, the kidneys become less able to concentrate urine, and the bladder has less capacity, becomes more irritable, and can hold residual urine (Kee, 1992). This leads to nocturia, frequency, urgency, and vulnerability to infection. The elderly person might not experience the sensation to void until the bladder is nearly full. Delayed sensation can lead to increased precipitancy and thus further compromise the time needed to get to a toilet. Decreased muscle tone in the pelvic floor and external sphincter can result in leakage caused by stress (Ulmsten, 1995; Wells, 1980). Furthermore, when the elder is at rest or sleeping, the kidneys can function more efficiently and increase the risk of nocturia. Consequently, there are more incontinent episodes among elders at night than during the day (O'Donnell, Beck, & Walls, 1990). The changes that accompany aging do not in and of themselves necessarily cause incontinence, but they make the balance between continence and incontinence for the elderly person more delicate so that other factors more easily precipitate incontinence.

The management of urinary incontinence in the elderly person has been constrained by the tendency to view incontinence as a single global problem. This has been partly because of a lack of research to describe more specific types of incontinence. However, nurses also have been slow to recognize their roles in diagnosis and treatment of incontinence and have lagged in the development and acquisition of the knowledge needed. As a result, it was not until the Classification of Nursing Diagnosis: Proceedings of the Seventh Conference that the North American Nursing Diagnosis Association (NANDA) classified five more specific incontinence diagnoses to their taxonomy (McLane, 1987): Stress Incontinence, Urge Incontinence, Reflex Incontinence, Functional Incontinence, and Total Incontinence. The AHCPR Guideline includes six types: Urge, Stress, Mixed, Overflow, Functional, and Reflex (Fantl et al., 1996). This chapter specifies eight distinct types of urinary incontinence, which can be grouped into three general categories. The category Incontinence Due to Problems With Bladder Filling includes Urge Incontinence, Reflex Incontinence, Stress Incontinence, and Mixed Incontinence. The category Incontinence Due to Problems With Bladder Emptying includes Overflow Incontinence and Total Incontinence. The category Incontinence Due to Spurious Functional and Environmental Maintenance Deficits includes Functional Incontinence and Iatrogenic Incontinence. These eight types of incontinence have differences in their etiologies, as well as in their defining characteristics (Table 22-1). Understanding the etiology of an elder's incontinence is critical for choosing interventions. Moreover, Tunink (1988) found that 16 of 17 male subjects had more than one type of incontinence, underscoring the importance of accurate assessment. Overflow and Iatrogenic Incontinence are not included in the NANDA classification.

Text continued on p. 257

	Suggested Nursing-Sensitive Outcomes and Nursing Interventions: Urge Incontinence; Stress Incontinence; Reflex Urinary Incontinence; Overflow Incontinence; Functional Urinary Incontinence; Total Incontinence; Iatrogenic Incontinence; Mixed Incontinence	
Table 22-1		

Nursing Diagnoses	Nursing-Sensitive Outcomes	Nursing Interventions
URGE INCONTINENCE ***Defining Characteristics*** Urinary urgency Frequency (void >q 2 hours) Bladder contracture/spasm Nocturia (>2 times per night) Voiding small amounts (>100 ml) Inability to reach toilet in time ***Related Factors/Etiologies*** Small bladder capacity/overdistension High caffeine/alcohol intake Medication effects (anticholinergic, diuretic, narcotic, beta-adrenergic) Bladder irritation Infection Detrusor instability Detrusor hyperreflexia	**URINARY CONTINENCE** ***Indicator*** Adequate time to reach toilet between urge and urination **INFECTION STATUS** ***Indicators*** White blood cell (WBC) elevation Pain/tenderness **KNOWLEDGE: TREATMENT PROCEDURE(S)** ***Indicators*** Description of treatment procedure Performance of treatment procedure **KNOWLEDGE: MEDICATION** ***Indicators*** Description of side effects of medication Description of self-monitoring techniques	**URINARY BLADDER TRAINING** ***Activities*** Determine ability to recognize urge to void Determine voiding pattern Establish toileting schedule based on voiding pattern Increase/decrease toileting intervals based on incontinence episodes **URINARY HABIT TRAINING** ***Activities*** Validate inability to cognitively recognize and act on urge Establish toileting schedule based on voiding pattern Assist to toilet and prompt to void at prescribed intervals Reinforce with staff importance of compliance with toileting schedule **PELVIC MUSCLE EXERCISE** ***Activities*** Instruct patient to tighten, then relax, the ring of muscle around urethra and anus Provide written instructions describing the intervention and the recommended number of repetitions Inform patient that it takes 6-12 weeks for exercises to be effective **FLUID MANAGEMENT** ***Activities*** Avoid caffeine/alcohol Promote fluid intake Keep accurate record of intake and output **PATIENT TEACHING** ***Activities*** Teach purpose of interventions Teach to actively hold urine Teach action/precautions with medications
STRESS INCONTINENCE ***Defining Characteristics*** Reported observed dribbling Urinary urgency Urinary frequency >q 2 hours ***Related Factors/Etiologies*** Weak pelvic muscles and structural supports High intraabdominal pressure (chronic cough, obesity, neoplasm, flatus) Incompetent bladder outlet Overdistention between voiding Rectocele/cystocele Atrophic vaginitis	**URINARY CONTINENCE** ***Indicator*** No urine leakage with increased abdominal pressure **COMPLIANCE BEHAVIOR** ***Indicator*** Reports following prescribed regimen	**PELVIC MUSCLE EXERCISE** ***Activities*** Instruct patient to tighten, then relax, the ring of muscle around urethra and anus Provide written instructions describing the intervention and the recommended number of repetitions Inform patient that it takes 6-12 weeks for exercises to be effective **BIOFEEDBACK** ***Activities*** Connect to instrumentation Assist to learn to modify responses to instrument cues Provide feedback of program after each session

| Table 22-1 | Suggested Nursing-Sensitive Outcomes and Nursing Interventions: Urge Incontinence; Stress Incontinence; Reflex Urinary Incontinence; Overflow Incontinence; Functional Urinary Incontinence; Total Incontinence; Iatrogenic Incontinence; Mixed Incontinence—cont'd |

Nursing Diagnoses	Nursing-Sensitive Outcomes	Nursing Interventions
		PATIENT TEACHING *Activities* Teach purpose of interventions Teach to actively hold urine Teach action/precautions with medications
REFLEX URINARY INCONTINENCE* *Defining Characteristics* No sensation of bladder filling No sensation of urge to void Sensation of urgency without voluntary inhibition of bladder contraction *Related Factors/Etiologies* Incomplete emptying with lesion above sacral micturition center Complete emptying with lesion above pontine micturition center Neural damage from radiation, inflammatory bladder, radical pelvic surgery, myomenigocele	**URINARY CONTINENCE** *Indicator* Predictable pattern to passage of urine	**URINARY BLADDER TRAINING** *Activities* Determine ability to recognize urge to void Determine voiding pattern Establish toileting schedule based on voiding pattern Increase/decrease toileting intervals based on incontinence episodes **URINARY CATHETERIZATION:** **INTERMITTENT** *Activities* Determine catheterization schedule based on a comprehensive urinary assessment Adjust frequency of catheterization to maintain output of 300 ml or less Teach patient/family purpose, supplies, methods, and rationale of intermittent catheterization **FLUID MANAGEMENT** *Activities* Maintain 1000 ml of fluid daily Keep accurate record of intake and output
OVERFLOW INCONTINENCE (AHCPR, 1996) *Defining Characteristics* Frequent or constant dribbling Urge or stress incontinence symptoms Palpable bladder Postvoid residual >100-200 ml *Related Factors/Etiologies* Outlet obstruction Underactive detrusor due to myogenic or neurogenic factors Pharmacologic interference with detrusor or sphincter activity	**URINARY CONTINENCE** *Indicator* Absence of postvoid residual >100-200 ml	**URINARY CATHETERIZATION:** **INTERMITTENT** *Activities* Determine catheterization schedule based on a comprehensive urinary assessment Adjust frequency of catheterization to maintain output of 300 ml or less Teach patient/family purpose, supplies, methods, and rationale of intermittent catheterization **FLUID MANAGEMENT** *Activities* Maintain 1000 ml fluid daily Keep accurate record of intake and output

Continued

*NANDA etiologies and related factors for Total Incontinence, neuropathy preventing transmission of reflex indicating bladder fullness and neurologic dysfunction triggering micturition of unpredictable times, are not included because they overlap with etiologies and related factors of Reflex Incontinence and therefore do not distinguish the two diagnoses.

Table 22-1	Suggested Nursing-Sensitive Outcomes and Nursing Interventions: Urge Incontinence; Stress Incontinence; Reflex Urinary Incontinence; Overflow Incontinence; Functional Urinary Incontinence; Total Incontinence; Iatrogenic Incontinence; Mixed Incontinence—cont'd	
Nursing Diagnoses	**Nursing-Sensitive Outcomes**	**Nursing Interventions**
FUNCTIONAL URINARY INCONTINENCE *Defining Characteristic* Senses need to void *Related Factors/Etiologies* Altered environmental factors (unfamiliar, inconvenient toilet, lack of privacy, lack of assistance, obstructive clothing) Sensory/cognitive/mobility deficits (impaired vision, gait/balance, dexterity, transfer, strength, endurance) Psychologic factors Weakened support/pelvic structures	**URINARY CONTINENCE** *Indicators* Able to manage clothing independently Able to manage toilet independently **SELF-CARE: TOILETING** *Indicators* Removes clothing Gets to and from toilet	**ENVIRONMENTAL MANAGEMENT** *Activities* Provide adaptive devices Provide accessible toilet, privacy, assistance, and clothing **URINARY HABIT TRAINING** *Activities* Validate inability to cognitively recognize and act on urge Establish toileting schedule based on voiding pattern Assist to toilet and prompt to void at prescribed intervals Reinforce with staff importance of compliance with toileting schedule **FLUID MANAGEMENT** *Activities* Promote fluid intake Keep accurate record of intake and output **SELF-CARE ASSISTANCE: TOILETING** *Activities* Encourage to perform to level of ability Assist to toilet at specified intervals
TOTAL INCONTINENCE* *Defining Characteristics* Constant flow of urine occurs Nocturia Lack of perineal or bladder filling Unawareness of incontinence *Related Factors/Etiologies* Anatomic (fistula) Surgical trauma of spinal cord Ectopic ureter Congenital ectopic urethral, bladder, or ureteral orifice Severe sphincter deficiency	**TISSUE INTEGRITY: SKIN & MUCOUS MEMBRANES** *Indicators* Color in expected range Skin intactness **URINARY ELIMINATION** *Indicators* 24-hour intake and output balanced Urine color and odor in expected range **SELF-CARE: HYGIENE** *Indicators* Cleans perineal area Free of urine odor	**URINARY INCONTINENCE CARE** *Activities* Provide protective garments Cleanse genital skin area at regular intervals **SELF-CARE ASSISTANCE: BATHING/HYGIENE** *Activities* Provide assistance until able to assume self-care Make needed supplies accessible Monitor for odor of urine
IATROGENIC INCONTINENCE *Defining Characteristics* Prescribed medications that affect urinary function Prescribed increase or decrease in medications Prescribed activity restriction Prescribed continence aids *Related Factors/Etiologies* Health caregiver prescriptions (restraints, fluid restrictions, bed rest, IV fluids, medications)	**KNOWLEDGE: MEDICATION** *Indicators* Description of side effects of medication Description of self-monitoring techniques **URINARY CONTINENCE** *Indicators* Free of medications that interfere with urinary control Fluid intake in expected range **MOBILITY LEVEL** *Indicator* Ambulation: walking	**PATIENT TEACHING** *Activities* Teach purpose of interventions Teach action/precautions with medications **REFERRAL** *Activities* Identify nursing/health care required Perform ongoing monitoring of need for referral **HEALTH CARE INFORMATION EXCHANGE** *Activities* Identify current medical and nursing diagnoses Describe nursing interventions being implemented

	Suggested Nursing-Sensitive Outcomes and Nursing Interventions: Urge Incontinence; Stress Incontinence; Reflex Urinary Incontinence; Overflow Incontinence; Functional Urinary Incontinence; Total Incontinence; Iatrogenic Incontinence; Mixed Incontinence—cont'd	
Table 22-1		
Nursing Diagnoses	**Nursing-Sensitive Outcomes**	**Nursing Interventions**
MIXED INCONTINENCE *Defining Characteristics* Urinary urgency Frequency (void >q 2 hours) Bladder contracture/spasm Nocturia (>2 times per night) Voiding small amounts (>100 ml) Inability to reach toilet in time Reported or observed dribbling	**URINARY CONTINENCE** *Indicators* Adequate time to reach toilet between urge and evacuation of urine Free of urine leakage between voidings	**PELVIC MUSCLE EXERCISE** *Activities* Instruct patient to tighten, then relax, the ring of muscle around urethra and anus, as if trying to prevent urination or bowel movement Provide written instructions describing the intervention and the recommended number of repetitions Inform patient that it takes 6-12 weeks for exercises to be effective **BIOFEEDBACK** *Activities* Connect patient to the instrumentation device, as needed Assist patient to learn to modify bodily responses to equipment cues Provide feedback of progress after each session **FLUID MANAGEMENT** *Activities* Maintain accurate intake and output record Maintain 1000 ml of fluid daily

RISK FACTORS

Older people are more apt to incur illnesses, injuries, and surgeries and are more vulnerable to urinary tract infections. In addition, the diminished efficiency of body systems and organs that often accompanies aging can predispose the elder to incontinence (see Chapter 28). Diminished sight and decreased mobility (flexibility, balance, strength) can increase the time taken to locate and reach the toilet. Chronic illnesses that often accompany aging (e.g., cerebrovascular accidents, parkinsonism, arthritis, dementia, diabetes mellitus) have the greatest impact on mobility, and the neurogenic consequences of many of these diseases (e.g., the neuropathy of diabetes mellitus) interfere with control of urine functions. Decreased facilitation and inhibition in cerebral function can make the control of urine unpredictable. The association of mental impairment and incontinence in the elders is common (James, 1979; Skelly & Flint, 1995).

Acute illness and hospitalization also can create risk factors that interfere temporarily with normal function. Quite often the acutely ill, hospitalized elder remains incontinent because of inappropriate assessment and treatment of the problem (Palmer, 1996). Factors that predispose elderly persons to urinary incontinence are (1) the prolonged use of indwelling catheters in an elder who could have regained continence had the catheter been removed earlier; (2) drug therapy such as diuretics, hyp-

notics, and tricyclic antidepressants that either increase the speed of urine production or dull sensations; and (3) environmental factors, including physical obstacles (e.g., bedrails) and staff attitudes and expectations. Nurses must have knowledge of all of these risk factors to assess, diagnose, and treat incontinence in elderly persons.

ASSESSMENT

See Table 22-1 for the etiologies and defining characteristics for the various types of incontinence (Carroll-Johnson, 1989; NANDA, 1999). Griffin (1983) outlined the categorization of incontinence as transient versus established to highlight the need for assessment to identify reversible causes amenable to treatment. The differential diagnosis of a definitive urinary incontinence requires careful and thorough assessment for the signs and symptoms that are associated with the specific etiologies for each of the eight incontinence diagnoses, with initial emphasis on reversible causes of transient incontinence (Fantl et al., 1996). Effective nursing intervention for incontinence is dependent on this critical first step because treatment must be directed at the underlying causes. Assessment Guide 22-1 presents a tool that nurses can use to gather assessment information.

Assessment information can be gathered through interviews with the elder, family member, or significant other,

Assessment Guide 22-1

Urinary Incontinence

Date _____ Assessed by _____

Name _____ D.O.B. _____ Sex _____

Marital Status _____ Race ____ _____

I. HISTORY
  A. Main Complaint _____
  B. Urinary Symptoms
     1. Frequency: How often do you urinate during the day? _____
     2. Nocturia: How often do you urinate during the night? _____
                          Do you awaken? _____ Number of nights per week? _____
     3. Urgency: Once you are aware you need to urinate, how long can you wait? _____
                          Can you tell when your bladder is full? _____
     4. Stress: Do you ever lose urine when you laugh, cough, sneeze, or change position? _____
                          Do you lose a little or a lot? _____
     5. Reflex: Can you tell when you have passed urine? _____
     6. Hesitancy: Do you have difficulty starting to urinate? _____
     7. Stream: Has the size of the stream changed recently? _____
                          Has the force of the stream changed recently? _____
                          Can you start and stop the stream? _____
     8. Straining: Do you ever strain to urinate? _____
                          Are you ever not able to urinate when you strain? _____
                          Do you use manual expression to help urinate? _____
     9. Postmicturition
        dribbling: Do you ever dribble urine after you have urinated? _____
    10. Dysuria: Do you have any pain or burning when you pass your urine? _____
    11. Turbidity: Is your urine clear? _____ Is it cloudy? _____
                          Does it appear to contain mucus? _____
    12. Hematuria: What color is your urine? _____
                          Does your urine ever have blood in it? _____
    13. Control: Do you ever have any problem controlling your urine? _____
                          If so, when did this begin? _____
                          How often does it occur? _____
                          How much urine is lost? _____
                          How do you manage this problem? _____
                          Is this effective? _____
                          Do you take any precautions to protect your skin? _____
                          What precautions? _____
                          Do you have any skin breakdown? _____
                          How has your daily living been changed because you have difficulty controlling your urine? _____
    14. Emptying: Do you feel like your bladder empties completely when you urinate? _____
  C. Fluid Intake
     1. Amount: How many cups of fluid do you drink in a day? _____
                          Do you restrict your fluids in any way? _____
     2. Kind: How much water do you drink daily? _____
                          Do you drink coffee? _____ Caffeinated? _____ Decaffeinated? _____
                          Tea? _____ Caffeinated? _____ Decaffeinated? _____
                          Cola? _____ Caffeinated? _____ Decaffeinated? _____
                          Chocolate drink? _____
                          Alcoholic beverages? _____
                          How much of each do you drink? _____
     3. Timing: Do you usually have fluids only with meals? _____
                          Do you drink fluids after supper or through the night? _____
  D. Bladder Record
     The client, family member, or significant other is asked to fill out the Urinary Continence Specification Record, _____
     which is presented in Assessment Guide 22-2. If this is not possible, nursing staff institutions should fill it out. The record is
     filled out daily for 1 week.

E. Medical History
  1. Relevant past health: Have you had any abdominal, genital, or gynecologic operations or treatments? _____
    Have you had any bladder or kidney infections? _____
    Have you had any brain or spinal cord disease or injury of any kind? _____
    (Women) Number of pregnancies? _____
    Number of live births? _____
    Have you reached menopause? _____
    How old were you? _____
    Do you have any history of stroke? _____
    Diabetes? _____
    Other chronic diseases? _____
    Did you have problem with bed-wetting at night as a child? _____
  2. Present health: What are your current health problems? _____
    Do you smoke? _____ How long? _____ How much? _____
  3. Medications: What medication(s) are you taking? _____
F. Bowels
  1. Habits: How often do you have a bowel movement? _____
    Any difficulty? _____
    Constipation? _____ Incontinence? _____ Diarrhea? _____
    Impactions? _____
  2. Treatment: Do you use any laxatives or other aids such as diet to assist with regularity? _____
G. Functional Abilities
  1. Mobility: Any difficulty getting to the toilet? _____
    Any difficulty getting on and off the toilet? _____
    Any problems with balance that affect your ability to use the toilet? _____
  2. Manual dexterity: Do you experience any difficulty removing or adjusting clothing to go to the toilet? _____
    Do you have difficulty cleaning yourself after toileting? _____
  3. Vision: Can you see well enough to get to the toilet and use the facilities? _____
    Is your vision more of a problem at night? _____
H. Environment Is your bathroom or toilet located in a convenient place? _____
  Is it available to you any time you need it? _____
  Is there any problem with the physical layout of the toilet? _____
  If dementia is present, are there environmental cues to assist in locating bathroom? _____
I. Psychologic State Describe your attitude and feelings about your incontinence. _____
J. Social Relationships Has incontinence restricted your usual activities or relationships in any way? _____
K. Goals What would you like to accomplish with treatment for your incontinence? _____

II. PHYSICAL EXAMINATION
A. TPR _____ Weight _____
B. Abdomen
  1. Bowel sounds _____
  2. Scars _____
  3. Bladder distention before and after voiding _____
C. Genitalia
  1. Skin _____
  2. Urethral meatus _____
    Stress test (stand with full bladder and see if any urine leaks out)
  3. Women:
    a. Labia, vaginal mucosae _____
      Dry _____ Moist _____
    b. Any protrusions from or in the vagina? _____
    c. Any objects in the vagina? _____
    d. Can the patient feel your finger in the vagina? _____
      Can she squeeze her vagina around it? _____
      Is the squeeze strong or weak? _____
  4. Men
    a. Penis circumcised? _____
    b. If not, is foreskin freely movable? _____
    c. Is the penis small and/or retracted? _____
    d. Is the scrotum enlarged? _____ Tender? _____ Hard? _____
      Hot? _____ Inflamed? _____ Other? _____
    e. Enlarged prostate? _____
    f. PSA _____ When done? _____ Results? _____

Continued

URINARY INCONTINENCE—CONT'D

D. Rectum
1. Hemorrhoids? _____
2. Anal tone firm? _____ Weak? _____
3. Stool soft? _____ Hard? _____ None? _____

E. Mental Function
1. Confused? _____ Oriented? _____ Forgetful? _____
2. Ability to recognize toilet articles and how to toilet? _____
3. Ability to perform familiar action, e.g., push down to defecate? _____
4. Is body perception intact? _____
   Test by touching contralateral buttock. _____

F. Urinalysis
1. Bacteria or fungi? _____
   WBCs? _____ Specific gravity? _____
   Other abnormalities? _____
2. Culture if significant bacteria? _____
3. Postvoid residual amount? _____

G. Mobility
1. Ambulate by self? _____
2. Transfer by self? _____
3. Manipulation of clothing? _____
4. Strength? _____ Endurance? _____
   Gait? _____ Balance? _____
5. Time needed to get to toilet after urge and before voiding? _____
6. Ability to get to toilet in time needed to avoid incontinence? _____

H. Urodynamic Studies _____

*Tools are available that expand the objective assessment of these items that should be used if there is reason to believe that the sub-
jective indicators are not reliable or valid or need further measurement.

through observation, through physical examination, and through consultation with other caregivers (Brink, 1980; Palmer, 1996). Establishing rapport, privacy, and a comfortable, unhurried environment will greatly influence the ability to gather accurate data about this sensitive area.

Medical literature often recommends urodynamic studies as essential for making an accurate diagnosis. Urodynamic studies measure the urine capacity of the bladder, bladder contraction, and urethral and sphincteric function. These studies can be complex and expensive, using computerized analog equipment. Although cystometry and urethral pressure profiles can assist with the identification of signs, they should be used with caution for elders (Specht, 1986). These procedures are complex and expensive, and elders can show abnormalities on urodynamic studies even when they are continent (Williams, 1983). Ouslander et al. (1988) found that alternative bedside procedures could be accurate in providing information for incontinence management decisions and were well tolerated by elders. Bedside cystometry, a less expensive option than urodynamic studies, consists of catheterization for postvoid residual followed by incremental filling of the bladder by gravity through a catheter-tipped syringe. The fluid level is observed for any rise in the meniscus, which is indicative of involuntary detrusor contractions. This procedure provides information about bladder capacity and the interval of time between initial contraction and bladder emptying (Wozniak-Petrofsky,

1996). Assessment of urine flow is a noninvasive alternative. A uroflowmeter can be used so that the patient can void in private. The uroflowmeter is a funnel-like device with electric sensors that measure flow rate and produce a graph of the individual's flow rate. Delays in starting to void or a long period of time to empty the bladder can indicate urinary retention. Another approach is to complete an evaluation of urinary incontinence using a history, physical examination, urinalysis, and postvoid residual urine to detect and track reversible causes, identify urge or stress incontinence, and treat the problem accordingly. If treatment does not succeed, more invasive assessment procedures can be considered (Weiss, 1998).

The literature includes a number of tools for assessing urinary incontinence. The Clinical Practice Guideline Panel (1992) and Fantl et al. (1996) provide principles for diagnostic evaluation and assessment and include sample voiding records and an algorithm to assist with assessment and diagnosis of the type of incontinence. The mandated Long Term Care Minimum Data Set (LTC MDS) and Resident Assessment Protocol for nursing homes provide a framework for assessment, with some decision support for the diagnosis of specific types of incontinence (Morris, Murphy, & Nonemaker, 1995). Some tools that are available, however, contain a variety of weaknesses. Some tools are very useful for collecting specific kinds of data but do not allow for the development of a database that is adequate to make decisions about specific etiologies and in-

URINARY CONTINENCE SPECIFICATION RECORD

Name _____ Date _____

Instructions:

1. In the first column mark the time of day each time you pass urine.

2. In the third and fourth columns mark every time you accidentally leak urine and the reasons/circumstances.

3. In the fifth column record your fluid intake for the hour.

Time Interval	Urinated in Toilet	Leaking or Large Accident	Reason for Accident	Fluids
6 AM				
7 AM				

terventions for all types of incontinence. A major weakness of many available tools is that the structures do not adequately assist the nurse with a logical progression of diagnostic decision making. Assessment guidelines should include tools that help the nurse gather data to screen for etiologies and to focus and structure the search for more detailed information in specific areas that are crucial for the effective treatment of incontinence. For example, the nurse needs to know whether the elder is ambulatory, whether the speed of ambulation is adequate to reach the toilet facility after the urge and before urination, and whether a bedside commode is needed. The assessment tool in Assessment Guide 22-1 was designed to overcome these weaknesses. Three gerontologic nursing specialists evaluated the content validity of the tool. The tool has been used for assessment in a large long-term care facility for 8 years. The tool refers to other instruments that are available to measure specific characteristics that can be used to augment data collection. The guide should be used in nursing homes to complete a more in-depth assessment if the Resident Assessment Protocol indicates that an incontinence problem exists. The assessment guide is not a questionnaire to be filled out. Rather, it is a guide that the nurse can use to prompt the framing of questions to fit each client and situation and as a reminder of data that are needed. It is important that the nurse use prompts to get the client (family) to describe subjective data and that the nurse follow patient cues for specific lines of questioning.

A critical part of assessment is the Urinary Continence Specification Record (Assessment Guide 22-2). This record helps to determine the number and pattern of incontinent episodes, as well as the associated relevant events, such as activity level and fluid intake. It is recommended that episodes of incontinence be recorded for 3 days or until a pattern can be identified (Iowa Intervention Project, 2000; Palmer, 1996; Robb, 1985).

The database that is gathered for making an accurate nursing diagnosis of incontinence must encompass the risk factors, physical causes, psychosocial causes, environmental causes, and information about how functional abilities are affecting continence for the elder (Brink, 1980; Brink, Wells, & Diokno, 1985; Fantl et al., 1996; Palmer, 1996; Specht, 1986; Wells & Brink, 1981). See Table 22-1 for the defining data for the specific types of incontinence. Assessment tools should be evaluated for adequacy by the extent that they guide the nurse to elicit these data. Nursing interventions that will assist with reestablishing continence cannot be determined without adequate and thorough assessment of the multiple factors contributing to specific types of incontinence (Penn, 1990; Rottkamp, 1985). Detailed information follows on the etiologies and defining characteristics associated with specific types of incontinence.

Urge Incontinence

Urge incontinence is involuntary urination that occurs soon after a strong sense of urgency to void (Carroll-Johnson, 1989). It also is defined as "an uncontrollable loss of urine preceded by an urge to void but failure to hold urine long enough to reach a toilet" (Diokno, 1983, p. 70). Urge incontinence is the most prevalent type of incontinence in nursing homes (Resnick, Yalla, & Laurino, 1989). The cardinal symptom of urge incontinence is strong urge to void with involuntary loss of urine, and it most often is associated with a urodynamic demonstration of detrusor instability (Fantl et al., 1996). However, Woodtli and Yocum (1994) found the most definitive characteristics of urge incontinence to be loss of urine before getting to toilet, sudden desire to pass urine, need to hurry to toilet, and inability to hold urine or suppress the desire to pass urine. Awad and McGinnis (1983) and Webster, Sihelnik, and Stone (1984) found a complex of symptoms similar to those described by Woodtli and Yocum more predictive of urge incontinence than urodynamic studies. Diokno (1983) says that the key question to ask is "Do you have a feeling of urge to void and leak urine before reaching the toilet?" (p. 72). Heightened urgency results from bladder irritation, reduced bladder capacity, or overdistention of the bladder. The irritation of the bladder stretch receptors causes spasms and emptying. The bladder, stretched to the limits of its capacity because of either a severely reduced capacity or overdistention, empties precipitously (Carroll-Johnson, 1989).

Urge incontinence is associated with cerebrovascular accidents (CVAs), incomplete suprasacral spinal cord injury, pelvic injury/trauma, multiple sclerosis (MS), brain tumor, previous brain trauma, enlarged prostate, interstitial cystitis, and smaller bladder capacity. When a neurologic lesion is confirmed as the cause, the underlying condition, formerly called uninhibited neurogenic bladder, is now considered to be detrusor hyperreflexia (Fantl et al., 1996; Palmer, 1996).

A problem with assessment and diagnosis of urge incontinence in elderly persons is that the signs and symptoms usually associated with detrusor instability in younger persons (urgency, diurnal, and nocturnal enuresis) are common in all diagnoses of incontinence for elders (Hilton & Stanton, 1981). Urine loss with urge incontinence is larger and more prolonged than with stress incontinence. With urge incontinence there is a tendency for urine loss to be greater in the morning than in the evening (Malvern, 1981). When detrusor hyperactivity is accompanied by impaired bladder contractility, the elder must strain to empty despite the involuntary contractions. This is why persons with urge incontinence also can have a postvoid residual. Thus, to be certain of appropriate diagnosis and intervention, urge incontinence must be distinguished from stress and overflow incontinence. Urgency and precipitancy are indicators of urge incontinence that are common to all etiologies. See Table 22-1 for other defining characteristics for the etiologies.

Reflex Incontinence

Reflex incontinence is the involuntary loss of urine caused by completion of the spinal cord reflex arc (bladder contraction) in the absence of higher neural control (Carroll-Johnson, 1989). As defined by the International Continence Society Committee on Standardization of Terminology (1990), reflex incontinence is "loss of urine due to detrusor hyperreflexia and/or involuntary urethral relaxation in the absence of sensation usually associated with the desire to micturate. Voiding often will occur as a specific and predictable volume is reached. This form of incontinence occurs with complete lesions of the spinal cord above the conus medullaris. There is no sensation of urgency or voiding. A reflex bladder contraction occurs with bladder filling or response to perineal or lower abdominal stimuli" (Wheatley, 1982, p. 77). One problem with this type of bladder is that the external sphincter, as well as the detrusor muscle, can be spastic, thereby preventing adequate emptying of the bladder. A major concern for these persons is the development of vesicoureteral reflux (urine backed from bladder into ureter) and hydronephro-

sis (urine backed into kidney), which lead to serious infections (Fantl et al., 1996). The person with reflex incontinence usually does not receive the message of the need to void. However, sensations such as sweating, restlessness, and abdominal discomfort can warn the person of the need to empty her bladder. The nurse can help this patient find "trigger areas" that initiate the voiding reflex when stimulated (Delehanty & Stravino, 1970). Digital stimulation of the anus and rectum is usually the most effective stimulus, but tapping the abdomen or doing push-ups on the commode chair also can be effective in precipitating voiding. See Table 22-1 for the etiologies and critical signs and symptoms for reflex incontinence.

Reflex incontinence and urge incontinence are often grouped together as neurogenic or uninhibited bladder. The distinction between reflex incontinence and urge incontinence is particularly difficult when the elderly person has an incomplete spinal cord lesion or damage to the cerebral cortex, as with dementia, CVA, or MS. In these situations partial sensation of urge to void and partial bladder control can result. Some sensation of urgency is a distinguishing characteristic for urge incontinence and is a positive prognostic indicator for regaining continence.

Stress Incontinence

Stress incontinence is leakage of urine related to increased intraabdominal pressure, often occurring with coughing, sneezing, or lifting (Carroll-Johnson, 1989). The International Continence Society on Standardization of Terminology (1990) defines stress incontinence as the involuntary loss of urine occurring when in the absence of a detrusor contraction the intravesical pressure (pressure in the bladder) exceeds the maximal urethral pressure. It is characterized by the sudden loss of a small amount of urine associated with increased physical activity (coughing, laughing, lifting) and with no other voiding symptoms present (Diokno, 1983). Women are more prone to stress incontinence because of a short urethra and loss of the urethrovesical angle resulting from a decrease in pelvic floor muscle tone (Palmer, 1996). Stress incontinence is most often associated with multiple incontinence surgical procedures, hypoestrogenism, and aging. Wells, Brink, and Diokno (1987), in a study of 200 community-dwelling older women, found that stress incontinence was the most common type of incontinence. Stress incontinence in men often is associated with prostatectomy and radiation (Fantl et al., 1996).

The etiologies for stress incontinence are weakened pelvic muscles and support structures, high intraabdominal pressure, overdistention, and incompetent bladder outlet or sphincter deficiency. Pregnancies, vaginal deliveries, surgical trauma, obesity, and chronic coughing are predisposing factors (McDowell, 1997). The following signs and symptoms are seen for all etiologies of stress incontinence: frequent leakage of small amounts of urine with activity, not preceded by urgency; gradual onset; low residual urine (less than 100 ml); and leakage when the bladder is full that is worse on standing. Wetting less at night than during the day is characteristic. Diokno (1983) suggests that the key question to ask the individual is "Do you lose urine when you cough or strain?" (p. 70).

When stress incontinence results from weakened pelvic muscles and support structures, the following additional critical signs and symptoms occur: incompetent levators ani, assessed by digital examination of the vagina; stretched pelvic floor fascia, assessed by digital examination; and ineffective muscle tone for bowel evacuation. Pelvic muscle strength can be evaluated through a simple test. The patient lies in a recumbent position with knees bent and apart. The gloved index and middle fingers of one hand are inserted into the patient's vagina. If there is stretching of the fascia, the downward thrust of "bearing down" will tend to push the fingers out of the vagina. When the fingers are withdrawn until the two distal phalanges are palpating the posterior vaginal wall, the strength of the levator ani muscles can be assessed. The patient is instructed, "Do not let me pull out my fingers." The levator ani muscles then act alone, and the strength of their action, from a flicker to a firm squeeze, can be assessed (Harrison, 1983). A digital test also has been developed by Brink, Sampselle, Wells, Diokno, and Gillis (1989) to rate the strength of pelvic muscle contraction on a scale of 0 to 4. This and other measures have been developed by nurses to standardize the quantification of pelvic muscle strength (Worth, Dougherty, & McKey, 1986).

Contributing factors to be assessed are obesity, multiple pregnancies, and vaginal deliveries (Thom & Brown, 1998); history of an occupation that required bouncing or heavy lifting; and history of constipation with straining to defecate. Studies have shown that the number of children has an effect on the risk for incontinence if it is greater than two; the risk does not continue to increase after five children (Norton, 1984). See Table 22-1 for additional signs and symptoms for etiologies of stress incontinence.

Mixed Incontinence

Mixed incontinence is defined as the leakage of urine associated with increased intraabdominal pressure (stress) and inability to delay voiding (urge) (Clinical Practice Guideline Panel, 1992). The prevalence of this type of incontinence is greatest among frail, elderly women and is common in both community-dwelling and nursing home elders. Persons present with symptoms of both urge and stress incontinence, with the symptom of one type usually predominating (Diokno et al., 1986; Ouslander, Staskin, Raz, Su, & Hepps, 1987; Woodtli, 1995).

Overflow Incontinence

Overflow incontinence occurs when the bladder becomes sufficiently overdistended that voiding attempts result in frequent small amounts of urine, often in the form of dribbling. Overflow incontinence is defined as involuntary loss of urine associated with overdistention of the bladder (Fantl et al., 1996; International Continence Society Committee on Standardization of Terminology, 1990). The terms *atonic bladder* and *lower motor neuron bladder* previously were used to describe overflow incontinence (Palmer, 1996). This type of incontinence is paradoxical because the inability to void occurs concurrently with incontinence. Overflow incontinence results either from bladder hypotonia caused by impaired bladder neuromusculature or from bladder outlet obstruction. Bladder hypotonia can be caused by diabetes mellitus, pelvic trauma, extensive pelvic surgery, lesions or injuries of the conus medullaris, herpes zoster, MS, tabes dorsalis, pernicious anemias, and poliomyelitis. The bladder reflex arc is lost, but parasympathetic innervation prevents vesicle hypersensitivity and hypertonicity. The external sphincter remains strong, but the detrusor loses its contractility. The bladder stores large volumes of urine at low pressure. Bladder outlet obstructions result from prostatic enlargement, bladder neck musculature hypertrophy, bladder neck contracture postsurgically, urethral stricture disease, and fecal impactions.

High levels of residual urine, hesitancy, slow stream, passage of infrequent small volumes of urine (dribbling), a feeling of incomplete bladder emptying, sudden leakage of urine related to bending or turning, dysuria, and a palpable full bladder more than two fingers above the symphysis pubis are common signs and symptoms seen with all etiologies of overflow incontinence.

Urodynamic studies often are necessary to distinguish obstruction from atonic causes of overflow incontinence (Griffin, 1983). Urodynamic studies are indicated if the critical signs and symptoms listed in Table 22-1 are not observed. The results of these studies are used to guide specific treatment. Ruling out outlet obstruction is especially important to prevent inappropriate and harmful bladder suppressant treatment of misdiagnosed detrusor hyperactivity or surgery to resolve an obstruction that does not exist (Resnick, 1990; Schaeffer, 1988).

Total Incontinence

Total incontinence is an unpredictable or continuous loss of urine resulting from neuropathy of bladder stretch receptors, damage to cerebral neuron control of urination, spinal cord or peripheral nerve lesions below the reflex arc, or anatomic fistulas from surgery, accidental trauma, or malformations (Carroll-Johnson, 1989). Total incontinence is often diagnosed after stress, urge, reflex, or functional incontinence has been ruled out. The diagnosis is distinguished from reflex incontinence by the unpredictable pattern of bladder emptying. Continuous flow of urine also can occur with predictable bladder emptying caused by fistula or congenital ectopic urethral bladder or ureteral orifice that circumvents the normal sphincter mechanisms (Wheatley, 1982).

Total incontinence is caused either by neuropathy of the bladder stretch receptors and spinal cord or by peripheral nerve lesions below the reflex arc. In these situations the reflex arc is interrupted and the brain does not receive the message that the bladder is full. Thus there is no reflex control of urination and the voiding pattern is not predictable. This has been referred to as lower motor neuron bladder or autonomous bladder (Delehanty & Stravino, 1970). With this etiology, controlled emptying can occur only if intraabdominal pressure is increased, either by contracting the abdominal and diaphragmatic muscles or by external suprapubic pressure (Crede's method).

Continuous incontinent urine flow usually results from an anatomic fistula caused by surgery or trauma or malformation such as ectopic urethral, bladder, or ureteral opening. With total incontinence, the reflex control is intact, but urination cannot be controlled because the urinary anatomy is impaired or misplaced. See Table 22-1 for etiologies and critical signs and symptoms for total incontinence.

Functional Incontinence

Functional incontinence is the inability to reach the toilet on time because of environmental barriers or disorientation to place. Functional incontinence refers to potentially continent individuals (frequently with compromised mobility) who cannot or will not reach the toilet in time to avoid an accident (Williams, 1983). Ouslander (1994) defines functional incontinence as urinary leakage associated with an inability to toilet because of impairment of cognitive and/or physical functioning, psychologic unwillingness, or environmental barriers. In general, the etiologies for functional incontinence are physical, cognitive/perceptual, or psychosocial deficits interacting with the environment that limit the individual's mastery of continence. A common etiology is the unavailability of caregivers to provide assistance to persons who have a functioning genitourinary system but compromised physical or cognitive function. Thus, involuntary loss of urine occurs even though there is normal bladder and urethral function. Large voidings with complete emptying of the bladder occur with all etiologies of functional incontinence. Ouslander (1981) and Ouslander, Kane, Vollmer, and Menezes (1985) suggested that functional incontinence might be the leading form of incontinence in nursing homes.

Environmental factors interact with physical, cognitive/perceptual, and psychosocial deficits to cause incontinence for elders. Much urinary incontinence results from the loss of the race between the bladder and legs. The following formula has been developed to assess the relationship between distance to the bathroom and bladder emptying (Fine, 1972):

$$\text{If } D/T2 > T1, \text{ incontinence will result,}$$

where:

T1 = Time interval between onset of desire for urination and arrival of uncontrollable urination

T2 = Rate of walking in feet per minute

D = Distance to the bathroom

D/T2 = Time taken by individual to reach toilet

Wyman, Elswick, Ory, Wilson, and Fantl (1993) tested the formula and found that the distance to the toilet was associated with frequency of incontinence, but distance divided by time to reach the toilet did not predict frequency of incontinence. Persons with slower mobility and shorter distances to the toilet had the highest number of incidences of incontinence.

Lack of privacy, lack of access to a toilet, poor lighting, inappropriate clothing, delays in answering "call lights," use of equipment that does not promote normal voiding, and caregivers who demean, punish, or accept incontinence as inevitable with aging can contribute to incontinence in elders who could be continent in a supportive environment. The critical signs and symptoms for physical, cognitive/perceptual, and psychosocial etiologies of functional incontinence are listed in Table 22-1 and must be evaluated along with the specific environmental conditions for each elderly person. For example, persons with dementia often can recognize picture symbols after word recognition is lost; so a picture of a toilet or a woman on a bathroom door is preferable to the word "toilet" or "women."

Iatrogenic Incontinence

Iatrogenic incontinence results from physician- and/or nurse-controlled factors, such as restraints, medications, fluid limitations, bed rest, and/or intravenous fluids. Without the treatment the elderly person would be continent. Although this diagnosis of incontinence is regrettable and we should seek to prevent its causes, iatrogenic incontinence often is easily reversed or compensated. A common cause of Iatrogenic Incontinence is drug therapy. Williams and Panill (1982) describe this type of incontinence and the common pharmaceutical treatments that are etiologies. Other authors often refer to this type of incontinence as a risk factor for transient forms of incontinence. Identification of Iatrogenic Incontinence emphasizes the importance of assessing these factors and maintaining vigilant assessment of treatments to ensure that they do not cause other serious problems for elders. See Table 22-1 for the etiologies and defining characteristics for Iatrogenic Incontinence.

CASE STUDY 1

C. Sanders is an 80-year-old man, widowed for 10 years, who is residing in his own home. Mr. Sanders had a cholecystectomy when he was 65 and a transurethral resection of the prostate for benign hypertrophy when he was 70. He has been treated for congestive heart failure for the past 5 years, and during the past 3 months he has been taking 80 mg of Lasix each morning. Mr. Sanders has had reduced activity because of his cardiac decompensation and has experienced loss of strength and mobility for self-care activities. He has particular difficulty with small-motor tasks, including putting on and removing his clothing. He often does not remove his clothing at night and resists changing his clothing more than once or twice a week. Frequently, the home health nurse or aide finds his underwear and trousers wet with urine. His voidings are usually in large amounts. He is a heavy coffee drinker and does not like decaffeinated coffee. Urinalysis revealed that the urine was clear of bacteria and fungi. Mr. Sanders reports that he knows when he has to urinate, but that emptying often comes before he has time to reach the toilet. He states that he has reduced his fluid intake other than coffee in an effort to reduce the need to urinate. Table 22-3 presents Mr. Sanders' significant signs and symptoms, those diagnoses that can be ruled out, and the additional data needed. Table 22-2 contains the nursing diagnoses, outcomes, and interventions used for the management of Mr. Sanders' incontinence.

Table 22-2 Nursing Diagnoses, Outcomes, and Interventions for MR. SANDERS

Nursing Diagnoses	Nursing-Sensitive Outcomes	Nursing Interventions
URGE INCONTINENCE *Defining Characteristics* Aware of need to void Voiding in large amounts	**URINARY CONTINENCE** *Indicators* Responds in timely manner to urge Predictable pattern to passage of urine	**URINARY HABIT TRAINING** *Activities* Establish toileting interval not <2 hours Maintain scheduled toileting **URINARY INCONTINENCE CARE** *Activities*
Low volume intake Large amount of coffee Underclothing frequently wet	Fluid intake in expected range Free of oral fluids containing caffeine Underclothing dry during day Underclothing/bedding dry at night Free of urine leakage between voidings	Instruct to drink not <1500 ml daily Limit ingestion of bladder irritants **PELVIC MUSCLE EXERCISE** *Activities* Instruct patient to tighten, then relax, the ring of muscle around the urethra and anus Instruct patient to void contracting the abdomen, thighs, and buttocks, and holding breath or straining down during the exercise Perform exercises 50-100 times each day, holding contractions for 10 seconds each Inform patient that it takes 6-12 weeks for exercise to be effective Discuss daily record of continence with patient to provide reinforcement
IATROGENIC INCONTINENCE *Defining Characteristic* Taking Lasix	**KNOWLEDGE: MEDICATION** *Indicator* Description of action of medications	**TEACHING: PRESCRIBED MEDICATION** *Activities* Instruct on purpose/action of each medicine Instruct criteria to alter dose/schedule
FUNCTIONAL URINARY INCONTINENCE *Defining Characteristics* Difficulty removing clothing Loss of strength/mobility	**SELF-CARE: TOILETING** *Indicators* Removes clothing Gets to and from toilet	**SELF-CARE ASSISTANCE: TOILETING** *Activities* Modify clothing Provide rails and riser for bathroom stool Monitor ambulation ability Prescribe strengthening exercises

Nursing Outcomes Classification (NOC) 5-point Likert measurement scales:

Urinary Continence: 1 = Never demonstrated; 2 = Rarely demonstrated; 3 = Sometimes demonstrated; 4 = Often demonstrated; 5 = Consistently demonstrated.

Knowledge: Medication: 1 = None; 2 = Limited; 3 = Moderate; 4 = Substantial; 5 = Extensive.

Self-Care: Toileting: 1 = Dependent, does not participate; 2 = Requires assistive person and device; 3 = Requires assistive person; 4 = Independent with assistive device; 5 = Completely independent.

Table 22-3 — Urinary Incontinence: Differential Diagnosis for MR. SANDERS

Significant Defining Characteristics	Nursing Diagnoses Ruled Out	Additional Data Needed
Aware of need to void Voiding large amounts Less intake/large amount coffee History BHP/TURP	REFLEX INCONTINENCE STRESS INCONTINENCE IRRITATED BLADDER* OBSTRUCTION	Time between urge and void Voiding pattern/schedule Intake pattern/amounts Relationship of medicine administration to incontinence episodes
Clear urine analysis Loss of strength/mobility	INFECTION FUNCTIONAL INCONTINENCE*	Ability to manipulate clothing and get to toilet in time
Denial of wetness	REFLEX INCONTINENCE*	Embarrassed or lack of sensation

TENTATIVE NURSING DIAGNOSES

General Types: Established Filling, Transient Spurious

- **Urge Incontinence** related to irritable bladder as evidenced by reduced fluid intake and coffee drinking
- **Iatrogenic Incontinence** related to prescribed medication as evidenced by Lasix therapy
- **Functional Incontinence** related to impaired mobility/dexterity as evidenced by inability to reach toilet and manipulate clothing after urge and prior to voiding

*Not ruled out by collecting additional data.

Table 22-4 — Urinary Incontinence: Differential Diagnosis for MRS. POST

Significant Defining Characteristics	Nursing Diagnoses Ruled Out	Additional Data Needed
Palpable bladder after voiding Voids small amounts	OBSTRUCTION STRESS INCONTINENCE	Check for prolapse/impaction Check for sphincter/pelvic muscle weakness
Bacteria in urine/vaginitis Diabetes with neuropathy Incontinent of bowel Dependence in activities of daily living (ADL) Unable to interpret urge	IRRITATED BLADDER* REFLEX INCONTINENCE STRESS INCONTINENCE FUNCTIONAL INCONTINENCE* REFLEX INCONTINENCE	Check onset of infection Amount of retention at void Check anal sphincter Voiding pattern/times/amount Voiding pattern/times/amount Any other indication of urge, e.g., restlessness
Pendulous abdomen/obesity Leakage with movement	STRESS INCONTINENCE STRESS INCONTINENCE	Voiding pattern/times/amount Types of activity leading to leakage

TENTATIVE NURSING DIAGNOSES

General Types: Established Emptying, Spurious; Transient Filling

- **Overflow Incontinence** related to impaired bladder neuromusculature as shown by no evidence of obstruction, evidence of weak musculature for bowel evacuation, absence of fecal impaction, high level of residual urine, and palpable bladder
- **Functional Incontinence** related to physical dependence and confusion as evidenced by inability to get to toilet facilities without help or to indicate need to void
- **Urge Incontinence** related to irritable bladder as evidenced by bacteria in urine, vaginitis/drainage

*Not ruled out by collecting additional data.

F. Post, age 79, recently has been widowed and admitted to a nursing home. She has a history of diabetes mellitus for the last 20 years, for which she takes daily insulin. For several years she has experienced neuropathy and pain in her legs and feet. She had a vaginal hysterectomy at age 55. She is very confused, which makes her dependent in all activities of daily living. Mrs. Post is quite obese, with a large pendulous abdomen. Her bladder is palpable after urination. She has been incontinent of both bowel and bladder for 2 years and dribbles urine when she moves in bed or transfers. Mrs. Post entered the nursing home wearing disposable briefs. Urinalysis revealed a large amount of bacteria in the urine. She also has an inflamed vagina with purulent drainage. Her intake is usually 2000 ml each day, and she takes fluids whenever they are offered. She is not able to interpret urge or say when she has to go to the bathroom. Table 22-4 presents Mrs. Post's significant signs and symptoms, those diagnoses that can be ruled out, and the additional data needed. Table 22-5 contains the nursing diagnoses, outcomes, and interventions used for the management of Mrs. Post's incontinence.

NURSING-SENSITIVE OUTCOMES

Following the determination of the diagnoses, the nurse selects the outcomes that are needed to select the appropriate nursing interventions and to monitor the impact of those nursing interventions. It is important that the patient or a family member participate in the selection of outcomes and that they reflect the patient's desired goals. The outcomes for urinary incontinence diagnoses are selected from the *Nursing Outcomes Classification (NOC)*, developed by the Iowa Outcomes Project (2000).

See Table 22-1 for NOC outcomes most appropriate for incontinence diagnoses. It is recommended that the anchors in the NOC measurement scale for Self-Care: Toileting be changed because a rating of 5 cannot be achieved if a person uses an assistive device but is nonetheless independent. The following anchors would be more useful: 1 = dependent, does not participate; 2 = requires assistive person and device; 3 = requires assistive person; 4 = independent with assistive device and supervision; and 5 = independent with or without assistive device.

All NOC outcomes and indicators selected for Mr. Sanders are in Table 22-2. Mr. Sanders and the nurse agreed that, as an outcome of nursing interventions, he should be able to (1) consistently demonstrate urinary continence; (2) have a totally adequate fluid intake; (3) be completely independent with self-care: toileting; and (4) have substantial knowledge about his medications. The primary NOC outcome for Mr. Sanders is Urinary Conti-

nence. Because the identified etiology of Mr. Sanders' incontinence is bladder irritation from caffeine, limited fluid intake, and the effects of the diuretic Lasix, the establishment of a predictable pattern of urination is most important to avoid an incontinent accident due to the inability to suppress urge. It also is important to monitor the timeliness of Mr. Sanders' response to urge and the adequacy of time needed to reach the toilet in the event a predictable pattern of voiding is not attained. Assessment of dryness of undergarments during the day and bedding at night provides data needed to determine if there are any incontinent episodes. Mr. Sanders' ability to manage clothing independently is evaluated periodically to assess whether it continues to interfere with the time it takes him to respond to the urge to urinate. Self-Care: Toileting is monitored to evaluate both his abilities to get to and from the toilet and remove clothing and to determine if any interventions are needed to prevent the loss of these abilities. Fluid intake is an essential outcome indicator to measure the dilution of urine and decreased bladder irritation. The amount of oral intake and avoidance of fluids that contain caffeine are important indicators for this outcome. "Free of oral fluids that contain caffeine" is not an indicator for the NOC outcome Urinary Continence but can be added as "other." Knowledge: Medication is an essential outcome because of the effect of Lasix on urine output and urgency and because of its role in the treatment of Mr. Sanders' congestive heart failure. Mr. Sanders' knowledge of his medication should be measured weekly until he achieves the goal of substantial understanding (Table 22-6). The other outcomes that are selected should be assessed weekly for the first month and, depending on his progress, potentially assessed monthly or at longer agreed-on intervals.

See Table 22-5 for NOC outcomes and indicators selected for Mrs. Post. Mrs. Post's daughter and the nurse agreed that, as a result of nursing interventions, Mrs. Post should be able to (1) have an infection-free status of urine and vagina; (2) sometimes demonstrate urinary continence; (3) have a fluid intake of 1500 ml daily; and (4) have tissue integrity not compromised. Infection Status was chosen as the primary NOC outcome because Mrs. Post's vaginal and urinary infections are easily reversible causes of incontinence. When the infections are cleared, the transient incontinence might be resolved sufficiently to enable treatment of the established overflow and functional incontinence. Monitoring Mrs. Post's infection status is as important because of her diabetes. It is important to monitor Mrs. Post's voiding amounts, leakage of urine between voidings, and postvoid residuals as indicators of the outcome Urinary Continence. It is essential to evaluate whether Mrs. Post's fluid intake is sufficiently large to discourage infection and promote a pattern of voiding, but no so large as to stretch the bladder and result in retention of urine and infection. The amount and timing of oral intake are important indicators for this outcome. Use

Table 22-5	Nursing Diagnoses, Outcomes, and Interventions for MRS. POST		

Nursing Diagnoses	Nursing-Sensitive Outcomes	Nursing Interventions
URGE INCONTINENCE ***Defining Characteristics*** Bladder infection Inflamed vagina with drainage Involuntary passage of stool	**INFECTION STATUS** ***Indicators*** Foul-smelling discharge Purulent drainage Pain/tenderness Bacteria in urine WBCs in urine	**MEDICATION ADMINISTRATION: TOPICAL** ***Activities*** Insert vaginal medication as prescribed Monitor irritation from medication **BOWEL INCONTINENCE CARE** ***Activities*** Wash perianal area after each stool Keep bed and clothing clean **MEDICATION ADMINISTRATION: ORAL** ***Activities*** Determine the patient's ability to swallow Assist with ingestion of medication Monitor for therapeutic/adverse effects **URINARY TRACT INFECTION MANAGEMENT** ***Activities*** Assist with fluid intake of 1500 ml Refer for medication prescription Monitor urinalysis for bacteria/WBCs
OVERFLOW INCONTINENCE ***Defining Characteristics*** Palpable bladder after voiding Voids small amounts Urine leakage with movement Unable to interpret urge	**URINARY CONTINENCE** ***Indicators*** Voids more than 150 ml each time Free of urine leakage between voidings Empties bladder completely Absence of post-void residual >100 to 200 ml Underclothing dry during day Underclothing/bedding dry at night Absence of urinary tract infection (<100,000 WBC)	**URINARY CATHETERIZATION: INTERMITTENT** ***Activities*** Maintain patient on prophylactic antibacterial therapy for 2 to 3 weeks at initiation of intermittent catheterization, as appropriate Maintain a detailed record of catheterization schedule, fluid intake and output Determine voiding pattern Adjust frequency of catheterization to maintain output of 300 ml or less for adults Use clean or sterile technique for catheterization Prompt to void prior to each catheterization Record amount of each voiding and catheterization output Determine catheterization schedule based on a comprehensive urinary assessment Complete a urinalysis about every 2 weeks to 1 month Teach family signs/symptoms of UTIs Monitor color, odor, and clarity of urine
FUNCTIONAL INCONTINENCE ***Defining Characteristics*** Cannot get to toilet without help Cannot indicate need to urinate	**TISSUE INTEGRITY: SKIN & MUCOUS MEMBRANES** ***Indicators*** Color in expected range Tissue lesion free Skin intactness	**URINARY INCONTINENCE CARE** ***Activities*** Inspect skin and mucous membranes for redness, heat, or drainage Monitor skin for areas of breakdown Cleanse perineal area regularly

Nursing Outcomes Classification (NOC) 5-point Likert measurement scales:

Infection Status:	1 = Severe; 2 = Substantial; 3 = Moderate; 4 = Slight; 5 = None.
Urinary Continence:	1 = Never demonstrated; 2 = Rarely demonstrated; 3 = Sometimes demonstrated; 4 = Often demonstrated; 5 = Consistently demonstrated.
Tissue Integrity: Skin & Mucous Membranes:	1 = Extremely compromised; 2 = Substantially compromised; 3 = Moderately compromised; 4 = Mildly compromised; 5 = Not compromised.

Table 22-6	Treatments URINARY INCONTINENCE		
Types of Treatment	**Examples**	**Mechanisms**	**Uses**
Drugs	Propantheline (Pro-Banthine)	Diminish bladder contractions	Urge incontinence associated with bladder instability
	Imipramine (Tofranil)	Diminish bladder contractions	Urge incontinence associated with bladder instability
	Oxybutynin (Ditropan)	Diminish bladder contractions	Urge incontinence associated with bladder instability
	Flavoxate (Urispas)	Diminish bladder contractions	Urge incontinence associated with bladder instability
	Ephedrine (Sudafed)	Strengthen bladder outlet	Stress incontinence associated with sphincter weakness
	Phenylpropranolamine (Ornade)	Strengthen bladder outlet	Stress incontinence associated with sphincter weakness
	Estrogen (Premarin)	Increase supporting tissue around urethra	Stress incontinence
	Oral or topical bethanechol (Urecholine)	Promotes bladder contraction	Overflow incontinence
Training procedures	Habit training	Caretaker determines individual's pattern of incontinence and gets him to toilet accordingly	Urge incontinence
	Bladder retraining	Caretaker establishes routine of fluid administration and toileting with progressive lengthening of toileting intervals to increase bladder capacity or initiate normal voiding	Urge incontinence after catheter use
	Pelvic floor exercises	Exercises to strengthen pelvic muscles	Overflow incontinence after overdistension, injury, or stress
	Biofeedback	With specialized equipment patient is trained to inhibit bladder contractions or contract pelvic muscles	Mainly urge incontinence associated with bladder instability and stress incontinence associated with sphincter weakness
	Behavioral modification	Caretaker rewards incontinent individual for staying dry	Incontinence associated with underlying mental or emotional discords; some forms of functional incontinence

Data from Ouslander, J. B., & Kane, R. L. (1984). The cost of urinary incontinence in nursing homes. *Medical Care, 22,* 69-79.

of the NOC outcome Urinary Continence requires that the nurse specify the amount and timing for the fluid intake indicator. Assessment of dryness of undergarments during the day and bedding at night provides data needed to evaluate whether leakage and incontinent episodes occur. Because of Mrs. Post's vaginitis and high risk for compromised tissue integrity, her skin and vaginal membranes must be monitored for color, lesions, and intactness. Outcomes are to be measured at the following recommended intervals: (1) Infection Status—weekly until urine is clear (<100,000 WBCs) and there is absence of vaginal foul smelling and purulent discharge, then monthly for maintenance, and if clear for 3 months, quarterly; (2) Urinary Continence—daily until a pattern of

voiding is established and residual is less than 200 ml, or after 1 month if further reduction of residual is not obtained, then monthly for 3 months, and quarterly if stabilization occurs; and (3) Tissue Integrity: Skin & Mucous Membranes—daily inspection and documentation until infection and incontinence are resolved, then at least monthly (Fantl et al., 1996).

NURSING INTERVENTIONS

Treatments for urinary incontinence include the use of devices to collect or prevent the flow of urine, medications or treatments to influence bladder function, surgical procedures that relieve obstruction or correct some other bladder pathology, and training procedures that alter the patient's behavior in some way (Ouslander et al., 1985). See Table 22-1 for a listing of primarily medical interventions for all types of incontinence. Surgical procedures, which are medical in nature, are not discussed in this chapter. Medications are discussed only as they relate to nursing interventions. Devices used to collect urine (such as condom catheters, bedpans, or disposable underpants) do not reduce the number or frequency of incontinent episodes, but merely manage urinary incontinence by containing and absorbing the urine (McCormick & Burgio, 1984). Thus the focus of this chapter is on nursing interventions, some of which are not listed in Table 22-1. When successful, these nursing interventions ultimately are expected to result in Urinary Continence or the reduction in the number or frequency of incontinent episodes.

A number of interventions available to nurses aim to control the number of incontinent episodes a client experiences. These include the following interventions from the *Nursing Interventions Classification (NIC):* Pelvic Floor Exercise; Urinary Habit Training; Urinary Bladder Training; and Urinary Catheterization: Intermittent (Iowa Intervention Project, 2000). Additional nursing interventions that have a less developed research base also are briefly described.

Pelvic Floor Exercises

Pelvic floor exercises involve the repetitive contraction of the pubococcygeal muscle, the muscle that forms the support for the pelvis and surrounds the vaginal, urethral, and rectal outlets of the pelvis (Newman & Smith, 1992; Taylor & Henderson, 1986). Pelvic floor exercises, often called Kegel exercises, were first described by Arnold H. Kegel as a treatment option for clients with stress incontinence (Kegel, 1948). The goal of this repetitive contraction is to strengthen the pubococcygeal muscle and decrease incontinent episodes. Associated exercises involve starting and stopping the urine stream while urinating, with a goal of strengthening the bladder outlet. Thus pelvic floor exercises are instituted to treat clients with stress incontinence related to weakened pelvic muscles and/or weakened bladder outlet.

Pelvic floor exercises also are recommended for individuals who experience urge incontinence. The exercises increase the tone of the pelvic floor muscles and raise the micturition threshold, resulting in decreased urgency (Newman & Smith, 1992). By strengthening the muscles of the pelvic floor at the time the urge to void is experienced, the individual might be able to increase the bladder capacity and delay the incontinent episode. This intervention often is paired with a bladder-training regimen that also serves to increase bladder capacity (Burgio, Whitehead, & Engel, 1985; Newman & Smith, 1992).

Researchers have used different exercise protocols in their studies. For instance, in one study the clients were instructed to tighten the pubococcygeal muscle for 10 seconds and then relax it, repeating the exercise 100 times throughout the day (Taylor & Henderson, 1986). In another study clients were instructed to practice 50 sphincter exercises daily in three positions (lying, sitting, and standing) and to contract their muscles after lifting or coughing (Burgio et al., 1985).

Several other studies have demonstrated the effects of pelvic floor exercises on pelvic muscle strength (Burns, Pranikoff, Nochajski, Desotelle, & Harwood, 1990; Henderson & Taylor, 1987; Tchou, Adams, Varner, & Denton, 1988; Wilson, Al Samarrai, Deakin, Kolbe, & Brown, 1987). Most studies recommend that clients need to be motivated and cognitively able to perform the exercises, and that several repetitions of the exercises are required each day. Taylor and Henderson recommended that clients continue the exercises for the rest of their lives. Although Burgio et al. (1985) did not include such a recommendation, they did note that two of three patients who reported fewer incontinent episodes at a 12-month posttreatment follow-up had continued their exercises.

Although the use of Kegel exercises to treat stress incontinence does not require the use of equipment to measure the muscle contraction, many research studies include biofeedback as part of the intervention strategy (Burgio et al., 1985; Burgio, Robinson, & Engel, 1986; Burns, Marecki, Dittmar, & Bullough, 1985; Taylor & Henderson, 1986). Kegel measured the strength of pubococcygeal muscle contraction with a perineometer, a compressible air chamber inserted in the vagina and attached to a manometer. The client contracted vaginal muscles, and the perineometer recorded the strength of the contraction. The client practiced the exercises and was able to measure progress with the perineometer objectively. Further evaluation of the success of the exercise regimen was measured as a reduction in incontinent episodes (Kegel, 1948). Although other biofeedback instruments have been designed, the basic principle of measuring the strength of muscle contraction remains the same (Dougherty, Abrams, & McKey, 1986; Olah, 1990; Peattie, Plevnik, & Stanton, 1988). Taylor and Henderson (1986) found that clients who received daily biofeedback while performing pelvic floor exercises achieved 100% continence, whereas the control group, who received biofeedback only at the beginning and end of the treatment period, achieved 67% continence. Other studies have shown that biofeedback-assisted exercise also yields more improvement in continence than exercise alone (Clinical News, 1986; Olah, 1990; Peattie et al., 1988). Electrical stimulation holds promise retraining, but studies are limited and too varied to generalize results. Thus more research is needed to determine the efficacy of electrical stimulation as an adjunct to pelvic muscle exercise (Newman & Smith, 1992).

As indicated earlier, pelvic floor raising is also a useful treatment for urge incontinence. Burgio et al. (1985) combined pelvic floor exercises with a program aimed at teaching clients more effective ways of handling bladder urgency. At a 6-month follow-up of eight clients treated with this regimen, five were totally continent and the remaining three showed, on average, an 84% improvement in frequency of incontinent episodes.

Implementing the Pelvic Exercise Intervention. Before elders can practice pelvic floor exercises, they must be aware of the muscles that are used in the exercises and then be able to tighten these muscles in a regularly scheduled exercise pattern. Written instructions are helpful. The following exercises will help identify the back portion of the pelvic floor:

- Sit or stand. Relax the muscles of legs, buttocks, and abdomen.
- Imagine you are trying to keep from passing a bowel movement by tightening the ring of muscle around the anus.

Awareness of the muscles in the front portion of the pelvic floor is enhanced by asking the older person to stop, then restart, urine flow. Performing this exercise with each urination ensures that it will be done regularly (Mandelstam, 1980; Newman & Smith, 1992). It usually takes 4 to 6 weeks of exercises to improve incontinence and up to 12 weeks for them to become maximally effective (Benvenuti et al., 1987; McCormick & Burgio, 1984; Newman & Smith, 1992). Feedback and encouragement are needed to help patients carry out the exercises long enough to make a difference.

Bladder Training and Habit Training

Although the terms are frequently used synonymously, *bladder training* and *habit training* represent two separate interventions. The goals of the two interventions are different, and they are used in different circumstances. Bladder training involves the gradual lengthening or shortening of periods between voidings, with the goal of restoring both normal voiding patterns and continence (Ouslander & Uman, 1985; Ouslander et al., 1985). Habit training involves adjusting the toileting schedule to the client's responses. The aim is to avoid incontinent episodes. There is no attempt to restore a normal pattern of voiding (Ouslander & Uman, 1985; Ouslander et al., 1985). Another term frequently used is *scheduled toileting*. Scheduled toileting is similar to habit training, except that the toileting schedule is fixed and is not based on the client's pattern of incontinence (Greengold & Ouslander, 1986).

Bladder training, also referred to as a bladder drill or bladder reeducation, is a treatment of choice for clients with urge incontinence related either to overdistention or to reduced bladder capacity (Ouslander & Uman, 1985).

When the bladder has a reduced capacity, the time between voidings is gradually extended until the client is able to void once every 2 to 4 hours without incontinence. When the bladder has been overdistended, possibly because of injury or medication use, the time between voidings is gradually reduced until a normal voiding pattern can be established. Candidates for bladder training must be mentally and physically capable of toileting themselves, and they must be motivated to do so (Greengold & Ouslander, 1986).

In a review of numerous research studies of bladder-training regimens, Hadley (1986) reported that cure rates ranged from 44% to 100%. Bladder-training protocols differed in a number of ways. Some allowed the clients to schedule their own voidings, whereas other studies had mandatory voiding schedules that ranged from ½ hour to 4 hours. Goal intervals, when identified, were 4 hours in length. Most of the studies were clinical trials, although a few included untreated controls. Several protocols included additional interventions, such as the use of concomitant drug therapy or the use of self-charting of voiding/incontinence pattern (Hadley, 1986). Other studies have reported increased continence following a bladder-training intervention (Fantl et al., 1991; Ferrie, Smith, Logan, Lyle, & Paterson, 1984; Jarvis & Millar, 1980; Pengelly & Booth, 1980).

Several other interventions also have been identified as part of a bladder-training protocol, including fluid intake of 1500 to 2000 ml daily, careful timing of fluid intake, complete bladder emptying, the use of techniques to inhibit or stimulate voiding, distraction, relaxation, and the use of reinforcement measures (Fantl et al., 1996; Ouslander & Uman, 1985; Specht, 1986). Although some of these interventions have been tested, additional research is needed to isolate and systematically test these adjuncts.

As indicated, habit training is used if the goal is to avoid incontinent episodes, but not to restore a normal voiding pattern. It can be very successful with physically or mentally impaired clients because it generally depends on the motivation of the staff to toilet the client rather than on the motivation of the client (Ouslander & Uman, 1985; Ouslander et al., 1985). For this reason, habit training is a treatment option in clients with functional incontinence related to physical or cognitive/perceptual deficits (Ouslander & Uman, 1985). Habit training is used frequently in long-term care institutions, although many nursing homes use a fixed (as opposed to flexible) 2-hour scheduled toileting protocol (Ouslander & Uman, 1985).

There are fewer research studies available that have examined the effectiveness of habit training or scheduled toileting. Hadley (1986) reviewed three studies that showed cure rates of 26% to 68%. These studies also included other interventions, such as staff reinforcement, aided toileting, scheduled fluids, or medication use. Long (1985) described a habit training intervention with elderly clients in a long-term care institution. The treatment included a flexible habit-training protocol, prescribed fluid intake, maintenance of an incontinence record, and prescribed (individualized) method of toileting. The author reported that the most difficult part of the study was orienting/motivating the staff to the training protocol. Results of the study indicated that successful habit training was linked to mental status. The greater the degree of mental impairment, the less likely the client would be successful in attaining continence. Schnelle and colleagues conducted a series of studies to test habit training combined with prompted voiding and positive reinforcement; the studies showed some success in reducing incidents of wetness and a reduction of costs of incontinence care (Schnelle, 1990; Schnelle, Newman, & Fogarty, 1990; Schnelle et al., 1989). However, Schnelle and colleagues also noted that improved continence was more likely due to the effects of positive reinforcement and increased opportunities to toilet, and thus is a more successful intervention for persons with functional incontinence. Prompted voiding has been demonstrated to be effective in improving dryness with moderately incontinent, cognitively intact and cognitively impaired, dependent nursing home residents (Burgio et al., 1994; Hu et al., 1989; McCormick, Burgio, Engel, Scheve, & Leahy, 1992; Schnelle, 1990). However, it can be difficult to sustain staff compliance with the intervention. Certified nursing assistants identified poor staffing, lack of staff education and support, and poor communication as reasons that voiding interventions were not sustained (Lekan-Rutledge, Palmer, & Belyea, 1998).

Colling, Ouslander, Hadley, Eisch, and Campbell (1992) demonstrated a significant reduction in incontinence in 86% of subjects in a controlled 3-month study of habit training. The investigators identified voiding patterns of 51 nursing home residents with an electronic monitoring device and taught nursing staff to toilet residents based on the individual's pattern of greatest voiding frequency. A 25% or greater reduction in incontinence over baseline occurred in the intervention group compared with an increase in incontinence in the control group. As with other studies, staff compliance with the intervention was difficult to sustain.

Implementing Bladder Training and Habit Training.

Although Bladder Training and Habit Training are two separate interventions, the methods used to implement them are similar. The major difference lies in the person who has major responsibility for implementing the intervention. Staff and caregivers have major responsibility in Habit Training, whereas the elder has major responsibility in Bladder Training. Also, Bladder Training ends with improved bladder function, whereas Habit Training requires an ongoing process of monitoring and reinforcing continence. However, Habit Training can result in increased predictability and a workable schedule for caregivers and the elderly person.

Long (1985) and Specht (1981) have used the following protocol, included in the NIC interventions Bladder Training and Habit Training:

1. Gather data on fluid intake pattern, voiding patterns (Urinary Continence Specification Record for 3 days; see Assessment Guide 22-2), sensation and awareness, underlying health problems, and potential for retraining (intact to mild cognitive impairment permits participation in the bladder-training program) (Long, 1985). Habit training is most successful with moderately incontinent, dependent persons.

2. Take or ask the person to go to the toilet, or have the elder use a bedpan upon waking. Assist or remind the person to toilet as scheduled during waking hours and as awake during the night. The elder should remain on the toilet no longer than 5 minutes. If voiding is not occurring, try measures to encourage micturition, for example, stroking inner aspect of thigh, deep breathing, bearing down, leaning forward at an acute angle, drinking water, and exerting manual pressure over the bladder area.

3. Repeat the previous step initially at the intervals established with the continence record and at bedtime. If incontinence occurs before the interval expires, reduce the interval by ½ hour. Do not toilet more often than 1 to 2 hours, as too frequent voiding causes chronic low-volume voiding, leading to reduced bladder capacity, increased detrusor tone, and bladder wall thickening (Long, 1985). Increase the toileting interval by ½ hour if the patient has no incontinence episodes in 48 hours or until the optimal schedule for the resident or a 4-hour schedule is achieved.

4. Maintain the agreed-on fluid schedule (see Increasing Fluids section).

5. Keep a record of continence and incontinence episodes.

6. Reward success (determine what constitutes reward for this person); support and encourage the person when there are incontinent episodes.

In Long's study (1985), the time required to establish a three to four toileting daily schedule without episodes of incontinence ranged from 4 days to 6 weeks, and at discharge 79% of the previously incontinent patients were continent. If using a prompted voiding adjunct to habit training, the essential activities are prompting and praising in addition to the toileting monitoring and assistance regimen (Fantl et al., 1996; Iowa Intervention Project, 2000).

Increasing Fluids as an Adjunct to Bladder and Habit Training

A regimen to increase fluids aims at increasing bladder capacity and decreasing detrusor activity (Colling, Owen, & McCreedy, 1994). Specific fluid intake activities are included in the NIC incontinence interventions. Older persons with incontinence normally reduce fluid intake, often down to 500 to 600 ml/day, in an effort to remain continent (Specht, 1981). Since older persons have reduced total body fluid and are at risk for dehydration, fluid intake is especially important (Davis & Minaker, 1994). A goal of 2000 ml is desirable. However, incontinence has been found to decrease when an intake of 1200 to 1800 ml/day is achieved and maintained (Spangler, Risely, & Bilyew, 1984; Specht, 1981). Certainly, contraindications for increasing fluids, such as when congestive heart failure is a comorbidity, must be considered in planning a fluid regimen. Planning daily living to increase fluid intake as a measure for improving continence includes the following elements, some of which are listed as NIC activities:

1. Explain how increasing fluids promotes continence.
2. Negotiate with the person or family caregiver to maintain an intake and output record.
3. Negotiate with the person or family caregiver to record incontinence episodes.
4. Negotiate an acceptable, workable fluid intake schedule of both amounts and kinds of fluids that will gradually move toward the agreed-on intake goal.
5. Reward and support the older person's efforts (determine what constitutes reward and support for the individual).
6. Work with spouses, family members, and companions so that their actions do not work against the plan.

Increased fluids should be used in conjunction with a scheduled toileting program, particularly if there are factors such as functional impairments or mental clouding as additional causes or contributors to the incontinency.

Intermittent Catheterization

Continuous indwelling catheterization is an appropriate management strategy for only a small number of incontinent clients: those with urinary retention who cannot be successfully treated by surgical or pharmacologic intervention or by intermittent catheterization; some persons who are terminally ill; and selected persons with severe impaired skin integrity (Fantl et al., 1996; Ouslander et al., 1985). Unfortunately, indwelling catheters are used in approximately 10% to 30% of incontinent individuals living in long-term care institutions and are a major cause of urinary tract infections (Ouslander et al., 1985). If indwelling catheters are used, the bulb should be inflated with 10 ml of fluid to avoid slippage and risk of obstruction (Fiers, 1994).

An alternative to indwelling catheters is the use of clean intermittent catheterization at regular intervals, either by patients or by caregivers. The technique can be recommended for use in clients with urinary retention related to a weak detrusor muscle (as in diabetic neuropathy) or blockage of the urethra (as in benign prostatic hypertrophy) and in clients with reflex incontinence related to spinal cord injury (Ouslander & Uman, 1985; Ouslander et al., 1985; Specht, 1986).

Intermittent catheterization was first introduced after World War II as a bladder-training technique for paraplegic and quadriplegic patients (Champion, 1976). At that time intermittent catheterization was conducted only under sterile conditions by a physician. Patients were catheterized at frequent intervals throughout the day. The procedure worked much as a bladder drill. Early studies showed that patients trained in such a manner for about 7 weeks were able to void at discharge from the hospital (Guttman & Frankel, 1966). Since that time, the procedure has been modified, and it is now taught as a clean, not sterile, self-catheterization. It is used for bladder training, as well as for other clients for whom nerve supply to the bladder has been disrupted (Champion, 1976; Sadowski & Duffy, 1988; Warren, 1990; Webb, Lawson, & Neal, 1990).

Bladder overdistention slows bladder circulation and predisposes the bladder to infection. Frequent catheterization of the bladder prevents overdistention and allows the bladder to fight infection (Horsley, Crane, & Haller, 1982). This technique has been shown to reduce the incidence of complications associated with indwelling catheter use (Oustander et al., 1985). The emphasis is not on maintaining sterility, but on frequent emptying of the bladder.

Clients or their caregivers can be taught the basic principles of catheterization and the procedure for catheterizing using clean technique. Patients are frequently maintained on antibacterial medications for a period of 2 to 3 weeks, as well as on anticholinergic or cholinergic medications to assist bladder control (Horsley et al., 1982). A candidate for clean intermittent self-catheterization must have the manual dexterity to manipulate the catheter and must be motivated to perform the technique frequently throughout the day (usually when the bladder has distended with approximately 300 ml of fluid) and in any number of settings. Caregivers must possess these same qualities.

Lapides and colleagues (1975) reported a review of 218 patients who were taught clean intermittent catheterization. The subjects' ages ranged from 4 to 84 years, with 145 subjects between 21 and 84 years of age. The subjects had a number of different diagnoses related to voiding difficulties and incontinence. The results of this study indicated that for clients experiencing incontinence related to reflex bladder contractions or overflow incontinence, clean intermittent catheterization combined with anticholinergic and alpha adrenergic medication alleviated incontinence, as well as chronic perineal dermatitis (Lapides, Diokno, Gould, & Lowe, 1975).

Intermittent catheterization is a clean, not a sterile, procedure. The emphasis is on frequency rather than sterility. However, a sterile procedure might be advisable for elderly persons with compromised immune systems (Fantl et al., 1996). The goal of intermittent catheterization is to maintain a volume of urine in the bladder of 300 ml or less. This requires catheterization every 2 to 3 hours while the person is awake and one to two times during the night. The NIC intervention includes the activities for implementing clean or sterile intermittent catheterization (Iowa Intervention Project, 2000).

Candidates for the self-catheterization procedure should meet the following criteria:

1. Sufficient manual dexterity and mental ability to perform the procedure in its entirety at frequent intervals, or availability of another person to do it
2. A bladder capacity of 100 ml or more
3. A urethra that is intact and free from stricture

This routine has been used successfully at the Iowa Veterans Home with residents who had atonic bladders. Nurses had difficulty in moving to a clean rather than sterile approach and did complain about the frequency of the treatment. It is essential for nurses, family, and the older person to understand the principles of this method. Although this approach needs further testing, it holds promise and is preferable to indwelling catheters. It should be noted, however, that clean intermittent catheterization has been researched far more extensively in the child and young adult than in the elderly client. It is presently unclear, for instance, whether complications might be more common in a geriatric population (Fantl et al., 1996). Although the theoretical principles supporting clean intermittent catheterization remain the same with elderly clients, further research with this intervention is needed to support its usefulness over time with older adults.

Other Treatment Options

Additional interventions might be indicated, depending on the client's type and etiology of urinary incontinence. For instance, a client experiencing functional incontinence related to physical deficits might benefit from a muscle-strengthening program and from environmental modification to reduce the obstacles between the client and the commode. Similarly, the elimination of fecal impactions can eliminate overflow incontinence related to an obstructed bladder outlet (Specht, 1986). Urge incontinence related to bladder irritation can be eliminated with a fluid intake of 1500 to 2000 ml if the irritation was due to highly concentrated urine in a dehydrated client (Colling et al., 1994; Specht, 1986). Further research is needed to determine which of these and other interventions commonly used to treat urinary incontinence are most useful, satisfactory, and cost-effective for elderly clients.

CASE STUDY 1

The nurse discussed the diagnoses of Urge, Iatrogenic, and Functional Incontinence with Mr. Sanders, explaining the factors that contributed to each, including the action of his medication. Mr. Sanders agreed that he desired to be continent. He and the nurse established a plan to achieve the goal of reducing his incidents of incontinence. After Mr. Sanders understood the roles of caffeine and reduced fluid intake in causing his bladder to be irritated, he agreed to limit his coffee intake to 2 to 3 cups each day and to increase his total fluid intake to at least 1500 ml daily. He volunteered to try decaffeinated coffee and to drink noncitric juices and a beer with his evening meal. With his approval, the nurse sent a pair of his trousers to the local laundry to have Velcro fasteners placed on the fly instead of a zipper. Mr. Sanders also agreed to toilet himself at least every 2 hours in an attempt to avoid urgency and precipitance of urination. The nurse also trained Mr. Sanders to regularly perform pelvic floor exercises each time he toileted.

Mr. Sanders and the nurse set up a weekly appointment to review his progress. At their third conference Mr. Sanders reported only one incontinence episode during the past week and that it had occurred when he had not been able to toilet for a period of 4 hours. He was having much better success with manipulating his clothing with the Velcro fasteners, so the nurse had his other trousers altered. He also reported that he thought he could extend his toileting interval to 3 hours. He said he was able to tolerate the decaffeinated coffee and that he was pleased to no longer have the discomforts of urge to void and being wet.

The nurse reviewed Mr. Sanders' outcomes and indicators with him, and together they rated his progress at each weekly visit. They agreed to monitor his progress monthly thereafter until otherwise agreed. Progress for Mr. Sanders' outcomes and indicators for the first 3 weeks of treatment are displayed in Table 22-7.

CASE STUDY 2

Mrs. Post's nurse first consulted with the physician, and Mrs. Post was given medication to relieve the infections. To support the medication therapy and prevent overflow incontinence, intermittent catheterization was initiated every 3 hours. The plan was to increase the interval of time to 4 hours between catheterizations after the infection cleared. Intermittent catheterization was continued for 8 weeks, during which time the urine remained free of infection. Mrs. Post was then placed on an every-3-hour voiding schedule and catheterized after each voiding. She continued to have residual urine of 70 to 100 ml and was unable to cooperate with the voiding schedule because of her confusion. As long as she remained infection free, she was maintained on a 4-hour intermittent catheterization schedule. The nurse did not consider the use of pelvic floor exercises to strengthen supporting musculature because of Mrs. Post's inability to understand and implement the exercises. Mrs. Post's progress toward outcomes and indicators for the first 8 weeks of intervention are presented in Table 22-8.

Table 22-7 Outcome and Indicator Ratings for **MR. SANDERS**	Base	1 week	2 weeks	3 weeks
URINARY CONTINENCE	3	3	4	5
• Responds in timely manner to urge	2	3	4	5
• Predictable pattern to voidings	2	4	4	5
• Oral fluid intake	2	5	5	5
• Free of oral fluids containing caffeine	1	2	5	5
• Underclothing dry during day	2	3	4	5
• Underclothing/ bedding dry at night	2	3	3	4
• Free of incontinence episodes	3	3	4	5
KNOWLEDGE: MEDICATION	2	4	4	4
• Description of action of medication	1	4	4	5
SELF-CARE: TOILETING	3	4	4	5
• Removes clothing	3	3	4	5
• Gets to and from toilet	3	4	5	5

Nursing Outcomes Classification (NOC) 5-point Likert measurement scales:

Urinary Continence:	1 = Never demonstrated; 2 = Rarely demonstrated; 3 = Sometimes demonstrated; 4 = Often demonstrated; 5 = Consistently demonstrated.
Knowledge: Medication:	1 = None; 2 = Limited; 3 = Moderate; 4 = Substantial; 5 = Extensive.
Self-Care: Toileting:	1 = Dependent, does not participate; 2 = Requires assistive person and device; 3 = Requires assistive person; 4 = Independent with assistive device; 5 = Completely independent.

Table 22-8 Outcome and Indicator Ratings for **MRS. POST**	Base	1 week	3 weeks	8 weeks
INFECTION STATUS	2	3	5	5
• Foul-smelling discharge	1	3	5	5
• Purulent drainage	2	3	5	5
• Pain and tenderness	3	3	4	5
• Bacteria in urine	1	2	5	5
• WBCs in urine	1	2	5	5
URINARY CONTINENCE	1	2	3	4
• Voids more than 150 ml each time	1	2	4	5
• Free of urine leakage between voidings	1	1	1	1
• Empties bladder completely	1	2	4	5
• Absence of postvoid residual >200 ml	1	2	4	5
• Underclothing dry during day	1	2	4	5
• Underclothing/ bedding dry at night	1	2	4	5
• Absence of urinary tract infection	1	2	3	5
TISSUE INTEGRITY: SKIN & MUCOUS MEMBRANES	3	3	4	5
• Color	2	2	4	5
• Tissue lesion free	3	3	5	5
• Skin intactness	5	5	5	5

Nursing Outcomes Classification (NOC) 5-point Likert measurement scales:

Infection Status:	1 = Severe; 2 = Substantial; 3 = Moderate; 4 = Slight; 5 = None.
Urinary Continence:	1 = Never demonstrated; 2 = Rarely demonstrated; 3 = Sometimes demonstrated; 4 = Often demonstrated; 5 = Consistently demonstrated.
Tissue Integrity: Skin & Mucous Membranes:	1 = Extremely compromised; 2 = Substantially compromised; 3 = Moderately compromised; 4 = Mildly compromised; 5 = Not compromised.

SUMMARY

Urinary Incontinence is a complex nursing diagnosis that requires detailed assessment data to differentiate the specific etiologies and type of incontinence. With elders, more than one etiology is often present and more than one type of incontinence must be treated. Specific etiologies, along with identified outcomes, should guide the selection of interventions. NOC provides standardized outcomes and indicators that are sensitive to nursing interventions and includes measurement scales for the nurse and patient to use in assessing progress. Nurses can use a number of the interventions standardized by NIC to treat incontinence successfully in elderly persons. However, the intervention chosen must be specific for the type of incontinence, and more than one may have to be tried before the desired outcomes of continence, increased comfort, and optimal independence are achieved. Nurses should anticipate that elders will need a considerable length of time to achieve success and that persistence, consistency of intervention, and regular monitoring of outcomes are essential. Including the elderly person and/or the family in determining desirable outcomes and strategies is fundamental to successful nursing intervention to resolve urinary incontinence. Resolute diagnosis, intervention, and monitoring of outcomes by nurses can both dispel the common misperception that incontinence in elders cannot be treated and improved and encourage assistive staff to comply with intervention protocols.

REFERENCES

Andrist, L., & Maillet, A. (1992). Vulvovaginal conditions: Social, psychological, and sexual considerations. *Nurse Practitioner Forum, 3*, 181-184.

Awad, S., & McGinnis, R. (1983). Factors that influence the incidence of detrusor instability in women. *Journal of Urology, 130,* 114-115.

Beheshti, P., & Fonteyn, M. (1998). Role of the advanced practice nurse in continence care in the home. *AACN Clinical Issues, 9*(3), 389-395.

Benvenuti, F., Caputo, G. M., Bandinelli, S., Mayer, F., Biagini, C., & Sommavilla, A. (1987). Reeducative treatment of female genuine stress incontinence. *American Journal of Physical Medicine, 66,* 155-168.

Brink, C. (1980). Assessing the problem. *Geriatric Nursing, 1,* 241-275.

Brink, C., Wells, T., & Diokno, A. (1985). The continence clinic for the aged. *Journal of Gerontological Nursing, 9,* 651-655.

Brink, C., Sampselle, C., Wells, T., Diokno, A., & Gillis, G. (1989). A digital test for pelvic floor muscle strength in older women with urinary incontinence. *Nursing Research, 38,* 196-199.

Burgio, K., Whitehead, W., & Engel, B. (1985). Urinary incontinence in the elderly. *Annals of Internal Medicine, 104,* 507-515.

Burgio, K., Robinson, J., & Engle, B. (1986). The role of biofeedback in Kegel exercise training for stress urinary incontinence. *American Journal of Obstetrics and Gynecology, 154*(1), 58-64.

Burgio, L. D., McCormick, K. A., Scheve, A. S., Engel, B. T., Hawkins, A., & Leahy, E. (1994). The effects of changing prompted voiding schedules in the treatment of incontinence in nursing home residents. *Journal of the American Geriatrics Society, 42*(3), 315-320.

Burns, P., Marecki, M. A., Dittmar, S. S., & Bullough, B. (1985). Kegel exercises with biofeedback: Therapy for treatment of stress incontinence. *Nurse Practioner, 10*(2), 28, 33-34, 46.

Burns, P. A., Pranikoff, K., Nochajski, T., Desotelle, P., & Harwood, M. K. (1990). Treatment of stress incontinence with pelvic floor exercises and biofeedback. *Journal of the American Geriatrics Society, 38,* 341-344.

Carroll-Johnson, R. (Ed.). (1989). *Classification of nursing diagnoses: Proceedings of the eighth conference.* Baltimore: Lippincott Williams & Wilkins.

Champion, V. (1976). Clean technique for intermittent self-catheterization. *Nursing Research, 25*(1), 13-18.

Clinical News. (1986). Lowering the nation's incontinence bill. *American Journal of Nursing, 86,* 1215-1216.

Clinical Practice Guideline Panel. (1992). *Urinary incontinence in adults* (AHCPR Pub #92-0038). Rockville, MD: Agency for Health Care Policy and Research, Public Health Service, U.S. Department of Health and Human Services.

Cohen, S. J., Robinson, D., Dugan, E., Howard, G., Suggs, P. K., Pearce, K. F., Carroll, D. D., McGann, P., & Preisser, J. (1999). Communication between older adults and their physicians about urinary incontinence. *Journals of Gerontology: Series A, Biological Sciences & Medical Sciences, 54*(1), M34-M37.

Colling, J., Ouslander, J., Hadley, B. J., Eisch, J., & Campbell, E. (1992). The effects of patterned urge response toileting (PURT) on urinary incontinence among nursing home residents. *Journal of the American Geriatrics Society, 40,* 135-141.

Colling, J. C., Owen, T. R., & McCreedy, M. R. (1994). Urine volumes and voiding patterns among incontinent nursing home residents. *Geriatric Nursing, 15*(4), 188-192.

Davis, K. M., & Minaker, K. L. (1994). Disorders of fluid balance: Dehydration and hyponatremia. In W. K. Hazzard, E. L. Bierman, J. P. Blass, W. H. Ettinger, & J. B. Walter (Eds.), *Prin-ciples of geriatric medicine and gerontology,* Hightstown, NJ: McGraw-Hill.

Delehanty, L., & Stravino, V. (1970). Achieving bladder control. *American Journal of Nursing, 70*(2), 312-316.

Diokno, A. C. (1983). Practical approach to the measurement of urinary incontinence in the elderly. *Comp Therapy, 9,* 67-75.

Diokno, A., Brock, B., Brown, M., & Herzog, A. R. (1986). Prevalence of urinary incontinence and other urological symptoms in the noninstitutionalized elderly. *Journal of Urology, 136,* 1022-1025.

Dougherty, M., Abrams, R., & McKey, P. L. (1986). An instrument to assess the dynamic characteristics of the circumvaginal musculature. *Nursing Research, 35*(4), 202-206.

Fantl, J. A., Wyman, J. F., McClish, D. K., Harkins, S. W., Elswick, R. K., Taylor, J. R., & Hadley, E. C. (1991). Efficacy of bladder training in older women with urinary incontinence. *Journal of the American Medical Association, 265*(5), 609-613.

Fantl, J., Newman, D., Colling, J., DeLancey, J., Keeys, C., Loughery, R., McDowell, B. J., Norton, P., Ouslander, J., Schnelle, J., Staskin, D., Tries, J., Urich, V., Vitousek, S. H., Weiss, B. D., & Whitmore, K. (1996). *Urinary incontinence in adults: Acute and chronic management.* Clinical practice guideline no. 2, 1996 update. Rockville, MD: Agency for Health Care Policy and Research, Public Health Service, U.S. Department of Health and Human Services.

Ferrie, B. G., Smith, J. S., Logan, D., Lyle, R., & Paterson, P. J. (1984). Experience with bladder training in 65 patients. *British Journal of Urology, 56,* 482-484.

Fiers, S. (1994). Indwelling catheters and devices: Avoiding the problems. *Urologic Nursing, 14*(3), 141-144.

Fine, W. (1972). Geriatric ergonomics. *Gerontological Clinics, 14,* 322-332.

Greengold, B., & Ouslander, J. (1986). Bladder retraining program for patients with post indwelling catheterization. *Journal of Gerontological Nursing, 12*(6), 31-35.

Griffin, D. (1983). Urinary incontinence in the elderly. *Postgraduate Medicine, 73*(2), 143-156.

Guttman, L., & Frankel, H. (1966). The value of intermittent catheterization in the early management of traumatic paraplegia and tetraplegia. *Paraplegia, 4,* 63-84.

Hadley, E. (1986). Bladder training and related therapies for urinary incontinence in older people. *Journal of the American Medical Association, 256*(3), 372-379.

Harrison, S. M. (1983). Stress incontinence and the physiotherapist. *Physiotherapy, 69,* 144-147.

Henderson, J., & Taylor, K. (1987). Age as a variable in an exercise program for the treatment of simple urinary stress incontinence. *Journal of Obstetrics Gynecology Neonatal Nursing, 16*(4), 266-272.

Herzog, A., Diokno, A., Brown, M. B., Normolle, D., & Brock, B. (1990). Two year incidence, remission, and change patterns of urinary incontinence in noninstitutionalized older adults. *Journal of Gerontology, 45*(2), 67-74.

Hilton, P., & Stanton, S. L. (1981). Algorithmic method for assessing urinary incontinence in elderly women. *British Medical Journal, 282,* 940-942.

Horsley, J. A., Crane, J., & Haller, K. B. (1982). *Intermittent catheterization: CURN Project, Michigan Nurses Association.* New York: Grune & Stratton.

Hu, T. W., Igou, J. F., Kaltreider, D. L., Yu, L. C., Rohner, T. J., Dennis, P. J., Craighead, W. E., Hadley, E. D., & Ory, M. G.

(1989). A clinical trial of a behavioral therapy to reduce urinary incontinence in nursing homes. *Journal of the American Medical Association, 261*(18), 2656-2662.

Hu, T. (1994). The cost impact of urinary incontinence on health care services. In National Multi-Specialty Nursing Conference on Urinary Continence, January, 1994, Phoenix, AZ.

International Continence Society Committee on Standardization of Terminology. (1990). The standardization of terminology of the lower urinary tract function. *British Journal of Obstetrics and Gynecology, 97*(Suppl. 6).

Iowa Intervention Project. J. C. McCloskey & G. M. Bulechek (Eds.). (2000). *Nursing interventions classification (NIC)* (3rd ed.). St. Louis, MO: Mosby.

Iowa Outcomes Project. M. Johnson, M. Maas, & S. Moorhead (Eds.). (2000). *Nursing outcomes classification (NOC)* (2nd ed.). St. Louis, MO: Mosby.

James, M. H. (1979, Nov.). Disorders of micturition in the elderly. *Age & Ageing, 8,* 286.

Jarvis, G. J., & Millar, D. R. (1980). Controlled trial of bladder drill for detrusor instability. *British Medical Journal, 281,* 1322-1323.

Jeter, K., & Wagner, D. (1990). Incontinence in the American home: A survey of 36,500 people. *Journal of the American Geriatrics Society, 38,* 379-383.

Kee, C. (1992, March/April). Age-related changes in the renal system: Causes, consequences, and nursing implications. *Geriatric Nursing,* 80-83.

Kirschner-Hermanns, R., Scherr, P. A., Branch, L. G., Wetle, T., & Resnick, N. M. (1998). Accuracy of survey questions for geriatric urinary incontinence. *Journal of Urology, 159*(6), 1903-1908.

Lapides, J., Diokno, A. C., Gould, F. R., & Lowe, B. S. (1975). Further observations on self catherization. *Transaction of the American Association of Genital Urinary Surgeons, 67,* 15-17.

Lekan-Rutledge, D., Palmer, M. H., & Belyea, M. (1998). In their own words: Nursing assistants' perceptions of barriers to implementation of prompted voiding in long-term care. *The Gerontologist, 38*(3), 370-380.

Long, M. (1985). Defining the nursing role. *Journal of Gerontological Nursing, 11*(1), 30-35.

Malvern, J. (1981). Incontinence of urine in women. *British Journal of Hospital Medicine, 25*(3), 224, 227, 229-231.

Mandelstam, D. (1980). Special techniques: Strengthening pelvic floor muscles. *Geriatric Nursing, 4,* 251-252.

McCormick, K., & Burgio, K. (1984). Incontinence: An update on nursing care measures. *Journal of Gerontological Nursing, 10*(10), 16-19, 22-23.

McCormick, K. (1991). From clinical trial to health policy—Research on urinary incontinence in the adult, Part II. *Journal of Professional Nursing, 7*(4), 202.

McCormick, K. A., Burgio, L. D., Engel, B. T., Scheve, A., & Leahy, E. (1992). Urinary incontinence: An augmented prompted void approach. *Journal of Gerontological Nursing, 18*(3), 3-10.

McDowell, B. (1997). Urinary incontinence. In M. M. Burke & M. B. Walsh (Eds.), *Gerontologic nursing: Wholistic care of the older adult* (2nd ed., pp. 348-368). St. Louis, MO: Mosby.

McLane, A. (Ed.). (1987). *Classification of nursing diagnoses: Proceedings of the seventh conference.* St. Louis, MO: Mosby.

Mohide, E. (1986). The prevalence and scope of urinary incontinence. *Clinics in Geriatric Medicine, 2,* 639-655.

Morris, J., Murphy, K., & Nonemaker, S. (1995). *Long term care facility assessment instrument (RAI) user's manual,* version 2.0. Rockville, MD: Health Care Financing Administration.

National Institutes of Health Consensus Development Conference. (1990). Urinary incontinence in adults. *Journal of the American Geriatrics Society, 38,* 265-272.

Newman, D. K., & Smith, D. A. (1992). Pelvic muscle reeducation as a nursing treatment for incontinence. *Urologic Nursing, 12*(1), 9-15.

North American Nursing Diagnosis Association. (1999). *Nursing diagnoses: Definitions and classification 1999-2000.* Philadelphia: Author.

Norton, C. (1984). The promotion of continence. *Nursing Times, 80*(Suppl. 14), 4, 6, 8.

O'Donnell, P., Beck, C., & Walls, R. (1990). Serial incontinence assessment in elderly inpatient males. *Journal of Rehabilitation Research, 27,* 1-8.

Olah, K. S. (1990). The conservative management of patients with symptoms of stress incontinence: A randomized prospective study comparing weighted vaginal cones and interferential therapy. *American Journal of Obstetrics and Gynecology, 162,* 87-92.

Ouslander, J. (1981). Urinary incontinence in the elderly. *Western Journal of Medicine, 135*(6), 482-491.

Ouslander, J., & Kane, R. (1982). *The costs of urinary incontinence in nursing homes,* Washington, DC: National Center for Health Services Research.

Ouslander, J. B., & Kane, R. L. (1984). The costs of urinary incontinence in nursing homes. *Medical Care, 22,* 69-79.

Ouslander, J., Kane, R., Vollmer, S., & Menezes, M. (1985). *Technologies for managing urinary incontinence.* Health Care Technology Case Study 33, 07A-HC533. Washington, DC: U.S. Congress, Office of Technology Assessment.

Ouslander, J., & Uman, G. (1985). Urinary incontinence: Opportunities for research, education, and improvements in medical care in nursing homes. In E. L. Schneider (Ed.), *The teaching nursing home* (pp. 173-190). New York: Raven Press.

Ouslander, J., Staskin, D., Raz, S., Su, H., & Hepps, K. (1987). Urological neurology and urodynamics. *The Journal of Urology, 137,* 68-71.

Ouslander, J., Leach, G., Abelson, S., Staskin, D., Blaustein, J., & Raz, S. (1988). Simple versus multichannel cystometry in the evaluation of bladder function in an incontinent geriatric population. *Journal of Urology, 140*(6), 1482-1486.

Ouslander, J., Palmer, M., Rovner, B., & German, P. (1993). Urinary incontinence in nursing homes: Incidence, remission, and associated factors. *Journal of the American Geriatrics Society, 41*(10), 1083-1089.

Ouslander, J. (1994). Incontinence. In R. Kane, J. Ouslander, & I. Abrass (Eds.), *Essentials of clinical geriatrics* (pp. 107-133). Hightstown, NJ: McGraw-Hill.

Palmer, M. H. (1993). Urinary incontinence. In V. Carrieri-Kohlman, A. M. Lindsey, & C. M. West (Eds.), *Pathophysiological phenomena in nursing* (pp. 221-244). Philadelphia: W. B. Saunders.

Palmer, M. (1996). Psychological impact. In *Urinary continence: Assessment and promotion* (pp. 111-121). Baltimore: Aspen.

Peattie, A. B., Plevnik, S., & Stanton, S. L. (1988). Vaginal cones: A conservative method of treating genuine stress incontinence. *British Journal of Obstetrics and Gynecology, 95,* 1049-1053.

Pengelly, A. W., & Booth, C. M. (1980). A prospective trial of bladder training as treatment for detrusor instability. *British Journal of Urology, 52,* 463-466.

Penn, C. (1990). *Incontinence assessment: Examining the reliability of a structured assessment tool in guiding staff nurses through a focused assessment and accurate nursing diagnosis.* Unpublished master's thesis. The University of Iowa, Iowa City.

Resnick, M. N., Wetle, T. T., Scherr, P., Branch, L., & Taylor, J. (1986). *Urinary incontinence in community dwelling elderly: Prevalence and correlates* (Abstract). In International Continence Society 16th Annual Meeting.

Resnick, N., Yalla, S., & Laurino, E. (1989). The pathophysiology of urinary incontinence among institutionalized elderly persons. *The New England Journal of Medicine, 320,* 1-7.

Resnick, N. (1990). Initial evaluation of the incontinent patient. *Journal of the American Geriatrics Society, 38*(3), 311-316.

Robb, S. (1985). Urinary incontinence verification on elderly men. *Nursing Research, 34,* 278-282.

Rottkamp, B. C. (1985). A holistic approach to identifying factors associated with an altered pattern of urinary elimination in stroke patients. *Neurosurgical Nursing, 17*(1), 37-43.

Sadowski, A., & Duffy, L. (1988). A survey of clean intermittent catheterization in long term care. *Urologic Nursing, 8,* 15-17.

Schaeffer, W. (1988). The value of free flow rate and pressure flow studies in routine investigation of BPH patients. *Neurourological Urodynamics, 7,* 219-221.

Schnelle, J. F., Traughber, B., Sowell, M. A., Newman, D. R., Petrilli, C. O., & Ory, M. (1989). Prompted voiding treatment of urinary incontinence in nursing home patients: A behavior management approach for nursing home staff. *Journal of the American Geriatrics Society, 37,* 1051-1057.

Schnelle, J. F. (1990). Treatment of urinary incontinence in nursing home patients by prompted voiding. *Journal of the American Geriatrics Society, 38,* 356-360.

Schnelle, J. F., Newman, D. R., & Fogarty, T. (1990). Management of patient continence in long term care nursing facilities. *The Gerontologist, 30,* 373-376.

Skelly, J., & Flint, A. J. (1995). Urinary incontinence associated with dementia. *Journal of the American Geriatrics Society, 43,* 286-294.

Spangler, P. F., Risley, T. R., & Bilyew, D. D. (1984). The management of dehydration and incontinence in nonambulatory geriatric patients. *The Journal of Applied Behavioral Analysis, 17,* 397-401.

Specht, J. (1981). *The effects of selected nursing interventions on incidents of incontinence of institutionalized elderly men.* Iowa City: The University of Iowa.

Specht, J. (1986). Genitourinary problems. In D. Carnivelli & M. Patrick (Eds.), *Nursing management for the elderly* (pp. 447-466). Baltimore: Lippincott Williams & Wilkins.

Taylor, K., & Henderson, J. (1986). Effects of biofeedback and urinary stress incontinence in older women. *Journal of Gerontological Nursing, 12*(9), 25-30.

Tchou, D., Adams, C., & Varner, R., & Denton, B. (1988). Pelvic floor muscular exercises in treatment of anatomical urinary stress incontinence. *Physical Therapy, 68*(5), 652-655.

Thom, D. H., & Brown, J. S. (1998). Reproductive and hormonal risk factors for urinary incontinence in later life: A review of the clinical and epidemiologic literature. *Journal of the American Geriatrics Society, 46*(11), 1411-1417.

Tunink, P. (1986). *Clinical usefulness of an assessment guide, a flowchart for diagnosis of urinary incontinence and critical indicators: A pilot study.* Unpublished paper. The University of Iowa, Iowa City.

Tunink, P. (1988). Alteration in urinary elimination. *Journal of Gerontological Nursing, 1*(4), 25-31.

Ulmsten, U. (1995). On urogenital ageing. *Maturitas, 21,* 163-169.

Warren, J. W. (1990). Urine collection devices for use in adults with urinary incontinence. *Journal of the American Geriatrics Society, 38,* 364-367.

Webb, R. J., Lawson, A. L., & Neal, D. E. (1990). Clean intermittent self-catheterization in 172 adults. *British Journal of Urology, 301,* 944-946.

Webster, G., Sihelnik, S., & Stone, A. (1984). Female urinary incontinence: The incidence, identification, and characteristics of detrition instability. *Neurourology and Urodynamics, 3,* 235.

Weiss, B. D. (1998). Diagnostic evaluation of urinary incontinence in geriatric patients. *American Family Physician, 57*(11), 2675-2684, 2688-2690.

Wells, T. (1980). Promoting urine control in older adults. *Geriatric Nursing, 1,* 236-241.

Wells, T., & Brink, C. A. (1981). Urinary continence: Assessment and management. In I. Burnside (Ed.), *Nursing and the aged* (pp. 519-548). Hightstown, NJ: McGraw-Hill.

Wells, T., Brink, C., & Diokno, A. (1987). Urinary incontinence in elderly women: clinical findings. *Journal of the American Geriatrics Society, 35,* 933-939.

Wheatley, J. (1982). Bladder incontinence: Four types and their control. *Postgraduate Medicine, 7,* 75-82.

Williams, M., & Panill, F. (1982). Urinary incontinence in the elderly: Physiology, pathophysiology, diagnosis, and treatment. *Annals of Internal Medicine, 97*(6), 895-907.

Williams, M. (1983). A critical evaluation of the assessment technology for urinary continence in older persons. *Journal of the American Geriatrics Society, 31,* 11.

Wilson, P. D., Al Samarrai, T., Deakin, M., Kolbe, E., & Brown, A. D. (1987). An objective assessment of physiotherapy for female genuine stress incontinence. *British Journal of Obstetrics and Gynecology, 94,* 575-582.

Woodtli, M., & Yocum, K. (1994). Urge incontinence: Identification and clinical validation of defining characteristics. In R. Carroll-Johnson & M. Paquette (Eds.), *Classification of nursing diagnosis: Proceedings of the tenth conference* (pp. 182-185). Baltimore: Lippincott Williams & Wilkins.

Woodtli, A. (1995). Mixed incontinence: A new nursing diagnosis? *Nursing Diagnosis, 6*(4), 135-142.

Worth, A., Dougherty, M., & McKey, P. (1986). Development and testing of the circumvaginal muscles rating scale. *Nursing Research, 35,* 166-168.

Wozniak-Petrofsky, J. (1996). Urodynamics for the primary care nurse. *Geriatric Nursing, 17*(3), 115-119.

Wyman, J., Elswick, R., Ory, M., Wilson, M., & Fantl, J. (1993). Influence of functional, urological, and environmental characteristics on urinary incontinence in community-dwelling older women. *Nursing Research, 42*(5), 270-275.

Yarnell, J., & St. Leger, A. (1979). The prevalence, severity, and factors associated with urinary incontinence in a random sample of the elderly. *Age and Ageing, 8*(2), 81-85.

PART IV

Activity-Exercise Pattern

OVERVIEW

Part Four begins with a look at the normal changes in activity-exercise patterns that result from aging. In Chapter 23 McAnaw, a physical therapist, overviews the age-related physiologic changes that occur in cardiovascular, respiratory, nervous, and musculoskeletal systems and points out common health conditions that affect activity level.

In Chapter 24 Dougherty provides an excellent overview of the diagnosis Decreased Cardiac Output. This diagnosis has stimulated controversy among proponents of the nursing diagnosis movement and among critical care nurses regarding whether nurses can independently treat actual and potential health problems related to this diagnosis, or whether they do so interdependently with medicine. Dougherty's chapter focuses on decreased cardiac output among the elderly, providing a model useful for linking conceptual parameters with clinical data and an assessment tool she developed. Dougherty also suggests specific nursing-sensitive outcomes and nursing interventions for this diagnosis in an older population.

Halm continues the discussion of circulation at the cellular level in Chapter 25, Altered Tissue Perfusion, noting that elderly persons are predisposed to decreased perfusion because of changes that occur in the cardiovascular system with aging. Halm focuses on five general etiologies related to altered renal, cerebral, cardiopulmonary, gastrointestinal, and peripheral tissue perfusion, identifying critical defining characteristics and nursing-sensitive outcomes appropriate for each. Several assessment tools are reviewed and evaluated. Both independent and interdependent nursing interventions are detailed to treat specific etiologies of Altered Tissue Perfusion.

In Chapter 26, Ineffective Breathing Pattern, Wakefield reviews the respiratory problems most likely to be experienced by elders and notes the importance of distinguishing between problems that tend to be associated with the aging process and those that are due to disease. The need for nurses to assess elderly patients systematically in order to identify risk factors and etiologies to guide treatment is emphasized. Use of the nursing-sensitive outcome Respiratory Status: Ventilation is discussed. Under the primary intervention Ventilation Assistance, *Nursing Interventions Classification (NIC)* activities related to education, monitoring, breathing exercises, exercise, medication administration, and energy conservation are described as treatments that nurses can independently use to treat Ineffective Breathing Pattern in the elderly.

In Chapter 27 Titler explicates the nursing diagnosis Activity Intolerance and identifies the most common etiologies and risk factors for elders. She notes that there is a limited research base for causative factors and clinical cues related to this diagnosis and points out that its complexity presents challenges for clinical use. She presents a useful critique of specific assessment tools and methods and describes commonly used physiologic measures related to Activity Intolerance. Nursing-sensitive outcomes are selected from the *Nursing Outcomes Classification (NOC)*. Nursing interventions suggested to treat this diagnosis are drawn primarily from the Activity and Exercise Management and the Immobility Management classes of the NIC. Titler offers a helpful review of principles and guidelines for exercise therapy with the elderly and suggests sources for further guidance.

In Chapter 28, Impaired Physical Mobility, Maas and Specht focus on a nursing diagnosis that has a high incidence among institutionalized elders and that is often the reason for admission to long-term care settings. Consequences of impaired mobility in this population are elaborated, suggesting that problems with mobility are a common etiologic factor among many of the diagnoses set forth in this book. Additionally, several separate etiologies for this diagnosis are discussed in terms of signs and symptoms that indicate specific types of impaired mobility. Nursing interventions focusing on specific etiologic factors and aimed at achieving desired outcomes are elaborated, and an assessment guide useful for diagnosing Impaired Physical Mobility among elders is presented.

Armer, Conn, Decker, and Tripp-Reimer, in Chapter 29, propose the use of a taxonomy of nursing diagnoses related to self-care based on activities needed for health. They broaden the definition of self-care as a phenomenon of nursing interest and reflect in the proposed taxonomy not only the traditional bodily care activities associated with self-care diagnoses but also social interaction, health protection, and health restoration. Armer and colleagues review and evaluate measures of self-care, including subjective measures based on the person's perception of ability and functional status measures using direct observation. They point out that most measures lack established psychometric properties for older persons across the health care continuum and among ethnically diverse populations, and they recommend areas for future research, including psychometric testing and theoretical development of health promotion and health restoration self-care categories. Nursing-sensitive outcomes are suggested for specific gerontologic case situations as well for the diagnosis Self-Care Deficit generally. Outcome criteria

developed by Carpentino are examined using NOC guidelines for the development of nursing-sensitive outcomes. Strategies for gerontologic nursing interventions with individuals with self-care deficits are outlined, including the use of NIC, and interventions suggested by research to encourage self-care and health promotion are elaborated.

Rantz and Popejoy, in Chapter 30, discuss the diagnosis Diversional Activity Deficit, which is closely related to many of the other diagnoses discussed within the activity-exercise pattern. They emphasize that failure to treat this problem in elders leads to multiple adverse consequences. Likewise, they provide compelling empirical support for the notion that treatment of this deficit can improve cognitive, affective, and physiologic status; increase socialization; and, in general, contribute to an enhanced quality of life for the elderly individual. A diversional assessment worksheet useful for nursing home residents and additional suggestions for assessment are presented. Leisure Participation is recommended as an appropriate primary nursing-sensitive outcome, and suggestions are offered for further development of this NOC outcome. Several other outcomes are suggested on the basis of research. Outcome measures that may be relevant to this diagnosis are listed. Activity Therapy is developed in some detail as the intervention of choice for this problem. Other rehabilitative therapies (e.g., reminiscence, pets, music, exercise) are also discussed, with special mention of use for persons with dementia.

CHAPTER 23

NORMAL CHANGES WITH AGING

Maire B. McAnaw

The cardiovascular, respiratory, nervous, and musculoskeletal systems function in an integrated manner to make activity and exercise possible. Consequently, age-related changes in one system will invariably affect the other systems. Aging is often complicated by the development of several diseases. At times, the distinction between normal aging changes and those changes associated with disease may be subtle and difficult to assess.

CARDIOVASCULAR SYSTEM

Several age-related changes reduce the efficiency of the cardiovascular system. Factors that contribute to the decreased compliance of the heart include sclerosis of the endocardium, fibrosis of the heart valves, increased myocardial stiffness, decreased muscle fibers, and reduced myocardial strength. An accumulation of lipofuscin develops in older myocardial cells (Lewis & Bottomley, 1994). The left ventricle stiffens and may become 25% thicker as it pumps harder to overcome the increased resistance of the aging aorta (Staab & Hodges, 1996). Diminished pacemaker cells and increased fibrosis of the sinoatrial (SA) node can lead to alterations in cardiac rhythm. Only 10% of the pacemaker cells seen in a 20 year old remain by age 75 (Rowe & Besdine, 1988).

Arterial stiffening occurs with advancing age as a result of thickening of the media, fibrosis of the intima, decreased smooth muscle cells, increased calcium deposits, increased collagen, and decreased elastic fibers. The media of the aorta becomes approximately 40% thicker after age 50 (Lewis & Bottomley, 1994). These changes increase peripheral vascular resistance, which increases the workload of the heart and decreases blood flow to various organs, especially the kidneys. Systolic and diastolic pressures are elevated as more force is required to pump blood through the narrowed lumen of the arteries. Veins thicken, dilate, and stretch. The valves of the large leg veins undergo structural changes that can contribute to impaired venous return (Gioiella & Bevil, 1985). Because of arterial stiffness and declining function of the autonomic nervous system, baroreceptors respond more slowly and become less capable of regulating blood pressure. Elders can experience orthostatic hypotension and an increased risk of vagal syncope (Fluckiger, Boivin, Quilliot, Jeandel, & Zannad, 1999). Consequently, a greater risk of falls and injuries exists for the elderly.

Although resting heart rate remains virtually unchanged, heart rate during exercise decreases slightly with age (Brocklehurst, Tallis, & Fillit, 1992). This attenuation is attributed to the growth of connective tissue in the SA node, atrioventricular (AV) node, and bundle branches. Longer periods of time are required for an older person's heart rate to return to normal after stress or exercise (Farrell, 1990; Gioiella & Bevil, 1985). Stroke volume declines, and resting cardiac output decreases approximately 20% by age 80 (Brocklehurst et al., 1992). A more significant decline in cardiac output is noted, however, during exercise, which results in reduced blood flow to the organs (Brocklehurst et al., 1992). Decreased blood flow to the coronary arteries reduces oxygen traveling to the heart and undermines the heart's ability to respond effectively to exercise. Dizziness and confusion can result from decreased cerebral blood flow during exercise. Maximal oxygen consumption declines with age and also contributes to reduced work capacity (Gioiella & Bevil, 1985).

RESPIRATORY SYSTEM

Several age-associated changes occur in the respiratory system, including atrophy of the respiratory musculature, increased rigidity of the rib cage, progressive postural kyphosis, and calcification of the costal cartilage. The anterior-posterior diameter of the chest increases because of flattening of the diaphragm and elevation of the ribs and results in a barrel-chested appearance. These factors reduce the compliance of the chest wall and negate its natural tendency to expand outward (Rowe & Besdine, 1988). Nevertheless, the elderly person is able to maintain adequate oxygenation during periods of health and moderate activity (Gioiella & Bevil, 1985).

With age, the decreased compliance of the chest wall is accompanied, to a lesser extent, by an increase in lung compliance. The alveoli lose elastic recoil, enlarge, and decrease in number, leading to collapse of these smaller airways during normal breathing. Consequently, partial inflation of the lungs occurs at rest. The alveolar surface area decreases 4% with each decade of life after age 30 (Brocklehurst et al., 1992). Reduced oxygen in the blood can result from incomplete ventilation and less surface area available for gas exchange. This reduced oxygenation can be exaggerated by low blood hemoglobin levels in persons with poor nutrition or anemia from other causes (Nesbitt, 1988).

Pulmonary blood flow decreases as a consequence of the decline in cardiac output. The capillaries surrounding the alveoli are reduced in number, and those that remain become thickened because of infiltrating fibrotic connective tissue. As a result, the pulmonary diffusion capacity of oxygen declines slightly with advancing age (Gioiella & Bevil, 1985). Nonuniform ventilation occurs with age as the small airways at the base of the lungs close while those larger airways toward the apex remain open. Since capillary blood flow to these upper regions is inadequate, a mismatch of areas of optimal ventilation and areas of optimal perfusion develops. Lowered red blood cell production and insufficient incorporation of iron into red blood cells can further compound problems with tissue oxygenation. Typical signs of activity intolerance can result from the composite of these physiologic changes (Nesbitt, 1988).

The altered pulmonary physiology that occurs with aging directly affects various lung volumes. Functional residual capacity increases. Expiratory and inspiratory reserve volumes decrease (Gioiella & Bevil, 1985). Total lung capacity declines, but inspiratory capacity remains virtually the same despite increasing age (Gioiella & Bevil, 1985; Lewis & Bottomley, 1994). Residual volume increases with age because of the loss of elastic recoil of the alveolar walls (Brocklehurst et al., 1992; Rowe & Besdine, 1988). Vital capacity, which equals total lung capacity minus residual volume, decreases (Farrell, 1990). The work of breathing increases 20% between the ages of 20 and 70 to overcome the stiffness of the chest wall (Gioiella & Bevil, 1985). Maximum ventilation during exhausting work decreases approximately 60% by the eighth decade (Gioiella & Bevil, 1985).

Epithelial atrophy causes ciliary action, the mechanism for mobilizing pulmonary secretions, to decline with age (Gioiella & Bevil, 1985). Mucus and foreign materials are less efficiently expelled from the lungs (Staab & Hodges, 1996). The cough reflex becomes less effective as a result of increased stiffness of the chest wall and reduced muscle strength. Poor physical mobility can accentuate normal aging changes and lead to the retention of pulmonary secretions (Staab & Hodges, 1996). Consequently, the elderly person becomes more vulnerable to reduced ventilation and the development of respiratory diseases.

CENTRAL NERVOUS SYSTEM

The central nervous system also demonstrates a number of age-related changes. By age 80, brain mass has declined 6% to 7% because of cell losses predominantly from the cerebellum and cerebral cortex (Lewis & Bottomley, 1994). Several neurotransmitters become less available in the senescent brain, slowing synaptic transmission (Lewis & Bottomley, 1994). The conduction of impulses particularly along the posterior spinal column tracts is decreased because of loss of large myelinated nerve fibers (Lewis & Bottomley, 1994). As a result, the transmission of proprioceptive input is slowed, which impedes one's ability to regain balance.

In the peripheral nervous system, neurons atrophy and are progressively lost. Heavily myelinated fibers decline more than thinly myelinated fibers. Motor units decrease in number, and larger numbers of motor units are required to produce a given force (Lewis & Bottomley, 1994). Delayed reaction time in elders is attributed to slowed nerve conduction velocity, which is more evident in sensory nerves than in motor nerves (Brocklehurst et al., 1992).

The internal thermostat of the hypothalamus becomes less sensitive with age, and faulty thermoregulation can result (Lewis & Bottomley, 1994). Higher rates of hypothermia and heatstroke are well documented among elders (Lewis & Bottomley, 1994). Sluggish autonomic vasomotor responses to warming and cooling directly affect activity tolerance and endurance (Lewis & Bottomley, 1994). Consequently, an elderly individual requires a longer cool-down period after exercise (Lewis & Bottomley, 1994).

All senses undergo degenerative changes and become less sensitive with advancing age. Balance is contingent on input from the visual, propioceptive, and vestibular systems (Bonder & Wagner, 1994; Newman, 1995). Visual acuity declines with age, which can significantly impede an individual's voluntary physical activity. Sensory receptors in the semicircular canals and otoliths of the vestibular system become less capable of monitoring head position and movements (Lewis & Bottomley, 1994). Propioceptive input is delayed as large myelinated fibers carrying this information are progressively lost with advancing age (Lewis & Bottomley, 1994). The decline of the visual, propioceptive, and vestibular systems results in increased postural sway, decreased balance, and a high incidence of falls in the elderly population (Newman, 1995).

MUSCULOSKELETAL SYSTEM

Age-associated changes in the musculoskeletal system contribute to activity intolerance and impaired physical mobility (Nesbitt, 1988). A decline in muscle strength is largely caused by muscle fiber atrophy and neurologic decline associated with aging. Many other age-related physiologic changes contribute on a smaller scale to muscle strength reduction.

Maximal muscular strength is achieved between 20 and 35 years of age (Metter, 1999). Noticeable decrements in muscle strength begin in the fifth decade, and by 80 years of age, 30% to 50% of muscle mass is lost (Brocklehurst et al., 1992; Sullivan, 1987). Muscle atrophy may be partially hidden by increased fat and collagen in the muscles of elderly individuals. A larger percent of type I fatigue–resistant muscle fibers remain in senescent muscles as a result of the preferential atrophy of type II, or fast-twitch, muscle fibers (Sullivan, 1987). This explains why muscle endurance only declines at a slow rate or not at all with advancing age (Sullivan, 1987). Muscles of the lower extremities demonstrate more atrophy and decreased strength than upper extremity muscles (Sullivan, 1987). It is believed that upper extremity muscles maintain their strength longer, since they are used more frequently for activities of daily living. An elderly individual may use only lower extremity muscles during bouts of short distance household ambulation but will continue to use upper extremity muscles throughout the day for personal hygiene, dressing, and eating.

Muscle atrophy alone cannot account for all of the strength reduction that is observed with aging (Yue, Ranganathan, Siemionow, Liu, & Sahgal, 1999). Yue et al. (1999) hypothesized that elderly individuals have an impaired ability to produce central nervous system commands to fully activate muscles. Older individuals were found to have a reduced ability to maximally activate the biceps brachii muscle when compared with young adults (Yue et al., 1999). Altered innervation patterns of aging muscles and reduced sensitivity of muscle to neural input might contribute to declining neuromuscular function (Gioiell & Bevil, 1985).

Other factors that might contribute to reduced muscle strength include insufficient dietary intake of potassium, decreased neurons, hormonal changes, and decreased mobilization of glucose with activity (Farrell, 1990). Senescent muscles use oxygen less efficiently. Slower gross movements result from reduced oxygen and nutrient perfusion to the muscles.

Although osteoblasts continue to lay down new bone until advanced old age, a progressive decline in bone mass starts between the ages of 35 and 40 (Brocklehurst et al., 1992). Fast absorption of the internal portions of long and flat bones outpaces the new bone growth on the outer surfaces. As a result, bone becomes hollow internally and more porous. Overall, women lose 25% to 30% of cortical bone mass from the shafts of long bones, whereas men typically lose 5% to 15% (Brocklehurst et al., 1992). Trabecular bone mass, found in the vertebrae, pelvis, and ends of long bones, is decreased by 35% to 50% in women and 15% to 45% in men by age 80 (Brocklehurst et al., 1992). Before the development of accurate bone mass measuring techniques, the distinction between normal skeletal aging and defined osteoporosis was vague. Although some bone loss with aging is universal, osteoporosis is viewed as a serious, pathologic condition because of the debilitating consequences of fractures in the elderly population.

Hyaline cartilage, which lines joint surfaces, frays and erodes with advancing age, and bones come in direct contact with each other. Tendons, ligaments, synovial membranes, and joint capsules stiffen and become less elastic. Pain and crepitus result. Limited joint range of motion also occurs and is more pronounced in those individuals who have worked in sedentary rather than active occupations (Brocklehurst et al., 1992). Intervertebral disks become dry and narrow and are more prone to tear (Brocklehurst et al., 1992; Staab & Hodges, 1996). The vertebrae of the spine become shorter and wider as a result of decreased bone mass and mineral content (Farrell, 1990). An individual's height decreases at the approximate rate of 1.2 cm for every two decades of life (Staab & Hodges, 1996). Vertebral osteophyte formation occurs, and, as a result, back pain is commonly experienced by the elderly (Newman, 1995).

Forward stooped posture results from increased flexion of the hips and knees, decreased lumbar lordosis, increased thoracic kyphosis, and rounded shoulders with protracted scapula (Bonder & Wagner, 1994). The head juts forward and tilts backward in an effort to maintain the gaze level (O'Hara-Devereaux, Andrus, & Scott, 1981). These postural deviations alter the older individual's center of gravity and lead to the development of a slower, shorter, cautious, wide-based gait pattern (Staab & Hodges, 1996). A fear of falling combined with these musculoskeletal changes reduces deliberate physical mobility.

SUMMARY

Numerous physiologic changes occur in the cardiovascular, respiratory, nervous, and musculoskeletal systems during the natural aging process. Strong evidence cites disuse caused by inactivity as the most important contributor to declining physical mobility and function (Sullivan, 1987). The heart and diaphragm demonstrate fewer changes with aging than voluntary muscles, a finding consistent with the belief that aging is not solely responsible for problems with activity in elders (Gioiella & Bevil, 1985; Harris, 1989). Theoretically, positive lifestyle modifications, such as moderate physical activity and proper nutrition, provide the physiologic foundation to optimize physical abilities and promote healthier aging.

REFERENCES

Bonder, B. R., & Wagner, M. B. (1994). *Functional performance in older adults.* Philadelphia: F. A. Davis.

Brocklehurst, J. C., Tallis, R. C., & Fillit, H. M. (1992). *Textbook of geriatric medicine and gerontology.* New York: Churchill Livingstone.

Farrell, J. (1990). *Nursing care of the older person.* Baltimore: Lippincott Williams & Wilkins.

Fluckiger, L., Boivin, J., Quilliot, D., Jeandel, C., & Zannad, F. (1999). Differential effects of aging on heart rate variability and blood pressure variability. *Journal of Gerontology, 54A*(5), B219-B224.

Gioiella, E. C., & Bevil, C. W. (1985). *Nursing care of the aging client: Promoting healthy adaptations.* Norwalk, CT: Appleton & Lange.

Harris, R. (1989). Exercise and physical fitness for the elderly. In W. Reichel (Ed.), *Clinical aspects of aging* (pp. 86-92). Baltimore: Lippincott Williams & Wilkins.

Lewis, C. B., & Bottomley, J. M. (1994). *Geriatric physical therapy: A clinical approach.* Norwalk, CT: Appleton & Lange.

Metter, E. J., Lynch, N., Conwit, R., Lindle, R., Tobin, J., & Hurley, B. (1999). Muscle quality and age: Cross-sectional and longitudinal comparisons. *Journal of Gerontology, 54A*(5), B207-B218.

Nesbitt, B. (1988). Nursing diagnosis in age-related changes. *Journal of Gerontological Nursing, 14*(7), 7-12.

Newman, L. A. (1995). *Maintaining function in older adults.* Boston: Butterworth-Heinemann.

O'Hara-Devereaux, M., Andrus, L. H., & Scott, C. D. (1981). *Eldercare: A practical guide to clinical geriatrics.* New York: Grune & Stratton.

Rowe, J. W., & Besdine, R. W. (1988). *Geriatric medicine.* Boston: Little, Brown.

Staab, A. S. & Hodges, L. C. (1996). *Essentials of gerontological nursing: Adaptation to the aging process.* Baltimore: Lippincott Williams & Wilkins.

Sullivan, M. (1987). Atrophy and exercise. *Journal of Gerontological Nursing, 13*(7), 26-31.

Yue, G. H., Ranganathan, V. K., Siemionow, V., Liu, J. Z., & Sahgal, V. (1999). Older adults exhibit a reduced ability to fully activate their biceps brachii muscle. *Journal of Gerontology, 54A*(4), M249-M253.

CHAPTER 24

DECREASED CARDIAC OUTPUT

Cynthia M. Dougherty

The function and viability of all body tissues depend on an adequate supply of oxygen and other nutrients from the circulating blood. This supply is primarily determined by the cardiac output, as indicated by the following formula:

$$CO = HR \times SV$$

where

CO = Cardiac output
HR = Heart rate
SV = Stroke volume

Stroke volume, in turn, is determined by preload, afterload, and contractility. When normal heart rate ranges from 60 to 100 beats/minute and is multiplied by a normal stroke volume of 60 to 130 ml, the product is a range of normal cardiac output of 4 to 8 liters/minute (Alexander, 1998). Cardiac index, or cardiac output divided by body surface area (CO/BSA), is a more individualized measure of cardiac function used in clinical practice, with normal ranges of 2.5 to 4 liters/minute (Alexander, 1998). The inability of the heart to supply the amount of oxygenated blood needed for the body's metabolic requirements is termed *pump failure* or *decreased cardiac output*. Methods to measure cardiac output have been perfected over the last 20 years using the Swan-Ganz catheter (Swan et al., 1970).

For many years it was thought that there was a marked age-associated decrease in overall left ventricular function and reduced coronary blood flow. This has not been supported in more recent investigations (Roffe, 1998). Cardiovascular changes with age occur selectively rather than globally as one ages. There is no general decline in overall cardiac functioning in the normal aging heart. The ability of the heart muscle to develop tension is well maintained with aging, as are global aspects of left ventricular function at rest. Response to beta sympathetic receptors in cardiac tissues decreases markedly and is manifested as a decrease in inotropic response of cardiac muscle to catecholamine stimulation, a decrease in heart rate response, and a decrease in arterial vasodilation. During exercise the aged exhibit an enhanced use of the Frank-Starling mechanism to compensate for the increased workload and lower inotropic state of the heart (Alexander, 1998). As one ages, there is evidence of prolonged relaxation and

contraction of cardiac muscle that produces a prolonged isovolumic phase of diastole and slowed diastolic left ventricular filling. In an aging heart with coronary artery disease, this can compromise subendocardial blood flow and produce ischemia.

In the older adult potential causes of reduced cardiac output can be related to fluid imbalances, dysrhythmias, and reduced contractility from previous myocardial infarction or myocardial injury (Davies, 1992). Systemic hypertension, myocardial ischemia, and infarction are more prevalent with advancing age and can contribute to reductions in diastolic function (Harizi, Bianco, & Alpert, 1988; Wong, Gold, Fukuyama, & Blanchette, 1989). Age-related changes at both the anatomic and cellular levels could be associated with decreases in both systolic and diastolic function. Changes in the cross-linking of intercellular connective tissue result in increased myocardial stiffness (Lakatta, 1990). Left ventricular hypertrophy and reduction in left ventricular cavity size are features of the aging heart, even in the absence of cardiovascular disease (Lakatta, 1990). The elder might be at higher risk for reductions in cardiac output for these reasons.

Although much has been written about decreased cardiac output, little of the work so far has explicated a conceptualization of cardiac output that reflects physiologic and pathophysiologic concepts within a framework that is workable for nurses. Parameters indicating right and left ventricular function can be calculated from hemodynamic data generated from monitoring. This concept is challenging and complex in delineation, since both the right and left heart are connected by two complex vascular systems. In clinical practice cardiac output is rarely allowed to fall below normal levels when individuals are hospitalized, so more information is required regarding defining characteristics in order for nurses to detect and adequately treat decreases in cardiac output effectively.

A model of altered cardiac output (Figure 24-1) is proposed that links conceptual parameters with hemodynamic and clinical data. The model clarifies that regulation of cardiac output is determined by factors controlling heart rate and stroke volume and that stroke volume, in turn, is determined by preload, afterload, and contractility. Using this model, components of altered cardiac output can then be applied in order to maintain an adequate cardiac output to meet the demands of the body.

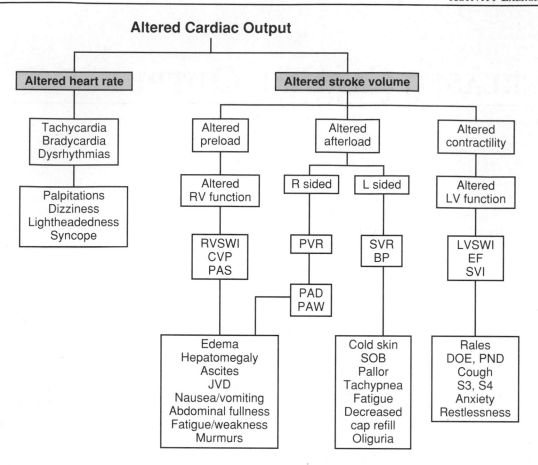

Altered Cardiac Output

RV = Right ventricle
RVSWI = Right ventricular stroke work index
CVP = Central venous pressure
PAS = Pulmonary artery systolic
JVD = Jugular venous distension
PVR = Pulmonary vascular resistance
PAD = Pulmonary artery diastolic
PAW = Pulmonary artery wedge
SVR = Systemic vascular resistance
BP = Blood pressure
SOB = Shortness of breath
LV = Left ventricle
LVSWI = Left ventricular stroke work index
EF = Ejection fraction
SVI = Stroke volume index
DOE = Dyspnea on exertion
PND = Paroxysmal nocturnal dyspnea

FIGURE **24-1**   Altered cardiac output.

RELATED FACTORS/ETIOLOGIES

Altered Heart Rate

Cardiac rate and rhythm are regulated by the rate of discharge from the SA node, discharges from the sympathetic and parasympathetic nervous systems, metabolic demands, and other neural mechanisms. Stimulation of the sympathetic nervous system will cause increases both in heart rate and in the strength of contraction through release of norepinephrine at nerve-ending sites throughout the heart muscle (Guyton, 1981). An increase in heart rate alone can increase cardiac output threefold within a limited time frame. Stimulation of the parasympathetic nervous system produces a decrease in heart rate only. Bradycardia does not always produce a decrease in cardiac output because stroke volume will increase to compensate for the drop. In patients with fixed stroke volume, decreases in heart rate will produce reductions in cardiac output, as in the patient who has suffered a myocardial infarction (Braunwald, 1997).

Heart rates that are too slow, too fast, or irregular can cause decreased cardiac output in patients with compromised cardiac function. Tachycardia (heart rate >100 beats/minute) results in decreased atrial and ventricular filling time and emptying. During diastole the coronary arteries fill with blood, with increased heart rates producing reduced oxygen supply to the myocardium. Bradycardia (heart rate <60 beats/minute) can result in decreased cardiac output if not compensated by increases in stroke volume. Dysrhythmias produce a loss in atrial-ventricular sequencing and can decrease cardiac output by as much as 30%. Individuals can experience alterations in heart rate as palpations, dizziness, lightheadedness, or syncope.

Altered Stroke Volume

Preload is the volume of blood that fills both ventricles during diastole, the right heart receiving blood from the systemic circulation and the left heart from the pulmonary circulation. Factors affecting preload include systemic venous return, venous pressure or tone, pulmonary venous volume, intrathoracic pressure, pericardial pressure, and atrial contraction (Braunwald, 1997).

A decrease in venous return caused by loss in intravascular volume (from hemorrhage, diuresis, or vomiting) or a loss of fluid into the interstitial space (caused by burns, sepsis, or electrolyte imbalances) will decrease preload. Venous capacity or tone decreases with vasodilatation of peripheral vessels and will, in turn, decrease preload. Pulmonary blood flow determines left ventricular preload and can be affected by right ventricular contractility or pulmonary embolism. During inspiration, intrathoracic pressure becomes slightly negative to enhance venous return, but with high inspiratory pressures as in mechanical ventilation, pulmonary hypertension, or tension pneumothorax, it will again decrease preload. Increases in pericardial pressure because of pericardial effusion, tamponade, or pericarditis prohibit blood from entering the right atrium and cause it to collapse; venous return to the heart and thus preload is decreased.

Under normal conditions, atrial contraction occurring at the end of ventricular diastole contributes 30% of the volume of ventricular filling. If this atrial kick is lost or absent, as in atrial dysrhythmias (atrial fibrillation, atrial flutter, paroxysmal atrial tachycardia), or is inappropriately timed, as in atrioventricular (AV) block, junctional rhythm, ventricular dysrhythmias, or paced rhythm of the ventricles, cardiac output will fall. Thus, factors that cause a decrease in preload have the potential for causing decreases in cardiac output.

Increases in preload occur when venous system pressure rises. The patient might experience edema in dependent body parts such as the sacrum and lower extremities and a weight gain of 10 lb or more. With advancing

decreases in cardiac output, fluid can accumulate in pericardial cavities. As the work and forcefulness of the right ventricle decrease, a lifting or heave in the chest wall along the sternal border can be produced. In either right ventricle (RV) or left ventricle (LV) failure, rising pressure within the heart produces apposition of valves, resulting in murmurs. Preload of the right heart is assessed by central venous pressure (CVP, normal 2 to 6 mm Hg), right ventricular stroke work index (RVSWI, normal 7 to 12 g/m²/beat), and pulmonary artery systolic pressure (PAS, normal 20 to 30 mm Hg). Preload of the LV is reflected as afterload of the RV. Alterations in RV function are manifested in the patient by peripheral edema, hepatomegaly, cool extremities, jugular venous distension, nausea and vomiting, abdominal fullness and pain, fatigue, and weakness.

Increases in pulmonary artery (PA) pressures will affect the right heart, resulting in decreased output from the right heart. As pressure in the right heart rises, congestion in the venous system, abdominal organs, and capillary interstitial spaces occurs. This rising pressure causes an increase in right ventricular end diastolic pressure (RVEDP), an increase in right atrium (RA) pressure, an increase in CVP, and backup of blood from the right heart into the venous system (Braunwald, 1997). Jugular venous distention (JVD) can be used to determine a general estimate of right heart venous return and RA pressure. An elevation of the JVD more than 1 to 2 cm above the angle of Louis at 45 degrees signals increased RA pressure and can produce observable venous pulsations. Increased pressure in the inferior vena cava causes the liver and spleen to become enlarged and congested. The patient might complain of abdominal pain, and the hepatojugular reflux might be positive. Ascites, edema of the bowel, nausea, vomiting, anorexia, and abdominal distension also can accompany venous congestion (Loeb & Gunnar, 1981).

Myocardial contractility is the inherent ability of the cardiac muscle to contract and is explained by the Frank-Starling law of the heart (Starling, 1926). Contractility is not readily measurable at the bedside but is indicative of LV function. The ability of the heart to contract is decreased by factors that increase myocardial oxygen consumption, such as tachydysrhythmias, an enlarged ventricular diameter, high afterload, primary myocardial disease (cardiomyopathy), coronary artery disease, and myocardial infarction; myocardial ischemia with a secondary decrease in contractility can result. Ventricular contractility is also affected by factors that decrease myocardial oxygen delivery, including hypoxemia, acidosis, narrowing of the coronary arteries, and low arterial pressure. Drugs known to affect the contractile state of the ventricle include lidocaine, quinidine, propranolol, pronestyl, and disopyramide (Loeb & Gunnar, 1981). Unless contractility is severely affected, the heart will pump whatever amount of blood that flows into it without significant changes in cardiac output.

A decreased pumping efficiency of the LV causes both backward and forward effects. The forward effect is decreased tissue perfusion to organs. The backward effect is increased volume and pressure in the pulmonary circulation. As the ventricle becomes less able to empty completely and effective cardiac output falls, blood remains in the LV at the end of systole. In an attempt to augment the amount of blood ejected from the LV, the heart enlarges and increases its rate and force of contraction (Starling, 1926). This compensatory mechanism, primarily governed by the sympathetic nervous system, can maintain cardiac output for a time, but eventually becomes ineffective and the heart decompensates. As decompensation progresses, more blood accumulates in the LV and causes further dilation and hypertrophy (Guyton, 1981). Tachycardia and pulsus alterans (alternation of one strong beat with one weak beat during sinus rhythm) can be noted. Consequently, left ventricular end diastolic pressure (LVEDP) increases and a third heart sound (S3) appears. The fourth heart sound (S4) is produced late in diastole and is created when the atria contract with resistance to ventricular filling, indicating decreased myocardial compliance and rising LV pressure (Braunwald, 1997).

As pressure continues to increase in the LV and blood backs up from the LV to the LA, a rise in LA pressure will be noted. Eventually PA and pulmonary venous pressures will increase, pulmonary artery wedge pressure will increase above plasma oncotic pressure in the lung, and signs of pulmonary vascular congestion will develop. As fluid begins to accumulate in the lungs, more specific symptoms such as dyspnea, orthopnea, paroxysmal nocturnal dyspnea, and Cheyne-Stokes respiration will appear (Poole-Wilson, 1988).

A dry cough develops early in the failure phase of decreased cardiac output as fluid becomes an irritant in the interstitial spaces. As the alveoli become filled with fluid, the cough will become productive, and occasionally pulmonary vessels will rupture, producing hemoptysis. Rales develop when pulmonary capillary pressure has exceeded normal plasma osmotic pressure and fluid moves from the pulmonary capillary to the alveoli (Chapman & Mitchell, 1965). Chest pain, wheezing, and pleural effusion can be noted. Rales are first noted in dependent lobes of lung tissue. As pulmonary edema develops, they will gradually become diffuse and bilateral. Myocardial contractility is indirectly measured by stroke volume index (SVI, normal 35 to 70 ml/beat/m^2 or SV/BSA), left ventricular stroke work index (LVSWI), normal 50 to 60 g/m^2 or

$$MAP - PAD/SVI \times 0.0136$$

where

MAP = Mean arterial pressure
PAD = Pulmonary artery diastolic
SVI = Stroke volume index

and ejection fraction (EF), normal 50% to 60% or

$$SV - EDV \times 100$$

where

SV = Stroke volume
EDV = End diastolic volume

Afterload is the resistance against which the heart must pump to eject blood. It is determined by the diameter of arterioles in the pulmonary and systemic circulation (Parmley, 1989). The following factors determine LV afterload: cold temperatures or any substance that causes vasoconstriction and increases systemic vascular resistance; drugs such as levophed, aramine, epinephrine, and dopamine in high doses; pulmonary artery hypertension; aortic valvular disease; and high mean arterial pressure (Dahlen & Roberts, 1996).

RV afterload is determined by the pulmonary circulation. If pulmonary vessels constrict or obstruction to pulmonary blood flow is present, an increase in pulmonary vascular resistance occurs with subsequent increase in afterload of the RV. This, in turn, will decrease preload of the left heart (Braunwald, 1997). The following factors affect RV afterload: any condition causing pulmonary constriction such as an increase in alveolar PO_2 or decrease in arterial PO_2; pulmonary embolism that causes obstruction to blood flow; pulmonary vascular defects; and vasoactive substances such as histamine, which increase pulmonary vascular resistance.

Afterload of the RV is determined by pulmonary vascular resistance (PVR), normal 150 to 250 dynes/sec/cm^{-5} or

$$PA\ mean - PAW/CO \times 80$$

where

PA = Pulmonary artery
PAW = Pulmonary artery wedge
CO = Cardiac output

PVR is the ratio of pressure drop across the pulmonary vascular system to total flow in the pulmonary circulation. An increase in intravascular volume or increase in venous return can overfill the LV and cause increased PVR and pulmonary edema. Pulmonary artery diastolic pressure (PAD, normal 10 to 20 mm Hg) and pulmonary artery wedge pressure (PAW, normal 4 to 12 mm Hg) are determinants of pulmonary vascular dynamics.

The forward effects of decreased cardiac output are primarily the result of decreased blood flow to organs and tissues and usually appear early in the cycle. A decrease in blood flow to the musculoskeletal system produces complaints of fatigue, weakness, and restlessness. The patient might complain that his energy level is gone and can exhibit changes in posture, gait, and speech. Blood flow to the heart and brain will be maintained by the sympathetic nervous system at the expense of the skin, kidneys, and muscle. Central nervous system signs of decreased perfusion are manifested by confusion, agitation, decreased attention span with memory lapse, and anxiety. The patient might complain of insomnia. As blood flow is decreased to the skin in response to vasoconstriction produced by the sympathetic nervous system, the skin becomes cold and clammy with slow capillary refill, diaphoretic, cyanotic, and pale. This redistribution of blood to the core organs will cause a decrease in skin temperature in peripheral areas, while the trunk remains warm (White & Roberts, 1992).

As vasoconstriction occurs in splanchnic, mesenteric, and renal vascular beds, a decrease in mean arterial pressure will decrease urine output. The glomerular filtration rate is decreased and is interpreted by the kidney as hypovolemia, which stimulates renin production, angiotensin, and further decreases in urine output. The kidney begins to conserve sodium and water via stimulation of the aldosterone and antidiuretic hormone mechanisms and will increase systemic blood volume.

Afterload of the LV is determined by systemic vascular resistance (SVR), normal 900 to 1200 dynes/sec/cm^{-5} or

$$\frac{MAP - CVP}{CO} \times 80$$

where

MAP = Mean arterial pressure
CVP = Central venous pressure
CO = Cardiac output

SVR reflects resistance to LV emptying and is affected by blood pressure and autonomic stimulation, producing catecholamines and angiotensin. Increased SVR is often an automatic response stimulated in an attempt to maintain blood pressure in patients with falling LV function. The patient with alterations in afterload with increased PVR and increased SVR will manifest shortness of breath (SOB), dyspnea, peripheral edema, anxiety, increased respiratory rate, confusion, cool skin, cyanosis, pallor, and fatigue.

As cardiac output becomes more severely decreased, the patient can begin to move toward cardiogenic shock, representing the most severe impairment of cardiac output. The exact cause is not known, but it can be predicted when greater than 40% of the heart muscle has become dysfunctional (White & Roberts, 1992). There are usually profound decreases in stroke volume and arterial pressure; therefore organs and tissues are severely deprived of oxygen. As a result, cells divert to anaerobic glycolysis, producing metabolic acidosis. For survival, the sympathetic nervous system maintains perfusion to vital organs, with widespread arteriole and venule constriction, tachycardia, increased forcefulness of contraction, and dilatation of coronary arteries. When cardiogenic shock is allowed to ensue and continue over an extended time period, compensatory mechanisms fail and death results.

ASSESSMENT

Tools for assessing decreased cardiac output based on clinical signs alone have not been developed. Assessment Guide 24-1 presents a cardiac output assessment tool developed for research purposes. The cardiac output tool is divided into two parts. The first section focuses on assessing the etiology of the diagnosis Decreased Cardiac Output. The second portion focuses on the defining characteristics and consists of subjective, objective, and laboratory assessments. Many of the items on the initial tool were included for research purposes and do not have clinical relevance for making the diagnosis Decreased Cardiac Output. However, significant differences in scores have been noted between patients with mild and severe reductions in cardiac output in a clinical population. The tool presented here has not been adapted for use in clinical settings or for an elderly population. An altered cardiac output assessment tool has also been published by Contrades (1987). This instrument was organized around theoretical concepts of Rogers' theory of unitary person. The tool is extremely lengthy and has not been systematically adapted for clinical use.

NURSING DIAGNOSIS

Decreased Cardiac Output has been defined by the North American Nursing Diagnosis Association (NANDA) as "a state in which the blood pumped by the heart is inadequate to meet the metabolic demands of the body" (NANDA, 1999, p. 29). For Decreased Cardiac Output, defining characteristics were developed by a panel of nurses at the Second Conference on the Classification of Nursing Diagnoses. Etiologies were not developed until the fifth national conference, at which time changes were made in the definition and defining characteristics as well. Subsequent NANDA publications now have eliminated etiologies for decreased cardiac output, with no further changes made in the other structural components of the diagnosis since 1982 (Table 24-1, p. 293).

Since its original listing in the NANDA taxonomy in the 1970s, a number of clinical papers have described nursing diagnoses associated with varying cardiac conditions, including decreased cardiac output (Brooks-Brunn, 1987; Buman & Speltz, 1989; Cardin, 1985; Contrades, 1987; Kelly, 1991; Rossi, 1979; Russell & Blake, 1989; Teplitz, 1990, 1991; Whitman & Hicks, 1988). Two papers have described the design of assessment tools for measuring the nursing diagnosis Decreased Cardiac Output (Contrades, 1987; Dougherty, 1986). Since the early 1980s a number of validation studies have suggested the need for revision in the original definition, etiologies, and defining characteristics listed by NANDA (Burke, Gabriel, Fischer, & Zemke, 1986; Dalton, 1985; Hubalik & Kim, 1984; Kern & Omery, 1992; Kim et al., 1984; Lazure & Cuddigan, 1987; Miller & Helander, 1979; Roberts,

1992; Scanlon, 1992). Investigations have used descriptive methods, contained small sample sizes, primarily focused on critically ill individuals, relied on medical records for data gathered, and used a variety of definitions of the concept. Despite these issues, research results reflect that NANDA's efforts at defining Decreased Cardiac Output had good beginnings. Recommended revisions in the definition and defining characteristics have been presented and incorporated into the NANDA taxonomy (NANDA, 1999).

Assessment Guide 24-1

CARDIAC OUTPUT ASSESSMENT TOOL

Study number _____   Age _____
ID number _____   Sex _____
Time/Date _____
General appearance and medical history:

1. **Etiology:**	Yes	No		2. **Subjective symptoms:**	Yes	No
Rheumatic fever	( )	( )		Chest pain	( )	( )
Heart murmur	( )	( )		Shortness of breath	( )	( )
Myocardial infarction	( )	( )		Fatigue	( )	( )
Pericarditis	( )	( )		Palpations	( )	( )
Pulmonary embolus	( )	( )		Anorexia	( )	( )
Phlebitis	( )	( )		Nausea	( )	( )
Stroke	( )	( )		Anxiety	( )	( )
Valvular disease	( )	( )		Cough	( )	( )
Dysrhythmia	( )	( )		Syncope	( )	( )
Cardiomyopathy	( )	( )		Orthopnea	( )	( )
Fluid overload	( )	( )		PND	( )	( )
Major trauma	( )	( )		Edema	( )	( )
Hypertension	( )	( )		Weight gain	( )	( )
Respiratory disorder	( )	( )		Wheezing	( )	( )
Other	( )	( )		Other	( )	( )

Total etiology _____   *Total symptoms* _____

Signs: Key: N = normal; A = abnormal; N/A = not applicable.

		N	A	N/A
3. Temperature _____ °C oral, rectal, core N = 37° C		( )	( )	( )
4. Heart rate _____ /min N = 60-80/min		( )	( )	( )
5. Respirations _____ /min N = 12-16/min		( )	( )	( )
6. Heart rhythm _____ N = sinus rhythm 60-80/min *see also ECG		( )	( )	( )

7. Arterial pressure   Cuff _____ Arterial line _____

		N	A	N/A
Systolic _____ mm Hg N = 90-140 mm Hg		( )	( )	( )
Diastolic _____ mm Hg N = 60-90 mm Hg		( )	( )	( )
Mean _____ mm Hg N = 70-90 mm Hg		( )	( )	( )

8. Pulmonary artery pressures		N	A	N/A
Systolic _____ mm Hg N = 20-30 mm Hg		( )	( )	( )
Diastolic _____ mm Hg N = 5-16 mm Hg		( )	( )	( )
Mean _____ mm Hg N = 10-15 mm Hg		( )	( )	( )
Wedge _____ mm Hg N = 4-12 mm Hg		( )	( )	( )
Cardiac output _____ L/min N = 4-8 L/min		( )	( )	( )
9. Skin color _____ N = pink		( )	( )	( )
A = pale, cyanotic, mottled, gray				
10. Skin temperature _____ N = warm/dry		( )	( )	( )
A = hot, cold, diaphoretic, cool, clammy				
11. Neck vein distension (JVD) external jugular _____ cm		( )	( )	( )
from angle of Louis at 45° elevation N = <1-2 cm (below)				

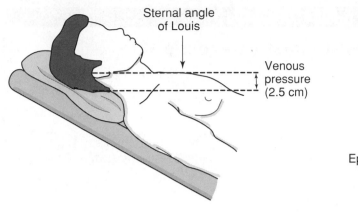

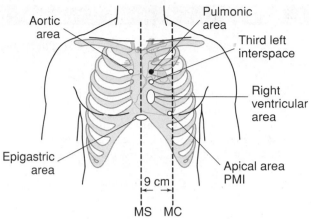

12. Heart sounds (above)
    S₁ _____ split _____   N = S₁>S₂ apex   ( )   ( )   ( )
    S₂ _____ split _____   N = S₁<S₂ base   ( )   ( )   ( )
    A = S₃, S₄, friction rub, murmur, heaves, thrills, lifts

    Describe _____
13. Peripheral pulses: O = absent; +1 = abnormal; +2 = normal.
    Carotid   R _____ L _____   R ( )   ( )   ( )
                                                          L ( )   ( )   ( )
    Brachial   R _____ L _____   R ( )   ( )   ( )
                                                          L ( )   ( )   ( )
    Radial   R _____ L _____   R ( )   ( )   ( )
                                                          L ( )   ( )   ( )
    Femoral   R _____ L _____   R ( )   ( )   ( )
                                                          L ( )   ( )   ( )
    Dorsalis pedis   R _____ L _____   R ( )   ( )   ( )
                                                          L ( )   ( )   ( )
    Posterior tibial R _____ L _____   R ( )   ( )   ( )
                                                          L ( )   ( )   ( )

14. Edema
    O = absent; +1 = slight indentation; +2 = indentation readily noticeable, disappears 10-15 seconds; +3 = deep indentation,
    disappears 1-2 minutes; +4 = deep indentation present at 5 minutes. (Grade by pressure for 5 seconds.)

                                                                          N   A   N/A
    Facial _____ N = O   ( )   ( )   ( )
    Hand _____   ( )   ( )   ( )
    Sacral _____   ( )   ( )   ( )
    Ankle _____   ( )   ( )   ( )
    Pretibial _____   ( )   ( )   ( )
15. Urine output _____ ml/hr   N = average 30 ml/hr   ( )   ( )   ( )
16. Emesis _____   N = none   ( )   ( )   ( )
17. Respiratory pattern: N = inspiration = expiration; A = Kussmall (hyperventilation),   ( )   ( )   ( )
    Cheyne-Stokes, Biots (shallow with apnea), labored, shallow, ventilator control.

    Describe _____
18. Accessory muscles to breathe _____ yes _____ no   ( )   ( )   ( )
    N = none; A = abdominal, thoracic, intercostal, neck.
19. Breath sounds: N = clear vesicular anterior & posterior;   R ( )   ( )   ( )
    A = rales, rhonchi, wheezes, rubs.   L ( )   ( )   ( )
    R _____ L _____
20. Sputum _____ yes _____ no   Color _____ N = none   ( )   ( )   ( )
21. Ascites _____ yes _____ no   Abdominal girth _____ N = none   ( )   ( )   ( )
                                                                          ( )   ( )   ( )

Continued

Assessment Guide 24-1—cont'd

CARDIAC OUTPUT ASSESSMENT TOOL—CONT'D

22. Neurologic: N = oriented to time, place, and person;
    A = anxious, restless, confused, slurred speech.
    If abnormal, see Glasgow Coma Scale below.
    Total Glasgow score (3-15) _____ N = 15   (   )   (   )   (   )
    Pupils: R size _____ reaction _____   R (   )   (   )   (   )
                                                                           (   )   (   )   (   )
             L size _____ reaction _____   L (   )   (   )   (   )
                                                                           (   )   (   )   (   )

Best Verbal Response		To Verbal Command Obeys	6	Open Eyes		Pupils	Reactive + Nonreactive − Closed C
Oriented and converses	5	**To Painful Stimulus Best Motor Response**		Spontaneously	4		
Disoriented and converses	4			To verbal command	3		
Inappropriate words	3	Localizes pain	5	To pain	2		
Incomprehensible sounds	2	Flexion-withdrawal	4	No response	1		
No response	1	Flexion-abnormal (decorticate rigidity)	3				
		Extension (decerebrate rigidity)	2				
		No response	1				

23. Significant Lab Data   N   A   N/A
    ECG: N = sinus rhythm, PR 0.12-0.20 QRS 0.06-0.10 QT 0.36-0.44, no ectopic beats, ST or T wave   (   )   (   )   (   )
    changes, no Q waves, rate 60-80/minute, with + P & T waves.
    Describe:

		N	A	N/A
Enzymes CPK _____	N = 40-200 IU/L	( )	( )	( )
LDH _____	N = 100-225 IU/L	( )	( )	( )
AST _____	N = 7.5-40 IU/L ·	( )	( )	( )
CPK-MB _____	N = <2%	( )	( )	( )
LDH Isos 1 _____ 2 _____ 3 _____ 4 _____ 5 _____	N = 1<2	( )	( )	( )

ABG N = pH 7.35-7.45, P_{CO_2} 35-45 mm, P_{O_2} 70-100 mm   (   )   (   )   (   )
HCO_3 22-26 mm.
pH _____ P_{CO_2} _____ P_{O_2} _____ HCO_3 _____

		N	A	N/A
Ejection Fraction _____ N = 60%		( )	( )	( )
Electrolytes Na _____ mEq/L	N = 136-142 mEq/L	( )	( )	( )
K _____ mEq/L	N = 3.5-5 mEq/L	( )	( )	( )
Cl _____ mEq/L	N = 95-103 mEq/L	( )	( )	( )
BUN _____ mg/dl	N = 8-18 mg/dl	( )	( )	( )
Creatinine _____ mg/dl	N = 0.6-1.2 mg/dl	( )	( )	( )
Hemoglobin _____ Gm/100 ml	N = 13.5-18♂ 12-16♀	( )	( )	( )
Hematocrit _____ %	N = 40-54%♂ 38-47%♀	( )	( )	( )

Chest film: N = normal heart size, clear lung fields, no pleural effusion, congestion, or interstitial edema.   (   )   (   )   (   )
Describe:

Total abnormal signs _____ *Total signs & symptoms* _____

	Suggested Nursing-Sensitive Outcome and Nursing Intervention	
Table 24-1	DECREASED CARDIAC OUTPUT	

Nursing Diagnosis	Nursing-Sensitive Outcome	Nursing Intervention
DECREASED CARDIAC OUTPUT *Defining Characteristics* Variations in blood pressure readings	**CARDIAC PUMP EFFECTIVENESS** *Indicators* Blood pressure IER*	**CARDIAC CARE** *Activities* Monitor vital signs frequently Recognize presence of blood pressure alterations
Elevated pulmonary artery pressures Dysrhythmias ECG changes	Cardiac index IER Dysrhythmias not present Heart rate IER	Document cardiac dysrhythmias Monitor for cardiac dysrhythmias Monitor pacemaker functioning, if appropriate Evaluate the patient's response to ectopy or dysrhythmias Provide antidysrhythmic therapy according to unit policy, as appropriate Monitor patient's response to antidysrhythmic medications
Decreased peripheral pulses	Peripheral pulses strong	Perform a comprehensive appraisal of peripheral circulation
Skin color changes Cold clammy skin Weight gain Edema Oliguria Jugular vein distention (JVD) Dyspnea	Skin color Profuse diaphoresis not present Peripheral edema not present Neck vein distension not present Pulmonary edema not present	Monitor fluid balance Monitor respiratory status for symptoms of heart failure
Orthopnea/paroxysmal nocturnal dyspnea Wheezing Increased respiratory rate Use of accessory muscles Abnormal chest x-ray (pulmonary vascular congestion) Chest pain	Heart size normal Angina not present	Monitor for dyspnea, fatigue, tachypnea, and orthopnea Evaluate chest pain Instruct the patient on the importance of immediately reporting any chest discomfort
Ejection fraction <40% Abnormal cardiac enzymes Increased heart rate Restlessness	Ejection fraction IER Abnormal heart sounds not present	Recognize psychologic effects of underlying condition Establish supportive relationship with patient and family Offer spiritual support to patient and/or family Promote stress reduction
Altered mental states Fatigue	Activity tolerance IER	Instruct the patient and family on activity restriction and progression Arrange exercise and rest periods to avoid fatigue Monitor the patient's activity tolerance
Other		Note signs and symptoms of decreased cardiac output Monitor cardiovascular status Monitor abdomen for indications of decreased perfusion

*IER, In expected range.

Nursing Outcomes Classification (NOC) 5-point Likert measurement scale: Cardiac Pump Effectiveness: 1 = Extremely compromised; 2 = Substantially compromised; 3 = Moderately compromised; 4 = Mildly compromised; 5 = Not compromised.

NURSING-SENSITIVE OUTCOMES

Outcomes associated with the diagnosis Decreased Cardiac Output will include a return to normal values in the defining characteristics found to be present when the diagnosis was made. Some of these outcomes could be associated with actions taken by the nurse when implementing nursing interventions, but others can be attributed to adaptive mechanisms in the body or medical interventions. As with nursing interventions associated with Decreased Cardiac Output, outcomes have been generally described (AACN, 1990) but not systematically studied in populations with varying cardiovascular conditions.

From the *Nursing Outcomes Classification (NOC)* (Iowa Outcomes Project, 2000), the two categories of outcomes most salient to the diagnosis Decreased Cardiac Output are Cardiac Pump Effectiveness and Circulation Status. Cardiac Pump Effectiveness is defined as "extent to which blood is ejected from the left ventricle per minute to support systemic perfusion pressure" and includes the following indicators: (1) blood pressure (BP), cardiac index, ejection fraction, heart rate, activity tolerance all within expected range; (2) peripheral pulses strong; (3) absence of neck vein distension, dysrhythmias, angina, abnormal heart sounds, peripheral edema, pulmonary edema, and diaphoresis; and (4) normal skin color and heart size (Iowa Outcomes Project, 2000, p. 136). Circulation Status is defined as the "extent to which blood flows unobstructed, unidirectionally, and at an appropriate pressure through large vessels of the systemic and pulmonary circuits" (Iowa Outcomes Project, 2000, p. 167). Indicators for Circulation Status that are in addition to those for cardiac pump effectiveness include a normal pulse pressure, mean BP, CVP, PWP, blood gases, A-V O_2 difference, peripheral tissue perfusion, and cognitive status; being free of orthostatic hypotension, adventitious breath sounds, large vessel bruits, ascites, and fatigue; balanced 24-hour intake and output; and strong and symmetrical peripheral pulses (Bumann & Speltz, 1989; Futrell, 1990; White & Roberts, 1992). Depending on the etiology and severity of the heart condition, any or all of these outcomes could be monitored and recorded.

The NOC (Iowa Outcomes Project, 2000) outcome to be achieved is Cardiac Pump Effectiveness that is adequate to meet the oxygen demands of the patient's body given the amount of functional myocardium that remains. Specific indicators that this goal has been achieved are vital signs within normal limits, absence of ankle edema, clear breath sounds, flat neck veins, absence of chest pain and dyspnea, and performance of activities of daily living (ADL). Corresponding NOC indicators of Cardiac Pump Effectiveness are blood pressure and heart rate in expected range, peripheral edema not present, pulmonary edema not present, neck vein distension not present, and activity tolerance in expected range (see Table 24-1). The NOC outcomes and indicators are measured on a 5-point scale (1 = extremely compromised to 5 = not compromised) (see Table 24-1).

CASE STUDY

R. Deere is an 86-year-old widower who has become a resident of a long-term care facility after a recent hospitalization. His wife died over 10 years ago, and he has had repeated admissions to the hospital for congestive heart failure (CHF) over the past 2 years. At his last hospitalization he was found to have digoxin toxicity, and his serum potassium level was 2.1. It was discovered after talking with Mr. Deere that he was not reliable in taking his medications or managing his finances. He has lost 44 lb since his last medical appointment 1 year ago. Mr. Deere is alert, but he is oriented to place and time only occasionally. His short-term memory is very poor.

Mr. Deere's past medical history is significant for a myocardial infarction 5 years ago, which was complicated by cardiogenic shock. His last ejection fraction was 28%, and his ECGs continue to demonstrate ST and T wave abnormalities with frequent PVCs. His skin is warm and dry. Mr. Deere has smoked three packs of cigarettes per day for 28 years and occasionally drinks alcohol at night to induce sleep. He is able to ambulate 50 feet without dyspnea but cannot climb stairs without chest pain.

Currently Mr. Deere has a productive cough of white sputum in small amounts. His chest has coarse rales bilaterally in the bases. His vital signs are stable. Both ankles are edematous, and his feet turn dark purple when in a dependent position. His heart sounds are normal. He sleeps with three pillows at night and frequently awakens because of coughing. On admission to the nursing home, Mr. Deere's priority nursing diagnosis was Decreased Cardiac Output related to myocardial destruction as evidenced by an ejection fraction less than 60%, cough, chest pain and dyspnea with minimal activity, rales in the chest, ankle edema, and three-pillow orthopnea. The outcome chosen for Mr. Deere was Cardiac Pump Effectiveness.

NURSING INTERVENTIONS

Nursing interventions for the treatment of decreased cardiac output have been described in clinical papers that outline nursing care for patients with coronary artery disease. Two research investigations (Dougherty, 1985; Wessel & Kim, 1984) have identified nursing interventions associated with decreased cardiac output by critical care nurses. These investigations are descriptive in nature. Clinical trials testing nursing interventions related to Decreased Cardiac Output with their associated outcomes have not been conducted.

In congestive heart failure and cardiogenic shock Dougherty (1985) identified both independent and collaborative interventions used by nurses when treating decreased cardiac output. Independent interventions included monitoring activity, responses to oxygen, arterial blood gases, intravenous (IV) fluids and intake, environment and laboratory values, planning frequent rest periods, bathing, feeding, assisting with deep breathing exercises, performing CPR and emergency drug administration, reassuring family members, changing dressings, providing positive support and frequent patient contact, starting IV fluids, encouraging rest, and allowing the patient to participate in care. Collaborative nursing interventions include calculating intake and output, daily weights, monitoring hemodynamic parameters, administering medications and oxygen, treating chest pain, and initiating bed rest.

Wessel and Kim (1984) outlined nursing interventions in a sample of 21 patients with congestive heart failure and decreased cardiac output. Twenty-six nursing interventions were developed from questionnaire data provided by staff nurses caring for this sample. Interventions were then classified as independent, collaborative, or dependent, based on nurses' opinions. Independent interventions included cardiovascular assessment, pulmonary assessment, physical assessment, interpretation of laboratory data, nutrition, ADL, skin care, therapeutic positioning, deep breathing/coughing, aseptic environment, IV therapy, patient teaching, psychologic support, family teaching and psychologic support, therapeutic environment, written communication, and overall evaluation. Collaborative interventions included vital signs, Swan-Ganz readings, ECG monitoring, fluid management, therapeutic activity, oxygen therapy, and collaboration with other health care providers. Dependent interventions included medication administration and regulating medications.

The goals of treatment for a person with decreased cardiac output are to (1) optimize the availability of oxygen and other nutrients to tissues, (2) optimize cardiovascular function, and (3) minimize fear, anxiety, and stress (Bumann & Speltz, 1989). Treatment strategies can be directed at determinants of cardiac output, namely, heart rate and rhythm, preload, afterload, and contractility. Four categories of nursing interventions have been described by Bumann and Speltz (1989): (1) rhythm monitoring and treatment; (2) hemodynamic monitoring and treatment; (3) reducing the workload of the heart; and (4) psychosocial interventions. The goal of rhythm monitoring and treatment is the establishment of an effective heart rate and rhythm to maintain cardiac output. Specific nursing interventions would include ECG monitoring, administration of antidysrhythmic treatments, monitoring activity, treating chest pain, and patient and family education (Bumann & Speltz, 1989; Futrell, 1990; White & Roberts, 1992).

The goal of hemodynamic monitoring and treatment is early detection and treatment of changes in cardiac output and prevention of complications. Astute observations, as well as accurate interpretations and clinical judgments by the nurse, are needed to maintain a stable cardiac output. This includes technical expertise in setup, maintenance, and troubleshooting of hemodynamic monitoring systems. Monitoring blood pressure and pulmonary artery pressure and calculating cardiac output, cardiac index, and other parameters are required. These hemodynamics must be correlated with physical data such as mentation, heart sounds, peripheral pulses, urine output, peripheral capillary refill, breath sounds, skin color and temperature, and fluid volume status to make correct judgments about the state of the heart. When hemodynamic parameters are abnormal, other nursing interventions are instituted, such as titrating medication drips, giving fluids, and monitoring side effects.

Reducing the workload of the heart is achieved by the monitoring of preload, afterload, and contractility. When preload is assessed to be reduced, crystalloids, colloids, and blood products will be used, depending on the needs of the person. Preload is reduced by the use of diuretics and vasodilating agents that the nurse must monitor. When afterload is elevated, the workload of the heart increases. Afterload is reduced by vasodilating agents and intraaortic balloon pumping, both of which require expert monitoring skills. Myocardial contractility must be maintained to improve ventricular emptying. This is achieved with titration of inotropic agents and monitoring clinical indicators of contractility. Reducing the workload of the heart is also achieved by eliminating activity and stressors that increase myocardial oxygen demands. Some of these interventions include planning rest periods, administering oxygen, positioning to optimize ventilation and bowel elimination, and evaluating the impact of activity.

Psychologic interventions will influence all other physiologic parameters of cardiac output. Cardiac-related illness produces cognitive and emotional responses that need to be assessed and monitored as well. Reducing stress associated with the critical care environment, assessing illness perceptions, and recognizing emotional responses will lead the nurse to facilitation of the expression of concerns and anxiety. Crisis management might be necessary for both patients and their family members (Bumann & Speltz, 1989; Futrell, 1990; White & Roberts, 1992).

A number of suggested nursing interventions have been linked to decreased cardiac output in the most recent *Nursing Interventions Classification (NIC)* (Iowa Intervention Project, 2000). The most salient of these intervention categories includes Cardiac Care, Circulatory Care, Hemodynamic Regulation, and Cardiac Shock Management, with many others identified as relevant. Cardiac Care has been defined as a "limitation in complications resulting from an imbalance between myocardial oxygen supply and demand for a patient with symptoms of impaired cardiac function" (Iowa Intervention Project, 2000, p. 195). Nursing activities associated with this intervention are included in Table 24-1. Cardiac Care also includes the activities associated with acute cardiac care and cardiac precautions. Acute cardiac care interventions are implemented to limit complications for a patient experiencing a recent cardiac event, whereas cardiac precautions are used to prevent an acute episode of impaired cardiac function.

Other nursing intervention categories relevant to the nursing diagnosis Decreased Cardiac Output include Hemodynamic Regulation, Fluid Management, Shock Management: Cardiac, Circulatory Care: Mechanical Assist Device, Dysrhythmia Management, and Electrolyte Management. Any or all of these interventions can be applied, depending on the severity of the impairment. The majority of the nursing activities within each intervention category contain monitoring interventions. Monitoring the defining characteristics of decreased cardiac output includes both the collection of data and the judgments made about the data that then lead the nurse to implement other interventions. The anticipation and prevention of complications in patients with acute cardiac disorders can be aided by these interventions.

CASE STUDY

The major nursing intervention put in place for Mr. Deere was Cardiac Care, instituted to prevent further bouts of Decreased Cardiac Output. The Cardiac Care activities that were implemented included monitoring of vital signs, lung and heart sounds, daily weight, cough and sputum production, jugular venous distension, ankle edema, activity tolerance, dyspnea, sleep patterns, number of cigarettes smoked, mental status, and reactions to medications. Serum potassium and digoxin levels were monitored when available.

Mr. Deere's living environment was also monitored and adjusted to reduce excessive activity and stair climbing. Mr. Deere moved from his current room to one that was across the hall from the dining room. He now is given a whirlpool bath instead of his regular shower. During the exercise class, Mr. Deere does mild arm and leg exercises while sitting in a chair. He has been asked to quit smoking. Siderails have been added to the walls of his room near his bed, in the bathroom around the stool and by the tub, and along the halls in the activity room. He is reminded to sit with his legs elevated when possible. During planned exercise periods and walking, Mr. Deere's vital signs and the occurrence of angina and dyspnea are monitored (see Table 24-1).

SUMMARY

Decreased Cardiac Output was first listed in the nursing diagnosis taxonomy in 1975. Since that time, discussions have focused on whether or not this diagnosis should continue to be included in the NANDA taxonomy. Current discussions now demonstrate that Decreased Cardiac Output is a nursing diagnosis frequently encountered by nurses in a variety of patient care settings. Interventions used by nurses to stabilize

and treat Decreased Cardiac Output have been designed through descriptive research methods. Nursing outcomes associated with Decreased Cardiac Output have been described in clinical papers but have not been systematically tested. Clinical trials testing nursing interventions have not been conducted. Future research therefore should be focused on the systematic testing of components of the conceptual model, linking the diagnosis with interventions and outcomes. It will be important to adopt a model in which theoretical concepts are linked with hemodynamic and clinical data. Only by doing so can the complex components of cardiac output be addressed effectively in order to promote an adequate supply of oxygen and nutrients to body tissues.

REFERENCES

Alexander, W. (1998). *Hurst's the heart* (9th ed.). New York: McGraw-Hill.

American Association of Critical Care Nurses. (1990). *Outcome standards for nursing care of the critically ill.* Laguna Niguel, CA: Author.

Braunwald, E. (1997). *Heart disease: A textbook of cardiovascular medicine* (5th ed.). Philadelphia: W. B. Saunders.

Brooks-Brunn, J. A. (1987). Formulating appropriate nursing diagnoses for the patient receiving tissue-type plasminogen activator. *Heart & Lung, 16*(6), 787-791.

Bumann, R., & Speltz, M. (1989). Decreased cardiac output: A nursing diagnosis. *Dimensions of Critical Care Nursing, 8*(1), 6-15.

Burke, I. J., Gabriel, L. M., Fischer, L. E., & Zemke, S. L. (1986). Nursing diagnoses, indicators and interventions in an outpatient cardiac rehabilitation program. *Heart & Lung, 15*(1), 70-76.

Cardin, S. (1985). A nursing diagnosis approach to the patient awaiting cardiac transplantation. *Heart & Lung, 14*(5), 499-504.

Chapman, C. B., & Mitchell, J. H. (1965). *Starling on the heart.* London: Dawsons of Pall Mall.

Contrades, S. (1987). Altered cardiac output: An assessment tool. *Dimensions of Critical Care Nursing, 6*(5), 274-283.

Dahlen, R., & Roberts, S. L. (1996). Acute congestive heart failure: Preventing complications. *Dimensions of Critical Care Nursing, 15*(5), 226-241.

Dalton, J. (1985). A descriptive study: Defining characteristics of the nursing diagnosis cardiac output, alterations in: Decreased. *IMAGE: Journal of Nursing Scholarship, 17*(4), 113-117.

Davies, M. J. (1992). Pathology of the aging heart. In J. C. Brocklehurst, R. C. Tallus, & H. M. Fillit (Eds.), *Textbook of geriatric medicine and gerontology* (4th ed., pp. 181-187). New York: Churchill Livingstone.

Dougherty, C. M. (1985). The nursing diagnosis decreased cardiac output. *Nursing Clinics of North America, 20*(4), 787-799.

Dougherty, C. M. (1986). Decreased cardiac output: Validation of a nursing diagnosis. *Dimensions of Critical Care Nursing, 5*(3), 182-188.

Futrell, A. (1990). Decreased cardiac output: Case for a collaborative diagnosis. *Dimensions of Critical Care Nursing, 9*(4), 202-209.

Guyton, A. C. (1981). The relationship of cardiac output and arterial pressure control. *Circulation, 64*(6), 1079-1088.

Harizi, R. C., Bianco, J. A., & Alpert, J. S. (1988). Diastolic function of the heart in clinical cardiology. *Archives of Internal Medicine, 148,* 99-109.

Hubalik, K., & Kim, M. J. (1984). Nursing diagnoses associated with heart failure in critical care nursing. Classification of nursing diagnoses: Proceedings of the fifth national conference (pp. 139-149). Baltimore: Lippincott Williams & Wilkins.

Iowa Intervention Project. J. C. McCloskey & G. M. Bulechek (Eds.). (2000). *Nursing interventions classification (NIC)* (3rd ed.). St. Louis, MO: Mosby.

Iowa Outcomes Project. M. Johnson, M. Maas, & S. Moorhead (Eds.). (2000). *Nursing outcomes classification (NOC)* (2nd ed.). St. Louis, MO: Mosby.

Kelly, D. J. (1991). The identification and clinical validation of the defining characteristics of alteration in cardiac tissue perfusion. In R. M. Carroll-Johnson (Ed.), *Classification of nursing diagnoses: Proceedings of the ninth national conference* (pp. 105-111). Baltimore: Lippincott Williams & Wilkins.

Kern, L., & Omery, A. (1992). Decreased cardiac output in the critical care setting. *Nursing Diagnosis, 3,* 94-106.

Kim, M. J., Seritella, R. A., Gulanick, M., Moyer, K., Parsons, E., Scheberel, J., Stafford, M. A., Suhayada, R. M., & Yocum, C. (1984). Clinical validation of cardiovascular nursing diagnoses. *Classification of nursing diagnoses: Proceedings of the fifth national conference* (pp. 128-138). St. Louis, MO: Mosby.

Lakatta, E. G. (1990). Cardiovascular disorders: Normal changes with aging. In W. B. Abrams & R. Berkow (Eds.), *Merck manual of geriatrics* (pp. 309-325). Rahway, NJ: Merck, Sharp, & Dohme Research Laboratories.

Lazure, L. L., & Cuddigan, J. (1987). (Abstract). Clinical validations of decreased cardiac output: Differentiation of defining characteristics according to etiology. In A. McLane (Ed.), *Classification of nursing diagnoses: Proceedings from the seventh national conference* (p. 275). St. Louis, MO: Mosby.

Loeb, H., & Gunnar, R. M. (1981). Treatment of pump failure in acute myocardial infarction. *Journal of the American Medical Association, 245,* 2093-2096.

Miller, J. C., & Helander, M. (1979). The 24-hour cycle and nocturnal depression of human cardiac output. *Aviation Space Environmental Medicine, 50,* 1139-1144.

North American Nursing Diagnosis Association. (1999). *Nursing diagnoses: Definitions and classification 1999-2000.* Philadelphia: Author.

Parmley, W. W. (1989). Pathophysiology and current therapy of congestive heart failure. *American College of Cardiology, 13*(4), 771-785.

Poole-Wilson, P. (1988). Current therapeutic principles in the acute management of severe congestive heart failure. *American Journal of Cardiology, 62,* 4C.

Roberts, S. (1992). Common nursing diagnoses for pulmonary alveolar edema patients. *Dimensions of Critical Care Nursing, 11*(1), 13-26.

Roffe, C. (1998). Aging of the heart. *British Journal of Biological Sciences, 55*(2), 136-148.

Rossi, L. P. (1979). Nursing diagnoses related to acute myocardial infarction. *Cardiovascular Nursing, 15*(3), 11-15.

Russell, A. C., & Blake, S. M. (1989). Aortic valvuloplasty: Potential nursing diagnoses. *Dimensions of Critical Care Nursing, 8*(2), 72-82.

Scanlon, L. M. (1992). The nursing diagnosis: Decreased cardiac output—a clinical diagnosis validation study. *Military Medicine, 157*(4), 166-168.

Starling, E. H. (1926). Regulation of the energy output of the heart. *Journal of Physiology, 62,* 243-261.

Swan, H. J. C., Ganz, W., Forrester, J., Marcus, H., Dimond, G., & Chonette, D. (1970). Catheterization of the heart in man with use of a flow-directed balloon-tipped catheter. *New England Journal of Medicine, 283,* 451-477.

Teplitz, L. (1990). Patients with ventricular assist devices: Nursing diagnoses. *Dimensions of Critical Care Nursing, 9*(2), 82-87.

Teplitz, L. (1991). Nursing diagnoses for automatic implantable cardioverter defibrillator patients. *Dimensions of Critical Care Nursing, 10*(4), 188-201.

Wessel, S., & Kim, M. J. (1984). Nursing functions related to the nursing diagnosis decreased cardiac output. In M. J. Kim, G. McFarland, & A. McLane (Eds.), *Classification of nursing diagnoses: Proceedings of the fifth national conference* (pp. 192-198). St. Louis, MO: Mosby.

White, B. S., & Roberts, S. L. (1992). Pulmonary alveolar edema: Preventing complications. *Dimensions of Critical Care Nursing, 11*(2), 90-103.

Whitman, G. R., & Hicks, L. E. (1988). Major nursing diagnoses following cardiac transplantation. *Journal of Cardiovascular Nursing, 2*(2), 1-10.

Wong, W. F., Gold, S., Fukuyama, O., & Blanchette, F. L. (1989). Diastolic dysfunction in elderly patients with congestive heart failure. *American Journal of Cardiology, 63,* 1526-1528.

CHAPTER 25

ALTERED TISSUE PERFUSION

Margo Halm

The circulation of blood is vital for the delivery of oxygen and nutrients to tissues and for the removal of metabolic waste products. Elders are especially prone to Altered Tissue Perfusion resulting from changes that occur in the cardiovascular system during aging. Nurses in both acute and long-term care settings must assess elderly clients for the defining characteristics of Altered Tissue Perfusion and institute a plan of care to modify the etiology. Health promotion interventions can help prevent Altered Tissue Perfusion, or, when alterations are already present, can help to maintain self-care abilities and functional health status among elders.

Altered Tissue Perfusion can involve local, regional, or compartmental disruptions in circulation (Hart, 1981). This chapter discusses only local reductions of blood.

RELATED FACTORS/ETIOLOGIES

Accurate diagnosis and management of Altered Tissue Perfusion in the elder must be based on both physiologic and psychosocial factors. A complete database is essential because age-related changes in the body's response to disease make diagnosis more difficult. Symptoms of illness vary in both quantity and quality and can include only a few or several of the following: fatigue, anorexia, confusion, incontinence, changes in ambulation, weight loss, or failure to thrive (Blake, 1976, p. 410).

Specification of etiologies and defining characteristics for the renal, cerebral, gastrointestinal, cardiopulmonary, and peripheral categories of Altered Tissue Perfusion aids differential diagnosis and helps nurses determine whether independent nursing interventions or referral for medical treatment is appropriate. Each general etiology and the associated defining characteristics for Altered Tissue Perfusion are listed in detail in Tables 25-1 through 25-3. The present discussion of etiologic factors is limited to those conditions that most commonly affect tissue perfusion in elders.

Interruption of Arterial Flow

An interruption of arterial blood flow decreases the oxygenated blood supply to body tissues. The two major factors that influence the adequacy of circulation are the amount of blood delivered to a tissue and its metabolic demands. Cerebral and coronary vessels are particularly sensitive to hypoxemia and dilate to restore tissue perfusion. Hypermetabolic states can precipitate ischemia when blood vessels cannot dilate or the cardiac pump cannot increase cardiac output to meet tissue needs. Redistribution of blood flow to meet tissue demands also can cause ischemia in regions where shunting occurs (Hart, 1981).

The patency of blood vessels can be compromised by conditions that obstruct vessel lumens, induce reflexive vasoconstriction, or produce mechanical pressure. Arterial blood flow in the elder is most often obstructed by arteriosclerosis, a group of diseases characterized by thickening and loss of elasticity of the arterial wall (Fagin-Dubin, 1977). Atherosclerosis is a major type of arteriosclerosis, which can affect any artery. Larger arteries like the abdominal aorta and renal artery and vessels in the lower extremities are more commonly involved (Fagin-Dubin, 1977; Sexton, 1977; Wagner, 1986). However, Sexton (1977) noted that peripheral involvement is only one facet of the atherosclerotic process. Often the heart, kidney, and brain are also affected to some degree.

The highest incidence of atherosclerosis occurs in postmenopausal women and males 50 to 70 years old (Jones, Dunbar, & Jirovec, 1982; Wagner, 1986). Precursor lesions in the intimal layer appear in the first decade of life as reversible, fatty streaks in the aorta and coronary arteries. Plaques composed of fibrous scar tissue and lipid cores form in early adulthood. Accumulated lipids, cell debris, complex carbohydrates, blood, calcium deposits, and fibrous tissue characterize the complex lesion by middle age (Fagin-Dubin, 1977; Wagner, 1986). Severity of symptoms depends on the extent of the lesion, the degree of obstruction, and the presence of collateral circulation. Thinning of the medial layer can lead to aneurysm formation in the aorta and in the iliac and femoral arteries (Wagner, 1986).

Intimal degeneration also can precipitate ulceration and thrombosis of the plaque and cause partial or complete arterial occlusion. This obstruction increases vascular resistance and turbulent blood flow, further damaging vessel walls and triggering thromboembolism (Hart, 1981; Jones et al., 1982). Stenosis commonly occurs at the carotid bifurcation and origin of the internal carotid artery, providing a source of emboli and/or compromised flow to the cerebral arteries (Gorelick, 1986).

Table 25-1　Suggested Nursing-Sensitive Outcomes and Nursing Interventions
ALTERED TISSUE PERFUSION RELATED TO INTERRUPTION OF ARTERIAL AND VENOUS FLOW

Nursing Diagnosis	Nursing-Sensitive Outcomes	Nursing Interventions
ALTERED TISSUE PERFUSION RELATED TO INTERRUPTION OF ARTERIAL AND VENOUS FLOW *Defining Characteristics* Renal • Decreased urine output • Hypertension • Edema	**TISSUE PERFUSION: CENTRAL** *Indicators* 24-hour intake and output balanced Systolic, diastolic and mean BP in expected range Free of peripheral edema	*Labels** VITAL SIGNS MONITORING FLUID MONITORING FLUID MANAGEMENT ELECTROLYTE MONITORING ELECTROLYTE MANAGEMENT FLUID/ELECTROLYTE MANAGEMENT URINARY CATHETERIZATION TUBE CARE: URINARY
Cerebral • Altered level of consciousness • Altered thought processes • Memory losses • Confusion/restlessness • Dizziness or faintness • ICP > 15 mm Hg • CPP < 50 mm Hg • Neurologic deficits • Papilledema/vomiting • Pupillary changes • Seizures/positive Babinski	**TISSUE PERFUSION: CENTRAL** *Indicators* Cognitive status in expected range Cerebral perfusion pressure > 50 mm Hg Neurologic findings in expected range	VITAL SIGNS MONITORING EMBOLUS PRECAUTIONS NEUROLOGIC MONITORING INTRACRANIAL PRESSURE (ICP) MONITORING CEREBRAL EDEMA MANAGEMENT
Cardiopulmonary • Hypotension • Cold, clammy skin • Slow capillary refill • Tachycardia • Angina (at rest or during activity) • Diaphoresis • Elevated or depressed ST segments, inverted T waves, Q waves of significant depth and range, R waves in precordial leads • Elevated CPK and LDH • Tachypnea • Dyspnea/orthopnea	**TISSUE PERFUSION: CENTRAL** *Indicators* Systolic, diastolic, and mean BP in expected range Skin color intact; brisk capillary refill Heart rate and rhythm in expected range Free of angina ECG manifestations of myocardial ischemia absent or reduced Cardiac enzymes in expected range Respiratory rate and rhythm in width diminished/absent	VITAL SIGNS MONITORING EMBOLUS PRECAUTIONS EMBOLUS CARE: PULMONARY PAIN MANAGEMENT CARDIAC PRECAUTIONS CARDIAC CARE CARDIAC CARE: ACUTE INVASIVE HEMODYNAMIC MONITORING HEMODYNAMIC REGULATION ACID-BASE MONITORING ACID-BASE MANAGEMENT DYSRHYTHMIA MANAGEMENT TUBE CARE: CHEST CARDIAC CARE: REHABILITATIVE SHOCK MANAGEMENT: CARDIAC RESUSCITATION CODE MANAGEMENT
Gastrointestinal • Abdominal distension • Positive guaiac findings of stool • Nausea • Thirst • Elevated serum enzymes (AST, LDH, CPK) • Constipation	**TISSUE PERFUSION: CENTRAL** *Indicators* Abdominal girth in expected range Guaiac findings of stool/nasogastric drainage negative Gastrointestinal symptomatology (nausea, vomiting, and constipation) absent Liver enzymes in expected range	VITAL SIGNS MONITORING EMBOLUS PRECAUTIONS GASTROINTESTINAL INTUBATION TUBE CARE: GASTROINTESTINAL SHOCK MANAGEMENT

Table 25-1	Suggested Nursing-Sensitive Outcomes and Nursing Interventions—cont'd ALTERED TISSUE PERFUSION RELATED TO INTERRUPTION OF ARTERIAL AND VENOUS FLOW—cont'd		
Nursing Diagnosis	**Nursing-Sensitive Outcomes**		**Nursing Interventions**
Peripheral • Diminished or absent peripheral pulses • Temperature of extremity cool (unilateral) • Pallor on elevation; dusky rubor and cyanosis on dependency (normal color does not return within 20 seconds) • Thin, shiny atrophic skin • Loss of hair on ankle, dorsum of feet, and toes • Slow-growing dry, thick, brittle nails • Slow healing of lesions • Intermittent claudication (specify) (at location of occlusion) or pain at rest (burning, throbbing, cramping, prickling feeling) • Loss of motor and sensory function (pressure, temperature, trauma) • Blood pressure changes in extremities • Bruits • Palpable pulsations • Muscle weakness • Paresthesias in affected part (numbness/tingling) • Edema • Decreased capillary refill • Poor resistance to infection • *Nonhealing painful ulcers:* Between or tips of toes, heels, and above lateral malleolus; deep cavernous and pale with even margins; necrotic or gangrenous tissue may be present with minimal granulation • Ankle edema; limb circumference asymmetric • Calf pain on dorsiflexion (positive Homan's sign) • Peripheral cyanosis with dependency • Brown pigmentation of skin around ankles and lower extremities • Skin temperature uniform (coolness or warmth) • Numbness and tingling • Leg heaviness and aching • Superficial veins enlarged and tortuous • *Venous stasis ulcers:* Ankle and pretibial regions; moderately painful; superficial with uneven edges, ruddy red granulated base; no gangrene	**TISSUE PERFUSION: PERIPHERAL** ***Indicators*** Capillary refill brisk Extremity bruits not present Peripheral edema not present Distal peripheral pulses strong Proximal peripheral pulses strong Distal peripheral pulses symmetric Proximal peripheral pulses symmetric Localized extremity pain not present Sensation level normal Skin color normal Muscle function intact Skin intact Extremity temperature warm Other _____		**SHOCK MANAGEMENT** **VITAL SIGNS MONITORING** **EMBOLUS PRECAUTIONS** **EMBOLUS CARE: PERIPHERAL** **FOOT CARE** **WOUND CARE** **CIRCULATORY PRECAUTIONS** **CIRCULATORY CARE: ARTERIAL INSUFFICIENCY**

*Refer to Iowa Intervention Project (2000) for list of specific nursing activities associated with each intervention label.

Data from Halm, M. (1991). Altered tissue perfusion. In M. Maas, K. Buckwalter, & M. Hardy (Eds.), *Nursing diagnosis and interventions for the elderly* (223-242). Reading, MA: Addison-Wesley Longman; American Association of Critical-Care Nurses. (1990). *Outcome standards for nursing care of the critically ill.* Laguna Niguel, CA: Author; Iowa Intervention Project. J. C. McCloskey & G. M. Bulechek (Eds.). (2000). *Nursing interventions classification (NIC)* (3rd ed.). St. Louis, MO: Mosby.

Table 25-2   Suggested Nursing-Sensitive Outcome and Nursing Interventions
ALTERED TISSUE PERFUSION RELATED TO EXCHANGE PROBLEMS

Nursing Diagnosis	Nursing-Sensitive Outcome	Nursing Interventions
ALTERED TISSUE PERFUSION RELATED TO EXCHANGE PROBLEMS *Defining Characteristics* Tachypnea Dyspnea Hypoxia Hypercapnia Pulmonary artery hypertension Cyanosis Apprehension Tachycardia Exertional angina	TISSUE PERFUSION: CENTRAL *Indicators* Respiratory rate and rhythm in expected range Blood gases in expected range Pulmonary artery pressures in expected range Skin color intact Anxiety absent or level reduced Heart rate in expected range Angina not present	*Labels** VITAL SIGNS MONITORING RESPIRATORY MONITORING EMBOLUS CARE: PULMONARY OXYGEN THERAPY AIRWAY SUCTIONING AIRWAY INSERTION AND STABILIZATION AIRWAY MANAGEMENT MECHANICAL VENTILATION MECHANICAL VENTILATORY WEANING PAIN MANAGEMENT

*Refer to Iowa Intervention Project (2000) for list of specific nursing activities associated with each intervention label.

Data from Halm, M. (1991). Altered tissue perfusion. In M. Maas, K. Buckwalter, & M. Hardy (Eds.), *Nursing diagnosis and interventions for the elderly*. Reading, MA: Addison-Wesley Longman; Iowa Intervention Project. J. C. McCloskey & G. M. Bulechek (Eds.). (2000). *Nursing interventions classification (NIC)* (3rd ed.). St. Louis, MO: Mosby.

Vasospastic conditions that reduce patency usually affect vessels that are regulated by the sympathetic nervous system and by local substances such as histamine, prostaglandins, and catecholamines. Raynaud's disease, for example, is manifested by episodic and symmetrical vasoconstriction of small peripheral arteries and arterioles, particularly in the hands. The vasospasms, often precipitated by cold or emotional stress, produce blanching, cyanosis, reactive hyperemia, and, if severe, may lead to ulceration and gangrene of the affected parts (Hart, 1981; Jones et al., 1982; Wagner, 1986).

Internal obstructive pressure can be exerted by exudate and collagen formation of the inflammatory process, extracellular fluid accumulation (ascites or edema), and rapid cell proliferation (tumor growth). However, the degree of ischemia is related to the involved vessels and site. In chronic inflammation, blood vessels are compressed by fibroblastic proliferation and extensive scarring (Hart, 1981).

Renal. Altered renal perfusion can result from any systemic condition that produces ischemia to the kidney: hypovolemia, sepsis, congestive heart failure, cardiac dysrhythmias, and myocardial infarction (Thompson, McFarland, Hirsch, & Tucker, 1998). Vasoconstriction, the normal response of the kidney to decreased tissue perfusion, produces further ischemia and, if prolonged, can lead to tissue death and renal failure.

Cerebral. Altered cerebral perfusion can result from reduced patency of the cerebral vessels and from internal mechanical pressure. Orthostatic hypotension can be related to sudden position changes (especially from lying or sitting to standing), prolonged bed rest, impaired skele-

tal muscle function, aging, severe varicose veins, decreased blood volume or dehydration, and medications such as antihypertensives, diuretics, vasodilators, and neuroleptics, especially tricyclic antidepressants (Carpenito, 1995).

Atherosclerosis is primarily responsible for progressive compromise of the cerebral circulation. Plaques form cerebral thromboses and embolic debris, reducing blood flow to the areas of the brain supplied by the compromised artery. Signs and symptoms depend on the location and extent of the ischemic area. Neurologic impairment can be minimized if collateral circulation is adequate to reestablish blood flow quickly after symptom onset (Gorelick, 1986). The risk of ischemic stroke is also increased post–myocardial infarction. The risk of a first-ever ischemic stroke is highest during the first few days after a myocardial infarction; however, the absolute number of stroke events is low (Mooe, Olofsson, Stegmayr, & Eriksson, 1999).

Saccular and congenital aneurysms can rupture spontaneously into the subarachnoid space or brain parenchyma, trigger cerebral infarction due to underlying vasospasm or emboli, or exert internal pressure. Accumulated subarachnoid blood obstructs cerebrospinal fluid absorption pathways and causes hydrocephalus, which further compresses arteries, veins, and brain tissue (Gorelick, 1986).

Cardiopulmonary. Atherosclerotic coronary artery lesions restrict the blood supply to the myocardium, producing angina and tachycardia or myocardial infarction with reduced cardiac output. Pulmonary emboli or infarction can interrupt blood flow to the pulmonary capillary bed, impeding alveolar gas exchange. Tissue necrosis and hemorrhage occur at the site of infarction (Thompson et al., 1998).

Suggested Nursing-Sensitive Outcomes and Nursing Interventions		
Table 25-3 ALTERED TISSUE PERFUSION RELATED TO HYPOVOLEMIA AND HYPERVOLEMIA		
Nursing Diagnosis	**Nursing-Sensitive Outcomes**	**Nursing Interventions**
ALTERED TISSUE PERFUSION RELATED TO HYPOVOLEMIA AND HYPERVOLEMIA *Defining Characteristics* Related to hypovolemia: • Cold, clammy skin • Ashen pallor to cyanosis • Decreased skin turgor • Normal serum sodium • Hypothermia • Weak, rapid pulse • Hypotension • Dysrhythmias • Tachypnea or air hunger • Decreased urine output • Intense thirst • Nausea/vomiting • Weight loss • Muscular weakness • Restlessness • Confusion • Memory losses • Altered levels of consciousness	TISSUE PERFUSION: CENTRAL *Indicators* Skin color intact Skin temperature and turgor in expected range Heart rate and rhythm in expected range Systolic, diastolic, and mean BP in expected range Body temperature in expected range Respiratory rate and rhythm in expected range 24-hour intake and output balanced Symptoms of dehydration (nausea/ vomiting, thirst, weight loss, muscle weakness) absent or reduced Cognitive status in expected range Serum electrolytes in expected range	*Labels** VITAL SIGNS MONITORING BLEEDING PRECAUTIONS BLEEDING REDUCTION BLEEDING REDUCTION: GASTROINTESTINAL BLEEDING REDUCTION: WOUND FLUID MANAGEMENT FLUID RESUSCITATION BLOOD PRODUCTS ADMINISTRATION HYPOVOLEMIA MANAGEMENT SHOCK MANAGEMENT SHOCK PREVENTION SHOCK MANAGEMENT: VOLUME
Related to hypervolemia: • Shortness of breath • Dyspnea • Moist crackles and rhonchi • Productive cough—pink frothy sputum • Puffy eyelids • Acute weight gain • Dependent pitting edema • Ascites—abdomen dull to percussion • Full bounding pulse • Increased central venous pressure • Reduced red blood cell count • Reduced hemoglobin and hematocrit	TISSUE PERFUSION: CENTRAL *Indicators* Respiratory rate and rhythm in expected range Free of adventitious breath sounds and productive cough Weight in expected range Peripheral edema not present Free of ascites Quality of peripheral pulses in expected range Central venous pressure in expected range Hemoglobin/hematocrit in expected range	VITAL SIGNS MONITORING FLUID MONITORING INVASIVE HEMODYNAMIC MONITORING FLUID MANAGEMENT

*Refer to Iowa Intervention Project (2000) for list of specific nursing activities associated with each intervention label.

Data from Halm, M. (1991). Altered tissue perfusion. In M. Maas, K. Buckwalter, & M. Hardy (Eds.), *Nursing diagnosis and interventions for the elderly.* Reading, MA: Addison-Wesley Longman; Iowa Intervention Project. J. C. McCloskey & G. M. Bulechek (Eds.). (2000). *Nursing interventions classification (NIC)* (3rd ed.). St. Louis, MO: Mosby.

Gastrointestinal. Atherosclerosis or postoperative complications can occlude the superior mesenteric vessels to reduce intestinal blood flow. As peristalsis decreases in the distal segments of the bowel, the gastrointestinal tract rids its contents through vomiting (Thompson et al., 1998).

Due to its high rate of metabolism and exposure to concentrated toxins, the liver is one of the first organs to

deteriorate with profoundly altered systemic perfusion. The pancreas responds by activating pancreatic enzymes and releasing toxins such as myocardial toxic factor, which reduces myocardial contractility. Ischemia of the liver also elevates the serum enzymes of serum glutamic-oxaloacetic transaminase (SGOT), serum glutamic-pyruvic transaminase (SGPT), and lactate dehydrogenase

(LDH) (Thompson et al., 1998). Yet Jeppesen (1986) noted that these enzymes are normally higher in elders. Further tissue damage eventually decreases the liver's ability to detoxify materials (Thompson et al., 1998).

Peripheral. Emboli can occlude peripheral arteries, particularly vessels in the brain, kidneys, spleen, and lower extremities. Emboli commonly originate from the mitral and aortic valves or from mural thrombi associated with atrial fibrillation and myocardial infarction (Hart, 1981; Jones et al., 1982; Sexton, 1977).

Buerger's disease (thromboangitis obliterans) is characterized by fibrotic thickening, segmental thrombi, and acute and chronic inflammatory responses in vessel walls. Gangrene can occur with significant occlusions (Hart, 1981; Jones et al., 1982; Thompson et al., 1998). Atherosclerosis remains an important etiology of altered peripheral tissue perfusion. Risk factors include hypertension, smoking, hyperlipidemia, and diabetes (McGee & Boyko, 1998; Santilli & Santilli, 1999).

Interruption of Venous Flow

The interruption of venous blood flow reduces blood returned to the heart. Reduced vessel patency and changes in blood composition are the two primary factors that impair venous circulation. Valve leaflets that are overstretched from prolonged or excessive pressure cannot close properly and promote reverse flow, a condition known as venous insufficiency or stasis (Wagner, 1986). Venous stasis also can be precipitated by decreased skeletal muscle activity (Hart, 1981).

Venous stasis is a major factor affecting thrombus formation but cannot individually precipitate thrombosis. Other predisposing factors, such as vessel wall damage, venous inflammation, hypercoagulability, and immobility, must be present for clot development (Carpenito, 1995; Doyle, 1986; Hart, 1981; Jones et al., 1982; Wagner, 1986). Thrombosis can occur in either superficial or deep veins and predominantly affects the lower extremities. The pulmonary arteries are common sites of emboli from venous origin (Doyle, 1986; Hart, 1981).

Conditions that increase the risk of thrombophlebitis in the aged client include major trauma, fractures of the long bones, severe burns, upper abdominal or pelvic surgery, congestive heart failure, varicose veins, cancer, prolonged bed rest, or immobilization of an affected part. Hypercoagulability and flow stasis are the major variables responsible for thrombosis in client populations with these conditions (Hart, 1981).

Exchange Problems

Exchange problems occur when oxygen diffusion across the alveolar capillary membrane is impaired. Alterations in diffusion develop when either the distribution of air (ventilation) or the flow of pulmonary capillary blood (perfu-

sion) to the alveolus is not adequate. The ventilation-perfusion (V/Q) ratio, normally 0.8, determines the alveolar gas composition (Thompson et al., 1998).

A low V/Q ratio (< 0.8) exists when there is less alveolar ventilation than perfusion. In contrast, high V/Q ratios (> 0.8) are directly related to shunting of blood from the pulmonary capillary bed (Thompson et al., 1998). This condition, known as wasted ventilation, causes hypoxia and hypercapnia (Roberts, 1987; Thompson et al., 1998).

A high V/Q ratio may be caused by blockage or infarction of the pulmonary vasculature, compression or destruction of the pulmonary capillary bed, decreased blood pH, shock, and decreased cardiac output resulting from cardiac dysrhythmias or a myocardial infarction (Thompson et al., 1998).

Hypovolemia

Hypovolemia, a decrease in the intravascular blood volume in relation to the size of the intravascular compartment, is associated with a blood volume deficit of at least 15% to 25% (Rice, 1981a). Internal losses can result from the sequestration of fluid into third spaces, leakage of fluid from capillaries into the intestinal lumen, long bone fractures, extravascular pooling of blood, and impaired venous return. Fluids lost externally may include (1) whole blood from trauma, bleeding disorders, and surgery; (2) plasma from burn injuries; and (3) body fluid from the gastrointestinal or genitourinary tract or diuresis (Frantz, 1981; Kelly, 1985; Rice, 1981a).

Reduction in intravascular volume produces a decrease in venous return, ventricular filling pressures, stroke volume, cardiac output, and blood pressure. Ultimately, hypovolemic shock results in decreased perfusion to body tissues and organs (Rice, 1981b). The tissue type and metabolic needs determine the length of time tissues can survive with inadequate perfusion (Carpenito, 1995; Jones et al., 1982).

Hypervolemia

Hypervolemia (circulatory overload) is an excessive increase in the intravascular blood volume that produces overload of all fluid compartments, including the intracellular space. Volume overload can occur when isotonic solutions are administered too rapidly, especially in the very young or old. Patients with renal, cardiac, or hepatic disease can retain body fluid with normal or reduced intake. Long-term use of corticosteroids also can result in the retention of water and sodium (Bruner & Suddarth, 1980; Kelly, 1985).

ASSESSMENT

Kane and Kane (1981) stated that measures of physical functioning were most important in long-term care. Measures of functional health status for the elder were categorized as general physical health and ability to perform ADL and IADL. Assessment of physical health includes items such as hospitalizations, pain, physiologic signs and symptoms, or self-ratings of health, whereas ability to perform ADL focuses on self-care and independent living activities. All three measures are essential for holistic assessment and management of Altered Tissue Perfusion in elders.

A few assessment tools are available to guide the diagnosis of Altered Tissue Perfusion in the elder. Most of these tools are broad in scope and focus primarily on general physiologic indicators of tissue perfusion. For instance, the topical outline frequently includes subjective assessment data related to past health history, risk factors, and pertinent symptoms, and objective data focuses on the review of biologic systems (Carnevali & Enloe, 1986; Carpenito, 1995). Therefore a major limitation of these assessment tools is their tendency to focus on the disease model rather than the whole person. Second, the tools often rely on the clinician's subjective interpretation of physiologic data collected by inspection, auscultation, palpation, and percussion.

Other assessment guides are directed at various alterations in tissue perfusion (Carpenito, 1995; Goetter, 1986; Herman, 1986; Quinless, 1986). Some of these tools are specific to a certain patient population or disease process, and others have a conceptual focus. Goetter (1986) used a review of systems to identify assessment cues for altered cerebral blood flow in the acute stroke patient population. A tool for orthostatic hypotension (cerebral) provided only a few subjective and objective cues for nursing assessment (Carpenito, 1995). In contrast, a guide for altered cardiopulmonary tissue perfusion focused only on assessing the symptom of angina (Quinless, 1986).

The assessment and diagnosis of Altered Tissue Perfusion also can be based on the typology of 11 functional health patterns. Gordon's health assessment guide (1994) provides a holistic approach for the collection of basic patient data that is appropriate for individuals, families, and communities across age-groups and nursing specialties. Gordon pointed out that nurses must assess each health pattern before they can understand how changes in one pattern are reflected in other areas. Herman (1986) identified that activity-exercise was the primary functional health pattern affected by altered peripheral tissue perfusion. Yet this assessment tool identified specific cues to assess the impact of altered peripheral blood flow on other patterns such as health perception–health management, nutritional-metabolic, and self perception–self concept. Focused cue searches were also provided to assess client problems related to social isolation, pain self-management, and ineffective individual coping.

Another tool incorporates critical assessment cues for each of the five categories of Altered Tissue Perfusion (Halm, 1991). These assessment cues could be further classified according to Gordon's functional health patterns to assist nurses to investigate the impact of Altered Tissue Perfusion on functional health status among elders. Other assessment tools provided by Guzetta, Bunton, Prinkey, Sherer, and Seifert (1989) are based on functional health patterns. Separate tools are available for assessing alterations in renal, cardiovascular, pulmonary, and cerebral tissue perfusion. In addition, a comprehensive critical care assessment tool incorporates assessment cues for all major body systems.

CASE STUDY 1

J. Meyer is a 70-year-old farmer with a past medical history of a myocardial infarction that was diagnosed at age 52, 3 days after a farm machinery accident with injury to his lower extremities. His cardiac condition was medically managed, and left ventricular function was preserved with an ejection fraction of 55%. In addition, Mr. Meyer also has a history of occupation-related restrictive lung disease. He denies ever having a smoking history.

In late January Mr. Meyer presented to the emergency room with complaints of increasing angina unrelieved by sublingual nitroglycerin. Cardiac catheterization revealed significant blockages in his left anterior descending and left circumflex arteries. As a result of these findings, he was scheduled for elective coronary artery bypass surgery. After surgery, Mr. Meyer was admitted to the intensive care unit (ICU) in stable condition. The electrocardiogram (ECG) revealed sinus bradycardia (rate 56 beats/min) without ectopy. Hemodynamic indices were measured by a right radial arterial line and a right internal jugular Swan-Ganz catheter. Blood pressure was stable at 100/58 with small doses of intravenous dopamine (3.5 μg/kg/min). Pulmonary artery pressure monitoring revealed slight pulmonary hypertension (48/30). The patient was mechanically ventilated on SIMV, rate 10, 40% and tidal volume 800. His postoperative course was complicated by the fact that he was unable to be weaned from the ventilator within the expected 12 hours after surgery because of his restrictive lung disease. After remaining on the ventilator for 1 week, his surgeon decided to extubate him one afternoon to see if he would "fly." Mr. Meyer's SaO$_2$ remained over 92%, and his arterial blood gases were within normal range; respiration was unlabored in the lower 20s. After transfer to the step-down unit, he developed atrial fibrillation and was given digitalis. Mr. Meyer was eventually discharged home on day 12.

Three days later Mr. Meyer had been recuperating at home and went upstairs for the night to retire. His daughter, home to help with his recovery, went to his room to check on him before going to bed. She opened the door to find her father gasping for air. She called his surgeon, who instructed her to contact the local emergency services. Within minutes the first responders arrived and placed him on oxygen, started an IV, and assessed his vital signs and overall condition. Mr. Meyer was then transported via AirCare to the university hospital's emergency room. On arrival, Mr. Meyer continued to complain of vague/non-specific signs and symptoms, including dyspnea, tachypnea, palpitations, pleuritic type chest pain, diaphoresis, syncope, and general apprehension (Box 25-1). Pulmonary assessment findings revealed respiratory rate 36/minute, decreased breath sounds, decreased chest wall excursion caused by splinting from pleuritic pain, asymmetric chest expansion, crackles bibasilarly, and a pleural friction rub. The ECG showed sinus tachycardia (rate 125 beats/min) with frequent unifocal PVCs, and his blood pressure was 90/52. His skin was diaphoretic with central cyanosis and jugular vein distention present.

As part of the diagnostic work-up phase, ABGs, chest x-ray, 12-lead ECG, and a V/Q scan were done. ABG results revealed hypoxemia with a PaO_2 of 60 mm Hg, hypocapnia with a $PaCO_2$ of 35 mm Hg, and respiratory alkalosis (pH 7.46). Although the initial chest x-ray examination was normal, the film at 24 hours revealed small bibasilar infiltrates secondary to atelectasis and an elevated hemidiaphragm. Nonspecific ECG changes were found with underlying sinus tachycardia (rate 125 beats/min) and frequent unifocal PVCs. No signs of acute pulmonary hypertension were present, ruling out a massive PE. Although not definitive, the V/Q scan indicated a high probability of pulmonary embolus, which most likely originated from the popliteal or ileofemoral veins. A high V/Q ratio (>0.8) was revealed, indicating normal ventilation with decreased perfusion. The following factors placed Mr. Meyer at increased risk for developing a pulmonary embolus: (1) age; (2) chronic pulmonary disease; (3) surgical procedure; (4) venous stasis caused by his congestive heart failure; (5) hypercoagulability resulting from his history of postoperative atrial fibrillation; and (6) immobility during the postsurgical and convalescent periods.

NURSING DIAGNOSIS

The North American Nursing Diagnosis Association (NANDA, 1999) has defined Altered Tissue Perfusion as "a decrease in oxygen resulting in the failure to nourish the tissues at the capillary level" (p. 25). Altered Tissue Perfusion is categorized according to renal, cerebral, cardiopulmonary, gastrointestinal, or peripheral systems (see Table 25-1) (NANDA, 1999). Similar definitions have been proposed by Carpenito (1995), Gordon (1987), and Rantz and LeMone (1994).

NURSING-SENSITIVE OUTCOMES

An essential task in the planning phase of the nursing process is the identification of desired client outcomes or goals. Desired outcomes are patient actions or behaviors that guide the selection of nursing interventions and also provide evaluation criteria for the effectiveness of treatments in achieving individualized client outcomes. The two fundamental outcomes desired for clients with Altered Tissue Perfusion are to reestablish adequate blood flow to meet metabolic tissue needs and to promote functional health status. First, it is proposed that Tissue Perfusion: Central be added to the Nursing Outcomes Classification (Iowa Outcomes Project, 2000) as a nursing-sensitive outcome for altered renal, cerebral, cardiopulmonary, and gastrointestinal tissue perfusion. This outcome could be defined as the "extent to which blood flows through the large vessels of the systemic and pulmonary circuits to maintain organ and tissue function." The desired indicators that would be used to measure whether this outcome for Altered Tissue Perfusion is met include the following:

- Heart rate and rhythm in expected range
- Respiratory rate and rhythm in expected range
- Body temperature in expected range
- Systolic, diastolic, and mean BP in expected range
- Pulmonary artery pressures in expected range
- Central venous pressure in expected range
- Cerebral perfusion pressure >50 mm Hg
- Skin color intact
- Skin temperature and turgor in expected range
- Capillary refill brisk
- Quality of peripheral pulses in expected range
- Peripheral edema absent
- Adventitious breath sounds and productive cough absent
- Cognitive status in expected range
- Neurologic findings in expected range

Box 25-1 | Case Study | MR. MEYER

Nursing Diagnosis

Altered Tissue Perfusion: Exchange problems related to ventilation-perfusion mismatch secondary to pulmonary emboli as evidenced by dyspnea, tachypnea, hypoxia, cyanosis, tachycardia, pulmonary artery hypertension, and apprehension.

Defining characteristics

Dyspnea and tachypnea
Hypoxia
Cyanosis
Tachycardia
Pulmonary artery hypertension
Apprehension/anxiety

Related factors/etiologies needed

Altered cardiopulmonary chemistries
Tissue perfusion related to exchange problems*

Other data

Blood
Hemodynamic measurements (CVP, PAP, PAW, CO)
Pulmonary angiography

---

*Unable to rule out.

- Anxiety absent or level reduced
- Angina absent
- ECG manifestations of myocardial ischemia absent or reduced
- Abdominal girth in expected range
- Guaiac findings of stool/nasogastric drainage negative
- GI symptomatology (nausea/vomiting and constipation) absent or reduced
- Ascites absent
- 24-hour intake and output balanced
- Symptoms of dehydration (nausea/vomiting, thirst, weight loss, muscle weakness) absent or reduced
- Weight in expected range
- Blood gases in expected range
- Cardiac enzymes in expected range
- Liver enzymes in expected range
- Serum electrolytes in expected range
- Hemoglobin/hematocrit in expected range

The second outcome label, Tissue Perfusion: Peripheral, is appropriate for altered peripheral perfusion. This outcome is defined as the "extent to which blood flows through the small vessels of the extremities and maintains tissue function" (Iowa Outcomes Project, 2000, p. 431). See Table 25-1 for the desired indicators for this outcome also. The desired indicators for both of these outcomes can be measured on a Likert scale from 1 to 5 in terms of clinical occurrence (i.e., 1 = never, 2 = rare, 3 = sometimes, 4 = often, and 5 = consistently). As a result, Tissue Perfusion: Central and Tissue Perfusion: Peripheral are variable states with levels of severity: extremely compromised (level 1), substantially compromised (level 2), moderately compromised (level 3), mildly compromised (level 2), and not compromised (level 1). In other words, the desired indicators for Tissue Perfusion: Central (or Peripheral), such as "mean blood pressure in expected range," will rarely (if ever) be present when tissue perfusion is extremely compromised.

Many methods exist to determine if the desired outcome indicators for Altered Tissue Perfusion have been achieved. The measurements that are available for this evaluation include assessment procedures such as vital sign assessment, blood pressure measurement (systolic, diastolic, orthostatic), hemodynamic monitoring indices, intake and output measurement, and blood gas assessment. In addition, physical assessment findings such as heart and lung sounds, peripheral pulses, presence of edema, ascites, and jugular vein distention, level of consciousness, and degree of pain also provide an indication of whether patient outcomes have been met.

CASE STUDY 2

F. Talbot is a 68-year-old Caucasian male with a history of type I insulin-dependent diabetes mellitus since the age of 8. He is admitted to the hospital to undergo a femoral-popliteal bypass of his lower left extremity. Over the past 5 years, he has complained of increasing claudication, which has progressed from pain occurring with walking to a throbbing, burning pain at rest. As a result, he opted to undergo the surgical procedure in an effort to prevent or hopefully altogether forestall the need for a lower extremity amputation in the future.

Preoperative physical assessment reveals rubor skin color of the lower left extremity. The skin is cool to the touch, and capillary refill is decreased. Pedal and posterior tibial pulses are diminished on the left compared with the right. Other signs of arterial insufficiency include thin and shiny skin of the lower extremities, with loss of hair on the dorsum of the feet and toes bilaterally. In addition, the patient's nails are thick and brittle. Because of his diabetes, Mr. Talbot also has a history of slow healing lesions, usually on the toes or heels of his feet.

After undergoing the surgical procedure, Mr. Talbot is admitted to the critical care unit for overnight observation and monitoring. Postoperative pain is controlled with a patient-controlled analgesia (PCA) pump with intravenous morphine. The nursing diagnosis for Mr. Talbot is shown in Box 25-2. Besides pain, the nurse assesses the following nursing-sensitive outcomes: (1) skin color and temperature; (2) capillary refill; (3) presence and symmetry of peripheral pulses; (4) presence of peripheral edema and bruits; and (5) muscle function. These outcomes are

---

Case Study
Box 25-2   MR. TALBOT

Nursing Diagnosis
Altered peripheral tissue perfusion related to interruption of arterial flow as evidenced by rubor skin, cool skin temperature of left lower extremity, diminished peripheral pulses and capillary refill, intermittent claudication progressing to pain at rest, thin, shiny skin with loss of hair on feet and toes, thick/brittle nails bilaterally, and slow healing lower extremity lesions.

Defining characteristics
Rubor skin color
Skin temperature cool unilaterally
Decreased capillary refill
Diminished peripheral pulses
Intermittent claudication progressing to pain at rest (burning and throbbing)
Thin, shiny skin of lower extremities with loss of hair on dorsum of feet and toes
Thick, brittle nails bilaterally
Slow healing lesions of lower extremities

Related factor/etiology needed
Altered peripheral tissue perfusion related to interruption of arterial flow*

Other data
Blood pressures in upper and lower extremities
Neurologic examination of motor and sensory components

*Unable to rule out.

assessed by systematic peripheral vascular assessment, and the clinical findings are ranked by the nurse on the following measurement scale: 1 = never present, 2 = rarely present, 3 = sometimes present, 4 = often present, and 5 = consistently present. In Mr. Talbot's case, his altered peripheral tissue perfusion improved from extremely compromised (level 1) in the preoperative period to mildly compromised (level 2) in the early postoperative period. This evaluation was based on the following clinical findings:

- Localized extremity pain controlled
- Skin color pink
- Skin warm and dry with moderately brisk capillary refill (approximately 4 seconds)
- Peripheral pulses (pedal and posterior tibials) present and symmetric bilaterally
- Peripheral edema absent
- Motor and sensory function of lower extremities intact bilaterally

NURSING INTERVENTIONS

The *Nursing Interventions Classification (NIC)* provides a taxonomy of 486 nursing interventions that nurses use to treat both physiologic and psychosocial nursing diagnoses. Each intervention label has a definition and set of defining nursing activities (Iowa Intervention Project, 2000). "A nursing intervention is any treatment based upon clinical judgment and knowledge, that a nurse performs to enhance patient/client outcomes. Nursing interventions include both direct and indirect care; those aimed at individuals, families, and the community; including nurse-initiated, physician-initiated, and other provider-initiated treatments" (Iowa Intervention Project, 2000, p. xix). Therefore nursing interventions include assessment, treatment, and evaluation activities.

Fifty-eight of the nursing intervention labels (see Tables 25-1 through 25-3) might be appropriate to treat specific instances of Altered Tissue Perfusion. These interventions include both monitoring activities and management-related activities.

Monitoring Interventions

Monitoring interventions are used for both assessment and evaluation purposes. These monitoring activities are used to assess for the defining characteristics of Altered Tissue Perfusion or for the development of complications. For instance, the three main monitoring-related nursing interventions that may be appropriate for altered cardiopulmonary tissue perfusion are Vital Signs Monitoring, Invasive Hemodynamic Monitoring, and Acid-Base Monitoring. Monitoring is also used to assess the effectiveness of nursing and medical interventions for the purposes of evaluation, not diagnosis. Therefore, in addition to monitoring the patient's physiologic status, the findings from

monitoring activities will provide an indication of how well the patient is responding to interventions aimed at modifying the altered perfusion state. For instance, Invasive Hemodynamic Monitoring often includes the use of a Swan-Ganz catheter for measurement of hemodynamic indices and cardiac output. These hemodynamic data, such as systemic vascular resistance and cardiac index, provide nurses with vital information regarding both the patient's physiologic status and the patient's response to various management interventions employed to enhance tissue perfusion (Cariou, Monchi, & Dhainaut, 1998; Gawlinski, 1998). The effectiveness of treatment can also be evaluated by changes observed in the client's signs and symptoms, such as amount of walking before the onset of pain, nutritional status, well-being, and ability to maintain personal care and engage in ADL, as well as the duration in which desired outcomes were achieved (Wild, 1986).

Management Interventions

Treatments for nursing diagnoses are directed toward altering the etiologic factor of the actual or potential health problem. The overall goals of nursing therapies for Altered Tissue Perfusion are to maintain tissue perfusion and cellular oxygenation (Hart, 1981; Thompson et al., 1998). Although nursing therapies are most successful when the etiology of the health problem can be modified, changing the etiologies of Altered Tissue Perfusion might not be possible in some situations. Such change can be especially difficult in the elderly client because alterations are often due to the interaction of pathologic processes and progressive physiologic changes associated with aging. Therefore management-related interventions can be implemented to either directly alter the etiology or to treat defining characteristics—such as pain—when the etiology cannot be changed.

Altered Tissue Perfusion can be influenced by one or more of the five etiologies and can affect multiple systems. Therefore the selection of nursing intervention(s) also varies according to the underlying etiology responsible for the altered state of tissue perfusion. Some nursing interventions will be the same regardless of the etiology, such as Vital Signs Monitoring (Interruption in Arterial Flow: Renal, cerebral, cardiopulmonary, gastrointestinal) and Circulatory Care (Interruption in Arterial Flow: Peripheral and Interruption of Venous Flow). However, most etiologies of Altered Tissue Perfusion require specific nursing interventions (see Tables 25-1 through 25-3). More than one nursing intervention may also be appropriate within a given etiology. Many of these nursing interventions are closely related, such as Invasive Hemodynamic Monitoring and Hemodynamic Regulation. For a detailed list of the specific nursing activities associated with each intervention label, refer to Iowa Intervention Project (2000).

Nursing interventions intended to alter etiologic factors must also consider the priority of the physiologic system(s) affected by the alteration. As a result, the nursing interventions selected depend on the severity of the altered state, that is, on how far the alteration in tissue perfusion has progressed and its effect on other body processes and systems. The impact of Altered Tissue Perfusion on other body systems would undoubtedly lead to the formulation of additional nursing diagnoses and appropriate selection of other nursing interventions. For instance, mechanical ventilation may or may not be necessary in a patient with Altered Tissue Perfusion related to exchange problems, as in the case study previously presented. In other words, nurses will use a core group of nursing interventions to treat a patient with a given alteration in tissue perfusion. In addition, secondary nursing interventions can be used to treat other associated health problems. For instance, the main management-oriented nursing interventions that would be used to treat altered cardiopulmonary tissue perfusion include the following: (1) Cardiac Precautions; (2) Embolus Precautions; (3) Embolus Care: Pulmonary; (4) Cardiac Care; (5) Cardiac Care: Acute; (6) Hemodynamic Regulation; (7) Acid-Base Management; (8) Dysrhythmia Management; (9) Pain Management; and (10) Cardiac Care: Rehabilitative. Other potential nursing interventions include Tube Care: Chest, Shock Management: Cardiac, Resuscitation, and Code Management, depending on how extensive the Altered Tissue Perfusion progresses, its impact on other body systems, and, consequently, the need for further medical intervention.

Other nursing interventions that are focused on altering the etiologic agent are collaborative in nature (dependent nursing function). Examples of these therapies might include the use of tissue plasminogen activator in the management of acute stroke (altered cerebral tissue perfusion) or the use of antiplatelet agents such as aspirin in secondary stroke prevention. Oral anticoagulant therapy is also used in the presence of venous thromboembolism, and current studies are exploring the role of anticoagulation in prophylaxis for both surgical and nonsurgical patients. Pharmacologic interventions for the treatment of altered peripheral tissue perfusion are also being investigated (Alberts, 1999; Bednar & Gross, 1999; Benavente & Hart, 1999; Calverley & Roth, 1998; Gallus, Nurmohammed, Kearon, & Prins, 1998; McNamara, Champion, & Kadowitz, 1998).

CASE STUDY 1

Mr. Meyer, diagnosed with a pulmonary embolism, was given 50% oxygen via facemask and monitored for signs and symptoms of increasing respiratory rate and dyspnea from baseline, cyanosis, and anxiety. ABGs were monitored for desired response to treatment (increased PaO_2 and correction of respiratory alkalosis). He received aggressive pulmonary care, including turning, coughing, and deep breathing, as well as analgesics to prevent splinting. The head of bed (HOB) was also elevated 30 degrees to ensure better V/Q match to improve PaO_2, and sequential compression devices were placed on his lower extremities bilaterally to enhance venous return. Mr. Meyer was instructed to avoid bending his knees, since this position impedes venous return from the legs and increases the risk of further emboli.

Among the other interventions focused on pharmacologic therapy, Mr. Meyer received a loading dose of 5000 U IV heparin over 10 minutes. This infusion was followed by a maintenance dose of 1000 U per hour IV. Coumadin was started 48 hours after the initiation of heparin at a dose of 10 mg PO per day. During this regimen, prothrombin time (PT) and partial thromboplastin time (PTT) were monitored daily to keep these values approximately 1.5 times normal. Seven days later IV heparin was discontinued and Mr. Meyer and his wife received Coumadin teaching. He was then discharged home and has recovered completely (see Box 25-1).

CASE STUDY 2

C. Young, a 76-year-old Caucasian woman, was seen in the Women's Cardiac Center for a personalized health and risk factor assessment. Assessment findings included HR 84 beats/min, BP 172/68, height 5 feet 5 inches, and weight 171 lb. Waist-hip ratio was 0.75, and skin fold calipers measured 42% body fat. Lipid profile included a total cholesterol of 239 mg/dl, high-density lipoprotein (HDL) 40 mg/dl, low-density lipoprotein (LDL) 159 mg/dl, ratio 5.9 mg/dl, and triglycerides 248 mg/dl. Fasting glucose was 79 mg/dl. Past medical history included cholecystectomy, hiatal hernia, hypothyroidism, arthritis, insomnia, and a long-standing history of ankle edema. The client also reported symptoms suspicious of sleep apnea. Based on this assessment, coronary risk factors were identified and the client was instructed on risk factor modification. The nursing intervention Cardiac Precautions used by the nurse was preventive in nature. As defined by McCloskey and Bulechek (Iowa Interventions Project, 2000), Cardiac Precautions is focused on "prevention of an acute episode of impaired cardiac function by minimizing myocardial oxygen consumption or increasing myocardial oxygen supply" (p. 199). The following nursing activities might be associated with this intervention:

- Identify the patient's readiness to learn lifestyle modification
- Restrict smoking
- Substitute artificial salt and limit sodium intake, if appropriate
- Identify the patient's methods of handling stress
- Promote effective techniques for reducing stress
- Perform relaxation therapy, if appropriate
- Instruct the patient on progressive exercise

Four months later Mrs. Young phoned the Women's Cardiac Center with complaints of anterior chest discomfort that radiated to her neck/jaw/back and that was accompanied by SOB. She was referred to the cardiology department and seen 3 days later. Based on the diagnostic findings, the client was referred for cardiac surgery. Two weeks later the client underwent a triple coronary artery bypass graft (CABG × 3) with internal mammary grafting. During surgery, she required AV sequential pacing, inotropic support with dobutamine and epinephrine, and, because of right heart failure, placement of an IABP via the right femoral artery. On the first postoperative day, the client remained in the ICU on the IABP and ventilator. Laboratory values showed a creatine kinase (CK) of 3113 and MB of 169.4. A bedside echocardiogram confirmed an inferior-posterior and RV infarct. Nursing interventions employed during the ICU phase included Vital Signs Monitoring, Invasive Hemodynamic Monitoring, Acid-Base Monitoring, Cardiac Care, Cardiac Care: Acute, Hemodynamic Regulation, Pain Management, and Tube Care: Chest.

The client was transferred to the cardiac surgical step-down unit on the third postoperative day, where she developed atrial fibrillation and was given digitalis. Oxygen was administered at 5 L via nasal cannula (NC), and her ambulation was significantly limited. In addition, a bruit was noted in her right groin. An echocardiographic Doppler test revealed a two-chamber pseudoaneurysm that was unsuccessfully compressed. On the sixth postoperative day the client went in and out of atrial fibrillation/flutter and converted to sinus rhythm by postoperative day 7. As a result, she was weaned from oxygen and progressed with independent ambulation. However, she remained hospitalized until postoperative day 12 for observation of her heart rhythm and right groin pseudoaneurysm. During the step-down phase, nursing interventions focused on Vital Signs Monitoring, Cardiac Care, Cardiac Care: Acute, Dysrhythmia Management, and Pain Management.

Two days after discharge the client received a follow-up phone call from the nursing staff to assess her condition. The client stated she was "feeling pretty good" yet indicated some difficulty with incisional pain, anorexia, fluid loss, insomnia, and confusion about her home-going medications. After recuperating at home, the client enrolled in a local Phase II cardiac rehab program. At this time the client reports no angina or chest discomfort since discharge. She is progressing in her exercise program and tolerating activity. Problems experienced since discharge include a urinary tract infection, depression, and increasing congestive heart failure. Her Lasix dosage has been increased, and she has obtained good relief of her symptoms. The primary nursing interventions during this phase of recovery focus on Cardiac Care: Rehabilitative (Iowa Intervention Project, 2000), the "promotion of maximum functional activity level for a patient who has suffered an episode of impaired cardiac function that resulted from an imbalance between myocardial oxygen supply and demand" (p. 198). Examples of nursing activities associated with this nursing intervention include the following:

- Instruct the patient on self-care of chest pain (e.g., take sublingual nitroglycerine every 5 minutes for 3 times; if chest pain unrelieved, seek emergency medical care).
- Instruct the patient and family on appropriate prescribed and over-the-counter medications.
- Instruct the patient and family on wound care and precautions (e.g., sternal incision or catheterization site), if appropriate.
- Instruct the patient and family on cardiac risk factor modification (e.g., smoking cessation, diet, exercise), if appropriate.
- Instruct the patient and family on the exercise regimen, including warm-up, endurance, and cool-down, as appropriate.
- Instruct the patient and family on any special considerations with ADL (e.g., isolate activities and allow rest periods), if appropriate.
- Monitor patient's activity tolerance.
- Instruct the patient and family on follow-up care.
- Instruct the patient and family on access of emergency services system available in their community, as appropriate.
- Coordinate patient referrals (e.g., dietary, social services, physical therapy).

The monitoring and management nursing interventions used during both the acute and convalescent periods

---

Box 25-3 Case Study MRS. YOUNG

Nursing Diagnosis
Altered Tissue Perfusion: Cardiopulmonary related to interruption of arterial flow secondary to atherosclerosis as evidenced by dyspnea, tachycardia, angina, and elevated creatine phosphokinase (CPK).

Defining characteristics
Dyspnea
Tachycardia
Angina
Elevated CPK

Related factor/etiology needed
Altered cardiopulmonary tissue perfusion related to interruption of arterial flow*

Other data
Blood pressure and other vital signs (e.g., respiratory rate)
12-lead ECG
Other physical assessment findings (e.g., capillary refill, skin temperature)

*Unable to rule out.

assisted the client in achieving the following desired outcomes related to altered cardiopulmonary tissue perfusion: (1) warm, dry skin with brisk capillary refill; (2) normal blood pressure; (3) normal heart rate (60 to 100 beats/min); (4) normal respiratory rate (12 to 24 breaths/min); (5) absent or decreased angina; and (6) ECG manifestations of myocardial ischemia absent or reduced (Box 25-3).

SUMMARY

Altered Tissue Perfusion is a common nursing diagnosis of elderly client populations in both acute and long-term care settings. Five general etiologies can be related to altered renal, cerebral, cardiopulmonary, gastrointestinal, and peripheral tissue perfusion. The critical defining characteristics associated with each of these alterations were identified, along with desired patient outcomes. Case studies were presented to illustrate the complex process of differential diagnosis and the selection of nursing interventions to treat Altered Tissue Perfusion in elders.

REFERENCES

Alberts, M. (1999). Diagnosis and treatment of ischemic stroke. *American Journal of Medicine, 106*(2), 211-221.

American Association of Critical-Care Nurses (AACN). (1990). *Outcome standards for nursing care of the critically ill.* Laguna Niguel, CA: Author.

Bednar, M. M., & Gross, C. E. (1999). Antiplatelet therapy in acute cerebral ischemia. *Stroke, 30*(4), 887-893.

Benavente, O., & Hart, R. G. (1999). Stroke: Part II. Management of acute ischemic stroke. *American Family Physician, 59*(10), 2828-2834.

Blake, D. (1976). Physical assessment of the aged: Differentiating normal and abnormal change. In I. Burnside (Ed.), *Nursing and the aged* (pp. 409-421). Hightstown, NJ: McGraw-Hill.

Bruner, L., & Suddarth, D. (1980). *Textbook of medical-surgical nursing.* Baltimore: Lippincott Williams & Wilkins.

Calverley, D. C., & Roth, G. J. (1998). Antiplatelet therapy: Aspirin, ticlopidine/clopidogrel, and anti-integrin agents. *Hematology-Oncology Clinics of North America, 12*(6), 1231-1249.

Cariou, A., Monchi, M., & Dhainaut, J. F. (1998). Continuous cardiac output and mixed venous oxygen saturation monitoring. *Journal of Critical Care, 13*(4), 198-213.

Carnevali, D., & Enloe, C. (1986). Assessment in the elderly. In D. Carnevali & M. Patrick (Eds.), *Nursing management for the elderly* (pp. 26-52). Baltimore: Lippincott Williams & Wilkins.

Carpenito, L. (1995). *Nursing diagnosis: Application to clinical practice.* Baltimore: Lippincott Williams & Wilkins.

Doyle, J. (1986). Treatment modalities in peripheral vascular disease. *Nursing Clinics of North America, 21*(2), 241-253.

Fagin-Dubin, L. (1977). Atherosclerosis: A major cause of peripheral vascular disease. *Nursing Clinics of North America, 12*(1), 101-108.

Frantz, R. (1981). Shock. In L. Hart, M. Fehring, & J. Reese (Eds.), *Concepts common to acute illness* (pp. 320-339). St. Louis, MO: Mosby.

Gallus, A. S., Nurmohammed, M., Kearon, C., & Prins, M. (1998). Thromboprophylaxis in non-surgical patients: Who, when and how? *Haemostasis, 28*(Suppl. 3), 71-82.

Gawlinski, A. (1998). Can measurement of mixed venous oxygen saturation replace measurement of cardiac output in patients with advanced heart failure? *American Journal of Critical Care, 7*(5), 374-380.

Goetter, W. (1986). Nursing diagnosis and interventions with the acute stroke patient. *Nursing Clinics of North America, 21*(2), 309-319.

Gordon, M. (1987). *Manual of nursing diagnosis.* Hightstown, NJ: McGraw-Hill.

Gordon, M. (1994). *Nursing diagnosis: Process and application.* Hightstown, NJ: McGraw-Hill.

Gorelick, P. (1986). Cerebrovascular disease: Pathophysiology and diagnosis. *Nursing Clinics of North America, 21*(2), 275-287.

Guzetta, C., Bunton, S., Prinkey, L., Sherer, A., & Seifert, P. (1989). *Clinical assessment tools for use with nursing diagnoses.* St. Louis, MO: Mosby.

Halm, M. (1991). Altered tissue perfusion. In M. Maas, K. Buckwalter, & M. Hardy (Eds.), *Nursing diagnosis and interventions for the elderly* (pp. 223-242). Reading, MA: Addison Wesley Longman.

Hart, L. (1981). Ischemia. In L. Hart, M. Fehring, & J. Reese (Eds.), *Concepts common to acute illness* (pp. 293-318). St. Louis, MO: Mosby.

Herman, J. (1986). Nursing assessment and nursing diagnosis in patients with peripheral vascular disease. *Nursing Clinics in North America, 21*(2), 219-231.

Iowa Intervention Project. J. C. McCloskey & G. M. Bulechek (Eds.). (2000). *Nursing interventions classification (NIC)* (3rd ed.). St. Louis, MO: Mosby.

Iowa Outcomes Project. M. Johnson, M. Maas, & S. Moorhead (Eds.). (2000). *Nursing outcomes classification (NOC)* (2nd ed.). St. Louis, MO: Mosby.

Jeppesen, M. (1986). Laboratory values for the elderly. In D. Carnevali & M. Patrick (Eds.), *Nursing management for the elderly* (pp. 102-142). Baltimore: Lippincott Williams & Wilkins.

Jones, D., Dunbar, C., & Jirovec, M. (1982). *Medical-surgical nursing: A conceptual approach.* Hightstown, NJ: McGraw-Hill.

Kane, A., & Kane, L. (1981). *Assessing the elderly: A practical guide to measurement.* Washington, DC: The Rand Corporation, Lexington Books, Health.

Kelly, M. (1985). *Nursing diagnosis sourcebook: Guidelines for clinical application.* Norwalk, CT: Appleton & Lange.

McGee, S. R., & Boyko, E. J. (1998). Physical examination and chronic lower-extremity ischemia: A critical review. *Archives of Internal Medicine, 158*(12), 1357-1364.

McNamara, D. B., Champion, H. C., & Kadowitz, P. J. (1998). Pharmacologic management of peripheral vascular disease. *Surgical Clinics of North America, 78*(3), 447-464.

Mooe, T., Olofsson, B. O., Stegmayr, B., & Eriksson, P. (1999). Ischemic stroke: Impact of a recent myocardial infarction. *Stroke, 30*(5), 997-1001.

North American Nursing Diagnosis Association. (1999). *Nursing diagnoses: Definitions & classification 1999-2000.* Philadelphia: Author.

Quinless, F. (1986). Assessing the client with acute cardiovascular dysfunction. *Topics in Clinical Nursing, 8*(1), 45-56.

Rantz, M., & LeMone, P. (Eds.). (1994). *Classification of nursing diagnoses: Proceedings of the eleventh national conference.* Glendale, CA: Cinahl Information Systems.

Rice, V. (1981a, March-April). Shock, a clinical syndrome. Part I: Definition, etiology, and pathophysiology. *Critical Care Nurse, 1,* 44-50.

Rice, V. (1981b, September-October). Shock, a clinical syndrome. Part IV: Nursing intervention. *Critical Care Nurse, 1,* 34-43.

Roberts, S. (1987). Pulmonary tissue perfusion altered: Emboli. *Heart & Lung, 16*(2), 128-137.

Santilli, J. D., & Santilli, S. M. (1999). Chronic critical limb ischemia: Diagnosis, treatment and prognosis. *American Family Physician, 59*(7), 1899-1908.

Sexton, D. (1977). The patient with peripheral arterial occlusive disease. *Nursing Clinics of North America, 12*(1), 89-99.

Thompson, J., McFarland, G., Hirsch, J., & Tucker, S. (1998). *Mosby's clinical nursing* (4th ed.). St. Louis, MO: Mosby.

Wagner, M. (1986). Pathophysiology related to peripheral vascular disease. *Nursing Clinics of North America, 21*(2), 195-205.

Wild, L. (1986). Cardiovascular problems. In D. Carnevali & M. Patrick (Eds.), *Nursing management for the elderly* (pp. 361-378). Baltimore: Lippincott Williams & Wilkins.

CHAPTER *26*

INEFFECTIVE BREATHING PATTERN

Bonnie Wakefield

Pulmonary function reaches its maximum level between ages 20 and 25 then declines progressively (Levitzky, 1984). The effects of aging, however, are difficult to separate from the effects of chronic exposure to air pollution, smoking, respiratory infections, and differences in lifestyle. The passage of time alone changes anatomy and the physiologic response to various stimuli. Normal loss can impede functional ability so that the results of aging can be additive or complicate existing pathology. For example, the incidence of emphysema increases with age so that by age 90 almost all individuals have some degree of obstructive lung disease (Petty, 1983). Attributing signs and symptoms such as dyspnea or fatigue solely to the aging process leads to lack of treatment and progressive worsening of pathology because of lack of treatment. Nurses need to understand the basic changes associated with aging because they are in a position to assess functional ability and the effects of normal and pathologic changes on activities of daily living (ADL).

RELATED FACTORS/ETIOLOGIES

Numerous changes in breathing patterns occur in the elderly, both as a result of aging and as a result of obstructive and restrictive lung diseases. These changes are summarized in Box 26-1 and compared with North American Nursing Diagnosis Association (NANDA)–proposed defining characteristics and related factors.

Physiologic Changes Associated With Aging

Two major functions of the respiratory system are ventilation and gas exchange. Other pulmonary system functions that can be affected by aging are neural control of breathing and defense mechanisms. Brandstetter and Kazemi (1983), Levitzky (1984), and Wahba (1983) provide excellent reviews of the effects of aging on respiratory system function.

Ventilation. The amount of effort required for ventilation is determined by compliance, airway resistance, and alveolar surface tension. Age-related changes occur in compliance and airway resistance but not in the surface tension of the alveoli.

Compliance. Ventilatory lung function deteriorates about two times faster after age 50 (Jedrychowski, 1983). Changes in lung volumes and mechanics are due to a decrease in the elastic recoil of the lung and a progressive stiffening of the chest wall (Brandstetter & Kazemi, 1983; Horvath & Borgia, 1984; Levitzky, 1984; Wahba, 1983). Collagen becomes more rigid, and cross linkage and rearrangement of collagen fibrils and elastin contribute to the loss of elastic recoil (Brandstetter & Kazemi, 1983; Levitzky, 1984; Wahba, 1983). Less pressure is required for lung expansion, and, in conjunction with alveolar dilation, an increased static pulmonary compliance results (Brandstetter & Kazemi, 1983; Wahba, 1983). Dynamic lung compliance (measured during active breathing) decreases and becomes frequency dependent with age, probably because of increased resistance to airflow in the small airways. In fact, most dynamic measurements of lung volume decrease with age (Levitzky, 1984; Wahba, 1983).

Whereas static pulmonary compliance increases, chest wall compliance decreases, resulting in a greater negative pleural pressure. Therefore elastic recoil of the chest wall shifts from outward to inward at a much lower volume. The closing volume or closing capacity (the lung volume at which small airways begin to close during forced expiration) increases from about 30% of total lung capacity at age 20 to about 55% at age 70. These two changes result in premature airway closure and poorly ventilated or unventilated alveoli at resting lung volumes. Small airways are more likely to collapse in the lower regions because of diminished elastic recoil and a higher gravity-dependent intrapleural pressure. These conditions can result in less efficient matching of ventilation and perfusion and in decreased arterial oxygen tension (Levitzky, 1984).

Airway Resistance. Decreased diameter of the small airways, decreased stability, and increased closing capacity contribute to premature closure on expiration. These small airway effects are exacerbated when the lungs are in the supine position. A coincident increase in the diameter of the larger and more central airways increases anatomic and physiologic dead space (Wahba, 1983). Dilation of the large airways concomitant with small airway constriction and closure results in gas trapping and increased dead space, leading to ventilation-perfusion imbalances.

313

Box 26-1	Comparison of Changes in the Pulmonary System With Aging, Obstructive Lung Disease, and Restrictive Lung Disease

Nursing Diagnosis
Ineffective Breathing Pattern
Defining characteristics
Dyspnea
Shortness of breath
Tachypnea
Fremitus
Respiratory depth changes
Pursed lip breathing
Prolonged expiratory phase
Use of accessory muscles
Altered chest excursion
Increased anteroposterior diameter
Assumption of three-point position
Abnormal arterial blood gases
Cyanosis
Cough
Nasal flaring

Related factors/etiologies
Neuromuscular dysfunction
Musculoskeletal impairment
Pain
Perception/cognitive impairment
Anxiety
Decreased energy/fatigue

Changes Associated With Aging
Ventilation
Decreased elastic recoil
Altered lung volumes
Decreased chest wall compliance
Premature airway closure
Ventilation-perfusion imbalance
Lack of basilar inflation
Diminished perception of airflow resistance

Gas exchange
Altered arterial blood gases

Neural control
Blunted response to hypoxia or hypercapnia
Diminished variability of rhythm and depth of respirations

Defense mechanisms
Decreased number of cilia
Less efficient cough

Structural changes
Kyphosis
Increased anterior-posterior (AP) diameter
Decreased total lung capacity
Diminished respiratory muscle strength

Changes Associated With Obstructive Disease
Cough
Wheezing
Sputum production
Mucus retention
Altered arterial blood gases (ABGs)
Cyanosis
Dyspnea and shortness of breath (SOB)
Increased work of breathing
Cachexia
Barrel chest

Changes Associated With Restrictive Disease
Decreased lung volume measures
Altered ABGs
Tachypnea
Shallow respirations
SOB
Fatigue
Cough
Weight loss

Perception of airflow resistance is blunted in elderly adults (Altose, Leitner, & Cherniack, 1985), making small changes in respiratory resistance more difficult to detect (Rubin, Tack, & Cherniack, 1982). Older individuals are less able to maintain a constant tidal volume (Altose et al., 1985). Prolonged airway obstruction, as is experienced with lung disease, decreases the ability to sense changes in resistance (Rubin et al., 1982), as does cigarette smoke (Morris, 1984). Closing volumes also increase disproportionately to age in smokers (Wahba, 1983).

Gas Exchange. Arterial oxygen tension decreases each decade, whereas alveolar P_{O_2} remains constant or increases slightly (Horvath & Borgia, 1984). As a result, arterial P_{O_2} decreases by 20 torr from age 20 to age 70

(Levitzky, 1984). This age-dependent widening of alveolar-arterial oxygen differences results from functional alterations in ventilation-perfusion dynamics (Horvath & Borgia, 1984). A physiologic shunt of alveolar ventilation becomes less uniform with age. Upper lung regions receive preferential ventilation without a corresponding increase of blood flow. The resulting alveolar dead space leads to underventilated pulmonary capillaries. Pulmonary diffusing capacity decreases 20% over the course of adult life because of decreased alveolar surface area and decreased pulmonary capillary blood volume (Levitzky, 1984). The end result is a decrease in the effective pulmonary-capillary area (Brandstetter & Kazemi, 1983). Although these changes affect the P_{O_2}, arterial CO_2 tension does not change with age (Levitzky, 1984).

Neural Regulation. Increased ventilation in response to hypoxia and hypercapnia is blunted, decreasing by one half between the ages of 25 and 70 (Brandstetter & Kazemi, 1983; Levitzky, 1984; Rubin et al., 1982; Wahba, 1983). Hypothesized causes for this decrease in response include diminished neural output to the respiratory muscle (Brandstetter & Kazemi, 1983), diminished sensitivity of the central and arterial chemoreceptors (Levitzky, 1984; Rubin et al., 1982) and changes in central respiratory control (Levitzky, 1984).

Observed differences in respiratory patterns can be caused as much by changes in the mechanics of the respiratory system as by changes in chemoreceptor sensitivity or the central nervous system (CNS) (Brandstetter & Kazemi, 1983; Levitzky, 1984; Rubin et al., 1982). Blunted perception of airflow resistance probably results from impaired central nervous system (CNS) processing (Altose et al., 1985). Patients with COPD, when compared with age-matched controls, have exhibited significantly less variable rhythm and depth of breathing, suggesting neural adjustments in breathing control (Loveridge, West, Anthonisen, & Kryger, 1984).

Defense Mechanisms. Decreased numbers of cilia lead to a diminished efficiency of the mucociliary elevator. The reflex response to mechanical or chemical stimulation of the upper airway is decreased. Coughing is less efficient in terms of volume, force, and flow rate because of decreased respiratory muscle strength and altered mechanics of the lung and chest wall (Levitzky, 1984).

Structural Changes. Alveolar ducts and respiratory bronchioles enlarge at the expense of the alveoli, leading to a decreased alveolar surface area. The number and size of interalveolar fenestrae increase with concomitant degeneration of adjacent elastic fibers. These changes appear to be the source of increased lung compliance and diminished pulmonary elastic recoil. Pulmonary vasculature is less distensible, but resting mean pulmonary arterial pressure and pulmonary vascular resistance change little with age. There is an increased thickness of the larger pulmonary arteries. The bronchial cartilage tends to calcify, leading to diminished chest wall compliance and increased dead space. Costal cartilages calcify, decreasing the mobility and compliance of the rib cage. Intervertebral spaces diminish in size, and kyphosis increases, resulting in a shorter thorax, increased anterior-posterior diameter, and reduced total lung capacity. Increased deposition of abdominal and thoracic adipose tissue also can contribute to decreased chest wall compliance. The muscles of breathing also lose strength (Levitzky, 1984).

Pulmonary Pathology in Aging

Pathophysiologic changes associated with pulmonary disease states will lead to ineffective breathing patterns, and these changes can be exacerbated by the changes associated with aging. Both obstructive lung disease (i.e., emphysema, asthma, and bronchitis involving increased airway resistance) and restrictive lung disease (i.e., tuberculosis involving a decrease in total lung capacity caused by structural or functional changes) produce symptoms of ineffective breathing patterns, albeit by different mechanisms. Both types of disease affect breathing mechanics. The changes associated with emphysema in particular mimic those associated with normal aging, as emphysematous changes are commonly found on autopsy in patients without documented chronic obstructive pulmonary disease (COPD). A review of these disease states is not possible in this chapter, but the hallmarks of each type of lung disease (obstructive and restrictive) are summarized in Box 26-1.

ASSESSMENT

York (1985) and McDonald (1985) have developed data collection tools that are essentially checklists of defining characteristics supporting a respiratory nursing diagnosis. Clinical assessment tools are published in textbooks and care planning guides, but are more broad based in scope. For example, Guzetta, Bunton, Prinkey, Sherer, and Seifert (1989) have published a collection of assessment tools. Three of these tools may be useful when assessing patients with an ineffective breathing pattern: the Pulmonary Assessment Tool, the Medical-Surgical Assessment Tool, and the Gerontologic Assessment Tool. Within each of these tools is a section addressing oxygenation/pulmonary function. Currently, all that is available are standard pulmonary assessment techniques. The frequency with which patients need to be assessed depends on whether their ineffective breathing pattern is an acute or chronic condition. For example, if pain causes shallow respirations, assessment would have to be carried out frequently, depending on the severity of the pain's effect on breathing patterns. If a more chronic condition such as a chronic respiratory disease causes an ineffective breathing pattern, assessments could be made much less frequently.

NURSING DIAGNOSIS

An ineffective breathing pattern occurs when an inhalation and/or exhalation pattern does not enable adequate pulmonary inflation or emptying (Rantz & LeMone, 1995). The three respiratory nursing diagnoses currently accepted by NANDA (1999) are Ineffective Airway Clearance, Ineffective Breathing Pattern, and Impaired Gas Exchange. The NANDA diagnosis Ineffective Breathing Pattern is defined as "inspiration and/or expiration that does not provide adequate ventilation" (NANDA, 1999, p. 31). The defining characteristics and related factors, related *Nursing Outcomes Classification (NOC)* outcomes (Iowa Outcomes Project, 2000), and *Nursing Interventions Classification*

| Box 26-2 | Suggested Nursing-Sensitive Outcome and Nursing Intervention INEFFECTIVE BREATHING PATTERN |

Nursing Diagnosis
Ineffective Breathing Pattern
Defining characteristics
Dyspnea
Shortness of breath
Tachypnea
Fremitus
Respiratory depth changes
Pursed lip breathing
Prolonged expiratory phase
Use of accessory muscles
Altered chest excursion
Increased anteroposterior diameter
Assumption of three-point position
Abnormal arterial blood gases
Cyanosis
Cough
Nasal flaring

Related factors/etiologies
Neuromuscular dysfunction
Musculoskeletal impairment
Pain
Perception/cognitive impairment
Anxiety
Decreased energy/fatigue

Nursing-Sensitive Outcome
Respiratory Status: Ventilation
Indicators
Respiratory rate IER*
Depth of inspiration
Chest expansion symmetric
Ease of breathing
Expulsion of air
Accessory muscle use not present
Pursed lip breathing not present
Dyspnea at rest not present
Orthopnea not present
Shortness of breath (SOB) not present
Tactile fremitus not present
Respiratory rhythm IER
Moves sputum out of airway

Vocalizes adequately
Adventitious breath sounds not present
Chest retraction not present
Percussed sounds IER
Auscultated breath sounds IER
Auscultated vocalizations IER
Bronchophony IER
Egophony IER
Whispered pectoriloquy IER
Tidal volume IER
Vital capacity IER
Chest x-ray findings IER
Pulmonary function tests IER

Nursing Intervention
Ventilation Assistance
Activities
Maintain a patent airway
Position to alleviate dyspnea
Position to facilitate ventilation/perfusion matching, as appropriate
Assist with frequent position changes, as appropriate
Position to minimize respiratory efforts
Encourage slow, deep breathing, turning, and coughing
Assist with incentive spirometry, as appropriate
Monitor the effects of position change on oxygenation: arterial blood gases (ABGs), SaO_2, SvO_2, end-tidal CO_2, Q_{sp}/Q_t, $A\text{-}aDO_2$ levels*
Auscultate breath sounds, noting areas of decreased or absent ventilation and presence of adventitious sounds
Monitor for respiratory muscle fatigue
Monitor respiratory and oxygenation status
Initiate a program of respiratory muscle strength and/or endurance training, as appropriate
Ambulate three to four times per day, as appropriate
Initiate and maintain supplemental oxygen, as prescribed
Administer medications (e.g., bronchodilators and inhalers) that promote airway patency and gas exchange
Teach pursed-lip breathing techniques, as appropriate
Teach breathing techniques, as appropriate
Administer appropriate pain medication to prevent hypoventilation
Initiate resuscitation efforts, as appropriate

*IER, In expected range; ABGs, arterial blood gases; SaO_2, saturation (arterial) oxygen; SvO_2, saturation (venous) oxygen; CO_2, carbon dioxide; Q_{sp}/Q_t, physiologic blood flow per minute/cardiac output per minute; $A\text{-}aDO_2$, alveolar arterial oxygen pressure difference.

(NIC) interventions (Iowa Interventions Project, 2000) are given in Box 26-2. Although all three NANDA diagnoses have existed for over 20 years, relatively little research has been conducted to investigate their validity. A computerized literature search covering the period of time from 1982 through 1999 revealed only four research-based articles and several clinical articles that discuss the application of Ineffective Breathing Pattern. Several clinically focused

(or overview) articles have been published either describing the application of this diagnosis (Humbrecht & Vanparys, 1982; Sjoberg, 1983) or giving an overview related to respiratory diagnoses (Kim & Larson, 1987). Many nursing textbooks also include a discussion of this diagnosis (Matteson, McConnell, & Linton, 1997).

Since publication of the book *Nursing Diagnoses and Interventions for the Elderly* (Maas, Buckwalter, & Hardy,

1991) two additional research studies focusing on validation of the diagnosis Ineffective Breathing Pattern have been published; this means that only four research studies have focused on this diagnosis. York (1985) presented a model for clinical validation of the nursing diagnoses Ineffective Airway Clearance and Ineffective Breathing Pattern. Clinical experts rated the appropriateness of the defining characteristics for each diagnosis, and clinical records were reviewed to identify the presence of the defining characteristics. McDonald (1985) measured the frequency of the defining characteristics of the three respiratory nursing diagnoses in 41 care plans and identified interventions used to treat these diagnoses. The recommendations of York and McDonald are compared with NANDA's related factors and defining characteristics in Table 26-1. As can be seen from the table, only some of the defining characteristics and related factors identified by NANDA were supported.

More recently, 100 registered nurses working on medical or surgical units in two acute tertiary care settings were surveyed about the three respiratory nursing diagnoses (Capuano, Hitchings, & Johnson, 1990). The patient population was described as including many who were elderly individuals. The nurses were given a checklist, based on the work of York (1985), and asked to check whether they agreed that a given defining characteristic was associated with one of the three respiratory nursing diagnoses. Defining characteristics selected by more than 50% of nurses in the sample are listed in Table 26-1. Consistent with the findings of earlier studies by York and McDonald, the investigators concluded that the overlapping of defining characteristics among the three diagnoses is problematic and that "critical clusters" of defining characteristics should be identified.

A weakness of these three studies is that the defining characteristics have to be validated from a systematically assessed group of patients who are likely to have one of these three diagnoses. This approach was used to validate three respiratory nursing diagnoses (Carlson-Catalano et al., 1998). A literature review identified 37 possible defining characteristics for the three diagnoses. Using these characteristics, 76 hospitalized patients with a mean age of 59 years were assessed by eight masters-prepared nurses. Data were collected on the presence or absence of the defining characteristics, the diagnosis(es) the patient was experiencing, the degree of importance of each defining characteristic for the diagnosis, etiologies for each diagnosis, and the degree of importance of 30 nursing interventions for each diagnosis and patient. For the diagnosis Ineffective Breathing Pattern, dyspnea and fatigue were the most frequent defining characteristics; fatigue, obstruction, pain, and anxiety were the most common etiologies; and 19 important nursing interventions were identified. Consistent with earlier work by McDonald (1985), in 45% of the cases two or more of the diagnoses were made supporting the cooccurrence of the three diagnoses. Since this study used hospitalized patients as a sample, it should be replicated in community-based and long-term care settings, where Ineffective Breathing Pattern is probably more prevalent and problematic.

For the NANDA diagnosis Ineffective Breathing Pattern, several of the defining characteristics are supported by the four studies of the diagnosis and by literature describing changes with aging and specific medical diagnoses, e.g., COPD. However, literature support for some of the current related factors and etiologies is weak or absent, e.g., perceptual impairment. As noted in the four studies, there is considerable overlap of the current defining characteristics with two other NANDA diagnoses: Ineffective Airway Clearance and Impaired Gas Exchange. Because so little work has been done on these diagnoses, it would be premature to recommend either the elimination of any one of them or the combining of all three into one diagnosis such as Altered Respiratory Function. The primary criticism of all three diagnoses and the work to date is the lack of validation of etiologies and defining characteristics in a sample of patients; this is needed to make the diagnoses more specific. Therefore current recommendations for Ineffective Breathing Pattern are shown in Box 26-2. Needless to say, these recommendations should be reviewed critically and tested in patients.

CASE STUDY

D. Klein, a 70-year-old white male, had frequent, shallow respirations and could not finish a sentence without significant shortness of breath. Further examination revealed the following findings: pulse 96 beats per minute, respiratory rate 28 at rest, and BP 138/82 mm Hg; increased anterior-posterior diameter of chest; clubbing of fingers with moderate cyanosis of nailbeds; height 6 feet and weight 170 lb; and orientation to time, place, and person. Mr. Klein verbalized fear of activity and fatigue, stating, "I just can't get around like I used to. I just can't get enough air. Most of the time, I just sit around watching TV." After smoking for 40 years, Mr. Klein quit 5 years ago because of increased breathing difficulty. He also reported decreased appetite caused by difficulty breathing while eating. He was diagnosed with emphysema, with the resultant nursing diagnosis Ineffective Breathing Pattern related to decreased lung expansion and anxiety, evidenced by dyspnea, shortness of breath, tachypnea, cyanosis, respiratory depth changes, increased anterior-posterior diameter, and fatigue.

NURSING-SENSITIVE OUTCOMES

The goals of treatment for patients with ineffective breathing patterns are to manage and/or avoid dyspnea, improve ability to perform ADL, enhance a sense of well-being,

Comparison of Defining Characteristics and Related Factors/Etiologies

Table 26-1 INEFFECTIVE BREATHING PATTERN

NANDA	York (1985)	McDonald (1985)	Capuano, Hitchings, & Johnson (1990)	Carlson-Catalano et al. (1998)
Defining Characteristics				
Dyspnea		Dyspnea/shortness of breath	Dyspnea	Dyspnea
Tachypnea		Tachypnea or bradypnea	Tachypnea	Fatigue
Cyanosis		Cyanosis	Cyanosis	
Cough				
Respiratory depth changes		Labored or shallow breathing	Respiratory depth changes	
Shortness of breath			Shortness of breath	
Fremitus	Fremitus			
Abnormal blood gases		Abnormal blood gases	Abnormal blood gases	
Nasal flaring			Nasal flaring	
Assumption of three-point position	Assumption of three-point position*	Assumption of three-point position	Assumption of three-point position	
Pursed lip breathing		Pursed lip breathing/prolonged expiratory phase	Pursed lip breathing/prolonged expiratory phase	
Prolonged expiratory phase				
Increased anterior-posterior (AP) diameter	Increased AP diameter	Increased AP diameter	Increased AP diameter	
Use of accessory muscles		Use of accessory muscles	Use of accessory muscles	
Altered chest excursion			Altered chest excursion	
Related Factors/Etiologies				
Neuromuscular dysfunction	Decreased lung expansion			Fatigue
Pain				Obstruction
Anxiety				Pain
Musculoskeletal impairment				Anxiety
Decreased energy/fatigue				
Perception/cognitive impairment				

*Considered a treatment modality by the nurses in the sample.

increase endurance time, and improve tolerance for exercise. The NOC (Iowa Outcomes Project, 2000) label Respiratory Status: Ventilation is defined as "movement of air in and out of the lungs" (p. 350). Ventilation is conceptualized as normal respiratory function within the limits imposed by aging. Outcome indicators are listed in Box 26-2.

The major function of the respiratory system is to supply the body with oxygen and rid the body of carbon dioxide. To accomplish this, air must be moved into and out of the lungs (ventilation), gas exchange must occur both in the lungs and at the capillary level (respiration), and oxygen and carbon dioxide must be moved between the lungs and body tissues via the cardiovascular system (transport). Of particular interest to this diagnosis and outcome is pulmonary ventilation, also referred to as the mechanics of breathing.

Ventilation, or breathing, is a mechanical process dependent on volume changes occurring in the thoracic cavity. When the thoracic cavity increases in size because of the activity of inspiratory muscles (diaphragm and external intercostal muscles), air rushes in (inspiration). Expiration, or exhalation, is usually a passive rhythmic process relying less on muscle contraction and is more a result of the elasticity of the lungs. As the inspiratory muscles relax, the lungs recoil, decreasing thoracic cavity volume and causing air to flow out of the lungs. During forced expiration, activating accessory muscles such as the sternocleidomastoid and pectoral muscles increases the capacity of the thorax.

Normally, breathing is quiet and easy and does not require thought. However, both the depth and rate of breathing can be affected by external factors (e.g., air pollution, carbon monoxide levels) and by internal factors (e.g., altered neural control, abnormal blood gases, lung disease, anxiety, pain, respiratory muscle fatigue, hemoglobin level, and temperature). Use of accessory muscles, such as the abdominal muscles in the adult, indicates respiratory distress. Localized intercostal retractions and paradoxical breathing are both abnormal findings in adults.

Energy is used for breathing, in the form of using muscles and overcoming airway resistance. Energy must be used to overcome the pressure gradient between the external atmosphere and the alveoli in order to move 500 ml of air (normal tidal volume) into and out of the lungs with each breath. The flow of air will decrease in direct proportion to resistance, and under normal circumstances airway resistance is insignificant. An example of increased airway resistance is the bronchoconstriction occurring during an acute asthma attack.

The volumes of air within and moved into and out of the lungs during breathing can be measured at several levels. The diagnostic significance of these parameters changes, depending on whether the individual has obstructive or restrictive lung disease. The effects of aging must also be taken into account. In a recent study of pulmonary function as measured by spirometry, differences as great as 20% from commonly used spirometry reference equations were found for a subgroup of "healthy" elders (Enright, Kronmal, Higgins, Schenker, & Haponik, 1993). This subgroup excluded smokers and those with lung disease or any other factor known to influence lung volume measurements. Clearly, recognition of the expected decrements in pulmonary function that accompany normal aging, as well as the effects of lung disease, is necessary to interpret these values.

A systematic physical assessment of the pulmonary system for the outcome indicators includes inspection, palpation, and auscultation. The person should be asked about his ability to breathe. Subjective reports of difficulty breathing are termed *dyspnea;* objectively, this is called shortness of breath. Persons with restrictive lung disease tend to take shallow, frequent breaths. Persons with obstructive lung disease tend to take slow, deep breaths with a prolonged expiratory phase, often accompanied by pursed-lip breathing (blowing out air with lips in an O shape). Orthopnea, the ability to breathe only in an upright position, is also abnormal.

The normal adult respiratory rate is 8 to 12 breaths per minute. Bradypnea is a respiratory rate of less than 8 breaths per minute; tachypnea is a rate in excess of the person's normal rate.

The ability to cough effectively is important to assess. The cough is a normal defense mechanism of the pulmonary system. Cough-related observations include frequency of coughing, activities that induce it, its effects on ADL, its nature, sources of relief, and its association with dyspnea, if present.

Skin color also should be observed. Since individual coloring is variable, changes in color should be assessed. Cyanosis is a diffuse bluish color of the skin that results from reduced levels of hemoglobin. The presence of cyanosis implies hypoxemia, but the absence of cyanosis does not preclude severe hypoxia, since cyanosis is not evident until 5 g of reduced hemoglobin are present per 100 ml of blood. Cyanosis is most easily observed in the lips and tongue. Cyanosis in the ears and nailbeds can be a response to a cold environment.

Chest configuration should be inspected. An increased anteroposterior diameter, equaling the transverse diameter of the chest, gives the patient a barrel-chested appearance. As noted earlier, this shape can result either from aging or from obstructive lung disease. Chest expansion should be symmetric.

Palpation is used to assess for several abnormalities, including crepitus and fremitus. Crepitus is recognized by a crackling or popping sound in response to touch and is caused by the presence of small air bubbles in the subcutaneous tissues. Fremitus is the sensation produced by moving air, such as when a person speaks. Fremitus will increase over a dense area, such as a lung tumor, and decrease in conditions that increase the amount of air in the chest, such as emphysema.

Auscultation involves listening to sounds made by air passing into and out of the airways, usually through a stethoscope. Several abnormal, or adventitious, breath sounds can occur. The absence of breath sounds can be caused by lack of ventilation to an area of the lung. Fine, or crepitant, rales are produced by moisture in the alveoli and small airways. Coarse rales are loud, gurgling noises caused by fluid in the large airways. Wheezing is a whistling noise caused by airway restriction. Bronchophony is the sound of the voice heard through a stethoscope over a healthy bronchus. Whispered pectoriloquy is the transmission of the sound of spoken words through the chest wall, indicating the presence of a cavity or solidification of pulmonary structures. Egophony is assessed by asking the patient to say *ee, ee, ee* while auscultating the chest. Over normal lung areas, the sound *ee* is auscultated; over areas of consolidation, an *aa* sound is heard.

The NOC label Respiratory Status: Ventilation (Iowa Outcomes Project, 2000) is inclusive of the indicators for ventilation. The NOC label includes some indicators (e.g., whispered pectoriloquy) that typically are used only by specialists in respiratory care. Several NOC indicators are the obverse of defining characteristics of the diagnosis, but some are not; these are identified for both the diagnosis and outcome in Box 26-2. However, this situation might indicate a problem with the diagnosis rather than with the outcome indicators. The activities identified by the NIC label address both the defining characteristics and outcome indicators well.

There is no rating scale other than the NOC scale for measuring the outcome Respiratory Status: Ventilation. There are rating scales, instruments, or measures for specific indicators, such as dyspnea (Lareau, Carrieri-Kohlman, Janson-Bjerklie, & Roos, 1994; Silvestri & Mahler, 1993); there also are measures of lung volume (Enright, Adams, Boyle, & Sherrill, 1995; Enright, Kronmal, Higgins, Schenker, & Haponik, 1993). Measures also exist for related outcomes, such as quality of life questionnaires specific to patients with pulmonary disease (Guyatt, Berman, Townsend, Pugsley, & Chambers, 1987; Jones, Quirk, Baveystock, & Littlejohns, 1992; Lareau, Breslin, & Meek, 1996; Larson et al., 1996; Pashkow et al., 1995).

Patients can be assessed for the NOC outcome indicators during routine assessment and monitoring. The frequency of assessment depends on the acuity of the ineffective breathing pattern. It is important to establish a baseline measurement, since serial measures are more informative than is an isolated assessment (Mahler, Tomlinson, Olmstead, Tosteson, & O'Connor, 1995; Rodarte, 1995).

NURSING INTERVENTIONS

Often the changes associated with Ineffective Breathing Pattern are not reversible because of the effects of aging or chronic disease. Since the problem associated with Ineffective Breathing Pattern is primarily one of inadequate ventilation, Ventilation Assistance, defined as the "promotion

of an optimal spontaneous breathing pattern that maximizes oxygen and carbon dioxide exchange in the lungs" (Iowa Interventions Project, 2000, p. 697), was chosen as the primary intervention. The large number of activities for the NIC intervention Ventilation Assistance can be grouped into categories that direct the nurse to other interventions in the taxonomy: education (Teaching: Disease Process, Teaching: Prescribed Medication, Health Education, Smoking Cessation Assistance, Nutritional Counseling), monitoring (Surveillance, Respiratory Monitoring), breathing exercises (Breathing Retraining Intervention, Cough Enhancement), exercise (Exercise Therapy: Ambulation, Exercise Promotion, Progressive Muscle Relaxation), medication administration (see Teaching: Prescribed Medication under education listed earlier), and energy conservation (Energy Management for Energy Conservation outcome). Each of these 13 interventions is supported by recent work for this diagnosis (Carlson-Catalano et al., 1998).

Education

Education in self-care is critical for stabilizing and preventing symptoms and for promoting optimal functional capacity. Pulmonary rehabilitation programs typically have the following goals: to reduce symptoms; to reestablish independence; to slow or arrest progress of disease; to reduce hospitalization; to increase exercise tolerance, appetite, and well-being; to improve psychologic status; and to prevent complications and decline in function (Bradley, 1983).

It is valuable for all patients to understand the disease process and treatments, when to seek medical assistance, and how to accomplish activities of daily living. The greatest benefit of structured pulmonary rehabilitation programs, however, seems to be in improving subjective well-being (Bebout, Hodgkin, Zorn, Yee, & Sammer, 1983; Bradley, 1983; McCord, 1985; Shenkman, 1985; Wright, Larsen, Monie, & Aldred, 1983). Other benefits include increased exercise tolerance and decreased number of hospital days (Wright et al., 1983). However, the usefulness of rehabilitation programs for elders has not been addressed.

The patient needs to be educated about the following components of pulmonary rehabilitation programs: breathing retraining, exercise, energy conservation, and general health maintenance, including adequate nutrition, smoking cessation, and stress management.

Breathing Exercises

Breathing retraining (BR) consists of education about COPD, chest wall muscle relaxation and movement synchronization, and pursed lip breathing. Resistive breathing training (RBT) consists of breathing continuously against a resistance several times a day (Ambrosino, Paggiaro, Roselli, & Contini, 1984). Breathing exercises (abdominal breathing, pursed lip breathing, and RBT) improve emptying of air from alveoli through coordinated use of the diaphragm and abdominal muscles. Use of pursed-lip breathing can be beneficial during periods of excitement or shortness of breath because it slows the respiratory rate and decreases the work of breathing. Respiratory muscle weakness can be a major factor limiting exercise and the ability to perform ADL (Martin, 1984).

Signs and symptoms of respiratory muscle fatigue include dyspnea, tachypnea, paradoxical chest wall and abdominal motion, altered chest excursion, and eventually elevated $PaCO_2$. Treatment includes increasing the energy supply through administration of oxygen or adequate nutrition, decreasing the work of breathing by decreasing airway resistance or congestion, decreasing energy requirements, or resting the respiratory muscles by mechanical ventilation (Braun, 1984). Breathing training can be an important aspect of therapy for elderly patients with compromised respiratory muscle function (Rochester, 1984). Further studies are needed, particularly with elders, to produce safe and consistent guidelines for respiratory muscle training prescriptions.

Exercise

Patients with breathing difficulties frequently limit activities for fear of inducing dyspnea. The deconditioning produced by inactivity results in dyspnea being induced at even lower intensity activities. With some limitations, improvement in exercise tolerance following exercise training programs in patients with COPD is fairly well established (Hughes & Davison, 1983). Specific physiologic correlates of enhanced exercise tolerance are not well defined. Studies consistently report, however, an enhanced sense of well-being following exercise training. The inability to exercise can have far-reaching negative consequences for physical independence and morale (Bradley, 1983). Mohsenifar, Horak, and Brown (1983) found significant changes in resting pulmonary function following exercise training and small but significant reductions in exercise heart rate and blood lactate levels. All patients in the study experienced a subjective enhancement of exercise tolerance and general sense of well-being, and endurance time at least doubled for every patient. Both respiratory and nonrespiratory (whole-body) muscle training have effected changes in resting pulmonary function gas exchange, exercise-induced hypoxemia, or VO_2max (Zack & Palange, 1985). A significant increase was noted in maximum workload, 12-minute walking distance, and endurance time, which, according to the cohort, translated into substantial improvements in quality of life. Tydeman, Chandler, Graveling, Culot, and Harrison (1984) found no improvement in physiologic parameters, but exercise tolerance improved as measured by the 12-minute walk test. Program participants were able to walk 1600 meters in their own time without stopping, a distance that should enable them to perform most social activities. The group took 26 to 51 weeks to reach peak performance, but the greatest improvement in performance occurred after approximately 4 weeks in the program. The exercises were easily tied to the home setting, and the improved level of functioning could be maintained at home. Because patients improved in the absence of changes in physiologic parameters, it was hypothesized that improvement was due to increased confidence and positive attitude and to the value of a group activity and support. Patients studied by Booker (1984) and by Niinimaa and Shephard (1978) also reported that, after training, they could do more, felt better, and were less afraid of becoming breathless, despite lack of clinically significant objective changes. The long-term hazards of exercise in COPD patients and all older subjects remain unclear but potentially include cardiac dysrhythmias, systemic hypotension, transient blood abnormalities, fatigue of the diaphragm, and right ventricular failure. Unresolved questions remain regarding exercise level, intensity, duration, frequency, and type. However, properly supervised exercise appears to carry little immediate risk when it is tailored to the patient's impairment, and it can substantially improve most participants' dyspnea, ADL performance, quality of life, and level of social and recreational activity (Bauldoff & Hoffman, 1977; Hughes & Davison, 1983; Zack & Palange, 1985). Improvements in social functioning could have far-reaching positive outcomes for elders.

Medication Administration

Several classes of medications are useful in patients with lung disease. Several of these medications are delivered via metered dose inhalers (MDI). An advantage of medication delivery with MDI is a reduction in the likelihood of systemic side effects (McConnell & Murphy, 1997). A reason for lack of maximal effectiveness is failure to use inhalers properly (Morris, 1990). This may be a particular problem in elders because of poor manual dexterity and cognitive impairment (McConnell & Murphy, 1997). Instruction can improve performance, and multiple sessions may be needed (McConnell & Murphy, 1997; Morris, 1990).

Oxygen also can be indicated for patients with Ineffective Breathing Pattern. Use of oxygen can prevent complications such as congestive heart failure, particularly in patients with severe hypoxia during sleep. The decision to use oxygen in the elder should be based on strict clinical and laboratory criteria. Disadvantages to home oxygen use include cost, limitation of physical activity, and the potential for CO_2 retention and oxygen toxicity (Morris, 1990).

Energy Conservation

Avoidance of dyspnea helps the elderly person to carry out ADL as independently as possible. Patients can be taught to simplify their daily routine and conserve energy through the following techniques: sitting for as many activities as possible, resting frequently during activities, alternating heavy and light tasks, breathing slowly with the diaphragm, carrying articles close to the body, and delegating tasks when possible (American Lung Association, 1995; D'Agostina, 1983).

Overall, the NIC label Ventilation Assistance is comprehensive and reflects appropriate activities for the diagnosis Ineffective Breathing Pattern. The primary criticism of the NIC label is the presence of "nesting." Specifically, several interventions seem to be included within this one intervention, as noted in Box 26-1 and in the discussion earlier in this section. This issue seems to be minor when applied to patients, that is, the patient will be unlikely to exhibit all of the defining characteristics of the diagnosis, nor will all the outcome indicators be appropriate for individual patients. Once the patient is assessed and outcome indicators are selected, the nurse selects activities within the NIC label. Should a patient require more intense or additional treatment in one area, e.g., exercise, then other appropriate NIC interventions can be prescribed, using an algorithm approach. It is recommended, however, that Breathing Retraining be added to NIC as an added intervention label.

CASE STUDY

The following NOC outcomes were chosen for Mr. Klein: Respiratory Status: Ventilation; Endurance; Anxiety Control; Energy Conservation; and Nutritional Status: Energy. Then the NIC interventions Teaching: Disease Process, Breathing Retraining, and Exercise Promotion were prescribed to promote adequate emptying of his lungs, to increase his energy level, and to reduce his anxiety level. Mr. Klein was also informed of the rationale for the interventions, of the need for adequate nutrition, and of techniques for energy conservation. The nurse instructed Mr. Klein in pursed lip breathing techniques, first while sitting and then while walking. He learned how to pace himself with this breathing technique while walking, taking two steps on inspiration and four steps on expiration. He also used a hand-held incentive spirometer four times a day for visual positive reinforcement. Mr. Klein's exercise program began with walking the length of the room and progressed to the length of the hallway 4 times per day after 1 month. Thus, for the outcome Endurance, he progressed from a rating of 1 (extremely compromised) to 2 (substantially compromised). Another client who enjoyed taking short walks began to walk with Mr. Klein, and the two would often play cards after the walking sessions. Six months later Mr. Klein was able to walk the length of the hallway without shortness of breath (endurance rated 4, mildly compromised), to stop his activity when dyspneic (energy conservation rating progressed from 1 to 5), and to use the pursed lip breathing maneuver deliberately. Although Mr. Klein's activity was still limited, he was less anxious about ambulating (Anxiety Control improved to 4, often demonstrated). He socialized more because he was able to converse without severe shortness of breath. A 5-lb weight gain was noted. Mr. Klein verbalized that he had not felt better in a long time (Nutritional Status: Energy improved to a rating of 3, moderately compromised).

SUMMARY

Nurses need to evaluate approaches to care in light of the increasing population of elders and the concomitant changes that occur with aging. Lack of awareness of these changes may lead to the assumption that pathologic changes are a part of aging and vice versa. Without an adequate knowledge base, assessment, diagnosis, and treatment may be unnecessary or inappropriate. Both practicing nurses and nursing students should receive education about the normal and pathologic changes that occur in the elder. In addition, existing treatments used in pulmonary rehabilitation programs must be tested for efficacy with elders.

REFERENCES

Altose, M. D., Leitner, J., & Cherniack, N. S. (1985). Effects of age and respiratory efforts on the perception of resistive ventilatory loads. *Journal of Gerontology, 40*(2), 147-153.

Ambrosino, N., Paggiaro, P., Roselli, M., & Contini, V. (1984). Failure of resistive breathing training to improve pulmonary function tests in patients with chronic obstructive pulmonary disease. *Respiration, 45,* 455-459.

American Lung Association. (1995). *Help yourself to better breathing.* Washington, DC: Author.

Bauldoff, G. S., & Hoffman, L. A. (1997). Teaching COPD patients upper extremity exercises at home. *Perspectives in Respiratory Nursing, 8*(2), 1-4.

Bebout, D. E., Hodgkin, J., Zorn, E., Yee, A., & Sammer, E. (1983). Clinical and physiological outcomes of a university hospital pulmonary rehabilitation program. *Respiratory Care, 28*(11), 1468-1473.

Booker, H. A. (1984). Exercise training and breathing control in patients with chronic airflow limitation. *Physiotherapy, 10*(7), 258-260.

Bradley, B. L. (1983). Rehabilitation of patients with chronic respiratory disease. *Respiratory Therapy, 13*(4), 15-21.

Brandstetter, R. D., & Kazemi, H. (1983). Aging and the respiratory system. *Medical Clinics of North America, 67*(2), 419-431.

Braun, N. (1984). Respiratory muscle dysfunction. *Heart & Lung, 13*(4), 327-332.

Capuano, T., Hitchings, K., & Johnson, S. (1990). Respiratory nursing diagnoses: Practicing nurses' selection of defining characteristics. *Nursing Diagnosis, 1*(4), 169-174.

Carlson-Catalano, J., Lunney, M., Paradiso, C., Bruno, J., Luise, B. K., Martin, T., Massoni, M., & Pachter, S. (1998). Clinical validation of ineffective breathing pattern, ineffective airway clearance, and impaired gas exchange. *IMAGE: The Journal of Nursing Scholarship, 30*(3), 243-248.

D'Agostina, J. S. (1983). You can breathe new life into your COPD patients. *Nursing, 13*(9), 72-77.

Enright, P., Adams, A., Boyle, P., & Sherrill, D. (1995). Spirometry and maximal respiratory pressure references from healthy Minnesota 65 to 85 year old women and men. *Chest, 108*(3), 663-669.

Enright, P., Kronmal, R., Higgins, M., Schenker, M., & Haponik, E. (1993). Spirometry reference values for women and men 65 to 85 years of age. *American Review of Respiratory Disease, 147,* 125-133.

Guyatt, G., Berman, L., Townsend, M., Pugsley, S., & Chambers, L. (1987). A measure of quality of life for clinical trials in chronic lung disease. *Thorax, 42,* 773-778.

Guzetta, C., Bunton, S., Prinkey, L., Sherer, A., & Seifert, P. (1989). *Clinical assessment tools for use with nursing diagnoses.* St. Louis, MO: Mosby.

Horvath, S. M., & Borgia, J. F. (1984). Cardiopulmonary gas transport and aging. *American Review of Respiratory Disease, 129,* S68-S71.

Hughes, R. L., & Davison, R. (1983). Limitations of exercise reconditioning in COPD. *Chest, 83*(2), 241-249.

Humbrecht, B., & Vanparys, E. (1982). From assessment to intervention: How to use heart and breath sounds as part of your nursing care plan. *Nursing, 12*(4), 34-41.

Iowa Intervention Project. J. C. McCloskey & G. M. Bulechek (Eds.). (2000). *Nursing interventions classification (NIC)* (3rd ed.). St. Louis, MO: Mosby.

Iowa Outcomes Project. M. Johnson, M. Maas, & S. Moorhead (Eds.). (2000). *Nursing outcomes classification (NOC)* (2nd ed.). St. Louis, MO: Mosby.

Jedrychowski, W. (1983). Biological meaning of the prospective epidemiological study on chronic obstructive lung disease and aging. *Archives of Gerontology and Geriatrics, 2,* 237-248.

Jones, P., Quirk, F., Baveystock, C., & Littlejohns, P. (1992). A self-complete measure of health status for chronic airflow limitation. *American Review of Respiratory Disease, 145,* 1321-1327.

Kim, M. J., & Larson, J. L. (1987). Ineffective airway clearance and ineffective breathing patterns: Theoretical and research base for nursing diagnosis. *Nursing Clinics of North America, 22*(1), 125-134.

Lareau, S., Breslin, E., & Meek, P. (1996). Functional status instruments: Outcome measure in the evaluation of patients with chronic obstructive lung disease. *Heart & Lung, 25,* 212-224.

Lareau, S., Carrieri-Kohlman, V., Janson-Bjerklie, S., & Roos, P. (1994). Development and testing of the pulmonary functional status and dyspnea questionnaire (PFSDQ). *Heart & Lung, 23*(3), 242-250.

Larson, J., Covey, M., Vitalo, C., Alex, C., Patel, M., & Kim, M. (1996). Reliability and validity of the 12-minute distance walk in patients with chronic obstructive pulmonary disease. *Nursing Research, 45,* 203-210.

Levitzky, M. G. (1984). Effects of aging on the respiratory system. *The Physiologist, 27*(2), 102-107.

Loveridge, B., West, P., Anthonisen, N., & Kryger, M. (1984). Breathing patterns in patients with chronic obstructive pulmonary disease. *American Review of Respiratory Disease, 130*(5), 730-733.

Maas, M., Buckwalter, K. C., & Hardy, M. (Eds.) (1991). *Nursing diagnoses and interventions for the elderly.* Redwood City, CA: Addison-Wesley Nursing.

Mahler, D., Tomlinson, D., Olmstead, E., Tosteson, A., & O'Connor, G. (1995). Changes in dyspnea, health status, and lung function in chronic airway disease. *American Journal of Respiratory and Critical Care Medicine, 151,* 61-65.

Martin, L. L. (1984). Respiratory muscle function: A clinical study. *Heart & Lung, 13*(4), 346-348.

Matteson, M., McConnell, E., & Linton, A. (1997). *Gerontological nursing: Concepts and practice* (2nd ed.). Philadelphia: W. B. Saunders.

McConnell, E., & Murphy, A. (1997). Nursing diagnoses related to physiological alterations. In M. Matteson, E. McConnell, & A. Linton (Eds.), *Gerontological nursing: Concepts and practice,* (2nd ed., pp. 407-551). Philadelphia: W. B. Saunders.

McCord, M. (1985). Nursing management of pulmonary health care services within a community hospital. *Nursing Administration Quarterly, 9*(4), 32-37.

McDonald, B. R. (1985). Validation of three respiratory nursing diagnoses. *Nursing Clinics of North America, 20*(4), 697-709.

Mohsenifar, Z., Horak, D., & Brown, H. (1983). Sensitive indices of improvement in a pulmonary rehabilitation program. *Chest, 83*(2), 189-192.

Morris, F. (1984). Pulmonary diseases. In C. K. Cassel & R. Walsh (Eds.), *Geriatric medicine* (Vol. 1, pp. 122-146). New York: Springer.

Morris, J. (1990). Pulmonary diseases. In C. Cassel, D. Riesenberg, L. Sorensen, & J. Walsh (Eds.), *Geriatric medicine* (2nd ed., pp. 362-382). New York: Springer.

Niinimaa, V., & Shephard, R. J. (1978). Training and oxygen conductance in the elderly. *Journal of Gerontology, 33*(3), 354-361.

North American Nursing Diagnosis Association. (1999). *Nursing diagnoses: Definitions & classification 1999-2000.* Philadelphia: Author.

Pashkow, R., Ades, P., Emery, C., Frid, D., Miller, N., Peske, G., Reardon, J., Shciffert, J., Southard, D., & ZuWallack, R. (1995). Outcome measurement in cardiac and pulmonary rehabilitation. *Journal of Cardiopulmonary Rehabilitation, 15,* 394-405.

Petty, T. L. (1983). Respiratory diseases. In F. U. Steinberg (Ed.), *Care of the geriatric patient* (6th ed., pp. 105-117). St. Louis, MO: Mosby.

Rantz, M., & LeMone, P. (1995). *Classification of nursing diagnoses: Proceedings of the eleventh conference.* Glendale, CA: Cinahl Information Systems.

Rochester, D. F. (1984). Respiratory muscle function in health. *Heart & Lung, 13*(4), 349-354.

Rodarte, J. (1995). The quest for normal values. *Chest, 108,* 594-595.

Rubin, S., Tack, M., & Cherniack, N. S. (1982). Effect of aging on respiratory responses to CO_2 and inspiratory resistive loads. *Journal of Gerontology, 37,* 306-312.

Shenkman, B. (1985). Factors contributing to attrition rates in a pulmonary rehabilitation program. *Heart & Lung, 14*(1), 53-58.

Silvestri, G., & Mahler, D. (1993). Evaluation of dyspnea in the elderly patient. *Clinics in Chest Medicine, 14*(3), 393-404.

Sjoberg, E. L. (1983). Nursing diagnosis and the COPD patient. *American Journal of Nursing, 83*(2), 245-248.

Tydeman, D. E., Chandler, A., Graveling, B., Culot, A., & Harrison, B. (1984). An investigation into the effects of exercise training on patients with chronic airway obstruction. *Physiotherapy, 70*(7), 261-264.

Wahba, W. M. (1983). Influence of aging on lung function—clinical significance of changes from age twenty. *Anesthesia Analgesia, 62,* 764-776.

Wright, R. W., Larsen, D. F., Monie, R. G., & Aldred, R. A. (1983). Benefits of a community-hospital pulmonary rehabilitation program. *Respiratory Care, 28*(11), 1474-1479.

York, K. (1985). Clinical validation of two respiratory nursing diagnoses and their defining characteristics. *Nursing Clinics of North America, 20*(4), 657-668.

Zack, M. B., & Palange, A. V. (1985). Oxygen supplement exercise of ventilatory and nonventilatory muscles in pulmonary rehabilitation. *Chest, 88*(5), 669-675.

CHAPTER 27

ACTIVITY INTOLERANCE

Marita G. Titler

As the population of the United States continues to age, maintenance of independent living among older adults becomes an increasingly broad challenge (Cherubini et al., 1998). In terms of medical dollars spent, the burden on the health care system caused by physical inactivity and its related cardiovascular morbidity is substantial. Some health care providers have shifted their emphasis from treating chronic disease to helping older adults maintain an independent lifestyle.

Activity Intolerance is a broad category of responses to various intensities of physical activity. Although functional aerobic capacity decreases with age, the rate of this decline is less for active persons than for sedentary persons (Larson & Bruce, 1987). Thus, determining those at risk for Activity Intolerance and providing early treatment are necessary to prevent functional decline.

Lack of physical activity is associated with increased morbidity and mortality and with decreased quality of life. The consequences of declining activity in elderly persons include increased cardiovascular and respiratory disease, increased falls and confusion, increased depression, decreased role performance and self-esteem, and premature institutionalization (Reynolds & Garrett, 1992).

Prevention of physical deterioration and care for those in physical decline are within the scope of nursing practice. The nursing diagnosis Activity Intolerance is applicable to those individuals who are at risk for or who are experiencing a decline in their ability to carry out required or desired daily activities.

RELATED FACTORS/ETIOLOGIES

Etiologies of Activity Intolerance can be conceptualized in several ways. The North American Nursing Diagnosis Association (NANDA) has listed the following related factors: (1) bed rest/immobility; (2) generalized weakness; (3) sedentary lifestyle; and (4) imbalance between oxygen supply and demand. Williams (1987) suggested two major categories of related factors for Activity Intolerance: (1) acute and chronic disease and (2) prior lifestyle behaviors. Chronic diseases common in elders include cardiovascular disease, respiratory disease, neoplastic disease, and neurologic impairment. Lifestyle behaviors, psychosocial factors, and situational limitations imposed by the individual's physical environment also have been explicated as etiologies of Activity Intolerance (Frantz & Ferrell-Torry, 1993; MacLean, 1989, 1992; Thompson, McFarland, Hirsch, & Tucker, 1997). This chapter conceptualizes etiologies and related factors for Activity Intolerance into the following categories: (1) acute or chronic illness, (2) lifestyle behaviors, (3) situational (environmental) limitations, and (4) psychologic factors (Box 27-1).

Acute and chronic illnesses contribute to Activity Intolerance via pathologic changes associated with the underlying disease. The pathology contributes to Activity Intolerance by interfering with energy production, by interfering with the neurologic control of mobility, and/or by compromising the musculoskeletal system directly (Frantz & Ferrell-Torry, 1993; Tang, Moore, & Woollacott, 1998). Cell function and activity require energy expenditure. Thus, activity is compromised when there is a critical imbalance between energy supply (e.g., cardiopulmonary disease) and demand (e.g., hyperthermia). Energy deficit is caused by limitations in oxygen and nutrients for production of adenosine triphosphate (ATP). Likewise, energy production is compromised when the byproducts of cellular metabolism are not eliminated properly through the gastrointestinal, renal, or cardiopulmonary system. Acute and chronic illnesses also contribute to activity intolerance by compromising neurologic functioning (e.g., Parkinson's disease) or the integrity of the musculoskeletal system (e.g., osteoarthritis) (Kaya, Krebs, & Riley, 1998). In addition to the underlying pathology, illness can contribute to Activity Intolerance through the treatment of side effects such as bed rest, immobility, pain, and adverse pharmacologic effects. Inappropriate use of physical restraints and medical immobilization are two additional treatment factors that limit activity in the elder.

Lifestyle behaviors that result in decreased activity tolerance include sedentary living (Schut, 1998), weight gain, obesity, poor nutrition, smoking, alcohol consumption, and high stress. These variables can contribute to the development of chronic disease and/or worsen an existing chronic illness, thereby contributing to Activity Intolerance.

Situational limitations (environmental factors) contribute to Activity Intolerance when, for example, appropriate structural supports, such as handrails, walkers, or other assistive devices, are not available to encourage par-

Box 27-1	Related Factors/Etiologies ACTIVITY INTOLERANCE

Acute or Chronic Illness
Imbalance between oxygen supply/demand

- Decrease in oxygen transport
- Decrease in nutrition
- Impaired elimination
- Increase in metabolic demand

Neurologic impairment

- Cognitive deficits
- Central nervous system changes
- Structural (e.g., atrophy of dendrites)
- Functional (e.g., neurotransmitters)

Decline or loss of peripheral nerve function

- Musculoskeletal impairment
- Alteration in muscle strength
- Degeneration in joint structures
- Joint pain
- Decline in bone mass

Treatment side effects

- Bed rest
- Immobility
- Pain
- Fatigue
- Physical restraints
- Medical immobilization
- Pharmacologic side effects

Lifestyle Behaviors
Sedentary living
Weight gain or loss
Obesity
Poor nutrition
Smoking
Alcohol consumption

Situational (Environmental) Limitations
Lack of structural supports
Climate extremes
Small living area
Limited access to exercise
Facilities

Psychologic Factors
Lack of social support

- Isolation
- Loneliness

Emotional factors

- Fear of falling
- Anxiety
- Hopelessness

Loss of autonomy and control

- Low self-efficacy regarding activity engagement
- Depression
- Cognitive impairment

ticipation in daily activities. Psychosocial factors such as lack of social support, isolation, fear of falling, low self-efficacy regarding activity engagement, depression, anxiety, hopelessness, loss of autonomy and control, cognitive impairment, and loneliness all contribute to Activity Intolerance in the elder. In addition, there is an overriding myth that minimal activity is the acceptable norm with aging, and thus sufficient economic resources are not committed to prevent and treat activity intolerance in elders (Cherubini et al., 1998; Mazzeo et al., 1998).

ASSESSMENT

A complete review of patient medical history and a thorough health assessment are essential to diagnosing Activity Intolerance (Fuller & Schaller-Ayers, 1990; Kane, Ouslander, & Abrass, 1994; Rubenfeld & McFarlane, 1988). The patient's previous experience with activity and difficulties related to increased activity levels provide critical information needed to evaluate the risk for development of Activity Intolerance. Health assessments should focus specifically on determining the presence of chronic or progressive conditions that place the patient at risk for

Activity Intolerance; these conditions must be considered during the development of an appropriate intervention program. Cardiovascular, respiratory, musculoskeletal, and neurologic conditions are particularly relevant to the development of activity deficits (Cherubini et al., 1998; Chyun, Ford, & Yursha-Johnston, 1991; Ignatavicius & Bayne, 1991; Kane et al., 1994; Lancaster & Rice, 1990; Mazzeo et al., 1998).

Although no comprehensive assessment forms measure activity tolerance directly, several related tools are helpful. These tools are based on self-report, observation, or caregiver reports of physical functioning with regard to activities of daily living (ADL) and instrumental activities of daily living (IADL). Grading of ADL performance is usually divided into three levels of dependency: (1) ability to perform tasks without human assistance; (2) ability to perform the task with some assistance; and (3) inability to perform even with assistance. The Katz Index and the Barthel Index are two tools commonly used to assess a person's ability to carry out basic tasks needed for self-care (Kane et al., 1994).

Tasks that require a combination of physical and cognitive ability (IADL) can be assessed using a variety of observation or self-report instruments (Kane & Kane, 1981). Reuben's Physical Performance Scale (Reuben, Siu, & Kimpau, 1992) and Lawton's Instrumental Activities of Daily Living Scale (Lawton & Brody, 1969) are examples of such instruments (Kane et al., 1994). Reuben's scale has been shown to have some predictive validity in terms of risk of decline and death in the geriatric population (Reuben et al., 1992).

Numerous other assessment tools incorporate self-reported ability to do specific activities such as walking on level ground, walking a flight of stairs, and participating in leisure activities (Cress et al., 1999; Kane & Kane, 1981; Spilker, 1996; Tang, Moore, & Woollacott, 1998). For example, the Iowa Self Assessment Inventory, a brief self-report instrument designed to measure the resources, needs, statuses, and abilities of older people, includes a mobility scale (Morris, Andrews, Gilmer, & Buckwalter, 1994). As noted by Kane and colleagues (1994), standard instruments are useful guides for assessment, but they also have certain pitfalls, insufficient sensitivity to measure change over time, and discrepancies in responses between different informants. In addition, the manner in which questions are asked (e.g., performance versus capability) is critically important and influences the response of elders and their family members.

The following physiologic tests are helpful in assessing activity tolerance: exercise stress test, 6-minute walk distance test, gait velocity test, and strength test. No single method is available to evaluate total body muscle strength and endurance because muscle strength and endurance are muscle group specific (Reimers, Harder, & Saxe, 1998; Topp, Mikesky, & Bawel, 1994).

Exercise stress testing is used to measure a variety of physiologic variables regarding physical fitness: resting, submaximal, and maximal heart rate; resting and submaximal blood pressure; maximum oxygen consumption; maximum exercise time; and maximum exercise workload. Exercise stress testing can be done on a cycle ergometer or treadmill. The exact protocol may vary by practitioner but usually involves an initial workload (e.g., 25 watts) and an increase in workload (e.g., 25 watts) every 2 minutes up to reported exhaustion or maximal heart rate (Pate et al., 1991; Stevenson & Topp, 1990). Tanji (1991) notes that not all persons over 65 require an exercise stress test before beginning an exercise program. Based on the American College of Sports Medicine guidelines (Pate et al., 1991), it is recommended that such testing be used with all symptomatic persons, with those who are asymptomatic but who have multiple cardiovascular risk factors, and with those who are asymptomatic with no cardiovascular risk factors but who plan to enter a vigorous exercise program. This screening test is probably not essential for asymptomatic persons without cardiovascular risk who pursue a moderate intensity exercise program such as walking. However, these individuals should obtain the consent of their health care provider before beginning even a moderate intensity exercise program (Tanji, 1991; Topp et al., 1994). Administering an exercise stress test provides an accurate assessment of maximal heart rate and fitness level. Maximal heart rate varies considerably from one person to another, and estimation using the standard equation (predicted maximal heart rate equals 220 beats per minute minus age) can be notoriously inaccurate (Tanji, 1991).

The 6-minute walk distance test requires that the individual walk on a flat surface such as an indoor track or hallway. Individuals proceed at their own pace but attempt to walk the greatest distance in 6 minutes. The distance walked in 6 minutes is measured. It is recommended that at least two practice sessions be performed before using this test as an assessment.

Gait velocity is the average speed (meters walked per second) walked over a 3-meter portion of a 10-meter course (Topp, Mikesky, Wigglesworth, Holt, & Edwards, 1993). The assessment protocol for measuring gait velocity is described elsewhere (Blanke & Hageman, 1989; Topp et al., 1993).

Muscle strength is commonly evaluated using various one-repetition maximum weight-lifting tests. Muscles in the hand are evaluated using a hand dynamometer, muscles in the arms and chest are evaluated using a bench press, and muscles in the legs are evaluated using a leg press (Topp et al., 1994).

NURSING DIAGNOSIS

Campbell (1978) categorized levels of activity that could be tolerated by an individual. A *minimum level* of activity tolerance was defined as "the inability to tolerate any physical activity without the presence of discomforts." A *mild level* of activity tolerance was defined as "the ability to tolerate only a very limited amount of physical activity without the presence of discomforts." A *moderate level* of activity tolerance was defined as "the ability to tolerate a moderate, but not a full day of physical activity without the presence of discomfort."

NANDA has chosen to focus not on activity tolerance but rather on activity intolerance. NANDA has formulated a nursing diagnosis Activity Intolerance and defined it as "a state in which an individual has insufficient physiological or psychological energy to endure or complete required or desired daily activities" (NANDA, 1999, p. 88). Activity Intolerance has been identified as an important area of nursing treatment in acute, rehabilitative, ambulatory, and long-term care settings (MacLean, 1992; McKeighen, Mehmert, & Dickel, 1991; Mol & Baker, 1991). However, there is little empirical work to guide nurses in the appropriate use of this diagnostic label, particularly in the aging population.

Box 27-2	Defining Characteristics ACTIVITY INTOLERANCE

Physiologic Measures
Blood pressure

- Change in 15 mm Hg or greater from baseline diastolic blood pressure
- Decrease in blood pressure
- Failure of blood pressure to increase with activity
- Diastolic blood pressure greater than 120 mm Hg
- Systolic blood pressure greater than 250 mm Hg

Heart rate

- Increase of 20 beats above baseline
- Change from regular to irregular heart rhythm
- Weakening pulse strength
- Decrease in heart rate
- Failure of heart rate to return to within 6 beats of resting by 3 minutes after ceasing activity

ECG changes

- Ventricular dysrhythmias
- Ventricular fibrillation
- Ventricular tachycardia more than 3 consecutive beats
- Second- or third-degree heart block
- Multifocal premature beats
- ST segment greater than 2.0 mm
- Couples premature ventricular contractions, three to four during exercise
- Premature ventricular contractions greater than 10%-20% of beats

Respiratory

- Labored breathing
- Excessive increase in respiratory rate
- Decrease in respiratory rate
- Cyanosis
- Pallor

Observational Cues
Confusion
Redness of skin
Change of skin temperature from warm to cool
Profuse diaphoresis
Syncope
Drooping shoulders
Progressive slowing of activity
Decreased dexterity
Worried or uneasy facial expression
Tremor
Irritability
Increase in number of requested rest periods
Sighing during activity
Decline in ADL
Decline in IADL

Self-Report Measures
Fatigue
Exertional dyspnea
Weakness
Chest pain/angina
Dizziness/vertigo

Adapted from Mol, V. J., & Baker, C. A. (1991). Activity intolerance in the geriatric stroke patient. *Rehabilitation Nursing, 16,* 337-342.
Italics = Critical as defined by NANDA.

Defining Characteristics

The critical defining characteristics of Activity Intolerance set forth by NANDA are (1) verbal report of fatigue or weakness, (2) abnormal heart rate or blood pressure response to activity, (3) exertional discomfort or dyspnea, and (4) electrocardiographic changes reflecting dysrhythmia or ischemia (NANDA, 1999, p. 89). Box 27-2 lists several defining characteristics of Activity Intolerance; critical cues, as defined by NANDA, are italicized. However, a reliable and valid list of cues for clinical use in diagnosing Activity Intolerance has not yet been achieved. Little research has been done to validate the defining characteristics of Activity Intolerance, and the majority of studies have focused on cardiac patients (MacLean, 1989; Mol & Baker, 1991).

Mol and Baker (1991) tested the defining characteristics of Activity Intolerance in a geriatric stroke population

($n = 32$ men, 1 woman). The following defining characteristics occurred with the highest frequency in this study: progressive slowing of ambulation; decreased dexterity with ambulation; failure of the heart rate to return to within 6 beats per minute of the baseline at 3 minutes postactivity; an increase of greater than 20 beats per minute in heart rate; and reported weakness. Decreased dexterity and progressive slowing of ambulation occurred regardless of the presence of other defining characteristics and often in conjunction with each other. Table 27-1 shows how the subjective characteristics dyspnea, required rest, dizziness, and weakness occurred with objective changes in blood pressure, heart rate, and respiratory rate (Mol & Baker, 1991).

Some elders who suffer from Activity Intolerance might not display some of the physiologic changes indicative of this diagnosis because of their pharmacologic treat-

Table 27-1	Association Between Significant Subjective and Objective Defining Characteristics
Significant Subjective Characteristics	**Associated Objective Characteristics**
Dizziness	Use of support Increased diastolic blood pressure (BP)
Dyspnea	Use of support Drooping shoulders Increased diastolic BP Increased heart rate Change from regular to irregular heart rhythm Failure of heart rate to return to resting rate within 3 minutes Irregular respiratory pattern
Required rest	Drooping shoulders Increased heart rate Increased respiratory rate Failure of heart rate to return to resting rate within 3 minutes Irregular respiratory pattern
Weakness	Increased respiratory rate Change from regular to irregular heart rhythm Irregular respiratory pattern

From Mol, V. J., & Baker, C. A. (1991). Activity intolerance in the geriatric stroke patient. *Rehabilitation Nursing, 16,* 337-342.

ment regimens (e.g., beta blockers). Further research will be needed to test diagnostic cues of Activity Intolerance both in well elders and in elders experiencing a variety of acute and chronic illnesses.

In addition, Activity Intolerance is a broad diagnostic label that overlaps with other diagnostic labels, including Decreased Cardiac Output, Altered Tissue Perfusion, and Impaired Physical Mobility. To clearly distinguish Activity Intolerance from these other diagnoses, clinicians will need clear guidelines regarding essential diagnostic cues.

CASE STUDY

T. Jones, a 70-year-old widowed housewife, was admitted to the ambulatory surgery center of a community hospital in preparation for a small bowel resection. Mrs. Jones had undergone an abdominal peritoneal resection in 1989 with follow-up radiation and chemotherapy for cancer. Subsequently, she managed her own colostomy and lived independently with minimal assistance from her children for strenuous activities such as mowing the grass, raking leaves, and washing the car. She played bridge 3 times per week, did her own grocery shopping, and was able to climb one flight of stairs with minimal difficulty. Mrs. Jones was 5 feet 7 inches tall, weighed 180 lb, and had a history of recurrent urinary tract infections. Mrs. Jones underwent the small bowel resection without apparent complications. She was discharged 1 week after surgery with instructions to increase her activity gradually over the next 2 weeks, to lift minimal weight less than 5 pounds, and to schedule an appointment to be seen in 1 week by her surgeon.

Within a week of discharge, Mrs. Jones was readmitted to the same hospital with peritoneal abscesses. She was weak and able to ambulate less than 100 feet without stopping to catch her breath. A tube was inserted through her gluteus maximus to drain the peritoneal abscess, and she was placed on intravenous antibiotic therapy. Mrs. Jones was permitted to undertake "activity as tolerated." She needed assistance with her bath because of fatigue and had difficulty moving about her room because of her intravenous and peritoneal drainage tubing. In preparation for discharge, the nursing staff decided to encourage Mrs. Jones to be out of bed more and to walk in the hall. However, when she walked to the door of her room and back to bed, Mrs. Jones complained of shortness of breath, "flip-flopping" of her heart, and feeling weak and dizzy. Nurses observed the following during this ambulation episode: sighing during walking; stopping three times to catch her breath; a change in blood pressure from 130/88 mm Hg before walking to 100/65 mm Hg during and following ambulation; an increase in heart rate from 100 beats per minute at rest to 140 beats per minute; an increase in respiratory rate from 26 to 40 breaths per minute; pallor, diaphoresis, and circumoral cyanosis. In a closer examination of her laboratory findings, the staff noted her hemoglobin was 8.0.

NURSING-SENSITIVE OUTCOMES

Nursing interventions for Activity Intolerance will vary depending on the patient outcomes that are desired. Patient outcomes can reflect changes in physiologic status (e.g., vital signs), changes in functional status, and changes in knowledge or behavior. Patient outcomes and associated indicators can be assessed through various methods, such as the use of nurse reports, patient record audits, patient self-reports, or family member reports. Self-reports of patients and/or family members are equally as important as physiologic indicators and provide some motivation for patients to continue their exercise program. Patient perceptions of less fatigue and weakness along with improvements in the ability to do ADL and IADL are important indications that activity tolerance is improving. This often leads to improved self-efficacy for activities, which in turn motivates patients to continue with their exercise program.

The *Nursing Outcomes Classification (NOC)* (Iowa Outcomes Project, 2000) provides a useful guide to the measurement of patient outcomes. The following NOC patient outcomes are useful to assess the effectiveness of interventions for Activity Intolerance:

- Vital Signs Status—Temperature, pulse, respiration, and blood pressure within expected range for the individual (p. 440)
- Symptom Severity—Extent of perceived adverse changes in physical, emotional, and social functioning (p. 420)
- Cardiac Pump Effectiveness—Extent to which blood is ejected from the left ventricle per minute to support systemic perfusion pressure (p. 136)
- Muscle Function—Adequacy of muscle contraction needed for movement (p. 308)
- Balance—Ability to maintain body equilibrium (p. 120)
- Endurance—Extent that energy enables a person to sustain activity (p. 204)
- Joint Movement: Active—Range of motion of joints with self-initiated movement (p. 251)
- Joint Movement: Passive—Range of motion of joints with assisted movement (p. 252)
- Ambulation: Walking—Ability to walk from place to place (p. 114)
- Ambulation: Wheelchair—Ability to move from place to place in a wheelchair (p. 115)
- Self-Care: Activities of Daily Living (ADL)—Ability to perform the most basic physical tasks and personal care activities (p. 379)
- Self Care: Instrumental Activities of Daily Living (IADL)—Ability to perform activities needed to function in the home or community (p. 385)
- Energy Conservation—Extent of active management of energy to initiate and sustain activity (p. 205)
- Knowledge: Energy Conservation—Extent of understanding conveyed about energy conservation techniques (p. 264)
- Knowledge: Prescribed Activity—Extent of understanding conveyed about prescribed activity and exercise (p. 289)
- Adherence Behavior—Self-initiated action taken to promote wellness, recovery, and rehabilitation (p. 110)

The reader is referred to the NOC text for a complete listing of indicators for each outcome.

Indicators for the outcomes Vital Signs Status, Symptom Severity, and Cardiac Pump Effectiveness should be monitored during an activity progression and exercise training as short-term measures of activity tolerance. These outcomes reflect improvements in the defining characteristics noted under physiologic measures, observational cues, and self-report measures in Table 27-1.

For example, it is imperative that nurses monitor blood pressure, heart rate, dyspnea, weakness, and other indicators as older adults increase their activity progression and exercise intensity to ensure that the increased workload is tolerated. The following patient outcomes and their associated indicators should improve over time as patients increase their progress in an exercise program: Muscle Function, Balance, Endurance, Joint Movement: Active, Joint Movement: Passive, Ambulation: Walking, Ambulation: Wheelchair, Self-Care: Activities of Daily Living (ADL), and Self-Care: Instrumental Activities of Daily Living (IADL). These are longer term outcomes and reflect that the defining characteristics noted in Table 27-1 are improving. For example, as the individual engages in more physical activity and if health is maintained, the individual will exhibit less postural limitation (e.g., the head and shoulders will droop less), muscles will exhibit stronger tone and flexibility, gait movements will show balance, and strength in the lower extremities will improve. The patient outcomes Energy Conservation, Knowledge: Energy Conservation, Knowledge: Prescribed Activity, and Adherence Behavior: Self-Initiated are useful for monitoring the effectiveness of interventions related to teaching, goal setting, contracting, and socialization.

NURSING INTERVENTIONS

Interventions to decrease Activity Intolerance are numerous and should be chosen to suit the needs of each individual. Characteristics to consider during the development of a tailored intervention program include age, previous physical activity history, individual preferences for type of activity, and physical and mental health status and comorbidity. It is essential that medical treatment for any underlying pathology contributing to Activity Intolerance be optimized before or in conjunction with initiating an exercise or ambulation program.

The major nursing interventions for treating Activity Intolerance in elders are classified within the Activity and Exercise Management Class of the *Nursing Interventions Classification (NIC)* (Iowa Intervention Project, 2000). This set of nursing interventions focuses on physical activity, energy expenditure, and use of an individualized exercise program. These interventions are as follows:

- Body Mechanics Promotion—Facilitating the use of posture and movement in daily activities to prevent fatigue and musculoskeletal strain or injury (Iowa Intervention Project, 2000, p. 184)
- Energy Management—Regulating energy use to treat or prevent fatigue and optimize function (p. 302)
- Exercise Promotion—Facilitation of regular physical exercise to maintain or advance to a higher level of fitness and health (p. 316)

- Exercise Promotion: Stretching—Facilitation of systematic slow-stretch-hold muscle exercises to induce relaxation, to prepare muscles/joints for more vigorous exercise, or to increase or maintain body flexibility (p. 319)
- Exercise Therapy: Ambulation—Promotion and assistance with walking to maintain or restore autonomic and voluntary body functions during treatment and recovery from illness or injury (p. 320)
- Exercise Therapy: Balance—Use of specific activities, postures, and movements to maintain, enhance, or restore balance (p. 321)
- Exercise Therapy: Joint Mobility—Use of active or passive body movement to maintain or restore joint flexibility (p. 322)
- Exercise Therapy: Muscle Control—Use of specific activity or exercise protocols to enhance or restore controlled body movement (p. 323)
- Teaching: Prescribed Activity/Exercise—Preparing a patient to achieve and/or maintain a prescribed level of activity (p. 648)

In addition, interventions in the Immobility Management Class (interventions to manage restricted body movement and the sequel) are important to prevent Activity Intolerance from developing in the elderly population (see Chapter 28). These interventions are as follows:

- Bed Rest Care—Promotion of comfort and safety and prevention of complications for a patient unable to get out of bed (Iowa Intervention Project, 2000, p. 158)
- Cast Care: Maintenance—Care of a cast after the drying period (p. 203)
- Cast Care: Wet—Care of a new cast during the drying period (p. 204)
- Physical Restraint—Application, monitoring, and removal of mechanical restraining devices or manual restraints that are used to limit physical mobility of patient (p. 510)
- Positioning—Deliberative placement of the patient or a body part to promote physiologic and/or psychologic well-being (p. 514)
- Positioning: Wheelchair—Placement of a patient in a properly selected wheelchair to enhance comfort, promote skin integrity, and foster independence (p. 518)
- Splinting—Stabilization, immobilization, and/or protection of an injured body part with a supportive appliance (p. 608)
- Traction/Immobilization Care—Management of a patient who has traction and/or a stabilizing device to immobilize and stabilize a body part (p. 670)
- Transport—Moving a patient from one location to another (p. 672)

For example, prolonged bed rest following a stroke with concomitant decreased muscle strength and disuse atrophy, decreased cardiopulmonary reserve, and depression can contribute to compromised oxygen transport, fatigue, and thus Activity Intolerance (Mol & Baker, 1991).

Research on Exercise and Older Adults

Despite the demonstrated benefits of Exercise Promotion and Exercise Therapy in elderly individuals (Cress et al., 1999; Ettinger, 1998; Mazzeo et al., 1998; Reimers, Harder, & Saxe, 1998), only 30% of persons over the age of 65 report exercising regularly (Kane et al., 1994). Studies on exercise in elderly persons have focused principally on endurance training, strength training, balance and movement, or some combination thereof. Studies on endurance training have consistently documented improvements in exercise endurance (relative aerobic requirements of functioning at any given submaximal level of exercise are less), function (ADL, IADL), range of motion, vitality (less fatigue), quality of life, well-being, and prolonged active life expectancy (Cress et al., 1999; Gillett et al., 1993; Hamdorf, Withers, Penhall, & Haslam, 1992; Jirovec, 1991; Misner, Massey, Bemben, Going, & Patrick, 1992; Naso, Carner, Blankfort-Doyle, & Coughey, 1990; Reimers, Harder, & Saxe, 1998; Stevenson & Topp, 1990). In addition, some evidence suggests that regular habitual exercise in elders lowers the age-specific incidence of falls (Reynolds & Garrett, 1992; Schnelle et al., 1996; Wolf et al., 1996). Studies vary in sample size, exercise intensity, type (groups versus single) and location (supervised and unsupervised). Despite these methodological issues, low and moderate intensity endurance training is beneficial for institutionalized and community-based elders (Hamdorf et al., 1992; Jirovec, 1991; Misner et al., 1992; Naso et al., 1990; Schnelle et al., 1996; Stevenson & Topp, 1990).

Similarly, the following beneficial effects of strength training in older adults have been demonstrated: improvements in dynamic strength, maximal workload capacity, dynamic balance, walking velocity, and functional mobility (Ettinger, 1998; Hunter et al., 1995; Mazzeo et al., 1998; Munnings, 1993; Topp et al., 1994; Topp et al., 1993; Wolf et al., 1996; Wolfson et al., 1996; Work, 1989). Older adults can reverse some of the declines in muscle strength that accompany aging through strength and balance training (Reimers, Harder, & Saxe, 1998; Topp et al., 1993; Topp et al., 1994; Wolfson et al., 1996).

A series of studies that combined strength and endurance training with balance and foot/hand-eye coordination exercises documented benefits in balance, neuromuscular control, and muscle strength (Cress et al., 1999; Lord & Castell, 1994; Lord, Castell, & Dip, 1994; Lord, Ward, & Williams, 1996). This series of studies, along with those previously cited, suggest that exercise programs offer older persons a means of keeping physically active and help prevent age-dependent impairments, even when they suffer from moderate disorders (Cherubini et al., 1998; Cress et al., 1999; Ettinger, 1998; Mazzeo et al., 1998; Reimers, Harder, & Saxe, 1998).

Principles and Guidelines for Exercise

Although a comprehensive discussion of how to prescribe and develop an exercise program for the elderly individual is beyond the scope of this chapter, basic principles are reviewed and the reader is referred to several sources for further information (Mazzeo et al., 1998; Pate et al., 1991; Siegel, Brackbill, & Heath, 1995; Swart, Pollock, & Brechue, 1996; Tanji, 1991; Topp et al., 1993; Topp et al., 1994). To improve cardiorespiratory fitness, an exercise program should include the following components: (1) maintaining rhythmic, aerobic use of large muscle groups for a period of time; (2) an exercise intensity between 40% and 85% of VO_2max or 55% to 90% of maximal heart rate; (3) a duration of 15 to 60 minutes of continuous or discontinuous aerobic activity; (4) a frequency of 3 to 5 days per week; and (5) a rate of progression to increase the amount of total work done per session. These components are interdependent (Pate et al., 1991).

Use of exercise to improve function should be guided by the following set of principles:

- Warm-up and cool-down phases (5 to 15 minutes) should be incorporated into all exercise programs.
- The training phase (20 to 30 minutes) should work the muscles beyond what is encountered in regular daily activities.
- Because muscles adapt to a given workload, the workload should be gradually increased to achieve and maintain a desired level of fitness.
- Muscle adaptation is specific to the muscles trained.
- Individual differences exist in how people respond to a training program.
- Self-assessment or assessment by a health care provider should be a part of the exercise program.

An exercise prescription for people over 65 consists of training in the areas of stretching, aerobics/endurance training, strength training, and coordination (Tanji, 1991). Stretching exercises consist of warm up by stretching muscles and joint rotation to decrease the incidence of muscle strain. Stretching exercises should be done for 5 to 15 minutes before and after each workout (Allan, 1992; Tanji, 1991). Aerobic training consists of 20 to 30 minutes of activity repeated 3 or 4 times per week at approximately 70% of the maximal heart rate. Deciding on the initial exercise intensity is important to improve function without causing injury or excessive fatigue. There is some evidence that a low-intensity exercise program is still beneficial in improving function for those over 65 years of age. Most experts in exercise with older adults suggest beginning exercise intensity at 50% to 60% of maximum heart rate and then gradually increasing the intensity to 60% to 70%. Achieving greater than 70% maximal heart rate is encouraged only when people are able to easily obtain 70% of their maximum heart rate.

Strength training in elders is beneficial to strengthen weakened muscles and, thereby, decrease falls and improve balance and mobility among older persons (Mazzeo et al., 1998; Munnings, 1993; Reimers, Harder, & Saxe, 1998; Topp et al., 1994; Work, 1989). One of the most important considerations in strength training is the amount of resistance used for a specific exercise (Munnings, 1993). An individual usually is started at some percent (30% to 80%) of repetition maximum (1 RM is the maximum resistance a person can lift once but cannot lift again). The standard recommendation is three resistance-training sessions per week for each muscle group, performed on alternate days (Munnings, 1993). Experts differ somewhat on whether to use machines, free weights, or elastic bands. Most importantly, a system must be available to progressively increase the resistance as the individual gets stronger. People also need to be taught how to breathe properly when performing strength training exercises to overcome the tendency to hold their breath while lifting the weight. This can be achieved by exhaling when the weight is lifted and inhaling when lowering the weight (Munnings, 1993). Strength training exercises designed specifically for older adults, detailing the muscle groups affected and associated improvements in function, are available (Topp et al., 1994). Guidelines for strength training are summarized in Box 27-3.

Box 27-3	Guidelines for Strength Training

Train selective muscle groups. Those used for mobility (e.g., hip and knee extensors) should be emphasized.
Establish goals related to improvement in functioning (ADL, IADL).
Warm up before and cool down after each training session.
Train 3 to 4 days per week with 1 day of rest in-between.
Use light weights to begin with and work up to heavier ones.
Train at a moderate intensity.
Learn proper exercise and breathing techniques.
If people are more than pleasantly tired the day after exercise, they are probably doing too much.

Data from Work, J. A. (1989). Strength training: A bridge to independence for the elderly. *The Physician and Sportsmedicine, 17*(11), 134-140.

Box 27-4 Nursing Treatments
ACTIVITY INTOLERANCE

Core NIC Labels	Consider Use of These NIC
Body Mechanics Promotion	Labels
Exercise Therapy:	Exercise Therapy: Balance
Ambulation	Exercise Therapy:
Exercise Therapy:	Muscle Control
Joint Mobility	Exercise Promotion:
Energy Management	Endurance
Teaching: Prescribed	Exercise Promotion: Strength
Activity/Exercise	Exercise Promotion:
Mutual Goal Setting	Coordination
Patient Contracting	Self-Modification Assistance
	Socialization Enhancement

Coordination training consists of exercises to improve hand-eye coordination and feet-eye coordination. Lateral moves, acceleration, and deceleration movements are examples of activities used to improve coordination.

Use of the *Nursing Interventions Classification (NIC)*

Nursing interventions applicable for most elderly people with the nursing diagnosis Activity Intolerance include Energy Management; Exercise Therapy: Ambulation; Exercise Therapy: Joint Mobility, and Body Mechanics Promotion (Iowa Intervention Project, 2000). These interventions are necessary to assist individuals to (1) space physical activities to avoid fatigue, (2) walk to improve or maintain mobility, (3) exercise joints to enhance joint flexibility, and (4) use appropriate sitting and movement in daily activities to avoid fatigue and prevent injury. The intervention Teaching: Prescribed Activity/Exercise should be considered for all older people to promote understanding of exercises to prevent and/or treat Activity Intolerance. Additionally, consideration should be given to the interventions Exercise Therapy: Balance and Exercise Therapy: Muscle Control, depending on the presence of comorbid conditions.

The nursing intervention Exercise Promotion is a broad intervention applicable both to older people who are in relatively good health and to those rehabilitating from illness. Consideration should be given to refining this single intervention into the following more specific interventions: Exercise Promotion: Endurance, Exercise Promotion: Strength, and Exercise Promotion: Coordination.

Adherence to an exercise regimen can have a major impact on recovery from Activity Intolerance. Nonadherence of individuals to medical recommendations also is a serious concern for all health care professionals. The reader is referred to Chapter 7 for a complete discussion of interventions to promote adherence behavior in elderly persons. In relation to exercise, Mutual Goal Setting is defined as "collaborating with patient to identify and prioritize care goals, then developing a plan for achieving those goals" (Iowa Intervention Project, 2000, p. 462), Self-Modification Assistance is the "reinforcement of self-directed change initiated by the patient to achieve personally important goals" (p. 581), Socialization Enhancement is the "facilitation of another person's ability to interact with others" (p. 604), Patient Contracting helps in "negotiating an agreement with a patient which reinforces a specific behavior change" (p. 494), and Teaching: Prescribed Activity/Exercise assists in "preparing a patient to achieve and/or maintain a prescribed level of activity" (p. 648). These interventions help promote adherence to activity progression in elders (Allan, 1992; Gillett et al., 1993). NIC interventions that are core or central for treatment of Activity Intolerance and interventions that, though not central, should be considered for use are distinguished in Box 27-4.

CASE STUDY

Mrs. Jones's nurse made the nursing diagnosis Activity Intolerance related to imbalance between energy supply and demand, treatment side effects (bed rest, limited mobility), and environmental limitations. The following outcomes were projected: Symptom Severity, Cardiac Pump Effectiveness, and Vital Signs Status. The interventions prescribed to meet these outcomes were Exercise Therapy: Ambulation, Energy Management, Body Mechanics Promotion, and Exercise Therapy: Joint Mobility. Specific activities for each intervention and specific indicators for each outcome are in Table 27-2. The interventions Mutual Goal Setting; Exercise Promotion: Endurance; and Teaching: Prescribed Activity/Exercise were added to the treatment plan over the next 4 days, as Mrs. Jones's activity tolerance improved (See Table 27-2).

Table 27-2	Nursing Diagnosis, Outcomes, and Interventions for MRS. JONES	
Nursing Diagnosis	**Nursing-Sensitive Outcomes**	**Nursing Interventions**
ACTIVITY INTOLERANCE RELATED TO: Imbalance between oxygen supply and demand (↓ decreased hemoglobin [Hgb]; infection) Treatment side effects (bed rest, limited mobility) Environmental limitations (intravenous [IV] tubing, drainage tubing, siderails)	**SYMPTOM SEVERITY** *Indicators* Symptom intensity Symptom frequency Symptom persistence Heart palpitations Associated fear Associated anxiety **CARDIAC PUMP EFFECTIVENESS** *Indicators* Blood pressure IER* Heart rate IER Skin color (pallor; cyanosis) Dysrhythmias not present Diaphoresis Hgb **VITAL SIGNS STATUS** *Indicators* Heart rate Respiration rate Systolic blood pressure Diastolic blood pressure Temperature **JOINT MOVEMENT: ACTIVE** *Indicators* Elbow (right and left [R&L]) Shoulder (R&L) Ankle (R&L) Knee (R&L) Hip (R&L) **AMBULATION: WALKING** *Indicators* Bears weight Walks with effective gait Walks at slow pace Walks at moderate pace Walks at fast pace Walks up steps Walks down steps Walks up inclines Walks down inclines Walks short distance (<1 block) Walks moderate distance (>1 block <5 blocks) Walks long distance (5 blocks or >)	**ENERGY MANAGEMENT** *Activities* Administer 2 units packed red blood cells (PRBCs) to correct low Hgb Monitor Hgb every other day Encourage diet of high-energy foods and iron Space walking (1100, 1500, 2000) Schedule AM and PM rest periods (1000-1100; 1300-1430) **EXERCISE THERAPY: AMBULATION** *Activities* Consult physical therapy about ambulation plan, as needed Ambulate increasing distances based on tolerance TID (1100, 1500, 2000) Assist to chair for two of three meals Administer pain medication as needed **BODY MECHANICS PROMOTION** *Activities* Instruct on proper techniques to get out of bed Demonstrate importance of body posture during ambulation **EXERCISE THERAPY: JOINT MOBILITY** *Activities* Administer active range of motion twice a day (ROM bid) Encourage patient to perform ROM Post pictures at bedside of active ROM exercises

Continued

Table 27-2	Nursing Diagnosis, Outcomes, and Interventions for MRS. JONES—cont'd	
Nursing Diagnosis	**Nursing-Sensitive Outcomes**	**Nursing Interventions**
	ENDURANCE *Indicators* Performance of usual routine Activity 6 minute walk distance test **ADHERENCE BEHAVIOR** *Indicators* Report exercises 4 times/week Monitors tolerance to exercise	**EXERCISE PROMOTION: ENDURANCE** *Activities* Consult with physical therapist about increasing distance walked/day after discharge Instruct on warm up and cool down Schedule exercise with patient 4 times/week Identify accessible area for walking Refer to local senior center for group walking
	KNOWLEDGE: PRESCRIBED ACTIVITY *Indicators* Description of prescribed activity Explanation of purpose of activity Description of expected effects of activity Description of activity restrictions Description of activity precautions Description of factors that lower activity tolerance Description of strategy for gradual activity increase Description of how to monitor activity Performance of self-monitoring activities Description of obstacles to implementing routine Description of realistic exercise plan Description of proper performance of exercise Proper performance of exercise	**MUTUAL GOAL SETTING** *Activities* Help patient identify 1-month functional goal and 3-month functional goal Help patient with types of routine activities important to her Give patient exercise diary and teach her how to complete it **TEACHING: PRESCRIBED ACTIVITY/EXERCISE** *Activities* Show video "Walking—A Good Exercise for You" Give exercise home-going instruction manual Teach and observe patient's ability to monitor heart rate Teach and question on symptoms indicating need to stop exercise; slow pace; and/or contact provider

*IER, In expected range.
Nursing Outcomes Classification (NOC) 5-point Likert measurement scales:

Symptom Severity: 1 = Severe; 2 = Substantial; 3 = Moderate; 4 = Slight; 5 = None.
Cardiac Pump Effectiveness: 1 = Extremely compromised; 2 = Substantially compromised; 3 = Moderately compromised; 4 = Mildly compromised; 5 = Not compromised.
Endurance: 1 = Extremely compromised; 2 = Substantially compromised; 3 = Moderately compromised; 4 = Mildly compromised; 5 = Not compromised.
Vital Signs Status: 1 = Extreme deviation from expected range; 2 = Substantial deviation from expected range; 3 = Moderate deviation from expected range; 4 = Mild deviation from expected range; 5 = No deviation from expected range.
Joint Movement: Active: 1 = No motion; 2 = Limited motion; 3 = Moderate motion; 4 = Substantial motion; 5 = Full motion.
Ambulation: Walking: 1 = Dependent, does not participate; 2 = Requires assistive person and device; 3 = Requires assistive person; 4 = Independent with assistive device; 5 = Completely independent.
Adherence Behavior: 1 = Never demonstrated; 2 = Rarely demonstrated; 3 = Sometimes demonstrated; 4 = Often demonstrated; 5 = Consistently demonstrated.
Knowledge: Prescribed Activity: 1 = None; 2 = Limited; 3 = Moderate; 4 = Substantial; 5 = Extensive.

SUMMARY

Acute and chronic illnesses, lifestyle behaviors, situational limitations, and psychosocial factors can decrease an older adult's ability to tolerate activity. Decreased activity, in turn, is associated with increased morbidity and mortality and with decreased quality of life. Decreased activity tolerance also makes it more difficult for older adults to maintain an independent lifestyle. The nursing diagnosis Activity Intolerance is a key element in caring for individuals who are at risk for or who are experiencing a decline in their ability to tolerate activity. It will be critical to develop clear research-based guidelines regarding use of this diagnosis so that it can be distinguished from other related diagnoses and so that it can be applied both to well elders and to elders experiencing a variety of acute and chronic illnesses. Research studies have demonstrated that exercise programs offer older persons a means of keeping physically active and help prevent age-dependent impairments. Stretching, aerobic training, strength training, and coordination can help improve overall levels of functioning in older adults. The nursing interventions Exercise Promotion, Energy Management, Exercise Therapy: Ambulation, Exercise Therapy: Joint Mobility, and Body Mechanics Promotion can be combined to improve both physiologic measures of activity tolerance and functional measures of movement and self-care. As nurses help older adults improve their tolerance of activity, they will also help them maintain a more independent lifestyle.

REFERENCES

Allan, J. D. (1992). Exercise promotion. In G. M. Bulechek & J. C. McCloskey (Eds.), *Nursing interventions. Essential nursing treatments* (2nd ed., pp. 406-424). Philadelphia: W. B. Saunders.

Blanke, D. J., & Hageman, P. A. (1989). Comparison of gait of young men and elderly men. *Physical Therapy, 69,* 144-148.

Campbell, C. (1978). *Nursing diagnosis and interventions in nursing practice.* New York: John Wiley & Sons.

Cherubini, A., Lowenthal, D. T., Williams, L. S., Maggio, D., Mecocci, P., & Senin, U. (1998). *Aging (Milano), 10*(1), 13-25.

Chyun, D., Ford, C. F., & Yursha-Johnston, M. (1991). Silent myocardial ischemia. *Focus on Critical Care, 18*(4), 295-302.

Cress, M. E., Buchner, D. M., Questad, K. A., Esselman, P. C., deLateur, B. J., & Schwartz, R. S. (1999). Exercise: Effects on physical functional performance in independent older adults. *Journals of Gerontology. Series A: Biological Sciences & Medical Sciences, 54*(5), M242-M248.

Ettinger, W. H., Jr. (1998). Physical activity, arthritis, and disability in older people. *Clinics in Geriatric Medicine, 14*(3), 633-640.

Frantz, R. A., & Ferrell-Torry, A. (1993). Physical impairments in the elderly population. *Nursing Clinics of North America, 28,* 363-371.

Fuller, J., & Schaller-Ayers, J. (1990). *Health assessment: A nursing approach.* Baltimore: Lippincott Williams & Wilkins.

Gillett, P. A., Johnson, M., Juretich, M., Richardson, N., Slagle, L., & Farikoff, K. (1993). The nurse as exercise leader. *Geriatric Nursing, 14*(3), 133-137.

Hamdorf, P., Withers, R. T., Penhall, R. K., & Haslam, M. V. (1992). Physical training effects on the fitness and habitual activity patterns of elderly women. *Archives of Physical Medicine and Rehabilitation, 73,* 603-608.

Hunter, G. R., Treuth, M. S., Weinsier, R. L., Kekes-Szabo, T., Kell, S. H., Rothe, D. L., & Nicholson, C. (1995). The effects of strength conditioning on older women's ability to perform daily tasks. *Journal of the American Geriatrics Society, 43,* 756-760.

Ignatavicius, D. D., & Bayne, M. V. (1991). *Medical-surgical nursing: A nursing process approach.* Philadelphia: W. B. Saunders.

Iowa Intervention Project. J. C. McCloskey & G. M. Bulechek (Eds.). (2000). *Nursing interventions classification (NIC)* (3rd ed.). St. Louis, MO: Mosby.

Iowa Outcomes Project. M. Johnson, M. Maas, & S. Moorhead (Eds.). (2000). *Nursing outcomes classification (NOC)* (2nd ed.). St. Louis, MO: Mosby.

Jirovec, M. M. (1991). The impact of daily exercise on the mobility, balance and urine control of cognitively impaired nursing home residents. *International Journal of Nursing, 28*(2), 145-151.

Kane, R. L., & Kane, R. A. (1981). *Assessing the elderly. A practical guide to measurement.* St. Charles, IL: Health, D. C. and Company.

Kane, R. L., Ouslander, J. G., & Abrass, I. B. (1994). *Essentials of clinical geriatrics* (3rd ed.). Hightstown, NJ: McGraw-Hill.

Kaya, B. K., Krebs, D. E., & Riley, P. O. (1998). Dynamic stability in elders: Momentum control in locomotor ADL. *Journals of Gerontology. Series A: Biological Sciences & Medical Sciences, 53*(2), M126-M134.

Lancaster, L. E., & Rice, V. (1990). Nursing care planning: Overview and application to the patient in shock. *Critical Care Nursing Clinics of North America, 2*(2), 279-286.

Larson, E. B., & Bruce, R. A. (1987). Health benefits of exercise in an aging society. *Archives of Internal Medicine, 147,* 353-356.

Lawton, M. P., & Brody, E. M. (1969). Assessment of older people: Self-maintaining and instrumental activities of daily living. *The Gerontologist, 9,* 179-186.

Lord, S., & Castell, S. (1994). Effect of exercise on balance, strength and reaction time in older people. *Australian Physiotherapy, 40*(2), 83-88.

Lord, S. R., Castell, S., & Dip, R. G. (1994). Physical activity program for older persons: Effect on balance, strength, neuromuscular control, and reaction time. *Archives of Physical Medicine and Rehabilitation, 75,* 648-652.

Lord, S. R., Ward, J. A., & Williams, P. (1996). Exercise effect on dynamic stability in older women: A randomized controlled trial. *Archives of Physical Medicine and Rehabilitation, 77,* 232-236.

MacLean, S. (1992). Activity intolerance. In M. Maas, K. Buckwalter, & M. A. Hardy (Eds.), *Nursing diagnoses and interventions for the elderly* (pp. 252-262). Reading, MA: Addison Wesley Longman.

MacLean, S. L. (1989). Activity intolerance: Cues for diagnosis. In R. M. Carroll-Johnson (Ed.), *Classification of nursing diagnoses: Proceedings of the eighth conference* (pp. 320-332). Baltimore: Lippincott Williams & Wilkins.

Mazzeo, R. S., Cavanagh, P., Evans, W. J., Fiatarone, M., Hagberg, J., McAuley, E., & Startzell, J. (1998, June). American College of Sports Medicine position stand: Exercise and physical activity for older adults. *Medicine & Science in Sports & Exercise, 30,* 992-1008.

McKeighen, R. J., Mehmert, P. A., & Dickel, C. A. (1991). Self-care deficit, bathing/hygiene: Defining characteristics and related factors utilized by staff nurses in an acute care setting. In R. M. Carroll-Johnson (Ed.), *Classification of nursing diagnoses. Proceedings of the ninth conference* (pp. 247-248). Baltimore: Lippincott Williams & Wilkins.

Misner, J. E., Massey, B. H., Bemben, M., Going, S., & Patrick, J. (1992). Long-term effects of exercise on the range of motion of aging women. *JOPST, 16*(1), 37-42.

Mol, V. J., & Baker, C. A. (1991). Activity intolerance in the geriatric stroke patient. *Rehabilitation Nursing, 16,* 337-342.

Morris, W. W., Andrews, P. H., Gilmer, J. S., & Buckwalter, K. C. (1994). *The Iowa self assessment inventory user's manual.* Iowa City: University of Iowa Press.

Munnings, F. (1993). Strength training. Not only for the young. *The Physician and Sportsmedicine, 21*(4), 133-140.

Naso, F., Carner, E., Blankfort-Doyle, W., & Coughey, K. (1990). Endurance training in the elderly nursing home patient. *Archives of Physical Medicine and Rehabilitation, 71,* 241-243.

North American Nursing Diagnosis Association. (1999). *Nursing diagnoses: Definitions & classification, 1999-2000.* Philadelphia: Author.

Pate, R. R., Blair, S. N., Durstine, J. L., Eddy, D. O., Hanson, P., Painter, P., Smith, L. K., & Wolfe, L. A. (1991). *Guidelines for exercise testing and prescription* (4th ed.). Philadelphia: Lea & Febiger, American College of Sports Medicine.

Reimers, C. D., Harder, T., & Saxe, H. (1998). Age-related muscle atrophy does not affect all muscles and can partly be compensated by physical activity: An ultrasound study. *Journal of the Neurological Sciences, 159*(1), 60-66.

Reuben, D. B., Siu, A., & Kimpau, S. (1992). The predictive validity of self-report and performance-based measures of function and health status. *Journal of Gerontology: Medical Sciences, 47,* 106-110.

Reynolds, B. J., & Garrett, C. J. (1992). Elderly exercise: Relationship to ambulatory function, fall behavior, and well-being. In S. G. Funk, E. M. Tornquist, M. T. Champagne, & R. A. Weise (Eds.), *Key aspects of elder care* (pp. 104-109). New York: Springer.

Rubenfeld, M. G., & McFarlane, E. A. (1988). Health assessment. In J. M. Flynn & P. B. Heffron (Eds.), *Nursing from concept to practice* (2nd ed.). Norwalk, CT: Appleton & Lange.

Schnelle, J. F., MacRae, P. G., Giacobassi, K., MacRae, H. S. H., Simmons, S. F., & Ouslander, J. G. (1996). Exercise with physically restrained nursing home residents: Maximizing benefits of restraint reduction. *Journal of the American Geriatrics Society, 44,* 507-512.

Schut, L. J. (1998). Motor system changes in the aging brain: What is normal and what is not. *Geriatrics, 53*(Suppl 1), S16-S19.

Siegel, P. Z., Brackbill, R. M., & Heath, G. W. (1995). The epidemiology of walking for exercise: Implications for promoting activity among sedentary groups. *American Journal of Public Health, 85,* 706-710.

Spilker, B. (Ed.) (1996). *Quality of life and pharmacoeconomics in clinical trials* (2nd ed.). Baltimore: Lippincott Williams & Wilkins.

Stevenson, J. S., & Topp, R. (1990). Effects of moderate and low intensity long-term exercise by older adults. *Research on Nursing and Health, 13,* 209-218.

Swart, D. L., Pollock, M. L., & Brechue, W. F. (1996). Aerobic exercise for older patients. *Activities, Adaptation & Aging, 20*(3), 9-25.

Tang, P. F., Moore, S., & Woollacott, M. H. (1998). Correlation between two clinical balance measures in older adults: Functional mobility and sensory organization test. *Journals of Gerontology. Series A: Biological Sciences & Medical Sciences, 53*(2), M140-M146.

Tanji, J. L. (1991, June). Exercise for adults over age 65. Recommendation in health and chronic disease. *Consultant,* 66-69.

Thompson, J. M., McFarland, G. K., Hirsch, J. E., & Tucker, S. M. (Eds.). (1997). Activity-exercise. In *Mosby's clinical nursing* (4th ed.). St. Louis, MO: Mosby.

Topp, R., Mikesky, A., & Bawel, K. (1994). Developing a strength training program for older adults: Planning, programming, and potential outcomes. *Rehabilitation Nursing, 19,* 266-273.

Topp, R., Mikesky, A., Wigglesworth, J., Holt, W., & Edwards, J. (1993). The effect of a 12-week dynamic resistance strength training program on gait velocity and balance of older adults. *The Gerontologist, 33,* 501-506.

Williams, T. F. (1987). The future of aging. *Archives of Physical and Medical Rehabilitation, 68,* 335-338.

Wolf, S. L., Barnhart, H., Kutner, N. G., McNeely, E., Coogler, C., Xu, T., and the Atlanta FICSIT Group. (1996). Reducing frailty and falls in older persons: An investigation of Tai Chi and computerized balance training. *Journal of the American Geriatrics Society, 44,* 489-497.

Wolfson, L., Whipple, R., Derby, C., Judge, J., King, M., Amerman, P., Schmidt, J., & Smyders, D. (1996). Balance and strength training in older adults: Intervention gains and Tai Chi maintenance. *Journal of the American Geriatrics Society, 44,* 498-506.

Work, J. A. (1989). Strength training: A bridge to independence for the elderly. *The Physician and Sportsmedicine, 17*(11), 134-140.

CHAPTER 28

IMPAIRED PHYSICAL MOBILITY

Meridean L. Maas and Janet P. Specht

Physical mobility is critical for the maintenance of health and quality of life of all persons and is especially important for the elder. Mobility is activity within an individual's environment (England, 1989). According to Milde (1988), mobility enables persons to move away from danger, to move to experiences that are enjoyable, and to maintain homeostasis. Mobility, care of one's person, and the performance of instrumental tasks to cope with the environment are behaviors that constitute functional health (Hogue, 1985; Tinetti, 1986). Many elders define their health status and physical fitness in terms of their mobility. Although ambulation is the expected mode of mobility, for the elderly person the use of assistive devices such as wheelchairs can provide greater mobility than ambulation (Kraft, 1991). When an elderly person is institutionalized, physical mobility may be impaired because of underlying illness and because of factors associated with the physical environment (Hogue, 1985). Clearly, preventive interventions are needed to maximize the functional abilities of the increasing numbers of elders in the population (Guralnik & Simonsick, 1993).

When physical mobility is viewed as an aspect of functional health, the consequences of impairment are broad, including physiologic, psychologic, and socioeconomic results (Table 28-1). These consequences are not inevitable, even though they are associated with the increased probability of physiologic decline with aging. The increment in functional dependence that accompanies Impaired Physical Mobility and its consequences can often be avoided, corrected, or minimized by astute nursing diagnosis and management (Johnson, Stone, Larson, & Hromek, 1992; Kochersberger, Hielema, & Westlund, 1994; Means, Currie, & Gershkoff, 1993). This makes the problem of Impaired Physical Mobility among elders a high priority for care, teaching, and research.

Falls

The elderly person with mobility limitations is prone to falls from gait changes, weakness, postural sway, and diminished reflexes (Woollacott, 1993). If a person falls once, she is more apt to fall again (Pendergast, Fisher, & Calkins, 1993; Tinetti & Powell, 1993). Fear of falling is common among elders, especially if they have fallen in the previous year (Tinetti et al., 1988). As noted above, many elderly individuals report that they avoid activity because of their fear of falling (Tinetti & Powell, 1993). Mobility limitations also can accompany chronic illnesses, which are more common among elders; mobility limitations can be exacerbated by medical treatments and medications. In addition, older persons, especially women, are more apt than younger persons to sustain fractures when they fall because of the high incidence of osteoporosis. One half or more of elderly persons who could walk before sustaining a hip fracture cannot walk afterward (Melton & Riggs, 1983). The treatment and rehabilitation for hip fractures has a first-year cost of about $40,000 per person (USDHHS, 1992). It is estimated that between $1 billion and $2 billion is spent yearly in the United States for the acute medical treatment of hip fractures in older adults (American Nurses Association, 1994). These circumstances, perhaps more than any others, are responsible for the high degrees of impaired mobility experienced by elders and lead to further physiologic, psychologic, and socioeconomic consequences. See Chapter 3 for further discussion of the relationship of falls and impaired mobility in elders.

Physiologic Consequences

In certain situations, decreased physical mobility is beneficial. When an individual is at rest, metabolism and oxygen consumption are lowered and the workload of the heart is reduced. Pain, tension, and venous pooling are often reduced when the musculoskeletal system relaxes with the body in a supine position. Many illnesses (e.g., congestive heart failure, fractures) require degrees of decreased mobility for effective treatment. The ability of a part of the body to function is decreased when it is injured or diseased. The physiologic requirements on the body part may be greater than its ability to respond. Thus rest may be necessary to maintain homeostasis and to prevent further injury. Rest may be functional in these cases because it equalizes metabolic capacity and demand and promotes healing. However, the body does not need to be immobile to rest (Monicken, 1991). Rather, the body and its organs will function optimally and the capacity to function will progress if demand is increased as ability and metabolic reserve increase. "The basis of the development of functional ability by any organ of the body is use" (Kottke,

Related Factors/Etiologies and Defining Characteristics Associated With Nursing-Sensitive Outcomes	
Table 28-1 IMPAIRED PHYSICAL MOBILITY	
Nursing Diagnosis	**Nursing-Sensitive Outcomes**
IMPAIRED PHYSICAL MOBILITY	
Related Factor/Etiology	
Muscle weakness	**ENDURANCE**
Defining Characteristics	***Indicators***
Decreased muscle strength/resistance from baseline	Performance of usual routine
Decreased muscle mass/size, circumference from baseline	Muscle endurance
Decreased muscle tone/tautness when relaxed from baseline	Exhaustion not present
Complaints of muscle heaviness	**MOBILITY LEVEL**
Related Factor/Etiology	***Indicator***
Altered cellular function	
Defining Characteristics	
Hypoxemia	Muscle movement
Decrease in tissue perfusion	
Dyspnea	**VITAL SIGNS STATUS**
Electrocardiogram (ECG)–ischemia dysrhythmias	***Indicators***
Fluid/electrolyte imbalance	Blood pressure
Acid-base imbalance	Pulse
Shared indicators	Respiration rate
• Complaints of fatigue or weakness	**MUSCLE FUNCTION**
• Decreased endurance	***Indicators***
• Tremors	Muscle tone
• Reluctance to engage in activity or to move	Steadiness of movement
• Abnormal rise in heart rate (HR), blood pressure (BP), respiratory rate (RR) with activity	
Related Factor/Etiology	
Pain	**COMFORT LEVEL**
Defining Characteristics	
Verbal complaints of pain/discomfort with movement	***Indicators***
Protective changes in posture/gait	
Reluctance to attempt movement	Willingness to move
Expressed feelings of helplessness/depression	Reported physical well-being
Moaning, crying, irritability with movement	
Facial grimace with movement; facial mask of pain	**PAIN LEVEL**
Diaphoresis	***Indicators***
Change in BP, HR, RR with movement	Muscle tension
Self-focusing	Protective body positions
Withdrawal from social contact	
Related Factors/Etiologies	
Cognitive/perceptual deficits	**COGNITIVE ABILITY**
Defining Characteristics	
Confusion	***Indicators***
Starts to move, forgets why or how	Demonstrates control over selected events and situations
Forgotten names/meaning of environmental stimuli	Orientation
Cannot choose between one or more movements	**SELF-CARE: ACTIVITIES OF DAILY LIVING (ADL)**
Cannot remember or follow instructions	***Indicators***
Receptive aphasia for language stimuli/descriptors of moving	Ambulation: walking
Reduced hearing, sight, touch, smell, proprioception	Transfer performance
Related Factor/Etiology	**NEUROLOGICAL STATUS: CENTRAL MOTOR CONTROL**
Neuromuscular impairment	
Defining Characteristics	***Indicators***
Diminished balance	
Impaired coordination	Balance

	Related Factors/Etiologies and Defining Characteristics Associated With Nursing-Sensitive Outcomes—cont'd
Table 28-1	IMPAIRED PHYSICAL MOBILITY—cont'd

Nursing Diagnosis	Nursing-Sensitive Outcomes
Decrease (weakness) or loss of muscle function	Gait effectiveness
Stiffness or rigidity of extremities	Maintenance of posture
Tremors	**MUSCLE FUNCTION**
Decreased muscle control	*Indicators*
	Control of movement
	Strength of muscle contraction
Related Factors/Etiologies	**JOINT MOVEMENT: ACTIVE**
Musculoskeletal disorders	
Defining Characteristics	*Indicators*
Structural	
• Limited range of motion	Specify joints _____
• Hypercalciuria	
• Hypercalcemia	
• Decreased density of bone	
• Contractures	
• Dislocation of joints	
Mechanical	
• External device that limits movement of any body part	
Related Factor/Etiology	**FEAR CONTROL**
Psychosocial impairment	
Defining Characteristics	*Indicators*
Anxiety	
Helplessness	Plans coping strategies for fearful situations
Hopelessness	Seeks information to reduce fear
Depression	**SOCIAL INVOLVEMENT**
Alienation	*Indicators*
Isolation	Interaction with family members
Decreased eye contact	Interaction with close friends
Lack of attention to dangerous stimuli	• Participation in leisure activities
Muscular rigidity	**HEALTH BELIEFS: PERCEIVED CONTROL**
Smaller scope of perceptions	*Indicator*
	Belief that own actions control health outcomes
Related Factors/Etiologies	**MOBILITY LEVEL**
Iatrogenic factors	
Defining Characteristics	*Indicators*
Use of physical or chemical restraints	
Use of drugs that sedate, provide analgesia, anesthetize	Balance performance
Bed rest without exercise, change of position, longer than 24 hrs	Body positioning performance
IV fluids, chest tubes, other treatments that keep person in bed	Transfer performance
Failure to prescribe mobility interventions	Joint movement
	Ambulation: walking
Related Factors/Etiologies	**PSYCHOSOCIAL ADJUSTMENT: LIFE CHANGE**
Social/physical impediments in environment	
Sociocultural	*Indicators*
• Inconsistent role expectations	Expressions of feeling empowered
• Lack of social relationships	Expressions of feeling socially engaged
• Altered power relationships	
Physical	**SAFETY BEHAVIOR: HOME PHYSICAL ENVIRONMENT**
• Presence of architectural barriers	*Indicators*
• Long distances to services, family, friends, activities	Provision of assistive devices in accessible location
• Lack of transportation	Arrangement of furniture to reduce risks

Continued

	Related Factors/Etiologies and Defining Characteristics Associated With Nursing-Sensitive Outcomes—cont'd
Table 28-1	**IMPAIRED PHYSICAL MOBILITY—cont'd**

Nursing Diagnosis	Nursing-Sensitive Outcomes
• Inadequate lighting • Absence of railings on stairs or in bathroom • Lack of or ill-fitting assistive devices for ambulation/self-care • Slippery surfaces • Obstructions: cords, rugs, furniture, clutter ***Related Factor/Etiology*** Lack of knowledge ***Defining Characteristics*** Expression of inaccurate facts about movement/exercise for health Inability to cite alternatives to and consequences of immobility Nonadherence with interventions for mobility Stated admission of lack of knowledge Lack of recall of instructions	**HEALTH BELIEFS: PERCEIVED ABILITY TO PERFORM** ***Indicators*** Perception that health behavior requires reasonable effort Perception of likelihood of performing health behavior over time **KNOWLEDGE: PRESCRIBED ACTIVITY** ***Indicators*** Description of prescribed activity Description of how to monitor activity **ADHERENCE BEHAVIOR** ***Indicators*** Performs activities of daily living (ADL) consistent with energy and tolerance Provides rationale for adopting a regimen

1965, p. 437; Pendergast et al., 1993). Thus, lack of use leads to a deterioration of functional ability. This is true for all body systems and organs.

The greater the impairment of physical mobility, the greater is the probability that physiologic problems will result. The kinds of physiologic deterioration that occur with Impaired Physical Mobility are wide ranging and include reduced range of motion (ROM) of joints, loss of muscular strength and endurance, loss of skeletal strength, cardiovascular deterioration, metabolic imbalances, ischemic ulcers, deterioration of urinary function, decreased gastrointestinal function, and respiratory deterioration.

Reduced Range of Motion of Joints.   Reduced ROM occurs with Impaired Physical Mobility because connective tissues around joint capsules and in muscle planes become dense (Harper & Lyles, 1988; Kottke, 1965; Matteson & McConnell, 1988). The fibers of the involved muscles shorten and atrophy because they do not regularly shorten and lengthen through their full range (Pendergast et al., 1993). Trauma, inflammation, and poor circulation interact with impaired mobility to accelerate the formation of dense connective tissue. Initially the joint loses flexibility and the effective ROM is constrained. Then, if the process continues, ROM is further curtailed, joints become stiffer, and contractures and ankylosis develop. The hip, knee, and ankle are most susceptible, although all joints can be affected. Restricted extension of joints is most apt to occur because of the greater strength of flexor muscles, the effects of gravity, and the difficulty in obtaining a full ROM of joints while lying down or sitting.

Loss of Muscle Strength and Endurance.   Reduced strength and endurance result when muscle contraction is less than 20% of maximum tension each day (Kottke, 1965). Maintenance of muscle strength and endurance is dependent on frequent maximum tension contractions. A few strong contractions each day are sufficient to maintain muscle mass and strength if protein nutrition is adequate. However, a completely resting muscle will lose 10% to 15% of strength each week and can lose as much as 5.5% per day, with the most rapid loss occurring in the early phase of immobility (Muller, 1970). Muscle endurance is largely a function of the circulation, nutrition, and removal of waste for the muscle. Immobilized muscles' venous pumps are more inactive, which leads to poorer circulation (Kottke, 1971). As circulation fails to meet the muscle's needs, endurance, strength, and muscle mass decrease because of lessened muscle oxidative capacity (Harper & Lyles, 1988; Monicken, 1991). The muscles most affected by immobilization are the gastrocnemius-soleus group, quadriceps, glutei, and erector spinae (Milde, 1981).

Loss of Skeletal Strength.   Loss of strength results from the increase in the reabsorption of bone that accompanies impaired mobility (Harper & Lyles, 1988). Normally, the skeletal structures are continually renewed through absorption and replacement of bone. This process depends on muscle contraction and stress to promote bone deposition. Osteoporosis occurs when bone destruction and reabsorption exceed bone production (Lueckenotte, 1996; Mehta & Nastasi, 1993). The greater the degree of impaired mobility, the greater the loss of bone matrix and minerals, especially calcium and phosphorous (Monicken, 1991). The long bones of the lower extremities, the os calcis, and the vertebrae are most susceptible to mineral loss. Loss of calcium increases rapidly from the first to the third week of immobility, reaches a peak at the fifth or sixth week, and then plateaus at a lower level, preventing further bone porosity (Deitrick, Whedon, & Shorr, 1948; Dunning & Plum, 1957). Elders are at increased risk for pathologic fractures, as the bone becomes increasingly fragile (Mehta & Nastasi, 1993).

Cardiovascular Deterioration.   Deterioration of the cardiovascular system is especially dramatic when impairment of mobility causes extended confinement in bed or chair. The deteriorating effect is even more pronounced if fever, injury, or disease is also present. Adaptability of circulation to an upright position deteriorates rapidly when the individual is in bed for extended periods. The normal sympathetic response of vasoconstriction to compensate for decreased arterial pressure and increased heart rate when the position is changed from supine to upright is not as effective. Rather, vasodilatation and venous pooling occur, resulting in reduced circulating volume, decreased venous return, decreased cardiac output, increased pulse rate, and decreased blood pressure (Browse, 1965; Harper & Lyles, 1988). After 21 days of bed rest, healthy young men in the classic study by Taylor et al. (1945) took more than 5 weeks after resumption of activity to regain cardiovascular response to the upright position. Elders can deteriorate even more rapidly and can require a longer period of activity to recover.

The longer the period of bed rest, the greater is the risk of venous thrombosis (Milde, 1988). Body movement no longer stimulates the pumping action of muscles and vessels; consequently, decreased emptying of vessels and increased stasis occur, especially in the calf, where the largest percent of thrombi originate (Clark, MacGregor, Prescott, & Ruckley, 1974). In addition, when the body is recumbent for long periods, the heart must work harder to achieve circulation because of altered distribution of blood and fluid in the body, decreased cardiac output, and decreased stroke volume (Monicken, 1991).

Metabolic Imbalances.   Reduced mobility results in breakdown of protein and excretion of nitrogen and, thereby, can result in other metabolic imbalances. There is a decreased metabolic rate, increased storage of fat or carbohydrate, negative nitrogen and calcium metabolic balance, decreased glucose tolerance, and metabolic alkalosis (Harper & Lyles, 1988; Milde, 1988; Monicken, 1991). Other electrolytes (e.g., potassium) also have been reported to go into a negative balance with immobility (Kottke, 1965). These assaults deprive the body of the energy that is necessary to fuel movement and maintain homeostasis. Hypercalcemia from disuse osteoporosis can cause a number of serious problems for the elderly person, including anorexia, malaise, nausea, vomiting, abdominal cramps, constipation, weight loss, and lethargy.

Ischemic Ulcers.   Ulcers of the skin and muscle can be a major consequence of Impaired Physical Mobility. Ischemic ulcers develop over body prominences (pressure points) where pressure prevents the flow of blood required to nourish cells. Ulcers also develop because of the shearing of soft tissues from being moved or moving while in bed. Ischemic ulcers can occur when the individual is in any position long enough to create sufficient pressure for cell necrosis (AHCPR, 1992). In addition, the circulation of blood, which is to some extent facilitated by the movement of muscles, is reduced when mobility is impaired. Impaired Skin Integrity: Pressure Ulcer is discussed in more detail in Chapter 11.

Deterioration of Urinary Function.   Decreased urinary function is most pronounced when impaired mobility results in the individual's confinement in a recumbent position. In an upright position, gravity assists the drainage of urine from the renal pelvis. In the recumbent position, urine flow from the kidney into the ureter is against gravity. Because peristalsis is not sufficient to overcome the force of gravity, the renal pelvis may completely fill before urine flows into the ureter. Thus, urinary stasis results, predisposing the individual to renal calculi or infection.

The inability to relax the perineal muscles and external sphincter easily during recumbency creates further urinary complications. Because of this difficulty, reflex action to micturate is not initiated even though the sensation to void is present. If voiding does not occur, the bladder becomes distended and the sensation to void may no longer be felt. Bladder distension can lead to overflow incontinence, pressure damage to the kidney, and infection.

If adequate drainage of urine from the kidney and bladder is maintained, the kidney nephron ordinarily is not damaged by prolonged confinement in a supine position (Olson, 1967). Therefore it continues to remove excess materials from the blood plasma. However, immobility is accompanied by renal insufficiency, decreased glomerular filtration rate, loss of ability to concentrate urine, lower creatinine tolerance, and increased nitrogen, phosphorus, total sulfur, sodium, potassium, and calcium secretion (Harper & Lyles, 1988; Monicken, 1991). Because of the metabolic changes that accompany immobility (protein breakdown and decalcification of bone), the kidney excretes large amounts of minerals and salts.

The excretion and precipitation of larger amounts of calcium salts create increased renal calculi in persons who are recumbent for long periods of time. Precipitation of calcium salts is encouraged by impaired urine drainage, which increases the time for precipitates to form; by the alkalization of urine caused by the absence of acidic byproducts of muscle metabolism; and from dehydration, which concentrates urine solids and increased stasis (Milde, 1988).

Decreased Gastrointestinal Function. Gastrointestinal problems associated with impaired mobility involve ingestion, digestion, and elimination. Prolonged immobility leads to a negative nitrogen balance (Means, Currie, & Gershkoff, 1993). Persons in negative nitrogen balance often are anorexic, which contributes to malnutrition and compounds other existing health problems. Lack of adequate nutrients, combined with impaired circulation and exchange of nutrients in the cells, interferes with food digestion and use. Reduced ingestion of fiber and fluid, impaired digestion, muscle weakness, and altered colonic motility are the major reasons that constipation is often a problem for persons with impaired mobility (Harper & Lyles, 1988). The muscles of fecal expulsion (abdominal, diaphragm, levator ani) atrophy with prolonged immobility, rendering the person less able to evacuate the lower bowel. Opiate and anticholinergic medications, lack of privacy, failure to heed the defecation reflex, and failure to provide the optimal defecation position (sitting erect or squatting) can also contribute to constipation. A more detailed discussion of constipation in elders is presented in Chapter 19.

Respiratory Deterioration. Respiratory deterioration from impaired mobility is caused primarily by reduced ventilation and inability to remove secretions. Full expansion of alveoli, which typically occurs with physical activity in the upright position, is compromised when mobility is impaired. Optimum gaseous exchange can take place only when the alveoli are full of air and in close proximity with circulating blood and when the air in the alveoli is being exchanged continuously (Olson, 1967). Vital capacity, tidal volume, carbon dioxide (CO_2) and oxygen (O_2) exchange, and the oxygen-carrying capacity of the blood decrease with age (Lueckenotte, 1996). When a person is in a supine position, vital capacity is reduced by about 4% (Browse, 1965) because of elevation of the diaphragm, changed contour of the chest, constraint on chest expansion, and redistribution of blood from the lower periphery.

Secretions are more difficult for the recumbent person to remove because of increased viscosity of mucus, dilated bronchi, reduced inspirational air volume and pressure, ineffective ciliary activity, reduced stimulation of the cough reflex, and weakness of the muscles that aid coughing. If there is any degree of alveolar collapse, the problem of removing secretions is compounded further, since secretions continue to form, increasing the likelihood of stasis, tracheitis, bronchitis, and pneumonia (Lueckenotte, 1996).

Sensory Deficits. Sensory impairments also accompany immobility for elders. There is a tendency for decreased kinesthetic, visual, auditory, and tactile stimuli when an individual is immobile, primarily caused by decreased activity and social interaction. Changes in affect, cognition, and perception also occur when the elderly person is immobile (Monicken, 1991).

Psychologic Consequences

Physical mobility influences the human being's self-concept, self-esteem, and ability to cope emotionally. The ability to interact physically with elements in the environment to meet human needs is closely allied with self-concept and feelings of worth. As discussed in Chapter 45, a part of self-concept and self-esteem includes the ability to move about at will (Parent & Whall, 1984; Simpson, 1986). Parent and Whall (1984) reported a strong positive correlation between increased activity and self-esteem and a negative correlation between high self-esteem and depression in elderly subjects. Impaired mobility alters the self-concept and self-esteem aspects of personality. As a result, immobility often leads to lack of interest and lack of motivation to learn and to solve problems. Drives and expectancies are diminished, and emotions can find expression in a variety of exaggerated or inappropriate ways, including apathy, anger, aggression, or regression (Miller, 1975; Olson, 1967). The magnitude of impairment, its visibility, and its prognosis all have potent effects on the elder (Schulz & Williamson, 1993). Fear, depression, and embarrassment can result in impairment of the elder's mobility.

Forced isolation and dependency deprive the person of intellectual and sensory stimulation that is needed for optimal perceptual behavior. As the quality and quantity of sensory information available to the elderly individual are reduced, the ability to interact with the environment is altered (see Chapter 37). Visual and somatosensory deficits (inaccuracies) have been shown to negatively affect the balance of healthy elders to a significantly greater degree than younger adults (Whipple et al., 1993). Sensory deprivation often leads to distortions of time, form, pattern, space, mass, and temperature. These aberrations affect the relevance that activities such as sleeping, working, having sex, eating, and playing have for the elderly person who has mobility impairment. If the threats to the ego and self are sufficiently overpowering, if high anxiety precipitates a turning inward of psychologic energy to protect the self, and if energy is withheld from interaction with people and realities in the environment, the elderly individual will be psychologically immobilized (Friedrich & Lively, 1981) and unable to cope effectively.

Socioeconomic Consequences

For the elder, the socioeconomic consequences of impaired mobility are often severe. The mobility impairment can change an individual's role activities as spouse, parent, employee, friend, and member of social groups and the community. Social responsibility usually requires physical activity and psychologic stability. With impaired mobility, social support networks are interrupted, leaving the elder with limited opportunity to maintain optimally functional social interactions and relationships. Impairment of mobility often is linked to the need for institutionalization in acute and long-term care settings. The chronic illnesses that tend to accompany aging further predispose the elderly person to mobility impairments and interact with the impairment to continue a progressive cycle of physical, psychologic, and socioeconomic deterioration. The descent into functional dependence with loss of work roles and income, loss of control of monetary assets, and the need for health care can be devastating for the elderly person. The cost of health care for the elder can be staggering even if mobility is not impaired and institutionalization is not required. Impaired mobility can initiate a cycle of events involving injuries and physiologic, psychologic, and social deterioration that adds greatly to an already substantial economic burden for the individual and society. Bone fractures are one of the most disabling frequent consequences of impaired mobility, with hip fractures the most disabling type. Six months after a hip fracture only 17% of 2806 community-living elders were able to walk independently (Marottoli, Berkman, & Cooney, 1992). Because hip fracture risk increases with age and the incidence of hip fractures is increasing, prevention of impairments in the elderly person to reduce the risk of hip fracture alone is imperative (Egan et al., 1992).

PREVALENCE

Impaired Physical Mobility occurs frequently among institutionalized elders, ranking along with falls, incontinence, and mental confusion as the most common problems of the elderly in long-term care settings (Joseph & Wanlass, 1993; Kane & Kane, 1981). However, surveys indicate a substantial amount of physical disability among community-dwelling elders as well. Wiener, Hanley, Clark, and Van Nostrand (1990) compiled the results of several national surveys and found that between 5% and 8.1% of noninstitutionalized elderly individuals age 65 and older received help with one or more ADL. Few reported studies document the incidence of the nursing diagnosis Impaired Physical Mobility in specific populations of institutionalized or noninstitutionalized elders. Hardy, Maas,

and Akins (1988), in a descriptive study of nursing diagnoses used in a state veterans home, found Impaired Physical Mobility to be the second most frequent nursing diagnosis both in 1983 (35% of a sample of 99 residents) and in 1985 (26% of a sample of 121 residents). Other studies have shown this nursing diagnosis to be the one most frequently used in long-term care facilities and hospitals for elders (Hallal, 1985; Leslie, 1981; Rantz, Miller, & Jacobs, 1985). In an analysis of physical disability among older people in the United States, Guralnik and Simonsick (1993) reported that 22% of women and 15% of men age 65 and older either need help to live at home or reside in an institution; however, this study did not distinguish physical reasons for inability to perform ADL from cognitive, emotional, or other influences.

RISK FACTORS/ETIOLOGIES

A number of factors associated with aging predispose elders to Impaired Physical Mobility (Tinetti, 1986). There is a general decrease in muscle strength, endurance, and agility (Aniansson, Hedberg, Henning, & Grimby, 1986; Oretel, 1986; Rikki & Busch, 1986). Muscle strength declines steadily after young adulthood (Bosco & Komi, 1980; Fiatarone & Evans, 1993; Hyatt, Whitelaw, Bhat, Scott, & Maxwell, 1990; Pendergast, Fisher, & Calkins, 1993), particularly in the legs (McDonagh, White, & Davies, 1984; Woollacott, 1993). Muscle strength, fiber number, and fiber size decrease in similar proportions. Although these decrements are somewhat more pronounced in men than women, men remain stronger (Hyatt et al., 1990). Clinical studies have suggested a model of spiraling decline in physical activity and motor ability among older women, with muscle strength playing a mediating role (Rantanen et al., 1999). Lower extremity muscles atrophy more than upper extremity muscles. Elders exhibit a 10% to 25% reduction in muscle strength compared with 25-year-olds (Monicken, 1991). Several studies have demonstrated age-related changes in muscle response synergies when balance is threatened (Manchester, Woollacott, Zederbauer-Hylton, & Marin, 1989; Woollacott, 1993; Woollacott, Inglin, & Manchester, 1988). In general, muscle endurance is affected less than strength (Sato et al., 1986), although muscles also lose oxidative potential with aging (Fiatarone & Evans, 1993). As muscles atrophy, joints become less flexible and more flexed, and the individual generally becomes more frail.

Reduced visual acuity, hearing impairments, arthritis, osteoporosis (especially in elderly women), decreased strength, poor balance, and mental confusion increase the elder's risk for falls; falls, in turn, often result in injuries that further reduce mobility (Tinetti & Powell, 1993; Whipple, Wolfson, Derby, Singh, & Tobin, 1993; Woollacott, 1993). Even if the elderly individual does not fall, he tends to curtail mobility to avoid accidents, compounding losses in muscle strength and joint movement. A substantial percentage of elderly persons who fall and those who do not fall report fear of falling and a decline in activity caused by their fear (Nevitt, Cummings, Kidd, & Black, 1989; Tinetti, Speechley, & Ginter, 1988; Vellas, Cayla, Bocquet, dePemille, & Albarede, 1987).

Elders also often experience changes in their social support systems that predispose them to impaired mobility (Schulz & Williamson, 1993). The loss of spouse, friends, and work role can eliminate many of the reasons for being active and mobile. Chronic illnesses increase the likelihood that the elderly person will receive treatments that restrict activity and mobility. Chronic illness itself can make activity even less desirable and more difficult. At home and in institutions, chronic illness and functional losses often interact with the physical and social environment to restrict mobility further (Czaja, Weber, & Nair, 1993; Daly & Berman, 1993; Egan, Warren, Hessel, & Gilewich, 1992; Kaplan, Strawbridge, Camacho, & Cohen, 1993; Weaver & Narsavage, 1992).

In general, the nurse can identify Impaired Physical Mobility, regardless of the specific etiology, by observing the client's limited activity and independent movement. Identifying signs and symptoms that indicate the specific cause(s) for decreased mobility allows the nurse to determine patient outcomes and to prescribe effective interventions. See Table 28-1 for etiologies and outcomes.

Activity Intolerance

Activity intolerance is a decrease in energy caused by loss of muscle mass and tone or to an alteration in cellular activity. Elders sustain loss of muscle mass and tone with normal aging, but also are at risk for further weakness from disuse related to chronic illness and decreased activity and movement. Respiratory muscles also weaken, and the lungs tend to become less elastic (Berry, Vitalo, Larson, Patel, & Kim, 1996). Thus, the elderly person has less tidal volume and reduced vital capacity. Chronic respiratory conditions such as chronic obstructive pulmonary disease (COPD) can compound normal respiratory changes so that even less oxygen is available for energy and movement (Harper & Lyles, 1988). Elders often experience social isolation and psychologic problems, which remove much of the motivation to be active.

Pain

Pain is a generalized or localized sensation of severe discomfort. Elders are predisposed to chronic and acute pain, both somatopathic and psychogenic, because of the higher incidence of chronic illnesses and their treatment, increased trauma from falls and fractures, and susceptibility to infections. Musculoskeletal conditions are among the most common of the chronic problems affecting elders, with an estimated 49% having some form of arthritis (Fowles, 1990). The elderly individual, like all individuals, responds to pain in a variety of ways. Responses are both physiologic and psychologic and are highly individual. See Chapter 36 for additional information about pain in elders.

Cognitive and Perceptual Deficits

Cognitive and perceptual deficits are the loss of ability to process sensory inputs mentally and/or the loss of sensations. Elders, more than any other age-group, experience diminished ability to receive sensory input. These deficits tend to accompany normal aging and also are secondary to illnesses that elderly persons more often incur. Elders also are more often subjected to environments that are socially and/or therapeutically restricted, largely because of mobility impairments. These environments reduce sensory inputs. Because sensory feedback is essential for optimum mobility (e.g., time and space orientation, reasons for movement and activity), restricted environments contribute to mobility impairment. Cognitive deficits are also common among elderly individuals, resulting primarily from reversible and irreversible dementias, transient cerebral ischemias, and cardiovascular accidents. Without adequate cognitive abilities, elders may not know how to move or why they should move and may be unable to relearn movement. Elders with mild cognitive impairment have been shown to have statistically significant poorer equilibrium and limb coordination performance than elders who are cognitively intact (Franssen, Souren, Torossian, & Reisberg, 1999).

Neuromusculature Impairment

Neuromuscular impairment is the loss of muscle movement caused by interrupted central nervous system or peripheral innervation (Creason et al., 1985). The nervous system controls innervation and the functions of all body parts; thus muscle contraction and reflexes are dependent on an intact neurologic system (Pendergast et al., 1993). Many conditions that elders are prone to develop result in impaired neurologic function. Some of the more common conditions are degenerative diseases, demyelinating diseases, vascular diseases, trauma, tumors, and drug treatment. Paralysis with flaccidity or spasticity and paresis of muscles are not uncommon.

Musculoskeletal Disorders

Musculoskeletal disorders are losses or decreases of function of muscles and skeletal support systems that may be mechanical or structural in origin (Creason et al., 1985). Mechanical origins are external devices, such as restraints or casts that restrict movement. Structural origins are physiologic limitations of movement. Chronic conditions such as osteoporosis, fractures, arthritis, tumors, and edema interfere with the structural stability or flexibility of the skeleton. Coimpairments of balance and strength particularly predispose elders to mobility disabilities

(Rantanen, Guralnik, Ferrucci, Leveille, & Fried, 1999). Finally, external devices, including the casts, splints, traction, slings, wheelchairs, and walkers commonly used to aid ambulation, comfort, and anatomic alignment, also can impair mobility.

Psychologic Impairment

Psychologic impairment is an emotional response that occurs when stress overwhelms an individual's ability to cope effectively (Carnevali & Brueckner, 1970). Fear and grief from the many losses sustained with aging can be immobilizing for the elder, who must often adjust to changes in lifestyle and environment without the benefit of her health and familiar support systems. Elders are especially vulnerable to losses that weaken their control over aspects of living that ordinarily are taken for granted by younger persons. These circumstances can be so overwhelming that they are psychologically immobilizing, which in turn promotes physical immobility.

Iatrogenic Factors

Iatrogenic factors associated with mobility impairment are treatment regimens that affect an elderly individual's movement. These include bed rest, pharmaceutic agents (sedatives, tranquilizers, analgesics, anesthetics), restrictive and unfamiliar health care environments, surgery, restraints, and other treatments that restrict activity such as IV fluids, suction, and catheters. Although these circumstances are usually necessary for the treatment of disease and injury, they can lead to serious problems, particularly for elders who have multiple predispositions to immobility and its consequences. Nurses should be vigilant about preventing or minimizing the effects of iatrogenic sources of immobility so that the elderly person is not compromised beyond what is absolutely necessary.

Barriers in the Sociocultural or Physical Environment

Barriers in the sociocultural or physical environment are social structures, processes, and/or cultural values and physical structures that limit activity and movement. Examples of sociocultural impediments are role conflicts and incongruencies, unbalanced power relationships, lack of social relationships, incompatible relationships, and incompatible cultural values. As mentioned previously, elderly persons are at risk both for loss of social relationships and for role change and transitions, such as retirement and dependence on others for assistance. Role conflicts and incongruencies are apt to result when role changes occur. Further, power relationships of parents and children often reverse, with the elder parent becoming dependent and having diminished control. Constraints on mobility of this type are usually present to some degree when elders enter institutions.

Staff caregivers are ordinarily younger and tend to have role expectations of elders and themselves that are not consistent with those held by the elders. Likewise, values are often divergent and the caregivers hold a definite power advantage over the elder. Incompatibilities in cultural values evolve from age-segregated subcultures, as well as from ethnic differences. Ageism, prejudiced negative stereotyping of older persons, not only is expressed by younger generations, but is also internalized by older persons as well, making a self-fulfilling prophecy of such myths as "Old people should rest" or "Old people have had their day for involvement and activity." Violence and crime are socioenvironmental conditions that are of concern to many elders. These circumstances tend to discourage mobility beyond immediate living quarters for many elderly persons who fear venturing out or who choose to avoid contacts that are uncomfortable. Physical constraints include stairs, distance, and lack of transportation. Older persons may not have the energy or ability to navigate stairs or walk long distances and may not be able to drive a car. Optimal mobility is thus inhibited.

Lack of Knowledge

It is not uncommon for persons to be unable to deal effectively with disease or injury because they lack knowledge about what to do (Carnevali & Brueckner, 1970). In addition, elders are more apt to have cognitive deficits caused by illnesses such as cardiovascular accidents and dementia. Many myths about how to deal with illness also constitute a lack of knowledge. The roles of exercise and movement to maintain function and health may be less familiar to elderly persons who grew up believing, along with many in the health care community, that bed rest was always necessary and beneficial for the treatment of illness or discomfort. Thus, elders may restrict their mobility because they are unaware of the need to maintain movement, of how to restore mobility, and of the resources that are available to assist them in order to prevent further impairment and the consequences that compromise their health and functioning. When elderly persons are knowledgeable, their involvement in decision making and their compliance are enhanced (Millar, 1983).

ASSESSMENT

Assessment of the elderly person for the diagnosis and management of Impaired Physical Mobility requires that data be collected regarding the individual's physiologic and psychologic capabilities, the individual's physical and social environment, and the individual's interface with the environment (Kane, 1993; Rockwood, Silvius, & Fox, 1998). This is because mobility (also functional health) is affected by a composite of factors, and the specific composite is different for each elderly person. A comprehensive and detailed database developed around these dimensions will allow the nurse to identify the specific factors that are associated with the client's mobility impairment and infer the extent, degree of control, and probable duration of the impairment. With these judgments, the nurse can proceed to the prescription of specific actions to treat the impaired mobility. Careful, comprehensive assessment by a skilled and experienced practitioner is especially important in the current health care environment, not only to ensure that the appropriate interventions are prescribed, but also to determine eligibility for needed health care services. Without careful assessment the elder can be deprived of services that are needed to maintain or improve function, resulting in further and more costly decline and need for assistance with activities of daily living.

To intervene effectively, it will be necessary for the nurse to distinguish specific etiologies and to describe the severity, probable duration, and potential to reverse the impairment. If available, the nurse will consult with the physician and/or physical therapist to clarify etiologies and to determine the outcomes to be monitored in order to assess the patient's progress following interventions. Several studies have validated the diagnosis Impaired Physical Mobility and its etiologies (Creason, Pogue, Nelson, & Hoyt, 1985; Johnson, Stone, Larson, & Hromek, 1992; Keenan, 1989; Kraft, 1991; Kraft, Maas, & Hardy, 1994; Mehmert &

Delaney, 1991; Ouellet & Rush, 1992). See Table 28-1 for signs and symptoms for Impaired Physical Mobility.

Various tools for assessing mobility in elders are available (Katz, Ford, Moskowitz, Jackson, & Jaffe, 1963; Shanas et al., 1968; Wolanin, 1976); however, none is entirely satisfactory (Hogue, 1985). Assessment of mobility is often a part of functional assessment. Measures reviewed by Kane and Kane (1981) include assessment of transfer, mobility, walking, bed activities, locomotion, ability to propel wheelchair, and physical condition of lower limbs. Some tools are broad in scope but have less detail for assessing specific aspects of mobility. Some require instrumentation, whereas others do not. Most depend on the clinician's subjective conclusions from observation of patient performance. Many focus almost entirely on dimensions of the physical act of movement and ignore or neglect psychosocial factors, environmental factors, and demands of the task that are associated with impaired mobility (Czaja et al., 1993). Some focus on the extent the impaired mobility interferes with the ability to perform ADL and do not provide the detailed assessment needed to identify etiologies and focus interventions. The tool in Assessment Guide 28-1 is designed to be broad enough to encompass the data needed to identify causes of

Assessment Guide 28-1

NURSING ASSESSMENT: IMPAIRED PHYSICAL MOBILITY

Name _____ Age _____ Date initial test _____
Address _____ Vocation _____ Gender _____

Reason for seeking care

General appearance _____

Ambulant: walking, in wheelchair; with assistance, without assistance
Chairbound: with assistance, without assistance
Bedbound
Body build
Skin condition
Skin coloration
Hair and nails condition
General impression of mental attitude to condition, activity, exercise

_____
_____
_____

Client's view of physical abilities and drawbacks

_____
_____

What does the client want to be able to do?

_____
_____

Family and social support system

_____
_____

Activities of Daily Living (see Chapter 29)

Activity/rest pattern
Bed activities
Wheelchair activities
Self-care activities
Miscellaneous hand activities
Walking activities
Standing and sitting down
Climbing and traveling activities

Cardiovascular Status (see Chapter 24)

(See Allan, J. (1992). Exercise program. In G. M. Bulechek & J. C. McCloskey (Eds.), *Nursing interventions: Essential nursing treatments* (2nd ed., pp. 406-424). Philadelphia: W. B. Saunders.
Simpson, W. (1986). Exercise: Prescriptions for the elderly. *Geriatrics, 41*(1), 95-100 for preexercise assessment parameters.)

Neurologic Integrity

Reflexes
Control: voluntary/conscious/purposeful?
Are automatic position changes made?

Proprioception/Perceptual (see Chapter 37)

Skin sensation: different types (blunt-sharp, hot-cold, hard-soft, two-point discrimination, numbness)
Joint position?
Stereognosis?

Vibration

Muscle contraction response?

Vision/Hearing

Can hear ordinary speech volume?
Can hear/see own feet on floor, body moving against bed, chair?
Visual fields? (Can be roughly tested by holding two different colored pencils different distances apart and asking the client to describe)
Pupil reaction?
Incoordinate eye movements (nystagmus)?
Double vision?

Cognitive/Mental Status

Orientation?
Short-term memory?

Communication/Speech/Language (cross-reference Impaired Communication)

Can use language to express needs, understand directions?

Laboratory Results

Urine calcium?
Blood calcium and other electrolytes?
Hemoglobin?
Blood gases?
Serum phosphotase?

Joint Function and Range/Flexibility

Imposed restrictions?
Passive range?
Active range?
Every joint?
Reason for limitation, if any? Fixed deformities?
Habitual posturing?

Muscle Activity/Strength/Tone/Mass

Weakness?
Fatigue?

Self-care abilities (see Chapter 29)

Grip? (use grip dynamometer)
How much weight can be lifted?

Lift to standing position?
Wheelchair?
Flaccid, spastic, normal tone?
Spastic when stimulated by touch or activity? Constant?
Superficial and tendon reflexes?
Fluctuation of tone?

Endurance

Distance can walk and/or use wheelchair?
Time can maintain sitting balance?
Heart rate, respiration, and blood pressure; response to activity?

Pain

Reluctance to attempt movement?
Quality?
Location?
How relieved?
Cramps? Tenderness?

Balance and Coordination

Help needed to maintain posture?
Response to balance disturbance with eyes open and closed?
Ability to stop and start movement?
Eye-hand coordination?
General posture and stance? Gait?
Frequency, type, precipitating factor of falls?
Injury from previous falls?
Results of "get-up-and-go" test?

Feet and Footwear

Any foot problems?
Type of shoes worn?

Psychosocial Status

Social interaction?
Depression?
Expressed feelings, outlook (hopelessness, powerlessness)?
Role relationships?
Social support?

Medications/Treatments

Physical or chemical restraints?
Sedatives, analgesics, psychotropics?
Prolonged bed rest?
Braces, prosthesis, splints?

Environmental Barriers

Stairs?
Curbs?
Available assistive devices?
Scatter rugs, cords?
Adequate lighting?
Color contrast of rug/tile on floors?

impaired mobility comprehensively and to be detailed enough to guide nursing interventions.

NURSING DIAGNOSIS

Impaired Physical Mobility is "a limitation in independent, purposeful physical movement of the body or of one or more extremities" (NANDA, 1999, p. 84), or the "decreased ability to move from one place or position to another" (Kelly, 1985). Impaired Physical Mobility is often defined as "potential or actual limitations of independent physical movement within the environment" (Ouellet & Rush, 1992, p. 76). Tinetti and Ginter (1988) coined ambulatory mobility to distinguish physical mobility from the broad concept of mobility. Although walking is a complicated function involving multiple maneuvers, the key components are balance and gait (Tinetti, 1986).

The diagnosis Impaired Physical Mobility is distinguished from physical immobilization, which is a total inability to move the body or any of its parts from place to place, to move from one body position to another, or to manipulate any physical environmental elements. When physical immobilization is present, nursing care focuses not on elimination of the problem, but rather on the management of problems that are probable sequelae (e.g., impaired skin integrity or constipation). Impaired Physical Mobility can vary in the extent of restricted movement, in the scope of affected body parts, in the length of time that movement is restricted, and in the amount of control the elderly individual has over the mobility impairment. Nursing interventions for Impaired Physical Mobility have several goals: to correct, compensate, or ameliorate the mobility impairment; to prevent further impairment; and to prevent or minimize the physiologic, psychologic, and socioeconomic consequences of impaired mobility. Thus, it is most useful for nurses to conceptualize impaired mobility as a phenomenon that has more than physical consequences and that affects the holistic health of the elderly person (Ouellet & Rush, 1992). In a nursing diagnosis framework, physical mobility is clearly important for carrying out ADL, maintaining body functions, and achieving physical fitness (Houldin, Salstein, & Ganley, 1987).

CASE STUDY 1

D. Lutz is a 73-year-old married man who has resided for the past 5 years in a long-term care facility. He experienced a left cerebrovascular accident (CVA) with resultant expressive aphasia 3 months before his admission. He is alert, follows simple commands, makes choices about his life situation through nonverbal nods of his head and facial expressions, and yells when upset or when his needs are blocked. Since his admission he has attended and enjoyed many agency programs and activities, including dances, bingo, and cookie socials. He is selective about the unit activities he attends, but does participate in music group and pet visits. Recently he has begun attending wheelchair bowling, but he watches and does not participate actively. He often comes and goes at activities and becomes upset and yells if hindered.

Mr. Lutz has right hemiparesis as a result of the stroke and ambulates independently in a wheelchair. Flexion in his right shoulder is 45 degrees (normal, 180 degrees), and the shoulder is slightly internally rotated. His right elbow flexes to 45 degrees; his right wrist is fixed and flexed; his fingers extend 90 degrees; right hip has partial flexion and 45-degree abduction and is slightly internally rotated; knee has −5 degrees of hyperextension. The right ankle has only 10 degrees of motion in any direction. All joints on the right side are stiffened, and passive range of motion causes a moderate amount of pain, which Mr. Lutz indicates by grimacing, yelling if motion is continued, or refusing treatment. Muscles on the right side are slightly atrophied. Muscles on the left side are strong with nearly full ROM. After a reminder, Mr. Lutz is able to turn himself about in bed with the help of the trapeze or side rail. He is able to remain in a chosen position without assistance. He is unable to walk. He uses a pivot transfer to the wheelchair with one staff person assisting. He has a stable sitting balance. Once he is in the wheelchair, he is able to propel himself about with his left arm and leg. His right leg is supported on the leg rest. In the last 6 months he has had difficulty keeping his right leg on the foot pedal, which has hindered his mobility and upsets him a great deal. He is able to wheel himself approximately two city blocks and up and down ramps without cardiac or respiratory difficulty.

Mr. Lutz awakens between 7:00 and 8:00 AM, leaves the unit when he chooses, and returns for lunch. He lies down for a nap in the afternoon and leaves the unit before supper or watches TV. After supper he goes to agency activities or watches TV and goes to bed between 8:00 and 9:00 PM. He needs some assistance with dressing, grooming, bathing, hygiene, and eating. He is able to wash his own face and axillae, comb his hair, shave, brush dentures, and insert them. Given a lot of time, he is able to put on his own shirt and button it. He feeds himself after his milk is open and his meat is cut. He uses a plate guard, a large tablespoon, and often his fingers. He is completely dependent in toileting, requiring staff to care for his indwelling catheter and involuntary stools. Table 28-2 presents the significant signs and symptoms and the additional data needed for this case study.

The following tentative diagnoses were formulated for Mr. Lutz:

1. Impaired Physical Mobility related to pain as evidenced by vocal expressions of pain and discomfort with ROM and occasional refusal to do ROM.
2. Impaired Physical Mobility related to musculoskeletal impairment as evidenced by stiffness in right upper extremity and limited ROM in right shoulder, elbow, wrist, hip, ankle, and knee.
3. Impaired Physical Mobility related to neuromuscular impairment as evidenced by loss of muscle tone, mass, control, and strength in right leg.

Table 28-2	Impaired Physical Mobility: Differential Diagnosis for MR. LUTZ		
Significant Defining Characteristics	**Nursing Diagnoses Ruled Out**	**Additional Data Needed**	
Sufficient muscle strength left side to propel wheelchair		Activity Intolerance	
Muscle resistance?			
Endurance (wheelchair) 2 blocks, up ramps			
Pain and discomfort with ROM	PAIN*	Frequency of refusing ROM?	
Occasional refusal of ROM			
Able to move about in environment	COGNITIVE/PERCEPTUAL	Effect of expressive aphasia on communicating response to ROM?	
Stiffness in right upper extremity	MUSCULOSKELETAL IMPAIRMENT*	Evidence of receptive deficits?	
Limited ROM: right shoulder, elbow, wrist, hip, ankle, knee		Potential to increase ROM? Spasticity present?	
Decreased muscle mass, control, strength right leg	NEUROMUSCULAR IMPAIRMENT*	Other neurologic disorders?	

*Unable to rule out.

CASE STUDY 2

P. Newton is an 89-year-old widow who lives alone in her apartment in a housing complex for elders. She has an enlarged heart with frequent episodes of shortness of breath, dizziness, occasional chest pain, and rapid fatigue with minimal activity. Mrs. Newton has osteoarthritis in the shoulders, elbows, wrists, hands, and knees. She can no longer feed herself with her right hand, and her flexion in the right shoulder is about 90 degrees (180 degrees maximum). She can manage to get her clothes on, but she cannot get them off unless they are very loose or have snaps or large buttons (1 inch or larger) clear down the front. She can no longer comb her hair, so she uses wigs. She has the most severe pain in her knees, which causes difficulty in going up and down stairs and in getting in and out of a chair.

Mrs. Newton is absolutely convinced that she has cancer, even though she has been examined repeatedly with negative results. She does not believe that arthritis could cause so much pain. She believes everything that she hears on the radio and nothing that health care personnel tell her in person. For example, she will not take any aspirin because she has heard that it is bad for you. In addition to her limited ROM, she has extreme weakness in her hands and is unable to open milk cartons, tightly screwed jar lids, or safety lid medicine containers. Mrs. Newton has a wide-based gait and loses her balance easily. She refuses to use a cane or walker but often needs the support of another person or rail to go distances. She has fallen a number of times around the apartment and has become increasingly frightened to venture out. Most of the time she sits alone with the TV or radio or sleeps in her apartment.

Mrs. Newton has been treated for hypertension for the past 20 years. Her blood pressure normally runs about 180/90 mm Hg, and if it falls below 160/80 mm Hg, she becomes so weak she can hardly move about at all. Her

vision has deteriorated markedly, and she can see only shadows, which increases her fright of walking around in unfamiliar surroundings. Her hearing is impaired, so she cannot participate in group social situations. She can hear the telephone ring and can hear fairly well to converse over the phone, which is her major means of socialization. She is fully oriented and listens regularly to current events on the TV and radio. Much of the time she is depressed and often says, "I can't figure out why I am still alive." Mrs. Newton has two sons and three grandchildren. One son lives a long distance away, but the other son lives in the same community, and he and his wife and daughter are very attentive. The son in town has power of attorney because of Mrs. Newton's visual problems and her inability to sign checks. Her relationship with her son has almost completely reversed. She appreciates the help he provides, but at the same time she resents being told what to do and often misinterprets his attempts to help as attempts to run her life. Table 28-3 presents the signs and symptoms and the additional data needed for this case study.

The following tentative diagnoses were developed for Mrs. Newton:

1. Impaired Physical Mobility related to activity intolerance as evidenced by shortness of breath with activity, weakness, and lack of endurance.
2. Impaired Physical Mobility related to pain as evidenced by verbal complaints of joint pain on movement, especially climbing stairs and getting in and out of a chair, and reluctance to move.
3. Impaired Physical Mobility related to psychologic impairment as evidenced by statements of hopelessness and fear of falling, moving, and venturing out.
4. Impaired Physical Mobility related to cognitive/perceptual deficit as evidenced by poor vision and hearing, poor balance, and reluctance to venture out.

Table 28-3	Impaired Physical Mobility: Differential Diagnosis for MRS. NEWTON		
Significant Defining Characteristics	**Related Factors/Etiologies Ruled Out**	**Additional Data Needed**
Weakness and lack of endurance	Activity Intolerance	Does regular exercise increase strength/endurance?
Shortness of breath (SOB) with activity		Amount of time required for SOB to abate?
Weakness when blood pressure (BP) <160/80	Iatrogenic factors	Should antihypertensive medication be reduced?
Limited ROM in shoulders	Musculoskeletal impairment	Effect of limited ROM on wrists, hands, knees, ambulation?
Wide-based, unsteady gait; frequent falls	Reason for refusing poor balance ambulation aids	Does ROM increase with exercise?
Joint pain in shoulders, hands, knees	Pain*	Extent pain limits mobility?
Refuses aspirin or other analgesic	Lack of knowledge	Explore and trial methods of pain relief?
Poor vision and hearing	Cognitive/perceptual deficits*	Vision/hearing examination; are deficits correctable?
Reluctance to move and venture out	Psychologic impairments*	Bases of fear?
Fear of falling		When does she feel secure?
Expressions of hopelessness	Depression	Evaluation of depression?
Difficulty with stairs	Physical/social barriers	Location of barriers? What overcomes difficulty with stairs?
Role conflict with son	Social barrier	How is mobility affected?

*Unable to rule out.

NURSING-SENSITIVE OUTCOMES

The most meaningful evaluation of the effectiveness of a nursing intervention is whether the desired outcome(s) for the client is achieved. See Table 28-1 for the nursing-sensitive outcomes for the etiologies of Impaired Physical Mobility. The desired outcomes are selected by the patient or a family member in consultation with the nurse, since the outcomes must be those that are most important to the patient. The outcomes selected for Impaired Physical Mobility diagnoses are selected from the standardized nursing-sensitive patient outcomes developed by the Iowa Outcomes Project (2000).

CASE STUDY 1

All *Nursing Outcomes Classification (NOC)* outcomes and indicators selected for Mr. Lutz are in Table 28-4. Mr. Lutz and the nurse agreed on the following goals for his care: (1) to achieve moderately compromised muscle function, strength, and control in his right leg; (2) to gain moderate flexibility (ROM) in the joints on his right side and maintain the ROM in the joints on the unaffected left side; and (3) to decrease pain with joint movement to a slight level. Before interventions can be applied to increase joint flexibility and muscle strength, Mr. Lutz's pain with movement must be controlled and monitored regularly. Daily evaluation of his pain level is recommended until it is no greater

than moderate; then it is monitored weekly before exercise intervention. When the desired response to interventions to control his pain is achieved, interventions to improve Mobility Level and Joint Movement: Active outcomes become the focus of treatment. Joint movement indicators should be assessed at least weekly for a minimum of 6 weeks or until movement is beyond moderate motion. After a moderate rating of ROM is realized, quarterly assessment of the range of each joint should be completed and documented. A more precise measurement of the actual degrees of ROM of joints is recommended for revision of the NOC scales using the percentage of the maximum range for each joint, and the use of a gonometer is advised. Addition of a muscle strength indicator to the Muscle Function outcome also is recommended. Table 28-5 presents the maximum ROM for joints (Cole & Tobis, 1982; Monicken, 1991; Swartz, 1989).

CASE STUDY 2

Mrs. Newton and the nurse mutually developed goals to optimize her functional ability and quality of life within the constraints of her current mobility and chronic conditions. NOC outcomes and indicators selected by Mrs. Newton and the nurse are in Table 28-6. The goals agreed on were to (1) increase endurance in performing activities to be only mildly compromised; (2) learn to pace self to accomplish important activities, thus conserving energy to a moderate extent; (3) maintain current moderate level

Table 28-4	Nursing Diagnosis, Outcomes, and Interventions for MR. LUTZ		

Nursing Diagnosis	Nursing-Sensitive Outcomes	Nursing Interventions
IMPAIRED PHYSICAL MOBILITY *Defining Characteristics* Pain/discomfort range of motion Occasionally refuses ROM	**PAIN LEVEL** *Indicators* Oral expressions of pain Facial expressions of pain Protective body positions	**PAIN MANAGEMENT** *Activities* Ensure that the patient receives appropriate analgesic care Teach the use of nonpharmacologic techniques Evaluate the effectiveness of pain control measures used throughout ongoing assessment of the pain experience
Joint stiffness	**MOBILITY LEVEL** *Indicator* Joint movement	**EXERCISE THERAPY: JOINT MOBILITY** *Activities* Perform passive PROM or assisted (AROM) exercises, as indicated Teach to perform PROM
Limited ROM of: • Right shoulder • Right elbow • Right wrist • Right hip • Right knee • Right ankle	**JOINT MOVEMENT: ACTIVE** *Indicators* Right shoulder Right elbow Right wrist Right hip Right knee Right ankle **MUSCLE FUNCTION** *Indicators* Muscle strength Control of movement	**EXERCISE THERAPY: MUSCLE CONTROL** *Activities* Assist patient to develop exercise protocol for strength, endurance, and flexibility Encourage patient to practice exercises independently, as indicated Evaluate patient's progress toward enhancement/restoration of body movement and function

Nursing Outcomes Classification (NOC) 5-point Likert measurement scales:

Pain Level:	1 = Severe; 2 = Substantial; 3 = Moderate; 4 = Slight; 5 = None.
Mobility Level:	1 = Dependent, does not participate; 2 = Requires assistive person and device; 3 = Requires assistive person; 4 = Independent with assistive device; 5 = Completely independent.
Joint Movement: Active:	1 = No motion; 2 = Limited motion; 3 = Moderate motion; 4 = Substantial motion; 5 = Full motion.
Muscle Function:	1 = Extremely compromised; 2 = Substantially compromised; 3 = Moderately compromised; 4 = Mildly compromised; 5 = Not compromised.

of joint movement with a slight level of pain; (4) improve balance measured by the "get-up-and-go" test to slightly unstable (Mathias, Nayak, & Isaacs, 1986); (5) improve behaviors to prevent falls to substantially adequate; and (6) assist to develop a substantial amount of hope. Rather than the NOC balance scale, use of the "get-up-and-go" test with scale anchors of stable to severely unstable is recommended. Because Mrs. Newton is in her own home, the nurse visits her weekly and measures each outcome during each visit for the first month or until the desired level of the outcomes is met. Thereafter, the nurse monitors the outcomes quarterly to maintain Mrs. Newton's level of function.

NURSING INTERVENTIONS

For persons with Impaired Physical Mobility, the ultimate desired outcome is increased activity and mobility. However, the elderly person's ability to be mobile is often complicated by several etiologies that make mobility too painful or too much effort. The elder can perceive mobility as purposeless or unattainable. Although some form of active exercise is the only intervention that will restore or maintain muscle tone and strength for optimum activity and mobility, the nurse might need to intervene with other etiologies of impaired mobility before the elderly person can or will engage in active exercise; the nurse will have to supply the exercise for the elderly person when there are

Table 28-5	Maximum Range of Joint Motion
Joint	**Direction/Degrees**
Neck	Flexion/45°
	Lateral bending/40°
	Rotation/70°
Back	Flexion/75°
	Extension/30°
	Lateral bending/35°
	Rotation/30°
Shoulder	Flexion/180°
	Extension/50°
	External rotation/90°
	Internal rotation/90°
	Abduction/180°
	Adduction/50°
Elbow	Flexion/160°
	Supination/90°
	Pronation/90°
Wrist	Extension/70°
	Flexion/90°
	Radial deviation/20°
	Ulnar deviation/20°
Fingers	Metacarpophalangeal hyperextension/30°
	Flexion/90°
	Proximal interphalangeal flexion/120°
	Distal interphalangeal flexion/80°
Hip	Flexion/90° (with knee at 120°)
	Hyperextension/15°
	Abduction/45°
	Internal rotation/40°
	External rotation/80°
Knee	Hyperextension/15°
	Flexion/130°
Ankle	Dorsiflexion/20°
	Plantarflexion/45°
	Inversion/30°
	Eversion/20°

From Monicken, D. (1991). Immobility and functional mobility in the elderly. In W. C. Chenitz, J. T. Stone, & S. A. Salisbury (Eds.), *Clinical gerontological nursing: A guide to advanced practice* (pp. 233-245). Philadelphia: W. B. Saunders.

deficits that prevent the person from engaging in any active exercise.

The nurse's decision concerning the interventions that should be used to treat impaired mobility rests on the delineation of all etiologies and the determination of outcome priorities. Based on the etiology and prognosis, the nurse can determine that active exercise will never be possible at all. In this case the nurse will need to plan for exercise and activity that requires no voluntary muscle movement on the part of the patient. A number of the interventions that are appropriate for treating elderly persons are described in other chapters in this book (e.g., Chapters 27, 35, 36, 37, 41, and 44). Because the overall desired outcomes of interventions for Impaired Physical Mobility are to maintain or increase mobility and to prevent or minimize the consequences of immobility, neither of which can be achieved without some form of exercise, we have selected exercise as the intervention of choice for Impaired Physical Mobility. Table 28-7 lists other useful interventions that the nurse will likely use in the comprehensive treatment of elderly persons with mobility impairments.

A number of factors that are usually not reversible with intervention have been shown to be associated with inactivity among community-dwelling elders (Hogue, 1996). These factors are age, female gender, rural dwelling, low socioeconomic status, and chronic illness. There are, however, many barriers to exercise and activity among elders for which interventions can be designed and tested. Some of the more prominent barriers are ageism with belief in the inevitability of decline, depression, incontinence, caregiver responsibilities, lack of transportation, lack of resources to enable participation in exercise instruction and exercise programs, inclimate weather, lack of knowledge, lack of early life experience with exercise, and fear of falling and concern for safety. The design of exercise interventions to increase activity and mobility in elderly persons is therefore a complex task that must take into account many factors, including the psychology of the elder, the individual's functional abilities, and the social, economic, and physical environment within which the elder lives. Many of the strategies that could be used to overcome barriers and thus increase activity and exercise among elderly persons have not been systematically tested. Self-efficacy and social support are exceptions that have been shown to be associated with increased exercise and maintenance of regular exercise in the elder (Conn, In press a & b; Hogue, 1996).

Exercise Prescriptions

In a study of adults who had an average age of 75 and who lived in a high-rise apartment, 37% claimed to have no exercise, and a majority claimed only limited or brief episodes of exercise (Perry, 1982). Only 7.5% of persons over age 65 meet the activity level defined in the 1990 National Physical Fitness and Exercise objectives, and fewer than 25% of community-dwelling adults age 65 and older participate in regular exercise (Caspersen, Christenson, & Pollard, 1986). No study was found that documented the incidence of exercise among institutionalized elders; however, it can be assumed to be quite low because of environmental and physical constraints on chronically ill, elderly persons in these settings. For example, studies have found that many residents become dependent on wheelchairs following admission to a nursing home (Pawlson, Goodwin, & Keith, 1986).

The outcomes of exercise are both physiologic and psychosocial. The benefits of regular physical exercise for the

Table 28-6	Nursing Diagnosis, Outcomes, and Interventions for MRS. NEWTON		

Nursing Diagnosis	Nursing-Sensitive Outcomes	Nursing Interventions
IMPAIRED PHYSICAL MOBILITY *Defining Characteristics* Shortness of breath with activity Weakness Lack of endurance	**ENDURANCE** *Indicators* Activity Exhaustion not present **ENERGY CONSERVATION** *Indicators* Balances activity and rest Endurance level adequate for activity	**ENERGY MANAGEMENT** *Activities* Determine what and how much activity is required to build endurance Encourage alternate rest and activity periods Teach pacing techniques
	JOINT MOVEMENT: ACTIVE *Indicators* Shoulder (left) Shoulder (right) Knee (left) Knee (right) Wrist (left) Wrist (right) Fingers (left) Fingers (right) Thumb (left) Thumb (right)	**EXERCISE THERAPY: JOINT MOBILITY** *Activities* Teach to perform active ROM Assist patient to develop a schedule for active ROM exercises Assist with regular rhythmic joint motion within limits of pain endurance and joint mobility
	MUSCLE FUNCTION *Indicator* Muscle strength	**EXERCISE THERAPY: MUSCLE CONTROL** *Activities* Evaluate sensory functions Assist patient to develop exercise protocols for strength, endurance, and flexibility Provide positive reinforcement for patient's efforts in exercise and physical activity
Pain on movement Reluctance to move	**PAIN LEVEL** *Indicators* Reported pain Length of pain episodes Protective body positions Muscle tension	**PAIN MANAGEMENT** *Activities* Teach use of nonpharmacologic techniques before/after activities Evaluate pain with activity
Poor vision, hearing Poor balance Reluctance to venture out	**BALANCE** *Indicators* Standing balance Walking balance	**EXERCISE THERAPY: BALANCE** *Activities* Instruct how to position and move Assist to sit, rock side to side Stand, eyes closed, regular schedule
Fear of falling, moving	**SAFETY BEHAVIOR: FALL PREVENTION** *Indicators* Elimination of clutter, spills, glare from floors Correct use of assistive devices Compensation for physical limitations	**FALL PREVENTION** *Activities* Remove hazards from environment Provide adequate lighting for increased visibility Teach use of assistive devices

Continued

Table 28-6	Nursing Diagnosis, Outcomes, and Interventions for MRS. NEWTON—cont'd	
Nursing Diagnosis	**Nursing-Sensitive Outcomes**	**Nursing Interventions**
	SAFETY STATUS: FALLS OCCURRENCE *Indicators* Number of falls per week	
Expressions of hopelessness	**HOPE** *Indicators* Expressions of reasons to live Expression of belief in self Expression of sense of self-control	**HOPE INSTILLATION** *Activities* Expand patient's coping methods Guided life review, reminiscence Emphasize sustaining relationships Assist with attainable goals

Nursing Outcomes Classification (NOC) 5-point Likert measurement scales:

Pain Level:	1 = Severe; 2 = Substantial; 3 = Moderate; 4 = Slight; 5 = None.
Joint Movement: Active:	1 = No motion; 2 = Limited motion; 3 = Moderate motion; 4 = Substantial motion; 5 = Full motion.
Muscle Function:	1 = Extremely compromised; 2 = Substantially compromised; 3 = Moderately compromised; 4 = Mildly compromised; 5 = Not compromised.
Endurance:	1 = Extremely compromised; 2 = Substantially compromised; 3 = Moderately compromised; 4 = Mildly compromised; 5 = Not compromised.
Energy Conservation:	1 = Not at all; 2 = To a slight extent; 3 = To a moderate extent; 4 = To a great extent; 5 = To a very great extent.
Balance:	1 = Dependent, does not participate; 2 = Requires assistive person and device; 3 = Requires assistive person; 4 = Independent with assistive device; 5 = Completely independent.
Safety Behavior: Fall Prevention:	1 = Not adequate; 2 = Slightly adequate; 3 = Moderately adequate; 4 = Substantially adequate; 5 = Totally adequate.
Safety Status: Falls Occurrence:	1 = Over 9; 2 = 7-9; 3 = 4-6; 4 = 1-3; 5 = None.
Hope:	1 = None; 2 = Limited; 3 = Moderate; 4 = Substantial; 5 = Extensive.

elderly person have been documented (Coats et al., 1992; Dustman et al., 1984; Fiatarone & Evans, 1993; Waldo, Ide, & Thomas, 1995). Benefits include a slower rate of physical and cognitive decline, increased energy, improved sleep, better appetite, less pain, increased vasodilatation, increased cardiac output, and less stress. Other benefits are strengthening and toning of muscles, enhanced ROM and flexibility, and decreased boredom and social isolation. In a study of the effects of an exercise program on older adults, Perri and Templar (1984) reported a significant increase in self-concept and perceived locus of control. Chandler, Duncan, Kochersberger, and Studenski (1998) documented gains in lower extremity strength, gait speed, mobility tasks, and confidence in mobility from exercise among community-dwelling older men and women.

In the Waldo, Ide, and Thomas (1995) study, although exercise improved cardiac output, there were no changes in the oxygen-carrying capacity of blood for the elderly participants. Further, studies have shown that non-strengthening exercise (e.g., walking) does not prevent the muscle atrophy and weakness that accompany normal aging (Fiatarone & Evans, 1993; Klitgaard et al., 1990).

Exercise also can reduce the risk of venous stasis, thrombosis, and embolism. However, these benefits often are not realized by elderly persons because of the fear of injury, lack of resources and opportunity, low motivation, and lack of knowledge on the part of the client and/or the caregiver. Although a number of studies (Agre, Pierce, Raab, McAdams, & Smith, 1988; Benestad, 1965; DeVries, 1970; Koroknay, Werner, Cohen-Mansfield, & Braun, 1995; Regensteiner, 1987; Seals, Hagberg, Hurley, Ensoni, & Hollsey, 1984; Waldo, Ide, & Thomas, 1995) have demonstrated benefits of exercise for elderly subjects, public perceptions persist that elders will not benefit and that elderly persons desire to be sedentary. Because family members may hold these attitudes, nurses should include the family in teaching and planning exercise interventions so that they will support and encourage the elderly person. Exercise is therapeutic when it reduces muscle pain; increases strength, endurance, and flexibility; creates relaxation; and improves circulation. It is not therapeutic when it increases discomfort, causes anxiety, or taxes the heart (Kamentz, 1971). Therefore preexercise screening and assessment are vital to the successful use of exercise. The elderly individual may be more prone to avoid preexercise screening by a physician than younger persons because of the cost of examination and because of an orientation that physician visits are for illness (Simpson, 1986). This makes it imperative that nurses be able to assess the need for exercise, screen for risk, and prescribe and evaluate an exercise program.

The findings of a study by Roberts and Palmer (1996) showed that aerobic walking is a safe exercise for sedentary elders who have no significant cardiovascular disease.

Table 28-7	Nursing Interventions for the Treatment of Impaired Physical Mobility
Nursing Interventions	**Related Factors/Etiologies**
SURVEILLANCE	
EXERCISE THERAPY: JOINT MOBILITY	Cognitive perceptual deficits
Activities	
Active ROM	Neuromuscular impairment
Passive ROM	Musculoskeletal impairment
Group exercise	
EXERCISE PROMOTION: STRETCHING	
EXERCISE THERAPY: MUSCLE CONTROL	Activity intolerance
Activity	
Resistive exercise	
EXERCISE PROMOTION	
Activity	
Aerobic exercise	
ENERGY MANAGEMENT	
EXERCISE THERAPY: AMBULATION	
Activity	
Transfer training	
EXERCISE THERAPY: BALANCE	
FALL PREVENTION	
TEACHING: PRESCRIBED ACTIVITY/EXERCISE	Lack of knowledge regarding value of physical activity
EXERCISE THERAPY: ISOMETRIC	Iatrogenic factors
POSITIONING	Pain
BODY MECHANICS PROMOTION	Neuromuscular impairment
	Musculoskeletal impairment
PROGRESSIVE MUSCLE RELAXATION	Psychologic factors
SIMPLE RELAXATION THERAPY	Pain
PAIN MANAGEMENT	Neuromuscular impairment
ENVIRONMENTAL MANAGEMENT	Cognitive perceptual deficits
MEMORY TRAINING	Environmental barriers
COGNITIVE STIMULATION	
REMINISCENCE THERAPY	Psychologic factors
SUPPORT GROUP	Social factors
SUPPORT SYSTEM ENHANCEMENT	
VALUES CLARIFICATION	
ROLE ENHANCEMENT	
HOPE INSTILLATION	

However, an increased heart rate among elderly persons who exercise is often associated with nonsymptomatic dysrhythmia, so the investigators recommend that elderly persons with significant cardiovascular disease should be evaluated before exercise is prescribed. Stress tests are advocated for anyone with a history of cardiovascular disease (Monicken, 1991). Simpson (1986) advises special monitoring of elders who are taking the following medications: beta blockers (decrease heart rate), antihypertensives (exercise may magnify effects), and antidepressants and neuroleptics (may produce postural blood pressure changes).

Prescriptions for exercise use both active and passive exercise. Active exercise involves muscle contraction for movement and includes aerobic and endurance exercise, flexibility exercise, and resistive and isometric exercise.

Passive exercise, the movement of joints with energy supplied by an external force (machine or therapist) that does not involve muscle contraction, is used to maintain flexibility of joint movement. Forms of exercise that require energy conservation or that are needed to regain balance or gait will involve one or more of the forms of active exercise. Their success often depends on the appropriate use of passive exercise during illnesses to maintain range of joint motion. All of these exercises can be used for individuals alone or in groups.

Exercise can be prescribed for persons who are ambulatory, in bed, in a chair, or on a stretcher. However, any form of exercise, passive or active, must be prescribed following a careful assessment of the cause(s) of impaired mobility, including an evaluation of musculoskeletal and cardiovascular pathology. This discussion of exercise interventions focuses on the rationale for using specific forms of exercise to treat impaired mobility in elders. The scope of the chapter does not allow a comprehensive discussion of exercise interventions. Milde (1988) offers important information about measurement of muscle tone, strength, size, endurance, and ROM as outcomes of interventions for impaired mobility.

Exercise for Fitness and Endurance

The goals of exercise must also be individualized based on the elderly person's assessed strengths, weaknesses, and interests. Ordinarily active exercise prescription will be to gradually achieve an increased activity level (Allan, 1992).

Active exercise for elderly persons should begin with a "warm-up" period to prepare joints and muscles. "Warm-up" exercise usually employs ROM and flexibility exercise, but may also include a period of gradual increase of the intensity of exercise. The warm up for aerobic and endurance exercise includes gentle stretching of muscles and avoids quick, forceful movements of all kinds. Warm up is also used to reinforce and establish breathing patterns that maximize ventilation. Warm up prepares the body for sustained activity and increased workload on the heart. If there is pain, the exercise should begin with motions of body parts where there is the least discomfort and move gradually, with the elder's willingness, to areas of the body where discomfort is greater. When specific motions are painful, it is usually helpful to hold the position following contraction and extension at the end points of available active range and then relax. Often it will be helpful to the client and will increase his willingness to perform if the therapist provides some physical support for the joint and body part during the active motion. It is important to taper off activity rather than abruptly stop. The "cool down" period following vigorous exercise should be 5 to 10 minutes. During the cool down, the individual exercises at a slower pace, using large muscle groups and ending with ROM, stretching, contracting, and relaxing to prevent syncope that results from a sudden decrease in the supply of blood to large muscle groups.

Any pain in the chest, arm, neck, or jaw, lightheadedness, pallor, or irregular or too rapid heart rate should be signals to cease exercise immediately and evaluate for the need to notify a physician. If breathlessness or rapid pulse persists for more than 10 minutes after exercise, if joint pain persists for more than 2 hours, or if there is prolonged fatigue or lethargy, there is need to reevaluate the exercise program.

Cardiovascular fitness is the primary aim of aerobic exercise. Running, walking, and jogging are most effective for fitness training with the most efficient cardiac output. Stair climbing also may be a useful form of aerobic training. Running and jogging, however, will be deleterious for many elderly persons. Thus, walking may be the most

likely form of aerobic exercise to be used. Swimming may also be an option for some elders who have access. Because more strenuous exercise may be contraindicated and because some elders will also not be able to walk or swim, Simpson (1986) suggests "jarming," jogging with the arms, as an alternative. It is important to emphasize that aerobic exercise is a desirable intervention for many elderly persons and often can be prescribed for institutionalized elders, as well as for elderly persons in the community.

A number of recent studies have demonstrated the advantages of walking for community-dwelling well elders, institutionalized elders, and elderly persons with chronic conditions, even those who are quite disabled, who have osteoarthritis, or who require a cane. Advantages include an increase in walking distance (Koroknay et al., 1995; Kovar et al., 1992), a decrease in fatigue (Gueldner & Spradley, 1988), and decreased use of pain medication (Kovar et al., 1992). However, MacRae et al. (1996) developed a walking program for cognitively impaired nursing home residents and was unable to demonstrate a statistically significant positive effect for walk endurance. The study did show that a walking program for the cognitively impaired could be implemented and integrated into the elderly persons' daily care. The requirement of few resources is a further advantage of walking as the exercise of choice for elders. Mall walking is described as adding social contacts and new roles and routines for the elder, along with exercise. It is inexpensive and can be done wherever the person lives (Travis, Duncan, & McAuley, 1996).

The aim of active exercise is to achieve an energy expenditure of 1000 to 2000 calories per week (Simpson, 1986). Thirty minutes of aerobic exercise can be expected to use about 300 calories when the heart rate is advanced to 70% of maximum. Target zones of 70% and 85% for heart rate have been established to guide the conduction of safe aerobic exercise. Active exercise for the elder will often never reach the aerobic point; however, these values for obtaining maximum training effects should be used to set goals, identify high-risk elders, and evaluate the effectiveness of interventions.

A fitness training program using aerobic exercise must be specified for each elderly person. Type of activity, intensity of activity, duration, frequency, warm-up and cooldown exercises, reasons to stop or modify the program, and the method for monitoring intensity should be specifically outlined (Fair, Allan-Rosenaur, & Thurston, 1979; Pollock & Wilmore, 1990). A drug history should be taken for accurate interpretation of heart rate response (American Nurses Association, 1994; DeVries, 1970). Beta blockers are probably the most common cause of diminished heart rate response to exercise, and the hypotensive effects of antihypertensive medications, antidepressants, and neuroleptics can be potentiated by exercise (Simpson, 1986). As noted previously, the description of aerobic exercise programs for fitness training in sufficient detail to guide their use by nurse clinicians is not possible within the scope of this chapter. The reader is referred to Allan (1992) for an excellent, detailed discussion of aerobic exercise prescription.

Exercise for Flexibility

Flexibility exercises aim to increase or maintain the ROM of a joint or joints. Active flexibility exercises are usually called calisthenics or active ROM exercises. Calisthenics of arm swings, neck rotation, hip and torso bending, leg swings, thigh abduction, and knee bends, in concert with a breathing pattern of deep inhalation and exhalation, are performed rhythmically, often to music. Passive flexibility exercises are the same as passive ROM exercises. These exercises commonly include stretching to increase the range of joint and muscle movements. The idea is to achieve maximum joint range, flexion, extension, inversion, eversion, rotation, adduction, and abduction where appropriate.

Usually a method of last resort, passive exercise, along with splinting, is used to prevent contractures that deform and deprive the client of joint movement, flexibility, and alignment. These joint functions are required for comfortable positioning, for the ability to perform ADL, and for the potential to increase activity, regain self-care abilities, and engage in active exercise for increased fitness. Elderly persons, especially those who are dependent on others for basic ADL and who have few other reasons for movement, will develop contractures of joints in the positions that are maintained for long periods of time. This often makes upper extremities at high risk because, even in sitting positions, the arms and hands are often not moved. Neck flexion contractures are also common among elderly persons who sit for long periods or who use too large a pillow while in bed. These contractures interfere with swallowing and social interaction. Joint contractures can occur within 3 to 7 days, so the nurse should be vigilant with exercise to prevent all forms. Passive exercise should not be prescribed when the elderly person can cooperate in a form of active exercise because of the risk of causing microtears in tissues that are already damaged and inelastic. Moreover, it is ordinarily a more painful form of exercise and has no effect on maintaining or increasing muscle tone and strength (Matson, 1985; Monicken, 1991). Elderly persons, in bed or not, need both active exercise to maintain physiologic integrity and passive exercise, judiciously prescribed, to prevent unnecessary loss of functional abilities.

Because there is a risk of tissue damage that can result in scar formation from increased fibrosis and thickening, a physical therapist or professional nurse who has a thorough knowledge of the anatomy and physiology of the neuromusculature and joints should always assess the client and prescribe the needed passive exercise intervention. One of these professionals should also perform the passive exercise until both the client and the therapist are assured that it can be carried out without undue discomfort and without tissue damage. Then it might be appropriate to delegate the implementation of the prescribed passive exercise to ancillary nursing personnel or to the family. In some instances, such as hemiplegia following stroke or paraplegia caused by spinal cord injury, the client might be able to perform passive ROM exercises on the affected extremities by using the unaffected ones.

When the potential exists to regain active exercise, the nurse should encourage the client to attempt to perform the ROM exercises. Then, as the elderly person regains the ability for active movement, the therapist can move from passive exercises to active-assistive exercises and then to active ROM exercises, providing the amount of support and assistance that is necessary to complete the movements. Finally, resistive exercises can be prescribed for strengthening of muscles. The advancement from passive to active movement and exercise can often be facilitated by exercising two or more joints simultaneously. This method invokes proprioceptive neuromuscular facilitation principles, and also reduces pain, decreases the chance of tissue damage, contributes to muscle tone, and reduces demands on the elderly person's endurance, as well as on the therapist's time.

The nurse should pay careful attention to the particular etiology and underlying disease that necessitates passive exercise. The prescription must be tailored to individual circumstances, as well as to other characteristics of the elderly client such as motivation, cognitive abilities, and condition of joints and muscles. For example, inflammation of the arthritic person's joints requires special attention to pain and possible trauma that movement will cause. Special attention should be given to the scheduling of analgesics and antiinflammatory medications before manipulations of the joints. Stroke victims with hemiplegia need special attention given to the affected arm, which is more vulnerable to contractures, and to the shoulder, which can subluxate easily because of gravitational pull of the arm on weakened muscles that support the shoulder joint. Joint integrity is always at risk when the supporting musculature for the joint is weakened as a result of disease or immobility.

Passive ROM exercise has been shown to have some positive effects on limited movement contractures in elders that result from extraarticular physiologic joint restriction secondary to neuromuscular dysfunction (Medeiros, Schmidt, Burmeister, & Soderberg, 1977; Tanigawa, 1972). When contracted joints are the object of intervention, the aim is to stretch and lengthen the shortened muscles and move the joint through its range before an ankylosed or permanently "frozen" joint results. The method of passive exercise used has traditionally been high-load brief stretch (Light, Nuzik, Personius, & Barstrom, 1984). Elderly persons are predisposed to limited movement contractures of many joints, and chronic knee flexion contractures are especially common because of inactivity and prolonged periods of sitting. In a study of nonambulatory residents of a nursing home who demonstrated gradually progressive bilateral knee contractures, low-load prolonged stretch using extension by skin traction was shown to be more effective than the traditional high-load brief stretch in reducing the knee contractures (Light et al., 1984). Nurses should consider this intervention for use with elderly patients, especially for the knee, hip, and neck flexion contractures that occur so often in this population.

Byers (1985) studied the effects of non–weight-bearing, active evening and morning exercise on measures of joint stiffness with 30 patients who had rheumatoid arthritis. Stiffness decreased and mobility increased significantly after performance of evening exercises, particularly for finger joints. Although the findings of the study are not conclusive for all joints and perceived stiffness did not always correlate with objective measures of stiffness, these results are encouraging for the use of evening exercise to treat impaired mobility associated with inflamed and arthritic joints.

Continuous passive ROM machines have been developed within the last several years. There are a number of different models of these machines, but they all consist of a motorized frame and a control that is used to turn the machine on and off and regulate the speed. When the machine is on and the client's limb is placed on it, the limb is flexed and extended continuously. Machines are available to exercise hand, shoulder, hip, knee, and ankle joints. They have essentially the same benefits as passive exercise performed by a therapist; that is, they prevent contractures, venous stasis, and thromboembolism and are most often used for total joint replacements, ligament reconstructions, fixations following joint fractures, and synovectomies. They are contraindicated for patients with arthritis, contracted joints, or muscle paralysis and for patients who are not competent mentally to turn the machine off when needed. Pain, potential injury to joints and muscles, and skin breakdown make the use of continuous passive motion hazardous (Johnson, 1983). The machines can be a useful adjunct for human energy to perform passive ROM exercise, but the nurse must be selective regarding their use and vigilant in surveillance when they are in use.

CASE STUDY 1

Because Mr. Lutz experiences considerable pain during ROM exercise, which makes him unwilling to do the exercises part of the time, Pain Management is the priority nursing intervention. The use of an analgesic and a muscle relaxant administered before each exercise session is discussed with the physician and ordered for the patient.

Nonpharmacologic relaxation therapy is also used to reduce Mr. Lutz's anxiety and to minimize further muscle tightening caused by tension. Exercise Therapy: Joint Mobility with passive ROM is performed by Mr. Lutz twice daily with the nurse's assistance to increase the ROM in his right shoulder, elbow, wrist, hip, knee, and ankle and to maintain the ROM in his other joints. Exercise Therapy: Muscle Control is prescribed, with Mr. Lutz encouraged to perform active ROM on the joints that have limited range one additional time during the day. He is able to do this by using his unaffected upper and lower extremities to assist the affected side. Resistive exercise is also prescribed for Mr. Lutz to strengthen the muscle in his right leg. This is accomplished by having him complete the full ROM of his right leg against some resistance provided by the therapist. When he is in bed, Mr. Lutz performs isometric exercises against the footboard and the bed for strengthening. Because Mr. Lutz propels his wheelchair a considerable distance without difficulty, additional strengthening exercises for his left arm and leg are not prescribed. Documentation of Mr. Lutz's progress for 3 weeks for the outcomes selected with the nurse are illustrated in Table 28-8. Isometric exercise is discussed following the case studies.

CASE STUDY 2

Mrs. Newton has a prescription for active ROM exercise once daily to maintain the flexibility of shoulders, wrists, hands, and knees. Because she refuses any analgesic and her pain is caused by osteoarthritis, increased flexibility of the affected joints is not a realistic outcome. Rather, the prescription is intended to prevent further loss of functional ROM. To promote strengthening, a small amount of resistance during active ROM exercises is also prescribed. Small weights (2 lb each), strapped to the upper and lower extremities, are worn while exercising. The weights can be gradually increased, if tolerated, to advance strengthening. After 4 weeks of exercise, improvement was noted in Mrs. Newton's balance and gait, and she has experienced no falls. Progress documented during a 4-week period with outcomes selected with the nurse is illustrated in Table 28-9.

Isometric and Resistive Exercise for Strength

Isometric exercise occurs when muscles contract or tense without shortening or joint movement. Isometric exercises are used for strengthening a muscle group. For the exercise to be most effective, the muscle should exert as much effort as possible against resistance for a prescribed period of 5 to 15 seconds (Daly & Berman, 1993; Sorenson & Ulrich, 1966). This form of exercise is used to prevent loss of muscle strength when persons are immobilized because of surgical procedures, such as orthopedic procedures, or injuries that require casting or traction. The ex-

Table 28-8 Mr. Lutz's Progress Using Selected Outcome and Indicator Ratings				
	Base	Day 7 of Week 1	Week 2	Week 3
PAIN LEVEL	1	3	3	4
Oral expression of pain	1	3	3	4
Facial expressions of pain	1	3	3	4
Protective body positions	2	3	4	4
MOBILITY LEVEL	1	2	2	4
Joint movement: right side	1	2	2	4
JOINT MOVEMENT: ACTIVE	1	2	2	3
Right shoulder: flexion	2	2	2	3
• Extension	2	2	2	3
• External rotation	1	2	2	3
• Internal rotation	1	2	2	3
• Abduction	1	2	2	3
• Adduction	2	2	2	3
Right elbow: flexion	2	2	3	3
• Extension	2	2	2	3
• Supination	1	2	2	3
• Pronation	2	3	3	3
Right wrist: flexion	1	2	2	2
• Extension	1	2	2	3
• Radial deviation	1	2	2	2
• Ulnar deviation	1	2	2	2
Right hip: flexion	1	1	2	3
• Hyperextension	1	1	2	2
• Abduction	1	1	1	3
• Internal rotation	1	1	2	3
• External rotation	1	1	2	3
Right knee: flexion	1	2	2	3
• Hyperextension	1	1	1	2
Right ankle: dorsiflexion	1	1	2	2
• Plantar flexion	1	2	3	3
• Inversion	1	1	2	2
• Eversion	1	1	2	2
MUSCLE FUNCTION	1	1	2	2
Strength in right leg	1	1	2	2
Control of movement of right leg	1	1	1	2

Nursing Outcomes Classification (NOC) 5-point Likert measurement scales:

Pain Level: 1 = Severe; 2 = Substantial; 3 = Moderate; 4 = Slight; 5 = None.
Mobility Level: 1 = Dependent, does not participate; 2 = Requires assistive person; 3 = Requires assistive person/device;
                   4 = Independent with assistive device; 5 = Completely independent.
Joint Movement: 1 = No motion (0% of maximum range); 2 = Limited motion (25% of maximum range);
                   3 = Moderate motion (50% of maximum range); 4 = Substantial motion (75% of maximum range);
                   5 = Full motion (100% of maximum range).
Muscle Function: 1 = Extremely compromised; 2 = Substantially compromised; 3 = Moderately compromised; 4 = Mildly compromised;
                   5 = Not compromised.

Table 28-9 Mrs. Newton's Progress Using Selected Outcome and Indicator Ratings	Base	Week 1	Week 2	Week 3	Week 4
ENDURANCE	1	1	2	2	2
Activity	2	2	2	2	3
Exhaustion not present	1	1	2	2	2
ENERGY CONSERVATION	2	2	2	3	3
Balances activity and rest	2	2	3	3	4
Endurance adequate for activity	2	2	2	3	3
JOINT MOVEMENT: ACTIVE	3	3	3	3	4
Left shoulder	3	3	3	3	3
Right shoulder	3	3	3	3	4
Left knee	3	3	3	3	4
Right knee	3	3	3	3	4
Left wrist	3	3	3	3	4
Right wrist	3	3	3	3	4
Left fingers/thumb	3	3	3	3	4
Right fingers/thumb	3	3	3	3	4
MUSCLE FUNCTION	2	2	2	2	3
Muscle strength	2	2	2	2	3
PAIN LEVEL	2	2	2	3	3
Reported pain	2	2	2	3	3
BALANCE	2	2	2	2	3
Standing balance	2	2	2	3	3
Walking balance	2	2	2	2	3
SAFETY BEHAVIOR: FALL PREVENTION	3	3	4	4	4
Free of clutter, spills, glare	3	3	4	5	5
Correct use of assistive devices	3	3	4	3	3
Compensation for limitations	2	3	3	3	3
SAFETY STATUS: FALLS	4	4	3	4	5
Number of falls per week	4	4	3	4	5
HOPE	2	2	1	2	3
Expressions of reasons to live	1	1	1	2	2
Expression of belief in self	2	2	2	2	3
Expression of sense of self-control	2	2	1	2	3

Nursing Outcomes Classification (NOC) 5-point Likert measurement scales:

Endurance:	1 = Extremely compromised; 2 = Substantially compromised; 3 = Moderately compromised; 4 = Mildly compromised; 5 = Not compromised.
Energy Conservation:	1 = Not at all; 2 = To slight extent; 3 = To moderate extent; 4 = To great extent; 5 = To very great extent.
Joint Movement: Active:	1 = 0%, 2 = 25%, 3 = 50%, 4 = 75%, 5 = 100%.
Muscle Function:	1 = Extremely compromised; 2 = Substantially compromised; 3 = Moderately compromised; 4 = Mildly compromised; 5 = Not compromised.
Pain Level:	1 = Severe; 2 = Substantial; 3 = Moderate; 4 = Slight; 5 = None.
Balance:	1 = Extremely unstable; 2 = Substantially unstable; 3 = Moderately unstable; 4 = Slightly unstable; 5 = Stable.
Safety Behavior:	1 = Not adequate; 2 = Slightly adequate; 3 = Moderately adequate; 4 = Substantially adequate;
Fall Prevention:	5 = Totally adequate.
Safety Status: Falls/week:	1 = Over 9; 2 = 7-9; 3 = 4-6; 4 = 1-3; 5 = None.
Hope:	1 = None; 2 = Limited; 3 = Moderate; 4 = Substantial; 5 = Extensive.

ercises are useful when the individual can participate in active exercise but for some reason cannot exercise in more normal activities. The exercises are also useful for muscles such as sphincters or perineal muscles that have more limited active movement during normal living.

Isometric exercises may be contraindicated for persons with abnormal cardiac function, although the effects are increased systolic and diastolic blood pressure during ex-

ercise rather than increased cardiovascular load (Nutter, Schlant, & Hurst, 1972). Lavin (1973) reported that isometric exercise accentuated left ventricular function in patients with abnormal cardiac function. Patients should be encouraged to breathe through their mouths to avoid the Valsalva maneuver—increased intrathoracic pressure from forced exhalation against a closed glottis. Isometric exercises are, however, convenient to use with cooperative clients and can be used to augment other active exercises periodically throughout the day. The client can implement these exercises without supervision or assistance by the nurse if the purpose, plan, and technique for the exercises are understood. Kegel exercises can help strengthen perineal musculature for relief of stress incontinence (Mandelstom, 1980). Isometric exercises have been used to treat other problems experienced by elders, including strengthening abdominal muscles to treat constipation, strengthening leg muscles before weight bearing following hip fracture, and strengthening the quadriceps in the person with arthritis who has knee involvement and finds weight bearing or other active joint movement too painful (Daly & Berman, 1993; Wolff, 1986).

Resistive exercise is used to strengthen muscles. Resistance can be added to isometric exercise by having the client push against something like the bed, footboard, or resistance provided by the therapist. Resistive exercise can vary from isometric resistance exercise, to having an elderly person who has had a stroke begin to lift small leg and arm weights in preparation for learning to balance, stand, transfer, and walk, to high-resistance weight lifting. Resistance is gradually increased as muscles acquire strength. Nurses can easily combine resistance exercise with active ROM exercise. A small sandbag strapped to the foot or grasped in the elderly person's hand is a simple example. The nurse can also supply resistance by pushing against the body part that is being exercised. The important point is that a plan be developed to strengthen muscle groups that are needed for regaining or preventing the loss of functional abilities.

The nurse should always be working to assist the elderly person to move to the highest level of functional ability. For maximum mobility, ambulation is the desired outcome. Although the maximum level of physical functional ability possible might not be walking, lesser levels of ability are still important achievements for maintaining mobility. A sequence of abilities leading to ambulation is required when illness, disability, and disuse have led to loss of the ability to ambulate. The first emphasis is on maintaining or regaining sufficient muscle strength and ROM. Next, attention is focused on the development of sitting balance. Then standing balance and transfer ability are developed. Training in shifting body weight and in achieving a specific gait pattern are the final steps. Often ambulation includes training in the use of walkers, canes, or crutches.

Even very frail elderly persons can improve muscle strength and endurance with a specifically prescribed muscle rehabilitation program. Progressive muscle rehabilitation programs have been shown to be effective with persons with symptomatic osteoarthritis when sustained for a 4- to 8-month period. Improvements in strength and functional performance of approximately 30%, as well as in degree of difficulty and pain during walking, standing, arising from a chair, and climbing stairs resulted (Fisher, Pendergast, & Calkins, 1991).

Common problems of exercise programs for all adults are motivation and consistency. Exercise groups are often useful to overcome these problems for elderly persons. Group exercise adds psychosocial benefits to exercise, which in turn increases the motivation of individuals to exercise (Travis, Duncan, & McAuley, 1996). Group exercise has been used successfully with elders in the community and in institutions.

There comes a time in rehabilitation programs when the person is no longer progressing with individual exercises. At this stage, group treatment is a valuable accessory to individual treatment. The person still receives a certain amount of individual attention, but learns to take some individual responsibility while working with others. As a group, elders can overcome their belief in the myths that old people naturally decline, that old people do not exercise, and that exercise is childish. Active exercises must be tailored to the particular population of elderly persons, as well as to individual capabilities.

Exercises have to be designed for sitting positions if the person is confined to a chair or has difficulty with balance. Mr. Lutz is encouraged to attend group exercise sessions for persons in wheelchairs. Since he began attending, his participation in the exercise prescription has increased. Exercises also should be designed for persons who are in bed or who cannot achieve sitting balance. Reference to motions in more familiar words, such as "picking cherries" instead of "reaching up," can assist elders who are too cognitively impaired to otherwise participate.

SUMMARY

Impaired Physical Mobility is a nursing diagnosis for many elderly persons in the community and in institutions. Because of the number of etiologies, the process of diagnosis, intervention, and evaluation of the efficacy of treatment is complex. Various signs and symptoms indicate specific types of impaired mobility. Accurate identification of types of impaired mobility allows for prescription of nursing interventions designed to achieve desired outcomes. Focused, standardized interventions that have clearly defined expected effects measured with standardized outcomes are needed for clinical nursing research. NIC interventions and NOC outcomes will promote nursing research and the development of research-based nursing clinical knowledge.

REFERENCES

Agency for Health Care Policy and Research (AHCPR). (1992). Pressure ulcers in adults: Prediction and prevention. *Clinical Practice Guideline No. 3.* Rockville, MD: Department of Health & Human Services.

Agre, J., Pierce, L. E., Raab, D. M., McAdams, M., & Smith, E. L. (1988). Light resistance and stretching exercises in elderly women: Effect upon strength. *Archives of Physical Medicine Rehabilitation, 69,* 273-276.

Allan, J. (1992). Exercise program. In G. M. Bulechek & J. C. Mc-
Closkey (Eds.), *Nursing interventions: Essential nursing treatments* (2nd ed., pp. 406-424). Philadelphia: W. B. Saunders.

American Nurses Association. (1994). *Clinician's handbook of
preventive services.* Waldorf, MD: American Nurses.

Aniansson, A., Hedberg, M., Henning, G., & Grimby, G. (1986).
Muscle morphology, enzymatic activity and muscle strength
in elderly men: A follow-up study. *Muscle and Nerve, 9,* 585-
591.

Benestad, A. M. (1965). Trainability of old men. *Acta Med Scandinavica, 178,* 321-327.

Berry, J. K., Vitalo, C. A., Larson, J. L., Patel, M., & Kim, M.
(1996). Respiratory muscle strength in elder adults. *Nursing
Research, 45*(3), 154-159.

Bosco, C., & Komi, P. (1980). Influence of aging on the mechanical behavior of leg extensor muscles. *European Journal of
Applied Physiology, 45*(2), 209-219.

Browse, N. (1965). *The physiology and pathology of bedrest.*
Springfield, IL: Charles C. Thomas.

Byers, P. H. (1985). Effect of exercise on morning stiffness and
mobility in patients with rheumatoid arthritis. *Research on
Nursing and Health, 8*(3), 275-281.

Carnevali, D., & Brueckner, S. (1970). Immobilization: Reassessment of a concept. *American Journal of Nursing, 70,* 1502-1507.

Caspersen, C., Christenson, G., & Pollard, R. (1986). Status of the
1990 physical fitness and exercise objectives—Evidence from
NHIS 1985. *Public Health Reports, 101*(6), 587-592.

Chandler, J. M., Duncan, P. W., Kochersberger, G., & Studenski, S.
(1998). Is lower extremity strength gain associated with improvement in physical performance and disability in frail,
community-dwelling elders? *Archives of Physical Medicine &
Rehabilitation, 79*(1), 24-30.

Clark, W., MacGregor, A., Prescott, R., & Ruckley, C. (1974).
Pneumatic compression of the calf and postoperative deep
vein thrombosis. *Lancet, 2,* 5.

Coats, A., Adamopoulos, S., Radaelli, A., McCance, A., Meyer, T.,
Bernardi, L., Solda, P., Davey, P., Ormerod, O., Forfar, C.,
Conway, J., & Sleight, P. (1992). Controlled trial of physical
training in chronic heart failure: Exercise performance, hemodynamics, ventilation, and autonomic function. *Circulation, 85,* 2119-2132.

Cole, T. M., & Tobis, J. S. (1982). Measurement of musculoskeletal function. In F. J. Kottke, G. K. Stillwell, & J. F. Lehmann
(Eds.), *Krusen's handbook of physical medicine and rehabilitation* (3rd ed., pp. 19-55). Philadelphia: W. B. Saunders.

Conn, V. (In press [a]). Older women and exercise: Theory of
planned behavior beliefs. *Nursing Research.*

Conn, V. (In press [b]). Exercise and older adults: Self-efficacy
constructs. *Nursing Research.*

Creason, N., Pogue, N., Nelson, A., & Hoyt, C. (1985). Validating
the nursing diagnosis of impaired physical mobility. *Nursing
Clinics of North America, 20,* 669-683.

Czaja, S. J., Weber, R. A., & Nair, S. N. (1993). A human factors
analysis of ADL activities: A capability-demand approach.
The Journals of Gerontology, 48, 44-48.

Daly, M., & Berman, B. (1993). Rehabilitation of the elderly
patient with arthritis. *Clinics in Geriatric Medicine, 9*(4), 783-
801.

Deitrick, J., Whedon, G., & Shorr, E. (1948). Effect of immobilization upon various metabolic and physiologic functions of
normal men. *American Journal of Medicine, 4,* 3.

DeVries, H. (1970). Physiological effects of an exercise training
regimen upon men aged 52 to 82. *Journal of Gerontology, 25,*
325-336.

Dunning, M., & Plum, M. (1957). Hypercalciuria following poliomyelitis: Its relationship to site and degree of paralysis.
Archives of Internal Medicine, 99, 716.

Dustman, R., Ruhling, R. O., Russell, E. M., Shearer, D. E.,
Bonekat, H. W., Shigeoke, J. W., Wood, J. S., & Bradford, D. C.
(1984). Aerobic exercise training and improved neuropsychological function of older individuals. *Neurobiological Aging,
5*(1), 32-42.

Egan, M., Warren, S. A., Hessel, P. A., & Gilewich, G. (1992). Activities of daily living after hip fracture: Pre- and post discharge. *The Occupational Therapy Journal of Research, 12*(6),
342-356.

England, M. (1989). Nursing diagnosis: A conceptual framework. In J. J. Fitzpatrick & A. L. Whall (Eds.), *Conceptual
models of nursing* (2nd ed., pp. 347-370). Norwalk, CT: Appleton & Lange.

Fair, J., Allan-Rosenaur, J., & Thurston, E. (1979, May/June). Exercise management. *Nurse Practitioner,* 13-18.

Fiatarone, M. A., & Evans, W. J. (1993). The etiology and reversibility of muscle dysfunction in the aged. *The Journals of
Gerontology, 48,* 77-83.

Fisher, N., Pendergast, D., & Calkins, E. (1991, March). Muscle
rehabilitation in impaired elderly nursing home residents.
Archives of Physical Medicine, 72, 181-185.

Fowles, D. G. (1990). *A profile of older Americans: 1990* (DHHS
Publication PF3029[1290]D996). Washington, DC: American
Association of Retired Persons, Association of Aging.

Franssen, E. H., Souren, L. E., Torossian, C. L., & Reisberg, B.
(1999). Equilibrium and limb coordination in mild cognitive
impairment and mild Alzheimer's disease. *Journal of the
American Geriatrics Society, 47*(4), 463-469.

Friedrich, R., & Lively, S. (1981). Psychological immobilization.
In L. Hart, M. Fehring, & J. Reece (Eds.), *Concepts common to
acute illness* (1st ed.). St. Louis, MO: Mosby.

Gordon, M. (1995). *Manual of nursing diagnosis 1995-1996.* St.
Louis, MO: Mosby.

Gueldner, S., & Spradley, J. (1988). Outdoor walking lowers
fatigue. *Journal of Gerontological Nursing, 14*(10), 6-12.

Guralnik, J. M., & Simonsick, E. M. (1993). Physical disability in older Americans. *The Journals of Gerontology, 48,*
3-10.

Hallal, J. (1985). Nursing diagnosis: An essential step to quality
care. *Journal of Gerontological Nursing, 11,* 35-38.

Hardy, M., Maas, M., & Akins, J. (1988). The prevalence of
nursing diagnoses among elderly and long term care residents: A descriptive comparison. *Recent Advances in Nursing,
21,* 144-158.

Harper, C. M., & Lyles, Y. M. (1988). Physiology and complications of bed rest. *Journal of the American Geriatrics Society, 36,*
1047-1054.

Hogue, C. (1985). Mobility. In E. L. Schneider, C. J. Wendland, A.
Zimmer, N. List, & M. Ory (Eds.), *The teaching nursing home*
(pp. 231-245). New York: Raven Press.

Hogue, C. (1996, Oct.). *State of the science: Interventions for physical mobility in the elderly.* Paper presented at the Gerontological Nursing Interventions: State of the Science, Gerontological Nursing Research Center, College of Nursing, Iowa City:
The University of Iowa.

Houldin, A., Salstein, S., & Ganley, K. (1987). *Nursing diagnosis for wellness.* Baltimore: Lippincott Williams & Wilkins.

Hyatt, R. H., Whitelaw, M. N., Bhat, A., Scott, S., & Maxwell, J. D. (1990). Association of muscle strength with functional status of elderly people. *Age and Ageing, 19,* 330-336.

Iowa Intervention Project. J. C. McCloskey & G. M. Bulechek (Eds.). (2000). *Nursing interventions classification (NIC)* (3rd ed.). St. Louis, MO: Mosby.

Iowa Outcomes Project. M. Johnson, M. Maas, & S. Moorhead (Eds.). (2000). *Nursing outcomes classification (NOC)* (2nd ed.). St. Louis, MO: Mosby.

Johnson, E. (1983, July). Continuous passive motion. *Journal of American Medical Association, 250,* 539.

Johnson, P. A., Stone, M. A., Larson, A. M., & Hromek, C. A. (1992, January/February). Applying nursing diagnosis and nursing process to activities of daily living and mobility. *Geriatric Nursing,* 25-27.

Joseph, C. L., & Wanlass, W. (1993). Rehabilitation in the nursing home. *Clinics in Geriatric Medicine, 9*(4), 859-871.

Kamentz, H. (1971). *Exercises for the elderly.* Washington, DC: American Pharmaceutical.

Kane, R. L. (1993). The implications of assessment. *The Journals of Gerontology, 48,* 27-31.

Kane, R. A., & Kane, R. L. (1981). *Assessing the elderly: A practical guide to measurement.* St. Charles, IL: Health, D. C.

Kaplan, G. A., Strawbridge, W. J., Camacho, T., & Cohen, R. D. (1993). Factors associated with change in physical functioning in the elderly. *Journal of Aging and Health, 5*(1), 140-153.

Katz, S., Ford, A. B., Moskowitz, R. W., Jackson, B., & Jaffe, M. (1963). Studies of illness in the aged. The index of ADL: A standardized measure of biological and psychosocial function. *Journal of American Medical Association, 185*(12), 914-919.

Keenan, K. (1989). Clinical validation of the etiologies and defining characteristics of the nursing diagnosis impaired mobility. In R. Carroll-Johnson (Ed.), *Classification of nursing diagnosis: Proceedings of the 8th conference.* Baltimore: Lippincott Williams & Wilkins.

Kelly, M. (1985). *Nursing diagnosis sourcebook: Guidelines for clinical application.* Norwalk, CT: Appleton & Lange.

Klitgaard, H., Mantoni, M., Schiaffino, S., Ausoni, S., Gorza, L., Laurent-Winter, C., Schnohr, P., & Saltin, B. (1990). Function, morphology, and protein expression of aging skeletal muscle: A cross-sectional study of men with different training backgrounds. *Acta of Physiology Scandinavica, 140,* 41-54.

Kochersberger, G., Hielema, F., & Westlund, R. (1994). Rehabilitation in the nursing home: How much, why, and with what results. *Public Health Reports, 109*(3), 372-376.

Koroknay, V., Werner, P., Cohen-Mansfield, J., & Braun, J. (1995). Maintaining ambulation in the frail nursing home resident: A nurse administered walking program. *Journal of Gerontological Nursing, 21*(11), 18-24.

Kottke, F. (1965). Deterioration of the bedfast patient, causes and effects. *Public Health Report, 80,* 437.

Kottke, F. (1971). Therapeutic exercise. In F. Krusen, F. Kottke, & P. Ellwood (Eds.), *Handbook of physical medicine and rehabilitation.* Philadelphia: W. B. Saunders.

Kovar, P., Allegrante, J., MacKenzie, C., Peterson, M., Gutin, B., & Charlson, M. (1992). Supervised fitness walking in patients with osteoarthritis of the knee: A randomized controlled trial. *Annals of Internal Medicine, 116,* 529-534.

Kraft, L. A. (1991). *Diagnostic content validity of the nursing diagnosis impaired physical mobility.* Unpublished Masters, Iowa City: The University of Iowa.

Kraft, L., Maas, M., & Hardy, M. (1994). Diagnostic content validity of impaired physical mobility in the older adult. In R. Carroll-Johnson (Ed.), *Classification of nursing diagnosis: Proceedings of the 10th conference* (pp. 197-199). Baltimore: Lippincott Williams & Wilkins.

Lavin, M. (1973). Bed exercises for acute cardiac patients. *American Journal of Nursing, 73,* 1226-1227.

Leslie, F. (1981). Nursing diagnosis: Use in long term care. *American Journal of Nursing, 81,* 1012-1014.

Light, K., Nuzik, S., Personius, W., & Barstrom, A. (1984). Low-load prolonged stretch versus high-load brief stretch in treating knee contractures. *Physical Therapy, 64*(3), 330-333.

Lueckenotte, A. G. (1996). *Gerontologic nursing.* St. Louis, MO: Mosby.

MacRae, P., Asplond, L. A., Schrelle, J. F., Ouslander, J. G., Abrahamse, A., & Morris, C. (1996). A walking program for nursing home residents: Effects on walk endurance, physical activity, mobility, and quality of life. *Journal of the American Geriatrics Society, 44,* 175-180.

Manchester, D., Woollacott, M. H., Zederbauer-Hylton, N., & Marin, O. (1989). Visual, vestibular and somatosensory contributions to balance control in the older adult. *Journal of Gerontology and Medical Science, 44,* M118-M127.

Mandelstom, D. (1980). Special techniques: Strengthening pelvic muscles. *Geriatric Nursing, 1,* 251-252.

Marottoli, R., Berkman, L., & Cooney, L. (1992). Decline in physical function following hip fracture. *Journal of the American Geriatrics Society, 40,* 861-866.

Mathias, S., Nayak, U., & Isaacs, B. (1986). Balance in elderly patients: The "get-up-and-go" test. *Archives of Physical Medicine Rehabilitation, 67,* 387-389.

Matson, K. (1985). Prevention of contracture deformities. *Clinical Management, 2,* 37-40.

Matteson, M. A., & McConnell, E. S. (1988). *Gerontological nursing: Concepts and practice.* Philadelphia: W. B. Saunders.

McDonagh, M., White, M., & Davies, C. (1984). Different effects of aging on mechanical properties of human arm and leg muscles. *Gerontology, 30,* 49-54.

Means, K., Currie, D., & Gershkoff, A. (1993). Geriatric rehabilitation: Assessment, preservation, and enhancement of fitness and function. *Archives of Physical Medicine Rehabilitation, 74*(5), 417-419.

Means, K. M., Currie, D. M., & Gershkoff, A. M. (1993). Geriatric rehabilitation. 4. Assessment, preservation, and enhancement of fitness and function. *Archives of Physical Medicine Rehabilitation, 74,* S417-S423.

Medeiros, J., Schmidt, G. L., Burmeister, L. F., & Soderberg, G. L. (1977). Influence of isometric exercise and passive stretch on hip joint motion. *Physical Therapy, 57,* 518-523.

Mehmert, M., & Delaney, C. (1991). Validation of defining characteristics of immobility using the computerized NMDS. *Nursing Diagnosis, 2*(4), 143-154.

Mehta, A. J., & Nastasi, A. E. (1993). Rehabilitation of fractures in the elderly. *Clinics in Geriatric Medicine, 9*(4), 717-730.

Melton, L., & Riggs, B. (1983). Epidemiology of age related fractures. In L. V. Avioli (Ed.), *The osteoporotic syndrome.* Orlando, FL: Grune & Stratton.

Milde, F. (1981). Physiological immobilization. In L. Hart, M. Fehring, & J. Reece (Eds.), *Concepts common to acute illness.* St. Louis, MO: Mosby.

Milde, F. (1988). Impaired physical mobility. *Journal of Gerontological Nursing, 14*(3), 20-25.

Millar, A. (1983). Influence of training and of inactivity on muscle strength. *Archives of Physical Medicine & Rehabilitation, 13,* 592-593.

Miller, S. (1975). The concept and measurement of mobility. In A. P. M. Coxon & C. L. Jones (Eds.), *Social mobility* (pp. 21-31). Bungary, Suffolk: Chaucer Press.

Monicken, D. (1991). Immobility and functional mobility in the elderly. In W. C. Chenitz, J. T. Stone, & S. A. Salisbury (Eds.), *Clinical gerontological nursing: A guide to advanced practice* (pp. 233-245). Philadelphia: W. B. Saunders.

Muller, E. (1970). Influence of training and of inactivity on muscle strength. *Physical Medicine Rehabilitation, 37,* 449.

Nevitt, M. C., Cummings, S. R., Kidd, S., & Black, D. (1989). Risk factors for recurrent nonsyncopal falls. *Journal of American Medical Association, 261,* 2663-2668.

North American Nursing Diagnosis Association. (1999). *Nursing diagnosis: Definitions & classification 1999-2000.* Philadelphia: Author.

Nutter, D., Schlant, R., & Hurst, J. (1972). Isometric exercise and the cardiovascular system. *Modern Concepts of Cardiovascular Disease, 41,* 11-15.

Olson, E. (1967). The hazards of immobility. *American Journal of Nursing, 70,* 779-797.

Oretel, G. (1986). Changes in human skeletal muscles due to aging. *Acts Neuropathologica, 69,* 309-313.

Ouellet, L. L., & Rush, K. L. (1992). A synthesis of selected literature on mobility: A basis for studying impaired mobility. *Nursing Diagnosis, 3*(2), 72-80.

Parent, C. J., & Whall, A. L. (1984). Are physical activity, self-esteem, and depression related? *Journal of Gerontological Nursing, 10*(9), 8-11.

Pawlson, G., Goodwin, M., & Keith, K. (1986). Wheelchair use by ambulatory nursing home residents. *Journal of the American Geriatrics Society, 34*(12), 860-864.

Pendergast, D. R., Fisher, N. M., & Calkins, E. (1993). Cardiovascular, neuromuscular, and metabolic alterations with age leading to frailty. *The Journals of Gerontology, 48,* 61-67.

Perri, S., & Templar, D. (1984). The effects of an aerobic exercise program on psychological variables in older adults. *International Journal of Aging and Human Development, 5*(20), 167-170.

Perry, B. (1982). Exercise patterns of an elderly population. *Journal of Family Medicine, 15,* 545-546.

Pollock, M., & Wilmore, J. (1990). *Exercise in health and disease: Evaluation and prescription for prevention and rehabilitation* (2nd ed.). Philadelphia: W. B. Saunders.

Rantanen, T., Guralnik, J. M., Ferrucci, L., Leveille, S., & Fried, L. P. (1999). Coimpairments: Strength and balance as predictors of severe walking disability. *Journals of Gerontology: Series A, Biological Sciences & Medicine Sciences, 54*(4), M172-M176.

Rantanen, T., Guralnik, J. M., Sakari-Rantala, R., Leveille, S., Simonsick, E. M., Ling, S., & Fried, L. P. (1999). Disability, physical activity, and muscle strength in older women: The Women's Health and Aging Study. *Archives of Physical Medicine & Rehabilitation, 80*(2), 130-135.

Rantz, M., Miller, T., & Jacobs, C. (1985). Nursing diagnosis in long term care. *American Journal of Nursing, 85,* 916-917, 926.

Regensteiner, J. (1987). Conditioning for elders. *Generations, 12*(1), 50-53.

Rikki, R., & Busch, S. (1986). Motor performance of women as a function of age and physical activity level. *Journal of Gerontology, 41,* 645-649.

Roberts, B., & Palmer, R. (1996). Cardiac response of elderly adults to normal activities and aerobic walking. *Clinical Nursing Research, 5*(1), 105-115.

Rockwood, K., Silvius, J. L., & Fox, R. A. (1998). Comprehensive geriatric assessment. Helping your elderly patients maintain functional well-being. *Postgraduate Medicine, 103*(3), 247-249, 254-258, 264.

Sato, T., Akatsuka, H., Kito, K., Tokoro, Y., Tauchi, H., & Kato, K. (1986). Age changes in myofibrils of human pectoral muscle. *Mechanisms of Aging Development, 34,* 297-304.

Schulz, R., & Williamson, G. M. (1993). Psychosocial and behavioral dimensions of physical frailty. *The Journals of Gerontology, 48,* 39-43.

Seals, D., Hagberg, J., Hurley, B., Ensoni, A., & Hollsey, J. (1984). Endurance training in older men and women: Cardiovascular responses to exercise. *Journal of Applied Physiology, 57,* 1024-1029.

Shanas, E., Townsend, P., Wedderburn, D., Friis, H., Milhoj, P., & Stenouwer, J. (1968). *Old people in three industrial societies.* New York: Atherton Press.

Simpson, W. M. (1986). Exercise: Prescriptions for the elderly. *Geriatrics, 41*(1), 95-100.

Sorenson, L., & Ulrich, P. (1966). *Ambulation: A manual for nurses.* Minneapolis, MN: American Rehabilitation Foundation.

Swartz, M. H. (1989). *Textbook of physical diagnosis.* Philadelphia: W. B. Saunders.

Tanigawa, M. (1972). Comparison of the hold-relax procedure and passive mobilization on increasing muscle length. *Physical Therapy, 52,* 725-735.

Taylor, H., Erickson, L., Henschel, A., & Keys, A. (1945). Effects of bedrest on the blood volume of normal young men. *American Journal of Physiology, 144,* 227-231.

Tinetti, M. E. (1986). Performance-oriented assessment of mobility problems in elderly patients. *Journal of the American Geriatrics Society, 34,* 119-126.

Tinetti, M. E., & Ginter, S. F. (1988). Identifying mobility dysfunctions in elderly persons. *Journal of American Medical Association, 259,* 1190-1193.

Tinetti, M. E., & Powell, L. (1993). Fear of falling and low self-efficacy: A cause of dependence in elderly persons. *The Journals of Gerontology, 48,* 35-38.

Tinetti, M. E., Speechley, M., & Ginter, S. F. (1988). Risk factors for falls among elderly persons living in the community. *New England Journal of Medicine, 319,* 1701-1707.

Travis, S., Duncan, H., & McAuley, W. (1996). Mall walking: An effective mental health intervention for older adults. *Journal of Psychosocial Nursing, 34*(8), 36-38.

United States Department of Health and Human Services. (1992). *Healthy people 2000: National health promotion and disease prevention objectives. Summary report.* Boston: Jones & Bartlett.

Vellas, B., Cayla, F., Bocquet, H., dePemille, F., & Albarede, J. L. (1987). Prospective study of activity in old people after falls. *Age & Ageing, 16,* 189-193.

Waldo, M., Ide, B., & Thomas, P. (1995). Postcardiac-event elderly: Effect of exercise on cardiopulmonary function. *Journal of Gerontological Nursing, 21*(2), 12-19.

Weaver, T. E., & Narsavage, G. L. (1992). Physiological and psychosocial variables related to functional status in chronic obstructive pulmonary disease. *Nursing Research, 41*(5), 286-291.

Whipple, R., Wolfson, L., Derby, C., Singh, D., & Tobin, J. (1993). Altered sensory function and balance in older persons. *The Journals of Gerontology, 48,* 71-76.

Wiener, J. M., Hanley, R. J., Clark, R., & Van Nostrand, J. F. (1990). Measuring the activities of daily living: Comparisons across national surveys. *Journal of Gerontological Social Science, 45,* S229-S237.

Wolanin, M. O. (1976). Nursing assessment. In I. Burnside (Ed.), *Nursing and the aged* (2nd ed., pp. 410-412). Hightstown, NJ: McGraw-Hill.

Wolff, H. (1986). Musculoskeletal problems. In D. Carnevali & M. Patrick (Eds.), *Nursing management for the elderly* (2nd ed., pp. 492-518). Baltimore: Lippincott Williams & Wilkins.

Woollacott, M. H. (1993). Age-related changes in posture and movement. *The Journals of Gerontology, 48,* 56-60.

Woollacott, M. H., Inglin, B., & Manchester, D. (1988). Response preparation and posture control in the older adult. In J. Joseph (Ed.), *Central determinants of age-related declines in motor function.* New York: Academy of Sciences.

CHAPTER 29

SELF-CARE DEFICIT

Jane M. Armer, Vicki S. Conn, Sheila A. Decker, and Toni Tripp-Reimer

A plethora of self-care definitions exist, both within and outside of nursing. Definitions vary in their breadth and in their differentiation of lay versus professional care activities. Levin's (1981) working definition of self-care is "a process by which people function on their own behalf in health promotion and prevention and in disease detection and treatment at the level of the primary health resource in the health care system" (p. 178). The World Health Organization's definition (1984) of self-care in health includes references to the activities undertaken by individuals, families, and communities with the intention of enhancing and restoring health, preventing disease, and limiting illness. Again, activities carried out by lay people on their own behalf, either separately or in cooperation with professionals, are targeted.

Medical self-care, as a component of self-care, is defined as what people do to recognize, prevent, treat, and manage their own health problems (Mettler & Kemper, 1993). More broadly, Dean (1989) stated that "self-care represents the range of behaviors undertaken by individuals to promote or restore their health" (p. 117). She further noted that in chronic illness, self-care, which often constitutes the bulk of the care of a given condition, often takes place in conjunction with care by health care professionals. There are those who propose a narrow definition of self-care as lay responses to illness versus professional care. Dean argued that a narrow illness-focused definition ignores the considerable body of evidence of the role of individual behaviors in health protection. Conceptualizing individual self-care as opposed to professional care, even with regard to illness, ignores the interaction and interface between lay behaviors and professional care. This interaction or interface is evident in a variety of behaviors, including the individual's monitoring of the healthy state, the recognition of symptoms, the decision to seek professional care, and the decision to apply professional recommendations. As numerous intervention studies have validated, in the presence of professional recommendations, prescriptions, and health education, actual performance still depends on the acceptance, motivation, and capacity of the individual (Dean, 1989). Reaching beyond the traditional view of medication compliance, Conn and colleagues' (1995) research documented the complex decision-making process inherent in medication management by elders and caregivers. Actual medication use, one self-care behavior, is reliant on the motivation and perceptions of the elder.

Orem (1995) espoused the more general notion of self-care as "the practice of activities that individuals initiate and perform on their own behalf in maintaining life, health, and well-being" (p. 104), which is among the earliest, best-known, and most fully developed nursing definitions of self-care. Orem (1980) viewed a primary nursing function to be that of helping an individual to maintain, restore, or increase the ability to provide self-care. Self-care Deficit refers to the person's inability to take appropriate actions for self-care. Orem identified three broad categories of actions that might be required: universal, developmental, and health deviation self-care requisites. Limitations in meeting self-care demands might be due to limited knowledge, motivation, or psychomotor skills or to such components as age, developmental stage, health state, and available resources (Orem's basic conditioning factors). Appropriate nursing intervention (in the form of acting or doing for, guiding, supporting, providing a developmental environment, and teaching) is provided by the nurse as the client(s) and nurse(s) collaborate to meet therapeutic self-care demands and eliminate self-care deficits (Penn, 1988). More recently, others, perhaps most notably Lipson and Steiger (1996), have attempted to place self-care theory in the broader context of cross-cultural and caring nursing theories and the broader social, political, and community context in which the person's self-care occurs.

ASSESSMENT

Several research instruments have been developed to assess self-care. Constructs from Orem's Self-Care Deficit Nursing Theory have provided the foundation for most of these instruments. Evaluation of each instrument requires assessing its conceptual foundation and reviewing its psychometric properties, including reliability and validity (Jacobson, 1988). Instruments that measure self-care fall naturally into two categories. In the first set, subjective measures of self-care are based on the person's "perception of ability to engage in actions to maintain life, health, and well-being" (Orem, 1995, p. 104). These instruments measure dimensions of self-care agency: foundational capabilities and dispositions, power components, and capabilities for care operations. For example, items such as "My endurance for doing physical work is good" or "I seek information to care for myself" reflect perception of self-care (McBride, 1991). Gast et al. (1989) reviewed seven self-care instruments to evaluate the operationalizations of self-care agency (Table 29-1). Self-care agency is broadly defined as the individual's ability or power to engage in self-care, that is, to carry out self-care activities for the maintenance and promotion of health. Several critical observations were reported. Measurement of the three dimensions of self-care agency (foundational capabilities and dispositions, power components, and capabilities for self-care operations) was inconsistent. The power components were best represented in the measure of self-care agency. The surveyed instruments measured foundational capabilities and dispositions and capabilities for self-care operations less adequately than power components. Reliability values for all of the self-care instruments were within an acceptable range (0.77 to 0.96) for new instruments. Content validity was reported for three of the seven instruments. Construct validity was reported for four instruments, of which three had no report of content validity. Factor analysis, an approach for assessing construct validity, was completed on three of the Gast-reviewed instruments, plus the Self-As-Carer Inventory (Geden & Taylor, 1991). Evers (1989) reported evaluation of intersubjectivity, internal consistency, stability, and discriminate validity for the Appraisal-of-Self-Care-Agency scale, with notable findings that self-appraisals were consistently higher than appraisals by others. Sample sizes for the seven tools ranged from 53 to 344 nonhospitalized individuals (Gast et al., 1989). Subjects' ages varied, with most participants being young to middle-age adults; very few older persons were represented. The Self-as-Carer Inventory (Geden & Taylor, 1991), a significant revision of the Perception of Self-Care Agency (Hanson & Bickel, 1995) and one of the more frequently used self-care instruments, measures perceived ability to care for self. Geden and Taylor (1991) included culturally diverse individuals, but they did not report examination of differences in self-care as influenced by age, gender, or ethnicity.

The second body of instruments builds on the concept of functional status as a measure of self-care. Functional status is measured by direct observation of the older person's ability to complete basic self-care tasks. Activities of daily living (ADL) refer to basic activities necessary for one's routine comfort and well-being: feeding, bathing, dressing, and so on. Instrumental activities of daily living (IADL) are more complex activities needed to carry out self-care activities, such as money management, laundering clothes, and acquiring and preparing food. Twenty-two scales used to assess independent living/daily living skills were reviewed by Kelley, Kawamoto, and Rubenstein (1991). As cited in Kane and Kane (1981) and Kane, Ouslander, and Abrass (1994), two commonly used measures

of functional ability are the Katz Index of ADL (Katz, Ford, Moskowitz, Jackson, & Jaffee, 1963) and the Barthel Index (Mahoney & Barthel, 1965) (Table 29-2). A third measure, Instrumental Activities of Daily Living, is a combination of physical and cognitive abilities reflecting performance of more complex activities (Kane, Ouslander, & Abrass, 1994). A team led by Pfeiffer (1981) developed and tested the Functional Assessment Inventory, a shortened revision of the OARS Multidimensional Functional Assessment Questionnaire, for use with elders in a variety of settings. The various dimensions of functional impairment, as measured by a series of five 6-point scales, correlated strongly with service setting. ADL scores most clearly distinguished between the settings (Pfeiffer, Johnson, & Chiofolo, 1981).

Jirovec and Kasno (1990) measured self-care agency using the Appraisal of Self-Care Agency with 83 nursing home residents. Residents included Caucasians ($n = 64$), African-Americans ($n = 18$), and an American Indian ($n = 1$), with ages ranging from 60 to 100. Jirovec and Kasno reported a Cronbach's alpha of 0.71 for this sample. Construct validity was examined through use of the data from the Dutch Elderly Study of nursing home residents.

Several limitations exist in the measurement of self-care, both subjective self-care and functional status. Few ethnic groups are represented in published reports. Essentially, the young to middle-age adults studied are healthy, revealing little about the influence of chronic illness on self-care agency. Few adults 65 years of age and older are included. Consequently, psychometric properties are lacking for older persons across the continuum of health care. The majority of gerontologic taxonomic development in the area of self-care focuses on the institutional setting and needs of the frail elder. A promising arena for future theoretical and research endeavors is the self-care behaviors of community-dwelling and ethnically diverse older persons.

The assessment tools already discussed were not constructed for the purpose of measuring nursing-sensitive patient outcomes, "a variable patient or family caregiver state, condition, or perception responsive to nursing intervention" (Maas, Johnson, & Moorhead, 1996, p. 297), nor were they constructed to measure the effectiveness of nursing interventions in enhancing self-care agency. This area of self-care measurement has its beginnings in the validation of taxonomic nomenclature discussed in the next sections (Iowa Intervention Project, 1992, 1993).

In the area of theoretical development of nursing diagnosis in self-care, much work remains to be done in the upper-level areas identified by Jenny (1989), most notably health promotion and health restoration. Future work also must be directed to examining differences and similarities among ethnic groups and with elders. Existing and future measurement tools must be examined for cultural, age, and gender appropriateness and sensitivity.

Table 29-1   Psychometrics of Eight Instruments Measuring Subjective Self-Care

Instrument's Title	Construct Measured	Sample	Reliability	Validity
Exercise of Self-Care Agency (ESCA); developers—Kirney & Fleischer (Gast et al., 1989)	Self-care agency: The power of an individual to engage in estimative and productive operations Identified four subconstructs that contribute to self-care	Nursing and psychology students	Test-retest reliability: 0.77 for nursing students **Split-half** 0.80, 0.81 for first and second testings with nursing students 0.77 for psychology students	Content validity Construct validity Factor analysis (Riesch & Hauk, 1988; Whetstone & Hansson, 1989)
Perceptions of Self-Care Agency; developers—Hanson & Bickel (Gast et al., 1989)	10 power components of self-care agency	Female and male nonhospitalized adults recruited from friends, relatives, acquaintances, church meetings, and senior citizen groups	Coefficient alpha = 0.96 (150 items) Coefficient alpha = 0.93 (53 items)	Check construct validity: Factor analysis (unstable across populations and lack of clarity regarding older persons)
Denyes Self-Care Agency Instrument (DSCAI); 35 items; developer—Denyes (Gast et al., 1989)	Limited development of self-care; used human development framework	Adolescents	Coefficient alpha ranges = 0.86 to 0.89	Content validity Construct validity: Factor analysis
Denyes Self-Care Practice Instrument (DSCPI); 22 items; developer—Denyes (Gast et al., 1989)	Limited development of self-care; used human development framework	Adolescents		Construct validity
Appraisal of Self-Care Agency Scale (ASA); 24 items; developer—Evers (Gast et al., 1989)	One's power to perform the productive operations of self-care	Elderly Dutch nursing home population		Construct validity
Health-related cognitive structure (HrCS); developer—Nevens (Gast et al., 1989)	Self-care: Needs, beliefs, attitudes, and intentions related to health care	Nonhospitalized adults		Construct validity: Factor analysis of HrCS
Health Self-Care (HSC) (needs reasons for performing or not performing common self-care actions); developer—Nevens (Gast et al., 1989)				
Self-As-Carer Inventory (SCI); 40 items; developers—Geden & Taylor (Geden & Taylor, 1991; Riesch & Hauk, 1988; Whetstone & Hansson, 1989)	Self-care: "Those things you do for yourself to maintain life; health and well-being"	56 students (reliability) 344 females, 241 males Age range: 18-94 Mean = 45 Range of ethnic groups	Test-retest reliability: 0.85 Subscale test-retest: 0.54-0.83 Cronbach's coefficient alpha = 0.96	Content validity: Construct validity; factor analysis

Table 29-2	Three Instruments Measuring Functional Status as Indicator of Self-Care Ability		
Instrument	**Tasks Measured**	**Reliability**	**Setting**
Katz Index of Activities of Daily Living	Bathing Dressing Toileting Transfer Continence Feeding	Coefficients of reproducibility: 0.948 and 0.976	Acute care Long-term care Community
Barthel Index	Feeding Moving to/from wheelchair/bed Personal toilet Getting on and off toilet Bathing self Walking on level surface Ascending and descending stairs Dressing Controlling bowels/bladder	Test-retest not reported Alpha reliabilities: 0.953-0.965 for hospital patients	Rehabilitation Long-term care Acute care
Instrumental Activities of Daily Living	Writing Reading Cooking Cleaning Shopping Doing laundry Climbing stairs Using telephone Managing medications Managing money Ability to perform Paid employment Duties or outside work Ability to travel		Community

NURSING DIAGNOSIS

Self-care deficits refer to the inability of a person to adequately perform self-care activities necessary for optimal health and function. Self-care deficits become the basis for nursing diagnoses, the judgments nurses make about patients and their unmet needs. Self-Care Deficit is the most common nursing diagnosis in rehabilitation (McCourt, 1987) and long-term care settings (Rantz & Miller, 1987; Rantz, Miller, & Jacobs, 1981). It ranks among the most common diagnoses among elderly and chronically ill clients in nursing homes (Hardy, Maas, & Akins, 1988) and in all nursing settings (Tracy, 1989). Chang and colleagues (1998) found that hospitalized patients diagnosed with Self-Care Deficit were significantly older, had more nursing diagnoses, required more assistance in activities of daily living, and were less mobile than those without the diagnosis label. As a person ages, abilities and deficits in the area of self-care take on increasing importance, often significantly affecting the choices available to the older person.

Self-care deficits are currently defined by the North American Nursing Diagnosis Association (NANDA) as impairments in certain bodily function abilities (Feeding Self-Care Deficit, Bathing/Hygiene Self-Care Deficit, Toileting Self-Care Deficit, Dressing/Grooming Self-Care Deficit) (NANDA, 1999; Tracy, 1989). These basic diagnoses and an additional diagnosis related to instrumental self-care deficits are outlined in Box 29-1, along with the defining characteristics for each (Carpenito, 1995). Carpenito (1995) suggested the consideration of an additional, more global category, Self-Care Deficit Syndrome (Box 29-2). Development of additional diagnostic categories related to the higher-level functions of health promotion and restoration is suggested in this chapter.

In 1982 Kim and Moritz listed several etiologic factors related to Self-Care Deficit: intolerance to activity; pain; uncompensated neuromuscular, musculoskeletal, or perceptual-cognitive impairment; and severe anxiety or depression (NANDA, 1986; Tracy, 1989). Carpenito (1995) listed related factors in the following categories: pathophysiologic, treatment-related, situational (personal, environmental), and maturational (Box 29-3). Carpenito (1995) developed assessment guides for Self-Care Deficit related factors (Assessment Guide 29-1) and defining characteristics associated with the self-care deficits of feeding, bathing, dressing/grooming, toileting,

Box 29-1	Defining Characteristics SELF-CARE DEFICIT

1. Self-feeding deficits
    Unable to cut food or open packages
    Unable to bring food to mouth
2. Self-bathing deficits (includes washing entire body, combing hair, brushing teeth, attending to skin and nail care, and applying makeup)
    Unable or unwilling to wash body or body parts
    Unable to obtain a water source
    Unable to regulate temperature or water flow
    Inability to perceive need for hygienic measures
3. Self-dressing deficits (including donning regular or special clothing, not nightclothes)
    Impaired ability to put on or take off clothing
    Unable to fasten clothing
    Unable to groom self satisfactorily
    Unable to obtain or replace articles of clothing
4. Self-toileting deficits
    Unable or unwilling to get to toilet or commode
    Unable or unwilling to carry out proper hygiene
    Unable to transfer to and from toilet or commode
    Unable to handle clothing to accommodate toileting
    Unable to flush toilet or empty commode
5. Instrumental self-care deficits
    Difficulty using telephone
    Difficulty accessing transportation
    Difficulty laundering, ironing
    Difficulty preparing meals
    Difficulty shopping
    Difficulty managing money
    Difficulty with medication administration

From Carpenito, L. J. (1995). *Nursing diagnosis: Application to clinical practice* (6th ed., pp. 771-772). Baltimore: Lippincott Williams & Wilkins.

Box 29-3	Related Factors/Etiologies SELF-CARE DEFICIT

Pathophysiologic
Related to lack of coordination secondary to (specify)
Related to spasticity or flaccidity secondary to (specify)
Related to muscular weakness secondary to (specify)
Related to partial or total paralysis secondary to (specify)
Related to atrophy secondary to (specify)
Related to muscle contractures secondary to (specify)
Related to comatose state
Related to visual disorders secondary to (specify)
Related to nonfunctioning or missing limb(s)
Related to regression to an earlier level of development
Related to excessive ritualistic behaviors
Related to somatoform deficits (specify)

Treatment-Related
Related to external devices (specify) (casts, splints, braces, intravenous [IV] equipment)
Related to postoperative fatigue and pain

Situational (Personal, Environmental)
Related to cognitive deficits
Related to pain
Related to decreased motivation
Related to fatigue
Related to confusion
Related to disabling anxiety

Maturational
Elderly
Related to decreased visual and motor ability, muscle weakness

From Carpenito, L. J. (1995). *Nursing diagnosis: Application to clinical practice* (6th ed., p. 772). Baltimore: Lippincott Williams & Wilkins.

instrumental abilities, and finances (Assessment Guide 29-2). Among related factors for Self-Care Deficit, consideration of mental status includes ability to remember, judgment, ability to follow directions, and ability to identify, express, or anticipate needs. Consideration of social supports includes the following factors: potential and actual support person(s); availability of help with IADL such as transportation, shopping, money manage-

Box 29-2	Self-Care Deficit Syndrome*:

The state in which the individual experiences an impaired motor function or cognitive function, causing a decreased ability in performing each of the five self-care activities: self-feeding, self-bathing, self-dressing, self-toileting, instrumental self-care.*

*Not currently on NANDA list, but suggested by Carpenito. (From Carpenito, L. J. (1995). *Nursing diagnosis: Application to clinical practice* (6th ed., p. 771). Baltimore: Lippincott Williams & Wilkins.)

ment, laundry, housekeeping, or food preparation; and availability of appropriate community resources. Other related factors include motivation and endurance.

There has been extensive theoretical development, albeit limited research, in identifying the etiologies and defining characteristics of the nursing diagnosis Self-Care Deficit as related to bodily function (toileting, bathing, dressing, eating) (Bulechek & McCloskey, 1985; Dickel & Mehmert, 1994; Hardy, Maas, & Akin, 1988). Less empirical evidence exists for the principles and rationale for nursing outcomes and interventions to alleviate, minimize, or reduce self-care deficits.

Validation of Bathing/Hygiene Self-Care Deficit

Validation of one specific self-care diagnosis, Bathing/Hygiene Self-Care Deficit (defined as impaired ability to perform or complete bathing/hygiene activities for oneself) (NANDA, 1999, p. 103), has been carried out by two sets of

Assessment Guide 29-1

RELATED FACTORS/ETIOLOGIES TO SELF-CARE DEFICIT

1. Mental status
   Ability to remember
   Judgment
   Ability to follow directions
   Ability to identify/express needs
   Ability to anticipate needs (food, laundry)
   Social supports
      Support person(s)

    Availability of help with transportation, shopping, money management, laundry, housekeeping, food preparation
    Community resources
2. Motivation
3. Endurance

From Carpenito, L. J. (1995). *Nursing diagnosis: Application to clinical practice* (6th ed., p. 774). Baltimore: Lippincott Williams & Wilkins.

Assessment Guide 29-2

DEFINING CHARACTERISTICS OF SELF-CARE DEFICIT

1. Self-feeding abilities
   Swallowing
   Chewing
   Using utensils and cutting food
   Drink from cup
   Selecting foods
   Seeing
   Open cartons
2. Self-bathing abilities
   Undressing to bathe
   Reaching water source
   Differentiating water temperatures
   Obtaining equipment (water, soap, towels)
   Washing body parts
   Performing oral care
3. Self-dressing/grooming abilities
   Putting on or taking off clothing
   Selecting appropriate clothing
   Washes and styles hair
   Shaves
   Uses deodorant
   Cleans/trims nails
   Brushes teeth
   Plug in cord
   Retrieving appropriate clothing
   Fastening clothing

4. Self-toileting abilities
   Getting to toilet and undressing
   Sitting on toilet
   Rising from toilet
   Cleaning self/flushing toilet
   Redressing
   Performing hygiene (washing hands)
   Can use tampon/sanitary napkin
5. Instrumental ADL
   Telephone
      Ability to dial
      Ability to answer
      Ability to talk, hear
   Transportation
      Ability to drive
      Access to transportation
   Food procurement and preparation
      Ability to cook
      Ability to select foods
      Ability to shop
   Medications
      Ability to remember
      Ability to administer
6. Finances
   Ability to write checks, pay bills
   Ability to handle cash transactions (simple, complex)

From Carpenito, L. J. (1995). *Nursing diagnosis: Application to clinical practice* (6th ed., pp. 773-774). Baltimore: Lippincott Williams & Wilkins.

nurse researchers. Metzger and Hiltunen (1987) retrospectively examined diagnostic content validity, critical and supporting defining characteristics, and support for NANDA-accepted critical defining characteristics for 10 frequently reported, NANDA-accepted nursing diagnoses. A nurse-validation model was used with a convenience sample of 76 registered nurses and a structured survey tool. Among the 10 most frequently reported nursing diagnoses was Bathing/Hygiene Self-Care Deficit. In the analysis of critical and supporting cues (validated with a weighted ratio of 0.75 or greater and 0.50 or greater, respectively), the cue with the highest score (0.962) among all potential cues for the 10 diagnostic categories was "inability to wash body or body parts" for the diagnostic category of Bathing/Hygiene Self-Care Deficit. This cue is listed as a defining characteristic in the latest NANDA revision (1999). This diagnostic category had three NANDA-accepted cues, with "inability to wash body or body parts" rated as a critical cue (as already noted) and "inability to obtain or get to a water source" (0.712) and "inability to regulate temperature or flow" (0.562) rated as supportive cues.

Dickel and Mehmert (1994) reported a replication study aimed at validating the diagnosis Bathing/Hygiene Self Care-Deficit for patients of all ages in an acute care setting. NANDA-identified defining characteristics and related factors were used, as well as one additional defining characteristic ("inability to perceive need for hygienic measures") and five inductively derived related factors ("ineffective coping," "knowledge deficit regarding affected body parts," "knowledge deficit regarding spatial relationships," "mobility impairment," and "maturational"). A systematic sampling procedure generated 212 clinical records from a potential pool of 859 patients with the self-care diagnosis who were discharged over a 9-month period. Findings supported the previous study. "Inability to wash body parts" was supported as a major defining characteristic (85%) and "inability to obtain or access water source" was supported as a minor defining characteristic (78%). "Inability to regulate temperature or flow," the third NANDA characteristic, occurred in 10% of the sampled records. A smaller percentage supported "inability to perceive need for hygienic measures." Related factors were supported as follows: decreased activity tolerance (50%); musculoskeletal impairment (19%); pain (9%); neuromuscular impairment (7%); perceptual or cognitive impairment (4%); and depression and anxiety (0.5%). Of the inductively derived related factors, "mobility impairment" demonstrated the strongest support (19%). "Ineffective coping" was supported by 1% and "maturational factor" by 0.5%. Knowledge deficit factors received no support. Dickel and Mehmert reported that the diagnosis appeared across all ages (14 to 94) and across 87 diagnosis-related groups (DRG), indicating substantial validity in a heterogeneous sample. In a measure of outcome, the diagnosis was unresolved at discharge in 44% of the sample with varying discharge destinations reported. The authors did not report the findings from two other research questions: length of stay for individuals with this diagnosis and discharge destination for individuals with the diagnosis unresolved.

Similar validation studies are needed for the other self-care diagnostic categories. As noted by Metzger and Hiltunen (1987), nurses appear to feel more comfortable with the biophysical, readily observable cues than with more subjective cues. Likewise, work has proceeded more rapidly with the bodily function self-care deficits than in other areas of self-care needs, such as health promotion and restoration. Very little work has been done to integrate nursing diagnosis with knowledge of the person's culture and health definitions (Herman, 1994). Further work with elders in a diversity of settings, from acute care to community, with a range of functional abilities and heterogeneous ethnic backgrounds is greatly needed.

Other Conceptualizations of Self-Care

Considering the domain of self-care behaviors needed to maintain and restore health and function, a vast array of nursing diagnoses and actual and potential self-care deficits exist. Concept analysis of existing nursing diagnoses by Jenny (1989) resulted in seven self-care diagnostic categories: Physiologic Homeostasis, Bodily Care, Ego Integrity, Social Interaction, Health Protection, Health Restoration, and Environmental Management (Figure 29-1).

Physiologic Homeostasis involves self-care activities of a largely involuntary basis. Maintenance of these self-care activities is essential to survival, with relatively little tolerance for malfunction as the individual adapts to environmental changes (Jenny, 1989). An example of a voluntary self-care activity aimed at improving or maintaining physiologic homeostasis is deliberate deep breathing and coughing to improve airway clearance after surgery.

The second category of self-care activities, and the one that is the prominent focus of nursing taxonomy efforts to date, is that of Bodily Care. This category includes self-care tasks such as bathing/hygiene, dressing/grooming, eating, and toileting. Nurturing, protective self-care tasks that maintain body integrity and personal comfort comprise this self-care domain (Jenny, 1989). Deficits in self-care abilities will result in discomfort but do not immediately threaten survival. Behaviors in this self-care category are deliberate and learned. They are also influenced by the life

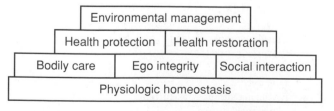

FIGURE **29-1**   Levels of diagnostic categories (non-NANDA). (From Jenny, J. [1989]. Classification of nursing diagnosis: A self-care approach. In R. M. Carroll-Johnson [Ed.], *Classification of nursing diagnoses: Proceedings of the eighth conference* [p. 153]. Baltimore: Lippincott Williams & Wilkins.)

ways and cultural patterns of the individual. Ego Integrity includes psychosocial self-care activities that support the individual's self-acceptance, identity, competence, emotional comfort, and self-development (Jenny, 1989). Social Interaction involves valued roles, communication, and relationships with family and others (Jenny, 1989). The second through fourth categories are seen as being on the same level hierarchically, as depicted in Figure 29-1.

The fifth and sixth categories, Health Protection and Health Restoration, are seen as being on the same level. These categories of self-care behaviors are deliberately practiced by the developing and mature person (Jenny, 1989). Behaviors in these categories are strongly influenced by the cultural environment, resources, and patterns of the individual. Adams (1986) documented the relative absence of gerontologic nursing research in the areas of health promotion or prevention and health maintenance and the deficiency in nurses' orientation to these areas of nursing practice. These categories have fewer developed nursing diagnoses and are areas of great importance for future nursing diagnoses, interventions, and outcomes development. Stolte (1994) made a strong case for the development of health-oriented nursing diagnoses. Further development in areas of special concern to the gerontologic population is needed.

Health Protection and Promotion encompass self-care activities that maintain and improve functional competence, well-being, and personal development and minimize risk for disease or injury. Jenny (1989) suggested that stress management be treated as a behavior falling within the Health Promotion category. Routine immunizations to reduce risk of influenza or pneumonia are another example of behaviors that promote health. Health Restoration, on the other hand, includes actions aimed at restoring health when illness has occurred and restoring function where impairment is present. Health Restoration can involve collaboration with health care professionals and use of health services.

The seventh category, Environmental Management, involves actions to provide and maintain a protective and nurturant environment and to ensure the availability of community resources (Jenny, 1989). This set of self-care behaviors requires the highest level of maturity and thus is seen as building on earlier categories and at the peak of the hierarchy.

Jenny's alternative self-care taxonomy (1989) differs from NANDA's Taxonomy I of nursing diagnoses in several ways. Categories of self-care are substituted for those of the original Human Response Patterns. Categories now "relate to tasks and activities required for health, not to 'parts' of a person" (Jenny, 1989, p. 154). Three ambiguous diagnostic categories were transformed into self-care categories: Self-Care and Health Maintenance were divided into categories of Bodily Care, Health Protection, and Health Restoration, and Social Interaction became a category, not a diagnosis. Self-care as an organizing principle creates a taxonomy that is congruent with the current nursing culture and accommodates key variables of current key nursing practice models, including Orem's self-care requisites, Roy's adaptive modes, Neuman's personal stressors, and Mazlow's human needs (Jenny, 1989). Self-Care Deficit: Medication Administration and Self-Care: Potential for Alteration are under review and in developmental staging.

CASE STUDY 1

S. Clark, an 85-year-old African-American, lives in her own home in a small rural community. She has been a widow for 23 years. She takes pride in her ability to continue to drive herself around the community. Mrs. Clark is active in community and church activities. A son and daughter-in-law live about five blocks away. Three other children and four grandchildren live 150 miles away. Mrs. Clark has osteoarthritis and hypertension. She takes aspirin and a blood pressure pill daily. Because of the pain in her hands, Mrs. Clark limits the amount of needlework she does and has some difficulty opening medication bottles. Her son and daughter-in-law take responsibility for all of the yard work, although Mrs. Clark still gets great pleasure from working with her roses. Recently, Mrs. Clark fell and broke her right proximal radius. She was discharged to home with assistance anticipated from her family and home health nurses. Her forearm is currently casted. Priority diagnoses for Mrs. Clark include the following:

- *Self-Care Deficit: Health Restoration (proposed):* Promotion of healing for a person who has experienced acute illness or injury
- *Self-Care Deficit: Environmental Management (proposed):* Provision and maintenance of a protective and nurturant environment and assurance of the availability of community resources
- *Self-Care Deficit: Non-Parenteral Medication Management (proposed):* Maintenance of safe and effective use of prescription and over-the-counter drugs

CASE STUDY 2

C. Morales, a 90-year-old person of Hispanic descent, was transferred to the nursing home after suffering a cerebral vascular accident. Mr. Morales has right hemiplegia, difficulty swallowing, difficulty with toileting, and impaired language function. Mr. Morales's family visits daily and is involved with his rehabilitation. Mrs. Morales hopes her husband can return home. Among Mr. Morales's self-care deficits are the following:

Self-Care Deficit Syndrome (proposed): Bathing/Hygiene Self-Care Deficit; Dressing/Grooming Self-Care Deficit; Feeding Self-Care Deficit; Toileting Self-Care Deficit;

In addition to deficits related to bodily functions, Mr. Morales is experiencing deficits related to IADL:

Self-Care Deficit: Instrumental (proposed): difficulty using telephone; difficulty accessing transportation; difficulty laundering, ironing; difficulty preparing meals;

difficulty shopping; difficulty managing money; difficulty in medication administration

CASE STUDY 3

P. Salas, a 79-year-old immigrant from Italy, decided to move to a congregate living center for older adults. Having never married, Mr. Salas thought it was time to turn the family restaurant over to the young people, his nieces and nephews. Mr. Salas has a history of recurrent bronchitis and has experienced pneumonia in 3 of the past 5 years. The public health department is offering an influenza and pneumonia immunization clinic in the building. Mr. Salas asks his gerontologic nurse practitioner if he should sign up for the vaccines. Mr. Salas is an example of an elder with the following diagnosis:

Self-Care Deficit: Health Promotion (proposed): Promotion of optimal state of health for a person who is not currently experiencing an acute health crisis

NURSING-SENSITIVE OUTCOMES

Today the majority of health problems are chronic long-term conditions that require individual self-care for health maintenance and restoration. Dean (1989) noted that research in the anthropologic, sociologic, and health services fields all document that the majority of illness care is self-care. Research has supported the effectiveness and appropriateness of the frequently lower-technology self-care (as compared with professional care). Self-care behaviors have been shown to effectively influence chronic headaches (Winkler, Underwood, Fatovich, James, & Gray, 1989), reduce pain and depression among arthritics (Lorig & Holman, 1993), and improve health decision making of mothers of small children (Rasmussen, 1989). As noted earlier, Conn and colleagues (1995) examined the complex set of self-care behaviors of elders and caregivers in managing medications. Other notable work by Conn (1991) examined the self-care behaviors of elders suffering from influenza and colds. Community-dwelling elders identified self-care behaviors in the areas of exercise, rest, fluids, and activity as strategies used in dealing with self-limiting illnesses.

Dean, Holst, and Wagner (1983) examined behavioral responses to six common illness conditions among Danish adults. Home remedy (nonmedication self-treatment) was practiced for 76% of 3100 reported illness episodes. Interaction differences in self-care behavior by gender, age, perceived health status, and attitude toward physicians were reported. Dean and colleagues' work documented how varying patterns of self-care behaviors are influenced by complex interactive sociocultural factors.

With the exception of those studies already noted, research support for individuals' self-care actions is limited. Research on self-care is fragmented and often fails to account for age, gender, or ethnic differences in self-care behaviors (Dean, 1989). Acceptable and appropriate self-care behaviors likely differ for persons of Hispanic versus African-American versus Anglo descent, as well as for persons of rural versus urban settings, young-old versus old-old, and younger versus older ages. Indeed, differences in patterns of self-care use by elders of different cultural groups have been reported (Haug, Akiyama, Tryban, Sonoda, & Wykle, 1991; Wykle & Haug, 1993). Behaviors examined are often limited to professional (nursing-centered) actions, even though the majority of self-care behaviors are initiated by the person, family, or friends. Further research examining the person's or the family/nonprofessional support system's care behaviors is needed.

Qualitative work in self-care also is limited and has often been treated less seriously (Dean, 1989). Work by Dill, Brown, Ciambrone, and Rakowski (1995) enriched the understanding of self-care by addressing the social context of health and aging, the meaning of common symptoms, and the relationship of health to self-identity. Based on data from in-depth interviews with 21 seniors, Dill and colleagues reported that elders' self-care responses are likely learned early in life, reinforced throughout the life cycle, and formed in collaboration with lay and professional persons. The researchers suggested that it is an oversimplification of symptom management to categorize care into mutually exclusive professional, informal, or self-care systems. Understanding of self-care must include the representation and interpretation of the self. Further qualitative work is essential to further understanding of self-care behaviors among elders.

Nursing-sensitive outcomes must consider measurable client outcomes in areas managed by client and family caregivers after appropriate education and guidance by nurses and other health care professionals. "To be useful for assessing the effectiveness of nursing, outcomes and indicators must be identified that are influenced by nursing and comprehensive enough to assess all aspects of nursing practice" (Maas, Johnson, & Moorhead, 1996, p. 299). As opposed to nursing interventions, which focus on phenomena related to nurse behaviors, nursing-sensitive outcomes are patient states or behaviors. A standardized taxonomy of nursing-sensitive outcomes has been developed and is being field tested at various clinical sites by the Iowa Outcomes Project (2000). As with nursing diagnostic categories, it will be essential to develop nursing-sensitive outcomes in the noninstitutional setting, with community-dwelling elders of diverse backgrounds who have a continuum of functional abilities.

Carpenito (1995, p. 777) outlined the following general outcome criteria for self-care deficits related to bodily function:

- Express preferences in self-care activities (time of day, location, hygiene products)
- Demonstrate optimal hygiene after appropriate assistance with care

- Participate verbally and physically in self-care: feeding, bathing, toileting, dressing activities

Using Carpenito's framework, Table 29-3 specifies outcome criteria for a client who is experiencing multiple self-care deficits in bodily functions. Carpenito's outcome criteria have several weaknesses. They apply to a broad clinical population and not specifically to the gerontologic population. The criteria are focused on a single level of abstraction. Carpenito's heading Self-Care Deficit (the NANDA diagnosis itself) contains a negative inference in the word deficit. Carpenito's outcome indicators lack specificity and comprehensiveness in comparison with the *Nursing Outcomes Classification (NOC)* indicators for Self-Care: Hygiene. Finally, Carpenito does not specify a timeline for outcome measurement. Overall, Carpenito's pioneering work will benefit from refinement according to the NOC guidelines and from further application to the specialized needs of the older population across the health care continuum.

Outcome criteria in the proposed diagnostic categories of Health Protection and Health Restoration suggested by Jenny (1989) include the following:

- Participate in decision making about level and duration of involvement of family and home health nurse in self-care: Be satisfied with level and duration of involvement.
- Return to former level of functioning (prefracture level), assuming responsibility for proper administra-

tion of daily medications; resume activities of interest such as driving short distances and tending roses.
- Participate in decision making about immunizations to prevent respiratory infection such as pneumonia: Understand value of immunization, decide on best course of action for this situation, act on this decision, and be content with results.
- Maintain adequate rest, exercise, and nutrition to support optimal state of health.

Other nursing-sensitive outcomes related to self-care include the following:

- *Self-Care: Activities of Daily Living (ADL):* Ability to perform the most basic physical tasks and personal care activities (Iowa Outcomes Project, 2000, p. 379)
- *Self-Care: Bathing:* Ability to cleanse own body (p. 380)
- *Self-Care: Dressing:* Ability to dress self (p. 381)
- *Self-Care: Eating:* Ability to prepare and ingest food (p. 382)
- *Self-Care: Grooming:* Ability to maintain kempt appearance (p. 383)
- *Self-Care: Instrumental Activities of Daily Living (IADL):* Ability to perform activities needed to function in the home or community (p. 385)
- *Self-Care: Non-Parenteral Medication:* Ability to administer oral and topical medications to meet therapeutic goals (p. 386)
- *Self-Care: Oral Hygiene:* Ability to care for own mouth and teeth (p. 387)

Table 29-3	Nursing Outcome Criteria SELF-CARE DEFICIT
Nursing Diagnoses	**Nursing Outcome Criteria**
Feeding Self-Care Deficit	Demonstrate increased ability to feed self
	Report that he is unable to feed self
	Demonstrate ability to make use of adaptive devices, if indicated
	Demonstrate increased interest and desire to eat
	Describe rationale and procedure for treatment
	Describe causative factors for feeding deficit
Instrumental Self-Care Deficit	Demonstrate use of adaptive devices, e.g., phone, cooking aids
	Describe a method to ensure adherence to medication schedule
	Report ability to call on and answer telephone
	Report regular laundering by self or others
	Report daily intake of two nutritious meals
	Identify transportation options to stores, physician, house of worship, social activities
	Demonstrate management of simple money transactions
	Identify individual(s) who will assist with money matters
Self-Care Deficit Syndrome	Identify preferences in self-care activities (e.g., time, products, location)
	Demonstrate optimal hygiene after assistance with care
	Participate physically and/or verbally in feeding, dressing, toileting, bathing activities

Adapted from Carpenito, L. J. (1995). *Nursing diagnosis: Application to clinical practice* (6th ed., pp. 777-778, 790). Baltimore: Lippincott Williams & Wilkins.

Table 29-4	Self-Care: Hygiene				
	Dependent, Does Not Participate 1	Requires Assistive Person & Device 2	Requires Assistive Person 3	Independent With Assistive Device 4	Completely Independent 5
SELF-CARE: HYGIENE *Indicators*					
Washes hands	1	2	3	4	5
Applies deodorant	1	2	3	4	5
Cleans perineal area	1	2	3	4	5
Cleans ears	1	2	3	4	5
Keeps nose blown and clean	1	2	3	4	5
Maintains oral hygiene	1	2	3	4	5
Other _____ (Specify)	1	2	3	4	5

Data from Cole, G. (1991). Hygiene and care of the patient's environment. In G. Cole (Ed.), *Basic nursing skills and concepts* (pp. 261-290). St. Louis, MO: Mosby; McKeighten, R. J., Mehmert, P. A., & Dickel, C. A. (1990). Bathing/hygiene self-care deficit: Defining characteristics and related factors across age groups and diagnosis-related groups in an acute care setting. *Nursing Diagnosis, 1*(4), 155-161; Ney, D. F. (1993). Cerumen impaction, ear hygiene practices, and hearing acuity. *Geriatric Nursing—American Journal of Care for the Aging, 14*(2), 70-73; Sorenson, K., & Luckmann, J. (1986). *Basic nursing: A psychophysiologic approach* (2nd ed.) Philadelphia: W. B. Saunders; Styker, R. (1977). *Rehabilitative aspects of acute and chronic nursing care.* Philadelphia: W. B. Saunders; Taylor, C. M. (1987). *Nursing diagnosis cards.* Springhouse, PA: Springhouse; Tracey, C. A. (1992). Hygiene assistance. In C. M. Bulechek & J. C. McCloskey (Eds.), *Nursing interventions: Essential nursing treatments* (2nd ed., pp. 24-33). Philadelphia: W. B. Saunders.

- *Self-Care: Parenteral Medication:* Ability to administer parenteral medications to meet therapeutic goals (p. 388)
- *Self-Care: Toileting:* Ability to toilet self (p. 389)
- *Self-Care: Hygiene:* Ability to maintain own hygiene (p. 384)
- *Health Promoting Behavior:* Actions to sustain or increase wellness (p. 232)

The nursing outcome Self Care: Hygiene is shown in its entirety in Table 29-4.

NURSING INTERVENTIONS

Sullivan (1980, p. 9) defined health:

as the state of being able to initiate and perform self-care activities which sustain life processes, maintain integrated functioning, promote normal growth and development, and prevent or control disease and disability and their effects. The healthy state occurs within the sociocultural expectations of the individual.

Sullivan also conceptualized a self-care model for nursing care of the aged that was based on Orem's (1995) five helping methods (acting or doing for another; guiding or directing; providing physical or psychologic support; providing or maintaining an environment that supports personal development; teaching). Sullivan incorporated the following system of four self-care levels for elders (and four corresponding nursing system levels):

1. The independents
2. The independents-threatened

3. The independents-delegated
4. The dependents

This model is based on the assumption that the aged, like other adults, desire and prefer self-care options whenever possible. The four levels represent a continuum, with movement occurring between and among the levels. Downward movement is feared by clients, and a goal of both self-care and nursing care is to prevent downward movement and to facilitate upward movement (Sullivan, 1980). There is a need for clients, families, and nurses to recognize the cues signaling immediate or imminent downward movement in order to take action to prevent or reverse the spiral. Sullivan's model also identifies the following four interpersonal subsystems:

1. The consuler/consultant system
2. The therapeutic alliance system
3. The delegated partial protective system
4. The relinquished fully protective system

Within each level there is an inverse relationship between the power of the nurse and that of the client. The client takes on the more active role in the consuler/consultant system; the nurse takes on the more active role in the fully relinquished system (Sullivan, 1980).

Nursing Interventions Classification (NIC)

The Iowa Intervention Team has reported the first two phases of a program of research designed to construct a taxonomy of nursing interventions. In the first phase an alphabetic list of 336 nursing interventions was developed and published in an effort to standardize the language of nursing interventions (Iowa Intervention Project, 1992). In the second phase the alphabetic classification was organized into a taxonomic structure (Iowa Intervention Project, 1993). In hierarchical clustering reported in 1993, Domain I, the Physiological: Basic domain, included care that supports physical functioning. This domain includes several classes of nursing interventions, including the class Self-Care Facilitation, interventions to provide, facilitate, or assist routine, basic, or daily living.

Also included in the physiologic domain are Elimination Management interventions to establish and maintain regular bowel and urinary elimination patterns and manage alterations caused by altered patterns. In cases where the underlying cause of an elimination problem is related to alterations in self-care abilities (i.e., ability to toilet self), it would be appropriate to select the nursing diagnosis Toileting Self-Care Deficit, the nursing-sensitive outcome Self-Care: Toileting (defined as the ability to toilet self) (Iowa Outcomes Project, 2000, p. 389), and the nursing intervention Self-Care Assistance: Toileting (defined as assisting another with elimination) (Iowa Intervention Project, 2000, p. 579). When the underlying problem is related to physiologic eliminatory dysfunction, the relevant nursing diagnosis is related to urinary and/or bowel dysfunction rather than to toileting self-care ability. In this case, the appropriate nursing-sensitive outcome would be Urinary Elimination (defined as ability of the urinary system to filter wastes, conserve solutes, and collect and discharge urine in a healthy pattern) (Iowa Outcomes Project, 2000, p. 437) and/or Bowel Elimination (defined as ability of the gastrointestinal tract to form and evacuate stool in a healthy pattern) (Iowa Outcomes Project, 2000, p. 127). In some cases both sets of diagnoses and outcomes might be relevant.

Other self-care interventions (Iowa Intervention Project, 2000) developed to date include the following:

- *Self-Care Assistance:* Assisting another to perform activities of daily living (p. 575)
- *Self-Care Assistance: Bathing/Hygiene:* Assisting patient* to perform personal hygiene (p. 576)
- *Self-Care Assistance: Dressing/Grooming:* Assisting patient* with clothes and make-up (p. 577)
- *Self-Care Assistance: Feeding:* Assisting a person to eat (p. 578)

Other Strategies

Penn (1988) identified five specific nursing strategies useful in compensating for clients' self-care deficits: reeducation; self-monitoring; contracting; self-help groups; and reminiscence therapy (Table 29-5). These categories of nursing interventions are admittedly not exhaustive in scope. Nursing interventions traditionally have been based

on clinical experience and knowledge as opposed to research. Development of research-based nursing interventions for aged persons in a diversity of settings is essential.

Population-Specific Interventions

Muchow (1993) suggested self-care strategies as a tool for rural elders. Rural people, particularly rural elders, are by tradition proud, independent, resilient, and self-sufficient. Rural people simultaneously have increased vulnerabilities: chronic health problems; diminished access to routine, acute, and emergency health care; less education; and fewer economic resources to affect health insurance, standard housing, and transportation. Muchow suggested a model of self-care based on the best of modern medical knowledge coupled with the tradition of self-reliance and "home remedies" characteristic of the struggle to survive in geographically and sometimes culturally remote areas. She suggested a program of health education based on assessment of group and individual needs, followed by tailoring of the health education program to the particular needs of rural people. Program costs, resource availability, and transportation are important issues for consideration. One successful large-scale example of such a self-care approach is the National Rural Health Network "Healthwise for Life" interactive video train-the-trainer program, in which over 15,000 rural residents were trained to teach others to fully participate in their own care (Muchow, 1993). This program has been modified and replicated in rural areas across the country.

Minority communities today find their members experiencing dependency that is encouraged by the overall social structure and health care system and that has replaced their historical self-sufficiency (Branch, 1985). Branch (1985) cited recommendations for restoration of self-care for members of African-American communities: lesser dependency on meager, overburdened existing facilities; individual responsibility for health; return to use of home remedies as appropriate; seeking medical care when necessary; development of first-line health leadership in African-American communities for after-hours and minor illness care; rediscovery of natural means of healing; renewed appreciation for holistic view of health; application of principles of prevention to physical and social ills; promotion of health through a total approach that includes environmental considerations; and elimination of harmful influences that undermine health teaching. Application of these principles in the promotion of autonomy and self-care among members of the African-American community, followed by research on effectiveness of the recommended approaches, has the potential to improve the health of this vulnerable population.

---

*Authors recommend changing "patient" to "person" (or "client") for consistency and to protect autonomy.

Table 29-5	Nursing Strategies to Manage Self-Care Deficit in Aged Clients	
Strategy	**Purpose**	**Considerations**
Reeducation	Focuses on teaching the older client psychomotor skills to maximize self-care in activities of daily living: feeding, toileting, bathing, dressing	One-on-one teaching, with teaching tailored to needs of individual client and specific deficit. Repetition, frequent, practice, and positive feedback essential.
Self-monitoring	Involves client's appraisal of cues, or signs and symptoms of etiologic factors that accompany the self-care deficit.	Client keeps a diary, journal, or chart of signs and symptoms, fluctuation in self-care deficit, and application of and response to intervention.
Contracting	Involves explicit identification of desired behavior in measurable terms acceptable to both client and nurse.	Desired behavior is broken down into small sequential measurable steps. Client chooses rewards or reinforcements for accomplishment of steps at specified dates. Progress is measured by achievement of short- and long-term goals.
Self-help groups	Comprise groups of elders who share a common deficit and come together to find mutual assistance in overcoming the deficit.	Based on the notion that an individual can best be helped by another individual experiencing similar events. Information, role models, and emotional support are provided.
Reminiscence therapy	Sharing of life experiences as a therapeutic modality in the treatment of depression, improvement of socialization, and stimulation of self-care activities.	May be carried out one-on-one or in small groups, including self-help groups.

Adapted from Penn, C. (1988). Promoting independence: The nurse can communicate an understanding of the self-care deficit, and elicit the client's perspective of the deficit and its meaning to daily living. *Journal of Gerontological Nursing, 14*(3), 14-19.

Elders can be supported in their self-care behaviors and overall empowerment through self-care handbooks and newsletters, workshops, and patient coaching/care counseling sessions (Mettler & Kemper, 1993). Written materials provide answers about common health concerns of elders, specific home care procedures or remedies, and when to seek professional help. Workshops can be used to increase self-care and consumerism skills, such as doctor-patient communication or caring for a frail spouse in the home setting. Tufts University researchers developed a program of coaching to help patients ask questions and play an active role in their professional care (Mettler & Kemper, 1993). Findings showed that coached patients got more information when seeing their doctor; they also reported fewer symptoms and rated their overall health better at the 4-month posttest, as compared with those who asked less questions. In another project, nurses prepared consumers by telephone to participate effectively in their health care by giving them the information they needed to understand their options and the encouragement to become actively involved with their physicians in treatment decisions (Mettler & Kemper, 1993). In an intervention study with adults with diabetes, experimental group patients trained to participate more actively in their medical care were twice as effective as control group patients at eliciting information from physicians, they reported fewer functional limitations, and they had lower mean glycosolated hemoglobin levels (Greenfield, Kaplan, Ware, Yano, & Harrison, 1988). Such nursing intervention strategies provide opportunity for the empowerment of older people through increased self-care and involvement in professional health care decision making, and have the added potential to create a health care system more relevant to the needs of elders.

Based on research findings from a study with 366 elders, Lantz (1985) characterized the profile of the older individual who has a significantly higher ability to assume self-care as including the following characteristics: female; self-perception of having "good" or "excellent" health, sense of self-worth and self-strength, and self-actualizing attributes; unwillingness to accept her weaknesses; high level of awareness; present oriented with a balance of past experiences and future expectations; and tendency toward rigidity and holding onto values to near-compulsiveness (p. 13). Further work in this area has the potential to guide gerontologic nursing assessment of self-care potential of clients, eventually leading to targeted interventions to increase self-care abilities.

Zauszniewski (1996) examined two forms of resourcefulness among 150 healthy elders: self-help and help-seeking strategies. She found that, unlike help-seeking behaviors, self-help strategies were significantly correlated with the adaptive functioning, life satisfaction, and absence of depressive cognitions. Neither set of strategies was associated with self-assessed health. The two strategies themselves were not strongly associated. Of those scoring high on self-help, help-seekers and non–help-seekers did not differ significantly. Further research examining the self-help and help-seeking behaviors of elders experiencing illness and impairment, as well as the normal challenges and losses of aging, is needed. Of particular interest is the potential differential benefit of certain strategies in situations involving acute and chronic conditions. The potential exists for gerontologic nurses to assess, teach, elicit, and/or guide strategies of self-help and help-seeking as a nursing intervention aimed at enhancing self-care.

Fiandt, Pullen, and Walker (1996) reported findings that provide a foundation for the development of a program of interventions focused on the modification of risk perceptions as a basis for improved preventive health self-care behaviors among older women. They found that a weak relationship existed between actual and perceived risk. Earlier research suggested that individuals' perceptions of risk are often inaccurate and that preventive health behaviors might be more closely correlated with the inaccurate perception of risk than with actual risk. This body of research points to a considerable opportunity for nurses, through assessment and education, to influence the practice of self-care health promotion behaviors that

have great potential to extend length of life and enhance control and quality of life for older people.

CASE STUDY 1

Mrs. Clark, having suffered a fractured radius, was diagnosed with Self-Care Deficit: Health Restoration, Self-Care Deficit: Environmental Management, and Self-Care Deficit: Non-Parenteral Medication Management. Care outcomes related to her self-care deficits included Self-Care: Activities of Daily Living (ADL), Self-Care: Instrumental Activities of Daily Living (IADL), and Self-Care: Non-Parenteral Medication. Related nursing interventions were Risk Identification (defined as the analysis of potential risk factors, determination of health risks, and prioritization of risk reduction strategies for an individual or group) and Medication Management (defined as the facilitation of safe and effective use of prescription and over-the-counter drugs). Details of Mrs. Clark's plan of care are given in Box 29-4.

Box 29-4 | Nursing Diagnosis, Outcomes, and Interventions for MRS. CLARK

Nursing Diagnosis
Self-Care Deficit: Health Restoration
Defining characteristics
Cast on right forearm limits flexibility and ability to be totally independent in ADL.
Assistance in procuring and preparing food needed.
Assistance with opening medication bottles required.

Nursing-Sensitive Outcomes
Self-Care: Activities of Daily Living (ADL)
Indicators
Eating
Dressing
Toileting
Bathing
Grooming
Hygiene
Oral hygiene

Self-Care: Instrumental Activities of Daily Living (IADL)
Indicators
Prepares meals
Opens containers
Manages medications

Self-Care: Non-Parenteral Medication
Indicators
Maintains needed supplies
Administers medication correctly
Stores medication properly
Disposes of medication appropriately

Nursing Interventions
Risk Identification
Activities
As part of risk analysis, assess and analyze causative factors contributing to deficit, including precipitating event and safety of home environment
Consult with physician, physical therapist, occupational therapist, home health nurse, family
With client and family, plan regimen of nutrition, rest, and exercise that will enable healing and restore former level of strength and flexibility

Medication Management
Activity
Explore use of alternative containers with lids for medications

Nursing Outcomes Classification (NOC) 5-point Likert measurement scales:

Self Care: Activities of Daily Living (ADL): 1 = Dependent, does not participate; 2 = Requires assistive persons and device; 3 = Requires assistive person; 4 = Independent with assistive device; 5 = Completely independent.
Self Care: Instrumental Activities of Daily Living (IADL): 1 = Dependent, does not participate; 2 = Requires assistive persons and device; 3 = Requires assistive person; 4 = Independent with assistive device; 5 = Completely independent.
Self Care: Non-Parenteral Medication: 1 = Dependent, does not participate; 2 = Requires assistive persons and device; 3 = Requires assistive person; 4 = Independent with assistive device; 5 = Completely independent.

| Table 29-6 | Nursing Diagnoses, Outcomes, and Interventions for MR. MORALES | | |

Nursing Diagnoses	Nursing-Sensitive Outcomes	Nursing Interventions
FEEDING SELF-CARE DEFICIT *Defining Characteristics* Inability to handle utensils (unable to hold utensil with right hand to carry food to mouth) Inability to chew food (difficulty chewing and swallowing foods of normal texture) Unable to express food preferences to staff 10-lb weight loss since illness onset Shows little interest in mealtime, turning head away when tray is brought to room	**SELF-CARE: EATING** *Indicators* Handles utensils Chews food Picks up cup or glass Gets food onto the utensil Client maintains weight within norms of age and height Client exhibits state of good nutritional balance, with adequate energy to participate in rehabilitation program	**SELF-CARE ASSISTANCE: FEEDING** *Activities* After assessing and analyzing causative factors contributing to deficit, consult with dietitian, speech therapist, occupational therapist, family Provide preferred foods of appropriate consistency in balanced diet with adequate caloric intake Provide only assistance needed, from feeding to verbal or physical cues Allow client to direct pace, sequence, amount of food/fluid taken Provide assistive devices, as helpful Provide privacy and nondistracting environment Involve family in creating a comfortable social environment and participation in assisting with feeding, as needed
BATHING/HYGIENE SELF-CARE DEFICIT *Defining Characteristics* Inability to wash body or body parts Inability to obtain or get to water source Inability to regulate temperature flow *Related Factors/Etiologies* Decreased or lack of motivation Weakness and tiredness Severe anxiety Inadequate to perceive body part or spatial relationship Perceptual or cognitive impairment Pain Neuromuscular impairment Musculoskeletal impairment Environmental barriers	**SELF-CARE: HYGIENE** *Indicators* Washes hands Applies deodorant Cleans perineal area Cleans ears Keeps nose blown and clean Maintains oral hygiene Other (specify)	**SELF-CARE ASSISTANCE: BATHING/HYGIENE** *Activities* Place towels, soap, deodorant, shaving equipment, and other needed accessories at bedside/bathroom Provide desired personal articles (e.g., deodorant, toothbrush, and bath soap) Facilitate patient's brushing teeth, as appropriate Facilitate patient's bathing self, as appropriate Monitor cleaning of nails, according to patient's self-care ability Facilitate maintenance of patient's usual bedtime routines, presleep cues/props, and familiar objects, as appropriate* Encourage parent/family participation in usual bedtime rituals, as appropriate* Provide assistance until patient is fully able to assume self-care

*Authors recommend deleting these nursing activities as a part of this nursing intervention and placing these activities with Sleep Enhancement facilitation of regular sleep/wake cycles, since a self-care deficit in bathing/hygiene is not necessarily accompanied by a sleep disturbance.
Nursing Outcomes Classification (NOC) 5-point Likert measurement scales:

Self Care: Hygiene: 1 = Dependent, does not participate; 2 = Requires assistive person and device; 3 = Requires assistive person; 4 = Independent with assistive device; 5 = Completely independent.
Self-Care: Eating: 1 = Dependent, does not participate; 2 = Requires assistive person and device; 3 = Requires assistive person; 4 = Independent with assistive device; 5 = Completely independent.

CASE STUDY 2

Mr. Morales, who had right hemiplegia, was diagnosed with the following self-care deficits: Self-Care Deficit Syndrome; Bathing/Hygiene Self-Care Deficit; Dressing/Grooming Self-Care Deficit; Feeding Self-Care Deficit; Toileting Self-Care Deficit; and Self-Care Deficit: Instrumental. Nursing outcomes and interventions that are appropriate for his feeding and bathing/hygiene deficits are given in Table 29-6.

CASE STUDY 3

Mr. Salas, the individual inquiring about influenza and pneumonia immunization, was given the nursing diagnosis Self-Care Deficit: Health Promotion. Desired nursing outcome was Health Promoting Behavior. The relevant nursing intervention was Risk Identification. Details are given in Box 29-5.

SUMMARY

Special aging considerations for nurses working with gerontologic clients with self-care deficits are listed in Box 29-6. The potential contribution to self-care of older persons by nurse clinicians, theoreticians, and researchers focusing on Self-Care Deficit across the continuum of settings and functional ability, across the diversity of age, ethnicity, and gender, is vast. As one of the most frequently encountered challenges in later life, Self-Care Deficit affects most elders to some degree in some aspect of health and lifestyle. Development of conceptually sound, research-based gerontologic nursing practice focused on restoring self-care abilities in the face of self-care deficits is a critically important, central aspect of nursing practice with the elderly population.

Box 29-5 | Nursing Diagnosis, Outcome, and Intervention for
MR. SALAS

Nursing Diagnosis
Self-Care Deficit: Health Promotion
Defining characteristics
No acute illnesses
History of chronic bronchitis and pneumonia

Nursing-Sensitive Outcome
Health Promoting Behavior
Indicators
Client will be able to maintain optimal state of health, free of preventable respiratory infection such as pneumonia
Upon consultation with primary care provider, chooses to obtain pneumonia/influenza immunizations from public health department clinic

Nursing Intervention
Risk Identification
Activities
Institute routine risk assessment, using reliable and valid instruments

Review past medical history and documents for evidence of existing or previous medical and nursing diagnoses
As part of risk analysis, assess and analyze causative factors contributing to deficit, including risk factors such as age, history of pneumonia and bronchitis, and residence in congregate setting
Consult with physician regarding prior medical history and possible contraindications with public health department nurse regarding scheduling of immunization clinic and costs, if any
Inform client of benefits and risks of immunizations, supporting client decision making in self-care behaviors that minimize health risks

Nursing Outcomes Classification (NOC) 5-point Likert measurement scale:

Health Promoting Behavior: 1 = Never demonstrated; 2 = Rarely demonstrated; 3 = Sometimes demonstrated; 4 = Often demonstrated; 5 = Consistently demonstrated.

Box 29-6	Age-Related Considerations With Self-Care Deficit Interventions

Increasing age itself does not cause self-care deficits. With increasing age, however, there is an increased incidence of chronic illnesses that are often accompanied by functional impairment and self-care deficit.

The community-dwelling older person must have the ability to perform or be assisted to perform six ADL, and may require assistance with other essential ADL. IADL such as activities related to housekeeping, shopping, food preparation, self-medication, money management, and transportation are even more complex than ADL and may particularly require outside assistance.

Functional status among older adults has substantially improved in the decades from the 1960s to the 1980s, and there is opportunity for further improvement with current knowledge and resources.

The majority, nearly three fourths of elders, rate their health as excellent. Only one fifth of those 65 to 74 and one fourth of those over 75 report limitations in ADL caused by chronic illness.

A small minority, estimated at 5%, of elderly are in institutions at any one time. Among those in nursing homes, 63% cannot perform basic ADL because of cognitive impairment. Those with dementia have varying abilities to perform self-care activities depending on memory deficits, ability to follow direction, and judgment. Among primary factors leading to institutionalization of older adults appears to be the exhaustion of their social support systems.

Cultural and family beliefs affect the self-caregiving potential of an older person. Caregivers who believe that dependency is the norm for aging people may promote excess disability, dependence, and deterioration in self-care abilities. Some cultures have a pattern of caregiving that involves doing as much for the ill person as possible in order to show concern.

Unnecessary assistance with activities such as feeding and bathing may prevent the elder's active participation in rehabilitation and self-care.

Assistance with bodily care may be restricted to certain persons (such as those with specific family roles) by spoken or unspoken cultural rules.

Maintaining older persons in community rather than institutions has significant value to society. Approximately one quarter of financial expenditures for health care for older adults in the United States goes to nursing homes. Medicaid funds 90% of publicly funded nursing home care. Most health care for older adults is provided in the community setting.

Beyond financial considerations, community living potentially strengthens family life, maintains autonomy, and affirms the value of older people in society. The nursing goal of maintaining the least restrictive environment for the older person contributes to the autonomy of the older individual and allows that older person to continue to contribute to society.

Adapted from Carpenito, L. J. (1995). *Nursing diagnosis: Application to clinical practice* (6th ed., pp. 776, 789). Baltimore: Lippincott Williams & Wilkins.

REFERENCES

Adams, M. (1986). Aging: Gerontological nursing research. In H. H. Werley, J. J. Fitzpatrick, & R. L. Taunton (Eds.), *Annual review of nursing research* (vol. 4, pp. 77-106). New York: Springer.

Branch, M. (1985). Self-care: Black perspective. In J. Riehl-Sisca (Ed.), *The science and art of self care* (pp. 181-188). Norwalk, CT: Appleton & Lange.

Bulechek, G. M., & McCloskey, J. C. (Eds.). (1985). Future directions. In *Nursing interventions: Treatments for nursing diagnoses* (pp. 401-408). Philadelphia: W. B. Saunders.

Carpenito, L. J. (1995). *Nursing diagnosis: Application to clinical practice* (6th ed.). Baltimore: Lippincott Williams & Wilkins.

Chang, B. L., Uman, G. C., & Hirsch, M. (1998). Predictive power of clinical indicators for self-care deficit. *Nursing Diagnosis, 9*(2), 71-82.

Cole, G. (1991). Hygiene and care of the patient's environment. In G. Cole (Ed.), *Basic nursing skills and concepts* (pp. 261-290). St. Louis, MO: Mosby.

Conn, V. S. (1991). Influenza and colds: Older adults' self-care actions. *Nursing Research, 40,* 176-181.

Conn, V. S., Taylor, S. G., & Messina, C. J. (1995). Older adults and their caregivers: The transition to medication assistance. *Journal of Gerontological Nursing, 21*(5), 33-38, 54-55.

Dean, K. (1989). Conceptual, theoretical and methodological issues in self-care research. *Social Science Medicine, 29,* 117-123.

Dean, K. J., Holst, E., & Wagner, M. G. (1983). Self-care of common illnesses in Denmark. *Medical Care, 21,* 1012-1032.

Dickel, C. A., & Mehmert, P. A. (1994). Self-care deficit: Bathing/hygiene replication study: Defining characteristics and related factors documented in acute care. In R. M. Carroll-Johnson & M. Paquette (Eds.), *Classification of nursing diagnoses: Proceedings of the tenth conference* (pp. 325-326). Baltimore: Lippincott Williams & Wilkins.

Dill, A., Brown, P., Ciambrone, D., & Rakowski, W. (1995). The measuring and practice of self-care by older adults: A qualitative assessment. *Research on Aging, 17,* 9-41.

Duncan, L. (Ed.). (1991). *Geriatric nursing care plans.* St. Louis, MO: Mosby.

Evers, G. C. M. (1989). *Appraisal of self-care agency ASA scale: Reliability and validity testing of the Dutch version of the A.S.A. scale measuring Orem's self-concept "self-care agency"* (pp. 19-31). Assen, The Netherlands: Van Gorcum & Comp.

Fiandt, K. L., Pullen, C. H., & Walker, S. N. (1996). Actual and perceived risk and utilization of preventive services in older woman (abstract). *Midwest Nursing Research Society: 20th Annual Research Conference.*

Gast, H. L., Denyes, M. J., Campbell, J. C., Hartweg, D. L., Schoot-Baer, D., & Isenberg, M. (1989). Self-care agency: Conceptualizations and operationalizations. *Advances in Nursing Science, 12*(1), 26-38.

Geden, E., & Taylor, S. (1991). Construct and empirical validity of the Self-As-Carer Inventory. *Nursing Research, 40,* 47-50.

Greenfield, S., Kaplan, S. H., Ware, J. E., Yano, E. M., & Harrison, F. J. L. (1988). Patient's participation in medical care: Effects on blood sugar control and quality of life in diabetes. *Journal of General Internal Medicine, 3,* 448-457.

Hanson, B. R., & Bickel, L. (1995). Development and testing of the questionnaire on perception of self-care agency. In J. Riehl-Sisca (Ed.), *The science and art of self-care* (pp. 271-278). Norwalk, CT: Appleton & Lange.

Hardy, M. A., Maas, M., & Akins, J. (Eds.). (1988). The prevalence of nursing diagnoses among elderly. In *Recent advances in nursing* (pp. 145-215). United Kingdom: Longman Group.

Haug, M. R., Akiyama, H., Tryban, G., Sonoda, K., & Wykle, M. (1991). Self-care: Japan and the U.S. compared. *Social Science Medicine, 33,* 1011-1021.

Herman, M. (1994). Integrating culture diversity into present nursing diagnosis taxonomy: Classification of nursing diagnosis. In R. M. Carroll-Johnson & M. Paquette (Eds.), *Proceedings of the tenth conference* (pp. 385). Baltimore: Lippincott Williams & Wilkins.

Iowa Intervention Project. (1993). The NIC taxonomy structure. *IMAGE: Journal of Nursing Scholarship, 25,* 187-192.

Iowa Intervention Project. J. C. McCloskey & C. M. Bulechek (Eds.). (1992). *Nursing interventions classification (NIC).* St. Louis, MO: Mosby.

Iowa Intervention Project. J. C. McCloskey & G. M. Bulechek (Eds.). (2000). *Nursing interventions classification (NIC)* (3rd ed.). St. Louis, MO: Mosby.

Iowa Outcomes Project. M. Johnson, M. Maas, & S. Moorhead (Eds.). (2000). *Nursing outcomes classification (NOC)* (2nd ed.). St. Louis, MO: Mosby.

Jacobson, S. F. (1988). Evaluating instruments for use in clinical nursing research. In M. Frank-Stromborg (Ed.), *Instruments for clinical research* (pp. 3-19). Norwalk, CT: Appleton & Lange.

Jenny, J. (1989). Classification of nursing diagnosis: A self-care approach. In R. M. Carroll-Johnson (Ed.), *Classification of nursing diagnoses: Proceedings of the eighth conference* (pp. 152-157). Baltimore: Lippincott Williams & Wilkins.

Jirovec, M. M., & Kasno, J. (1990). Self-care agency as a function of patient-environment factors among nursing home residents. *Research in Nursing & Health, 13,* 303-309.

Kane, R. A., & Kane, R. L. (1981). *Assessing the elderly: A practical guide to measurement.* Lexington, MA: Lexington Books.

Kane, R. L., Ouslander, J. G., & Abrass, I. B. (1994). *Essentials of clinical geriatrics* (3rd ed.). Hightstown, NJ: McGraw-Hill.

Katz, S., Ford, A. B., Moskowitz, R. W., Jackson, B. A., & Jaffee, M. W. (1963). Studies of illness in the aged. The index of ADL: A standardized measure of the biological and psychosocial function. *Journal of American Medical Association, 185,* 914-919.

Kelley, F. A., Kawamoto, T. T., & Rubenstein, L. Z. (1991). Assessment of the geriatric patient. In J. M. Kiernat (Ed.), *Occupational therapy and the older adult: A clinical manual* (pp. 76-98). In the Aspen Series in Occupational Health. Baltimore: Aspen.

Kim, M. J., & Moritz, D. E. (1982). *Classification of nursing diagnosis: Proceedings of the third (1978) and fourth (1980) national conferences.* Hightstown, NJ: McGraw-Hill.

Lantz, J. M. (1985). In search of agents for self-care. *Journal of Gerontological Nursing, 11*(7), 10-14.

Levin, L. S. (1981). Self-care in health: Potentials and pitfalls. *World Health Forum, 2*(2), 177-184.

Lipson, J., & Steiger, N. (1996). *Self-care in a multicultural context.* Thousand Oaks, CA: Sage.

Lorig, K., & Holman, H. (1993). Arthritis self-management studies. A twelve year review. *Health Education Quarterly, 20*(1), 17-28.

Maas, M., Johnson, M., & Moorhead, S. (1996). Classifying nursing-sensitive patient outcomes. *Image—Journal of Nursing Scholarship, 28*(4), 295-301.

Mahoney, F. I., & Barthel, D. W. (1965). Functional evaluation: The Barthel Index. *Maryland State Medical Journal, 14,* 61-65.

McBride, S. H. (1991). Comparative analysis of three instruments designed to measure self-care agency. *Nursing Research, 40,* 12-16.

McCourt, A. E. (1987). Implementation of nursing diagnoses through integration with quality assurance. *Nursing Clinics of North America, 22*(4), 899-905.

McKeighten, R. J., Mehmert, P. A., & Dickel, C. A. (1990). Bathing/hygiene self-care deficit: Defining characteristics and related factors across age groups and diagnosis-related groups in an acute care setting. *Nursing Diagnosis, 1*(4), 155-161.

Mettler, M., & Kemper, D. W. (1993). Self-care and older adults: Making healthcare relevant. *Generations, 17,* 7-10.

Metzger, K. L., & Hiltunen, E. F. (1987). Diagnostic content validation often frequently reported nursing diagnoses. In A. M. McLane (Ed.), *Classification of nursing diagnoses: Proceedings of the seventh conference* (pp. 144-153). St. Louis, MO: Mosby.

Muchow, J. A. (1993). Self-care as a rural healthcare strategy. *Generations, 17,* 29-32.

Ney, D. F. (1993). Cerumen impaction, ear hygiene practices, and hearing acuity. *Geriatric Nursing—American Journal of Care for the Aging, 14*(2), 70-73.

North American Nursing Diagnosis Association. (1986). *Nursing diagnoses: Definitions & classification.* Philadelphia: Author.

North American Nursing Diagnosis Association. (1999). *Nursing diagnoses: Definitions and classification 1999-2000.* Philadelphia: Author.

Orem, D. E. (1980). *Nursing: Concepts of practice* (2nd ed.). Hightstown, NJ: McGraw-Hill.

Orem, D. E. (1995). *Nursing: Concepts of practice* (5th ed.). St. Louis, MO: Mosby.

Penn, C. (1988). Promoting independence: The nurse can communicate an understanding of the self-care deficit, and elicit the client's perspective of the deficit and its meaning to daily living. *Journal of Gerontological Nursing, 14*(3), 14-19.

Pfeiffer, E., Johnson, T. M., & Chiofolo, R. C. (1981). Functional assessment of elderly subjects in four service settings. *Journal of the American Geriatrics Society, 39,* 433-443.

Rantz, M., & Miller, T. (1987). How diagnoses are changing in long-term care. *American Journal of Nursing, 87,* 306-361.

Rantz, M., Miller, T., & Jacobs, C. (1981). Nursing diagnosis in long-term care. *American Journal of Nursing, 85,* 916-926.

Rasmussen, F. (1989). Mother's benefit of a self-care booklet and a self-care educational session at child health center. *Social Science & Medicine, 29*(2), 205-212.

Riesch, S., & Hauk, M. (1988). The exercise of self-care agency: An analysis of construct and discriminate validity. *Research in Nursing and Health, 11,* 245-255.

Sorenson, K., & Luckmann, J. (1986). *Basic nursing: A psychophysiologic approach* (2nd ed). Philadelphia: W. B. Saunders.

Stolte, K. (1994). Health oriented nursing diagnoses: Development and use. In R. M. Carroll-Johnson & M. Paquette (Eds.), *Classification of nursing diagnoses: Proceedings of the tenth conference* (pp. 143-147). Baltimore: Lippincott Williams & Wilkins.

Styker, R. (1977). *Rehabilitative aspects of acute and chronic nursing care.* Philadelphia: W. B. Saunders.

Sullivan, T. J. (Ed.). (1980). Self-care model for nursing. In *New Directions for Nursing in the 80's* (pp. 57-68). Kansas City, MO: American Nurses Association.

Taylor, C. M. (1987). *Nursing diagnosis cards.* Springhouse, PA: Springhouse.

Tracey, C. A. (1992). Hygiene assistance. In C. M. Bulechek & J. C. McCloskey (Eds.), *Nursing interventions: Essential nursing treatments* (2nd ed., pp. 24-33). Philadelphia: W. B. Saunders.

Tracy, C. A. (1989). Etiologies of the nursing diagnosis of self-care deficit. In R. M. Carroll-Johnson (Ed.), *Classification of nursing diagnoses* (pp. 349-351). Baltimore: Lippincott Williams & Wilkins.

Whetstone, W., & Hansson, A. (1989). Perceptions of self-care in Sweden: A cross cultural replication. *Journal of Advanced Nursing, 14,* 962-969.

Winkler, R., Underwood, P., Fatovich, B., James, R., & Gray, D. (1989). A clinical trial of self-care approach to the management of chronic headache in general practice. *Social Science & Medicine, 29*(2), 213-219.

World Health Organization. (1983). Scientific consultations. In *Health education in self-care possibilities and limitations.* Geneva: World Health Organization.

Wykie, M. L., & Haug, M. R. (1993, Fall). Multicultural and social-class aspects of self-care. *Self-Care and Older Adults,* 25-28.

Zauszniewski, J. A. (1996). Measurement of two forms of resourcefulness in health elders. *Midwest Nursing Research Society: 20th Annual Research Conference.*

CHAPTER 30

DIVERSIONAL ACTIVITY DEFICIT

Marilyn J. Rantz and Lori Popejoy

The central ideas of diversional activity are change and enjoyment or pleasure. Diversion as change simply means activities that are different from one's usual activities. Diversion as enjoyment or pleasure means activities that are recreational and pursued during leisure time for the purpose of personal amusement or satisfaction. Leisure time is time that is free from obligations (Rubenfeld, 1993). Diversional Activity Deficit is "the state in which an individual experiences a decreased stimulation from or interest or engagement in recreational or leisure activities" (NANDA, 1999, p. 93). The central ideas of change or enjoyment and pleasure are not clearly indicated in the North American Nursing Diagnosis Association (NANDA) definition. However, they are inherent in the words of the diagnostic label Diversional Activity Deficit.

The foundation for the diagnosis Diversional Activity Deficit in elders can be traced to aging theories proposed in the 1950s and 1960s and a subsequent proliferation of studies targeted to support or refute the theories. As a result of these efforts, negative outcomes of withdrawal from society were identified and positive outcomes of strategically planned interventions were demonstrated. These theories include activity theory (Havighurst & Albrecht, 1953), disengagement theory (Cummings & Henry, 1961), and continuity theory (Neugarten, Havighurst, & Tobin, 1968). More recent theoretical endeavors (Burbank, 1986; Burnside & Haight, 1992, 1994) support an individualized phenomenologic approach, which explores the meanings of activities and events in older persons' lives using the techniques of life review and reminiscence.

These sometimes controversial theoretical explorations must continue. They will provide a foundation to guide the development of effective care for elderly people. Intervention and outcome research generated by theory development can provide practical direction for nursing interventions targeted to address the diagnosis Diversional Activity Deficit. To date, no specific empirical testing of this diagnosis has been published in the literature, although considerable research has been conducted regarding applicable interventions (Abraham, Neundorfer, & Currie, 1992; Buckwalter et al., 1995; Clark, Lipe, & Bilbrey, 1998; Koroknay, Werner, Cohen-Mansfield, & Braun, 1995; Moore, 1992) and subsequent outcomes (Aldridge,

1994; Francis, 1991; Kovach & Magliocco, 1998; Stevens-Ratchford, 1993), particularly in elders.

Diversional activity deficits are not unique to elderly persons; however, older persons are particularly vulnerable to developing these deficits. Compared with younger persons, elders usually have more time that is free from obligations. In one study, elders spent about half of their waking hours in leisure activities such as watching television or reading (Horgas, Wilms, & Baltes, 1998). Typically, most elders are retired from employment or family obligations, although many provide care for other elderly relatives or young children. Elders in independent living arrangements frequently experience chronic illness, limited income, lack of transportation, social isolation, impaired mobility, impaired sensory functions, fear of neighborhood crime, and other exertional physical limitations that increase their risk for diversional activity deficits (Ebersole & Hess, 1998; Lawton, Moss, & Moles, 1984; Rubenfeld, 1993). Many of these same factors impede the involvement of institutionalized elders in diversional activities. In institutional settings, involvement can be diminished further by care delivery routines, space constraints, lack of encouragement to develop new or to enhance interests, accessibility to resources, availability of staff to provide individualized assistance, lack of a peer group with similar interests or cognitive capability, lack of encouragement from staff and families to be involved in recreational activities, and limited activities because staff offer activities that are familiar and comfortable for them.

Failure to diagnose and treat diversional activity deficits in elders can result in several negative outcomes: social isolation, withdrawal, depression, hostility, poor self-esteem, decreased life satisfaction, and further declines in physical endurance, coordination, and cognitive ability (Rantz, 1991).

Empirically supported positive outcomes related to diagnosing and treating diversional activity deficits include the following: improved cognitive function (Aldridge, 1994; Stones & Dawes, 1993); improved learning capacity (Yesavage, 1984); focused discussion with peers (Baker, 1985; Beck, 1982; Cook, 1984); increased and improved social interaction or involvement (Fick, 1993; Francis, 1991; Moore, 1992; Sambandham & Schirm, 1995); decreased depression (Francis, Turner, & Johnson, 1985;

Ruuskanen & Parkatti, 1994); improved self-esteem (Baker, 1985; Parent & Whall, 1984; Stevens-Ratchford, 1993); decreased hostility (Robb & Stegman, 1983); reduced agitated behavior for dementia patients (Casby & Holm, 1994; Clark, Lipe, & Bilbrey, 1998; Gerdner & Swanson, 1993; Goddaer & Abraham, 1994); increased engagement and psychosocial well-being (Greene & Monahan, 1982; McCormack & Whitehead, 1981; Wikstrom, Theorell, & Sandstrom, 1993); lowered blood pressure and improved survival independent of health status (Baun, Bergstrom, Langston, & Thoma, 1984); increased muscle strength, endurance, and joint flexibility (Allen, 1992; MacRae et al., 1996; Schnelle et al., 1996); and improved mobility (Jirovec, 1991; Wolfson et al., 1996). These impressive outcomes are highly significant to nurses caring for elderly persons.

Elderly individuals are vulnerable to Diversional Activity Deficit regardless of their independent or institutional living arrangements. The magnitude of negative outcomes if the diagnosis is unrecognized and untreated, as well as the magnitude of the positive outcomes if the diagnosis is identified and treated, establishes Diversional Activity Deficit as a significant nursing diagnosis.

RELATED FACTORS/ETIOLOGIES

Although time for leisure activities can increase as family and work obligations lessen with age, other factors can interfere with pursuing activities of one's choice. Declining health status, impaired mobility, impaired vision, and fear of falling can lead to an inability to attend previously enjoyed activities in community settings (Ebersole & Hess, 1998). The elder simply might not have developed leisure interests because of economic constraints during the Depression era or because of cultural and religious values related to work. The elder might have experienced a lack of leisure time during younger years when today's time-saving devices were not available. Strong work values may be a major factor in their decisions not to engage in diversional activities. Deciding not to engage in activities that involve other people results in social isolation that can be compounded by family members living some distance from them and the loss of lifelong friends and neighbors through institutionalization, relocation, or death.

Rantz and Miller (1993) have grouped factors related to diversional activity deficits in elders into three categories: personal preference, sensory deficit, or former lifestyle. Carpenito (1992) lists four categories of related factors: pathophysiologic factors (such as pain), treatment-related factors (such as length and frequency), situational factors (such as loss of social network or monotonous environment), and maturational factors (such as sensory/motor deficits). McFarland and McFarlane (1997) also list four categories of related factors: time factors (major life changes such as long-term illness or retirement), environ-

mental factors (such as space constraints), factors related to functional abilities (such as impaired mobility), and factors related to interest in activities (such as lack of knowledge of options). All of these related factors are applicable to elders.

ASSESSMENT

Radziewicz and Schneider (1992) developed and published in its entirety a diversional assessment instrument for cancer patients. By specifically assessing for this diagnosis, they wanted to improve relationships and enhance coping for those experiencing long hospitalization. The instrument includes a comprehensive list of staff and activities available for patients on their cancer unit. A specific question is asked about the patient's major concern during the current hospitalization and if any of the activities can help with the concern. Rantz and Miller (1993) identified the relevant items from the Minimum Data Set for Resident Assessment and Care Screening for Nursing Homes (MDS) and constructed a therapeutic recreation resident assessment work sheet for nursing home residents. Assessment Guide 30-1 illustrates this assessment tool. Other items that would be important to assess include the following: previous interests, values, and lifestyle; functional abilities, mobility, and endurance; depression, social support, and anxiety; and chronic illnesses, sensory impairments, and cognitive impairment. In some cases, assessment information may need to come from family and friends.

NURSING DIAGNOSIS

The diagnosis, related factors, and defining characteristics of Diversional Activity Deficit were first identified at the Fourth National Conference for Classification of Nursing Diagnosis in 1980 (Kim & Moritz, 1982). A definition of Diversional Activity Deficit was not advanced until the seventh conference in 1986 (McLane, 1987). The definition, related factors, and defining characteristics have remained unchanged since their original acceptance: "Patient statement's regarding: boredom, wish there was something to do, to read, etc.; usual hobbies cannot be undertaken in hospital" (NANDA, 1999, p. 93). Although there are no reported validation studies of the nursing diagnosis Diversional Activity Deficit, some authors have reported the use of this diagnosis for elderly nursing home residents (Rantz & Miller, 1987; Rantz, Miller, & Jacobs, 1985; Rantz, Miller & Matson, 1995) and for patients hospitalized for long periods of time (Radziewicz & Schneider, 1992).

Rantz and Miller (1993) reported additional defining characteristics from a content analysis of the care plans of their nursing home residents. Other authors (Carpenito, 1992; McFarland & McFarlane, 1997) have listed addi-

THERAPEUTIC RECREATION RESIDENT ASSESSMENT BASED ON MINIMUM DATA SET

Instruction: Select all items that apply during last 7 days.

Sense of Initiative/Involvement

_____ a. At ease interacting with others
_____ b. At ease doing planned or structured
activities
_____ c. At ease doing self-initiated activity
_____ d. Establishes own goals

_____ e. Pursues involvement in life of facility (e.g.,
makes/keeps friends; involved in group activities;
responds positively to new activities; assists at
religious services)
_____ f. Accepts invitations into most group
activities
_____ g. NONE OF THE ABOVE

Average Time Involved in Activities

_____ a. Most—more than 2/3 of time
_____ b. Some—1/3 to 2/3 of time

_____ c. Little—less than 1/3 of time
_____ d. None

Preferred Activity Setting

_____ a. Own room
_____ b. Day/activity room
_____ c. Inside nursing home/off unit

_____ d. Outside facility
_____ e. NONE OF THE ABOVE

General Activities Preference (Adapted to Resident's Current Abilities)

Instructions: Select all preferences whether or not activity is currently available to resident.
_____ a. Cards/other games
_____ b. Crafts/art
_____ c. Exercise/sports
_____ d. Music
_____ e. Reading/writing
_____ f. Spiritual/religious activities
_____ g. Trips/shopping

_____ h. Walking/wheeling outdoors
_____ i. Watching television
_____ j. Gardening or plants
_____ k. Talking or conversing
_____ l. Helping others
_____ m. NONE OF THE ABOVE

Prefers Change in Daily Routine

Instructions: Code for resident preferences in daily routines.
a. Type of activities in which resident is currently involved
_____ 0 = No change
_____ 1 = Slight change
_____ 2 = Major change
b. Extent of resident involvement in activity
_____ 0 = No change
_____ 1 = Slight change
_____ 2 = Major change
Activity interest before admission: _____
_____
_____

Personal preferences for activities: _____
_____
_____

Plan for meeting desired activities: _____
_____
_____

Box 30-1	Defining Characteristics DIVERSIONAL ACTIVITY DEFICIT

Rantz & Miller, 1993
Daytime napping
Refuses to go to off-unit therapeutic recreation activities
Refuses to go to therapeutic recreation activities
Needs verbal direction to therapeutic recreation program and location
Needs assistance to therapeutic recreation program and location
Elective in therapeutic recreation involvement
Fatigues easily
Lacks interest in therapeutic recreation programs
No independent hobbies
Prefers privacy
Expresses desire to spend leisure time alone
Does not refer to therapeutic recreation unit calendar
Needs special invitation or encouragement to therapeutic recreation activities
Limited activity tolerance
Minimal peer interaction
Negative about activities and staff suggestions
Lack of self-direction
Hearing impairment
Visual impairment
Onset of disability limiting or preventing leisure involvement
Lack of knowledge of leisure skills
Lack of leisure skills
Considers leisure skills frivolous and unimportant
Disinterested in surroundings
Confusion or forgetfulness
Unaware of surroundings or activities

McFarland & McFarlane, 1997
Frequent yawning
Flat affect
Overeating or eating too little
Inattentiveness
Restlessness
Daytime napping (seemingly unwarranted)

Hostility/irritation
Perception of time passing slowly
Perception of time passing too quickly
Statement of boredom
Statement of missing recreational activity
Statement of frustration
Little or no unobligated time
Increase in unobligated time
No pattern of leisure activities
Pre-illness (or before life changes) leisure activities impossible since illness
No post-illness (or after life changes) substitute activities defined
Statement of desire for something to do
Unavailability (actual or perceived) of resources for desired activity
Confined space
Disinterest in television
Refusal to attend planned recreational programs
Selective attendance at planned recreational programs

Carpenito, 1992
Major (Must Be Present)
Observed and/or statements of boredom/depression due to inactivity

Minor (May Be Present)
Constant expression of unpleasant thoughts or feelings
Yawning or inattentiveness
Flat facial expression
Body language (shifting body away from speaker)
Restlessness/fidgeting
Immobile (on bed rest or confined)
Weight loss or gain
Isolation
Hostility
Physical/emotional handicap

tional defining characteristics, many of which are applicable to the elder. Box 30-1 displays the defining characteristics provided by these authors. Additional validation studies of the defining characteristics and related factors of this diagnosis are needed.

Examples of diagnostic statements for Diversional Activity Deficit include the following:

- Diversional Activity Deficit related to sensory deficits as manifested by visual impairment, hearing impairment, and statements regarding boredom, wishing there was something they could do.
- Diversional Activity Deficit related to loss of social network as manifested by no community-dwelling

family or close friends, statements of time passing slowly, and no pattern of leisure activities.
- Diversional Activity Deficit related to personal preference as manifested by refusing to attend activities, expressing desire to spend leisure time alone, and considering leisure activities available to be a "waste of time."
- Diversional Activity Deficit related to cognitive impairment as manifested by disinterest in surroundings, not participating in organized activities, and short attention span.

Diversional activities are important to the well-being of the elderly person. Involvement in diversional activities can enhance quality of life (Wikstrom, Theorell, & Sandstrom, 1993), improve mobility and strength (Koroknay, Werner, Cohen-Mansfield, & Braun, 1995; Skelton, Young, Greig, & Malbut, 1995; Wolfson et al., 1996), and enhance self-esteem (Parent & Whall, 1984; Stevens-Ratchford, 1993). To facilitate involvement in diversional activities, it is important that nurses learn about assessment and interventions for the elderly individual in community-based and institutional settings.

CASE STUDY

C. James, an 88-year-old man, has lived in the nursing home for 1 year. Mr. James is well educated and worked as a journalist before retirement. He enjoyed traveling and kept a journal of travel activities. He has a complex medical history that includes recent pneumonia, congestive heart failure, arthritis, and diabetes. His wife, who suffers from Alzheimer's disease, was recently moved from their room in the nursing home to the Special Care Unit in the same facility. He has one living child who resides in town, but she has not visited her father for 6 months.

Mr. James can propel himself in a wheelchair to the dining room when he chooses to. He requires moderate support with most activities of daily living and is frequently incontinent of both urine and stool. He has difficulty controlling his anger, has a tendency to be verbally abusive of nursing home personnel, and believes that most staff and other residents are "stupid." He will visit his wife in the Special Care Unit, but becomes frustrated with the other men in the unit and frequently gets angry and strikes out at them.

Recent interdisciplinary assessment of Mr. James using MDS Version 2.0 identified several items that indicated Mr. James had a diversional activity deficit. He is not at ease interacting with others or doing planned or structured activities. He does not pursue active life in the facility. His preferred place to be is alone in his room, and he refuses to attend recreational activities in the nursing home. He isolates himself from others in the nursing home and will often become frustrated and verbally aggressive with confused residents. Mr. James's behavior has led to staff intervention to control his verbal aggression with other residents. Mr. James resents being reprimanded by staff, has developed a dislike of the nurses, and is rude to them and other residents. The situation has accelerated to the point that he has further limited contact with other residents and staff. He frequently states that he hates being in the nursing home and that he "doesn't have anything to do that's worth doing."

NURSING-SENSITIVE OUTCOMES

Promoting involvement in diversional activities is an important dimension of nursing interventions for older adults. The central outcome concept for caring for elders with this diagnosis is Leisure Participation (Iowa Outcomes Project, 2000). Leisure Participation is defined by the Iowa Outcomes Project (p. 296) as the "use of restful or relaxing activities as needed to promote well-being." This definition may have been developed with younger people in mind. The central focus of leisure activities as restful/relaxing may not be of major concern when obligations of work and family are no longer major stressors in the older person's life. The definition needs to be enhanced for older people by adding "meaningful, interesting, and enjoyable" to "restful/relaxing."

In addition to the central outcome of participation in leisure activities, several other outcomes can be anticipated from successfully intervening with this diagnosis. These are of major interest for nursing and have been used as outcome measures for numerous research efforts with older adults. Nursing-sensitive outcomes from the Iowa Outcomes Project (2000) that appropriately fit the diagnosis of Diversional Activity Deficit include the following:

- *Cognitive Ability:* "Ability to execute complex mental processes" (p. 170)

  Cognition has been shown to improve for elderly nursing home residents using an exercise intervention (Stones & Dawes, 1993) or group therapy (Abraham, Neundorfer, & Currie, 1992). Cognition improved with music therapy for elders with dementia (Aldridge, 1994; Sambandham & Schirm, 1995). On the other hand, cognitive decline is associated with the use of restraints (Burton, German, Rovner, & Brant, 1992).
- *Endurance:* "Extent that energy enables a person to sustain activity" (p. 204)

  Endurance can improve for nursing home residents with walking programs (MacRae et al., 1996) and specific exercise protocols (Schnelle et al., 1996).
- *Mobility Level:* "Ability to move purposefully" (p. 305)

  Daily exercise improves the mobility and balance of cognitively impaired nursing home residents (Jirovec, 1991); balance and strength training improved the mobility of elders living in the community (Wolfson et al., 1996); and resistance training improved the strength for older women living in the community (Skelton, Young, Greig, & Malbut, 1995). Koroknay, Werner, Cohen-Mansfield, and Braun (1995) demonstrated the positive results of improved ambulation and reduced falls from a walking program for nursing home residents.
- *Quality of Life:* "An individual's expressed satisfaction with current life circumstances" (p. 347)

  Improved life satisfaction has been demonstrated with pet therapy involvement for those living in adult homes (Francis, 1991; Francis et al., 1985); improved attitude toward aging and improved morale resulted from activity therapy for nursing home residents (Goldberg & Fitzpatrick, 1980); and improved satisfaction and positive mood resulted from art therapy (Wikstrom et al., 1993).

- *Self-Esteem:* "Personal judgment of self-worth" (p. 391)

    Self-esteem improved as a result of reminiscence (Baker, 1985; Stevens-Ratchford, 1993) and activity involvement for elders living in the community (Parent & Whall, 1984).

- *Social Interaction Skills:* "An individual's use of effective interactive behaviors" (p. 404)

    Social interaction improved as a result of pet therapy (Francis, 1991; Francis et al., 1985), music therapy for elders with dementia (Aldridge, 1994), and reminiscence (Baker, 1985; Cook, 1984).

- *Social Involvement:* "Frequency of an individual's social interactions with persons, groups, or organizations" (p. 405)

    Social interactions and involvement have been shown to improve with interventions involving pets (Fick, 1993; Kongable, Buckwalter, & Stolley, 1989), music (Sambandham & Schirm, 1995), art therapy (Goodwin, 1983; Rugh, 1985), and reminiscence (Moore, 1992).

Other Outcomes

A review of the literature for outcomes relevant to the diagnosis of Diversional Activity Deficit identified additional outcomes that have not been classified by the Iowa Outcomes Project (2000): positive physiologic effects, reduction in depression, and reduction in agitated behavior. Positive physiologic effects included reduction in blood pressure resulting from pet therapy (Baun et al., 1984; Baun, Oetting, & Bergstrom, 1991; Harris, Rinehart, & Gerstman, 1993) and a decrease in urinary incontinence in cognitively impaired nursing home residents who participated in exercise (Jirovec, 1991). Reducing depression has been demonstrated through pet therapy (Francis et al., 1985), reminiscence groups (Moore, 1992; Stevens-Ratchford, 1993), and physical activity (Ruuskanen & Parkatti, 1994). Agitated behavior was reduced in residents with dementia through the use of music (Casby & Holm, 1994; Clark, Lipe, & Bilbrey, 1998; Gerdner & Swanson, 1993; Goddaer & Abraham, 1994) and hand massage (Snyder, Egan, & Burns, 1995a, 1995b).

Establishing Goals to Meet the Outcomes

The nurse, the elderly person, and the family may agree on a variety of goals when designing activities to address this diagnosis. Goals may be related to promoting leisure, interaction, or involvement in specific structured activity programs. A plan might specify, for example, that a person will accomplish the following goals:

- Join peers in conversation and therapeutic activities.
- Initiate conversation.
- Express an interest in attending therapeutic recreation programs.
- Participate in therapeutic recreation activities.
- Be receptive to trying new therapeutic recreation groups.
- Continue to plan own leisure activities.

Although no unique instrument has been developed to measure diversional activity outcomes specifically, multiple measures have been employed to measure outcomes that are likely to be affected by intervening in this diagnosis. Table 30-1 displays instruments that have been used to measure the effectiveness of interventions for Diversional Activity Deficit in elders.

NURSING INTERVENTIONS

Nurses and other interdisciplinary team members can design multiple interventions for the diagnosis Diversional Activity Deficit in elders. Following an assessment of interests, values, capabilities, motivation, availability, and desire, goals are mutually established. Then interventions are considered in light of assessment information, desired goals, and access to activities. A variety of interventions are available, most of which have a relatively strong research base that establishes their credibility and effectiveness with the elderly.

Human beings need to be active and involved with activities and interactions that are of value and that have meaning for them; the elder is no exception. Literature on interventions for the diagnosis Diversional Activity Deficit repeatedly addresses the concept of volunteerism for older adults. Volunteerism may be a natural phenomenon pursued to fill unobligated time. In that way, volunteerism can be an intervention that elders actually design and implement for themselves to prevent Diversional Activity Deficit. While 47% of people ages 70 to 74 participate in volunteer activities (Chambre, 1993), participation drops to 39% for those 75 to 79 and to 27% for those 80 and over; yet older adults are spending a considerable amount of their time in volunteer activities. Could it be that pursuing volunteer activities is a phenomenon sparked to fill unobligated time in a meaningful way? Are volunteer activities a way to boost self-esteem by doing for others and maintaining the valued work role? In one study of those age 60 and older, 52% were involved in volunteer work for organizations, 42% volunteered services to individuals, and 59% volunteered in helping families (Fischer, Mueller, & Cooper, 1991).

Working as a volunteer is not limited to community-dwelling elders. Successful programs for those who are

Table 30-1	Instruments Used to Measure Effectiveness of Interventions Applicable to Diversional Activity Deficit

Measurement (Author)	Intervention
Education Tool for Reminiscence Group Therapy (Baker, 1985)	ACTIVITY THERAPY
Geriatric Depression Scale, Life Satisfaction (Abraham, Neundorfer, & Currie, 1992)	ACTIVITY THERAPY
Philadelphia Geriatric Center Morale Scale, Rosenberg Self-Esteem Scale (Goldberg & Fitzpatrick, 1980)	ACTIVITY THERAPY
Psychogeriatric Dependency Rating Scale, Cohen-Mansfield Agitation Scale, Mini-Mental State Exam, Resource Utilization Groups (Rovner, Steele, Shmuely, & Folstein, 1996)	ACTIVITY THERAPY
Blood Pressure (Baun, Bergstrom, Langston, & Thoma, 1984)	ANIMAL-ASSISTED THERAPY
Blood Pressure, General Well-Being Scale (Harris, Rinehart, & Gerstman, 1993)	ANIMAL-ASSISTED THERAPY
Health Concept Index, Life Satisfaction, Affect Balancing Scale, Observed Patient Behavior Scale, Psychosocial Function Scale, Geriatric Rating Scale, Beck Depression Inventory (Francis, Turner, & Johnson, 1985)	ANIMAL-ASSISTED THERAPY
Lawton's revised Philadelphia Geriatric Center Morale Scale, Rotter's Locus of Control Scale, Duke University's Older Americans Resources and Services Multi-Dimensional Functional Assessment Questionnaire (Robb & Stegman, 1983)	ANIMAL-ASSISTED THERAPY
Social Behavior Checklist (Kongable, Buckwalter, & Stolley, 1989)	ANIMAL-ASSISTED THERAPY
Human Activity Profile, Tokyo Metropolitan Institute of Gerontology Index of Social Competence, Isometric Extension and Flexor Strength, Handgrip Strength (Skelton, Young, Greig, & Malbut, 1995)	EXERCISE PROMOTION
Mini-Mental State Examination, Center for Epidemiologic Studies—Depression, ADL's, IADL's, Status of Physical Health (Wolfson et al., 1996)	EXERCISE PROMOTION
Physical Self-Maintenance Scale (Koroknay, Werner, Cohen-Mansfield, & Braun, 1995)	EXERCISE PROMOTION
Quitlet Index of Body Mass, Mini-Mental State Exam, Geriatric Depression Scale, Bodily Pain Scale, COOP Chart of Physical Work, Caltrac Personal Activity Monitor, Timed-Up-and-Go Test, Tinetti Mobility Assessment, Handgrip Strength (MacRae, Asplund, Schnelle, Ouslander, Abrahamse, & Morris, 1996)	EXERCISE PROMOTION
Rosenberg Self-Esteem Scale, Beck Depression Inventory Scale (Parent & Whall, 1984)	EXERCISE PROMOTION
Glynin Music Therapy Assessment Tool, Global Deterioration Scale, Mini-Mental State Exam (Sambandham & Schirm, 1995)	MUSIC THERAPY
Mini-Mental State Exam, Cohen-Mansfield Agitation Inventory (Goddaer & Abraham, 1994)	MUSIC THERAPY
Mini-Mental State Exam, Modified Hartsock Music Preference Questionnaire, Modified Cohen-Mansfield Agitation Inventory (Gerdner & Swanson, 1993)	MUSIC THERAPY
Folstein Mini-Mental State Exam, Psychogeriatric Dependency Rating Scale (Burton, German, Rovner, & Brant, 1992)	PHYSICAL RESTRAINT
Mini-Mental State Exam, SAFE Assessment, Rowing Assessment, Handgrip Strength (Schnelle, MacRae, Giacobassi, MacRae, Simmons, & Ouslander, 1996)	PHYSICAL RESTRAINT
Beck Depression Inventory Scale, Rosenberg Self-Esteem Scale (Stevens-Ratchford, 1993)	REMINISCENCE THERAPY
Geriatric Depression Scale, Mental Status Questionnaire, Set Tests for Dementia (Brink & Curran, 1985)	REMINISCENCE THERAPY
Life Satisfaction in the Elderly Scale, Sheltered Care Environment Scale, Physical Functioning Index (Gould, 1992)	SOCIALIZATION ENHANCEMENT
Norbeck Social Support Questionnaire, Brief Symptom Inventory (Sutherland & Murphy, 1995)	SOCIALIZATION ENHANCEMENT
Perceptions of Affection and Immediacy, Mini-Mental State Exam (Moore & Gilbert, 1995)	TOUCH
Speilberger State-Trait Anxiety Inventory (Simington & Laing, 1993)	TOUCH
Haycox Rating Scale for Dementia, Relaxation Checklist (Snyder, Egan, & Burns, 1995b)	TOUCH

residents in institutional settings have also been described (Goodwin, 1985; Seville, 1985). As acuity rises in nursing homes, the number of elders physically and mentally capable of doing some volunteer work might decline. However, creative efforts can effectively involve those who can engage in meaningful volunteer activities that can address the diagnosis Diversional Activity Deficit.

Nursing interventions identified and classified by the Iowa Nursing Intervention Classification Project (Iowa Intervention Project, 2000) that are potentially effective to address the diagnosis and desired outcomes for Diversional Activity Deficit include the following:

- *Activity Therapy:* "Prescription of and assistance with specific physical, cognitive, social, and spiritual activities to increase the range, frequency, or duration of an individual's (or group's) activity" (p. 128)

  Group therapeutic activities are common interventions recommended for the elders. The focus of group activities varies, depending on interest and capabilities. Examples include cognitive-behavioral discussion groups (Abraham et al., 1992); reminiscence discussion groups (Baker, 1985; Burnside, 1990; Moore, 1992); structured activity with music, exercise, crafts, relaxation, reminiscences, word games, and food preparation (Rovner, Steele, Shmuely, & Folstein, 1996); movement therapy group (Goldberg & Fitzpatrick, 1980); and intergenerational activities (Perschbacher, 1985; Schelinder, 1985; West & Hutchinson, 1992). Activity Therapy is the primary intervention for Diversional Activity Deficit.
- *Animal-Assisted Therapy:* "Purposeful use of animals to provide affection, attention, diversion, and relaxation" (p. 144)

  Pets have been used in a variety of settings: with elderly clients in nursing homes (Fick, 1993; Gammonley & Yates, 1991; Kongable et al., 1989); with persons who are homebound (Harris et al., 1993); in adult homes (Francis et al., 1985); in hospitals (Carmack & Fila, 1989); and in most settings where nursing care is given (Haggerty-Davis, 1988).
- *Art Therapy:* "Facilitation of communication through drawings and other art forms" (p. 148)

  The positive effects of art therapy as an intervention have been examined in nursing home residents (Rugh, 1985), in nursing home residents with mental illnesses (Goodwin, 1983), and specifically with elderly women (Wikstrom et al., 1993).
- *Exercise Promotion:* "Facilitation of regular physical exercise to maintain or advance to a higher level of fitness and health" (p. 316)

  Exercise is a highly recommended intervention for elderly persons (Glick, 1992; Rooney, 1993). Positive results of exercise have noted in several groups: cognitively impaired nursing home residents (Jirovec, 1991); nursing home residents using objects

to facilitate movement (Lang, Nelson, & Bush, 1992); a cross section of all residents in one nursing home (Ruuskanen & Parkatti, 1994); ambulatory nursing home residents (Koroknay et al., 1995; MacRae et al., 1996); and community-dwelling elders (Parent & Whall, 1984; Wolfsen et al., 1996). Elders respond to exercise with endurance and to resistance training with higher levels of fitness (Skelton et al., 1995).
- *Humor:* "Facilitating the patient to perceive, appreciate, and express what is funny, amusing, or ludicrous in order to establish relationships, relieve tension, release anger, facilitate learning, or cope with painful feelings" (p. 380)

  The benefits of humor have been explored in nursing as a stress release (Wooten, 1996), as an adaptive coping mechanism (Davidhizar & Bowen, 1992), as a means to facilitate education and communication with the elder (Hulse, 1994), and specifically as an intervention with Alzheimer's patients and their families (Buckwalter et al., 1995).
- *Music Therapy:* "Using music to help achieve a specific change in behavior, feeling, or physiology" (p. 461)

  The use of music therapy has had the most attention as an effective intervention for elders who have dementia (Aldridge, 1994; Casby & Holm, 1994; Clark, Lipe, & Bilbrey, 1998; Gerdner & Swanson, 1993; Goddaer & Abraham, 1994; Sambandham & Schirm, 1995).
- *Physical Restraint:* "Application, monitoring, and removal of mechanical restraining devices or manual restraints which are used to limit physical mobility of a patient" (p. 510)

  The use of physical restraints is associated with cognitive decline (Burton et al., 1992) and other documented health risks (Evans & Strumpf, 1989). Reducing physical restraint use can contribute to increased interactions and increased participation in activities. Conversely, effective diversional activities can contribute to reduced restraint use. Rovner, Steele, Shmuely, and Folstein (1996) were effective in reducing behavior problems and the use of physical and chemical restraints in nursing home residents through a creative structured activities program. Residents who use physical restraints should not be precluded from exercise programs because they can physically benefit from exercise and because exercise programs may facilitate the success of restraint reduction efforts (Schnelle et al., 1996).
- *Reminiscence Therapy:* "Using the recall of past events, feelings, and thoughts to facilitate pleasure, quality of life, or adaptation to present circumstances" (p. 554)

  Reminiscence is highly recommended as a therapeutic and worthwhile intervention for elders (Burnside & Haight 1992, 1994; Soltys & Coats, 1994; Stevens-Ratchford, 1993). Use of reminiscence is effective because it helps people find meaning in their memories and come to terms with unresolved life conflicts (Lashley, 1993). Reminiscence has been found to be a major activity in the lives of nursing home residents (Liukkonen, 1995).

- *Socialization Enhancement:* "Facilitation of another person's ability to interact with others" (p. 604)

The importance of social supports and networks has been explored with elders living in nursing homes (Gould, 1992; Powers, 1988), as well as with elders living in the community (Sutherland & Murphy, 1995). Windriver (1993) recommends unit-based activities to enhance socialization and intervene with social isolation experienced by institutionalized older people.

- *Touch:* "Providing comfort and communication through purposeful tactile contact" (p. 669)

Touch has been explored as an intervention with elders (McCann & McKenna, 1993; Moore & Gilbert, 1995; Routasalo, 1996; Simington & Laing, 1993). Touch is likely to be an aspect of most diversional activities and may be a central focus of some. Hand massage has been recommended as a therapeutic activity for elderly patients with dementia as a calming intervention (Snyder et al., 1995a, 1995b).

Other Interventions

A recent development as a diversional activity is SNOEZE-LEN therapy, a sensory experience for people with dementia (Moffat, Barker, Pinkney, Garside, & Freeman, 1993). A total sensory experience with gentle lights, sounds, smells, and soft objects to touch is guided by a nurse as a therapeutic activity. Residents frequently experience a calming effect and at times improved cognition. Residents, their families, and staff commonly report positive responses to the activity. Testing of the effectiveness of the intervention is promising (Maria Strickland, personal communication, 1996).

Special Applications for Persons With Dementia

Many of the interventions for Diversional Activity Deficit have been studied and found useful for persons who have chronic cognitive impairment such as Alzheimer's and related dementia. Structured group and individual activities with music, exercise, relaxation, reminiscence, and pets improve socialization, reduce agitation, and maintain mobility (Aldridge, 1994; Buckwalter et al., 1995; Casby & Holm, 1994; Clark, Lipe, & Bilbrey, 1998; Gerdner & Swanson, 1993; Goddaer & Abraham, 1994; Jirovec, 1991; Kovach & Magliocco, 1998; Kongable, Buckwalter, & Stolley, 1989; Magliocco, 1996; Moffat et al., 1993; Weaver,

1995). Touch is important, but some persons with dementia react negatively to touch that they do not understand or perceive as threatening (Snyder, Egan, & Burns, 1995a, 1995b). For those with memory loss that makes it difficult or impossible to experience joy in recalling the past, activities that help them experience pleasure in the immediate moment are essential (Ryden & Feldt, 1992).

CASE STUDY

Part of the interdisciplinary team approach to Mr. James's outbursts, withdrawal, and isolation are to offer him activities directed at reestablishing his desire to be involved in things he previously enjoyed. Group activities with residents who are cognitively intact were encouraged, so that Mr. James could build relationships with people with similar interests. Mr. James agreed to participate in a reminiscence group for nursing home residents who are cognitively intact after receiving strong encouragement to do so from his primary nurse and social worker. Initially he was reluctant to speak in the group, but after he realized that many of the group members were alert and quite intelligent, he began to open up with stories about his travels. The reminiscence group found his stories to be very interesting and offered Mr. James positive reinforcement for sociable behaviors.

The reminiscence group offered Mr. James an avenue to build new friendships in the nursing home. Over time, Mr. James was able to build positive relationships with several group members. His self-esteem improved as a result of interests others expressed about his stories. Mr. James encouraged several other residents to begin a journal as a way to document their life experiences. Through reminiscence Mr. James was able to place value on past achievements and make an adaptation to his present circumstances. Mr. James no longer isolated himself from others in the facility. Although he was still easily irritated by confused people and at times became angry, outbursts and verbally abusive behavior markedly decreased after he joined the reminiscence group. Box 30-2 summarizes the nursing diagnosis, nursing-sensitive outcomes, and nursing interventions that are applicable for Mr. James.

SUMMARY

Elderly persons have much to gain when health care professionals successfully address the nursing diagnosis Diversional Activity Deficit. Activities provide meaning and meet basic human needs for interaction, socialization, and feeling involved in life. The institutionalized elder may find that life is tedious and controlled by rules imposed by others. He may experience a sense of loss of control, depression, and reduced self-esteem. Well-planned, meaningful diversional activities can moderate the effect of institutional life. Community-dwelling elders may find themselves isolated from others by virtue of poor health,

| Box 30-2 | Diversional Activity Deficit Related to Situational Changes Interfering With Prior Interests |

Nursing Diagnosis
Diversional Activity Deficit
Defining characteristics
Refuses to go to off-unit therapeutic recreation activities
Refuses to go to therapeutic recreation activities
Minimal peer interaction
Negative about activities and staff suggestions
Hostility and irritation
Isolation

Nursing-Sensitive Outcomes
Quality of Life
Indicators
Satisfaction with social circumstances
Satisfaction with environmental circumstances

Self-Esteem
Indicator
Feelings about self-worth

Social Involvement
Indicators
Interaction with close friends
Interaction with neighbors
Interaction with family members

Interaction with members of work group(s)
Participation as member of church
Participation in active church work
Participation as club member
Participation as a volunteer group member
Performance of volunteer activities
Participation in leisure activities
Other _____

Nursing Interventions
Activity Therapy
Activity
Participate in discussion group to increase interests in
    available activities and living situation

Reminiscence Therapy
Activity
Join group to facilitate adaptation to present circumstances
    and enhance self-esteem

Socialization Enhancement
Activity
Facilitate Mr. James's ability to interact with others and reduce
    social isolation

---

absence of family and friends, or lack of transportation. The effects of diversional activities on low physical and emotional well-being are documented in the literature. Engaging individuals in activities can reduce depression and illness. Preventing Diversional Activity Deficit should be a priority for nurses caring for elderly people.

REFERENCES

Abraham, I. L., Neundorfer, M. M., & Currie, L. J. (1992). Effects of group interventions on cognition and depression in nursing home residents. *Nursing Research, 41*(4), 196-202.

Aldridge, D. (1994). Alzheimer's disease: Rhythm, timing and music as therapy. *Biomedicine & Pharmacotherapy, 48,* 275-281.

Allen, J. D. (1992). Exercise program. In G. M. Bulechek & J. C. McCloskey (Eds.), *Nursing interventions: Essential nursing treatments* (2nd ed., pp. 406-424). Philadelphia: W. B. Saunders.

Baker, N. J. (1985). Reminiscing in group therapy for self worth. *Journal of Gerontological Nursing, 11*(7), 21-24.

Baun, M. M., Bergstrom, N., Langston, N. F., & Thoma, L. (1984). Physiological effects of human/companion animal bonding. *Nursing Research, 33*(3), 126-129.

Baun, M. M., Oetting, K., & Bergstrom, N. (1991). Health benefits of companion animals in relation to the physiologic indices of relaxation. *Holistic Nursing Practice, 5*(2), 16-23.

Beck, P. (1982). Two successful interventions in nursing homes: The therapeutic effects of cognitive activity. *The Gerontologist, 22,* 378-383.

Brink, R., & Curran, M. (1985). Geriatric depression scale reliability: Order, examiner and reminiscence effects. *Clinical Gerontologist, 3,* 57-60.

Buckwalter, K. C., Gerdner, L. A., Richards-Hall, G., Stolley, J. M., Kudart, P., & Ridgeway, S. (1995). Shining through: The humor and individuality of person's with Alzheimer's disease. *Journal of Gerontological Nursing, 21*(3), 11-16.

Burbank, P. M. (1986). Psychosocial theories of aging: A critical evaluation. *Advances in Nursing Science, 9*(1), 73-86.

Burnside, I. (1990). Reminiscence: An independent nursing intervention for the elderly. *Issues in Mental Health Nursing, 11,* 33-48.

Burnside, I., & Haight, B. (1994). Reminiscence and life review: Therapeutic interventions for older people. *Nurse Practitioner, 19*(4), 55-61.

Burnside, I., & Haight, B. K. (1992). Reminiscence and life review: Analyzing each concept. *Journal of Advanced Nursing, 17,* 855-862.

Burton, L. C., German, P. S., Rovner, B. W., & Brant, L. J. (1992). Physical restraint use and cognitive decline among nursing home residents. *Journal of the American Geriatrics Society, 40,* 811-816.

Carmack, B. J., & Fila, D. (1989). Animal-assisted therapy: A nursing intervention. *Nursing Management, 20*(5), 96-101.

Carpenito, L. J. (1992). *Nursing diagnosis: Application to clinical practice.* Baltimore: Lippincott Williams & Wilkins.

Casby, J. A., & Holm, M. B. (1994). The effect of music on repetitive disruptive vocalizations of persons with dementia. *The American Journal of Occupational Therapy, 48*(10), 883-889.

Chambre, S. M. (1993). Volunteerism by elders: Past trends and future prospects. *The Gerontologist, 33*(2), 221-228.

Clark, M. E., Lipe, A. W., & Bilbrey, M. (1998). Use of music to decrease aggressive behaviors in people with dementia. *Journal of Gerontological Nursing, 24*(7), 10-17.

Cook, J. B. (1984). Reminiscing: How it can help confused nursing home residents. *Social Casework: The Journal of Contemporary Social Work, 103,* 90-93.

Cummings, E., & Henry, W. E. (1961). *Growing old.* New York: Basic Books.

Davidhizar, R., & Bowen, M. (1992). The dynamics of laughter. *Archives of Psychiatric Nursing, VI(2),* 132-137.

Ebersole, P., & Hess, P. (1998). *Toward healthy aging: Human needs and nursing response* (5th ed.). St. Louis, MO: Mosby.

Evans, L. K., & Strumpf, N. E. (1989). Tying down the elderly: A review of the literature on physical restraint. *Journal of the American Geriatrics Society, 37*(1), 65-74.

Fick, K. M. (1993). The influence of an animal on social interactions of nursing home residents in a group setting. *American Journal of Occupational Therapy, 47*(6), 529-534.

Fischer, L. R., Mueller, D. P., & Cooper, P. W. (1991). Older volunteers: A discussion of the Minnesota senior study. *The Gerontologist, 31*(2), 183-194.

Francis, G. M. (1991). "Here come the puppies": The power of the human-animal bond. *Holistic Nursing Practice, 5*(2), 38-41.

Francis, G., Turner, J. T., & Johnson, S. B. (1985). Domestic animal visitation as therapy with adult home residents. *International Journal Nursing Studies, 22*(3), 201-206.

Gammonley, J., & Yates, J. (1991). Pet projects: Animal assisted therapy in nursing homes. *Journal of Gerontological Nursing, 17*(1), 12-15.

Gerdner, L. A., & Swanson, E. A. (1993). Effects of individualized music on confused and agitated elderly patients. *Archives of Psychiatric Nursing, VII*(5), 284-291.

Glick, O. J. (1992). Interventions related to activity and movement. *Nursing Clinics of North America, 27*(2), 541-568.

Goddaer, J., & Abraham, I. L. (1994). Effects of relaxing music on agitation during meals among nursing home residents with severe cognitive impairment. *Archives of Psychiatric Nursing, VII*(3), 150-158.

Goldberg, W. G., & Fitzpatrick, J. J. (1980). Movement therapy with the aged. *Nursing Research, 29*(6), 339-346.

Goodwin, D. (1985). Innovative "resident volunteer" programming. *Activities, Adaptation & Aging, 6*(3), 69-71.

Goodwin, M. E. (1983). Art therapy in an interdisciplinary program: For long-term institutionalized mental patients. *American Journal of Art Therapy, 22,* 87-92.

Gould, M. T. (1992). Nursing home elderly: Social environmental factors. *Journal of Gerontological Nursing, 18*(8), 13-20.

Greene, V., & Monahan, D. (1982). The impact of visitation on patient well-being in nursing homes. *The Gerontologist, 22,* 418-423.

Haggerty-Davis, J. (1988). Animal-facilitated therapy in stress mediation. *Holistic Nursing Practice, 2*(3), 75-83.

Harris, M. D., Rinehart, J. M., & Gerstman, J. (1993). Animal-assisted therapy for the homebound elderly. *Holistic Nursing Practice, 8*(1), 27-37.

Havighurst, F. J., & Albrecht, R. (1953). *Older people.* Reading, MA: Addison Wesley Longman.

Horgas, A. L., Wilms, H. U., & Baltes, M. M. (1998). Daily life in very old age: Everyday activities as expression of successful living. *The Gerontologist, 38*(5), 556-568.

Hulse, J. R. (1994). Humor: A nursing intervention for the elderly. *Geriatric Nursing, 15*(2), 88-90.

Iowa Intervention Project. J. C. McCloskey & G. M. Bulechek (Eds.). (2000). *Nursing interventions classification (NIC)* (3rd ed.). St. Louis, MO: Mosby.

Iowa Outcomes Project. M. Johnson, M. Maas, & S. Moorhead (Eds.). (2000). *Nursing outcomes classification (NOC)* (2nd ed.). St. Louis, MO: Mosby.

Jirovec, M. M. (1991). The impact of daily exercise on the mobility, balance and urine control of cognitively impaired nursing home residents. *International Journal of Nursing Studies, 28*(2), 145-151.

Kim, M. J., & Moritz, D. A. (1982). *Classification of nursing diagnosis: Proceedings of the third and fourth conferences.* Hightstown, NJ: McGraw-Hill.

Kongable, L. G., Buckwalter, K. C., & Stolley, J. M. (1989). The effects of pet therapy on the social behavior of institutionalized Alzheimer's clients. *Archives of Psychiatric Nursing, 3*(4), 191-198.

Koroknay, V. J., Werner, P., Cohen-Mansfield, J., & Braun, J. V. (1995). Maintaining ambulation in the frail nursing home resident: A nursing administered walking program. *Journal of Gerontological Nursing, 21*(11), 18-24.

Kovach, C. R. & Magliocco, J. S. (1998). Late-stage dementia and participation in therapeutic activities. *Applied Nursing Research, 11*(4), 167-173.

Lang, E. M., Nelson, D. L., & Bush, M. A. (1992). Comparison of performance in materials-based occupation, imagery-based occupation, and rote exercise in nursing home residents. *The American Journal of Occupational Therapy, 46*(7), 607-611.

Lashley, M. E. (1993). The painful side of reminiscence. *Geriatric Nursing, 14*(3), 138-141.

Lawton, M., Moss, M., & Moles, E. (1984). Pet ownership: A research note. *The Gerontologist, 24,* 208-210.

Liukkonen, A. (1995). Life in a nursing home for the frail elderly. *Clinical Nursing Research, 4*(4), 358-372.

MacRae, P. G., Asplund, L. A., Schnelle, J. F., Ouslander, J. G., Abrahamse, A., & Morris, C. (1996). A walking program for nursing home residents: Effects on walk endurance, physical activity, mobility, and quality of life. *Journal of the American Geriatrics Society, 44*(2), 175-180.

Magliocco, J. S. (1996). Therapeutic activities for low functioning older adults with dementia. In C. R. Kovach (Ed.), *Late-stage dementia care: A basic guide* (pp. 135-145). Washington, DC: Taylor & Francis.

McCann, K., & McKenna, H. P. (1993). An examination of touch between nurses and elderly patients in a continuing care setting in northern Ireland. *Journal of Advanced Nursing, 18,* 838-846.

McCormack, D., & Whitehead, A. (1981). The effect of providing recreational activities on the engagement level of long-stay geriatric patient. *Age & Ageing, 10,* 287-291.

McFarland, G. K., & McFarlane, E. A. (1997). *Nursing diagnosis & intervention* (3rd ed.). St. Louis, MO: Mosby.

McLane, A. M. (Ed.). (1987). *Classification of nursing diagnosis: Proceedings of the seventh conference.* St. Louis, MO: Mosby.

Moffat, N., Barker, P., Pinkney, L., Garside, M., & Freeman, C. (1993). *SNOEZELEN: An experience for people with dementia.* Derbyshire, Australia: Rompa.

Moore, B. G. (1992). Reminiscing therapy: A CNS intervention. *Clinical Nurse Specialist, 6*(3), 170-173.

Moore, J. R., & Gilbert, D. A. (1995). Elderly residents: Perceptions of nurses' comforting touch. *Journal of Gerontological Nursing, 21*(1), 6-13.

Neugarten, B. L., Havighurst, R. J., & Tobin, S. S. (1968). Personality and patterns of aging. In B. L. Neugarten (Ed.), *Middle age and aging* (pp. 173-177). Chicago: University of Chicago Press.

North American Nursing Diagnosis Association. (1999). *Nursing diagnoses: Definitions & classification 1999-2000.* Philadelphia: Author.

Parent, C. J., & Whall, A. L. (1984). Are physical activity, self-esteem, and depression related? *Journal of Gerontological Nursing, 10*(9), 8-10.

Perschbacher, R. (1985). Making connections between the school system and the nursing home. *Activities, Adaptation & Aging, 6*(3), 37-41.

Powers, B. A. (1988). Social networks, social support, and elderly institutionalized people. *Advances in Nursing Science, 10*(2), 40-58.

Radziewicz, R. M., & Schneider, S. M. (1992). Using diversional activity to enhance coping. *Cancer Nursing, 15*(4), 293-298.

Rantz, M. (1991). Diversional activity deficit. In M. Maas, K. C. Buckwalter, & M. Hardy (Eds.), *Nursing diagnosis and interventions for the elderly* (pp. 299-312). Reading, MA: Addison Wesley Longman.

Rantz, M. J., & Miller, T. V. (1987). How diagnoses are changing in long-term care. *American Journal of Nursing, 87,* 360-361.

Rantz, M. J., & Miller, T. V. (1993). *Quality documentation for long-term care: A nursing diagnosis approach.* Baltimore: Aspen.

Rantz, M. J., Miller, T. V., & Jacobs, C. (1985). Nursing diagnosis in long-term care. *American Journal of Nursing, 85*(8), 916-917, 926.

Rantz, M., Miller, T. V., & Matson, S. (1995). Nursing diagnosis in long-term care: A longitudinal perspective for strategic planning. *Nursing Diagnosis, 6*(2), 57-62.

Robb, S., & Stegman, C. (1983). Companion animals and elderly people: A challenge for evaluators of social support. *The Gerontologist, 23,* 277-282.

Rooney, E. M. (1993). Exercise for older patients: Why it's worth your effort. *Geriatrics, 48*(11), 68-77.

Routasalo, P. (1996). Non-necessary touch in the nursing care of elderly people. *Journal of Advanced Nursing, 23,* 904-911.

Rovner, B. W., Steele, C. D., Shmuely, Y., & Folstein, M. F. (1996). A randomized trial of dementia care in nursing homes. *Journal of the American Geriatrics Society, 44*(1), 7-13.

Rubenfeld, M. (1993). Diversional activity deficit. In J. Thompson, G. McFarland, J. Hirsh, & S. Tucker (Eds.), *Clinical nursing* (3rd ed., pp. 1509-1511). St. Louis, MO: Mosby.

Rugh, M. M. (1985). Art therapy with the institutionalized older adult. *Activities, Adaptation & Aging, 6*(3), 105-120.

Ruuskanen, J. M., & Parkatti, T. (1994). Physical activity and related factors among nursing home residents. *Journal of the American Geriatrics Society, 42*(9), 987-991.

Ryden, M. B., & Feldt, K. S. (1992). Goal-directed care: Caring for aggressive nursing home residents with dementia. *Journal of Gerontological Nursing, 18*(11), 35-41.

Sambandham, M., & Schirm, V. (1995). Music as a nursing intervention for residents with Alzheimer's disease in long-term care. *Geriatric Nursing, 16*(2), 79-83.

Schelinder, K. D. (1985). Intergenerational mixing. *Activities, Adaptation & Aging, 6*(3), 43-45.

Schnelle, J. F., MacRae, P. G., Giacobassi, K., MacRae, H. S. H., Simmons, S. F., & Ouslander, J. G. (1996). Exercise with physically restrained nursing home residents: Maximizing benefits of restraint reduction. *Journal of the American Geriatrics Society, 44*(5), 507-512.

Seville, J. (1985). The good Samaritan program: Patients as volunteers. *Activities, Adaptation & Aging, 6*(3), 73-78.

Simington, J. A., & Laing, G. P. (1993). Effects of therapeutic touch on anxiety in the institutionalized elderly. *Clinical Nursing Research, 2*(4), 438-450.

Skelton, D. A., Young, A., Greig, C. A., & Malbut, K. E. (1995). Effects of resistance training on strength, power, and selected functional abilities of women aged 75 and older. *Journal of the American Geriatrics Society, 43*(10), 1081-1087.

Snyder, M., Egan, E. C., & Burns, K. R. (1995a). Efficacy of hand massage in decreasing agitation behaviors associated with care activities in persons with dementia. *Geriatric Nursing, 16*(2), 60-63.

Snyder, M., Egan, E. C., & Burns, K. R. (1995b). Interventions for decreasing agitation behaviors in persons with dementia. *Journal of Gerontological Nursing, 21*(7), 34-40.

Soltys, F. G., & Coats, L. (1994). The SolCos model: Facilitating reminiscence therapy. *Journal of Gerontological Nursing, 20*(11), 11-16.

Stevens-Ratchford, R. G. (1993). The effect of life review reminiscence activities on depression and self-esteem in older adults. *American Journal of Occupational Therapy, 47*(5), 413-420.

Stones, M. J., & Dawes, D. (1993). Acute exercise facilitates semantically cued memory in nursing home residents. *Journal of the American Geriatrics Society, 41*(5), 531-534.

Sutherland, D., & Murphy, E. (1995). Social support among elderly in two community programs. *Journal of Gerontological Nursing, 21*(2), 31-38.

Weaver, D. (1995). Activity interventions. In J. Rader & E. M. Tornquist (Eds.), *Individualized dementia care* (pp. 197-207). New York: Springer.

West, M., & Hutchinson, S. (1992). Intergenerational geriatric motivation. *Clinical Nursing Research, 1*(3), 221-235.

Wikstrom, B. M., Theorell, T., & Sandstrom, S. (1993). Medical health and emotional effects of art stimulation in old age. A controlled intervention study concerning the effects of visual stimulation provided in the form of pictures. *Psychotherapy & Psychosomatics, 60*(3-4), 195-206.

Windriver, W. (1993). Social isolation: Unit based activities for impaired elders. *Journal of Gerontological Nursing, 19*(3), 15-21.

Wolfson, L., Whipple, R., Derby, C., Judge, J., King, M., Amerman, P., Schmidt, J., & Smyers, D. (1996). Balance and strength training in older adults: Intervention gains and tai chi maintenance. *Journal of the American Geriatrics Society, 44*(5), 498-506.

Wooten, P. (1996). Humor: An antidote for stress. *Holistic Nursing Practice, 10*(2), 49-56.

Yesavage, J. (1984). Relaxation and memory training in 39 elderly patients. *American Journal of Psychiatry,* 778-781.

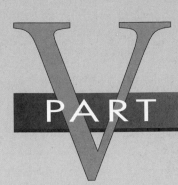

PART V

Sleep-Rest Pattern

OVERVIEW

Sleep disturbances are among the chief complaints of elders, with estimates of over half of persons over 65 years of age living at home and two thirds of those in long-term care facilities having some sleep difficulty. Part Five begins with a review of factors—biologic, environmental, and psychosocial—that affect sleep/wake patterns in normal aging. In Chapter 31 Bunten reviews the normal sleep cycle and normal age-related changes, noting that most severe disturbances are related to sleep disorders, chronic health problems, or their treatment rather than aging itself. She suggests that anticipatory guidance concerning sleep patterns and sleep habit education offered by nurses can effectively resolve many expressed sleep complaints.

In Chapter 32, Sleep Pattern Disturbance, Schoenfelder and Culp explore the related factors of this diagnosis in two categories, internal and external. Internal related factors include worry, stress, body temperature, dementia, and other medical problems, whereas external related factors include noise, excessive daytime napping, interruptions of sleep by institutional caregivers, and intake of caffeine and alcohol. Authors advocate greater use of the diagnosis Sleep Pattern Disturbance with elders, since clinical validation appears adequate. Several measures of sleep are presented, and nursing-sensitive outcomes and indicators are selected from the *Nursing Outcomes Classification (NOC)* (Iowa Outcomes Project, 2000). Schoenfelder and Culp identify several interventions from *Nursing Interventions Classification (NIC)* (Iowa Intervention Project, 2000) useful for this diagnosis, and intervention research findings are reviewed. Additional research to test effectiveness of sleep-promoting interventions is identified as a major need.

CHAPTER 31

NORMAL CHANGES WITH AGING

Donna Bunten

Sleep is a time for restoration of the body and mind and is essential for good health (Foreman & Wykle, 1995; Spencely, 1993). Much research has been directed toward increasing our understanding of the mechanism of arousal and sleep in relation to aging. Although sleep and arousal represent opposite extremes on a behavioral spectrum, they are thought to be regulated at least in part by common physiologic and neurochemical mechanisms. Changes in the aging brain produce changes in the excitation and inhibition of the nervous system. The frontal cortex of the brain has now been implicated as having an inhibitory function on the arousal system; this inhibitory function declines with advancing age. The frontal cortex is also instrumental in the regulation of sleep (Bliwise, 1994). Age changes in the frontal lobe may account at least in part for arousal and sleep changes observed in elders.

Other simultaneous changes occur in the brain of the elderly person, including cell loss in various areas other than the frontal cortex. Declines in blood flow and alterations in neurotransmitters and synaptic mechanisms are undoubtedly involved in changes in sleep and arousal associated with advancing age. Extrinsic factors such as retirement, normally an age-related experience, can cause an abrupt change in the demand for daily physical activity and energy and lead to changes in demands for sleep. Social and psychologic events involving loss also can predispose the elder to depression, which can profoundly affect sleep/wake patterns. Thus sleep patterns may be at least in part a product of environmental demands or psychosocial circumstances and not totally a function of biologic changes of aging (Garcia-Garcia & Drucker-Colin, 1999).

SLEEP CYCLE

Carskadon and Dement (1994) define sleep as "a reversible behavioral state of perpetual disengagement from and unresponsiveness to the environment" (p. 16). There are two distinct components of the sleep cycle: non–rapid eye movement (NREM) sleep and rapid eye movement (REM) sleep, which can be differentiated by physiologic characteristics. Sleep begins with the NREM state, which progresses through four stages. Stage 1 NREM is the transitional period of drifting to sleep when one can be easily

aroused. Stage 2 NREM is considered to be a period of light sleep with somewhat greater relaxation. Stage 3 NREM is the first stage of deep sleep. Stage 4 NREM is the deepest and most restorative period of sleep. Decreases in pulse, blood pressure, and metabolism occur during stage 4 NREM sleep. Stages 3 and 4 NREM are sometimes called "slow-wave sleep" because of the slow waves exhibited in electroencephalographic (EEG) activity (Carskadon & Dement, 1994; Spenceley, 1993).

The four stages of NREM sleep are followed by REM sleep. The deepest level of relaxation of the body occurs during REM sleep, but EEG activity is similar to the pattern seen during wakefulness. REM sleep is accompanied by bursts of rapid eye movements (giving this phenomenon its name) and dreaming. Respiratory rate, heart rate, and blood pressure become highly variable, irregular, and frequently elevated during REM sleep. Ebersole and Hess (1998) note that loss of REM sleep has been associated with an increase in irritability and anxiety and a decrease in the ability to concentrate. Disturbed behavior occurs with severe deprivation of REM sleep. These authors also point out that "elderly individuals with pulmonary or cardiac disorders may be severely compromised during REM sleep" (p. 166).

A typical sleep cycle consists of NREM 1 followed by NREM 2, 3, and 4, with possible drifting back through previous stages of NREM 3 and 2 before the REM stage starts (Kedas, Lux, & Amodes, 1989). The NREM stage of the sleep cycle accounts for 75% to 80% of total sleep time. REM sleep accounts for the remaining 20% to 25% of total time asleep. The REM component of the cycle begins approximately 60 minutes into the sleep cycle, and typically four to six cycles of NREM to REM sleep activity occur per night (Carskadon & Dement, 1994).

Aging makes sleep more fragile for even the extremely healthy older person. A 1990 National Institute of Health Consensus Development Conference estimated that more than half of persons over 65 years of age living at home and about two thirds of those in long-term care facilities experience some difficulties in their sleep. Sleep disorders become more common with advancing age, and age-related changes in sleep structure may mask their recognition (Foreman & Wykle, 1995; Webb, 1989).

SLEEP IN ELDERS

Difficulty falling to sleep once in bed is often reported by elders, and research has shown the validity of these complaints. Webb (1989) reported that sleep onset delay occurred in one of three elderly women and one of five elderly men. The elderly participants in his study averaged 30 minutes in bed trying to fall asleep. Sleep latency, as this delay in sleep onset is sometimes called, can be affected by changes in the elderly individual's circadian cycle (Buysse et al., 1992). A reduction in the strength of the circadian response has been found in senescent sleep studies (Carskadon & Dement, 1994; Dijk & Duffy, 1999; Wooten, 1992). Trouble falling to sleep also might be related to easily corrected causes such as consuming caffeine or eating a heavy meal too close to bedtime (Lankford, 1994).

Research by Pressman and Fry (1988) and Lankford (1994) demonstrated an increase in stage 1 NREM sleep in the elderly. Elders are easily aroused during this time by sounds, touch, or light. Disruption in stage 1 NREM produces fragmentation of sleep (Garcia-Garcia & Drucker-Colin, 1999). The sleep of the elderly person can be further fragmented by frequent awakenings, which can result from pain, nocturia, or institutional regimens and routines. Webb (1989) reported sex differences in awakenings, with consistently higher numbers of awakenings recorded in elderly men than in elderly women. Comments by elders identifying themselves as "light sleepers" and/or of being awake during the night parallel these research findings. Stages 3 and 4 NREM sleep have been found to decrease in both amount and density in the elderly person. The most striking difference reported by Wooten (1992), Prinz, Vitiello, Raskind, and Thorpy (1990), and Bliwise (1994) is the near-absence of stage 4 NREM sleep. These changes all affect the efficiency of sleep in elders.

Researchers agree that the distribution of REM sleep throughout the night changes with advancing age (Bliwise, 1994; Pressman & Fry, 1988). The first REM period occurs earlier during the elder's sleep. Subsequent periods of REM are equal in length during the night instead of increasing in duration, as is normally seen in younger adults. This shift of REM sleep and the reduction of stages 3 and 4 NREM alter the efficiency of the older person's sleep.

Many elders report daytime sleepiness or increased time napping during the day. However, napping is not a pervasive activity among elders (Webb, 1989). Those older persons who do nap may be attempting to increase total sleep time. Increases in the frequency of napping episodes in healthy older adults may be related to having more opportunities to nap and not associated with unfulfilled sleep need (Bliwise, 1994; Webb, 1989). The question of whether napping interferes with night sleeping is frequently raised. The research of Hayter (1985) and Floyd (1995) indicated that napping does not displace nighttime sleep, but rather supplements total sleep time. Naps less than an hour in length were found by Aber and Webb (1986) not to affect sleep on the subsequent night and to have a desirable relationship to daytime alertness.

A slight increase in sleep demand has been noted in the elderly population, especially in those over 80 years of age. However, Bachman (1992) and Bliwise (1994) have reported substantial subgroups of elders who sleep either more than 10 hours or less than 5 hours in a 24-hour period. These two subgroups demonstrate the increased variability of the elderly person's need for sleep. In general, sleep can be considered to be adequate regardless of the overall amount if one awakens refreshed and feels rested.

Monk (1989) reports a slight tendency toward earlier bedtimes and waking times in elderly individuals. Again, this pattern may result from changes in behavior patterns, such as experiencing less rigid schedules. The redistribution of sleep times during a 24-hour period by some elderly people also fits well with reports of a decline in the amplitude of circadian rhythms (Ancoli-Israel, 1997; Bliwise, 1994).

Other salient factors in geriatric populations can cause sleep changes: heightened autonomic activity and greater susceptibility to external arousal, simple inactivity, anxiety, depression, bereavement, retirement, fear of death during sleep, and reduced exposure to outdoor light (Bliwise, 1994).

SUMMARY

Severe sleep disturbance in an otherwise healthy person is most likely secondary to sleep disorders, chronic health problems, or their treatment rather than to aging itself (Bliwise, 1994). Age-related physiologic and socioeconomic changes that affect the elder's sleep should not cause insomnia and daytime sleepiness, two of the most common symptoms of sleep disorders (Prinz et al., 1990). Age-related differences in the elderly person's sleep lead to lighter and more interrupted sleep but do not usually interfere with the person's ability to achieve the restorative value of sleep. The differences in the elderly person's sleep architecture, however, may become problematic in the context of illness (Vitiello, 1997).

Nurses can effectively advise many elderly persons on improving sleep habits. Nurses also can educate elderly clients about the changes in sleep structure that occur with aging, reassuring the older person and changing his expectation regarding what is normal sleep in elders.

REFERENCES

Aber, R., & Webb, W. B. (1986). Effects of a limited nap on night sleep in older subjects. *Psychology and Aging, 1*(4), 300-302.

Ancoli-Israel, S. (1997). Sleep problems in older adults: Putting myths to bed. *Geriatrics, 52*(1), 20-30.

Bachman, D. L. (1992). Sleep disorders with aging: Evaluation and treatment. *Geriatrics, 47*(9), 53-61.

Bliwise, D. L. (1994). Normal aging. In M. H. Kryger, R. Roth, & W. C. Dement (Eds.), *Principles and practice of sleep medicine* (2nd ed., pp. 26-39). Philadelphia: W. B. Saunders.

Buysse, D., Browman, K., Monk, T., Reynolds, C., Fasiczka, A., & Kupfer, D. (1992). Napping and 24-hour sleep-wake patterns in healthy elderly and young adults. *Journal of the American Geriatrics Society, 40*(8), 779-786.

Carskadon, M. A., & Dement, W. C. (1994). Normal human sleep; an overview. In M. H. Kryger, R. Roth, & W. C. Dement (Eds.), *Principles and practice of sleep medicine* (2nd ed., pp. 16-25). Philadelphia: W. B. Saunders.

Dijk, D. J., & Duffy, J. F. (1999). Circadian regulation of human sleep and age-related changes in its timing, consolidation and EEG characteristics. *Annals of Medicine, 31*(2), 130-140.

Ebersole, P., & Hess, P. (1998). *Toward healthy aging: Human needs and nursing response* (5th ed.). St. Louis, MO: Mosby.

Floyd, J. A. (1995). Another look at napping in older adults. *Geriatric Nursing, 16*(3), 136-138.

Foreman, M. D., & Wykle, M. (1995). Nursing standard-of-practice protocol: Sleep disturbances in elderly patients. *Geriatric Nursing, 16*(5), 238-243.

Garcia-Garcia, F., & Drucker-Colin, R. (1999). Endogenous and exogenous factors on sleep-wake cycle regulation. *Progress in Neurobiology, 58*(4), 297-314.

Hayter, J. (1985). To nap or not to nap? *Geriatric Nursing, 6,* 104-106.

Kedas, A., Lux, W., & Amodes, L. (1989). A critical review of aging and sleep research. *Western Journal of Nursing Research, 11*(2), 196-206.

Lankford, S. R. (1994). Sleep loss in the elderly: Understanding the reasons. *Journal of Gerontological Nursing, 20*(8), 49-52.

Monk, R. H. (1989). Circadian rhythms. *Clinical Geriatric Medicine, 5,* 331.

National Institutes of Health Consensus Development Conference. (1990, March 26-28). *The treatment of sleep disorders of older people.*

Pressman, M. R., & Fry, J. M. (1988). What is normal sleep in the elderly? *Clinics in Geriatric Medicine, 4*(1), 71-81.

Prinz, P. N., Vitiello, M. V., Raskind, M. A., & Thorpy, M. J. (1990). Geriatrics: Sleep disorders and aging. *The New England Journal of Medicine, 323*(8), 520-526.

Spenceley, S. M. (1993). Sleep inquiry: A look with fresh eyes. *IMAGE: Journal of Nursing Scholarship, 25*(3), 249-256.

Vitiello, M. V. (1997). Sleep disorders and aging: Understanding the causes. *Journals of Gerontology: Series A, Biological Sciences & Medical Sciences, 52*(4), M189-M191.

Webb, W. B. (1989). Age-related changes in sleep. *Clinics of Geriatric Medicine, 5*(2), 275-287.

Wooten, D. (1992). Sleep disorders in geriatric patients. *Clinics in Geriatric Medicine, 8*(2), 427-439.

CHAPTER 32

SLEEP PATTERN DISTURBANCE

Deborah Perry Schoenfelder and Kennith R. Culp

Sleep is a basic human need. When that need is unmet either in quantity or in quality, undesirable consequences are likely to result. Older adults are susceptible to sleep pattern disturbances (Almeida, Tamai, & Garrido, 1999; Bundlie, 1998; Maggi et al., 1998; Middelkoop, Smilde-van den Doeil, Neven, Kamphuisen, & Springer, 1996), especially those who are hospitalized (Gall, Petersen, & Riesch, 1990), those who are placed in long-term care facilities (Ancoli-Israel, 1989; Gentili, Weiner, Kuchibhatil, & Edinger, 1997), those who are diagnosed with depression or Alzheimer's disease (Ancoli-Israel, Kaluber, Gillin, Campbell, & Hofstetter, 1994; Beck-Little & Weinrich, 1998; Maggi et al., 1998), and those who are functioning as informal caregivers (Wilcox & King, 1999). Common sleep complaints in older adults include difficulty falling asleep, difficulty staying asleep, early-morning awakening, and excessive sleepiness (Neubauer, 1999). Maggi and colleagues (1998) found that night awakenings, cited by two thirds of the study participants, was the most common sleep disturbance.

Sleep is important for health and quality of life. Poor sleep is characteristic of many medical conditions in the elderly, including somatic and psychiatric illnesses. Also, unfavorable habits and lifestyle factors increase the probability of sleep problems in older persons (Asplund, 1999). In a survey of 427 community-dwelling older adults, 19% of the subjects reported being somewhat or very troubled with their sleep, 21% felt they got too little sleep, 24% reported trouble falling asleep at least once per week, and 39% reported experiencing excessive daytime sleepiness (Ancoli-Israel et al., 1991). In a sample of community-dwelling older adults, only 26% of men and 21% of women reported no sleep complaints (Maggi et al., 1998).

Objective sleep measures also confirm the existence of sleep disruption in older adults. In a comprehensive review of sleep in normal aging and dementia, Bliwise (1993) found general uniformity in age differences in most polysomnographic measures (electroencephalogram [EEG], electromyogram [EMG], electrooculogram [EOG]), with sleep efficiency decreasing to about 70% to 80% in older adults.

This chapter provides a theoretical presentation of the nursing diagnosis Sleep Pattern Disturbance (SPD), outcome indicators related to SPD, and nursing interventions identified to treat SPD in older adults. For background information on sleep and sleep in older adults, the reader is referred to Chapter 31 and several review articles (Beck-Little & Weinrich, 1998; Bliwise, 1993; Clark, 1992; Jensen & Herr, 1993; Neubauer, 1999).

RELATED FACTORS/ETIOLOGIES

The harmonious interrelationship of the immune, neuroendocrine, and sleep-wake systems establishes a circadian pattern of sleep and wakefulness (Moldofsky, 1994). Sleep pattern disturbances result from interacting psychosocial, psychophysiologic, neurodevelopmental, and health-altering factors that disrupt this balance. Circadian rhythmicity is challenged with aging (Copinschi & Van Cauter, 1995), and there is a disruption in the cycle of sleep and wakefulness in the elderly person (Pascoe, 1994).

Factors related to sleep pattern disturbances can be categorized as internal (illness, psychologic stress) and external (environmental changes, social cues) (Kim & Moritz, 1982). Alternatively, factors related to sleep pattern disturbances can be grouped into the following categories: alterations in sleep-wake patterns, physical illnesses, psychologic factors, and medications (Hoch & Reynolds, 1986) (Figure 32-1).

Internal Related Factors

Worry and anxiety can delay sleep, usually for only a few nights. However, bouts may recur frequently in elders (Feinsilver & Hertz, 1993). In particular, hospitalized elderly patients do not get sufficient sleep, which adds to their worries and pain (Spenceley, 1993). Possible related factors for older adults experiencing a critical illness are pain, acute stress, depression, alterations in body temperature, respiratory distress, and urinary frequency (Davis-Sharts, 1989). Acute pain is known to impact negatively on sleep patterns, especially pain following a surgical procedure (Closs, 1992). For elderly nursing home residents experiencing a sleep pattern disturbance, deterioration of the circadian sleep-wake rhythm, sleep apnea, and dementia are common related factors (Ancoli-Israel, 1989). Nocturia and pain are also common factors that disturb the sleep of elderly nursing home residents (Gentili et al., 1997).

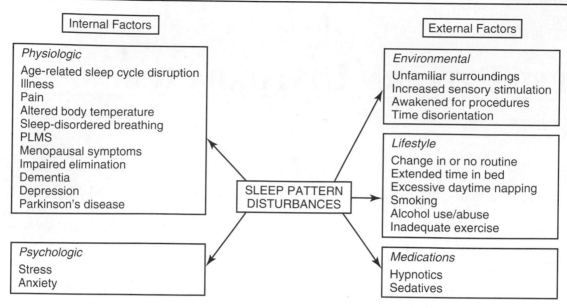

FIGURE **32-1**   Proposed model for Sleep Pattern Disturbance in the elderly.

It has been hypothesized that host defense factors might play a role in sleep regulation (Pollmacher, Mullington, Korth, & Hinze-Selch, 1995). Non–rapid eye movement (NREM) sleep might have an immunosupportive function, although the link is not clearly understood. There may also be an influence of certain cytokines such as interleukin-1 on the sleep-wake cycle (Moldofsky, 1994). In elders, mean cortisol levels are increased, and the immune system declines in effectiveness (Copinschi & Van Cauter, 1995). These physiologic changes can precipitate sleep pattern disturbances in elders and are exacerbated with illness, especially when a fever is present.

The occurrence of breathing problems in sleep seems to increase with age (Bliwise, 1993). Sleep apnea, a disorder in which people repeatedly stop breathing during sleep, is commonly seen in elderly clients (Beck-Little & Weinrich, 1998). Obstructive sleep apnea (OSA) is an upper airway disorder that tends to produce apnea during rapid eye movement (REM) sleep (Okabe, Hida, Kikuchi, Taguchi, Takishima, & Shirato, 1994). One type of OSA is Pickwickian syndrome or "fat neck," a condition where the obstruction of the upper airway by soft tissue leads to apnea in the obese person (Solow, Ovesen, Nielsen, Wildschiodtz, & Tallgren, 1993). During REM, oxygen desaturation causes episodes of apnea and an increase in blood pressure (Garpestad, Ringler, Parker, Remsburg, & Weiss, 1995). In patients with chronic obstructive pulmonary disease (COPD), periods of hypopnea occur during REM sleep; the mechanisms involved are not clear (White, Drinnan, Smithson, Griffiths, & Gibson, 1995). Hypopnea during REM sleep in patients with COPD is associated with reduced inspiratory muscle activity. The pattern of hypopnea may be either "obstructive" or "central" and is generally consistent within an individual. However, severe

sleep-related O_2 desaturation is only observed in patients who exhibit a marked daytime hypoxemia (Weitzenblum, Chaouat, Charpentier, & Krieger, 1995).

Ancoli-Israel and associates (1991) surveyed community-dwelling older adults and found a prevalence rate for sleep-disordered breathing of 24% for the Apnea Index ($\geq$ 5 apnea periods per hour of sleep) and 62% for the Respiratory Disturbance Index ($\geq$ 10 apnea periods and hypopnea periods per hour of sleep, hypopnea periods measured by a portable recording of 50% to 90% decrease in respiratory signal). They concluded that sleep-disordered breathing contributes to excessive daytime sleepiness and disturbed sleep at night in the elderly person.

Periodic leg movements in sleep (PLMS), a disorder in which people kick or jerk their legs every 20 to 40 seconds for periods throughout the sleep period, can contribute to sleep complaints (Hanly & Zuberi-Khokhar, 1996). The prevalence of PLMS is high in older adults (Beck-Little & Weinrich, 1998; Bliwise, 1993).

Menopausal symptoms can disrupt sleep patterns (Gass & Rebar, 1990). During menopause there is a tremendous change in the neuroendocrine system, most likely hypothalamic in origin, causing perimenopausal women to have trouble sleeping (Shaver & Paulsen, 1993; Stone & Pearlstein, 1994).

Sleep pattern disturbances frequently are observed in patients with dementia of the Alzheimer's type (DAT), a disease with progressive degeneration of the cortical and subcortical neurons. Sleep problems are similar to those experienced in healthy older adults but more pronounced, including increased awakenings at night, more wakeful time during the night, and increased daytime sleeping (Bundlie, 1998). This disturbance in rhythm is most frequently precipitated by delirium and by the cardinal "sundowning" presentation (Vitiello, Bliwise, & Prinz, 1992). Exacerbation of this behavior usually occurs in the late afternoon or at night. The underlying neurologic basis for this symptom is altered cerebral metabolism. Specifically, the amount of REM sleep is lower in patients with DAT (Bahro, Riemann, Stadtmuller, Berger, & Gattaz, 1993).

Abnormal sleep-wake organization is also frequently seen in Parkinson's disease (PD) and other parkinsonism syndromes (Dowling, 1995; Louden, Morehead, & Schmidt, 1995; Smith, Ellgring, & Oertel, 1997). During REM sleep, parkinsonian tremors disappear (Askenasy & Yahr, 1990). However, there is evidence to suggest a shorter time to REM, particularly when the PD patient is depressed (Kostic, Susic, Covickovic-Sternic, Marinkovic, & Jankovic, 1989).

External Related Factors

Sleep can be interrupted by noise and other environmental stimuli. Beyerman (1987) interviewed 100 hospitalized patients (mean age 68 years) to ascertain what they believed were the causes of their hospital-induced sleep pattern disturbances. The most frequently identified cause of sleep pattern disturbance was noise, followed by being awakened by nurses and the strangeness of the hospital environment. Sleep problems are also common in intensive care units and may often be due to environmental noise (Aaron et al., 1996; Freedman, Kotzer, & Schwab, 1999; Shilo et al., 1999).

Related factors for sleep disturbances in nursing home patients include external noisy environments, extended time in bed, and excessive daytime napping. Schnelle and associates (1998) found strong evidence that the nighttime sleep of nursing home residents was adversely affected by environmental noise and light. A study by Gentili and colleagues (1997) reported that environmental noise or light disturbed residents' sleep three or more times per week.

Daytime napping may or may not be helpful, either serving as compensation for poor sleep quality or disturbing nighttime sleep patterns (Creighton, 1995; Frisoni, De Leo, Rozzini, & Trabucchi, 1996). In a sample of healthy elderly persons, total duration of daytime sleep averaged about 1 hour (Evans & Rogers, 1994). Another study reported daytime napping by 50% of the men and 31% of the women in a sample of community-dwelling elders (Gislason, Reynisdottir, Kristbjarnarson, & Benediktsdottir, 1993).

Cigarette smokers are more likely than nonsmokers to report problems going to sleep, problems staying asleep, problems with daytime drowsiness, and a higher daily caffeine intake (Lexcen & Hicks, 1993; Phillips & Danner, 1995). At low concentrations, nicotine has a biphasic effect on sleep that leads to relaxation and sedation; at high concentrations, nicotine inhibits sleep (Onen, Onen, Bailly, & Parquet, 1994). Sleep disturbance may be more prevalent among smokers due to the increased prevalence of breathing disorders over those who do not smoke and an association with more stress (Wetter & Young, 1994).

Alcohol can act as a relaxing, sedative agent when consumed just before sleeping, but nighttime awakening can be a problem with moderately high blood alcohol levels due to sympathetic activation (Onen et al., 1994). One study suggests that sleep-disordered breathing in older male alcoholics is more prevalent than among normal elderly men (Aldrich, Shipley, Tandon, Kroll, & Brower, 1993). There is evidence that patients with alcohol dependency show a decrease in stage 4 or slow-wave sleep, especially in alcoholics with clinical depression (Hatzinger, Kocher, Hemmeter, Ladewig, & Holsboer-Trachsler, 1995).

Sleep medications can cause sleep disturbances such as increasing time to fall asleep and increasing number of awakenings (Almeida, Tamai, & Garrido, 1999; Krska & MacLeod, 1995; Maggi et al., 1998). Sleep architecture can be disrupted, especially REM sleep. Thus such medications should be used with caution, and the effects of hypnotics and sedatives should be considered when searching for what is contributing to sleep pattern disturbances in the elder.

ASSESSMENT

Two types of methods typically used to assess sleep are subjective and objective measurements of physiologic and psychologic factors associated with sleep. Subjective methods (perceptions reported by the individual) include visual analogue scales, subjective rating scales, questionnaires, interviews, and daily sleep charting. Objective methods of measurement include polysomnography, direct observation of the sleeper, observing body movements, and assessing vigilance and sleepiness.

Subjective Measures

A visual analogue scale requires the sleeper to place a mark on a 100 mm horizontal line that ranges at one end from "best sleep ever" to the other end with "worst sleep ever." The distance of the mark along the line is then measured in millimeters to supply a numerical value for the person's evaluation of the previous night's sleep. Bond and Lader (1974) found the use of analogue scales effective in rating subjective feelings.

The Verran and Snyder-Halpern Sleep Scale (VSH) is a well-known visual analogue to assess sleep. The 100 mm response line asks subjects about their previous night's sleep on these sleep factors: mid-sleep awakenings, movement during sleep, total sleep period, sleep onset latency, soundness of sleep, rest upon awakening, method of awakening, and subjective quality of sleep (Snyder-Halpern & Verran, 1987). Each item can be scored, and a total score can be calculated. The higher the total score, the better is the quality of sleep. The scale was tested with a sample of young, middle-aged, and older adults, and a theta reliability of 0.82 was computed, indicating "adequate reliability for a new instrument" (Snyder-Halpern & Verran, 1987). In addition, the investigators compared the VSH to two other sleep quality measures and found evidence of convergent construct validity.

Subjective rating scales can be used to ask subjects to compare one night of sleep with the next in order to ascertain which night the individual perceived as better. Another subjective scale might ask subjects to describe their previous night's sleep or their overall sleep as excellent, good, fair, or poor. In a large-scale study, participants were asked how often (never, sometimes, often, always) they had trouble with falling asleep, with waking up during the night, or with waking up too early and not being able to fall asleep again and how often they feel really rested when they wake up in the morning. The sleep complaint score is the sum of the score for all four questions. In addition, the variable *insomnia* included those who reported often or always having trouble falling asleep and/or waking up too early. Night awakeners were those who reported often or always waking up during the night. Those respondents characterized as awakened not rested included those who reported that they never or rarely feel rested when they wake up in the morning (Maggi et al., 1998).

Self-administered questionnaires and sleep logs are useful in establishing subjects' sleep patterns (Neubauer, 1999). For instance, asking what time one usually goes to bed could be followed by a list of time ranges from which to choose. An often-used questionnaire is the Sleep Log developed by Baekeland and Hoy (1971). Three questions to be completed just before going to bed assess state of fatigue, state of mind at bedtime, and what time the subject got into bed. Seven additional questions, answered immediately on awakening, assess perceptions of time to sleep onset, number of nocturnal awakenings, total sleep time, soundness of sleep, movement during sleep, feelings of refreshment on awakening, and satisfaction with sleep. For all 10 questions, subjects are given responses to choose from that are on a continuum. In comparing subjects' reports and EEG and EOG recordings, subjects correctly estimated the time it took them to fall asleep and the number of body movements during sleep (Baekeland & Hoy, 1971). Concurrent validity and satisfactory test-retest reliability have been established (Johnson, 1991b). Snyder-Halpern and Verran (1987) found a theta reliability for the Sleep Log of 0.76.

A modified version of the Sleep Log, the Sleep Pattern and Daytime Behavior Questionnaire (SPDBQ), was expanded to include items about drug side effects, bedtime drug-taking behavior, and daytime napping behaviors. Content validity was established by four nurse experts, and the tool was found to have stability for the variables across three data collection times with significant Pearson product-moment correlations ($p < 0.01$) (Johnson, 1988).

The Bedtime Routine Questionnaire contains six items that assess whether subjects have a usual time to go to sleep, whether subjects have a bedtime routine, what that routine is, how important a bedtime routine is, and how the sleeper feels when he does not get enough sleep. For those who are not living in their own home, subjects are asked how much their bedtime routine changed since moving and the reasons for a change in bedtime routine (Johnson, 1986). The author reported that the questionnaire is reliable and valid but did not provide the statistical results for the psychometrics.

Daily sleep charting, usually in the format of a diary, requires sleepers to record certain sleep-related information over a period of time. It can be done by the sleeper at home and then used by individuals and health professionals to gain insight into their sleep patterns. Rogers, Caruso, and Aldrich (1993) compared sleep diary data with polysomnographic readings and found the percentage agreement acceptable (kappa = 0.87).

The authors recommend the use of a valid and reliable sleep tool such as the VSH or Sleep Log in addition to the nurse's observations of sleep and waking patterns for older adults in acute or long-term care settings. For community-dwelling elders, keeping a sleep diary is a recommended method for assessing sleep patterns, especially when supplemented by observations of the nurse regarding wakefulness and relevant complaints voiced by the individual.

Objective Measures

Polysomnography includes EEGs, EOGs, and EMGs. An EEG is a tracing of electrical activity of the brain, an EOG is a recording of the electrical currents produced by eye movements, and an EMG is a recording of muscular contraction as a result of electrical stimulation (Beck-Little & Weinrich, 1998). These assessments, conducted while the person is asleep in a laboratory, provide information about the onset, progression, and depth of sleep and sleep stages. Polysomnography can be costly and is usually reserved for relatively severe sleep disorders such as sleep apnea. In addition, electrodermal activity can be measured by applying an electrode to the skin. Predictable patterns during sleep have been established. Another objective measure can be obtained through the use of devices or recorders that detect body movements while in bed. Such measures provide information about restfulness rather than sleep itself.

Observation of sleep by a trained observer at regular intervals is useful to detect sleep patterns. Gress, Bahr, and Hassanein (1983) used this method and developed a coding system to record nighttime behaviors of elderly patients on a skilled care unit. Behaviors were coded as sleeping, restless, awake (with subcodes such as eliminating, complaining of pain, crying), or up (i.e., out of bed). There was 93.9% agreement on the observations between two nurse researchers. In addition, how one functions during awake time is an important reflection of sleep quality and quantity. Vigilance, the ability to maintain attention, may be tested by asking persons to perform some sort of repetitive task. Sleepiness can be assessed by asking subjects to describe their level of sleepiness or by measuring the time taken to fall asleep while attached to an EEG monitor.

NURSING DIAGNOSIS

The nursing diagnosis Sleep Pattern Disturbance (SPD) was first developed in 1980 by the North American Nursing Diagnosis Association (NANDA) and defined as the "disruption of sleep time that causes discomfort or interferes with desired lifestyle" (Kim & Moritz, 1982). The following critical defining characteristics were identified: verbal complaints of difficulty falling asleep, awakening earlier or later than desired, three or more nighttime awakenings, and verbal complaints of not feeling well rested. Other defining characteristics (not designated as critical) were the following: changes in behavior and performance (increasing irritability, restlessness, disorientation, lethargy, listlessness); physical signs (mild fleeting nystagmus, slight hand tremor, ptosis of eyelid, expressionless face, dark circles under eyes, frequent yawning,

changes in posture); and thick speech with mispronunciation and incorrect words.

Lo and Kim (1986) established construct validity of SPD through expert and clinical validation. Thirty-three defining characteristics for SPD emerged from the literature review, with fifteen of those being retained through the validation procedures. They are similar to those enumerated by NANDA in the initial development and are presented for comparison in Table 32-1.

CASE STUDY

S. Clark is a 72-year-old woman who lives alone in her own home in a rural community. At a well elderly clinic sponsored by the local Visiting Nurses Association, Mrs. Clark described her health as "pretty good for my age." Her only complaints are having to take "those expensive pills" for her high cholesterol level and often feeling sleepy during the day.

On further questioning by the nurse, the following information was obtained about Mrs. Clark's sleep patterns:

- Sleeps about 5 hours per night.
- When asked how well she sleeps, she responds, " 'So-so'; I just don't sleep all that well."
- Has no established bedtime routine.

Table 32-1	Defining Characteristics SLEEP PATTERN DISTURBANCE	
NANDA (Kim & Moritz, 1982)	**Lo & Kim (1986)**
Critical Defining Characteristics	
Verbal complaints of difficulty falling asleep	Difficulty falling asleep
Awakening earlier or later than desired	Awakening earlier or later than desired
Interrupted sleep	Interrupted sleep
Verbal complaints of not feeling well rested	Not feeling well rested
Other Defining Characteristics	
Changes in behavior and performance	
• Increasing irritability	Irritability
• Restlessness	Restlessness
• Lethargy	Lethargy
• Listlessness	Listlessness
• Disorientation	
Physical signs	
• Mild fleeting nystagmus	Apathy
• Slight hand tremor	Slow reaction
• Ptosis of eyelid	Feeling of floating
• Expressionless face	Disturbed bodily sensation
• Dark circles under eyes	Malaise
• Frequent yawning	Tiredness
• Changes in posture	Sensitivity to pain and discomfort
Thick speech with mispronunciation and incorrect words	

- When asked about sleep efficiency (ratio of sleep time to total time trying), she responds, "That's frustrating for me. I feel I spend a lot of time in bed trying to sleep, especially when I wake up during the night."
- States she often does not feel rested on awakening and arising in the morning.
- Says she awakens almost every night after going to sleep "for no reason that I can think of" and has great difficulty falling back to sleep. "The longer I stay awake, the more frustrated I get so I can't relax and get to sleep. I also start thinking about what I have to do the next day, and then I'm even less relaxed."
- Naps almost every day for 2 to 3 hours; reports feeling groggy for several hours after napping.
- Caffeine intake: drinks 4 to 5 cups of coffee (not decaffeinated) per day, having 2 of those cups around 8 PM nightly.

NURSING-SENSITIVE OUTCOMES

Indicators for sleep are the patient states, behaviors, or perceptions that are responsive to nursing intervention(s) and that are used for determining the sleep-related outcome(s). Sleep studies use various objective and subjective instruments, described earlier, to measure the phenomenon of sleep in terms of indicators.

Asking the sleeper or caregiver about time to sleep onset, number of nocturnal awakenings, soundness of sleep, and total sleep time provides information about sleep. Other indicators are sleep complaints, feelings of refreshment on awakening, and satisfaction with sleep. Daytime behavior also furnishes cues about the quality and quantity of sleep. Specifically, the ability to perform daytime activities, feelings of daytime sleepiness, and reports of fatigue are indicators of sleep. Polysomnography and vital signs are used in sleep laboratories to determine the architecture of sleep. In addition, having an established bedtime routine is an important indicator of sleep. These indicators are measurable and provide a way to gauge the outcome of sleep.

The *Nursing Outcomes Classification (NOC)* research team, through concept analysis and validation by expert surveys, has developed the outcome "Sleep." Field testing is under way to provide further validation and to assess the clinical usefulness of this outcome. NOC defines the outcome Sleep as the "extent and pattern of natural periodic suspension of consciousness during which the body is restored" (Iowa Outcomes Project, 2000, p. 403). The following are indicators for the outcome Sleep: hours of sleep; observed hours of sleep; sleep pattern; sleep quality; sleep efficiency (ratio of sleep time to total time trying); uninterrupted sleep; sleep routine; feelings of rejuvenation after sleep; napping appropriate for age; wakeful at appropriate times; EEG in expected range; EMG in expected range; EOG in expected range; and vital signs in expected range.

These indicators, which reflect the physiologic and functional nature of sleep, are measured by questioning individuals' or significant others' perceptions about their sleep, by direct observation, and through the use of instrumentation. Choosing indicators appropriate for the individual and rating the individual for those particular indicators will help determine the person's status for the outcome Sleep.

The outcome Sleep and its indicators are measured on a scale as follows: 1 = extremely compromised; 2 = substantially compromised; 3 = moderately compromised; 4 = mildly compromised; and 5 = not compromised (Iowa Outcomes Project, 2000, p. 403). This outcome and its indicators have been approved by NOC for clinical testing, and the measurement scales will be refined based on the feedback from clinical testing. Refer to the earlier discussion of sleep assessment methods and specific tools for example measurement procedures for the outcome Sleep and its indicators. An important aspect of the outcome and indicators is their responsiveness to nursing intervention(s), which clinical testing will confirm or point to the need for modification of the outcome and/or indicators.

NURSING INTERVENTIONS

Suggested interventions to promote sleep abound in the nursing literature: educating the individual and/or family about age-related changes in sleep; shortening or eliminating naps; avoiding strenuous exercise close to bedtime; avoiding heavy meals or spicy foods before bedtime; avoiding caffeine and alcohol; and avoiding smoking and other tobacco use (Beck-Little & Weinrich, 1998; Cohen & Merritt, 1992; Dinner, Erman, & Roth, 1992; Landolt, Werth, Borbely, & Dijk, 1995; Morin, Mimeault, & Gagne, 1999; Neubauer, 1999; Vgontzas & Kales, 1999). For the symptoms of OSA, proper positioning (e.g., elevating the head of the bed) and continuous positive airway pressure via a nasal mask may be recommended (Beck-Little & Weinrich, 1998; Engleman, Martin, Deary, & Douglas, 1994; Neubauer, 1999; Pevernagie & Shepard, 1992).

Regular exercise can be helpful in promoting sleep and is often suggested to improve sleep quality (Edinger et al., 1993; Neubauer, 1999; O'Connor & Youngstedt, 1995). Daytime exercise appears to slightly increase slow-wave sleep (O'Connor & Youngstedt, 1995). For example, one study found weight-lifting exercise was effective in improving subjective sleep quality (Singh, Clements, & Fiatarone, 1997). The mechanism(s) that underlie exercise-associated increases in slow-wave sleep is unknown. However, elevations in daytime core body temperature, which appears to increase slow-wave sleep and decrease REM sleep, might be related. Kohsaka and colleagues (1998) exposed healthy elderly subjects to bright light for 6 days and found the light to be effective in maintaining sleep without changing daytime activity.

The importance of a bedtime routine, including establishing a consistent bedtime and arising time, is emphasized in the literature (Cohen & Merritt, 1992; Dinner, Erman, & Roth, 1992). Establishing a bedtime routine to promote sleep was supported in a study by Johnson (1991a). Fifty-four percent of the subjects reported having a bedtime routine, and all of those subjects indicated that their routine was very important to them. Subjects with a bedtime routine had fewer sleep complaints than those without a routine. Based on these findings, the investigator recommended that, for those who have an established bedtime routine, the maintenance of these activities on a nightly basis should be encouraged. For those with no routine, it would seem logical that the nurse should assist the individual to identify appropriate routine pre-sleep activities and incorporate them into a nightly pattern.

Altering the environment to make it more restful is important in promoting adequate sleep (Cohen & Merritt, 1992; Dinner, Erman, & Roth, 1992). For instance, providing adequate blankets and a warm environment is a simple but effective intervention to promote sleep (Finlay, 1991). It is absolutely necessary to decrease environmental stimuli at night in order to provide supportive care for elderly patients in intensive care (Richards, 1994). This same principle applies to the long-term care setting, where a careful evaluation of sleep problems in elderly residents must be addressed in the plan of care (Swales, Friedman, & Sheikh, 1993). Execution of early morning nursing staff activities, such as checking vital signs or changing linens, is generally problematic in these institutions, and an effort should be made to accommodate sleeping elders whenever possible.

Finally, there is agreement in the literature that drug therapy for the treatment of sleep disturbances should be used judiciously (Cohen & Merritt, 1992; Neubauer, 1999).

Intervention Research

Although the literature contains numerous recommendations to promote sleep, only a small number of these recommendations have been tested through research. Castor and associates (1991) examined the effect of sunlight on the sleep patterns of elderly institutionalized demented patients. Twelve subjects (mean age 75.2 years) participated in the study for 3 weeks. Sleep-wake status was assessed through hourly observer report using predetermined behavioral criteria. Subjects were exposed to sunlight 2 hours daily during the second week of the study. Beneficial effects from sunlight exposure were manifest in increased mean sleep hours, increased uninterrupted night sleep hours, decreased night wake hours, and decreased daytime sleep hours. Disrupted sleep patterns resumed in the first 24 hours after sunlight deprivation in the third week of the study. The results were not influenced by length of residence, medications, or age.

Johnson (1991b) used progressive relaxation with a sample of noninstitutionalized older women. Using a pretest-posttest same subject design, subjects perceived a significant decrease in the time to sleep onset, a decrease in the number of nighttime awakenings, sleeping more soundly, feeling more refreshed upon awakening, and feeling more satisfied with their sleep after using progressive relaxation. Polysomnography (EEG, EMG, and EOG) indicated a significantly reduced time to sleep onset, a decreased number of nocturnal awakenings, less time in light sleep during the first 3 hours of the sleep time, and more time in slow-wave sleep during the first 3 hours of the sleep time.

Pickett and colleagues (1989) tested the effect of combined progestin and estrogen on sleep-disordered breathing in postmenopausal women. The combined hormone therapy decreased the number of sleep-disordered breathing episodes by an average of 15 ± 4 to 3 ± 1 per subject. This study was conducted on a small sample ($n = 9$), and the investigators suggested that sleep-disordered breathing is not particularly pronounced in healthy, postmenopausal women. In another sample of 242 postmenopausal women, the group that received transdermal estradiol replacement therapy experienced a significant decrease in sleep disturbances when compared with a placebo treatment group (Wiklund, Karlberg, & Mattsson, 1993).

Individuals with dementia often experience nighttime sleep interruptions. Sundowning may be defined as the differential nighttime exacerbation of disruptive behaviors and agitation. For demented elderly individuals living at home and suffering from sundowning, Bliwise (1993) suggested night respite as a possible intervention to offer relief to exhausted caregivers. For those institutionalized older adults with dementia and sleep disruptions, the author suggested the possibility of a regularly scheduled nocturnal activities time (e.g., 2:00 to 4:00 AM) with an occupational therapist brought in for this purpose. Although creative, this intervention is questionable, since the behavior might have a physiologic basis and therefore warrant an intervention aimed at resolving or at least diminishing the contributing physiologic factor(s).

Pharmacologic interventions to promote sleep are considered much less desirable than nonpharmacologic interventions. A study of 375 subjects, most age 60 years or older, revealed that those subjects using benzodiazepine hypnotics estimated their average sleep time as less than that of controls; sleep onset latency was significantly longer for the hypnotic users in comparison with the controls (Krska & MacLeod, 1995). Sleep tablet use has been associated with subjective sleep difficulties, difficulties falling asleep, and frequent awakening during the night (Almeida, Tamai, & Garrido, 1999). Maggi and colleagues (1998) found significant relationships between use of sleep medications and insomnia (defined as reporting often or always having trouble falling asleep and/or waking up too early) and between use of sleep medications and not feeling rested upon awakening.

Exogenous melatonin, taken in the form of an over-the-counter medication currently available as a dietary supplement, is able to influence the endogenous secretion of the hormone according to a phase-response curve. In normal physiology, melatonin is secreted principally by the pineal gland, mostly at night and under normal environmental conditions (Geoffriau, Brun, Chazot, & Claustrat, 1998). There are practical implications for melatonin in situations when biologic rhythms are disturbed (e.g., jet-lag syndrome, delayed sleep phase syndrome, SPD in blind people, and shift-work). However, there are also impractical uses for melatonin, portrayed by the consumer media as a formidable weapon against disease and aging; these media claims are unfounded (Kendler, 1997).

The efficacy of melatonin in the treatment of sleep disorders remains under scrutiny. In one study, patients were classified according to three groups: those with sleep disturbances alone, those with sleep disturbances and signs of depression, and those with sleep disorders and dementia (Brusco, Fainstein, Marquez, & Cardinali, 1999). Each subject received 3 mg melatonin orally for 21 days at bedtime. After 2 to 3 days of treatment, melatonin significantly augmented sleep quality and decreased the number of awakening episodes in patients with sleep disturbances with or without depression. Estimates of next-day alertness improved significantly only in patients with primary insomnia. Among the dementia patients group, agitated behavior at night decreased significantly.

Although the results from the Brusco et al. study suggest that melatonin may be useful in treating sleep disturbances in elderly patients, other researchers disagree about its effectiveness or the appropriateness of its use in the elderly (Youngstedt, Kripke, & Elliott, 1998). Certainly more clinical research needs to be done in evaluating the role of melatonin in patients with Alzheimer's disease. While reductions in melatonin secretion have been associated with many disorders including cardiovascular disease, Alzheimer's, and diabetes, melatonin's role in the etiology and/or pathophysiology of these disorders is unproven. Primary health care providers should be aware of the proposed uses of melatonin and which are supported by biomedical research (Kendler, 1997).

The nursing interventions recommended by *Nursing Interventions Classification (NIC)* reflect the state of knowledge about strategies to promote sleep. The primary nursing intervention identified by NIC for Sleep Pattern Disturbances (SPD) is Sleep Enhancement, which is defined as "facilitation of regular sleep/wake cycles" (Iowa Intervention Project, 2000, p. 602). There are 24 activities listed under Sleep Enhancement. Two examples of those activities are "encourage patient to establish a bedtime routine to facilitate transition from wakefulness to sleep" and "instruct patient how to perform autogenic muscle relaxation or other nonpharmacologic forms of sleep inducement." Besides Sleep Enhancement, the following nursing interventions are suggested for resolution of SPD (Iowa Intervention Project, 2000):

- Dementia Management: provision of a modified environment for the patient who is experiencing a chronic confusional state (p. 249).
- Environmental Management: manipulation of the patient's surroundings for therapeutic benefit (p. 305).
- Environmental Management: Comfort: manipulation of the patient's surroundings for promotion of optimal comfort (p. 308).
- Medication Administration: preparing, giving, and evaluating the effectiveness of prescription and nonprescription drugs (p. 434).
- Medication Management: facilitation of safe and effective use of prescription and over-the-counter drugs (p. 451).
- Medication Prescribing: prescribing medication for a health problem (p. 453).
- Security Enhancement: intensifying a patient's sense of physical and psychologic safety (p. 571).
- Simple Relaxation Therapy: use of techniques to encourage and elicit relaxation for the purpose of decreasing undesirable signs and symptoms such as pain, muscle tension, or anxiety (p. 598).
- Touch: providing comfort and communication through purposeful tactile contact (p. 669).

In addition, a nurse could select from 18 additional optional NIC interventions, including Anxiety Reduction, Exercise Promotion, Music Therapy, and Simple Massage. Intervention(s) are selected that are suitable for the identified related factor(s) and defining characteristics for an individual experiencing SPD.

Diagnosis-Intervention-Outcome Linkages

In 1998 the nursing diagnosis Sleep Pattern Disturbance was revised. Sleep Pattern Disturbance is now defined as "time limited disruption of sleep (natural, periodic suspension of consciousness) amount and quality" (NANDA, 1999, p. 90). In addition, the defining characteristics and related factors/etiologies have been expanded. To facilitate treatment of SPD and the use of standardized nursing language, linkages among diagnoses, interventions, and outcomes are necessary. Now that outcomes and indicators for Sleep have been developed and are in clinical testing, the three components of standardized nursing language can be linked. The linkages are presented in Table 32-2. The authors recognize that outcomes other than Sleep and nursing interventions other than Sleep Enhancement may be appropriate for SPD. For purposes of this chapter, however, the linkages are illustrated for SPD, the NOC outcome Sleep and its indicators, and the NIC nursing intervention Sleep Enhancement and its activities.

Table 32-2	Suggested Nursing-Sensitive Outcome and Nursing Intervention SLEEP PATTERN DISTURBANCE		

Nursing Diagnosis	Nursing-Sensitive Outcome	Nursing Intervention
SLEEP PATTERN DISTURBANCE *Defining Characteristics* Prolonged awakenings Sleep maintenance insomnia Self-induced impairment of normal pattern Sleep onset greater than 30 minutes Early morning insomnia Awakening earlier or later than desired Verbal complaints of difficulty falling asleep Verbal complaints of not feeling well rested Increased proportion of stage 1 sleep Dissatisfaction with sleep Less than age-normed total sleep time Three or more nighttime awakenings Decreased proportion of stages 3 and 4 sleep Decreased proportion of REM sleep Decreased ability to function *Related Factors/Etiologies* Psychologic • Age-related sleep shifts • Body temperature • Depression • Anxiety • Illness • Pain • Sleep-disordered breathing • Periodic leg movements in sleep • Menopausal symptoms • Impaired urinary elimination • Impaired bowel elimination • Dementia • Parkinson's disease • Stress Environmental • Noise • Unfamiliar sleep furnishings • Ambient temperature, humidity • Lighting • Other-generated awakening • Excessive stimulation • Physical restraint • Lack of sleep privacy/control • Nurse for therapeutics, monitoring, lab tests • Sleep partner • Noxious odors • Unfamiliar environment • Increased environment • Time disorientation • Change in or lack of sleep routine	**SLEEP** *Indicators* Hours of sleep Observed hours of sleep Sleep pattern Sleep quality Sleep efficiency Uninterrupted sleep Feelings of rejuvenation after sleep Wakeful at appropriate times EEG IER* EMG IER EOG IER Vital signs IER Sleep routine Napping appropriate for age	**SLEEP ENHANCEMENT** *Activities* Determine patient's sleep/activity pattern Explain the importance of adequate sleep during pregnancy, illness, psychosocial stresses, and so on Monitor/record patient's sleep pattern and number of sleep hours Monitor patient's sleep pattern and note physical and/or psychologic circumstances that interrupt sleep Monitor bedtime food and beverage intake for items that facilitate or interfere with sleep Instruct patient how to perform autogenic muscle relaxation or other nonpharmacologic forms of sleep inducement Initiate/implement comfort measures of massage, positioning, and affective touch Promote an increase in number of hours of sleep, if needed Provide for naps during the day, if indicated, to meet sleep requirements Instruct the patient and significant others about factors that contribute to sleep pattern disturbances Discuss with patient and family comfort measures, sleep-promoting techniques, and lifestyle changes that can contribute to optimal sleep Assist to eliminate stressful situations before bedtime Encourage patient to establish a bedtime routine to facilitate transition from wakefulness to sleep Facilitate maintenance of patient's usual bedtime routine, presleep cues/props, and familiar objects, as appropriate Approximate patient's regular sleep/wake cycle in planning care Adjust environment to promote sleep Group care activities to minimize number of awakenings; allow for sleep cycles of at least 90 minutes Instruct patient to avoid bedtime foods and beverages that interfere with sleep Adjust medication administration schedule Regulate environmental stimuli to maintain normal day-night cycles Assist patient to limit daytime sleep by providing activity that promotes wakefulness, as appropriate

*IER, In expected range.

Continued

Table 32-2	Suggested Nursing-Sensitive Outcome and Nursing Intervention—cont'd SLEEP PATTERN DISTURBANCE—cont'd		
Nursing Diagnosis	**Nursing-Sensitive Outcome**		**Nursing Intervention**

• Extended time in bed
• Excessive daytime napping
• Smoking
• Alcohol use/abuse
• Inadequate exercise
Effects of medications
  • Hypnotic
  • Sedatives
			Determine the effects of the patient's medications on sleep pattern
			Encourage use of sleep medications that do not contain REM sleep suppressor(s)

CASE STUDY

The nurse identified for Mrs. Clark a nursing diagnosis of Sleep Pattern Disturbance related to lack of a bedtime routine, inability to relax at bedtime, and excessive caffeine intake. The nurse identified the outcome Sleep as appropriate for evaluating the effectiveness of nursing care. Then the nurse selected and rated the indicators important for Mrs. Clark, as shown in Table 32-3.

The nurse offered several suggestions to help Mrs. Clark obtain a better quantity and quality of sleep. First, verbal and written information about expected changes with aging was provided. Next, Mrs. Clark and the nurse identified relaxing and enjoyable activities for Mrs. Clark to incorporate into a bedtime routine. Mrs. Clark's caffeine intake was identified as excessive. A plan was worked out to gradually reduce Mrs. Clark's caffeine intake to the point of drinking decaffeinated coffee only. In addition, Mrs. Clark and the nurse agreed that a program of simple relaxation become a part of her newly established bedtime routine. The nurse referred Mrs. Clark to a relaxation therapy class at the local Senior Center where she could learn the technique and purchase an audiotape to guide her through simple relaxation therapy. Finally, Mrs. Clark was asked to keep a sleep diary for 3 sequential days the first week of each month until she returned to the well elderly clinic in 6 months. These interventions were selected as appropriate for the nursing diagnosis Sleep Pattern Disturbance and the outcome Sleep.

At the next well elderly clinic 6 months later, Mrs. Clark brought her completed sleep diary and reported the following: sleeping 6 to 6½ hours per night, good to excellent quality sleep, high sleep efficiency, adequate uninterrupted sleep, sleeping with the established routine, verbalizing feelings of being refreshed, naps no more than 45 minutes per day, and wakefulness at appropriate times. Based on these data, the nurse again rated Mrs. Clark for the selected indicators to evaluate the effectiveness of the intervention Sleep Enhancement (Table 32-4).

Table 32-3	Sleep Pattern Disturbance: Selected and Rated Assessment Indicators for MRS. CLARK				
Sleep	**Extremely compromised** 1	**Substantially compromised** 2	**Moderately compromised** 3	**Mildly compromised** 4	**Not compromised** 5
INDICATORS					
Hours of sleep			X		
Sleep quality		X			
Sleep efficiency		X			
Uninterrupted sleep		X			
Sleep routine	X				
Feelings of rejuvenation after sleep		X			
Napping appropriate for age		X			
Wakeful at appropriate times		X			

Table 32-4 Sleep Enhancement: Nurse-Rated Outcome Indicators for MRS. CLARK	Extremely compromised 1	Substantially compromised 2	Moderately compromised 3	Mildly compromised 4	Not compromised 5
INDICATORS					
Hours of sleep				X	
Sleep quality					X
Sleep efficiency					X
Uninterrupted sleep					X
Sleep routine					X
Feelings of rejuvenation after sleep					X
Napping appropriate for age				X	
Wakeful at appropriate times					X

SUMMARY

Sleep is necessary for physical and psychosocial well-being. The importance of "healthy" sleep for older adults must not be underestimated. Inadequate sleep can leave the older individual feeling fatigued and frustrated. Nurses can play a key role in promoting optimal sleep among elders with no current sleep problems as well as those with potential or actual sleep pattern disturbances. This is accomplished through linking the nursing diagnosis SPD with relevant nursing interventions to achieve the desired outcomes. Making those linkages will enhance clinical practice, nursing education, and nursing research in the area of sleep problems among older adults.

REFERENCES

Aaron, J. N., Carlisle, C. C., Carskadon, M. A., Meyer T. J., Hill, N. S., & Millman, R. P. (1996). Environmental noise as a cause of sleep disruption in an intermediate respiratory care unit. *Sleep, 19*(9), 707-710.

Aldrich, M. S., Shipley, J. E., Tandon, R., Kroll, P. D., & Brower, K. J. (1993). Sleep-disordered breathing in alcoholics: Association with age. *Alcoholism, Clinical & Experimental Research, 17*(6), 1179-1183.

Almeida, O. P., Tamai, S., & Garrido, R. (1999). Sleep complaints among the elderly: Results from a survey in a psychogeriatric outpatient clinic in Brazil. *International Psychogeriatrics, 11*(1), 47-56.

Ancoli-Israel, S. (1989). Epidemiology of sleep disorders. *Clinics in Geriatric Medicine, 5*, 347-362.

Ancoli-Israel, S., Kaluber, M. R., Gillin, J. C., Campbell, S. S., & Hofstetter, C. R. (1994). Sleep in non-institutionalized Alzheimer's disease patients. *Aging, 6*, 451-458.

Ancoli-Israel, S., Kripke, D., Klauber, M., Mason, W., Fell, R., & Kaplan, O. (1991). Sleep disordered breathing in community dwelling elderly. *Sleep, 14*, 486-495.

Askenasy, J. J., & Yahr, M. D. (1990). Parkinsonian tremor loses its alternating aspect during non-REM sleep and is inhibited by REM sleep. *Journal of Neurology, Neurosurgery & Psychiatry, 53*(9), 749-753.

Asplund, R. (1999). Sleep disorders in the elderly. *Drugs & Aging, 14*(2), 91-103.

Baekeland, F., & Hoy, P. (1971). Reported vs. recorded sleep characteristics. *Archives of General Psychiatry, 24*, 548-551.

Bahro, M., Riemann, D., Stadtmuller, G., Berger, M., & Gattaz, W. F. (1993). REM sleep parameters in the discrimination of probable Alzheimer's disease from old-age depression. *Biological Psychiatry, 34*(7), 482-486.

Beck-Little, R., & Weinrich, S. P. (1998). Assessment and management of sleep disorders in the elderly. *Journal of Gerontological Nursing, 24*(4), 21-29.

Beyerman, K. (1987). Etiologies of sleep pattern disturbance in hospitalized patients. In A. M. McLane (Ed.), *Classification of nursing diagnoses: Proceedings of the seventh conference* (pp. 193-198). St. Louis, MO: Mosby.

Bliwise, D. (1993). Sleep in normal aging and dementia. *Sleep, 16*, 40-81.

Bond, A., & Lader, M. (1974). The use of analogue scales in rating subjective feelings. *British Journal of Medical Psychology, 47*, 211-218.

Brusco, L. I., Fainstein, I., Marquez, M., & Cardinali, D. P. (1999). Effect of melatonin in selected populations of sleep-disturbed patients. *Biological Signals & Receptors, 8*(1-2), 126-131.

Bundlie, S. R. (1998). Sleep in aging. *Geriatrics, 53*(Suppl. 1), S41-S43.

Castor, D., Woods, D., Pigott, K., & Hemmes, R. (1991). Effect of sunlight on sleep patterns of the elderly. *Journal of the American Academy of Physician Assistants, 4*, 321-326.

Clark, H. M. (1992). Sleep. In M. M. Burke & M. B. Walsh (Eds.), *Gerontologic nursing: Care of the frail elderly* (pp. 334-354). St. Louis, MO: Mosby.

Closs, S. J. (1992). Post-operative patients' views of sleep, pain and recovery. *Journal of Clinical Nursing, 1*(2), 83-88.

Cohen, F. L., & Merritt, S. L. (1992). Sleep promotion. In G. M. Bulechek & J. C. McCloskey (Eds.), *Nursing interventions: Essential nursing treatments* (pp. 109-119). Philadelphia: W. B. Saunders.

Copinschi, G., & Van Cauter, E. (1995). Effects of aging on modulation of hormonal secretions by sleep and circadian rhythmicity. *Hormone Research, 43*(1), 20-24.

Creighton, C. (1995). Effects of afternoon rest on the performance of geriatric patients in a rehabilitation hospital: A pilot study. *American Journal of Occupational Therapy, 49*(8), 775-779.

Davis-Sharts, J. (1989). The elder and critical care: Sleep and mobility issues. *Nursing Clinics of North America, 24,* 755-767.

Dinner, D. S., Erman, M. K., & Roth, T. (1992). Help for geriatric sleep problems. *Patient Care, 26,* 166-168.

Dowling, G. A. (1995). Sleep in older women with Parkinson's disease. *Journal of Neuroscience Nursing, 27*(6), 355-362.

Edinger, J. D., Morey, M. C., Sullivan, R. J., Higginbotham, M. B., Marsh, G. R., Dailey, D. S., & McCall, W. V. (1993). Aerobic fitness, acute exercise and sleep in older men. *Sleep, 16,* 351-359.

Engleman, H. M., Martin, S. E., Deary, I. J., & Douglas, N. J. (1994). Effect of continuous positive airway pressure treatment on daytime function in sleep apnoea/hypopnoea syndrome. *Lancet, 343,* 572-575.

Evans, B. D., & Rogers, A. E. (1994). 24-hour sleep/wake patterns in healthy elderly persons. *Applied Nursing Research, 7,* 75-83.

Feinsilver, S. H., & Hertz, G. (1993). Sleep in the elderly patient. *Clinics in Chest Medicine, 14*(3), 405-411.

Finlay, G. (1991). Sleep and intensive care. *Intensive Care Nursing, 7,* 61-68.

Freedman, N. S., Kotzer, N., & Schwab, R. J. (1999). Patient perception of sleep quality and etiology of sleep disruption in the intensive care unit. *American Journal of Respiratory and Critical Care Medicine, 159*(4PT1), 1155-1162.

Frisoni, G. B., De Leo, D., Rozzini, R., & Trabucchi, M. (1996). Napping in the elderly and its association with night sleep and psychological status. *International Psychogeriatrics, 8*(3), 477-487.

Gall, K., Petersen, T., & Riesch, S. K. (1990). Night life: Nocturnal behavior patterns among hospitalized elderly. *Journal of Gerontological Nursing, 16,* 31-38.

Garpestad, E., Ringler, J., Parker, J. A., Remsburg, S., & Weiss, J. W. (1995). Sleep stage influences the hemodynamic response to obstructive apneas. *American Journal of Respiratory & Critical Care Medicine, 152*(1), 199-203.

Gass, M. L. S., & Rebar, R. W. (1990). Management of problems during menopause. *Comprehensive Therapy, 16,* 3-10.

Gentili, A., Weiner, D. K., Kuchibhatil, M., & Edinger, J. D. (1997). Factors that disturb sleep in nursing home residents. *Aging (Milano), 9*(3), 207-213.

Geoffriau, M., Brun, J., Chazot, G., & Claustrat, B. (1998). The physiology and pharmacology of melatonin in humans. *Hormone Research, 49*(3-4), 136-141.

Gislason, T., Reynisdottir, H., Kristbjarnarson, H., & Benediktsdottir, B. (1993). Sleep habits and sleep disturbances among the elderly—An epidemiological survey. *Journal of Internal Medicine, 234,* 31-39.

Gress, L. D., Bahr, R. T., & Hassanein, R. S. (1983). Nocturnal behavior of selected institutionalized adults. *Journal of Gerontological Nursing, 7,* 86-92.

Hanly, P. J., & Zuberi-Khokhar, N. (1996). Periodic limb movements during sleep in patients with congestive heart failure. *Chest, 109*(6), 1497-1502.

Hatzinger, M., Kocher, R., Hemmeter, U., Ladewig, D., & Holsboer-Trachsler, E. (1995). Sleep and addiction. *Schweiz Rundsch Med Prax, 84*(15), 450-453.

Hoch, C. C., & Reynolds, C. F. (1986). Sleep disturbances and what to do about them. *Geriatric Nursing, 7,* 24-27.

Iowa Intervention Project. J. C. McCloskey & G. M. Bulechek (Eds.). (2000). *Nursing interventions classification (NIC)* (3rd ed.). St. Louis, MO: Mosby.

Iowa Outcomes Project. M. Johnson, M. Maas, S. Moorhead (Eds.). (2000). *Nursing outcomes classification (NOC)* (2nd ed.). St. Louis, MO: Mosby.

Jensen, D. P., & Herr, K. A. (1993). Sleeplessness. *Nursing Clinics of North America, 28,* 385-405.

Johnson, J. E. (1986). Sleep and bedtime routines of noninstitutionalized aged women. *Journal of Community Health Nursing, 3,* 117-125.

Johnson, J. E. (1988). Effect of benzodiazepines on older women. *Journal of Community Health Nursing, 5,* 119-127.

Johnson, J. E. (1991a). A comparative study of the bedtime routines and sleep of older adults. *Journal of Community Health Nursing, 3,* 129-136.

Johnson, J. E. (1991b). Progressive relaxation and the sleep of older noninstitutionalized women. *Applied Nursing Research, 4,* 165-170.

Kendler, B. S. (1997). Melatonin: Media hype or therapeutic breakthrough? *Nurse Practitioner, 22*(2), 66-67.

Kim, M. J., & Moritz, D. A. (Eds.). (1982). *Classification of nursing diagnoses: Proceedings of third and fourth national conferences.* Hightstown, NJ: McGraw Hill.

Kohsaka, M., Fukuda, N., Kobayashi, R., Honma, H., Sakakibara, S., Koyama, E., Nakano, O., & Matsubara, H. (1998). Effects of short duration morning bright light in healthy elderly. II: Sleep and motor activity. *Psychiatry & Clinical Neurosciences, 52*(2), 252-253.

Kostic, V. S., Susic, V., Covickovic-Sternic, N., Marinkovic, Z., & Jankovic S. (1989). Reduced rapid eye movement sleep latency in patients with Parkinson's disease. *Journal of Neurology, 236*(7), 421-423.

Krska, J., & MacLeod, T. N. (1995). Sleep quality and the use of benzodiazepine hypnotics in general practice. *Journal of Clinical Pharmacy and Therapeutics, 20*(2), 91-96.

Landolt, H. P., Werth, E., Borbely, A. A., & Dijk, D. J. (1995). Caffeine intake (200 mg) in the morning affects human sleep and EEG power spectra at night. *Brain Research, 675,* 67-74.

Lexcen, F. J., & Hicks, R. A. (1993). Does cigarette smoking increase sleep problems. *Perceptual & Motor Skills, 77*(1), 16-18.

Lo, C. K., & Kim, M. J. (1986). Construct validity of sleep pattern disturbance: A methodological approach. In M. E. Hurley (Ed.), *Classification of nursing diagnoses: Proceedings of the sixth conference* (pp. 197-206). St. Louis, MO: Mosby.

Louden, M. B., Morehead, M. A., & Schmidt, H. S. (1995). Activation by selegiline (Eldepryle) of REM sleep behavior disorder in parkinsonism. *West Virginia Medical Journal, 91*(3), 101.

Maggi, S., Langlois, J. A., Minicuci, N., Grigoletto, F., Pavan, M., Foley, D. J., & Enzi, G. (1998). Sleep complaints in community-dwelling older persons: Prevalence, associated factors, and reported causes. *Journal of the American Geriatrics Society, 46*(2), 161-168.

Middelkoop, H. A., Smilde-van den Doeil, D. A., Neven, A. K., Kamphuisen, H. A., & Springer, C. P. (1996). Subjective sleep characteristics of 1,485 males and females aged 50-93: Effects of sex and age, and factors related to self-evaluated quality of sleep. *Journals of Gerontology. Series A, Biological Sciences & Medical Sciences, 51*(3), M108-115.

Moldofsky, H. (1994). Central nervous system and peripheral immune functions and the sleep-wake system. *Journal of Psychiatry & Neuroscience, 19*(5), 368-374.

Morin, C. M., Mimieault, V., & Gagne, A. (1999). Nonpharmacological treatment of late-life insomnia. *Journal of Psychosomatic Research, 46*(2), 103-116.

Neubauer, D. N. (1999). Sleep problems in the elderly. *American Family Physician, 59*(9), 2551-2560.

North American Nursing Diagnosis Association. (1999). *Nursing diagnoses: Definitions & classification 1999-2000.* Philadelphia: Author.

O'Connor, P. J., & Youngstedt, S. D. (1995). Influence of exercise on human sleep. *Exercise & Sport Sciences Reviews, 23,* 105-134.

Okabe, S., Hida, W., Kikuchi, Y., Taguchi, O., Takishima, T., & Shirato, K. (1994). Upper airway muscle activity during REM and non-REM sleep of patients with obstructive apnea. *Chest, 106*(3), 767-773.

Onen, S. H., Onen, F., Bailly, D., & Parquet, P. (1994). Prevention and treatment of sleep disorders through regulation of sleeping habits. *Presse Medicale, 23*(10), 485-489.

Pascoe, P. A. (1994). Drugs and the sleep-wakefulness continuum. *Pharmacology & Therapeutics, 61*(1-2), 227-236.

Pevernagie, D. A., & Shepard, J. W. Jr. (1992). Relations between sleep stage, posture and effective nasal CPAP levels in OSA. *Sleep, 15*(2), 162-167.

Phillips, B. A., & Danner, F. J. (1995). Cigarette smoking and sleep disturbance. *Archives of Internal Medicine, 155*(7), 734-737.

Pickett, C. K., Regensteiner, J. G., Woodward, W. D., Hagerman, D. D., Weil, J. V., & Moore, L. G. (1989). Progestin and estrogen reduce sleep-disordered breathing in postmenopausal women. *Journal of Applied Physiology, 66,* 1656-1661.

Pollmacher, T., Mullington, J., Korth, C., & Hinze-Selch, D. (1995). Influence of host defense activation on sleep in humans. *Advances in Neuroimmunology, 5*(2), 155-169.

Richards, K. C. (1994). Sleep promotion in the critical care unit. *AACN Clinical Issues in Critical Care Nursing, 5*(2), 152-158.

Rogers, A. E., Caruso, C. C., & Aldrich, M. S. (1993). Reliability of sleep diaries for assessment of sleep/wake patterns. *Nursing Research, 42,* 368-372.

Schnelle, J. F., Cruise, P. A., Alessi, C. A., Ludlow, K., al-Samarrai, N. R., & Ouslander, J. G. (1998). Sleep hygiene in physically dependent nursing home residents: Behavioral and environmental intervention implications. *Sleep, 21*(5), 515-523.

Shaver, J. L., & Paulsen, V. M. (1993). Sleep, psychological distress, and somatic symptoms in perimenopausal women. *Family Practice Research Journal, 13*(4), 373-384.

Shilo, L., Dagan, Y., Smorjik, Y., Weinberg, U., Dolev, S., Komptel, B., Balaum, H., & Shenkman, L. (1999). Patients in the intensive care unit suffer from severe lack of sleep associated with loss of normal melatonin secretion pattern. *American Journal of the Medical Sciences, 317*(5), 278-281.

Singh, N. A., Clements, K. M., & Fiatarone, M. A. (1997). A randomized controlled trial of the effect of exercise on sleep. *Sleep, 20*(2), 95-101.

Smith, M. C., Ellgring, H., & Oertel, W. H. (1997). Sleep disturbances in Parkinson's disease patients and spouses. *Journal of the American Geriatrics Society, 45*(2), 194-199.

Snyder-Halpern, R., & Verran, J. A. (1987). Instrumentation to describe subjective sleep characteristics in health subjects. *Research in Nursing and Health, 10,* 155-163.

Solow, B., Ovesen, J., Nielsen, P. W., Wildschiodtz, G., & Tallgren, A. (1993). Head posture in obstructive sleep apnoea. *European Journal of Orthodontics, 15*(2), 107-114.

Spenceley, S. M. (1993). Sleep inquiry: A look with fresh eyes. *Image: The Journal of Nursing Scholarship, 25*(3), 249-256.

Stone, A. B., & Pearlstein, T. B. (1994). Evaluation and treatment of changes in mood, sleep, and sexual functioning associated with menopause. *Obstetrics & Gynecology Clinics of North America, 21*(2), 391-403.

Swales, P., Friedman, L., & Sheikh, J. (1993). Interrelationship of anxiety and sleep disorders in the elderly. In P. A. Szwabo & G. T. Grossberg (Eds.), *Problems in long-term care* (pp. 70-80). New York: Springer.

Vgontzas, A. N., & Kales, A. (1999). Sleep and its disorders. *Annual Review of Medicine, 50,* 387-400.

Vitiello, M. V., Bliwise, D. L., & Prinz, P. N. (1992). Sleep in Alzheimer's disease and the sundown syndrome. *Neurology, 42*(S6), 83-93.

Weitzenblum, E., Chaouat, A., Charpentier, C., & Krieger, J. (1995). Sleep and COPD. *Revue du Praticien, 45*(10), 1257-1260.

Wetter, D. W., & Young, T. B. (1994). The relation between cigarette smoking and sleep disturbance. *Preventive Medicine, 23*(3), 328-334.

White, J. E., Drinnan, M. J., Smithson, A. J., Griffiths, C. J., & Gibson, G. J. (1995). Respiratory muscle activity during rapid eye movement (REM) sleep in patients with chronic obstructive pulmonary disease. *Thorax, 50*(4), 376-382.

Wiklund, I., Karlberg, J., & Mattsson, L. (1993). Quality of life of postmenopausal women on a regimen of transdermal estradiol therapy: A double-blind placebo-controlled study. *American Journal of Obstetrics and Gynecology, 168,* 824-830.

Wilcox, S., & King, A. C. (1999). Sleep complaints in older women who are family caregivers. *Journal of Gerontology: Series B, Psychological Sciences & Social Sciences, 54*(3), P189-P198.

Youngstedt, S. D., Kripke, D. F., & Elliott, J. A. (1998). Melatonin excretion is not related to sleep in the elderly. *Journal of Pineal Research, 24*(3), 142-145.

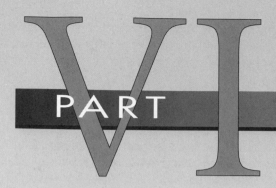

PART VI

Cognitive-Perceptual Pattern

OVERVIEW

Part Six begins with a look at the normal changes in cognition and perception associated with aging, emphasizing that a decline in cognition is not universal among the aging and that not all areas of cognition are affected. Bunten reviews the evidence in Chapter 33, suggesting specific recommendations to assist elders to compensate with cognitive and sensory-perceptual changes. She points out the importance of distinguishing between the normal changes in these areas and difficulties that should be investigated further.

Alterations in cognition and perception affect many elders and can precipitate institutionalization. In Chapter 34 Gerdner and Hall describe a conceptual model, Progressively Lowered Stress Threshold (PLST), to guide the practitioner in four levels of assessment and intervention with clients who experience the nursing diagnosis Chronic Confusion: Alzheimer's Disease and Related Disorders (ADRD). The PLST model, developed by Hall from the cluster of losses and behavioral states associated with this diagnosis, is contrasted with the NANDA diagnosis. Authors present detailed suggestions on institutional and home assessment and care planning, incorporating NIC interventions from the *Nursing Interventions Classification (NIC)* (Iowa Intervention Project, 2000) with special attention to the problems of combative reactions and wandering. The chapter concludes with a discussion of client outcomes identified by the PLST model contrasted with the *Nursing Outcomes Classification (NOC)* outcomes.

In Chapter 35 Wakefield and colleagues discuss current research pertinent to the nursing diagnosis Acute Confusion, observing that most studies have been done in hospitals rather than community or long-term care settings, and pointing out the difficulties in establishing a credible esti-

mate of prevalence. They discuss the defining characteristics and etiologic factors, contrasting those found in the literature with the NANDA diagnosis, and present suggestions for nursing assessment, intervention, and analysis of client outcomes using standardized language classifications. NIC interventions and NOC outcomes are analyzed and critiqued for their usefulness for this specific diagnosis.

Although the topic of pain in elderly persons could consume a book itself, Mobily and Herr provide a salient overview of this important and often overlooked topic in Chapter 36, Pain. The authors identify and discuss biologic, chemical, physical, and psychologic sources of pain and address the particular challenges of assessment of pain in older adults. The NANDA diagnosis Pain, particularly the defining characteristics, is critiqued, and a number of clinically useful assessment tools are set forth and evaluated for use with elders. Authors also evaluated the usefulness of NIC interventions for this population. The section describing interventions highlights the importance of theory in targeting appropriate nursing activities and presents both pharmacologic and nonpharmacologic approaches. Finally, client outcomes are identified and authors recommend subjective and objective evaluation techniques, including the measurement of NOC outcomes at specific points in time.

In Chapter 37 Swanson and Drury explicate the diagnosis Sensory/Perceptual Alterations. They discuss points of controversy associated with this and related diagnoses proposed by NANDA and Gordon, suggesting that the diagnoses may require further refinement to make this complex area wholly amenable to nursing practice. Authors discuss environmental and physiologic causative factors in normal aging and present the NANDA defining characteristics, suggesting a variety of assessment techniques for detecting alterations in the elderly person's vision, hearing, kinesthesia, and senses of taste, smell, and touch. The authors recommend NIC interventions useful for alterations in any of these senses and select NOC outcomes most appropriate for older adults.

Weitzel discusses the related diagnosis Unilateral Neglect in Chapter 38. She emphasizes that Unilateral Neglect is the result of pathology and not normal aging, which largely differentiates the diagnosis from other altered sensory perceptions. Weitzel compares defining characteristics she identified with those of the NANDA diagnosis and suggests that two separate diagnoses are most useful for practice with elderly clients: Unilateral Neglect: Inattention, and Unilateral Neglect: Denial. She describes etiologies and related deficits for the diagnoses and presents a specific assessment guide developed for clients with brain injury. NOC safety and self-care outcomes are iden-

tified. NIC interventions, including environmental structuring to compensate for the elderly person's neglect of stimuli and specific intervention strategies for inattention and denial, are discussed.

In Chapter 39 Conn and colleagues address Knowledge Deficit, a common problem among elders. The authors review the defining characteristics and related factors of the diagnosis and elaborate on assessment parameters in the areas of client knowledge, learning readiness, previous learning experiences, and culture. Nursing interventions are selected from the Teaching domain of the NIC. Authors briefly review principles of teaching and learning and discuss the common learning challenges encountered by older adults. They recommend specific teaching strategies that may enhance learning among elders and identify a number of NOC outcomes useful for evaluation.

CHAPTER 33

NORMAL CHANGES WITH AGING

Donna Bunten

Cognition refers to the processes by which information is acquired, stored, shared, and used. Intellectual tasks such as thinking, remembering, perceiving, communicating, calculating, and problem solving are all examples of cognitive function. Many people hold the view that all cognitive abilities inevitably decline in old age. These persons (and unfortunately some of them are elders themselves) believe that older people cannot think clearly and have poor memories; they would agree with the old adage that you can't teach old dogs new tricks. These generalizations are extremely inappropriate. Experience and research both demonstrate that only some elderly persons experience only some deficits in some areas of cognition; the onset of decline occurs at different times in their lives. In this area of gerontologic research, as in most areas of study of the aged, individual differences are of extreme importance and must be considered before making any generalizations about cognitive abilities (Cunningham & Haman, 1992; Dellasega, 1998).

COGNITION

General intelligence tests measure a combination of several cognitive abilities. The type of change in performance that might be associated with aging depends on the specific ability being measured. Scores on vocabulary and information tests typically show no appreciable changes with aging, but perceptual-integrative abilities and comprehension of numerical symbols decline more rapidly (Cerella, DiCara, Williams, & Bowles, 1986). These slight decrements in some intellectual variables occur during the 60s and 70s in healthy older adults and have little significance for competent behavior in this young aging group (Schaie, 1994). Research has demonstrated that, even in the oldest age groups, many subjects maintain their intellectual functions. Matthews, Cauley, Yaffe, and Zmuda (1999) found that formal education protects against age-related cognitive decline even if the education had taken place many years earlier. Formal education also was found to be a powerful predictor of cognitive functions in old age (Zhu, Viitanen, Guo, Winblad, & Fratiglioni, 1998). Many elders are able to improve intellectual performance with training and with experience in performing various tasks (Schaie & Willis, 1986).

Decrements in intellectual functioning have been found to be significantly greater in subjects who have arteriosclerotic cardiovascular disease than in healthy elderly persons (Zhu et al., 1998). In addition, emphysema, acute infections, poor nutrition, injuries, and surgery can temporarily or permanently affect intelligence in elderly individuals by reducing the blood supply to the brain (Aiken, 1995; Cohen, 1990). Another exception to the conclusion that intellectual abilities do not decline dramatically in healthy elders is a phenomenon referred to as "terminal drop." Researchers found declines in various areas of cognitive and sensorimotor functioning and in the ability to cope with environmental demands in patients who died within 1 or 2 years of being tested (Aiken, 1995). The same examinees showed no drop in physical function when tested. Since illness affects intellectual functioning, significant changes in function should be investigated and not simply attributed to aging.

Standard laboratory testing of intelligence does not evaluate how successfully elders are able to perform in everyday situations. Some older persons who do poorly in the laboratory are found to be well adjusted and able to successfully perform real-life activities. This ability to perform familiar and ongoing activities, called "cognitive competence" by Salthouse (1990), is thought to be the product of repeated applications of cognitive processes to various situations. Cattell's (1963) term, "crystallized intelligence" describes much the same concept. Crystallized intelligence is used when the task at hand calls for knowledge that has been acquired during one's lifetime and shows little or no change with advancing age. Intelligence that relies on accumulated experience sets elderly individuals apart from younger age-groups. On the other hand, fluid intelligence, as described by Cattell, is required when doing tasks not related to previous experiences or knowledge and is thought to decline in elders. Whether cognitive competence is determined by a different type of cognition than is evaluated by laboratory tasks and psychometric testing is being debated (Schaie & Willis, 1986).

A common fear among the soon-to-be aged and a common complaint of older people is memory loss. Why aging may affect the ability to remember is not entirely clear. But minor memory difficulties do appear to be associated with advancing age. There are at least three phases in learning and remembering: acquisition of the material, encoding or storing the material to be remembered, and recall or retrieval of stored material. Acquisition of material is accomplished by the sensory systems. Once acquired, information is stored in short-term or primary memory, where it is held for only a few seconds or minutes. Learning a telephone number only long enough to dial it and then immediately forgetting it is an example of information stored only in short-term memory. If material is to be remembered for an extended period of time, it must be taken out of short-term memory, encoded in some way by using some mechanism to facilitate remembering, and then stored in long-term memory.

Long-term memory, or secondary memory as it is sometimes called, is a more permanent type of information storage. The process of encoding information for storage in long-term memory can be jeopardized for older persons who may have never learned or used information association techniques (mnemonics, visual associations, etc.) and who might not organize new material for remembering as efficiently or as quickly as younger persons. Once information is stored in long-term memory, the elderly person still can face problems in retrieval, since he must sort through secondary memory for the piece required (Hultsch & Dixon, 1990). The retrieval process is slower and recall is less accurate in elders (Aiken, 1995). An increase in response time can be misinterpreted both as a deficit in learning and as a deficit in memory. Furthermore, the acquisition, encoding, and retrieval processes can all be affected by distractions, fatigue, grief, depression, stress, illness, medications, alcohol use, vision or hearing loss, lack of concentration, or an attempt to remember too many details at once (Ebersole & Hess, 1998). One can also deduce that elders with uncompensated sensory deficits would be at a disadvantage when asked for information; a stronger stimulus might be needed to attract and hold their attention.

Age-associated memory impairment (AAMI) is a term being used to describe deficiencies in recall that occur in aging (Ebersole & Hess, 1998; Rinn, 1988). It may be quite reassuring to the elderly client for the nurse to point out that AAMI, unlike some dementias, is neither progressive nor disabling. AAMI is most noticeable when a person is under pressure. Once the person is more relaxed, he is usually able to remember the forgotten material. No treatment has been discovered for AAMI. Using written reminders and lists, repeating information to be remembered out loud, learning to use mnemonics or other mechanisms to associate materials, and allowing plenty of time to remember information are frequently helpful to elders. Memory loss associated with AAMI can usually be compensated for by using these suggestions and should not interfere with normal activities of daily living. When normal activities are interrupted by forgetfulness of short-term events, there is cause for concern and investigation (Rinn, 1988).

Excellent guidelines for comprehensive evaluation of cognition in the elderly may be found in "Assessment of Cognition in the Elderly: Pieces of a Complex Puzzle" (Dellasega, 1998).

SENSORY-PERCEPTUAL CHANGES

Uncompensated age changes in the sensory systems of the elderly person impact intelligence, learning, and memory processes. An overall slowing is experienced in all areas of sensory reception, with some decrease in, but not total loss of, efficiency (Nusbaum, 1999). The senses provide the means by which elderly individuals interact with and interpret the world. Consequently, a decrease in functional ability frequently has a marked impact on behavior and the quality of life experienced by older persons. A decline in sensory ability also can simulate an intellectual decline that is not in fact present (Nusbaum, 1999).

A mild loss of visual acuity called presbyopia occurs with advancing age. Presbyopia involves the loss of the ability to focus on near objects, and onset may be noticed around 40 years of age (Carter, 1994). Presbyopia is caused by the loss of elasticity of the lens, which can no longer be shaped to focus on close objects. The image then appears behind the retina, blurring close vision. Adding an extra lens such as reading glasses or bifocals will focus the image appropriately on the retina (Meltzer, 1983). With this gradual loss of accommodation, more time is needed for the elder to refocus when looking from one distance to another; the ability to discriminate details also becomes more difficult. Some loss of rods and cones in the retina (which convert light waves to electrical impulses) also results in less distinct images being sent to the brain. Increasing illumination will assist the elder in seeing when lighting is poor or when there is poor contrast in material.

Light and dark adaptation also become problematic for the elderly person. The light-sensing thresholds for both rods and cones is significantly affected by aging, slowing adaptation. Pupil size also becomes smaller, which affects the amount of light reaching the retina and limits the efficiency of pupillary constriction and dilation (Saxon & Etten, 1994; Tallis, Fillit, & Brocklehurst, 1998). The elderly person should be advised that this change affects activities like night driving or moving from a dark room to one with greater illumination and that extra time should be allowed to adapt to new lighting conditions before continuing activities (Carter, 1994).

The crystalline lens of the eye becomes denser, more yellow, and less elastic with aging (Castor & Carter, 1995). With yellowing of the lens and impaired transmission of light through the retina, color discrimination becomes less acute, especially in the blue, green, and violet color tones (Tallis, Fillit, & Brocklehurst, 1998). This age change should be considered when planning the environment of elderly individuals.

Increasing opacity of the lens of the eye is also associated with a decreased tolerance for glare. The vitreous, a jellylike substance behind the lens of the eye, is supported by a fibrous network that normally distributes that substance evenly within the eyeball. With aging, the fibers thicken and gather into bundles that scatter light within the eyeball and contribute to glare and to the production of floaters. Elders are susceptible not only to the reflection of sunlight when outdoors, but also to the glare from highly polished surfaces on walls and floors and the glare produced by fluorescent lighting. Suggestions to wear hats and visors, to use sunglasses, or to have the lenses of glasses tinted or coated with antireflective material can assist elders in addressing this problem. Sensitivity to glare can indicate a developing cataract, especially if the elderly person experiences symptoms such as headache, eye fatigue, or a burning sensation of the eyes. These symptoms obviously warrant further investigation (Mayo Medical Essay, 1995).

Peripheral vision, the useful field of vision when the eyes are centrally fixed, also decreases with age (Schieber, 1992). This loss is associated with diminished pupil size and can be further compromised by decreased muscle tone, causing drooping or ptosis of the upper eyelid. If there is a sudden development of ptosis, immediate evaluation and treatment should be advised, as this may be associated with a stroke or other acute neurologic problem. Peripheral vision can be slightly lessened by a phenomenon called arcus senilis. The arcus senilis, a grayish or cloudy arc or circle at the outer edge of the iris in some elderly individuals, is caused by an age-related deposition of calcium and cholesterol salts (Castor & Carter, 1995).

Older persons often complain of symptoms of dry eyes such as burning or stinging. A decreased production of tears by the lacrimal gland is associated with aging. Some medications such as anti-anxiety preparations, soporifics, antihistamines, decongestants, and certain arthritis and hypertensive drugs can worsen this condition (Ebersole & Hess, 1994). Preservative-free artificial tear products can be used to soothe dry eyes. Conversely, excessive amounts of tears can be produced in response to dry and irritated eyes. In the elderly person the eyelid tissue gets thin and wrinkled and the underlying muscles are weak, so tears flow out rather than lubricating the eyes.

Vision is an obvious and important link to the world we live in. Awareness of the gradual changes that occur with aging in this system should motivate elders to seek preventative care. They should be encouraged to have a regular eye examination every 1 to 2 years after age 65 or more frequently if there is a history of eye disease in the family or if they suffer from a chronic condition that can affect the eyes (Mayo Medical Essay, 1995).

Some type of hearing loss affects approximately one third of adults over 65 years of age. Although hearing loss is one of the most prevalent chronic health problems of elders in the United States, it is known to be underreported by professionals as well as by hearing-impaired elders and their families (Ciurlia-Guy, Cashman, & Lewsen, 1993). Elders who do report hearing difficulties usually complain of difficulties understanding speech, especially the high-pitched voices of women and children, and/or difficulty conversing in large groups, especially when there is background noise (restaurants, receptions, etc.). Loneliness, depression, and/or paranoid tendencies can result if affected persons are self-conscious about their hearing limitation and avoid interactive situations (Chenitz, Stone, & Salisbury, 1991).

Auditory changes begin to be noticed at approximately age 40 (Schieber, 1992). Onset may be significantly affected by a variety of factors other than aging: exposure to noise (jets, traffic, guns, occupational noises), recurrent otitis media or trauma, ototoxic drugs (anti-inflammatory drugs including aspirin, loop diuretics, aminoglycosides, etc.), genetic conditions, or circulatory deficits to the vital structure of the inner ear (Eliopoulos, 1993).

The most common hearing deficit in older age is called presbycusis, a sensorineural hearing loss that progresses from a high-tone loss to a generalized loss of hearing at all frequencies (Wiley et al., 1998). Presbycusis occurs gradually; the resulting hearing loss is bilateral. Several pathophysiologic types of presbycusis have been described. Sensory presbycusis is associated with atrophy of the organ of Corti and the impaired audibility of high-frequency sounds. Neural presbycusis is associated with the degeneration of hair cells and the loss of cochlear neurons. Neural loss includes both limitations in hearing high-frequency sounds and a loss of speech discrimination (Schieber, 1992).

Conductive hearing loss is also prevalent in the elderly person. Conductive hearing loss generally involves a mechanical problem in the transfer of sound waves through the outer and middle ear to the eardrum, where they are converted to electrical impulses. This type of loss can be caused by environmental damage to the outer ear (pinna), arthritic stiffening of the joints of the ossicular bones, or decreased flexibility of the conductive membranes, eardrum, or oval window. Conductive loss is often reversible if associated with a treatable disorder such as cerumen impaction (Mahoney, 1993). Ear wax or cerumen is less copious in elders but is harder in consistency because of the greater amount of keratin present. The cilia of the aging ear show increased coarseness and stiffness and become less effective in propelling residue to the external canal opening (Andresen, 1989). Hearing impairment resulting from cerumen impaction has been demonstrated to be significantly improved after removal of the cerumen obstruction (Mahoney, 1993).

Treatment of presbycusis varies according to the audiometric patterns exhibited. Although elders with good discrimination ordinarily benefit from amplification of sound, those with severe loss of discrimination might not benefit as significantly. In sensorineural loss, sound is distorted especially when speech is very fast or contains high-frequency consonants such as *s, z, th, f, k,* and *g* (Chenitz et al., 1991; Corso, 1971). The elderly person may have unconsciously become adept at some lip reading, and hearing can improve when appropriate visual clues are presented with conversation. Gaining the older person's attention and facing her directly when speaking to her assists in communication efforts. Mahoney (1993) points out, "If ignored, a hearing impairment can cause older adults to become inappropriately labeled as 'confused' or 'uncooperative' when they misinterpret communication and respond improperly" (p. 24). Vision and hearing complement each other, and a deficit in one may not be compensated for by the other when decrements exist in both systems. Hearing and/or vision loss is frustrating and threatens the security and self-esteem of the elder (Chen, 1994).

Research in the areas of taste and smell is sparse, perhaps because of the abstract nature of these sensations and the difficulties in trying to quantify them. The senses of taste and smell play an important role in the regulation of eating behaviors and the maintenance of health and pleasure for everyone.

The sense of taste depends on the number of taste buds stimulated by the soluble form of a substance. Conflicting reports appear in the literature about whether the number of taste buds decreases with aging, although it appears that the sense of taste does decline with age (Schieber, 1992). Stronger solutions of salt, sweet, sour, and bitter substances have been found to be needed to stimulate the taste buds, with sweet showing the greatest loss (Eliopoulos, 1993; Yen, 1996). Shklar (1966) noted that the tongue of the elderly person is smoother than that of a younger adult, resulting in less aqueous access to the taste buds. Saliva is necessary to liquefy substances. Saliva production is decreased in the elderly person and becomes thicker, affecting the ability to taste (Eliopoulos, 1993). Long-term exposure to toxic substances, such as smoking, is known to decrease gustatory sensation. Other factors affecting the ability to taste include the temperature of foods, oral hygiene, the prevalent use of dentures among elders, and the intactness of the sense of smell.

Changes in the sense of smell in the aged are attributed to loss of cells in the olfactory bulb in the brain and loss of sensory cells in the lining of the nasal passages (Schieber, 1992). A longitudinal study of smell identification in elders found that smell identification diminished with progressive aging, that women consistently outperformed men in identifying various odors, and that the sense of smell has more to do with age-related problems in the recognition and enjoyment of food than with taste (Ship, Pearson, Cruise, Brant, & Metter, 1996). The results of this study were not affected by either medical problems or medication usage by some participants. The ability to smell is affected by long-term exposure to toxic substances

like dust, pollen, and smoke. It is important to note that elderly persons who neglect personal hygiene may simply not be able to smell themselves and not recognize the need to bathe. Decrements in the sense of smell also present an associated safety risk for elders, as harmful odors (gas, smoke, etc.) may be unrecognized.

Tactile sensitivity (somesthetics) decreases with advancing age due to thinning of the epidermal layers and loss of a large number of nerve endings. According to Verillo (1980), this is particularly significant in the fingertips, palms of the hands, and lower extremities. The skin also loses elasticity, and more pressure is needed to deform the skin tissue and enable recognition of touch, pressure, and vibration (Colavito, 1978). Some loss in the ability of the adult to recognize vibration begins to emerge around age 50, and more loss accompanies advancing age. Decrements in vibratory sensation appear to be more severe in the lower as opposed to the upper extremities (Schieber, 1992). The ability of the elderly individual to regulate body temperature is also decreased, as the small blood vessels that supply blood to the epidermis are decreased in number. Lessened fat deposits and lessened sweat gland production, in addition to the vascular changes, predispose older persons to altered regulation of body temperature and a greater inability to adjust to extremes in environmental temperatures (Saxon & Etten, 1994).

There is general confusion about any association between aging and pain perception as opposed to pain related to coexisting disease in elders (Ferrell & Ferrell, 1990). There is no evidence that aches and pains are a normal accompaniment of aging. Decreases in the number of neurons, dendritic connections, and neurotransmitters within the central nervous system have been found in elders, but there is still little evidence to suggest that pain or the perception of pain is altered by aging (Forrest, 1995). However, older persons are in far greater jeopardy of suffering from both acute and chronic pain and have been found to be less likely to report pain or to request pain relief (Closs, 1996; Ferrell, 1991). The belief that pain is an unavoidable consequence of aging is likely to lead to neglect in treating pain in elders.

The kinesthetic sense allows us to be aware of and to monitor muscular control of limbs and trunk movements. The receptors for kinesthetic sensation are located in muscles, joints, bone, ligaments, and tendons. They give information to the brain about the state of muscle contraction, the angle of rotation of our joints, and the position of our limbs in space. Colavito (1978) stated that deterioration of muscle fiber and decreased feedback from kinesthetic receptors resulted in decreased coordination in elders. Perception of the movement and placement of body parts in space are critical to performing skilled activities. A decline in the kinesthetic sense has implications for the elderly person. Minor injury can result from accidents with wheelchairs or from stumbles; severe injuries can result from falls.

SUMMARY

Despite the numerous changes commonly experienced by elders, most are able to function admirably and to lead satisfying lives. Nurses must develop expertise in recognizing age-related changes in cognition and perception and in helping the elderly to compensate for losses. Maximizing the elderly client's achievable independence and assisting him in experiencing a healthy, safe, and satisfactory aging process are critical goals for nursing practice.

REFERENCES

Aiken, L. R. (1995). *Aging: An introduction to gerontology* (pp. 100-133). Thousand Oaks, CA: Sage.

Andresen, G. P. (1989). A fresh look at assessing the elderly. *RN, 56*(6), 28-40.

Carter, T. L. (1994). Age-related vision changes: A primary care guide. *Geriatrics, 49*(9), 37-45.

Castor, T. D., & Carter, T. L. (1995). Low vision: Physician screening helps to improve patient function. *Geriatrics, 50*(12), 51-58.

Cattell, R. B. (1963). Theory of fluid and crystallized intelligence: A critical experiment. *Journal of Educational Psychology, 54*, 1-22.

Cerella, J., DiCara, R., Williams, D., & Bowles, N. (1986). Relations between information processing and intelligence in elderly adults. *Intelligence, 10*, 75-91.

Chen, H. L. (1994). Hearing in the elderly: Relation of hearing loss, loneliness and self-esteem. *Journal of Gerontological Nursing, 6*, 22-28.

Chenitz, W. C., Stone, J. T., & Salisbury, S. A. (1991). *Clinical gerontological nursing: A guide to advanced practice.* Philadelphia: W. B. Saunders.

Ciurlia-Guy, E., Cashman, M., & Lewsen, B. (1993). Identifying hearing loss and hearing handicap among chronic care elderly people. *The Gerontologist, 33*(5), 644-649.

Closs, S. J. (1996). Pain and elderly patients: A survey of nurse's knowledge and experiences. *Journal of Advanced Nursing, 23*, 237-242.

Cohen, G. D. (1990). Normal changes and patterns of psychiatric disease. In W. B. Abrams & R. Berkow (Eds.), *Merck manual of geriatrics* (pp. 995-996). Rahway, NJ: Merck, Sharp, & Dohme Research Laboratories.

Colavito, F. B. (1978). *Sensory changes in the elderly.* Springfield, IL: Charles C. Thomas.

Corso, J. (1971). Sensory processes and age effects in normal adults. *Journal of Gerontology, 26*(1), 90-103.

Cunningham, W. R., & Haman, K. L. (1992). Intellectual functioning in relation to mental health. In J. E. Birren, R. B. Sloan, & G. D. Cohen (Eds.), *Handbook of mental health and aging* (2nd ed., pp. 339-354). San Diego, CA: Academic Press, Inc.

Dellasega, C. (1998). Assessment of cognition in the elderly: Pieces of a complex puzzle. *Nursing Clinics of North America, 33*(3), 395-405.

Ebersole, P., & Hess, P. (1998). *Toward healthy aging: Human needs and nursing response* (5th ed.). St. Louis, MO: Mosby.

Eliopoulos, C. (1993). *Gerontological nursing* (3rd ed.). Baltimore: Lippincott Williams & Wilkins.

Ferrell, B. A. (1991). Pain management in elderly people. *Journal of the American Geriatrics Society, 39*, 64-73.

Ferrell, B. R., & Ferrell, B. A. (1990). Easing the pain. *Geriatric Nursing, 4*, 175-178.

Forrest, J. (1995). Assessment of acute and chronic pain in older adults. *Journal of Gerontological Nursing, 10*, 15-20.

Hultsch, D. F., & Dixon, R. A. (1990). Learning and memory in aging. In J. E. Birren & K. W. Schaie (Eds.), *Handbook of psychology of aging* (3rd ed., pp. 258-290). San Diego, CA: Academic Press.

Mahoney, D. F. (1993). Cerumen impaction: Prevalence and detection in nursing homes. *Journal of Gerontological Nursing, 4*(19), 23-30.

Matthews, K., Cauley, J., Yaffe, K., & Zmuda, J. M. (1999). Estrogen replacement therapy and cognitive decline in older community women. *Journal of the American Geriatrics Society, 47*(5), 518-523.

Mayo Medical Essay Supplement to Mayo Clinic Health Letter. (1995). *Vision and your eyes: Managing common problems.* Rochester, MN: Mayo Foundation for Medical Education and Research.

Meltzer, D. W. (1983). Ophthalmic aspects. In F. U. Steinberg (Ed.), *Care of the geriatric patient* (6th ed., pp. 450-461). St. Louis, MO: Mosby.

Nusbaum, N. J. (1999). Aging and sensory senescence. *Southern Medical Journal, 92*(3), 267-275.

Rinn, W. E. (1988). Mental decline in normal aging: A review. *Journal of Geriatric Psychology and Neurology, 1*, 144-148.

Salthouse, T. A. (1990). Cognitive competence and expertise in aging. In J. E. Birren & K. W. Schaie (Eds.), *Handbook of the psychology of aging* (3rd ed., pp. 310-319). San Diego, CA: Academic Press.

Saxon, S. V., & Etten, M. J. (1994). *Physical change and aging* (3rd ed.). New York: Tiresias Press.

Schaie, K. W. (1994). The course of adult intellectual development. *American Psychologist, 49*(4), 304-313.

Schaie, K. W., & Willis, S. L. (1986). Can decline in adult cognitive function be reversed? *Developmental Psychology, 22*, 223-232.

Schieber, F. (1992). Aging and the sense. In J. E. Birren, R. B. Sloane, & G. D. Cohen (Eds.), *Handbook of the mental health and aging* (2nd ed., pp. 251-306). San Diego, CA: Academic Press.

Ship, J. A., Pearson, J. D., Cruise, L. J., Brant, L. J., & Metter, E. J. (1996). Longitudinal changes in smell identification. *Journal of Gerontology: Medical Science, 51A*(2), M86-M91.

Shklar, G. (1966). The effects of aging on oral mucosa. *Journal of Investigative Dermatology, 47*, 115-120.

Tallis, R., Fillit, H., & Brocklehurst, J. C. (Eds.). (1998). *Brocklehurst's textbook of geriatric medicine and gerontology* (5th ed.). New York: Churchill Livingstone.

Verillo, R. T. (1980). Age-related changes in sensitivity and vibration. *Journal of Gerontology, 35*, 185-190.

Wiley, T. L., Cruickshanks, K. J., Nondahl, D. M., Tweed, T. S., Klein, R., Klein, R., & Klein, B. E. (1998). Aging and high-frequency hearing sensitivity. *Journal of Speech, Language, & Hearing Research, 41*(5), 1061-1072.

Yen, P. (1996). When food doesn't taste good anymore. *Geriatric Nursing, 17*, 44-45.

Zhu, I., Viitanen, M., Guo, Z., Winblad, B., & Fratiglioni, L. (1998). Blood pressure reduction, cardiovascular diseases, and cognitive decline in the mini-mental state examination in a community population of normal very old people: a three-year follow-up. *Journal of Clinical Epidemiology, 51*(5), 385-391.

CHAPTER 34

CHRONIC CONFUSION

Linda A. Gerdner and Geri Richards Hall

Alzheimer's disease (AD) is the most common dementia among elderly persons; however, chronic confusion is characteristic of persons with Alzheimer's Disease and Related Disorders (ADRD). ADRD includes AD and a number of other dementias, such as multiinfarct dementia and Pick's disease. In 1997, AD was reported to affect 2.32 million people in the United States (range 1.09 to 4.58 million). It is projected that this number will quadruple by 2050 (Brookmeyer, Gray, & Kawas, 1998). Because of the prolonged duration of the disease and the lack of funding for professional nursing services, 80% to 90% of people with ADRD are cared for in their homes by family members (OTA, 1987).

Many persons with ADRD exhibit a state of chronic confusion, which greatly complicates their care. Care of persons with chronic confusion usually occurs in the home, since hospital care is limited to short periods of time and to persons who have acute conditions. Caring for a relative with chronic confusion is among the most difficult of family responsibilities. Caregivers often receive inadequate support and training and can experience significant emotional, physical, and financial stress. The stress associated with caring for someone with ADRD has been linked to a number of adverse outcomes, including depression (Cohen & Eisdorfer, 1988; Dura, Stukenberg, & Kiecolt-Glaser, 1990, 1991; Gallagher, Rose, Rivera, Lovett, & Thompson, 1989; Gallagher-Thompson & Powers, 1997; Pearson, Teri, Wagner, Truax, & Logsdon, 1993), high psychotropic drug use (Kuhlman, Wilson, Hutchinson, & Wallhagen, 1991; Mort, Gaspar, Juffer, & Kovarna, 1996; Pruchno & Potashnik, 1989), decline in physical health (Bergman-Evans, 1994; Chenoweth & Spencer, 1986; Pruchno & Potashnik, 1989; Schulz, O'Brien, Bookwala, & Fleissner, 1995); and compromised immune response (Esterling, Kiecolt-Glaser, Bodnar, & Glaser, 1994; Kiecolt-Glaser, Dura, Speicher, Trask, & Glaser, 1991; Kiecolt-Glaser et al., 1987).

A reduction in the patient's environmental stress can result in a slower rate of physical and behavioral deterioration, reduced anxiety and catastrophic behavior, and increased quality of life for both patients and caregivers. The Progressively Lowered Stress Threshold (PLST) model can serve as a conceptual framework for nursing interventions and individualization of care.

RELATED FACTORS/ETIOLOGIES

Chronic confusion due to progressive degeneration of the cerebral cortex indicates a lack of integration among stimuli, perception, and memory to assign meaning and responses to stimuli. The pathologies causing degeneration of the cerebral cortex are varied; however, the resulting behaviors are relatively similar for many of the dementing illnesses. The most common cause is Alzheimer's disease (AD), characterized by an insidious onset and inexorable progression. AD is thought to cause between 60% and 75% of diagnosed dementias (Hull, 1996; Jellinger, Danielczyk, Fischer, & Gabriel, 1990).

AD involves several chemically specific neural systems, or networks of nerve cells in the brain, that produce neurotransmitters. Research has shown that nerve cells in selected parts of the brain are particularly vulnerable to AD. The greatest neurotransmitter losses occur in the cholinergic system, which produces acetylcholine (ACh) and affects learning and memory functions. In fact, a 75% reduction in ACh cells in the nucleus basalis of Meynert and a 50% reduction of norepinephrine cells in the locus ceruleus have been reported in persons with AD (Coyle, Price, & DeLong, 1983). The degree of deficit in choline acetyltransferase (CHAT) correlates with the degree of dementia and the extent of cortical neuritic plaque formation (Davie, 1983). Research also suggests that excitotoxins, such as the amino acids glutamate and aspartate, might be related to AD in that they can damage or even destroy brain cells (Olney, Wozniak, & Farber, 1997).

Other investigators have focused their studies on an abnormal fibrous protein called amyloid that accumulates in the neuritic plaques that are characteristic of AD. There are several known steps in the process by which a normal brain cell protein degenerates into the beta amyloid fragments that form the core of the neuritic plaques. Investigation is now underway to determine how other brain proteins undergo phosphorylation, producing the molecular changes to form neurofibrillary tangles (Advisory Panel on Alzheimer's Disease, 1991).

Neuritic plaques are an important target of research because they cluster near the brain's communication points. The number of plaques has been shown to be positively correlated with disturbances in memory and intellectual functioning. Scientists are looking at both the function of amyloid and the mechanism(s) that cause its breakdown in AD (Advisory Panel on Alzheimer's Disease, 1991). Of note is the recent finding that the gene that codes for the amyloid precursor protein is located on the twenty-first chromosome, near the region of trisomy 21. Interestingly in Down's syndrome, AD-like pathologic changes occur in the brain by middle age, and this pathology is attributed to triplication of the twenty-first chromosome. Diffuse amyloid plaques have also been noted in adolescents with Down's syndrome.

Researchers have reported that genes on the nineteenth (Roses et al., 1990) and twenty-first chromosomes might be associated with a familial (hereditary), early-onset type of AD (FAD) that affects 5% to 10% of persons with AD (St. George-Hyslop et al., 1987). The exact mechanism of gene action in FAD is as yet unknown. Population genetic studies have also offered strong evidence of a familial factor in some cases of AD (Huff, Auerback, Chakravarti, & Boller, 1988). However, studies of AD in identical twins indicate that environmental as well as genetic factors contribute to the onset of the disorder (Gatz et al., 1997; Raiha, Kaprio, Koskenvuo, Rajala, & Sourander, 1996, 1998).

Apolipoprotein E (APOE) genotype on the nineteenth chromosome has been identified as a major risk factor for late-onset FAD (Morrison-Bogorad, 1993). APOE has three major allelic variants: e2, e3, and e4. Individuals with an APOE genotype e4/e4 combination (derived from both parents) are at a dramatically higher risk for developing AD than individuals with the APOE genotype e2/e3 (Corder et al., 1995).

In 1992 researchers reported genetic linkage of FAD to a locus on chromosome 14 (Mullan et al., 1992; Schellenberg et al., 1992). Almost 70% of persons with FAD have this chromosome 14 linkage (Peskind, 1996). In addition, research has shown an association between AD and loci on chromosome 1 (Bird et al., 1996; Levy-Lahad, Wasco et al., 1995; Levy-Lahad, Wijsman et al., 1995).

Because several dementing disorders (e.g., kuru, Creutzfeldt-Jakob disease) are caused by viral or infectious agents, it has been suggested that AD also might be caused by a virus or infectious agent (Prusiner, 1984). Recent studies suggest that herpes simplex virus (HSV1) might be a cofactor in the pathogenesis of AD (Itzhaki et al., 1997; Lin, Casas, Wilcock, & Itzhaki, 1997).

Theories related to heavy metal intoxication, especially from aluminum, manganese, and silicon, are plausible; the neurofibrillary tangles and neuritic plaques found in the brains of persons with AD have been associated with high levels of aluminum (Perl & Brody, 1980). However, research in this area is quite inconsistent, and aluminum and silicon deposits might be the result of cell degradation and death rather than the cause (Belojevic & Jakovljevic, 1998; Strunecka & Patocka, 1999).

A second major cause of degenerative decline in the cerebral cortex is multiple infarctions, or strokes. North

American Nursing Diagnosis Association (NANDA) continues to refer to this condition as multiinfarct disease (MID). However, in 1994 the American Psychiatric Association relabeled this condition "vascular dementia" (p. 143). Consequently, NANDA terminology is not systematically linked with the *Diagnostic and Statistical Manual of Mental Disorders,* fourth edition (DSM-IV), which is the primary basis for both diagnosis and reimbursement for psychiatric care.

Vascular dementia has been reported to account for 15% to 20% of dementing illness (Malone, 1994; Mirsen & Hachinski, 1988). Although the onset of the disease can be slow, vascular dementia is characterized by a step-like progression as each new infarction occurs. Combinations of AD and vascular dementia have been reported to account for another 7% to 18% of dementing illnesses (Malone, 1994; Mirsen & Hachinski, 1988). Variations in prevalence statistics may be due to changes in diagnostic criteria and terminology over time (Jorm, 1990).

Environmental factors also have been implicated in the onset of AD. In particular, brain trauma has been postulated as a major risk factor of AD (Graves et al., 1990; Nemetz et al., 1999; O'Meara et al., 1997; Schofield et al., 1997). It is thought that head trauma (especially trauma resulting in loss of consciousness), anoxia, or other insults to the brain (such as alcohol) might lead to the production of excess amounts of the amyloid precursor and the development of neuritic plaques. For example, the brains of prizefighters that suffer from dementia pugilistica contain diffuse plaques and neurofibrillary tangles, although the latter are distributed differently than in AD.

The last 13% of dementing illnesses are rare. A few of these illnesses may be amenable to treatment. Pick's disease is a progressive dementia characterized by the formation of Pick's cells, primarily in the frontal and temporal lobes. The patient exhibits amnesia, aphasia, and losses of socially appropriate behavior and inhibitions.

Creutzfeldt-Jakob disease (CJ disease) is an infectious disease thought to be caused by a slow virus and characterized by a rapid onset and progression. The patient exhibits myoclonus in addition to the demented behaviors. Life span is usually 12 to 18 months after symptoms appear. Because of the viral nature of the disease, the patient should be placed on blood and secretion/excretion precautions. However, to date there are no documented cases of nursing personnel contracting the disease from an infected patient.

Normal pressure hydrocephalus (NPH) is a treatable dementia characterized by the early onset of aphasia, incontinence, and ataxia. The excess accumulation of fluid in the cranial cavity causes the ventricles to enlarge, compressing the cortex. The disease is treated by implanting a shunt in a ventricle to drain excess fluid.

Toxic substance ingestion, including ingestion of alcohol, barbiturates, opioids, cocaine, amphetamines, hallucinogens, caffeine, and tobacco, can cause dementia.

Carbon monoxide and some metals, such as lead, also can cause dementia. In some cases the dementia resolves with the cessation of substance use.

Emotional disorders such as depression are frequently called "pseudodementia" because they tend to mimic the symptoms. Depression is a treatable disorder.

Degenerative neurologic diseases such as Parkinson's disease, Friedreich's ataxia, progressive supranuclear palsy, Wilson's disease, multiple sclerosis, and Huntington's disease can cause cognitive loss. Diffuse Lewy body syndrome initially presents as AD, yet is caused by the formation of Lewy bodies in the parietal lobes rather than subcortically. As the dementia progresses, patients increasingly develop parkinsonian signs and symptoms as well as florid psychotic symptoms that may not respond to antipsychotic medications.

Tumors, subdural hematomas, trauma, and conditions causing insufficient oxygenation affect the structure or integrity of the brain. Some of these conditions may be amenable to medical treatment.

Fungal, bacterial, and viral infections, including tuberculosis, meningitis, and encephalitis, can produce dementia. Persons with acquired immune deficiency syndrome (AIDS) may develop an encephalitis in the later stages of the disease (Bell, 1998). Autoimmune diseases such as temporal arteritis and lupus erythematosus can also cause dementia-like syndromes (Caselli & Hunder, 1997; Camdessanche et al., 1997).

Finally, alterations in confusion can result from pathophysiologic changes in biologic compounds; these alterations are reversible if treated. Usually referred to as delirium or acute confusion, these alterations in behavior have a rapid onset, are transient, and result in an altered state of awareness that renders the patient cognitively and socially inaccessible. Figure 34-1 demonstrates the relationship of acute confusion to chronic confusion as conceptualized by Wolanin and Phillips (1981). Refer to Chapter 35 (Acute

Confusion) for an in-depth discussion of acute confusion. It is interesting to note that NANDA has identified age greater than 60 years as a related factor for acute confusion, but not for chronic confusion (Gordon, 1995).

ASSESSMENT

In the 1960s the symptoms associated with ADRD were categorized into three groups of losses: cognitive, affective, and conative (planning) or functional. The presence of several behavioral symptoms in each group or cluster appeared to be indicative of a dementing illness. However, the symptoms still allowed for enormous variety in clinical presentation among individuals (Ballinger, 1982; Gottfries, Barnes, & Steen, 1982; Venn, 1983). Researchers noted the presence of other symptoms, such as confusion, agitation, night wakening, wandering, and combative behavior, but failed to incorporate these into existing clusters or to create a new cluster. Hall and Buckwalter (1987) incorporated these symptoms into a separate cluster entitled "progressively lowered stress threshold." The symptom clusters for Chronic Confusion are listed in Table 34-1.

These behaviors are consistent with the deterioration found on positron emission tomography (PET) scans and on autopsy. Researchers report that scans demonstrate significant deterioration in the posterior parietal and occipital lobes of the brain and in the hippocampus. These areas are responsible for receiving stimuli, assigning meaning, and coordinating responses. This function is called cerebral integration, and damage in this area helps to explain the clusters of symptoms presented by patients with ADRD (Burns & Buckwalter, 1988).

Identification of patients suffering from cognitive loss assists nurses in determining which patients would benefit from environments and programs that promote safety and maximize function (Rader & Doan, 1985). Nurses are often expected to provide care to patients experiencing

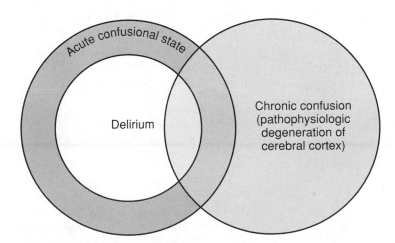

FIGURE **34-1**   The relationship of etiologies of alterations in thought processes. (Adapted from Wolanin, M. O., & Phillips, L. [1981]. *Confusion: Prevention and care.* St. Louis, MO: Mosby.)

Defining Characteristics and Related Factors/Etiologies	
Table 34-1 CHRONIC CONFUSION	
Chronic Confusion (NANDA, 1999)	**Chronic Confusion: Alzheimer's Disease and Related Disorders (Hall, 1991)**
DEFINING CHARACTERISTICS	
Altered interpretation/response to stimuli; clinical evidence of organic impairment; progressive/long-standing cognitive impairment; altered personality; impaired memory (short- and long-term); impaired socialization; no change in level of consciousness	Irreversible dementing illness • Cognitive or intellectual losses: Loss of memory, initially for progressive degeneration of the cerebral cortex (SDAT) recent events; loss of time sense; inability to abstract such as understanding safety needs; inability to make choices and decisions, to problem solve and reason; poor judgment; altered perceptions; loss of language abilities • Affective or personality losses: Loss of affect; diminished inhibitions, characterized by emotional lability, spontaneous conversation and loss of tact, loss of control of temper; inability to delay gratification; decreased attention span; social withdrawal; loss of recognition of others, environment, and, eventually, self (agnosia); increasing self-preoccupation; antisocial behavior; confabulation, perseveration, psychotic features such as paranoia, delusions, and pseudohallucinations; increased fatigue with exertion or cognition, loss of energy reserve • Conative or planning losses: Loss of general ability to plan activities, especially those requiring thought to set goal, organize, and carry out; functional loss starting with high level and transportation and progressing to losses in ADL in generally the following order: bathing, grooming, choosing clothing, dressing, mobility, toileting, communicating, and eating (Reisberg et al., 1982); motor apraxia (the inability to plan and coordinate voluntary motor activity) • Progressively lowered stress threshold: Catastrophic behaviors characterized by cognitive and social inaccessibility; purposeful wandering; violent, agitated, or anxious behavior, purposeless behavior; withdrawal or avoidance behavior such as belligerence; compulsive repetitive behavior; other cognitively or socially inaccessible behaviors
RELATED FACTORS/ETIOLOGIES	
Alzheimer's disease; Korsakoff's psychosis; multiinfarct dementia; cerebral vascular accident; head injury	Irreversible dementing illness (progressive degeneration of the cerebral cortex) • Alzheimer's disease • Vascular dementia • Head trauma Rare and/or occasionally reversible dementing illnesses • Pick's disease • Creutzfeldt-Jakob disease • Normal pressure hydrocephalus • Toxic substance ingestion • Emotional disorders • Degenerative neurologic disease • Diffuse Lewy body syndrome • Conditions affecting the structure or integrity of the brain • Metabolic disorders • Infections • Autoimmune disease (AIDS, temporal arteritis, lupus erythematosus) • Subcortical dementia, including Parkinson's disease (American Psychiatric Association, 1994; Jorm, 1990; Mace & Rabins, 1991; Morris, 1996; Office of Technological Assessment, 1987; Weiner, 1996)

cognitive decline when no medical diagnosis of dementia has been established. In many settings where gerontologic nurses practice, administration of cognitive assessment instruments is required for screening and development of an appropriate plan of care.

Environmental factors affect nursing judgments about confusion. Morgan (1985) reported that patient and setting characteristics influenced nurses' perceptions of mental confusion. Subjects were less likely to be assessed as confused when residing in a large institution than when residing in a small one. Nurses were more likely to perceive confusion and communication difficulties if a subject was dependent in activities of daily living (ADL) or if the patient was older than the median age for patients in that home. Results of these studies are strengthened by attitudinal surveys suggesting that nurses stereotype older people, preferring to care for younger patients. These ageist attitudes can affect the care provided and goals set regarding quality of life (Knowles & Sarver, 1985).

The nursing, medical, and allied health care literature contains numerous assessment instruments and scales for evaluating cognitive impairment. The Short Portable Mental Status Questionnaire (SPMSQ) and the Mini-Mental Status Examination (MMSE) are brief evaluations of current mental status. These tools were developed to assist health professionals screen patients for altered mental status, thereby determining the need for further medical evaluation. Both instruments test recent and past memory, temporal orientation, quick recall, and ability to abstract and calculate. The MMSE also asks patients to carry out simple motor tasks. The scores of both instruments indicate the severity of cognitive impairment. Each instrument has limitations (Blessed, Tomlinson, & Roth, 1968; Folstein, Folstein, & McHugh, 1975; Hays, 1984; Isaacs & Akhtar, 1972; Isaacs & Kennie, 1973; Pfeiffer, 1975). Short assessments evaluating mental status changes can yield false positive results with their use (Mattis, 1976; Morgan, 1985; Nagley, 1986; Palmateer & McCarthy, 1985; Winograd, 1984). These instruments rely on the person's ability to respond verbally and in writing. In addition, mental status examination are limited in their ability to detect sensitivity in the disease process over time (Reisberg, 1988). Studies show that scores on the MMSE are related to education, age, and ethnicity (Anthony, LeResche, Niaz, VonKorff, & Folsteen, 1982; Bohnstedt, Fox, & Kohatsu, 1994; Crum, Anthony, Bassett, & Folstein, 1993; Escobar et al., 1986; Fillenbaum, Hughes, Heyman, George, & Blazer, 1988; Hill et al., 1993; Jorm, Scott, Henerson, & Kay, 1988).

Most brief screening tests for dementia focus on verbal memory and orientation. However, the Clock Drawing assesses cognitive function specific to visuospatial aspects, constructional abilities, and abstract thinking (Sunderland et al., 1989). This quick, easy-to-administer instrument produces a numeric score to establish a severity rating of dementia. Recent studies have been conducted to establish the instrument's psychometric properties (Ferrucci et al., 1996; Rouleau, Salmon, & Butters, 1996).

The Global Deterioration Scale (GDS) is used to assess clinically identifiable stages of ADRD (Reisberg, Ferris, de Leon, & Crook, 1982). However, late-stage disease presents problems for this assessment (as well as for the MMSE and SPMSQ), as patients score "0" long before death. This phenomenon is termed the "floor effect."

The "floor effect" limitation has been addressed successfully by the Functional Assessment Staging Test (FAST), which was developed to correspond to the seven stages of the Global Deterioration Scale (Reisberg et al., 1984). The FAST was designed to characterize aspects of the patient's daily functioning through 16 ordinal functioning assessment stages ranging from normality to severe dementia of the Alzheimer's type (Reisberg et al., 1984). The progression of deficits on the FAST was designed to mirror the characteristic progression of functional loss in dementia of the Alzheimer's type. FAST has undergone extensive testing to establish validity and reliability (Auer, Sclan, Yaffee, & Reisberg, 1994; Franssen, Kluger, Torossian, & Reisberg, 1993; Reisberg et al., 1984; Sclan & Reisberg, 1992; Souder, Saykin, & Alavi, 1995; Williams & Smith, 1994). FAST can stage in relative detail dementia patients who, because of the severity of their deficits, achieve only bottom scores on the MMSE. In addition, FAST can stage mild dementia patients who may appear normal or achieve perfect or near-perfect scores on widely used mental status measures (Reisberg, 1988; Auer et al., 1994).

The Alzheimer's Disease Assessment Scale (ADAS) is a widely used instrument to assess the severity of cognitive and noncognitive behavioral dysfunction characteristic of persons with AD (Rosen, Mohs, & Davis, 1984). Importantly, the ADAS, like the FAST, is sensitive to detecting changes in the disease process over time. These and other assessment instruments can be used by nurse clinicians and researchers to plot the trajectory of the patient's cognitive impairment.

Home Assessment

In-home assessment provides the opportunity to observe the interaction between the impaired person and the environment in relation to symptom presentation. Nurses should evaluate the following factors: Is the home noisy, cluttered, quiet, and/or generally safe? If there are family members living with the patient, what are the living arrangements? Does the patient spend much time alone? Are family members supportive, or do they challenge the patient's losses, finding them embarrassing or annoying? What are the interactions like between patient and family members?

An initial history of mental status changes should be obtained. Determining the patient's premorbid personality, including educational level, occupation, hobbies, relationships with family prior to illness, daily routine, and methods used for relaxation, helps the nurse and staff in identifying the meaning of behavioral patterns and responses after admission. The onset of mental status changes and any medical or psychiatric conditions that might be contributing to those changes, such as a history of heart disease or hypothyroidism, will help to determine the need for further medical evaluation prior to admission (Hall & Buckwalter, 1991). Despite their importance, NANDA does not address premorbid conditions.

As part of the assessment process, nurses should discuss the defining characteristics or symptom clusters with the family (see Table 34-1), as they cue additional information. For example, many families assume memory loss is a normal part of the aging process and attribute other symptoms, such as inability to inhibit behavior, as willfulness. By providing behavioral examples for the family, the nurse will develop a comprehensive understanding of the patient's symptom clusters and the global nature of the illness.

The family should be encouraged to describe dysfunctional behaviors, as the person with ADRD will tend to repeat the same pattern. The nurse will want to determine the onset and duration of stress-related behaviors and any triggers, such as large social gatherings or concerns about money. Stress-related events should be described, such as characteristics of wandering or combativeness. Measures

to relieve these events should also be discussed. This will assist family caregivers in coping with problematic behaviors. It also assists the nursing staff to determine if the impaired person can be cared for in the nursing home environment and to prevent and/or prepare for such events in the future.

The patient's functional level should be assessed both for basic ADL and for maintenance activities such as socialization and daily routine. The nurse will use this information to determine the level of supervision, direction, and assistance required to accomplish bathing, dressing, ambulating, toileting, and eating. The family should be encouraged to share any special techniques or management strategies they use to ensure success.

Assessment of the family and/or caregiver should also take place. The psychosocial history of the family, how they coped with past problems, and perceptions of nursing home placement all will affect patient behavior and thus the plan of care. If the family perceives placement as a catastrophe, as failure on their part to care for a family member, or as the breakup of a family, the nurse and social worker can develop special measures to assist the family in resolving these issues.

Ongoing assessment is required for community-based care as well as for admission to long-term care. The numerous aspects of a patient's life that need to be assessed and techniques for assessment are summarized in Table 34-2.

Table 34-2	Ongoing Assessment for Community-Based or Facility-Based Care	
Level	Title	Technique
1	Getting to know the impaired person	Time: Early in the day or reported best time of day
		Location: Quiet area away from others
		Speak clearly in a low-pitched voice; use simple sentences
		Patient requires more time to process information and respond
		Use of family data from psychosocial history
2	Observe nonverbal behavior	Gestures, eye contact, motor skills, response time
3	Environmental comprehension	Help the patient express her fears
4	Functional level and social participation	Resident's participation in activities
		Socialization with other residents
		Instrumental ADL
		Favorite activities
		ADL—level of direction/supervision/assistance
5	Psychologic status	Assessment of physical health at baseline and every time confusion increases or other symptoms present
		Evaluate medication regularly
6	Stress-related behaviors	Describe antecedents, behaviors, and consequences
		Try to identify causative factors
		Modify plan of care to prevent future occurrence
7	Continued assessment of caregivers and families	Frequency and quality of family visits and interaction
		Family may provide counseling and additional support
		Conflict with other family members
		Relationship with staff
		Describe antecedents, behaviors, and consequences

CHRONIC CONFUSION
Alzheimer's Disease and Related Disorders

In 1973 NANDA developed the nursing diagnosis Altered Thought Processes, defined as "a state in which an individual experiences a disruption in cognitive operations and activities" (Carroll-Johnson, 1989, p. 553; NANDA, 1999, p. 120). Defining characteristics include inaccurate interpretation of the environment, cognitive dissonance, distractibility, memory deficit/problems, egocentricity, hypervigilance, and hypovigilance. Historically, persons with dementia most closely fit this diagnosis. In 1994 NANDA added Chronic Confusion to their list of nursing diagnoses specifically tailored for persons with ADRD. NANDA defines Chronic Confusion as "an irreversible, long-standing and/or progressive deterioration of intellect and personality characterized by decreased ability to interpret environmental stimuli, decreased capacity for intellectual thought processes and manifested by disturbances of memory, orientation, and behavior" (Carroll-Johnson & Paquette, 1994; Gordon, 1995, p. 281; NANDA, 1999, p. 119). Related factors and defining characteristics of Chronic Confusion as identified by NANDA (1999) are listed in Table 34-1 and compared to those identified by Hall (1991). The NANDA behaviors tend to be less specific and provide less direction for the development of a care plan that incorporates the pathophysiology of cortical degeneration.

Hall (1988) has identified four distinct stages of functional decline with ADRD that can be used in planning care (Box 34-1). In comparison, NANDA does not describe disease staging.

Persons with a chronic dementing illness experience losses in four cognitive domains or clusters: cognitive, affective, conative, and stress threshold. Behavioral symptoms from each cluster will be present in all persons with ADRD. However, symptoms will be exhibited differently depending on the size and location of lesions within the cerebral cortex, the premorbid personality, cultural and ethnic affiliations, and external demands and resources (Hall & Buckwalter, 1987). Most patients exhibit three main types of affective behavior: baseline, anxious, and dysfunctional or catastrophic.

Baseline behavior is functional behavior that is characterized by two features. The patient is cognitively accessible, meaning there is a basic awareness of the environment and an ability to interact calmly and function within the limits of the neurologic deficit. The patient is also socially accessible, meaning he or she is able to communicate needs and respond to the communications of others. Baseline or normative behavior is generally a calm state incorporating the cognitive, affective, and conative behav-

---

| Box 34-1 | Stages of Chronic Confusion: Alzheimer's Disease and Other Related Disorders |

1. Forgetful—The client has begun to forget and lose things, expressing awareness of the problem and compensating for losses. This might compromise job performance, but a problem is not diagnosable at this time. Problems are usually attributed to stress, illness, or fatigue. Depression is not uncommon.
2. Confused—The client has difficulty with maintenance activities such as money management, legal affairs, occupational affairs, transportation and driving, home maintenance, housekeeping, and cooking. Family members are aware of problems and may seek medical attention for the client. Client may deny problem but gives frequent "clues" about "losing my mind." Client may become depressed and withdraw from occupational and social activities. Personality changes become evident. Client has difficulty functioning in strange environments, such as on vacation. Behaviors related to lowered stress threshold occur when under extreme stress, fatigue, change, or illness. Clients living alone may be placed in daycare or long-term care because of compromised safety or inability to manage necessary tasks.
3. Ambulatory dementia—Functional losses in ADL occur in approximately the following order: loss of bathing; grooming; choosing clothing; dressing; gait and mobility; toileting; communication; reading; and writing skills. The client begins to withdraw from the family group, becoming increasingly self-absorbed. Depression resolves, and the person appears to be unaware of losses at times. Stress threshold behaviors are common, and the person may be up at night, wandering, confused, agitated, pacing, and/or belligerent. Client may become combative or withdraw. Communication becomes increasingly difficult as the client has increasing difficulty in understanding written and spoken language and in finding words. The client may return to using a primary language, which also may be distorted. Frustration is very common. The client's ability to reason, recognize others, and plan for safety is impaired. Families usually place the client in long-term care during the ambulatory-dementia stage.
4. End stage—The client no longer ambulates and has little purposeful activity. Recognition of family, self in a mirror, or body parts is generally gone; however, the client may experience moments of lucidity. The client is mute or may scream or yell spontaneously. The client forgets how to eat and loses much of his body weight. Problems associated with immobility, such as decubitus ulcers, urinary tract infections, contractures, and aspiration pneumonia are common. As the client becomes more vegetative, death usually results from pneumonia or another complication.

Data from Hall, G. R. (1988). Care of the patient with Alzheimer's disease living at home. *Nursing Clinics of North America,* 23(1), 31-46.

ioral losses with the premorbid personality and lifelong cultural and coping patterns. However, baseline behavior deteriorates with the progression of the disease and is replaced by increasing amounts of anxious and dysfunctional behavior.

Anxious behavior occurs when the patient experiences stress. The patient might complain of feeling uneasy. Eye contact is usually lost, and there is a perceptible increase in psychomotor activity as the patient attempts to avoid offending stimuli. For example, the patient might attempt to leave or return to his room. Although anxious, the patient is still able to communicate with staff and family.

Dysfunctional behavior results if the stress level is allowed to continue or increase. Catastrophic events are sudden changes from baseline behavior characterized by cognitive and social inaccessibility. The patient is unable to communicate effectively with others and is unable to use the environment in a functionally appropriate manner (Wolanin & Phillips, 1981). Most catastrophic episodes are characterized by fearfulness, panic, and vigorous attempts to avoid offensive stimuli (Hall, Kirschling, & Todd, 1986). Examples of additional catastrophic behavior include confusion, purposeful wandering, night wakening, "sundowner's syndrome," agitation, combativeness, or sudden withdrawal. These behaviors usually appear suddenly and last a relatively short period of time, presenting a tremendous challenge to caregivers. Caregivers often cite dysfunctional or catastrophic episodes as reasons to institutionalize patients in nursing homes or acute care facilities.

Catastrophic behaviors were recognized to be stress related in the early 1960s. Research has shown that internal stressors such as pain (Cohen-Mansfield, 1986; Cohen-Mansfield et al., 1990; Ferrell & Ferrell, 1995) or infection (Cohen-Mansfield, Werner, & Marx, 1990; Ragneskog, Gerdner, Josefsson, & Kihlgren, 1998) can cause disfunctional behavior. In a survey of relocated elders, Aldrich and Mendkoff (1963) identified the role of stress in producing dysfunctional behavior. Lawton and Nahemow (1973) suggest that functional behavior is likely to occur when the external demands (stressors) on the older individual are adjusted to the level to which the person has adapted. It is logical that persons with ADRD need their environmental demands modified to compensate for their declining ability to adapt.

Verwoerdt (1980) described catastrophic behaviors as primary anxiety resulting from an overwhelming influx of external or internal stimuli. The stimuli create psychologic states of stress to deal with the stressors when mastery is unobtainable, resulting in altered mental mechanisms and behavior patterns. Verwoerdt (1980) described the behavior created by primary anxiety as a "primitive response of diffuse painful pleasure" (p. 370). Mild cases can include restlessness, tension, or irritability. Severe cases are manifested by rage and defensive attempts to reestablish a stimulus barrier by avoidance behaviors such as repression, denial, magical thinking, and acting out. Frequently, the

concept of what is dangerous is impaired, affecting higher-order activities such as driving, operating machinery, and making patients susceptible to financial scams. Verwoerdt (1980) cites Cannon's concept of "fight or flight," suggesting that the situation might be resolved by adjusting and organizing the environment for the patient so that spatiotemporal relations remain constant and the loss of sense of mastery is minimized.

NANDA (1999) identifies "altered interpretation/response to stimuli" as a defining characteristic of Chronic Confusion (p. 120). The effect of stressors, an important factor in planning care, is not identified.

Adams and Lindemann (1974) identified four biologic mechanisms required for coping: movement, energy production, sensing, and cerebral integrating. If any of these mechanisms are compromised, individuals become disabled in their ability to cope with the environment. The first three mechanisms are normally somewhat compromised with the aging process. However, most changes occur slowly, and the person develops compensatory mechanisms. ADRD initially compromises the fourth mechanism. As the disease progresses, all mechanisms become deficient, placing the individual at progressively higher risk for dysfunctional coping. Although a key concept, NANDA does not address dysfunctional coping in relation to chronic confusion.

The role of stressors in producing dysfunctional behavior in the healthy person is diagrammed in a conceptual model in Figure 34-2. The model has been adapted for use with persons with ADRD (Hall & Buckwalter, 1987). As the disease progresses and brain cells are lost, the victim becomes less able to receive and process stimuli and information. This, coupled with losses in special senses, mobility, slowed synaptic responses, and diminished energy-producing hormones associated with normal aging, acts to compromise the patient's ability to adapt to stress and stimuli. A concomitant progressive decline in the stress threshold, which relies heavily on intact cerebral function, modifies the model as shown in Figure 34-3.

Persons with ADRD report increased levels of stress due to planning deficits, intolerance to multiple stimuli, and increased fatigue from processing information in their environment. This heightens the potential for anxiety, avoidance behavior, and catastrophic behavior (Hall & Buckwalter, 1987).

Numerous early studies involved manipulation of the environment of ADRD patients to produce increased levels of socialization or other desired responses (Hall, Kirschling, & Todd, 1986; Maas & Buckwalter, 1990; Negley & Manley, 1990). Those researchers who decreased environmental stimuli, such as moving the ADRD patients to small groups or decreasing the size of dining groups, noted increases in functional or baseline behavior. Researchers who increased stimuli by moving more chairs into a conversational circle found decreased functional behavior. In fact, patients repeatedly moved the additional

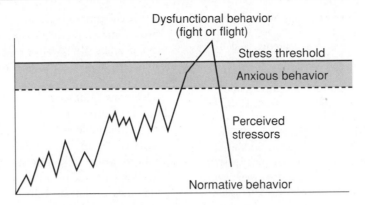

FIGURE **34-2**   Stress threshold in a "healthy" individual. (From Hall, G., & Buckwalter, K. [1987]. Progressively lowered stress threshold: A conceptual model for care of adults with Alzheimer's disease. *Archives of Psychiatric Nursing, 1*[6], 399-406.)

chairs out of the circle, returning them to the wall (Peterson, Knapp, Rosen, & Pither, 1977). Lawton (1980) reported similar effects on the ADRD unit at the Philadelphia Geriatric Center when ADRD patients spent 20% of their time alone in their room: socialization and social contact increased the remaining 80% of the time, and patients exhibited decreased incidence of catastrophic behavior, increased interest in external surroundings, increased meaningful nonsocial behavior, and decreased need for nursing care. Lawton's findings correspond to the "Environmental Docility Hypothesis" (Lawton & Simon, 1968), which states that external environmental factors become increasingly important determinants of behavior and affect as competence decreases.

CASE STUDY

K. Norman was a 72-year-old retired English professor who resided with his wife in their home of 40 years in a small midwestern college town. Over a period of 3 years, Mrs. Norman noticed Mr. Norman becoming increasingly forgetful, disorganized, and distant. Previously methodical, Mr. Norman began to make mistakes in the checkbook, miss appointments, and lose possessions. His

driving and temper became erratic, problems he blamed on his wife. He stopped paying bills, fearful that "they" would take his money. One day, while trying to discuss an article in the newspaper, Mrs. Norman came to the realization that her husband could no longer read. Fearful of the worst, she sought medical attention for him.

A local physician diagnosed Mr. Norman with ADRD. Mrs. Norman took Mr. Norman to a tertiary medical center for a second opinion, where the diagnosis of ADRD was confirmed. After their daughter, Sue, convinced her parents to move to her town, Mrs. Norman sold her home and she and her husband moved to a small apartment near their daughter.

The move caused Mr. Norman's symptoms to worsen. In familiar surroundings he had been able to manage on a daily basis without having to plan all activities. Within 6 months of moving, he required assistance with bathing and dressing. The unpacked boxes from the move made Mr. Norman fearful, so his wife stayed up nights to unpack while he slept. To rest, Mrs. Norman located a companion to stay with her husband during the day, but after the first day he refused to allow the companion in the house.

Mr. Norman began to think that pictures of people on the wall were real. Television made him think there were children in the room. In fear, he broke two mirrors. One night Mr. Norman woke his wife repeatedly, fearful that

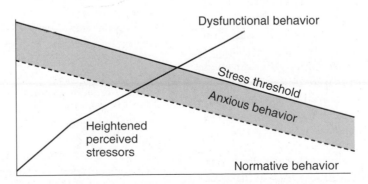

FIGURE **34-3**   Progressively lowered stress threshold. (From Hall, G., & Buckwalter, K. [1987]. Progressively lowered stress threshold: A conceptual model for care of adults with Alzheimer's disease. *Archives of Psychiatric Nursing, 1*[6], 399-406.)

the apartment was on fire. After 3 days of this fearful be-havior, he handed her a book in which he had found a picture of children sitting around a campfire, and he screamed "Fire, fire!"

In the next 2 weeks, Mr. Norman began to wander away from the apartment. Fearful for his safety and ex-hausted from lack of sleep, Mrs. Norman contacted a local nursing home. After much anguish and without the support of friends or children, she decided she had to place her husband in a care facility. The nurse and social worker made the initial assessment at the couple's apart-ment. A thorough assessment and social history were also completed and a nursing diagnosis of Chronic Confusion was identified.

NURSING-SENSITIVE OUTCOMES

The goals of nursing care for persons with Chronic Con-fusion are to maximize patient safety, comfort, and func-tion; to prevent complications associated with chronic illness and increasing immobility; and to improve quality of life for both patients and caregivers. The Progressively Lowered Stress Threshold (PLST) model (Hall & Buck-walter, 1987) provides as a conceptual framework in which outcomes of care for persons with Chronic Confusion are linked to levels of stress. According to the PLST model, re-duction of environmental stress through the caregiver training intervention should result in a slower rate of physical and behavioral deterioration. Because people with ADRD have less demand on their cognitive process-ing abilities in an environment with reduced sensory stimuli, they are expected to use remaining cognitive abil-ities more effectively. In turn, this should result in slower decline and greater retention of functional abilities such as dressing, grooming, toileting, and eating. Likewise, it is hy-pothesized that diminished stress on cognitive processing will result in reduced anxiety and catastrophic behaviors. Improved nutritional status is also expected, which would be reflected through stabilization in weight at least until the endstage of the disease. These outcomes should allow a person with ADRD to remain at home for a longer period of time, thus reducing overall costs of care. The ultimate goal is increased quality of life for both caregivers and pa-tients (Buckwalter et al., 1992; Gerdner, Hall, & Buckwal-ter, 1996). In one study conducted by Hall and colleagues (1986), after a 3-month intervention, the following changes in behavior of patients were observed: increased socialization, stable weight or gain in weight, and reduc-tion of psychotropic or neuroleptic medications, seda-tives, and tranquilizers. Residents appeared calm, and agi-tation and wandering episodes decreased.

In addition, it is expected that family caregiver train-ing based on the PLST model will increase the caregiver's knowledge of ADRD and the family's competence in managing problematic behaviors. Research has shown

that such training results in improved mood, affect, sense of mastery, and satisfaction and in decreased care-giver burden (Buckwalter et al., 1999). More specifically, caregivers report less depression (Buckwalter et al., 1999).

Nursing Outcomes Classifications (NOC) have not been established for the nursing diagnosis of Chronic Confusion. Table 34-3 includes nursing classification out-comes consistent with the PLST model and family inter-ventions. Both strive for a safe environment that compen-sates for patients' cognitive and functional impairments. Outcomes associated with the PLST model focus on a quantifiable decrease in problematic behaviors; in con-trast, NOC (Iowa Outcomes Project, 2000) addresses symptom control in relation to emotional functioning and mood equilibrium. Both strive to improve the quality of life for the patient through improved nutrition, sleep, and social interaction. Both address improved quality of life for family members. Outcomes based on the PLST model state improved mood, sense of mastery/satisfaction, and decreased burden. They are as follows:

Safety Behavior: Home Physical Environment—"Individ-ual or caregiver actions to minimize environment factors that might cause physical harm or injury in the home" (Iowa Outcomes Project, 2000, p. 373).
Nutritional Status: Food & Fluid Intake—"Amount of food and fluid taken into the body over a 24 hour prior" (p. 323).
Sleep—"Extent and pattern natural periodic suspension of consciousness during which the body is restored" (p. 403).
Comfort Level—"Extent of physical and psychological ease" (p. 173).
Communication Ability—"Ability to receive, interpret, and express spoken, written, and nonverbal message" (p. 174).
Social Interaction Skills—"An individual's use of effective interaction behaviors" (p. 404).
Coping—"Actions to manage stressors that tax an individ-ual's resources" (p. 192).
Symptom Control—"Personal actions to minimize per-ceived adverse changes in physical and emotional func-tioning" (p. 419).
Mood Equilibrium—"Appropriate adjustment of prevail-ing emotional tone in response to circumstances" (p. 306).
Leisure Participation—"Use of restful or relaxing activi-ties as needed to promote well-being" (p. 296).
Self-Care: Activities of Daily Living (ADL)—"Ability to perform the most basic physical tasks and personal care activities" (p. 379).
Quality of Life—"An individual's expressed satisfaction with current life circumstances" (p. 347).

Outcomes associated with NOC focus on the physical and psychologic health of the caregiver. The outcomes that

Table **34-3** Care of Patient With Chronic Confusion		
Principles of PLST Model (Hall & Buckwalter, 1987)	*Nursing Interventions Classification (NIC) (Iowa Intervention Project, 2000)*	*Nursing Outcomes Classification (NOC) (Iowa Outcomes Project, 2000)*
Maximize the level of safe function by supporting all areas of loss in a prosthetic manner	**DEMENTIA MANAGEMENT** ***Activities*** Identify and remove potential dangers in environment for patient Place identification bracelet on patient Provide space for safe pacing and wandering Provide finger foods to maintain nutrition for patient who will not sit and eat Monitor nutrition and weight Provide rest periods to prevent fatigue and reduce stress	SAFETY BEHAVIOR: HOME PHYSICAL ENVIRONMENT NUTRITIONAL STATUS: FOOD & FLUID INTAKE SLEEP
Provide patients with unconditional positive regard	Provide unconditional positive regard Avoid use of physical restraints Address patients distinctly by name when initiating interaction and speak slowly Introduce self when initiating contact Speak in a clear, low, warm, respectful tone of voice Prepare for interaction with eye contact and touch as appropriate	COMFORT LEVEL COMMUNICATION ABILITY SOCIAL INTERACTION SKILLS
Use behaviors indicating anxiety and avoidance to determine limits of levels of activity and stimuli	Determine behavioral expectations appropriate for patient's cognitive status Seat patients at small table in groups of three to five at meals as appropriate Allow to eat alone if appropriate Avoid frustrating patient by quizzing with orientation questions that cannot be answered Monitor carefully for physiologic causes for increased confusion, which may be acute and reversible Ask family and friends to see a patient one or two at a time if needed to reduce stimulation Limit choices patient has to make to number that does not cause anxiety Give one simple direction at a time Avoid touch and close proximity if this causes stress or anxiety Use distraction rather than confrontation to manage behavior	COPING SYMPTOM CONTROL MOOD EQUILIBRIUM LEISURE PARTICIPATION
Teach caregivers to "listen" to the patient, evaluating verbal and nonverbal responses	Determine type and extent of cognitive deficit(s), using standardized assessment tool Monitor cognitive functioning using a standardized assessment tool Identify usual patterns of behavior for such activities as sleep, medication use, elimination, food intake, and self-care	SELF-CARE: ACTIVITIES OF DAILY LIVING (ADL)
Modify environment to support losses and enhance safety	Provide a low-stimulation environment (e.g., quiet, soothing music, nonvivid and simple, familiar patterns in decor, performance expectations that do not exceed cognitive processing ability, dining in small groups) Decrease noise levels by avoiding paging systems and call lights that ring or buzz Provide a consistent physical environment and daily routine	QUALITY OF LIFE

Continued

Table 34-3	Care of Patient With Chronic Confusion—cont'd	
Principles of PLST Model (Hall & Buckwalter, 1987)	*Nursing Interventions Classification (NIC)* (Iowa Intervention Project, 2000)	*Nursing Outcomes Classification (NOC)* (Iowa Outcomes Project, 2000)
Provide ongoing education, support, care, and problem-solving for caregivers	Provide a patient with a general orientation to the season of the year by using appropriate cues (e.g., holiday decorations, seasonal decorations and activities, access to contained out-of-doors area) Provide cues such as current events, seasons, location, and names to assist orientation Select artwork for patient rooms featuring landscapes, scenery, or other familiar images Use symbols other than written signs to assist patient to locate room, bathroom, etc. Remove or cover mirrors if patient is frightened or agitated by them Provide boundaries, such as red or yellow tape on the floor, when low-stimulus units are not available Place a patient's name in large block letters in his room and on his clothing as needed Label familiar photos with names of the individuals in photos Provide caregivers who are familiar to the patient (e.g., avoid frequent rotations of staff assignment) Avoid unfamiliar situations when possible Select television or radio activities based on cognitive processing abilities and interests Provide adequate but nonglare lighting Include family members in planning, providing, and evaluating care to the extent desired Assist family to understand it may be impossible for patient to learn new material Determine physical, social, and psychologic history of patient, usual habits, and routines Discuss with family members and friends how best to interact with the patient	CAREGIVER PERFORMANCE: DIRECT CARE CAREGIVER PERFORMANCE: INDIRECT CARE CAREGIVING ENDURANCE POTENTIAL CAREGIVER STRESSORS CAREGIVER WELL-BEING CAREGIVER EMOTIONAL HEALTH GRIEF RESOLUTION CAREGIVER ADAPTATION TO PATIENT INSTITUTIONALIZATION PARTICIPATION: HEALTH CARE DECISIONS QUALITY OF LIFE

provide ongoing education, support, care, and problem-solving for caregivers are as follows:

Caregiver Performance: Direct Care—"Provision by a family care provider of appropriate personal and healthcare for a family member or significant other" (p. 146).

Caregiver Performance: Indirect Care—"Arrangement and oversight of appropriate care for a family member or significant other by a family care provider" (p. 148).

Caregiving Endurance Potential—"Factors that promote family care provider continuance over an extended period of time" (p. 152).

Caregiver Stressors—"The extent of biopsychosocial pressure on a family care provider caring for a family member or a significant other over an extended period of time" (p. 150).

Caregiver Well-Being—"Primary care provider's satisfaction with health and life circumstances" (p. 151).

Caregiver Emotional Health—"Feelings, attitudes, and emotions of a family care provider while caring for a member or significant other over an extended period of time" (p. 140).

Grief Resolution—"Adjustment to actual or impending loss" (p. 223).

Caregiver Adaptation to Patient Institutionalization—"Family caregiver adaptation of role when the care recipient is transferred outside of the home" (p. 138).

Participation: Health Care Decisions—"Family involvement in decision making, delivery and/or evaluation of care provided by health care personnel" (p. 335).

Major research has supported the outcomes associated with the PLST-based intervention (Buckwalter et al., 1992). However, the outcomes associated with NOC still need empirical testing.

NURSING INTERVENTIONS

Dementia Management

Dementia Management is the primary nursing intervention for persons with chronic confusion related to ADRD. Dementia Management is defined as "provision of a modified environment for the patient who is experiencing a chronic confusional state" (Iowa Intervention Project, 2000, pp. 249). The PLST model (Hall & Buckwalter, 1987) serves as a conceptual framework for the nursing intervention Dementia Management. This model provides an intervention upon which both formal and informal caregivers can base logical planning of care and problem solving. Caregivers can use the PLST model to individualize care by determining the type and levels of activity. The model is currently being used in homes, intermediate care facilities, special care units, acute care facilities, and adult daycare programs.

The PLST conceptual framework for Dementia Management is based on the following principles*:

1. Maximize the level of safe function by supporting all areas of loss in a prosthetic manner—that is, to replace what has been lost. For example, if the patient's judgment has been compromised, a caregiver could act "prosthetically" by turning down the temperature on the water heater so that the demented person would not scald herself.
2. Provide patients with unconditional positive regard.
3. Anxious behavior, demanding to leave, or seeking an exit are indications that either a single activity or sequence of events has produced stress that threatens to exceed the patient's coping capacity.
4. Teach caregivers to listen to patients, evaluating verbal and nonverbal responses.
5. Modify the environment to support losses and enhance safety.

*Adapted from Hall & Buckwalter, 1987, p. 404.

6. Provide ongoing education, support, care, and problem-solving for caregivers.

These principles of care can be implemented by both professional and family caregivers in a variety of settings. Table 34-3 correlates these principles with the Dementia Management activities identified by the Iowa Intervention Project (2000).

Interventions for persons with chronic confusion are based on the provision of a supportive environment that maximizes their level of safe function and comfort within the nursing home community without compromising the needs, rights, and quality of life for lucid patients. This includes enhancing the quality of visits by family and friends through interventions that increase their awareness, understanding, and comfort. Increased visitor comfort will diminish stressors for patients and staff.

Maximizing functional level is obtained by reducing stress, thus preventing excess disability. Excess disability may be defined as a reversible deficit that is more disabling than the primary condition. Excess disability exists when the disturbance in functioning is greater than might be accounted for by basic physical illness or cerebral pathology (Dawson, Kline, Wiancko, & Wells, 1986). The most common causes of excess disability for patients with chronic confusion are listed in Box 34-2. These can occur alone or in combination. Interestingly, NIC identifies ways to decrease excess disability, but does not actually use this term.

Although most dementing illnesses that cause chronic confusion are progressive, the rate of behavioral change is not consistent across individuals. Most patients exhibit good and bad days rather than a single behavioral pattern. "Bad days" may be attributed to the presence of internal or external stressors that serve to worsen symptoms, most without worsening the pathophysiology of the disease. These stressors produce excess disability and can be controlled by nursing interventions to prevent or eliminate behavioral complications.

The goals of maximizing patient safety, comfort, and function and preventing complications associated with chronic illness and increasing immobility require attention to all details within the patient's environment. To accomplish this, the staff must assume a helping posture, compensating for the patient's losses rather than increasing the patient's stress levels by encouraging reeducation or rehabilitation for lost abilities. When the staff assumes responsibility for compensating for lost abilities, patient stress is diminished and some spontaneous increase in level of function is observed. This increase may be attributed to the resolution of excess disability by elimination of stress (Dawson et al., 1986; Hall & Buckwalter, 1987).

One method of gaining staff and family understanding of the impact of excess disability is to use an analogy of an amputee. Most adults can imagine a person who has lost a leg. When asked to envision the amputee being instructed to walk without benefit of a prosthesis, crutches, or other devices, most will understand the frustration and anger the amputee would experience after repeated falls. Residents with chronic confusion experience the loss of cerebral cortex functions, which impairs their ability to integrate sensory input, use intellect, and respond to their environment in the manner expected by society. When these losses are challenged rather than supported, patients experience frustration, anger, fear, and increased awareness of their limitations.

This prosthetic/orthotic approach to care begins in the confused stage of the illness. During this phase, patients rely on memory aids such as lists, calendars, and clocks to negotiate in their environment. As the disease progresses, patients must rely increasingly on others to provide cues that remind them of when, where, and how to function appropriately.

Short-range goals are developed to compensate for specific losses and to prevent behavioral complications. During the confused phase of the disease, patients begin to experience frustration, anxiety, and an occasional stress reaction. Therefore, in planning care for the patient, the nurse can decide how many stimuli and how much stress the patient is able to manage by listening to patient reactions and observing for anxiety-related behavior. Anxiety-related behavior might include an increase in psychomotor activity, increased or decreased verbalization, loss of eye contact, complaints of feeling uncomfortable or nervous, and/or an attempt to avoid or retreat from the offensive situation (Nowakowski, 1985).

In planning care for the person with chronic confusion, the caregiver makes the following assumptions:

1. The patient exists in a 24-hour continuum. Care cannot be planned or evaluated on an 8-hour shift basis. If the patient has a problem during the night, some changes need to be implemented during the day.
2. The patient who is confused or agitated is not comfortable and should be regarded as frightened. All patients have the right to be comfortable.
3. All behavior is rooted and has meaning; therefore, all catastrophic and stress-related behaviors have a cause.
4. All humans require some control over their person and their environment and need some degree of unconditional positive regard.
5. There are certain basic caring functions that, because of the need to consider the good of all patients, the institution cannot always provide. Therefore the institution must coordinate care with the societal structure (e.g., family unit) that can provide for those unmet needs, for example, the provision of special celebrations for a patient on a religious holiday (Buckwalter & Hall, 1987).

The caregiver should plan interventions that are consistent for the patient's level of coping. The use of a consistent routine has been shown to be effective in reducing stress, as the patient does not need to rely on planning skills for most activities (Hall, Gerdner, Zwygart-Stauffacher, & Buckwalter, 1995). Regular rest periods are important, and they do not potentiate night wakening. Without measures to diminish stress and fatigue, the patient's day might be characterized by increasingly anxious behavior and cycling between dysfunctional and anxious behavior as diagrammed in Figure 34-4.

During a typical day the patient experiences high stress levels when performing the morning ADL. Rather than being afforded the opportunity to rest, compensating for fatigue and high stress, the patient might be sent (by well-meaning staff) to activities or a therapy session. At lunchtime the patient enters the communal dining room where there can be 50 or more patients. Nurses are passing medications; dietary personnel are passing trays; assistants are feeding other patients; others are collecting trays; and the general noise level is loud. The fatigued patient with chronic confusion often attempts to leave, an example of avoidance behavior stemming from anxiety. A nursing assistant returns the patient to the table where there are three or four people talking and a tray with multiple food choices. The overly stressed patient eats little of the meal and then attempts to leave again.

The patient might get some opportunity for rest in the afternoon, but could have visitors or be scheduled for another activity or facility event. Late in the day or during the night, the patient crosses the already lowered stress threshold and becomes dysfunctional. The patient is confused, agitated, combative, or up at night.

Using a care plan that compensates for fatigue and other losses, the patient's stress level fluctuates but does not become dysfunctional, as diagrammed in Figure 34-5. The patient's stress level is reduced in accordance with his ability to tolerate activity without anxiety. Stress-related dysfunctional behavior is prevented if the stress threshold is not surpassed.

The PLST-based intervention is theoretically and empirically grounded. Theory is essential to develop knowledge, conduct research, and guide practice. Although there is a growing consensus for the importance of applying nursing theory to practice and testing its effectiveness, few examples exist in the literature (Silva & Sorrell, 1992). The PLST model provides a framework for formal and informal caregivers to provide individualized care. In contrast, care based on the *Nursing Interventions Classification (NIC)* is atheoretical. A list of NIC interventions provides a range of options but no basis for selection. NIC does address methods of incorporating family members in the planning and provision of care.

Interventions With Family Members

Patients with Chronic Confusion often are unable to give helpful input into decision making or may refuse in-home

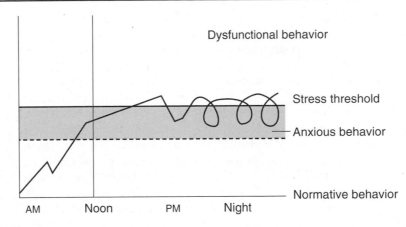

FIGURE **34-4**   Effects of stress during a 24-hour day in the person with chronic confusion: ADRD. (From Hall, G., & Buckwalter, K. [1987]. Progressively lowered stress threshold: A conceptual model for care of adults with Alzheimer's disease. *Archives of Psychiatric Nursing, 1*[6], 399-406.)

services, nursing home placement, or any help from family or professionals. Consequently, family members can experience moral dilemmas regarding placement, advocacy, and decision-making (Mace & Rabins, 1991). Many long-term care facilities have found that support groups for family members help to ease their stress. Peer counseling from one trained family member to others is another successful intervention. Staff must continuously be aware of the family burden and offer empathy and support throughout the admission process and thereafter. Some families find tips on how to visit helpful, such as preplanning an activity to use during the visit. Others might want to attend care-planning meetings. It can be helpful to have one primary nurse interact with a patient's family, developing a bond that will help both family and staff to provide better care for the patient and to resolve conflicts more readily.

Placement in long-term care is also made difficult when a family member has been the primary caregiver for an extended period of time and is suddenly faced with a sudden and drastic change in role. The Family Involvement in Care protocol was developed as a means of easing this transition, promoting a cooperative relationship between family and staff and enhancing the quality of care of the resident (Maas, Buckwalter, Swanson, Specht, Tripp-Reimer, & Hardy, 1994; Maas & Swanson, 1992). This is achieved by negotiating the family member's role through a clearly defined process.

Special Problems

Although a care plan is identified, the caregiver should anticipate that additional problems and needs will arise for the patient with chronic confusion as the pathophysiologic process progresses. One of the more common problems to arise in the long-term care setting is the combative reaction. Combative episodes create the potential for injury to patient, staff, other patients, and visitors. They

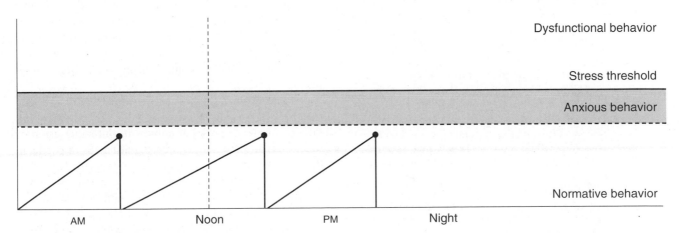

FIGURE **34-5**   Planned activity levels for the person with chronic confusion: ADRD. (From Hall, G., & Buckwalter, K. [1987]. Progressively lowered stress threshold: A conceptual model for care of adults with Alzheimer's disease. *Archives of Psychiatric Nursing, 1*[6], 399-406.)

also increase fear of all patients with chronic confusion. The following consequences can occur: permanent isolation of the combative patient from other patients and visitors; exclusion of combative patients from normative social activities; increased use of tranquilizing medications, which tend to limit function; increased use of soft tie restraints, which limit mobility and worsen patient fear; and increased staff fear of the patient, which may limit the amount of contact staff have with the combative patient. In some states, a combative patient must be discharged from the long-term care center once an episode involving another patient has occurred.

In assessing a combative episode the nurse should recognize that combative behavior is the last resort many patients with Chronic Confusion have for coping with fear and frustration. The cause of the episode should be determined and eliminated, if possible. Common causes of combative episodes, in addition to those listed in Box 34-2, are listed below:

- Negative, restrictive feedback from staff, patients, and visitors
- Restraints
- Misinterpretation of environmental stimuli, especially material on television
- Misinterpretation of boundaries and ownership
- Nonrecognition of familiar persons or mistaking other patients for spouse, family members, or persons who trouble them
- Fear of water or resistance to an activity such as bathing

Box 34-2	Common Causes of Excess Disability

1. Fatigue
2. Change in routine, caregiver, or environment, such as holiday decorations or a visit home
3. Competing or misleading stimuli, or high stimulus activity, such as a band concert, lunch in the crowded dining room, prolonged visit from family, television, mirror images, or potentially frightening pictures of people or animals
4. Stress or frustration from trying to function beyond limits imposed by Chronic Confusion: ADRD or others, such as trying to participate in reality orientation therapy; trying to bathe, choose clothing, or dress when no longer able to accomplish independently; having other residents, staff, or others constantly telling resident she is wrong or to try harder; trying to relearn lost skills; or being physically restrained
5. Affective response to perception of loss
6. Physical illness, discomfort, pain, or medication reaction

Data from Hall, G. R., Gerdner, L. A., Zwygart-Stauffacher, M., & Buckwalter, K. C. (1995). Principles of nonpharmacological management: Caring for people with Alzheimer's disease using a conceptual model. *Psychiatric Annals, 25*(7), 432-440.

It is essential to assess the combative situation and control it quickly to prevent injury and minimize the amount of intervention required, such as medication. The combative patient should be quickly separated from offensive stimuli with minimal physical contact. For example, if the combative patient is in another patient's room, the other patient might be asked to step outside while the staff works with the combative patient. If the incident involves a staff member, it is best to have another staff member deal with the crisis calmly under the direction of the nurse.

The combative patient should be regarded as frightened, and interventions should focus on removing fear. The combative patient should be allowed to maintain a sense of personal control through the use of retained social graces. Statements by staff such as "I know this doesn't look familiar, but this is the room I reserved for you this evening" can help the patient to regain a sense of mastery without reinforcing that they are confused or wrong again.

Another successful technique is to focus on the feeling behind the action. For example, statements such as "It must be frustrating to have people tell you you're wrong," or "Mrs. Jones does resemble your wife. Are you lonely for her now?" provide the patient with an opportunity to state feelings and needs that may have been buried. It is often surprising how articulate a patient with a communication deficit can be when agitated. Residents who repeatedly become combative or agitated, despite reductions in stimuli and increases in rest periods, might require use of a tranquilizer or might benefit from a special care environment designed for persons with chronic confusion.

Persons who have used violent behavior as a lifelong coping mechanism for stress can present a significant, ongoing problem in terms of combative behavior. The patient who has a history of spouse abuse, child abuse, or other regular violent acts can use aggression as a method of controlling others and coping with the environment. These patients usually express no fear when combative and tend to be combative with people as they become more familiar. Lifelong patterns of violence should be identified prior to the patient's admission to the facility and a determination made concerning the facility's ability to provide care without compromising the rights of other patients or staff.

Another special care problem is wandering. Wandering is generally considered to be leaving the nursing unit, nursing home, or personal home without supervision or sanctions from the staff. Wandering differs from pacing in that the patient actually elopes from the specified environment and is generally considered to be at risk for injury. Patients wander for several reasons (Goldsmith, Hoeffer, & Rader, 1995; Rader & Doan, 1985). They may be following environmental cues, acting on a reminiscent delusion such as needing to go to work, or feeling frightened and trying to escape. Care must be taken to assess the behavioral characteristics of the patient who wanders in order to determine appropriate interventions that do not impose excessive restraint.

Interventions from the nursing diagnosis Risk for Injury should be reviewed (see Chapter 3); however, the nurse must educate staff and family that the patient is unable to assess and self-monitor for danger and potential injury. Regular inservice programs need to be presented on the safety needs of patients with chronic confusion. Wandering drills can provide experience and provide staff with practical application of protocols under a timed, simulated situation.

CASE STUDY

Mr. Norman's nurse met with both the day shift staff and the evening shift staff on the unit where he would be residing. The staff was briefed on Mr. Norman's background and behavioral symptoms, and a tentative care plan was identified to assist him in coping with his new residence. The plan consisted of having Mr. Norman spend the first several days in a consistent routine on the nursing unit until he adapted to the stimulus level within the facility. He was admitted to a special unit for persons with ADRD, as he had a history of wandering. Mr. Norman had rest periods scheduled for 9:30 AM and 1:30 PM in his own recliner in his room. His room was kept free of misleading pictures and television, and all mirrors were removed.

The morning of admission, Sue brought her father's recliner and personal belongings to the facility. Mr. Norman was admitted before lunch, his optimal time of day. The staff oriented Mr. Norman to his room and hall, serving lunch to him and Mrs. Norman in his room. To promote family caregiver adaptation to institutionalization, the director of nursing provided a family orientation for Mrs. Norman and Sue. They were encouraged to visit freely, but to choose which time of day was best and incorporate it into Mr. Norman's routine. Mrs. Norman was introduced to a family member of another patient with chronic confusion who would remain her peer counselor throughout her husband's stay. To facilitate participation in health care decisions, Mrs. Norman was encouraged to attend care-planning sessions and the monthly family support group. She was encouraged to bring any care problems to the attention of the director of nursing, social worker, and/or administrator without fear of repercussions.

On admission, Mr. Norman was taking large doses of the antipsychotic medication, Mellaril, 225 mg per day. When shown the unit, he had difficulty walking and became incontinent of urine. That night he was awake and confused. The next day he left the facility repeatedly. To promote a safe (physical) environment, the nurses placed two strips of yellow tape at either end of the hallway to his nursing unit. Mr. Norman stopped the director of nursing in the hall and pointed to the tapes, saying, "At last, I know my boundaries. I won't wander off now." Mr. Norman did not wander again.

The night wakening continued. The nurses made a decision to feed Mr. Norman at a small table in his room with two other patients. Night wakening diminished over time and eventually ceased. Over the months that ensued, Mr. Norman's Mellaril was slowly decreased until he became agitated without it when stimulus and activity levels could no longer be reduced. He was then maintained on 25 mg of Mellaril at bedtime. As the medication was reduced, Mr. Norman's gait and continence improved. This improvement, however, was not permanent.

Two years later Mr. Norman stopped walking. After 10 more months of dependent care, he became unable to eat. Mrs. Norman agonized over the decision to pass a nasogastric tube. With support from the staff and her daughter, she decided on the tube. One year later, Mr. Norman died. Mrs. Norman was unable to sever her ties with the nursing home staff. She was surprised by her grieving at Mr. Norman's death, for which she had prayed so long. As a means of grief resolution, she has become a peer counselor, helping other families.

SUMMARY

Care of the patient with Chronic Confusion due to progressive degeneration of the cerebral cortex is one of the largest challenges for geriatric nurses. Few techniques used to manage Chronic Confusion have been substantiated consistently by nursing or other research. Such research, when undertaken, is compromised because of the difficulty of evaluating results in subjects with communication and reasoning deficits. Subject selection and attrition problems occur because patients are often unable to consent to be studied or regress beyond a point where they can participate in a study.

It is helpful in planning nursing care for these patients to use a conceptual model that links interventions and outcomes to the patient's level of stress. The Progressively Lowered Stress Threshold model encourages caregivers to individualize care by using patient responses to determine activity tolerance. The model is being used extensively in homes, integrated nursing homes, special care units, hospitals, and adult day programs throughout the United States and Australia. The model has been shown to be an effective guide for increasing patient comfort and minimizing behaviors that might otherwise require medication or physical restraint.

REFERENCES

Adams, J., & Lindemann, E. (1974). Coping with long term disability. In G. Coelho, D. Hamburg, & J. Adams (Eds.), *Coping and adaptation* (pp. 127-138). New York: Basic Books.

Advisory Panel on Alzheimer's Disease. (1991). *Second report of the advisory panel on Alzheimer's disease, 1990* (DHHS Pub. No. (ADM) 91-1791). Washington, DC: Superintendent of Documents, U.S. Government Printing Office.

Aldrich, C., & Mendkoff, E. (1963). Relocation of the aged and disabled: A mortality study. *Journal of the American Geriatrics Society, 11*(3), 185-194.

American Psychiatric Association. (1994). *Diagnostic and statistical manual of mental disorders* (4th ed.). Washington, DC: American Psychiatric Association.

Anthony, J. E., LeResche, L., Niaz, U., VonKorff, M. R., & Folstein, M. F. (1982). Limits of the "mini-mental state" as a screening test for dementia and delirium among hospital patients. *Psychological Medicine, 12*, 397-408.

Auer, S. R., Sclan, S. G., Yaffee, R. A., & Reisberg, B. (1994). The neglected half of Alzheimer's disease: Cognitive and functional concomitants of sever dementia. *Journal of the American Geriatrics Society, 42*, 1266-1272.

Ballinger, B. (1982). Cluster analysis of symptoms in elderly demented patients. *British Journal of Psychiatry, 140*(3), 257-262.

Bell, J. E. (1998). The neuropathology of adult HIV infection. *Revue Neurologique, 154*(12), 816-829.

Belojevic, G., & Jakovljevic, B. (1998). Aluminum and Alzheimer's disease. *Srpski Arhiv Za Celokupno Lekarstvo, 126*(7-8), 283-289.

Bergman-Evans, B. (1994). A health profile of spousal Alzheimer's caregivers: Depression and physical health characterisics. *Journal of Psychosocial Nursing, 32*(7), 25-30.

Bird, T. D., Levy-Lahand, E., Poorkay, P., Sharman, V., Nemens, E., Lahad, A., Lampe, T. H., & Schellenberg, G. D. (1996). Wide range in age of onset for chromosome 1—related to familial Alzheimer's disease. *Annals of Neurology, 40*(6), 932-936.

Blessed, G., Tomlinson, B., & Roth, M. (1968). The associations between quantitative measures of dementia and senile change in the cerebral gray matter of elderly subjects. *British Journal of Psychiatry, 114* (3), 797-811.

Bohnstedt, M., Fox, P. J., & Kohatsu, N. D. (1994). Correlates of mini-mental status examination scores among elderly demented patients: The influence of race-ethnicity. *Journal of Clinical Epidemiology, 47*(12), 1381-1387.

Brookmeyer, R., Gray, S., & Kawas, C. (1998). Projections of Alzheimer's disease in the United States and the public health impact of delaying disease onset. *American Journal of Public Health, 88*(9), 1337-1342.

Buckwalter, K., & Hall, G. (1987). Families of the institutionalized older adult: A neglected resource. In T. Brubaker (Ed.), *Aging, health, and family: Long term care* (pp. 176-196). Thousand Oaks, CA: Sage.

Buckwalter, K. C., Gerdner, L. A., Hall, G. R., Kelly, A., Kohout, F., Richards, B., & Sime, M. (1999). Effects of family caregiver home training based on the progressively lowered stress threshold model. In S. H. Gueldner & L. W. Poon (Eds.), *Gerontological nursing issues for the 21st century: A multidisciplinary dialogue commemorating the international year of older persons* (pp. 81-98). Sigma Theta Tau International: Center Press.

Buckwalter, K. C., Gerdner, L. A., Kohout, F., Hall, G. R., Kelly, A., Richards, B., & Sime, M. (1999). A nursing intervention to decrease depression in family caregivers of persons with dementia. *Archives of Psychiatric Nursing, 13*(2), 80-88.

Buckwalter, K. C., Hall, G. R., Kelly, A., Sime, A. M., Richards, B., & Gerdner, L. A. (1992). *PLST model—Effectiveness for rural ADRD caregivers* (5R01NR03234). Bethesda, MD: National Institute of Health/National Institute of Nursing Research.

Burns, E., & Buckwalter, K. (1988). Pathophysiology and etiology of Alzheimer's disease. *Nursing Clinics of North America, 23*(1), 11-29.

Camdessanche, J. P., Michel, D., Cathebras, P., Thomas-Anterion, C., Antonine, J. C., Barral, F. G., & Rousset, H. (1997). Neurolupus with dementia manifestations. *Revue Neurologique, 153*(6-7), 398-405.

Carroll-Johnson, R. M. (1989). *Classification of nursing diagnoses: Proceedings of the eighth conference.* Baltimore: Lippincott Williams & Wilkins.

Carroll-Johnson, R. M., & Paquette, M. (1994). *Classification of nursing diagnoses: Proceedings of the tenth conference.* Baltimore: Lippincott Williams & Wilkins.

Caselli, R. J., & Hunder, G. G. (1997). Giant cell (temporal arteritis). *Neurologic Clinics, 15*(4), 893-902.

Chenoweth, B., & Spencer, B. (1986). Dementia: The experience of family caregivers. *The Gerontologist, 26*(3), 267-272.

Cohen, D., & Eisdorfer, C. (1988). Depression in family members caring for a relative with Alzheimer's disease. *Journal of the American Geriatrics Society, 36*, 885-889.

Cohen-Mansfield, J. (1986). Agitated behaviors in the elderly II. Preliminary results in the cognitively deteriorated. *Journal of the American Geriatrics Society, 34*(10), 722-727.

Cohen-Mansfield, J., Billig, N., Lipson, S., Rosenthal, A. S., & Pawlson, L. G. (1990). Medical correlates of agitation in nursing home residents. *Geronotology, 36*(6), 150-158.

Cohen-Mansfield, J., Werner, P., & Marx, M. S. (1990). Screaming in nursing home residents. *Journal of the American Geriatrics Society, 38*(7), 785-792.

Corder, E. H., Saunders, A. M., Strittmatter, W. J., Schmechel, D. E., Gaskell, P. C., Rimmler, J. B., Locke, P. A., Conneally, P. M., Schmader, K. E., Tanzi, R. E., Gusella, J. F., Small, G. W., Roses, A. D., Pericak-Vance, M. A., & Haines, J. L. (1995). Apolipoprotein E, survival in Alzheimer's disease patients, and the competing risks of death and Alzheimer's disease. *Neurology, 45*, 1323-1328.

Coyle, J. T., Price, D. L., & DeLong, M. R. (1983). Alzheimer's disease: A disorder of cortical cholinergic innervation. *Science, 219*(4589), 1184-1190.

Crum, R., Anthony, J., Bassett, S., & Folstein, F. (1993). Population-based mini-mental state examination by age and education level. *Journal of the American Medical Association, 269*(18), 2386-2421.

Davie, P. (1983). An update on the neurochemistry of Alzheimer's disease. In R. Mayeux & W. G. Rosen (Eds.), *The dementias* (pp. 75-86). New York: Raven Press.

Dawson, P., Kline, K., Wiancko, D. C., & Wells, D. (1986). Preventing excess disability in patients with Alzheimer's disease. *Geriatric Nursing, 7*(6), 298-330.

Dura, J. R., Stukenberg, K. W., & Kielcolt-Glaser, J. K. (1990). Chronic stress and depressive disorders in older adults. *Journal of Abnormal Psychology, 99*, 284-290.

Dura, J. R., Stukenberg, K. W., & Kielcolt-Glaser, J. K. (1991). Anxiety and depressive disorders in adult children caring for demented parents. *Psychology and Aging, 6*, 467-473.

Escobar, J. I., Burnam, A., Karno, M., Forsythe, A., Landsverk, J., & Golding, J. M. (1986). Use of the mini-mental state examination (MMSE) in a community population of mixed ethnicity. *Journal of Nervous Mental Disease, 174*(10), 607-614.

Esterling, B. A., Kiecolt-Glaser, J. K., Bodnar, J. C., & Glaser, R. (1994). Chronic stress, social support, and persistent alterations in the natural killer cell response to cytokines in older adults. *Health Psychology, 13*(4), 291-298.

Ferrell, B. A., & Ferrell, B. R. (1995). Pain in cognitively impaired nursing home patients. *Journal of Pain & Symptom Management, 10*(8), 591-598.

Ferrucci, L., Cecchi, F., Guralnik, J. M., Giampaoli, S., LoNoce, C., Salani, B., Bandinelli, S., & Baroni, A. (1996). Does the clock drawing test predict cognitive decline in older persons independent of the mini-mental state? *Journal of the American Geriatrics Society, 44*(11), 1326-1331.

Fillenbaum, G. G., Hughes, D. C., Heyman, A., George, L. K., & Blazer, D. G. (1988). Relationship of health and demographic characteristics to mini-mental state examination score among community residents. *Psychological Medicine, 18,* 719-726.

Folstein, M., Folstein, S., & McHugh, P. (1975). Mini-mental state: A practical method for grading the cognitive state of patients for the clinician. *Journal of Psychiatric Research, 12*(3) 189-198.

Franssen, E. H., Kluger, A., Torossian, C. L., & Reisberg, B. (1993). The neurologic syndrome of severe Alzheimer's disease. *Archives of Neurology, 50,* 1029-1039.

Gallagher, D., Rose, J., Rivera, P., Lovett, S., & Thompson, L. W. (1989). Prevalence of depression in family caregivers. *The Gerontologist, 29*(4), 449-456.

Gallagher-Thompson, D., & Powers, D. V. (1997). Primary stressors and depressive symptoms in caregivers of dementia patients. *Aging & Mental Health, 1*(3), 248-255.

Gatz, M., Pedersen, N. L., Berg, S., Johansson, B., Johansson, K., Mortimer, J. A., Posner, S. F., Viitanen, M., Winblad, B., & Ahlbom, A. (1997). Heritability for Alzheimer's disease: The study of dementia in Swedish twins. *Journals of Gerontology: Series A, Biological Sciences & Medical Sciences, 52*(2), M117-M125.

Gerdner, L. A., Hall, G. R., & Buckwalter, K. C. (1996). Caregiver training for people with Alzheimer's based on a stress threshold model. *IMAGE: Journal of Nursing Scholarship, 28*(3), 241-246.

Goldsmith, S. M., Hoeffer, B., & Rader, J. (1995). Problematic wandering behavior in the cognitively impaired elderly. *Journal of Psychosocial Nursing, 33*(2), 6-12.

Gordon, M. (1995). *Manual of nursing diagnosis 1995-96.* St. Louis, MO: Mosby.

Gottfries, C. G., Barnes, G., & Steen, G. (1982). A new rating scale for dementia syndromes. *Gerontology, 28*(Suppl. 2), 20-31.

Graves, A. B., White, E., Koepsell, T. D., Reifler, B. V., Belle, G. V., Larson, E. B., & Raskind, M. (1990). The association between head trauma and Alzheimer's disease. *American Journal of Epidemiology, 131*(3), 491-501.

Hall, G. R. (1988). Care of the patient with Alzheimer's disease living at home. *Nursing Clinics of North America, 23*(1), 31-46.

Hall, G. R. (1991). Altered thought processes: Dementia. In M. Maas, K. C. Buckwalter, & M. Hardy (Eds.), *Nursing diagnoses and interventions for the elderly* (pp. 332-347). Reading, MA: Addison Wesley Longman.

Hall, G. R., & Buckwalter, K. C. (1991). Whole disease care planning: Fitting the program to the client with Alzheimer's disease. *Journal of Gerontological Nursing, 17*(3), 38-41.

Hall, G. R., Gerdner, L. A., Zwygart-Stauffacher, M., & Buckwalter K. C. (1995). Principles of nonpharmacological management: Caring for people with Alzheimer's disease using a conceptual model. *Psychiatric Annals, 25*(7), 432-440.

Hall, G., & Buckwalter, K. (1987). Progressively lowered stress threshold: A conceptual model for care of adults with Alzheimer's disease. *Archives of Psychiatric Nursing, 1*(6), 399-406.

Hall, G., Kirschling, M., & Todd, S. (1986). Sheltered freedom: The creation of a special care Alzheimer's unit in an intermediate level facility. *Geriatric Nursing, 7*(3), 132-136.

Hays, A. (1984). The set test to screen mental status quickly. *Geriatric Nursing, 5*(2), 96-97.

Hill, L. R., Klauber, M. R., Salmon, D. P., Yu, E. S. H., Liu, W. T., Zhang, M., & Katzman, R. (1993). Functional status, education, and the diagnosis of dementia in the Shanghai survey. *Neurology, 43*(1), 138-145.

Huff, F. J., Auerback, J., Chakravarti, A., & Boller, F. (1988). Risk of dementia in relatives of patients with Alzheimer's disease. *Neurology, 38,* 786-790.

Hull, M. (1996). Oral presentation at an Alzheimer's conference. Friday Center at Duke University. Chapel Hill, North Carolina.

Iowa Intervention Project. J. C. McCloskey & G. M. Bulechek (Eds.). (2000). *Nursing interventions classification (NIC)* (3rd ed.). St. Louis, MO: Mosby.

Iowa Outcomes Project. M. Johnson, M. Maas, & S. Moorhead (Eds.). (2000). *Nursing outcomes classification (NOC)* (2nd ed.). St. Louis, MO: Mosby.

Isaacs, B., & Akhtar, A. (1972). The set test: A rapid test of mental functions in old people. *Age & Ageing, 1*(11), 222-226.

Isaacs, B., & Kennie, A. (1973). The set test as an aid to detection of dementia in old people. *British Journal of Psychiatry, 123*(10), 467-470.

Itzhaki, R. F., Lin, W. R., Shang, D., Wilcock, G. K., Faragher, B., & Jamieson, G. A. (1997). Herpes simplex virus type 1 in brain and risk of Alzheimer's disease. *Lancet, 349*(9047), 241-244.

Jellinger, K., Danielczyk, W., Fischer, P., & Gabriel, E. (1990). Clinicopathological analysis of dementia disorders in the elder. *Journal of Neurological Science, 95,* 239-258.

Jorm, A. F. (1990). *The epidemiology of Alzheimer's disease and related disorders.* London: Chapman & Hall.

Jorm, A. F., Scott, R., Henderson, A. S., & Kay, D. W. K. (1988). Educational level differences on the mini-mental state: The role of test bias. *Psychological Medicine, 18,* 727-731.

Kiecolt-Glaser, J. K., Dura, J. R., Speicher, C. E., Trask, O. J., & Glaser, R. (1991). Spousal caregivers of dementia victims: Longitudinal changes in immunity and health. *Psychosomatic Medicine, 53,* 345-362.

Kiecolt-Glaser, J. K., Glaser, R., Shuttleworth, E. E., Dyer, C. S., Ogracki, P., & Speicher, C. E. (1987). Chronic stress and immunity in family caregivers of Alzheimer's disease patients. *Psychosomatic Medicine, 49,* 523-535.

Knowles, L., & Sarver, V. (1985). Attitudes affect quality of care. *Journal of Gerontological Nursing, 11*(8), 35-39.

Kuhlman, G. J., Wilson, H. S., Hutchinson, S. A., & Wallhagen, M. (1991). Alzheimer's disease and family caregiving: Critical synthesis of the literature and research agenda. *Nursing Research, 40*(6), 331-338.

Lawton, M. P. (1980). Psychosocial and environmental approaches to the care of senile dementia patients. In J. Cole & J. Barrett (Eds.), *Psychopathology in the aged* (pp. 265-278). New York: Raven Press.

Lawton, M. P., & Nahemow, L. (1973). Ecology and the aging process. In C. Eisdorfer & M. P. Lawton (Eds.), *The psychology of adult development and aging* (pp. 619-674). Washington, DC: American Psychological Association.

Lawton, M. P., & Simon, B. (1968). The ecology of social relationships in shared housing for the elderly. *The Gerontologist, 8*(2), 108-115.

Levy-Lahad, E., Wasco, W., Poorkaj, P., Romano, D. M., Oshima, J., Pettingell, W. H., Yu, C. E., Jondro, P. D., Schmidt, S. D., Wang, K., Crowley, A. C., Ying-Hui, F., Guenette, S. Y., Galas, D., Nemens, E., Wijsman, E. M., Bird, T. D., Schellenberg, G. D., & Tanzi, R. E. (1995). Candidate gene for the chromosome 1 familial Alzheimer's disease locus. *Science, 269*(5226), 973-977.

Levy-Lahad, E., Wijsman, E. M., Nemens, E., Anderson, L., Goddard, K. A., Weber, J. L., & Bird, T. D. (1995). A familial Alzheimer's disease locus on chromosome 1. *Science, 269*(5226), 970-973.

Lin, W., Casas, I., Wilcock, G. K., & Itzhaki, R. (1997). Neurotropic viruses and Alzheimer's disease: A search for varicella zoster virus DNA by the polymerase chain reaction. *Journal of Neurology, Neurosurgery, & Psychiatry, 62*(6), 586-589.

Maas, M., & Buckwalter, K. C. (1990). *Nursing evaluation research: Alzheimer's care unit* (Final Report) (R01NR01689). Bethesda, MD: National Institute of Health/National Institute of Nursing Research.

Maas, M., Buckwalter, K. C., Swanson, E., Specht, J., Tripp-Reimer, T., & Hardy, M. (1994). The caring partnership: Staff and families of persons institutionalized with Alzheimer's disease. *American Journal of Alzheimer's Care and Related Disorders and Research, 9*(6), 21-30.

Maas, M. L., & Swanson, E. (1992). *Nursing Interventions for Alzheimer's Family Role Trials*, Rockville, MD: National Institutes of Health/National Institute of Nursing Research (R01NR01689).

Mace, N. L., & Rabins, P. V. (1991). *The 36 hour day* (revised ed.). Baltimore: The Johns Hopkins University Press.

Malone, M. J. (1994). Multi-infarct dementia (MID). *The Journal of the South Carolina Medical Association, 90*(11), 539-542.

Mattis, S. (1976). Mental status examination for organic mental syndrome in the elderly patient. In R. Bellack & B. Karasu (Eds.), *Geriatric psychiatry* (pp. 77-121). Philadelphia: Grune & Stratton.

Mirsen, T., & Hachinski, V. (1988). Epidemiology and classification of vascular and multi-infarct dementia. In J. S. Meyer, H. Lechner, J. Marshall, & J. F. Toole (Eds.), *Vascular and multi-infarct dementia* (pp. 61-76). Mount Kisco, NY: Futura.

Morgan, D. (1985). Nurses' perceptions of mental confusion in the elderly: Influence of resident and setting characteristics. *Journal of Health and Social Science, 26*(2), 102-112.

Morris, J. C. (1996). Classification of dementia and Alzheimer's disease. *ACTA Neurologica Scandanavica* (Suppl. 165), 41-50.

Morrison-Bogorad, M. (1993). *Scientists discover possible risk factor for Alzheimer's disease* (Press Release). Seattle, WA: Alzheimer's Disease Research Center, University of Washington.

Mort, J. R., Gaspar, P. M., Juffer, D. I., & Kovarna, M. B. (1996). Comparison of psychotropic agent use among rural elderly caregivers and noncaregivers. *Annals of Pharmacotherapy, 30*(6), 583-585.

Mullan, M., Houlden, H., Windelspecht, M., Fidani, L., Lombardi, C., Diaz, P., Rossor, M., Crook, R., Hardy, J., & Duffy, K. (1992). A locus for familial early-onset Alzheimer's disease on the long arm of chromosome 14, proximal to the alpha 1-antichymotrypsin gene. *Nature Genetics, 2*(4), 340-342.

Nagley, S. (1986). Predicting and preventing confusion in your patients. *Journal of Gerontological Nursing, 12*(3), 27-31.

Negley, E., & Manley, J. (1990). Environmental interventions in assaultive behavior. *Journal of Gerontological Nursing, 16*(3), 29-33.

Nemetz, P. N., Leibson, C., Naessens, J. M., Beard, M., Kokmen, E., Annegers, J. F., & Kurkland, L. T. (1999). Traumatic brain injury and time to onset of Alzheimer's disease: A population-based study. *American Journal of Epidemiology, 149*(1), 32-40.

North American Nursing Diagnosis Association. (1999). *Nursing diagnoses: Definitions & classification 1999-2000.* Philadelphia: Author.

Nowakowski, L. (1985). Accent capabilities in disorientation. *Journal of Gerontological Nursing, 11*(9), 15-20.

Office of Technological Assessment. (1987). *Losing a million minds: Confronting the tragedy of Alzheimer's disease and other dementia.* Washington, DC: U.S. Congress, U.S. Printing Office.

Olney, J. W., Wozniak, D. F., & Farber, N. B. (1997). Excitotoxic neurodegeneration in Alzheimer's disease: New hypothesis and new therapeutic strategies. *Archives of Neurology, 54*(10), 1234-1240.

O'Meara, E. S., Kukull, W. A., Sheppard, L., Bowen, J. D., McCormick, W. C., Teri, L., Pfanschmidt, M., Thompson, J. D., Schellenberg, G. D., & Larson, E. B. (1997). Head injury and risk of Alzheimer's disease by apolipoprotein E genotype. *American Journal of Epidemiology, 146*(5), 373-384.

Palmateer, L., & McCarthy, J. (1985). Do nurses know when patients have cognitive deficits? *Journal of Gerontological Nursing, 11*(2), 6-17.

Pearson, J., Teri, L., Wagner, A., Truax, P., & Logsdon, R. (1993). The relationship of problem behavior in dementia patients to the depression and burden of caregiver spouses. *The American Journal of Alzheimer's Disease and Related Disorders and Research, 8*(1), 15-22.

Perl, D. P., & Brody, A. R. (1980). Alzheimer's disease: X-ray spectometric evidence of aluminum accumulation in neurofibrillary tangle-bearing neurons. *Science, 208*, 297-299.

Peskind, E. (1996). Neurobiology of Alzheimer's disease. *Journal of Clinical Psychiatry, 57*(Suppl. 14), 5-8.

Peterson, R. F., Knapp, T. J., Rosen, J. C., & Pither, B. F. (1977). The effects of furniture arrangements on the behavior of geriatric patients. *Behavior Therapy, 8*(3), 464-467.

Pfeiffer, E. (1975). A short portable mental status questionnaire for assessment of organic brain deficit in the elderly patients. *Journal of the American Geriatrics Society, 23*(10), 433-441.

Pruchno, R. A., & Potashnik, S. L. (1989). Caregiving spouses: Physical and mental health in perspective. *Journal of the American Geriatrics Society, 37*, 697-705.

Prusiner, S. B. (1984). Prions. *Scientific American, 251*, 50-59.

Rader, J., & Doan, J. (1985). How to decrease wandering, a form of agenda behavior. *Geriatric Nursing, 6*(4), 196-199.

Ragneskog, H., Gerdner, L. A., Josefsson, K., & Kihlgren, M. (1998). Probable reasons for expressed agitation in persons with dementia. *Clinical Nursing Research, 7*(20), 189-206.

Raiha, I., Kaprio, J., Koskenvuo, M., Rajala, T., & Sourander, L. (1996). Alzheimer's disease in Finnish twins. *Lancet, 347*(9001), 573-578.

Raiha, I., Kaprio, J., Koskenvuo, M., Rajala, T., & Sourander, L. (1998). Environmental differences in twin pairs discordant for Alzheimer's disease. *Journal of Neurology, Neurosurgery & Psychiatry, 65*(5), 785-787.

Reisberg, B. (1988). Functional assessment staging (FAST). *Psychopharmacology Bulletin, 24*(4), 653-655.

Reisberg, B., Ferris, S. H., Anand, R., de Leon, M. J., Schneck, M. K., Buttinger, C., & Borenstein, J. (1984). Functional staging of dementia of the Alzheimer's type. *Annals of the New York Academy of Science, 435,* 481-483.

Reisberg, B., Ferris, S. H., de Leon, M. J., & Crook, T. (1982). The global deterioration scale for assessment of primary degenerative dementia. *American Journal of Psychiatry, 139*(9), 1136-1139.

Rosen, W. G., Mohs, R. C., & Davis, K. L. (1984). A new rating scale for Alzheimer's disease. *American Journal of Psychiatry, 141,* 1356.

Roses, A. D., Debout, J., Yamaoka, L. H., Gaskell, P. C., Hung, W. Y., Walker, A. P., Alberts, M. J., Clark, C., Welch, K., Earl, N. L., Heyman, A. L., & Pericak-Vance, M. A. (1990). Linkage of late-onset familiar Alzheimer's disease on chromosome 19. *Society of Neuroscience Abstracts, 16,* 149.

Rouleau, I., Salmon, D. P., & Butters, N. (1996). Longitudinal analysis of clock drawing in Alzheimer's disease patients. *Brain & Cognition, 31*(1), 17-34.

Schellenberg, G. D., Boehnke, M., Wijsman, E. M., Moore, D. K., Martin, F. M., Bird, T. D., Nemens, L., White, J. A., Alonso, M. E., & Ball, M. J. (1992). Genetic association and linkage analysis of the apolipoprotein CII locus and familial Alzheimer's disease. *Annals of Neurology, 31*(2), 223-227.

Schofield, P. W., Tang, M., Marder, K., Bell, K., Dooneief, G., Chun, M., Sano, M., Stern, Y., & Mayeus, R. (1997). Alzheimer's disease after remote head injury: An incident study. *Journal of Neurology, Neurosurgery & Psychiatry, 62*(2), 119-124.

Schulz, R., O'Brien, A. T., Bookwala, J., & Fleissner, K. (1995). Psychiatric and physical morbidity effects of dementia caregiving. Prevalence, correlates, and causes. *The Gerontologist, 35*(6), 771-791.

Sclan, S. G., & Reisberg, B. (1992). Functional assessment staging (FAST) in Alzheimer's disease: Reliability, validity, and ordinality. *International Psychogeriatrics, 4*(suppl. 1), 55-69.

Silva, M. C., & Sorrel, J. M. (1992). Testing of nursing theory: Critique and philosophical expansion. *Advances in Nursing Science, 14*(4), 12-23.

Souder, E., Saykin, A. J., & Alavi, A. (1995). Multi-modal assessment in Alzheimer's disease, ADL in relation to PET, MRI and neuropsychology. *Journal of Gerontological Nursing, 21*(9), 7-13.

St. George-Hyslop, P. H., Tanzi, R. E., Polinsky, R. J., Haines, J. L., Nee, L., Watkins, P. C., Myers, R. H., Feldman, R. G., Pollen, D., Drachman, D., Growdon, J., Bruni, A., Foncin, J. F., Salmon, D., Frommelt, P., Amaducci, L., Sorbi, S., Piacentini, S., Stewart, G. D., Hobbs, W. J., Conneally, P. M., & Gusella, J. F. (1987). The genetic defect causing familial Alzheimer's disease maps on chromosome 21. *Science, 235,* 885-890.

Strunecka, A., & Patocka, J. (1999). Reassessment of the role of aluminum in the development of Alzheimer's disease. *Ceskoslovenska Fysiologie, 48*(1), 9-15.

Sunderland, T., Hill, J. L., Mellow, A. M., Lawlor, B. A., Gundersheimer, J., Newhouse, P. A., & Grafman, J. H. (1989). Clock drawing in Alzheimer's disease: A novel measure of dementia severity. *Journal of the American Geriatrics Society, 37*(8), 725-729.

Venn, R. (1983). The Sandoz clinical assessment geriatric (SCAG) scale: A general purpose psychogeriatric rating scale. *Gerontology, 29*(3), 185-198.

Verwoerdt, A. (1980). Anxiety, dissociative and personality disorders in the elderly. In E. Busse & D. Blazer (Eds.), *Handbook of geriatric psychiatry.* New York: Van Nostrand Reinhold.

Weiner, M. F. (1996). *The dementias: Diagnosis, management and research* (2nd ed.). Washington, DC: American Psychiatric Press, Inc.

Williams, R. B., & Smith, M. B. (1994). Comments on a process for identifying stages of dementia in residents of nursing facilities. *Psychological Reports, 75,* 743-746.

Winograd, C. (1984). Mental status tests and the capacity for self care. *Journal of the American Geriatrics Society, 32*(1), 49-55.

Wolanin, M. O., & Phillips, L. (1981). *Confusion: Prevention and care.* St. Louis, MO: Mosby.

CHAPTER 35

ACUTE CONFUSION

Bonnie Wakefield, Janet Mentes, Paula Mobily, Toni Tripp-Reimer, Kennith R. Culp, Carla Gene Rapp, Phyllis Gaspar, Mary Kundrat, Karen R. Wadle, and Jackie Akins

Acute confusion can occur in any age-group or any setting, but it is most common among elders in hospitals and long-term care settings. Although it can be reversible when the underlying cause is diagnosed and successfully treated, it is a sign of impending death in 25% of cases (Rabins & Folstein, 1982). Acute confusion is characterized by a disturbance in consciousness and a change in cognition that develops over a short period of time (usually hours to days), and that can be attributed to a physiologic cause (American Psychiatric Association, 1994). In fact, acute confusion is often *the* major or only presenting feature of an acute illness, an exacerbation of a chronic illness, or a drug toxicity in the elderly person (Lipowski, 1990). Given the aging of the population, the incidence of acute confusion will likely continue to increase in the coming decade.

While nurses have commonly used the term *acute confusion,* numerous other terms, including *acute brain failure, altered mental status,* and *subacute befuddlement* have been used to describe this problem (Foreman, 1993). Acute confusion is differentiated from chronic confusion (chronic cognitive impairments such as Alzheimer's disease) primarily by its sudden onset and reversible nature, usually lasting from several hours to no longer than 1 month (Foreman, 1993; Lipowski, 1990). Controversy exists as to whether acute confusion and delirium are the same phenomenon (Vermeersch, 1992). For the purposes of this chapter, the terms *acute confusion* and *delirium* are assumed to be interchangeable.

PREVALENCE

Most studies of acute confusion are conducted on elderly populations in hospital settings, since advanced age and hospital admissions seem to be associated with acute confusion. Because over one third of hospital beds in the United States are occupied by persons aged 65 and older, the diagnosis of acute confusion in any general hospital is likely to be high (Lipowski, 1989). Comparisons among studies of hospitalized clients are difficult because investigators have used varying methods and criteria to diagnose acute confusion. Estimated prevalence rates at time of admission range from 10.5% of elderly medical-surgical patients in a teaching hospital (Levkoff et al., 1992) to 18% of patients admitted on a geriatric assessment unit targeted for frail elders (Rockwood, 1993). Incidence rates vary from 7% of patients in a geriatric assessment unit for frail elders (Rockwood, 1993) up to 47.5% of elderly general medical patients (Foreman, 1990). Very few studies have assessed the persistence of acute confusion at discharge from the hospital. Levkoff et al. (1992) found that only 4% of their sample of elderly medical-surgical patients had experienced resolution of all new symptoms of acute confusion prior to discharge, and only 17% and 21%, respectively, had resolution of all new symptoms at 3 and 6 months after discharge.

An estimated 45% of all nursing home residents are confused or disoriented at some point (Roberts & Lincoln, 1988), although this figure probably represents a mix of chronic and acute confusion. However, reports vary dramatically from about 5% (Katz, Parmelee, & Brubaker, 1991) to 84% (Teitelbaum, Ginsburg, & Hopkins, 1991). In a recently completed study of 37 residents in two veteran's facilities, the prevalence rate was 40.5% over a 14-day period (Culp et al., 1997).

As is the case with studies in long-term care settings, community-based studies of acute confusion are also rare. In one study designed to sample the community prevalence of all psychiatric disorders in adults, six cases of acute confusion were found among 810 adults (Folstein, Bassett, Romanoski, & Nestadt, 1991). The estimated prevalence of acute confusion was 0.4% in the adult population and 1.1% among those 55 years of age and older, with the age-specific rate rising dramatically for those over 85 years of age. Factors that differentiated these six cases from individuals who did not have a psychiatric diagnosis or who had dementia included a greater number of current medical conditions, higher use of prescription medications, and greater functional impairment; findings that are consistent with studies of hospitalized patients (Folstein et al., 1991).

RELATED FACTORS/ETIOLOGIES

Etiologies of acute confusion vary depending on what was measured in individual studies and how risk factors were conceptualized. By and large, acute confusion is a phenomenon of elderly individuals (Marcantonio et al., 1994; Rockwood, 1989; Schor et al., 1992), although it can occur at any age. In fact, two of the three established predisposing factors (age of 60 years or older, brain damage, and chronic brain disease such as Alzheimer's) are clearly relevant to elders (Lipowski, 1990). This is not to suggest that acute confusion does not occur in children; however, no prevalence or incidence studies of acute confusion in children have been published and evidence is largely anecdotal.

Foreman (1993) summarized the most frequently identified etiologies in the literature to date. In order of frequency of identification, these etiologies are medications, infections (particularly urinary tract and upper respiratory infections), fluid and electrolyte imbalance, and metabolic disturbances (e.g., pH, nutrition). While each etiology probably predisposes the individual to acute confusion through different physiologic mechanisms, discussion of these is beyond the scope of this chapter. Lipowski (1990) categorized etiology according to predisposing factors, facilitating factors, and precipitating factors. While the presence of one or more precipitating factors (which include the four most frequently identified etiologies noted by Foreman above) is necessary for the occurrence of acute confusion, these factors alone may not be a sufficient cause.

RISK FACTORS

The probability of developing acute confusion is increased if certain predisposing (advanced age, dementia, brain damage) and facilitating (sensory over or underload, immobilization, sleep deprivation, psychosocial stress) factors are present (Lipowski, 1990). Risk factors found to be associated with increased rates of acute confusion are listed in Table 35-1. The prevalence of acute confusion is likely to be higher among females because of their greater longevity. However, male gender has been identified as a risk factor in at least one study (Schor et al., 1992). To date, differences among ethnic and cultural groups have not been studied, nor have familial tendencies been identified.

The related factors specified by North American Nursing Diagnosis Association (NANDA) are listed in Box 35-1. The NANDA related factors advanced age and dementia are consistent with the literature. The NANDA factors alcohol abuse and drug abuse have not been identified in studies of risk factors for acute confusion. It is not clear why NANDA includes delirium as a related factor. It would be interesting to know how acute confusion and delirium were differentiated by the individual who submitted this diagnosis to NANDA. Finally, NANDA omits important risk factors, including infection and metabolic disturbances such as hypoxia or dehydration (Mentes, Culp, Maas, & Rantz, 1999).

ASSESSMENT

Acutely confused patients can exhibit a wide range of behaviors, complicating the process of making a diagnosis and planning interventions. Several behaviors exhibited in

acute confusion are similar to those found in elderly persons with dementia or depression. The presenting features of these three diagnoses are summarized and compared in Box 35-2.

Lipowski (1983) identified three variants of acute confusion based on verbal and nonverbal behaviors exhibited by the patient. These variants are distinguished by the labels *hyperkinetic, hypokinetic,* and *mixed.* Patients with the hyperkinetic variant exhibit behaviors most commonly recognized as acute confusion: psychomotor hyperactivity, marked excitability, and a tendency toward hallucinations. The patient with the hypokinetic variant can be lethargic, somnolent, and apathetic and can exhibit reduced psychomotor activity; this is the "quiet" patient for whom the diagnosis of acute confusion is often missed. The third, a mixed variant, involves behavior that fluctuates between the hyperactive and hypoactive variants (Liptzin & Levkoff, 1992). In a study comparing the three presentations in a hospital setting, patients in the hyperactive group had shorter lengths of stay and a lower mortality rate than patients in either the hypoactive or mixed groups, although the reasons for this are unclear (Liptzin & Levkoff, 1992).

In most studies of acute confusion, the subtypes are not described. As a result, etiologies cannot be related to specific subtypes and proposed interventions remain globally defined. Linking clinical subtypes to antecedent conditions could improve recognition of acute confusion, facilitate clinical trials to test interventions targeted toward specific subtypes, and identify subtype-specific outcomes as well. For example, if hypoxic conditions were more likely to precipitate a hyperactive presentation, the nurse might be more likely to assess oxygen saturation as opposed to applying physical or chemical restraints. Two diagnostic algorithms have been published (Foreman, 1984; Mentes, 1995) to facilitate diagnosis and discernment of etiology. However, since intervention research is sparse, these are to be considered clinically developed protocols that need to be systematically tested.

The subtypes, as well as the *Diagnostic and Statistical Manual of Mental Disorders* (DSM-IV) behaviors and NANDA defining characteristics, are included in Box 35-3. DSM-IV behaviors focus on a disturbance in consciousness and reflect cognitive behaviors, while NANDA defining characteristics are more consistent with DSM-III-R behaviors, e.g., disturbed sleep-wake cycle. NANDA defining characteristics may also focus more on the hyperkinetic variant of acute confusion, e.g., agitated or restless behavior, although it is currently believed that elderly patients are more likely to exhibit hypoactive behaviors when acutely confused (Inouye, 1993).

Assessment Scales

The combination of an initial health history and physical assessment, mental status assessment, and ongoing use of a

Table 35-1	Significant Risk Factors ACUTE CONFUSION		
Risk Factor	**Author(s)**	**Risk Factor**	**Author(s)**
Increased age*	Gustafson et al. (1988)	Infection:	
	Levkoff et al. (1992)		
	Marcantonio et al. (1994)	• Admission prevalence	Levkoff, Cleary, et al. (1991)
	Rockwood (1989, 1993)		Rockwood (1989, 1993)
	Schor et al. (1992)	• Incident acute	Francis, Martin, & Kapoor
	Williams et al. (1985)	confusion (AC)	(1990)
	Williams-Russo et al. (1992)		Rockwood (1989, 1993)
Education	Foreman (1989, 1990)		Schor et al. (1992)
Depression	Foreman (1989)	Fluid/electrolyte imbalance	Foreman (1989)
	Pompei et al. (1994)		Francis, Martin, & Kapoor
Race	Foreman (1990)		(1990)
Gender:			Inouye (1993)
			Levkoff et al. (1988)
• Female	Foreman (1990)		Levkoff, Cleary, et al. (1991)
• Male	Schor et al. (1992)		Marcantonio et al. (1994)
	Williams-Russo et al., (1992)		Rockwood (1989, 1993)
Residence before	Levkoff et al. (1992)	Pain	Schor et al. (1992)
admission	Schor et al. (1992)		Williams et al. (1985)
Fracture on admission	Rockwood (1989)	Medications (number and/	Foreman (1989)
	Schor et al. (1992)	or type)	Francis, Martin, & Kapoor
	Williams et al. (1985)		(1990)
Physical functional status	Marcantonio et al. (1994)		Gustafson et al. (1988)
	Williams et al. (1985)		Rockwood (1993)
Dementia/cognitive	Francis, Martin, & Kapoor		Rogers et al. (1989)
impairment*	(1990)		Schor et al. (1992)
	Gustafson et al. (1988)		Williams et al. (1985)
	Inouye (1993)	Hypotension, hypoxemia	Gustafson et al. (1988)
	Levkoff et al. (1992)		Rockwood (1989, 1993)
	Marcantonio et al. (1994)	Alcohol intake*	Gustafson et al. (1988)
	Pompei et al. (1994)		Pompei et al. (1994)
	Rockwood (1989)		Williams-Russo et al. (1992)
	Schor et al. (1992)	Visual deficits	Inouye (1993)
Severity of illness	Francis, Martin, & Kapoor		
	(1990)		
	Inouye (1993)		
	Pompei et al. (1994)		
	Rockwood (1989)		

*Included in NANDA list of related factors.

standardized acute confusion rating tool will assist in differentiating acute confusion from other states of altered cognition (i.e., depression or dementia). However, detecting acute confusion in a person with dementia is difficult unless the nurse is familiar with the patient's baseline behaviors. Since, by definition, acute confusion is a recent and *acute* change in behavior, gathering information from proxy sources, i.e., the family or other care providers, is critical if the patient is unfamiliar to the nurse or in cases where the patient is unable to respond to interview questions.

Several investigators have used standard mental status questionnaires such as the Mini Mental Status Examination (MMSE) and the Short Portable Mental Status Questionnaire (SPMSQ) to assess for acute confusion.

However, these instruments assess general cognitive function and are not specific for acute confusion (Levkoff, Cleary, Liptzin, & Evans, 1991; Levkoff, Liptzin, Cleary, Reilly, & Evans, 1991). While standard mental status instruments can provide useful data to assist in diagnosing acute confusion, several acute confusion-specific scales are currently available (Rapp et al., 2000). These instruments, including the NEECHAM, Confusion Assessment Method (CAM), Delirium Rating Scale (DRS), Delirium Symptom Interview (DSI), and Clinical Assessment of Confusion (CAC), are listed in Table 35-2. Of these, the NEECHAM and CAC were developed from a nursing perspective. The NEECHAM is recommended because it has been tested more extensively, is easy to administer, and provides a nu-

| Box 35-1 | Suggested Nursing-Sensitive Outcomes and Nursing Interventions
ACUTE CONFUSION |

Nursing Diagnosis
Acute Confusion
Defining characteristics
Fluctuation in cognition
Fluctuation in sleep-wake cycle
Fluctuation in level of consciousness
Fluctuation in psychomotor activity
Increased agitation or restlessness
Misperceptions
Lack of motivation to initiate and/or follow through with goal-directed or purposeful behavior
Hallucinations

Related factors/etiologies
Over 60 years of age
Dementia
Alcohol abuse
Drug abuse
Delirium

Nursing-Sensitive Outcome
Cognitive Ability
Indicators
Communicates clearly and appropriately for age and ability
Demonstrates control over selected events and situations
Attentiveness
Concentration
Orientation
Demonstrates immediate memory
Demonstrates recent memory
Demonstrates remote memory
Processes information
Weighs alternatives when making decisions

Nursing Interventions
Delirium Management
Activities
Identify and treat etiology

- Identify etiologic factors causing delirium
- Initiate therapies to reduce or eliminate factors causing the delirium

Maintain patient safety

- Maintain a well-lit environment that reduces sharp contrasts and shadows
- Maintain a hazard-free environment
- Place identification bracelet on patient
- Provide appropriate level of supervision or surveillance to monitor patient and to allow for therapeutic actions, as needed
- Encourage use of aids that increase sensory input (e.g., eyeglasses, hearing aids, and dentures)
- Use physical restraints, as needed

- Administer medications as needed (PRN) for anxiety or agitation

Provide psychologic support and comfort

- Provide unconditional positive regard
- Verbally acknowledge the patient's fears and feelings
- Provide optimistic but realistic reassurance
- Allow the patient to maintain rituals that limit anxiety
- Avoid demands for abstract thinking, if patient can think only in concrete terms
- Limit need for decision making, if frustrating or confusing for patient
- Encourage visitation by significant others, as appropriate
- Recognize and accept the patient's perceptions or interpretation of reality (hallucinations or delusions)
- State your perception in a calm, reassuring, and nonargumentative manner
- Respond to the theme/feeling/tone, rather than the content, of the hallucination or delusion
- Remove stimuli, when possible, that create misperception in a particular patient (e.g., pictures on wall, television)
- Avoid frustrating patient by quizzing with orientation questions that cannot be answered
- Inform patient of person, place, and time, as needed
- Provide a consistent physical environment and daily routine
- Provide caregivers who are familiar to the patient
- Use environmental cues (e.g., signs, pictures, clocks, calendars, color coding of environment) to stimulate memory, reorient, and promote appropriate behavior
- Provide a low-stimulation environment for patient in whom disorientation is increased by overstimulation
- Provide patient with information about what is happening and what can be expected to occur in the future
- Approach patient slowly and from the front
- Address the patient by name when initiating interaction
- Reorient the patient to the health care provider with each contact
- Communicate with simple, direct, descriptive statements
- Prepare patient for upcoming changes in usual routine and environment prior to their occurrence
- Provide new information slowly and in small doses, with frequent rest periods
- Focus interpersonal interactions on what is familiar and meaningful to the patient

Monitor/support physical status

- Monitor neurologic status on an ongoing basis
- Assist with needs related to nutrition, elimination, hydration, and personal hygiene

Box 35-2	Features of Delirium (Acute Confusion), Dementia, and Depression

Dimension	Dementia
Onset	Insidious
24-hour course	Stable
Consciousness	Clear
Attention	Usually normal
Cognition	Globally impaired
Hallucinations	Often absent
Orientation	Often impaired
Psychomotor	Often normal, but may
Speech	be reduced or shift
Recent memory	Difficulty finding words,
Physical illness or drug	perseveration
toxicity	Impaired, confabulation
	Often absent
Delirium	
Sudden	**Depression**
Fluctuating	Weeks
Reduced	Worse in morning
Diminished	Intact
Globally disoriented	Withdrawn
Visual or auditory	Slowed
Usually impaired	Delusions
Increased activity	Intact
Incoherent, slow, or	Flat affect, apathy
rapid	Normal or slowed
Patchy	Normal, or recent impaired
One or both present	Absent

Data from Lipowski, Z. J. (1990). *Acute confusion: Acute confusional states*. New York: Oxford University Press; Mezey, M., Rauckhorst, L., & Stokes, S. (1993). *Health assessment of the older individual*. New York: Springer.

merical score that can be used to track a patient's trajectory of confusion.

The NEECHAM Confusion Scale was developed to differentiate normal information processing, early cues preceding confusion, and acute confusion. Scores range from 0 to 30, with a score of 0 to 19 representing acute confusion. The NEECHAM is correlated with the MMSE, but is more sensitive to impending confusion (Champagne, Neelon, McConnell, & Funk, 1987). NEECHAM scores are significantly related to key clinical indicators of acute confusion development (Neelon, Funk, Carlson, & Champagne, 1989). According to the developers of the NEECHAM, the correlation for inter-rater reliability is 0.96, test-retest coefficient is 0.98, Cronbach's alpha for internal consistency is 0.86, and correlation with the MMSE is 0.78 (Neelon, Champagne, Carlson, & Funk, 1996).

CASE STUDY

S. Zitmyer, a widowed 73-year-old male from Los Angeles was visiting his adult niece in Chicago when he was admitted to the county hospital with suspected appendicitis at 8:00 AM. Because Mr. Zitmyer was a veteran and normally

received much of his care at the Veterans' Administration (VA) medical center in California, the doctor had his medical summary records faxed to the admission department and sent to the unit with his admission work-up. From this record, the admitting nurse learned that Mr. Zitmyer was a prisoner of war (POW) in Japan during World War II and had been receiving treatment for peptic ulcer disease (PUD). He was divorced and had no adult children.

After a brief admission history, the nurse measured Mr. Zitmyer's baseline mental status and determined that he was oriented to person, place, and time. Mr. Zitmyer's niece, Maggie, noted that he was fine when she picked him up at the airport the day before and they had stayed up late the night before recalling family memories. As the nurse completed her assessment, she noted that Mr. Zitmyer appeared somewhat unkempt from the nausea and vomiting and somewhat slow in responding to questions, but answered appropriately when she rephrased the question a second time. He had poor eye contact, as he was very focused on receiving an injection to make the pain go away. Mr. Zitmyer's preoperative urinalysis, complete blood cell count (CBC), and serum electrolyte levels were all within normal limits, with the exception of a 151mEq/dL serum sodium level.

At 9:00 AM, Mr. Zitmyer was quickly rushed off to surgery where an appendectomy was performed. After 2 hours in the recovery room, Mr. Zitmyer returned to his room. The nurse noted a dry and intact abdominal dressing, a nasogastric (NG) tube set to low intermittent suction, a Foley catheter with dark amber urine, an intravenous (IV) pump infusing lactated Ringer's solution at 100 ml/hr, oxygen at 1 L per nasal prongs (NP), and patient-controlled analgesia (PCA) programmed with morphine sulfate at 1 mg/hour continuous infusion and a PCA dose set for 1 mg every 10 minutes.

At 12:00 PM, Mr. Zitmyer's vital signs were stable, with the exception of a 38.5° C temperature. The nurse emptied the drainage canister and noted 450 ml of dark brown NG drainage. Because of his history of PUD, cimetidine 300 mg IV was ordered. Mr. Zitmyer was lethargic from his anesthesia and did not seem to follow her directions for using the incentive spirometer. At 2:30 PM, Mr. Zitmyer asked to stand up to void, but the nurse politely explained to him that a catheter was in place and asked him to stay in bed. Mr. Zitmyer also began to complain of pain and the nurse instructed him on using the PCA. His niece, Maggie, was at his bedside, but extremely tired.

At 5:45 PM, Mr. Zitmyer became rather adamant that he needed to void and asked for assistance in standing up. The nurse noted that his Foley bag contained 500 ml of clear yellow urine during the last 2 hours and once again reinforced her prior instructions about having a catheter, but Mr. Zitmyer did not seem to understand. He began to pull at his Foley device and demanded to have his NG tube removed. Mr. Zitmyer was significantly more restless. He verbalized references to being at the neighborhood gas station and asked for a key to the restroom. Mr. Zitmyer's attention was noticeably altered and he did not know the nursing assistant came into the room at 8:45 PM to drain the Foley bag, which contained another 500 ml of clear yellow urine.

Box 35-3	Summary of Behavior Subtypes and DSM Behaviors

Hyperactive Behaviors
Restlessness
Fast or loud speech
Irritability
Wandering
Distractability
Impatience
Uncooperativeness
Persistent thoughts
Hypervigilance
Combativeness
Swearing
Singing
Laughing
Euphoria
Anger
Easy startling
Fast motor responses
Tangentiality
Nightmares

Hypoactive Behaviors
Lethargic
Decreased alertness
Sparse or slow speech
Slowed movements
Staring
Unawareness
Apathy

DSM-IV
Diminished ability to focus, sustain, or shift attention, including:

- Difficult to engage in conversation
- Attention wanders
- Easily distracted
- Perseverates

Change in cognition:

- Disoriented to time, place, person
- Speech (rambling, incoherent, pressured, irrelevant)
- Perceptual disturbances (hallucinations, delusions)
- Recent memory impairment
- Language disturbance (naming objects, sentences, switching between subjects)

NANDA Defining Characteristics
Major:

- Fluctuation in cognition
- Fluctuation in sleep/wake cycle
- Fluctuation in level of consciousness
- Fluctuation in psychomotor activity
- Increased agitation or restlessness
- Misperceptions
- Lack of motivation to initiate and/or follow through with goal-directed or purposeful behavior

Minor:

- Hallucinations

Data from Liptzin, B., & Levkoff, S. E. (1992). An empirical study of delirium subtypes. *British Journal of Psychiatry, 161,* 843-845; American Psychiatric Association (APA). (1994). *Diagnostic and statistical manual of mental disorders* (4th ed.). Washington, DC: Author; Rantz, M., & LeMone, P. (1995). *Classification of nursing diagnoses: Proceedings of the eleventh NANDA conference.* Glendale, CA: Cinahl Information Systems.

Table 35-2	Acute Confusion Rating Scales
Rating Scale	**Dimension Measured**
Delirium Rating Scale (DRS)	Temporal onset of symptoms, perceptual disturbances, hallucination type, delusions, psychomotor behavior, cognitive status during testing, physical disorder, sleep-wake cycle disturbances, lability of mood, variability of symptoms (Trzepacz, Baker, & Greenhouse, 1988)
Confusion Assessment Method (CAM)	Acute onset, inattention, disorganized thinking, altered level of consciousness, disorientation, memory impairment, perceptual disturbances, psychomotor agitation, psychomotor retardation, altered sleep-wake cycle (Inouye et al., 1990; Levkoff, Cleary, et al., 1991; Levkoff, Liptzin, et al., 1991)
Delirium Symptom Interview (DSI)	Disorientation, disturbance of consciousness, disruption of sleep-wake cycle, perceptual disturbances, incoherence of speech, change in psychomotor activity, fluctuating behavior (Albert et al., 1992)
Clinical Assessment of Confusion	Cognition, general behavior, motor activity, orientation, and psychotic/neurotic behavior (CAC-A); for CAC-B, the following were added: level of consciousness, behaviors that threaten safety of patient, and ability to interact, perform ADL, speech content (Vermeersch, 1990, 1992)
NEECHAM	Processing: neurosensory, motor, verbal; performance: appearance/hygiene, motor, verbal; vital function stability, oxygen saturation stability, urinary continence control (Champagne et al., 1987; Neelon et al., 1989; Neelon et al., 1996)

NURSING DIAGNOSIS

The nursing diagnosis Acute Confusion was approved by NANDA in 1994 (Rantz & LeMone, 1995). NANDA defines Acute Confusion as "the abrupt onset of a cluster of global, transient changes and disturbances in attention, cognition, psychomotor activity level of consciousness, and/or sleep/wake cycle" (NANDA, 1999, p. 119). Previously, either Altered Thought Processes or Sensory Perceptual Alteration would have been chosen as the nursing diagnosis in the presence of acute confusion. An additional potential diagnosis proposed by Gordon (1987) is Potential Cognitive Impairment. While there is overlap among the defining characteristics of the three diagnoses with the DSM indicators for delirium, none of these diagnoses are particularly descriptive of the etiologies and defining characteristics of acute confusion. Therefore the focus of this discussion will be the nursing diagnosis of Acute Confusion.

Current NANDA work on the diagnosis Acute Confusion has several weaknesses. The diagnosis, as submitted, is not consistent with current DSM-IV terminology. Delirium (which is synonymous with acute confusion) is presented as an etiology. The defining characteristics do not reflect hypoactive presentations. Finally, the related factors need to be modified, as they reflect both predisposing factors and one etiology, i.e., substance abuse, but ignore other medical conditions/physiologic-based causes.

NURSING-SENSITIVE OUTCOMES

Suggested goals for the acutely confused person are (1) correction of the underlying physiologic alteration; (2) diminished or resolution of confusion; (3) family member verbalization of understanding of confusion; and (4) pre-

vention of injury (Zimberg & Berenson, 1990). Although resolution of the confusion is the primary goal, the nurse makes important contributions toward achievement of all four goals. While the primary goal will be to identify and treat the cause of confusion, the effectiveness of the intervention is measured by improvement in cognition. Cognitive mental health has been defined by Rubenstein and Rubenstein (1992) as "the degree to which the person is alert, oriented, able to concentrate, and able to perform complex mental tasks, such as learning" (p. 153). This is differentiated from affective mental health, defined as "the degree to which the person feels anxious, depressed, or generally happy" (Rubenstein & Rubenstein, 1992). The corresponding NOC outcome label Cognitive Ability is defined as the "ability to execute complex mental processes" (Iowa Outcomes Project, 2000, p. 170). Indicators for Cognition Ability are shown in Table 35-2.

Cognitive function has been conceptualized in various ways. In general, cognition is reflected by an individual's level of consciousness, orientation, ability to pay attention and concentrate, and ability to perform complex mental tasks (Rubenstein & Rubenstein, 1992). For the purpose of this chapter, cognition will be discussed as a combination of perception (including attention and interpretation), memory (both retention and recall), and thinking (a conscious process of awareness, ability to understand, reason, make decisions, and apply judgment) (Lipowski, 1990). In acute confusion, all of these functions are compromised. These indicators of cognition are compared to the NOC indicators in Table 35-3.

Perception

Perception refers to a process of extracting, interpreting, and integrating information in a meaningful way

Table 35-3 Comparison of Outcome Indicators	
Indicators of Cognition	**NOC Cognition Indicators**
PERCEPTION Sustained attention (able to concentrate) Selective attention (ability to extract relevant information)	Communicates clearly and appropriately for age and ability Demonstrates control over selected events and situations Attends
MEMORY Short-term memory intact Long-term memory intact	Concentrates Is oriented Demonstrates immediate memory Demonstrates recent memory Demonstrates remote memory
THINKING Able to engage in: problem solving, abstract thinking, computation	Processes information Weighs alternatives when making decisions

(Lipowski, 1990). To do this first requires attention. Alertness is required for attention, but the alert patient may not necessarily be able to attend. The person's ability to maintain attention must be established before other more complex functions can be assessed (Strub & Black, 1993). Attention has two aspects: sustained attention (vigilance or concentration) and selective attention (the ability to extract relevant from irrelevant information). Numerous studies indicate that elders normally perform well on tests of both sustained and selective attention. Earlier findings of poor performance on tests of selective attention have been attributed to lack of control for perceptual difficulties (Albert, 1994). The most common cause of decreased attention is diffuse brain dysfunction, usually caused by metabolic disturbances, drug intoxication, infections, post-surgical states (relevant to acute confusional states) or extensive bilateral cortical damage of any etiology (Strub & Black, 1993). Perceptual disorders also include misperceptions (such as illusions and hallucinations), which are sometimes experienced by the acutely confused person (Lipowski, 1990).

Memory

Other than overall intelligence, age-related memory alterations have been more widely studied than any other aspect of cognition. Primary memory, or short-term (recent, immediate) memory, is the ability to retain a small amount of information over a brief period of time. Secondary memory, or long-term (remote) memory, is a memory store containing an unlimited amount of information over an indefinite period of time. Both types of memory may be impaired in acute confusion, which clouds the diagnosis of acute confusion in the person with a pre-existing dementia. While some assert that primary memory shows few, if any, losses with aging (Albert, 1994), others believe there are striking age-related differences in performance on short-term memory tasks (Morris & McManus, 1991; Verhaeghen, Marcoen, & Goossens, 1993). Age decrements are greater when subjects are asked to recall information than when they are asked to recognize stimuli they were previously exposed to (Albert, 1994).

Memory deficits in later life are believed to be due to problems in encoding, or "getting" the information in the first place. This can be due to sensory problems, to not paying attention, or to a general failure either to link the "to-be-remembered" information to existing knowledge through association or to strengthen the memory through repetition. It is important, however, not to confuse decline with deficit. While a decline in memory ability can be frustrating for older individuals, it does not necessarily hamper their ability to function day to day. Threats to memory include medications, depression (impairs concentration and attention), poor nutrition, infection, heart and lung disease (lack of oxygen), thyroid problems (can cause symptoms of depression or confusion that mimic memory loss), alcohol use, sensory loss (interferes with perception), and multiple competing stimuli. Several of these threats to memory are risk factors for acute confusion.

Thinking

Thinking, or higher integrative cognitive function, includes such abilities as problem solving, abstract thinking, and computation. With the exception of the period immediately preceding death (called terminal drop), intelligence is stable over the life span in the absence of disease. The learning abilities of older persons, however, can be more selective, requiring motivation, meaning, and familiarity with the content. As noted earlier, the inability to pay attention precludes many learning activities. Additionally, lack of motivation or apathy is a common finding in acutely confused individuals (Lipowski, 1990). Level of education needs to be considered in evaluating responses to mental status examinations. It can serve as a proxy measure for socioeconomic status and occupation, both of which are positively correlated with performance on mental status examinations (Frisoni, Rozzini, Bianchetti, & Trabucchi, 1993; Launer, Dinkgreve, Jonker, Hooijer, & Lindeboom, 1993).

As aging occurs, reaction time slows (Salthouse, 1993), affecting how quickly the elder responds to questions. Hurrying elders to answer questions can decrease their ability to provide the correct answer. In a "speed-accuracy shift," elderly individuals focus more on accuracy than on speed in responding (Hertzog, Vernon, & Rympa, 1993). Caution tends to increase with age, while risk-taking behavior tends to decrease. As a result, older adults are more likely to make errors of omission (leaving an answer out) than errors of commission (making a guess) (Cerella, 1990). Therefore a slowed reaction time should not necessarily be attributed to diminished attention.

In summary, changes in cognition as aging occurs are most likely accounted for by anatomic and physiologic changes in the brain. Anatomic and physiologic alterations are probably highly specific, since age-related indicators of cognitive decline are very specific and many abilities are preserved. Moreover, external factors such as activity level, socioeconomic status, education, personality, and overall health can modify the development or expression of age-related changes in cognition (Albert, 1994; Hultsch, Hammer, & Small, 1993; Inouye, Albert, Mohs, Sun, & Berkman, 1993). These factors must be taken into account when assessing the acute cognitive changes associated with acute confusion.

Overall, the outcome label Cognitive Ability is inclusive of the indicators for cognition. One criticism concerns the inclusion of both immediate and recent memory as indicators; this should be considered in future revisions of the label. The outcome indicators do not directly reflect the obverse of the NANDA defining characteristics for acute confusion as currently accepted. However, this more likely indicates that the NANDA defining characteristics need to be updated and changed. The outcome indicators also are not directly linked to the *Nursing Interventions Classification (NIC)* (Iowa Intervention Project, 2000) activities. However, with the exception of the first two activities aimed at identifying and treating the cause of the AC, the remaining activities are supportive interventions during an episode of AC. Treating the cause, whether it be interventions for dehydration or changing the person's medications, will lead most directly to the identified outcome. However, the supportive activities are important during the acute confusional episode.

Outcome Rating Scales

As noted earlier, there are several excellent mental status rating scales available; choice of a scale will depend on the particular cognitive problem being measured. No rating scale exists to operationalize the outcome indicators for cognition. Therefore the rating scales discussed earlier; in particular the NEECHAM scale, are recommended to monitor cognition in the acutely confused person.

The NEECHAM has certain advantages over other scales. It does not place the patient in a "testing" situation with repeated demanding questions and, therefore, minimizes response burden (Miller et al., 1997; Neelon et al., 1996). The first subscale measures the three aspects of cognition discussed earlier and is given the most weight in scoring the scale (from 0 to 14 points). The second subscale (0 to 10 points) measures verbal and motor behaviors associated with neuromotor manifestations of toxic or metabolic disturbances. The third subscale measures physiologic parameters, including vital signs, oxygen stability, and urinary continence (range 0 to 6); this subscale can both help detect early physiologic signs of confusion and indicate the pathophysiology of ensuing confusion (Neelon et al., 1996). Overall, the NEECHAM Confusion Scale is quick and easy to use.

NURSING INTERVENTIONS

The appropriate NIC intervention for acute confusion is Delirium Management, which is the "provision of a safe and therapeutic environment for the patient who is experiencing an acute confusional state" (Iowa Interventions Project, 2000, p. 245) (Table 35-1). This intervention is global in nature and reflects the current state of knowledge about interventions for acutely confused persons. As noted earlier, it would be preferable to have interventions that are targeted at specific subtypes of AC with their associated etiologies, but research in this area is limited. As the knowledge base develops, more specific interventions can be developed. Of course, other NIC interventions might be appropriate for the acutely confused patient depending

on how the syndrome is manifested, i.e., interventions for specific electrolyte imbalances or drug toxicity. As with all patients requiring nursing interventions, the approach needs to be individualized according to patient needs.

Management of acute confusion occurs at two levels: (1) elimination or correction of the underlying cause and (2) symptomatic and supportive measures (e.g., adequate rest, comfort promotion, environmental support and cues such as lighting and family pictures, maintenance of fluid and electrolyte balance, and protection from injury) (Lipowski, 1990). Cronin-Stubbs (1996) reviewed nine experimental or quasi-experimental studies testing interventions for acutely confused persons age 65 and older. Seven of these were found in published articles; two were dissertations. Of the seven published studies, two focused on pain management techniques (Egbert, Parks, Short, & Burnett, 1990; Williams-Russo, Urquhart, Sharrock, & Charlson, 1992) and one focused on interventions primarily under the control of physicians (e.g., timing of surgery, preoperative pharmacologic thrombosis prophylaxis, anesthetic technique) (Gustafson et al., 1991). The remaining published studies evaluated "usual" nursing or medical activities (e.g., orientation of the patient) and environmental manipulations (e.g., adequate lighting); these four studies are summarized in Table 35-4. Clearly, the theoretical and empirical base for confusion-specific interventions is weak. Tested interventions have not been significantly unique or different from usual care. Tested interventions have tended to be highly individualized for patients. Finally, the dose of the intervention has not been measured.

Rabins (1991) suggests three broad actions that can be taken to improve the care of the patient with acute confusion. These suggestions are consistent with the interventions tested in the studies listed in Table 35-4 and should accompany the process of identification and treatment of the physiologic cause(s) of acute confusion (infection, medications, or fluid and electrolyte imbalances). First, provide a predictable, orienting environment. Staff should have frequent interaction with the patient and explain that they are confused and may be hallucinating. This allows the patient to express his fears and discomforts. Adequate lighting, easy-to-read calendars and clocks, a reasonable noise level, along with frequent verbal orientation, can lessen this frightening experience for patients. If the patient wears eyeglasses or uses a hearing aid, these devices should be used by the patient. Including familiar personal possessions in the environment also can help. Second, physical restraint should be avoided *if possible* and used only to prevent potential self-injury from agitated behavior. Third, proper diagnosis of acute confusion can be used to explain the patient's behavior to family members. Families can work with staff in reorienting the patient and providing a supportive environment. Families will need to understand that important decisions requiring the patient's input should be delayed, if at all possible, until

Table 35-4	Summary of Intervention Studies			
Author	**Sample**	**Intervention**	**Outcome Measures**	**Findings**
Williams et al. (1985)	Hip fracture patients age ≥60 Control *n* = 170 Treatment *n* = 57	Nursing care directed at patient symptoms, at the discretion of the nursing staff; use of a nurse-visitor	Incidence of acute confusion, length of hospital stay	Significantly lower incidence of confusion in the treatment group
Wanich, Sullivan-Marx, Gottlieb, & Johnson (1992)	Hospitalized general medicine patients age ≥70 Control *n* = 100 Treatment *n* = 135	Nursing staff education; caregiver education; patient orientation and communication, mobilization, environmental modifications, medication management, and discharge planning	Incidence of acute confusion, complications (e.g., urinary tract infection, cardiac arrest, decubiti), hospital mortality, discharge to nursing home, length of stay, change in functional status	Intervention group had greater improvement and less deterioration in functional status compared to control group; no significant differences in acute confusion incidence or other measures
Nagley (1986)	Hospitalized general medicine patients age ≥65 Control *n* = 30 Treatment *n* = 30	Sixteen nursing actions directed at the environment, patient interaction, and monitoring	Investigator developed AC measure and the Short Portable Mental Status Questionnaire	No significant differences between the two groups on development of AC on day 4 of hospitalization
Cole et al. (1994)	Hospitalized general medicine patients with acute confusion on admission age ≥75 Control *n* = 46 Treatment *n* = 42	Consultation by physician with follow-up by nurse	Mental status score, behavior rating scale, use of restraints, length of stay, discharge to higher level of care than admission	Short-term improvement in mental status, improved behavior rating scores

the patient is recovered. While patients might be able to participate in decision making, they might not remember this later; therefore it is important to have several witnesses present (Rabins, 1991). Most of Rabins' suggestions are included in the NIC activities. It will be important to add support for and communication with family members during the acute confusional episode to the activity list. Finally, one helpful "systems" intervention is the use of specially trained resource nurses to identify and manage acutely confused individuals (Rapp et al., 1998).

Although the literature on interventions is sparse, four themes emerge: identifying and treating the etiology; ensuring the safety of the patient; providing psychologic support and comfort; and maintaining physiologic homeostasis. In Box 35-1 the activities of Delirium Management are organized under these four categories. In an effort to be inclusive and applicable to as many practice settings as possible, many NIC interventions include a large number of activities. This intervention includes 36 activities. Of the 36 activities, 25 fall under psychologic support and comfort, even though by definition acute confusion has a physiologic cause. To facilitate use of this intervention, the 25 activities under psychologic support and comfort should be condensed. As noted, because there are several physiologic causes for acute confusion, the appropriate NIC intervention should also be selected for that cause, for example, Fluid/Electrolyte Management for a suspected fluid and electrolyte etiology. This reasoning extends to choice of the NOC outcome indicator (Iowa Outcomes Project, 2000). That is, more than one outcome label may be chosen in addition to Cognitive Ability, depending on the physiologic cause of acute confusion.

CASE STUDY

The nurse became concerned about losing the NG tube and phoned the physician, who gave an order for Haldol 1 mg IM and soft restraints. As his NG output had increased 100 ml in the last hour, serum electrolytes and a complete blood count (CBC) were also obtained. The nurse initiated these measures and found Mr. Zitmyer much more distressed when his hands were tied to the bed frame. He no longer seemed to look when someone walked into the room. He tugged at the restraints and begged the nurse to release him.

At 9:30 PM, the serum potassium level came back as 3.1 mEq/dL and the hematocrit was 42.4%. His serum sodium level was now normal. The nurse changed the IV to normal saline with 20 mEq KCl/dL per written instructions. However, there was still no improvement in Mr. Zitmyer's mental status change. The oxygen per nasal pronges (NP) had been displaced from his nares several times during the night, and the nurse found his oxygen-hemoglobin saturation to be 88%. The oxygen was repositioned and promptly increased to 3 L per NP. The follow-up reading with the pulse oximeter was 95%. His niece, Maggie, was quite distressed over his change in status.

Maggie stayed with her elderly uncle throughout the night. She felt so concerned that he might be in pain that she pressed the PCA button for him. Knowing the button could be pressed as frequently as every 10 minutes she tried to keep up a schedule throughout the night. By 7:00 AM the night nurse found Maggie asleep in the lounge chair by Mr. Zitmyer. The NG output was now light green and had decreased to <20 ml over 2 hours. The nurse assessed the abdomen for bowel sounds, which were now hypoactive. At 8:00 AM the surgical team made rounds and discontinued Mr. Zitmyer's NG tube. The cloth restraints were removed and Mr. Zitmyer reached up to rub his nose. The doctor also discontinued the PCA and started Tylenol with Codeine 60 mg PO for pain.

At 11:00 AM Mr. Zitmyer's mental status had markedly improved. Maggie asked him if he knew where he was; all Mr. Zitmyer could remember was his admission through the emergency room and knowing he was going to have surgery. When Maggie explained how he had tried to pull all of his tubes out the night before, he could not remember doing so.

SUMMARY

Although acute confusion is a significant problem among elders, the effectiveness of nursing interventions to prevent and treat this problem has yet to be established. Nurses are familiar with patients' usual behaviors and are intimately involved in basic care procedures such as ensuring adequate hydration and monitoring responses to medication. Nurses also must be knowledgeable about the assessment and treatment of acute confusion. Those activities included in NIC intervention Delirium Management reflect current thinking about potentially effective approaches. However, much work is needed to precisely define effective interventions for both prevention and treatment of acute confusion.

REFERENCES

Albert, M., Levkoff, S., Reilly, C., Liptzin, B., Pilgrim, D., Cleary, P., Evans, D., & Rowe, J. (1992). The delirium symptom interview: An interview for the detection of delirium symptoms in hospitalized patients. *Journal of Geriatric Psychiatry and Neurology, 5*, 14-21.

Albert, M. S. (1994). Cognition and aging. In W. R. Hazzard, E. L. Bierman, J. P. Blass, W. H. Ettinger, & J. B. Halter (Eds.), *Principles of geriatric medicine and gerontology* (3rd ed., pp. 1013-1019). Hightstown, NJ: McGraw-Hill.

American Psychiatric Association (APA). (1994). *Diagnostic and statistical manual of mental disorders* (4th ed.). Washington, DC: Author.

Cerella, J. (1990). Aging and information-processing rate. In J. E. Birren & K. W. Schaie (Eds.), *Handbook of the psychology of aging* (3rd ed., pp. 201-221). San Diego, CA: Academic Press.

Champagne, M., Neelon, V., McConnell, E., & Funk, S. (1987). The NEECHAM confusion scale: Assessing acute confusion in the hospitalized and nursing home elderly. *The Gerontologist, 27,* 4A.

Cole, M. G., Primeau, F. J., Bailey, R. F., Bonnycastle, M. J., Masciarelli, F., Engelsmann, F., Pepin, M. J., & Ducie, D. (1994). Systematic intervention for elderly inpatients with acute confusion: A randomized trial. *Canadian Medical Association Journal, 151*(7), 965-970.

Cronin-Stubbs, D. (1996). Delirium intervention research in acute care settings. *Annual Review of Nursing Research, 14,* 57-73.

Culp, K., Tripp-Reimer, T., Wadle, K., Wakefield, B., Akins, J., Mobily, P., & Kundrat, M. (1997). Acute confusion in elderly nursing home residents. *Journal of Neuroscience Nursing, 29*(2), 86-88, 95-100.

Egbert, A., Parks, L., Short, L., & Burnett, M. (1990). Randomized trial of postoperative patient-controlled analgesia vs intramuscular narcotics in frail elderly men. *Archives of Internal Medicine, 150,* 1897-1903.

Folstein, M. F., Bassett, S. S., Romanoski, A. J., & Nestadt, G. (1991). The epidemiology of acute confusion in the community: The Eastern Baltimore mental health survey. *International Psychogeriatrics, 3*(2), 169-176.

Foreman, M. (1984). Algorithm for the assessment of confusional states. *Dimensions in Critical Care Nursing, 3*(4), 208-215.

Foreman, M. (1989). Confusion in the hospitalized elderly: Incidence, onset, and associated factors. *Research in Nursing and Health, 12,* 21-29.

Foreman, M. (1990). The cognitive and behavioral nature of acute confusional states. *Scholarly Inquiry for Nursing Practice, 5*(1), 3-16.

Foreman, M. (1993). Acute confusion in the elderly. *Annual Review of Nursing Research, 11,* 3-30.

Francis, J., Martin, D., & Kapoor, W. (1990). A prospective study of acute confusion in hospitalized elderly. *Journal of the American Medical Association, 263,* 1097-1101.

Frisoni, G. B., Rozzini, R., Bianchetti, A., & Trabucchi, M. (1993). Principal lifetime occupation and MMSE score in elderly persons. *Journal of Gerontology, 48*(6), S310-S314.

Gordon, M. (1987). *Manual of nursing diagnosis.* Hightstown, NJ: McGraw-Hill.

Gustafson, Y., Berggren D., Brannstrom, B., Bucht, G., Norberg, A., Hansson L., & Winblad B. (1988). Acute confusional states in elderly patients treated for femoral neck fracture. *Journal of the American Geriatrics Society, 36,* 525-530.

Gustafson, Y., Brannstrom, B., Berggren, D., Ragnarsson, J., Sigaard, J., Bucht, G., Reiz, S., Norberg, A., & Winblad, B. (1991). A geriatric-anesthesiologic program to reduce acute confusional states in elderly patients treated for femoral neck fractures. *Journal of the American Geriatrics Society, 39,* 655-662.

Hertzog, C., Vernon, M. C., & Rympa, B. (1993). Age differences in mental rotation task performance: The influence of speed/accuracy tradeoffs. *Journal of Gerontology, 48*(3), P150-P156.

Hultsch, D. F., Hammer, M., & Small, B. J. (1993). Age differences in cognitive performance in later life: Relationships to self-reported health and activity life style. *Journal of Gerontology, 48*(1), P1-P11.

Inouye, S. (1993). Delirium in hospitalized elderly patients: Recognition, evaluation, and management. *Connecticut Medicine, 57*(5), 309-315.

Inouye, S., VanDyck, C., Alessi, C., Balkin, S., Siegal, A., & Horvitz, R. (1990). Clarifying confusion: The confusion assessment method. A new method for detection of delirium. *Annals of Internal Medicine, 113,* 941-948.

Inouye, S., Viscoli, C., Horwitz, R., Hurst, L., & Tinetti, M. (1993). A predictive model for acute confusion in hospitalized elderly medical patients based on admission characteristics. *Annals of Internal Medicine, 119*(6), 474-481.

Inouye, S. K., Albert, M. S., Mohs, R., Sun, K., & Berkman, L. F. (1993). Cognitive performance in a high-functioning community-dwelling elderly population. *Journal of Gerontology, 48*(4), M146-M151.

Iowa Intervention Project. J. C. McCloskey & G. M. Bulechek (Eds.). (2000). *Nursing interventions classification (NIC)* (3rd ed.). St. Louis, MO: Mosby.

Iowa Outcomes Project. M. Johnson, M. Maas, & S. Moorhead (Eds.). (2000). *Nursing outcomes classification (NOC)* (2nd ed.). St. Louis, MO: Mosby.

Katz, I. R., Parmelee, P., & Brubaker, K. (1991). Toxic and metabolic encephalopathies in long-term care patients. *International Psychogeriatrics, 3,* 337-347.

Launer, L., Dinkgreve, M., Jonker, C., Hooijer, C., & Lindeboom, J. (1993). Are age and education independent correlates of the mini-mental state exam performance of community-dwelling elderly? *Journal of Gerontology, 48*(6), P271-P277.

Levkoff, S., Cleary, P., Liptzin, B., & Evans, D. (1991). Epidemiology of acute confusion: An overview of research issues and findings. *International Psychogeriatrics, 3*(20), 149-68.

Levkoff, S., Evans, D., Liptzin, B., Cleary, P., Lipsitz, L., Wetle, T., Reilly, C., Pilgrim, D., Schor, J., & Rowe, J. (1992). Acute confusion: The occurrence and persistence of symptoms among elderly hospitalized patients. *Archives of Internal Medicine, 152,* 334-340.

Levkoff, S., Liptzin, B., Cleary, P., Reilly, C., & Evans, D. (1991). Review of research instruments and techniques used to detect acute confusion. *International Psychogeriatrics, 3*(2), 253-271.

Lipowski, Z. J. (1983). Transient cognitive disorders (delirium/acute confusional states) in the elderly. *American Journal of Psychiatry, 140,* 1426-1436.

Lipowski, Z. J. (1989). Delirium in the elderly patient. *New England Journal of Medicine, 320,* 578-582.

Lipowski, Z. J. (1990). *Acute confusion: Acute confusional states.* New York: Oxford University Press.

Liptzin, B., & Levkoff, S. E. (1992). An empirical study of delirium subtypes. *British Journal of Psychiatry, 161,* 843-845.

Marcantonio, E. R., Goldman, L., Mangione, C. M., Ludwig, L., Muraca, B., Haslauer, C. M., Donaldson, M. C., Whittemore, A. D., Sugarbaker, D. J., Poss, R., Haas, S., Cook, E. F., Orav, J., & Lee, T. H. (1994). A clinical prediction rule for acute confusion after elective non-cardiac surgery. *Journal of the American Medical Association, 271,* 134-139.

Mentes, J., Culp, K., Maas, M., & Rantz, M. (1999). Acute confusion indicators: Risk factors and prevalence using MDS data. *Research in Nursing & Health, 22*(2), 95-105.

Mentes, J. C. (1995). Nursing protocol to assess causes of delirium: Identifying delirium in nursing home residents. *Journal of Gerontological Nursing, 2,* 26-30.

Mezey, M., Rauckhorst, L., & Stokes, S. (1993). *Health assessment of the older individual.* New York: Springer.

Miller J., Neelon, V., Champagne, M., Bailey, D., Ng'andu, N., Belyea, M., Jarrell, E., Montoya, L., & Williams, A. (1997). The assessment of acute confusion as part of nursing care. *Applied Nursing Research, 10*(3), 143-151.

Morris, J. C., & McManus, D. Q. (1991). The neurology of aging: Normal versus pathologic change. *Geriatrics, 46*(8), 47-54.

Nagley, S. (1986). Predicting and preventing confusion in your patients. *Journal of Gerontological Nursing, 12*(3), 27-31.

Neelon, V., Champagne, M., Carlson, J., & Funk, S. (1996). The NEECHAM confusion scale: Construction, validation, and clinical testing. *Nursing Research, 45*(6), 324-330.

Neelon, V. J., Funk, S. G., Carlson, J. R., & Champagne, M. T. (1989). The NEECHAM confusion scale: Relationship to clinical indicators of acute confusion in hospitalized elders. *The Gerontologist, 29,* 65A.

North American Nursing Diagnosis Association. (1999). *Nursing diagnoses: Definitions & classification 1999-2000.* Philadelphia: Author.

Pompei, P., Foreman, M., Rudberg, M. A., Inouye, S. K., Braund, V., & Cassel, C. K. (1994). Acute confusion in hospitalized older persons: Outcomes and predictors. *Journal of the American Geriatrics Society, 42,* 809-815.

Rabins, P. (1991). Psychosocial and management aspects of acute confusion. *International Psychogeriatrics, 3*(2), 319-324.

Rabins, P., & Folstein, M. F. (1982). Acute confusion and dementia: Diagnostic criteria and fatality rates. *British Journal of Psychiatry, 140,* 149-153.

Rantz, M., & LeMone, P. (1995). *Classification of nursing diagnoses: Proceedings of the eleventh NANDA conference.* Glendale, CA: Cinahl Information Systems.

Rapp, C. G., Onega, L. L., Tripp-Reimer, T., Mobily, P., Wakefield, B., Kundrat, M., Wadle, K., Mentes, J., Culp, K., Meyer, J., & Waterman, J. (1998). Unit-based acute confusion resource nurse: An educational program to train staff nurses. *The Gerontologist, 38*(5), 628-632.

Rapp, C. G., Wakefield, B., Kundrat, M., Mentes, J., Tripp-Reimer, T., Culp, K., Mobily, P., Akins, J., & Onega, L. (2000). Acute confusion assessment instruments: Clinical versus research utility. *Applied Nursing Research 13*(1), 37-45.

Roberts, B. C., & Lincoln, R. (1988). Cognitive disturbance in hospitalized and institutionalized elders. *Research in Nursing & Health, 11,* 309-311.

Rockwood, K. (1989). Acute confusion in elderly medical patients. *Journal of the American Geriatrics Society, 37,* 150-154.

Rockwood, K. (1993). The occurrence and duration of symptoms in elderly patients with acute confusion. *Journal of Gerontology: Medical Sciences, 48*(4), M162-M166.

Rogers, M. P., Liang, M. H., Daltroy, L. H., Eaton, H., Peteet, J., Wright, E., & Albert, M. (1989). Delirium after elective orthopedic surgery: Risk factors and natural history. *International Journal of Psychiatry in Medicine, 19*(2), 109-121.

Rubenstein, L. Z., & Rubenstein, L. V. (1992). Multidimensional geriatric assessment. In J. C. Brocklehurst, R. C. Tallis, & H. M. Fillit (Eds.), *Geriatric medicine and gerontology* (4th ed., pp. 150-159). New York: Churchill Livingstone.

Salthouse, T. A. (1993). Attentional blocks are not responsible for age-related slowing. *Journal of Gerontology, 48*(6), P263-P270.

Schor, J., Levkoff, S., Lipsitz, L., Reilly, C., Cleary, P., Rowe, J., & Evans, D. (1992). Risk factors for acute confusion in hospitalized elderly. *Journal of the American Medical Association, 267,* 827-831.

Strub, R., & Black, B. (1993). *The mental status examination in neurology* (3rd ed.). Philadelphia: F. A. Davis.

Teitelbaum, L., Ginsburg, M., & Hopkins, R. (1991). Cognitive and behavioral impairment among elderly people in institutions providing different levels of care. *Canadian Medical Association Journal, 144,* 169-173.

Trzepacz, P., Baker, R., & Greenhouse, J. (1988). A symptom rating scale for delirium. *Psychiatry Research, 23,* 89-97.

Verhaeghen, P., Marcoen, A., & Goossens, L. (1993). Facts and fiction about memory aging: A quantitative integration of research findings. *Journal of Gerontology, 48*(4), P157-P171.

Vermeersch, P. (1990). The clinical assessment of confusion-A. *Applied Nursing Research, 3,* 128-133.

Vermeersch, P. (1992). Clinical assessment of confusion. In S. Funk, E. Tornquist, M. Champagne, & R. Wiese (Eds.), *Key aspects of elder care: Managing falls, incontinence, and cognitive impairment* (pp. 251-261). New York: Springer.

Wanich, C., Sullivan-Marx, E., Gottlieb, G., & Johnson, J. (1992). Functional status outcomes of a nursing intervention in hospitalized elderly. *IMAGE: Journal of Nursing Scholarship, 24*(3), 201-207.

Williams, M., Holloway, J., Winn, M., Wolanin, M., Lawler, M., Westwick, C., & Chin, M. (1985). Nursing activities and acute confusional states in elderly hip-fractured patients. *Nursing Research, 28,* 25-35.

Williams-Russo, P., Urquhart, B., Sharrock, N., & Charlson, M. (1992). Post-operative delirium: Predictors and prognosis in elderly orthopedic patients. *Journal of the American Geriatrics Society, 40,* 759-767.

Zimberg, M., & Berenson, S. (1990). Delirium in patients with cancer: Nursing assessment and intervention. *Oncology Nursing Forum, 17*(4), 529-538.

CHAPTER 36

PAIN

Paula Mobily and Keela A. Herr

Management of pain in the elder poses an important and unique challenge for nurses. Pain is the most common complaint in the physician's office, the most common symptom of disease, and one of the nursing diagnoses most often used in nursing practice, regardless of setting. Because of the increased incidence of chronic diseases, falls, and other health problems associated with aging, older adults are at increased risk for experiencing both acute and chronic pain that can seriously impact their day-to-day functioning and quality of life. Although Browning (1895) wrote "Grow old along with me—the best is yet to be," the quality of life for older adults experiencing pain, and particularly chronic pain, can be seriously jeopardized. Nurses knowledgeable about the management of pain in this population can make a significant difference in promoting functional activity and quality of life.

There are many definitions of pain, both conceptual and operational, that attempt to describe this unique and subjective phenomenon. The International Association for the Study of Pain (1986) defines pain as "an unpleasant sensory and emotional experience associated with actual or potential tissue damage" (p. S216). Although widely accepted, this medical definition of pain is limited by its focus on pain only as an indicator of actual or potential tissue damage. Some types of pain, such as psychogenic pain, and some forms of headache pain are not associated with tissue damage. The definition proposed by McCaffery and Beebe (1989) focuses on the individual's experience of pain: "Pain is whatever the experiencing person says it is, existing whenever he says it does." The importance of this definition, which serves as the basis for nursing assessment and care of clients with pain, is that it acknowledges the client as the only person who can accurately define and describe her own pain experience.

As implied in these definitions, pain is a complex and multidimensional phenomenon. The experience of pain is not mediated solely by specific sensory processes or nociceptive events, but is influenced by social history, cultural expectations, individual differences concerning the meaning of pain, and effectiveness of personal and social coping resources (Harkins & Price, 1992; Melzack & Wall, 1965; Turk & Rudy, 1988). The scope and complexity of the pain experience are evident in the conceptualization of pain proposed by Ahles, Blanchard, and Ruckdeschel (1983) and expanded by McGuire (1992). Reflective of pain as a multidimensional, subjective, and uniquely personal experience, six dimensions of the pain experience are proposed: physiologic, sensory, affective, cognitive, behavioral, and sociocultural. The physiologic dimension incorporates the organic etiology, physiologic processes, anatomic factors, type of pain, and pain parameters such as location, onset, and duration. The sensory dimension is related to the actual perception of pain and includes components such as intensity, quality, and pattern. The affective dimension incorporates the feelings of the individual experiencing pain and includes anxiety, depression, mood state, and sense of well-being. The cognitive dimension is concerned with the meaning of pain to the individual and includes coping strategies and attitudes and beliefs that impact the pain experience. Behavioral activities directed toward decreasing pain include physical activity, communication, medications, and sleep, among others. Finally, the sociocultural dimension of pain incorporates a broad range of ethnocultural, demographic, spiritual, social, and other factors related to the perception of and response to pain; both the individual and supporters or caregivers are incorporated in this dimension. Recognition of the complex nature of pain and use of this broad conceptualization provide caregivers with a more comprehensive framework for the assessment of pain and, ultimately, for the evaluation of outcomes following the use of intervention strategies.

PREVALENCE

Although there has been limited epidemiologic investigation, population-based studies of community-dwelling elders estimate that 25% to 86% of older adults experience pain (Brattberg, Mats, & Anders, 1989; Crook, Rideout, & Brown, 1984; Mobily, Herr, Clark, & Wallace, 1994). In long-term care facilities, it is estimated that 49% to 83% of elderly residents experience pain (Brody & Kleban, 1983; Ferrell, Ferrell, & Osterweil, 1990; Ferrell, Ferrell, & Rivera, 1995; Lau-Ting & Phoon, 1988; Mobily, Herr, Rapp, & Ansley, 1999; Roy & Thomas, 1986; Sengstaken & King, 1993). Although pain is not an inevitable concomitant of aging, elders are at greater risk for many disorders associated with pain. More than 80% of the geriatric population have identifiable degenerative joint disease associated with significant pain (Davis, 1988), and 60% of all cancers occur in this age group (Silverman & Temple, 1992). Significant pain is reported by one third of all cancer patients and two thirds of those with advanced disease (Foley, 1987). Other common conditions associated with pain in the elderly include atherosclerotic peripheral vascular disease, herpes zoster, trigeminal neuralgia, diabetic neuropathy, temporal arteritis, polymyalgia rheumatica, osteoporosis with vertebral compression, and lumbar spinal stenosis. Also, injuries such as falls and hip fractures are more common in this population and may result in both acute and chronic pain.

The impact of pain on older adults, particularly chronic pain, can be significant. Pain can adversely affect a wide range of activities, resulting in impaired functional abilities, social interactions, sleep, nutritional status, and cognitive function. Not surprisingly, studies have demonstrated significant relationships between pain, mood or depression, and overall quality of life (Brown, Nicassio, & Wallston, 1989; Cohen-Mansfield & Marx, 1993; Doan & Wadden, 1989; Haley, Turner, & Romano, 1985; Haythornthwaite, Seiber, & Kerns, 1991; Herr, Mobily, & Smith, 1993; Scudds & Robertson, 1998; Weiner, Pieper, McConnell, Martinez, & Keefe, 1996).

Myths and misconceptions about pain in the elderly can seriously affect the quality of care provided. One of the major misconceptions is the belief that pain is a natural and expected outcome of aging. In fact, pain is not an inevitable consequence of growing old; unfortunately, this pain-related ageism often leads to lack of aggressive assessment and intervention for pain experienced by older adults. Another important misconception is that pain sensitivity or perception decreases with aging. However, results of experimental studies on pain perception in the elderly fail to conclusively demonstrate age-related differences in pain perception (Harkins, Price, & Martelli, 1986; Tucker, Andrew, Ogle, & Davison, 1989). Although older adults may be slower to perceive or respond to pain, research does not support that they perceive pain less intensely. There are instances of atypical presentations of clinical pain in the elderly, including silent myocardial infarction and the absence of abdominal pain with peptic ulcer disease. However, these exceptions cannot be generalized to all disorders that result in pain or to all older adults who experience these conditions. Assuming that elders experience less pain most certainly results in needless suffering and decreased quality of life.

RELATED FACTORS/ETIOLOGIES

The etiology of pain can be attributed to four major injuring agents: (1) biologic; (2) chemical; (3) physical; and (4) psychologic (psychogenic).

Biologic Agents

A number of etiologies related to pain can be classified as biologic agents, including inflammatory, neurologic, ischemic, and musculoskeletal conditions. Pain often results from the occurrence of multiple pathologic processes and biologic agents. Pain related to cancer provides an excellent illustration of this point. The following five leading causes of cancer-induced pain have been described by Matthews, Zarrow, and Osterholm (1973): (1) bone destruction; (2) infiltration or compression of nerves; (3) obstruction of a viscus or vessel; (4) infiltration or distension of integument or tissues; and (5) inflammation, infection, or necrosis of tissue.

Inflammatory Conditions. Inflammatory pain is due to a combination of factors, including sensitization, pressure, temperature changes, and chemicals released from injured cells. For example, the pain associated with rheumatoid arthritis results from the inflammatory processes within the involved joints. The tissue destruction associated with the disease process results in inflammation amplified by a variety of mediators, including prostaglandins and a number of cytokines released by synovial and infiltrating cells (Bonica, 1990; Wigley, 1991). Any disease process initiating the inflammatory response will result in pain. Other disorders common to the elderly that result in pain from inflammatory processes include gout and temporal arteritis.

Neurologic Conditions. Pain that is neurologic in origin can be seen in a number of pathologic conditions common to the elderly, including herpes zoster, trigeminal neuralgia, and peripheral neuropathies such as diabetic neuropathy. With herpes zoster, also known as shingles, pain is related to a latent infection by the varicella zoster virus of dorsal root ganglia of the spinal nerves, the sensory ganglia of a cranial nerve, and occasionally the anterior horn cells of the spinal cord. An intense necrotizing reaction results from the infection, causing inflammation, hemorrhage, demyelination, fibrosis, and cellular infiltration in the affected portions of the nervous system (Loeser, 1990a).

Trigeminal neuralgia, also known as tic douloureux, is a facial pain syndrome affecting one or more branches of the fifth cranial nerve and resulting in intense recurring episodes of sudden, severe, paroxysmal, lancinating pain. Although the exact etiology of this disorder is unknown, microneuromas and vascular compression of the nerve are thought to be possible causes.

The pain associated with diabetic neuropathy is neurologic in origin as well. Although the exact mechanism of pain associated with this is neuropathy unclear, it is thought to be related either to abnormal activity in peripheral nerve axons that are degenerating or becoming demyelinated or to entrapment or compression of peripheral nerves by adjacent structures (Corse & Kuncl, 1991; Loeser, 1990b).

Ischemic Conditions. Ischemia of tissues results from an imbalance between oxygen supply and demand. Ischemic pain is caused by a buildup of lactic acid in ischemic tissues or by the release of chemicals such as bradykinins and histamines from cells damaged by ischemia. Common disorders associated with ischemic pain include myocardial ischemia, which results in angina, and peripheral vascular disease, which results in intermittent claudication.

Musculoskeletal Conditions. Musculoskeletal conditions are a significant etiology of pain in the elder. Musculoskeletal conditions associated with pain that are common in the elderly include osteoarthritis and low back pain.

Osteoarthritis or degenerative joint disease is characterized by deterioration of articular cartilage that occurs as a result of accumulated joint stress and trauma. Breakdown products from the cartilage are thought to stimulate an inflammatory response and perpetuate a continuous cycle of joint destruction (Jacobson, 1996). As the disease progresses, there are many potential sources of pain, including periosteal irritation, denuded bone, compression of soft tissues, microfractures of subchondral bone, stress on ligaments resulting from loss of cartilage and joint incongruity, low-grade synovitis, effusion, and spasm of surrounding muscles (Townes, 1991).

Pathologic conditions associated with back pain in the elderly include lumbar osteoarthritis (also known as degenerative disk disease), osteoporosis, and spinal stenosis. Pain is reported in the back, buttocks, or lower extremities, usually as a result of muscle spasm or irritation of spinal nerve roots.

Chemical Agents

With any pathologic condition causing tissue trauma and cellular damage, various chemical substances are released that mediate pain by affecting the sensitivity of nerve endings or pain receptors. Chemicals known to increase the transmission or perception of pain include histamine, bradykinin, serotonin, potassium, and norepinephrine. Similarly, prostaglandins, leukotrienes, and substance P are chemical substances known to increase the sensitivity of pain receptors (Bonica, 1990).

Physical Agents

Diminished sensory perceptions and loss of mobility make many elders more susceptible to injury, with a resultant increase in the incidence of injuries related to physical trauma. Poor vision and altered mobility can lead to falls and subsequent fractures. Hip fractures are the primary cause of more than 200,000 hospital admissions each year, with persons over age 65 sustaining 84% of all such fractures (Baker, O'Neill, & Karpf, 1984). The pain that accompanies traumatic injury can be due to a variety of injurious agents, including the release of irritating chemicals at the site of tissue damage, nerve compression, or the stretching or tearing of tissue. In response to physical injury, splinting movements initiated to protect the injured site can cause muscle contraction. If the splinting continues, anaerobic metabolism within the muscle tissue causes an accumulation of lactic acid that irritates small fibers and results in further pain.

Psychologic Agents

Although all pain is real, regardless of its cause, typically there are both physiologic and psychologic components at work. Pure psychologic pain, or psychogenic pain, may be defined as a localized sensation of pain caused solely by mental events, with no physical findings to initiate or sustain the pain (McCaffery & Beebe, 1989). Most often, psychogenic pain is associated with a long history of complaints of severe pain. It is postulated that pain sensations are prompted by emotional needs and may result from interpersonal conflicts, from a need for support from others, or from a desire to avoid stressful or traumatic situations. Depression is often present as well, complicating the diagnosis of this type of pain. Regardless of cause, it is important to keep in mind that psychogenic pain is real, not pretended; psychogenic pain, in turn, can lead to physiologic changes such as muscle tension that produce further pain.

ASSESSMENT

Pain in older adults is often poorly assessed (Bernabei et al., 1998; Dalton, 1989; Faherty & Grier, 1984; Ferrell et al., 1990; Ferrell, Ferrell, & Rivera, 1995; Parmalee et al., 1993; Rankin & Snider, 1984; Sengstaken & King, 1993; Teske, Daut, & Cleeland, 1983; Yates, Dewar, & Fentiman, 1995). Lack of knowledge related to pain assessment and management by health professionals and lack of clinical skills to assess and manage pain are key factors impacting unsatisfactory assessment.

The assessment process allows the nurse to identify subjective and objective defining characteristics that indicate a diagnosis of pain. Gathering verbal information from elders regarding their pain can be difficult. Often the older adult will not verbalize pain, leading to an incorrect assumption that he must not have pain. A variety of factors interfere with reports of pain: age-related stoicism; belief that pain is to be expected with aging and that nothing can be done to relieve it (Ferrell et al., 1990; Foley, 1985; Gagliese & Melzack, 1997; McCaffery & Beebe, 1989;

Melding, 1991); fear of the consequences of acknowledging pain such as the need for hospitalization, diagnostic tests, or loss of independence (Copp, 1990; Hofland, 1992; Portenoy, 1988); fear that pain might be indicative of more serious illness or even impending death (Nishikawa & Ferrell, 1993); expectations that health professionals know when patients hurt and will initiate appropriate interventions (Hickey, 1988); not wanting to be a bother (Ferrell et al., 1990); and feeling tired of continually asking for help with their pain (Yates, Dewar, & Fentiman, 1995). Anticipating some of the barriers to reporting pain can provide opportunities to explore the older adult's concerns and beliefs and, hopefully, move to a more open sharing of information regarding pain.

Many health professionals assume that older clients who are cognitively intact can accurately and succinctly describe their pain. The elderly client may respond negatively to a query regarding "pain," but openly share sensations of discomfort when asked about an "ache," "soreness," or "hurt." Perceptual deficits are common in several neurologic problems (e.g., stroke, dementia) and can severely limit the elderly client's ability to describe pain verbally. If subjective data cannot be obtained reliably from the elder, family and caregivers will be an important source of information.

Pain intensity is just one component of assessment data. However, information regarding the impact of pain on a variety of life activities is often critical when working with the older adult in chronic pain. Disrupted social and family relationships, changes in eating and sleeping patterns, altered ability to continue previous activities, and altered mood may best reflect the severity of chronic pain.

Due to uniquely individual patterns of pain responses, each older adult may present with subtle, yet definitive signs of pain. The nurse must observe carefully and consider changes in the daily routines. This is especially important when evaluating those unable to verbalize their pain. When the patient is unable to communicate pain complaints, vocalizations such as crying, moaning, and whimpering might indicate discomfort. However, in the elder with chronic pain, vocalizations might be absent; nonverbal pain behaviors, such as guarding and protective posturing, are commonly seen. A statement by the nurse such as "You seem to be limping. Is your leg bothering you?" invites the elder to respond and demonstrates the nurse's observation of the individual's difficulty. Withdrawal and restlessness might also be noted and indicate the need for further assessment. For the noncommunicative older adult, observation of pain behavior and deviations from normal behavior patterns can be essential (Marzinski, 1991). While older adults with acute pain will exhibit readily observable autonomic responses, these responses will be altered or diminished for those with chronic pain.

Finally, older adults in chronic pain can exhibit self-focusing behavior that can be misinterpreted as being reclusive or uncaring of others. Either through their own withdrawal from relationships or because of avoidance by significant others, social interactions can become very limited.

Chronic pain significantly impacts quality of life. Although there is no universally accepted definition of quality of life, most agree that physical, emotional, social, and spiritual aspects are important. All of these can be impacted by the presence of pain. Gathering information on key quality of life variables from a variety of sources, including the older adult, significant others, other health care workers, roommates, and activity therapists, will be important in determining the impact of pain on the elder's life.

Because of the high prevalence of depression among older adults (Blazer, Hughes, & George, 1987) and the significant impact on functioning when depression and pain coexist (Haythornthwaite, Seiber & Kerns, 1991; Herr & Mobily, 1992; Herr, Mobily, & Smith, 1993), the topic of depression warrants additional comment. The health care provider and the family caregiver need to be particularly aware of the possibility that depression can be a consequence of pain and that pain can be a symptom of an underlying depressive disorder. Differentiating between chronic pain and depression is not easy. The symptoms are similar (e.g., sleep disturbance, fatigue, loss of appetite, loss of interest, inability to feel pleasure, pessimism, social incapacity), and careful exploration of etiologies is needed.

Complexities of Assessment

Many factors complicate the collection and interpretation of pain data in this population, including sensory impairment, cognitive impairment, sociocultural factors, and polypharmacy. Although key recommendations are presented here, the reader is referred to Herr and Mobily (1991) for more detailed information.

Asking the older adult to describe his pain or read an assessment tool may provide a basic indicator of sensory ability or impairment. Hearing impairment, common in the elder, can be accommodated through proper positioning, lighting, tone, pacing, and speed; through reduction of extraneous noises; or through use of other communication modes (i.e., written questions). To make adjustment for decreases in visual acuity, rate of accommodation, and color discrimination, it is recommended to use assessment tools with large, simple lettering and adequate line spacing, nonglare paper (e.g., buff-colored), and nonglare lighting.

Cognitive impairment, present in 37% to 80% of elders in long-term care facilities (Ferrell et al., 1990; Rovner et al., 1990), presents serious barriers to accurate assessment of pain. Cognitive impairment can result in underreporting of pain due to problems recalling, interpreting, or communicating pain symptoms or lead to exaggeration or fabrication of pain complaints (Parmalee, Smith, & Katz, 1993). For the older adult with minimal to mild cognitive impairment, efforts should be made to first obtain self-report. Recent studies document that standard assessment techniques can be used effectively on older adults with mild to moderate cognitive impairment (Feldt, Ryden, & Miles, 1998; Ferrell et al., 1995; Ferrell, Cronin-Nash, & Warfield, 1992; Parmalee et al., 1993; Porter, Malhotra, Wolf, Morris, & Smith, 1996). It is important to be sure you have the elder's attention and validate understanding of what is being asked. Helpful strategies include keeping the content of assessment simple, providing clear explanations that clarify any medical terminology, using examples and demonstrations of assessment activities, and providing more time to assimilate questions and respond.

For cognitively impaired elders unable to reliably report the presence of pain, other strategies must be used. Nonverbal pain behaviors, such as grimacing, guarding, facial expressions, and posturing often are indicators of discomfort. Another useful approach is to observe for sudden changes in the elder's typical behavior patterns, such as decreased activity, decreased social interactions, difficulty sleeping, agitation (American Geriatrics Society Panel on Chronic Pain in Older Persons, 1998; Cleary & Carbone, 1997; Gagliese & Melzack, 1997). Several scales have been developed to assist with observation of behavior indicative of pain in cognitively impaired older adults (Feldt et al., 1998; Hurley, Volicer, Hanrahan, Houde, & Volicer, 1992; Miller et al., 1996; Simons & Malabar, 1995). Most of these tools have undergone only limited testing or need adaptation to make them clinically useful in daily practice.

Although studies show that surrogate judgments of pain intensity, such as that from health care providers and family members, do not accurately represent the patient's perception of pain (Cleeland et al., 1994; Ferrell et al., 1995; Madison & Wilkie, 1995; Weiner, Peterson, & Keefe, 1999), gathering information from family and caregivers can assist in assessing pain in those unable to advocate for themselves.

Because sociocultural background can influence the way in which an individual interprets pain, tolerates pain, and reacts verbally and nonverbally to pain, this must be considered when assessing pain-related experiences. Cultural standards also teach individuals how much pain to tolerate, what types of pain to report, and to whom to report their pain. Many of the current cohort of older adults in the United States are immigrants or first generation U.S.-born, and research has demonstrated that these individuals often maintain stronger ethnic and cultural ties that may influence response to pain (Bates, Edwards, & Anderson, 1993; Zatzick & Dimsdale, 1990). Although sociocultural influences certainly can impact pain assessment, it is important to keep in mind that behaviors can also vary within cultures and from generation to generation. More research is needed to identify variables that most influence an individual's response to pain. Nonetheless, recognition of potential cultural differences will provide a greater understanding of an individual's pain and will foster more accurate assessment of pain and pain-related behaviors.

A final factor complicating pain assessment is polypharmacy. Perception of pain and ability to report pain experience can be impacted by drug interactions and side effects resulting from multiple drug use. A thorough drug history and consideration of possible impacts from polypharmacy is an important component of the overall assessment.

Measurement of Pain in the Elderly

The importance of obtaining accurate data in an organized manner that will provide a complete picture of the older adult's pain cannot be overstated. In addition to qualitative assessment of pain and its related components, use of selected measurement instruments can help to quantify the pain experience and provide outcome indicators useful in evaluating response to nursing intervention. The use of a standard pain scale to record self-report of pain should be attempted with older patients (American Geriatrics Society Panel on Chronic Pain in Older Persons, 1998). Criteria for choosing an assessment tool include the elderly individual's verbal, physical, and cognitive capabilities. As suggested earlier, it may be necessary to adapt a particular tool to accommodate any limitations that are present. Both single-item scales that quickly evaluate the sensory intensity of pain (e.g., visual analog scale, verbal descriptor scale, and numeric rating scale) and multidimensional measures are available.

Single-Item Pain Scales. To gather information on pain intensity, verbal and visual pain scales that are quick to administer and interpret are commonly used (Figure 36-1). The verbal descriptor scale (VDS) consists of a set of numbers with words representing different levels of pain; the patient selects the word or number that best represents her pain intensity. The numeric rating scale (NRS), providing a series of numbers to represent level of pain with variations from 0 to 10 or 0 to 100, is more sensitive to change because of the increased levels of scaling (Downie et al., 1978; Jensen, Karoly, Riordan, Bland, & Burns, 1989). A commonly used variant is the verbal numeric rating scale in which the patient is asked to rate his pain from 0 to 10, with 0 representing "no pain" and 10 representing "the worst pain possible" (Murphy, McDonald, Power, Unwin, & MacSullivan, 1988). The benefit of this approach is the elimination of visual and motor components involved in determining a score. The visual analogue scale (VAS), a more sophisticated assessment tool consisting of a 10 cm line with extremes of pain at either end of the continuum, may be too abstract for elders who have lower educational levels or impaired

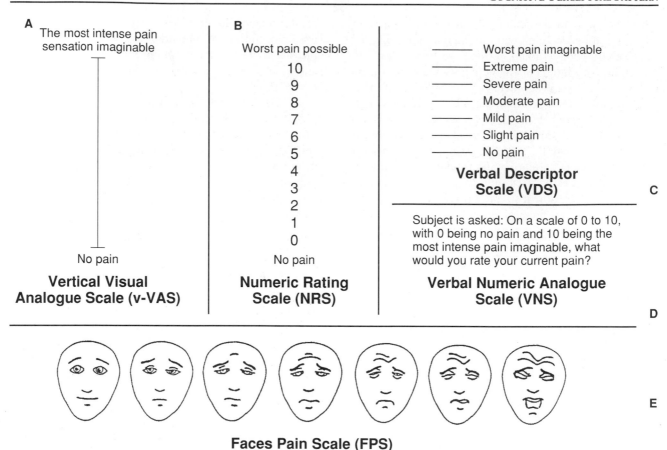

Faces Pain Scale (FPS)

FIGURE **36-1**   Illustrations of pain intensity measures. (*E* from Bieri, D., Reeve, R., Champion, G., Addicoat, L., & Ziegler, J. [1990]. The Faces Pain Scale for the self-assessment of the severity of pain experienced by children: Development, initial validation, and preliminary investigation for ratio scale properties. *Pain 41,* 139-150.)

motor coordination; however, well-educated elders have been able to successfully complete the VAS (Herr & Mobily, 1993). Vertical presentations of scales, such as a pain thermometer, can be easier for older subjects to respond to than those displayed horizontally (Herr & Mobily, 1993). Facial scales developed for assessment of pain intensity with children (Beyer & Aradine, 1986; Bieri, Reeve, Champion, Addicoat, & Ziegler, 1990; McGrath, DeVeber, & Hearn, 1985; Tyler, Tu, Douthit, & Chapman, 1993) might also be appropriate for older adults (Herr, Mobily, Kohout, & Wagenaar, 1998). Adaptation of these instruments might provide alternatives for working with those with impaired communication skills. Careful and often repeated instructions may be needed, particularly with the VAS, to ensure proper understanding and use of the pain scales (Ferrell et al., 1995; Weiner et al., 1999).

The utility or usability and preference for a given tool are issues that are not often addressed but that certainly are relevant when determining interest in and use of a selected tool. Although there is interindividual variability in several studies with older adults, we have found that most older adults preferred to use a verbal description scale, a

pain thermometer, or a numeric rating scale (Herr & Mobily, 1993; Herr, Mobily, Richardson, & Spratt, 1998). Offering a choice in tool selection may yield more positive results than choosing the tool for the older adult.

Multidimensional Pain Scales. The McGill Pain Questionnaire (MPQ) (Melzack, 1975), which assesses location of pain, pattern of pain over time, sensory, affective, evaluative, and miscellaneous components of pain, and intensity, is one of the best-known multidimensional assessment tools. However, the MPQ is often perceived as complex and time-consuming, with an overwhelming number of descriptors that may be difficult for the elder to understand. The short-form MPQ (Melzack, 1987), which includes drawings of the human body for location of pain, a 20-word descriptor list, a section assessing pain pattern, and finally, a pain intensity scale, may be a more suitable alternative for the elder. For those with limited language abilities, a human body drawing may facilitate identification of the pain location and quality.

A diary can be useful for recording various postures and activities, pain intensity level, use of pain relief measures, time spent in pain relief activities, use of analgesics, and factors that exacerbate or mediate the pain experience (McCaffery & Beebe, 1989). Inconsistencies between pain report and recorded pain and activities also can provide useful information.

Although impact on quality of life might be the most important indicator of pain control, especially for those with chronic pain conditions, nurses often fail to gather data about the effect of pain on quality of life (Dalton, 1989). The Multidimensional Pain Inventory (MPI) (Kerns, Turk, & Rudy, 1985) and the Pain Disability Index (PDI) (Tait, 1993) are instruments used successfully with the elder to provide a comprehensive evaluation of several quality of life domains related specifically to pain.

Pain-Related Measurements

Complete assessment should elicit information about functional health as well. Identifying tools that address the specific components involved in overall functioning is important, as intervention is often directed at increasing mobility or independence. Although scales used to evaluate basic ADL and instrumental activities may be used, advanced or elective activities may be more sensitive to changes in pain (Turk & Melzack, 1992). Instruments targeting specific functional domains include the Katz ADL scale (Katz, Ford, Moskowitz, Jackson, & Jaffe, 1963), the Instrumental Activities of Daily Living scale (Lawton & Brody, 1969), and the Barthel Index (Mahoney & Barthel, 1965), among others.

The presence of dysphoria or depression, earlier shown to be of concern for the older adult with chronic pain, can be evaluated through the use of several scales, including the Geriatric Depression Scale (Yesavage et al., 1983), the Beck Depression Inventory (Beck, Ward, Mendelson, Mock, & Erbaugh, 1961), and the Center for Epidemiologic Studies Depression Scale or CES-D (Radloff, 1977), among others.

The use of a pain flow sheet can be invaluable in assessing and monitoring pain status. Various flow sheets are available in the literature (McCaffery & Beebe, 1989), but one could be developed to meet the needs of individual agency or patient needs. Aside from the obvious merits in evaluating response to intervention, flow sheets can be used as a positive reinforcer of progress toward pain relief, can identify peculiar patterns or situations that exacerbate pain, and can facilitate communication related to pain problems among health care providers.

CASE STUDY

T. Green is a 79-year-old retired farmer with osteoarthritic hip and back pain. He describes his pain as "deep, gnawing, and aching" and states that the pain is always worse when it rains or is cold outside. The pain from his back radiates into his right buttock and calf and into the side of his foot. He notes that the pain gets worse with activity and is relieved somewhat by rest. He complains of "stiffness" in his hips and lower back, particularly upon arising or after a period of rest or decreased activity. Upon inspection, there is local tenderness in the lower back over the area of pain with spasm of the surrounding muscles. Mr. Green takes nabumetone (Relafen) daily for his osteoarthritis. He reports that the pain from his hips and back has a severe impact on his daily activities and on his ability to fully enjoy them.

NURSING DIAGNOSIS

The multidimensional nature of pain has led to the adoption of two accepted North American Nursing Diagnosis Association (NANDA) nursing diagnoses related to pain: Pain and Chronic Pain (NANDA, 1999). These two diagnoses reflect basic differences with respect to duration, defining characteristics, and related factors of the pain. Reflective of acute pain, Pain as defined by NANDA is "an unpleasant sensory and emotional experience arising from actual or potential tissue damage or described in terms of such damage (International Association for the Study of Pain, 1986); sudden or slow onset of any intensity from mild to severe with an anticipated or predictable end and a duration of less than 6 months" (p. 122). Chronic Pain is defined as "an unpleasant sensory and emotional experience arising from actual or potential tissue damage or described in terms of such damage (International Association for the Study of Pain, 1986); sudden or slow onset of any intensity from mild to severe, constant or recurring without an anticipated or predictable end and a duration of greater than 6 months" (p. 123). These two diagnoses are delineated with respect to defining characteristics and related factors in Box 36-1.

As noted by Simon, Nolan, and Baumann (1995), it is important that nurses be able to both diagnose pain and differentiate between acute and chronic pain. Typically, acute and chronic pain are differentiated according to onset, duration, and cause of pain. Acute pain is associated with recent, sudden onset and is limited in duration. It is also associated with acute illness or disease, treatment or operative procedures, or trauma. Acute pain typically subsides as healing occurs. Conversely, chronic pain is caused by chronic pathologic processes, by prolonged and sometimes permanent dysfunction of the peripheral or central nervous system, or by both. Also, in contrast with acute pain, the primary cause of chronic pain can be psychologic mechanisms and/or environmental factors (Bonica, 1990). Other characteristics distinguishing chronic pain are that the pain area often becomes less easily differentiated, the intensity of the pain becomes more difficult to evaluate, suffering usually increases over time, defining characteristics are less obvious, and the

Suggested Nursing-Sensitive Outcomes and Nursing Interventions

Box 36-1 PAIN AND CHRONIC PAIN

Nursing Diagnoses
Pain
Defining characteristics
Verbal or coded report
Observed evidence
Antalgic position
Protective behavior
Guarding behavior
Antalgic gestures
Facial mask
Sleep disturbance (eyes lack luster, "beaten look," fixed or
    scattered movement, grimace)
Self-focus
Narrowed focus (altered time perception, impaired thought
    processes, reduced interaction with people and
    environment)
Distraction behavior (e.g., pacing, seeking out other people
    and/or activities)
Autonomic responses (e.g., diaphoresis, blood pressure,
    respiration, pulse change, pupillary dilation)
Autonomic alteration in muscle tone (may span from listless
    to rigid)
Expressive behavior (e.g., restlessness, moaning, crying,
    vigilance, irritability, sighing)
Changes in appetite and eating

Related factors/etiologies
Injury agents (biologic, chemical, physical, psychologic)

Chronic Pain
Defining characteristics
Verbal or coded report or observed evidence of protective
    behavior
Fear of reinjury
Physical and social withdrawal
Altered ability to continue previous activities
Anorexia
Weight changes
Changes in sleep patterns
Verbal or coded report of observed evidence of facial mask
Verbal or coded report of observed evidence of guarded
    behavior

Related factors/etiologies
Chronic physical/psychosocial disability

Nursing-Sensitive Outcomes
Pain Level
Indicators
Reported pain
Percent of body affected
Frequency of pain
Length of pain episodes
Oral expressions of pain
Facial expressions of pain
Protective body positions
Restlessness
Muscle tension

Change in respiratory rate
Change in heart rate
Change in blood pressure
Change in pupil size
Perspiration
Appetite loss

Pain Control
Indicators
Recognizes causal factors
Recognizes pain onset
Preventive measures
Uses nonanalgesic relief measures, uses analgesics
    appropriately; uses warning signs to seek care
Uses available resources; uses pain diary
Reports pain controlled

Pain: Disruptive Effects
Indicators
Impaired interpersonal relationships
Impaired role performance
Compromised play
Compromised leisure activities
Compromised work
Compromised life enjoyment
Compromised sense of control
Impaired concentration
Compromised sense of hope
Impaired mood
Lack of patience
Disrupted sleep
Impaired physical mobility
Impaired self-care
Lack of appetite
Difficulty eating
Impaired elimination

Comfort Level
Indicators
Reported physical well-being
Reported satisfaction with symptom control
Reported psychologic well-being
Expressed contentment with physical surroundings
Expressed contentment with social relationships
Expressed spiritual contentment
Reported satisfaction with level of independence
Expressed satisfaction with pain control

Nursing Intervention
Pain Management
Activities
Perform a comprehensive assessment of pain to include
    location, characteristics, onset/duration, frequency,
    quality, intensity or severity of pain, and precipitating
    factors
Observe for nonverbal cues of discomfort, especially in those
    unable to communicate effectively

Box 36-1	Suggested Nursing-Sensitive Outcomes and Nursing Interventions—cont'd PAIN AND CHRONIC PAIN—cont'd

Assure patient attentive analgesic care

Use therapeutic communication strategies to acknowledge the pain experience and convey acceptance of the patient's response to pain

Consider cultural influences on pain response

Determine the impact of the pain experience on quality of life (e.g., sleep, appetite, activity, cognition, mood, relationships, performance of job, and role responsibilities)

Evaluate past experiences with pain to include individual or family history of chronic pain or resulting disability, as appropriate

Evaluate, with the patient and the health care team, the effectiveness of past pain control measures that have been used

Assist patient and family to seek and provide support

Use a developmentally appropriate assessment method that allows for monitoring of change in pain and that will assist in identifying actual and potential precipitating factors, (e.g., flow sheet, daily diary)

Determine the needed frequency of making an assessment of patient comfort and implement monitoring plan

Provide information about the pain, such as causes of the pain, how long it will last, and anticipated discomforts from procedures

Control environmental factors that may influence the patient's response to discomfort (e.g., room temperature, lighting, and noise)

Reduce or eliminate factors that precipitate or increase the pain experience (e.g., fear, fatigue, monotony, and lack of knowledge)

Consider the patient's willingness to participate, ability to participate, preference, support of significant others for method, and contraindications when selecting a pain relief strategy

Select and implement a variety of measures (e.g., pharmacologic, nonpharmacologic, and interpersonal) to facilitate pain relief, as appropriate

Consider type and source of pain when selecting pain relief strategy

Encourage patient to monitor own pain and to intervene appropriately

Teach the use of nonpharmacologic techniques (e.g., biofeedback, transcutaneous electrical nerve stimulation (TENS), hypnosis, relaxation, guided imagery, music

therapy, distraction, play therapy, activity therapy, acupressure, hot/cold application, and massage) before, after, and, if possible, during painful activities; before pain occurs or increases; and along with other pain relief measures

Collaborate with the patient, significant other, and other health professionals to select and implement nonpharmacologic pain relief measures, as appropriate

Provide the person optimal pain relief with prescribed analgesics

Implement the use of patient-controlled analgesia (PCA), if appropriate

Use pain control measures before pain becomes severe

Medicate prior to an activity to increase participation, but evaluate the hazard of sedation

Ensure pretreatment analgesia and/or nonpharmacologic strategies before painful procedures

Verify level of discomfort with patient, note changes in the medical record, and inform other health professionals working with the patient

Evaluate the effectiveness of the pain control measures used through ongoing assessment of the pain experience

Institute and modify pain control measures on the basis of the patient's response

Promote adequate rest/sleep to facilitate pain relief

Encourage patient to discuss his pain experience, as appropriate

Notify physician if measures are unsuccessful or if current complaint is a significant change from patient's past experience of pain

Inform other health care professionals/family members of nonpharmacologic strategies being used by the patient to encourage preventive approaches to pain management

Utilize a multidisciplinary approach to pain management, when appropriate

Consider referrals for patient, family, and significant others to support groups, and other resources, as appropriate

Provide accurate information to promote family's knowledge of and response to the pain experience

Incorporate the family in the pain relief modality, if possible

Monitor patient satisfaction with pain management at specified intervals

likelihood of complete relief is diminished (McFarland & McFarlane, 1997).

Although NANDA has defined Chronic Pain as pain that continues for more than 6 months, respected experts in the field of pain management argue that this time designation is inappropriate. The International Association for the Study of Pain (1986) defines chronic pain as "that pain which persists past the normal time of healing" (p. S216). They further note that, in practice, healing may be less

than a month or more than 6 months and have chosen to define the time frame for chronic pain as pain of 3 months' duration "as the most convenient point of division." Although these differences in definition might appear arbitrary, they have clinical relevance in terms of choosing and implementing the most effective therapy (Bonica, 1990).

Chronic pain is frequently subdivided into two categories—chronic malignant and chronic nonmalignant pain (National Institutes of Health, 1986). Whereas chronic malignant pain is associated with cancer, chronic nonmalignant pain typically refers to pain in which tissue injury is nonprogressive or healed.

The following discussion of defining characteristics emphasizes deviations in assessment data pertinent to elders; factors common to adults in general have been omitted. Considerations for gathering and interpreting assessment data from the elder and specific tools for measuring constructs related to pain in the elder follow.

Several studies provide validation of the nursing diagnosis Pain (Gyldenvand & Tunick, 1989; Riordan, 1991; Simon et al., 1995). However, there are no studies noted that address the validity of the diagnostic criteria for the elderly. Defining characteristics are necessary to guide nurses in determining the nursing diagnosis of pain and differentiating whether the pain is acute or chronic. The research of Simon and colleagues (1995), although providing support for differentiation between acute and chronic pain, demonstrated inadequacies in the defining characteristics currently used in NANDA for pain, in that less than half of the defining characteristics found in this study were included in NANDA. There appears to be a particular lack in the clinical indicators for chronic pain, with five of the top eight rated defining characteristics absent from NANDA, including disruption of social and family relationships, irritability, physical inactivity or immobility, depression, and rubs painful part. These behaviors are commonly seen with the elder in chronic pain. Further revision of the NANDA diagnoses of acute and chronic pain is warranted, with emphasis on identifying the most relevant defining characteristics and clustering of defining characteristics for acute and chronic pain. Studies with elders would also enhance the use of NANDA diagnoses with this population.

NURSING-SENSITIVE OUTCOMES

Evaluation of client outcomes is an important aspect of the nursing process. Some form of evaluation of pain must be used to obtain baseline data, initially as well as periodically, to determine the effectiveness of pain management interventions. The nurse should not overlook the client's involvement in evaluating pain relief measures, underscoring the advantages of mutual goal setting.

The timing and use of several evaluative criteria to judge the success or failure of interventions for pain is important. For acute pain, the evaluation may occur very quickly (e.g., in 10 to 30 minutes). For chronic pain problems, outcome measurement at admission, discharge, 1 month, 3 months, and 6 months post-discharge is common practice (Wielde, 1996). Reassessing the status of the defining characteristics used to identify pain as a problem is a simple approach to evaluating the outcome of the interventions attempted.

Subjective Evaluation

Successful interventions should result in decreased use of pain references during conversations and an overall decrease in specific complaints of pain. Although pain might not be entirely eliminated, the nurse should listen carefully for qualitative descriptions that indicate a lessening of intensity of the pain. As a part of the planning process, the older adult should have been asked to determine what level of pain is acceptable. For example, on a 0-to-10 scale of pain, what level of pain would allow the elder to do what she wants to do. Once the goal for pain relief is established, the nurse can reevaluate to determine whether the interventions have achieved the acceptable level of pain. It is also important to determine whether the location and quality of the pain are the same or different, as changes may reflect an alteration in the etiology and necessitate further evaluation.

Objective Evaluation

The nurse should look and feel for a relaxation of skeletal muscles, which indicates decreased muscle tension and decreased fear and anxiety. Elimination of pain postures is also indicative of pain relief, in that the older adult no longer needs to protect a joint or a limb with a rigid posture. As muscles relax, rigid posturing should continue to decrease with an accompanying increase in activity level and mobility. Increased participation in activities, such as recreational and leisure activities, work, and sexual relations, might also reflect relief of pain or, at least, increased coping with the stress of pain. It is important to remember that the older adult with chronic pain might not experience complete relief, but rather a decrease to a level that is compatible with increasing quality of life reflected in the elder's ability to perform the activities he desires. Once the fearful grip of pain is broken, there should be an almost immediate increase in the ability to rest, relax, or sleep. It is not uncommon for a person who has been experiencing excruciating pain of long duration to sleep for quite extended periods of time.

Another approach to evaluation of patient outcomes related to pain incorporates the use of standardized measures. As noted in the assessment section, measurement scales currently available range from simple, single-item scales measuring pain intensity (e.g., VAS or numeric rating scales) to more complex measures that address quality of life, productivity, physical health, mental health, satisfaction, and health perceptions (e.g., Pain Disability Index, Sickness Impact Profile, Multidimensional Pain Inventory, Beck Depression Inventory). Reevaluation using these same assessment instruments provides the nurse with indications of improvement in patient outcomes that relate to pain and its impact.

A third approach to measuring patient outcomes is to identify nursing-sensitive patient outcomes (Iowa Outcomes Project, 2000) that provide a quantitative method of communicating outcomes in a way that transfers across settings and individual practitioner use. For the diagnosis of Pain and Chronic Pain, several outcomes would be appropriate: Pain Level is defined as "severity of reported or demonstrated pain" (Iowa Outcomes Project, 2000, p. 328); Pain Control is the "personal actions to control pain" (p. 326); Pain: Disruptive Effects is the "observed or reported disruptive effects of pain on emotions and behavior" (p. 327); and Comfort Level is the "extent of physical and psychological ease" (p. 173) (see Box 36-1). The indicators identified in the outcome reflect a change in some of the defining characteristics identified in the NANDA definitions.

The outcome Pain Level is especially useful to evaluate the effect of interventions for Acute Pain, since most of the defining characteristics identified by NANDA are incorporated into the indicators of the outcome. The outcomes could be more inclusive if verbal expression clearly indicated moaning and crying, as well as speech, and if pacing, self-focusing, and narrowed focus were incorporated. Three indicators that are not noted as defining characteristics in NANDA, including percentage of body affected, frequency of pain, and length of pain episodes, would provide additional data to support a change in the pain state.

The outcome Pain Control (Iowa Outcomes Project, 2000) is especially important for intervention effectiveness for those with chronic pain. Because of the nature of chronic pain and the long-term need for behavior change, compliance or adherence to the treatment regimen is often a problem. This outcome addresses the client behaviors that are necessary for a successful outcome and provides indicators that are important in promoting compliance.

The outcome Pain: Disruptive Effects (Iowa Outcomes Project, 2000) is also particularly useful when dealing with the client with chronic pain. The indicators clearly identify the many areas of life activities that are often interrupted by pain. NANDA's defining characteristics address these factors minimally, so the outcome is clearly a more comprehensive approach to evaluating the results with chronic pain patients.

Finally, the outcome Comfort Level (Iowa Outcomes Project, 2000) provides a broad indicator of pain control by addressing overall feelings of psychologic and physical comfort that are often impacted by pain, particularly chronic benign and malignant pain.

These four outcome measures could be useful in clinical practice in focusing evaluation of intervention outcome and providing a consistent method of documenting response to pain treatment. However, these NOC outcome measures are relatively new, and empirical testing of these measurement scales is needed to determine procedures for implementation and to determine psychometric properties that support their validity and reliability for use with all ages.

NURSING INTERVENTIONS

Older adults can benefit tremendously from a wide variety of interventions in the management of pain, particularly chronic pain. Advances in the conceptualization and treatment of pain support the use of a multimodal approach, incorporating both pharmacologic and nonpharmacologic interventions that exert their effect at different levels of the peripheral and central nervous system (Butler & Gastel, 1980; Ferrell & Ferrell, 1991; Haley & Dolce, 1986; Harkins, Kwentus, & Price, 1984; Jay & Miller, 1990).

To date, research examining the effects of various pain control modalities with the elderly is limited, and strategies for effective pain control in this population are based mostly on the theoretical underpinnings of the interventions, clinical experience, and application of pain control methods found to be useful with younger adults. There is a serious need for research in all areas of pain control for the elderly, particularly with respect to identifying adaptations in interventions most useful for this population.

The Nursing Interventions Classification (NIC) (Iowa Intervention Project, 2000) provides a number of global and specific interventions that address the majority of nursing interventions for the person in pain. The major intervention Pain Management is defined as the "alleviation of pain or a reduction in pain to a level of comfort that is acceptable to the patient" (Iowa Intervention Project, 2000, p. 485). Pain Management provides a comprehensive perspective on nursing activities that ultimately alleviate or reduce pain (see Box 36-1). Within this intervention, nurses are referred to more specific interventions, including those focusing on physical techniques to promote comfort (e.g., Acupressure; Cutaneous Stimulation; Environmental Management: Comfort; Heat/Cold Application; Progressive Muscle Relaxation; Simple Massage; Therapeutic Touch; Transcutaneous Electrical Nerve Stimulation [TENS]), those focusing on psychologic techniques to promote comfort (Anxiety Reduction; Autogenic Training; Biofeedback; Calming Technique; Distraction; Hypnosis; Meditation Facilitation; Simple Guided Imagery; Simple Relaxation Therapy), and those related to pharmacologic intervention (Analgesic Administration; Analgesic Administration: Intraspinal).

References in the activity lists to "developmental appropriateness" and the use of the modifier "as appropriate" suggest that the activities need to be tailored to the individual client situation. The NIC pain interventions do not provide the specificity or information on adaptations that must be considered for older adults with pain. The following presentation of nursing interventions, both pharmacologic and nonpharmacologic, addresses some of the knowledge needed to implement the NIC interventions for pain with the elderly population.

Many theories have been proposed to explain the phenomenon of pain. Early theories, such as the specificity theory and the pattern theory, emphasized the recognition of specific pathways of pain transmission; later theories, such as the gate control theory, have attempted to uncover the complexity of central processing and modulation of pain in specific areas of the brain and nervous system. Because of the complexity of the pain experience, no single theory to date fully explains the transmission or perception of pain, the complexity of the pathways that affect transmission of pain impulses, the actual sensation of pain, or individual differences in pain sensation.

Although the state of scientific knowledge related to pain continues to evolve, the gate control theory, proposed and later modified by Melzack and Wall (1965, 1982), is one of the most widely accepted theories of pain and provides the clinician with a theoretical foundation for employing both pharmacologic and nonpharmacologic interventions for pain management. Essentially, this theory recognizes pain as a complex, multidimensional experience interrelating three dimensions of the individual's perception: the sensory-discriminative (physical); the affective-motivational (psychologic); and the cognitive-interpretive (cognitive) dimension. A gating mechanism in the dorsal horn of the spinal column allows pain to be reduced or modulated at four points: (1) at the peripheral site of pain; (2) in the spinal cord itself; (3) in the brainstem; and (4) in the cerebral cortex. At the peripheral site of pain, nonopioid analgesics, application of heat and cold, and local anesthetics alter the release of nociceptive substances and decrease accompanying muscle spasm. In the spinal cord, application of heat and cold, massage, and direct electrical stimulation activate large nerve fibers and interfere with the transmission of pain impulses. Interventions that can effectively reduce or eliminate the transmission of pain impulses in the brainstem include electrical stimulation, acupuncture, and administration of opioid analgesics. Finally, administration of opioid and opioid antagonist analgesics and cognitive-behavioral techniques such as relaxation, imagery, distraction, music therapy, hypnosis, and cognitive therapy work primarily through action in the cerebral cortex (Donovan, 1989).

Pharmacologic Interventions

Although pharmacologic intervention might not be the sole intervention of choice for the older adult, it plays an important role in managing acute and both malignant and benign chronic pain. The NIC intervention Analgesic Administration provides a list of activities to guide pharmacologic interventions. Information essential to tailor these to the specific needs of older adults follows.

Lack of knowledge and skill in pharmacologic intervention is a barrier to optimal pain management in the elderly. When pharmacologic strategies are tried, they are often less than adequate in controlling pain due to ineffective dosing and ineffective patterns of administration by both physicians and nurses (Ferrell et al., 1990; Roy & Thomas, 1986).

Two specific concerns, noted by the older adult, significant others, and health care providers, can create barriers to successful pharmacologic intervention and need to be addressed. An unreasonable fear of opiate addiction and respiratory depression contributes to undertreatment of pain with opioids in this population (Faherty & Grier, 1984; McCaffery & Ferrell, 1991; Short, Burnett, Egbert, & Parks, 1990). Research, however, indicates that addiction is rare (less than 0.1%) (Angel, 1982) and is most likely to occur in those with a past history of drug abuse. Similarly, the incidence of respiratory depression is also quite low (Miller & Jick, 1978). With initial reduction and careful titration of doses/and or interval between doses and frequent assessments of the elder's response, opioids can be safely administered to elderly patients (Acute Pain Management Guideline Panel, 1992).

Safe and effective use of analgesic drugs in the elderly requires an understanding of age-related changes that can impact pharmacokinetics and pharmacodynamics. The heterogeneity of the older population, resulting in physiologic aging that might not coincide with chronologic aging, as well as the increased incidence of chronic diseases in the elder, can impact drug effect and toxicity and make the process of pharmacologic management challenging. Understanding the general physiologic changes that occur with aging can alert the nurse to anticipated adverse effects of analgesic administration.

In general, an increased proportion of body fat, decreased circulating proteins, decreased hepatic metabolism, and decreased glomerular filtration and drug clearance all contribute to potential alterations in the older adult's response to pharmacologic intervention. The effect of these physiologic changes can result in increased sensitivity to the effect of analgesics, with a higher peak and longer duration of pain relief, as well as greater risk of toxic effect (Kaiko, Wallenstein, Rogers, Grabinski, & Houde, 1982; Kwentus, Harkins, Lignon, & Silvermann, 1985; Moore, Vilderman, Lubenskyi, McCans, & Fox, 1990; Zaccharias, Pfeifer, & Herbison, 1990). For more detailed explanation of the changes in pharmacokinetics and pharmacodynamics related to the older adult, the reader is referred to Popp and Portenoy (1996).

Although a detailed review of individual drugs is beyond the scope of this chapter, several important generalizations and principles related to the administration of opioid and nonopioid analgesics will be addressed. First, drug selection should be based on the older adult's report of pain and directed at choosing the drug that is least invasive, most cost-effective, with the least side effects that can alleviate the reported level of pain. One strategy is to use the World Health Organization (1990) "analgesic ladder" for managing chronic cancer pain. The ladder advocates selecting an analgesic based on the usual severity of pain. A nonopioid, such as aspirin or a nonsteroidal anti-inflammatory drug (NSAID), is recommended for the initial trial if pain is generally mild to moderate. For more moderate, persistent pain, adding a weak opioid, such as codeine, hydrocodone, or oxycodone, is advocated. More severe pain often requires use of a pure agonist opioid (e.g., morphine). Adjuvant drugs can be included at any step of the ladder and may act to enhance the effect of the analgesic. There are basic guidelines for using analgesics in the three categories of drugs (opioid, nonopioid, adjuvant) with the elder that need to be addressed.

Opioids.   Codeine is probably the most important weak opioid that can be used safely with the elder for management of moderate pain. Oxycodone, a moderate opioid with good analgesic properties, also is relatively safe for the older adult. Giving either of these agents in combination with a nonopioid, such as aspirin or acetaminophen, allows the opioid dosage to be reduced, thus decreasing the significant constipating effects associated with opioids.

Morphine, the most used and most predictable opioid for the older patient, is the choice for severe pain due to its short half-life, which allows for the rapid dose adjustments necessary when titrating to effective pain control. Because of the large variability in response to different opioids in older adults, switching from one opioid to another when pain relief is not achieved is advocated (de Stoutz, Bruera, & Suarez-Almazor, 1995). Alternative opioids commonly used in this population include hydromorphone, oxycodone, levorphanol, fentanyl, and methadone. Opioids with long half-lives, such as methadone, fentanyl, and levorphanol, can be used, but require caution and careful monitoring, since they can result in delayed toxicity (Popp & Portenoy, 1996). Sustained-release opioids offer increased convenience for patients and caregivers and may increase compliance with the medication regimen (American Geriatrics Society Panel on Chronic Pain in Older Persons, 1998; Hofmann, Farnon, Javed, & Posner, 1998; Leland, 1999). These agents may be considered with the patient in chronic pain who has been stabilized on short-acting agents. Monitoring for side effects is always essential.

An analgesic to be avoided for chronic opioid therapy in the elder is meperidine (Ferrell, 1996; Jacox et al., 1994). Meperidine produces an active toxic metabolite, normeperidine, that can accumulate in older adults, causing tremulousness, dysphoria, myoclonus, and seizures, and is recommended only for acute pain. Meperidine should be used for 2 to 3 days at most.

Although opioids are widely used for acute and malignant pain management, controversy continues over the use of long-term opioid therapy to manage chronic nonmalignant pain. Although the role of opioid therapy in the elderly chronic pain population has not yet been defined, current guidelines suggest that opioids might be considered after other "reasonable" analgesic therapies have failed (Portenoy, 1994). It is logical that there are many older adults who could benefit from long-term opioid therapy with careful management.

Propoxyphene, although widely used, is no more effective than aspirin and acetaminophen, but has increased risks for dependence and central nervous system side effects (Ferrell, 1996; McCue, 1998; Schnitzer, 1998). The American Pain Society's and the American Geriatrics Society's guidelines recommend avoiding the use of this drug with the elderly (American Geriatrics Society Panel on Chronic Pain in Older Persons, 1998; American Pain Society, 1999).

Nonopioids.   Nonopioid analgesics, including acetaminophen and nonsteroidal anti-inflammatory drugs (NSAIDs), are often chosen for the treatment of acute or chronic pain in elders. Acetaminophen is safer than NSAIDs and should be tried first, then followed by NSAID therapy when pain management is inadequate (American Geriatrics Society Panel on Chronic Pain in Older Persons, 1998). Acetaminophen is the easiest agent to take, but its lack of anti-inflammatory properties minimizes its usefulness for many pain conditions associated with aging. All drugs in this class have a ceiling effect, and toxic side effects can occur when used at high dosages over a extended period.

Aspirin is not a desirable drug for older adults because of its potential for gastritis and gastrointestinal bleeding and diminished renal function. Salicylate salts, such as choline magnesium trisalicylate (Trilisate) and salsalate, have fewer gastrointestinal side effects, do not affect bleeding time or platelet aggregation, and are renal sparing, making them a good choice for older adults.

Although NSAIDs, such as ibuprofen, naproxen and indomethacin, can be effective for short-term management of mild to moderate pain, the use of NSAIDs with older adults requires special considerations. In addition to common concerns related to gastric ulceration, renal toxicity, and inhibition of platelet aggregation, unusual drug reactions including cognitive impairment, constipation, and headache (Roth, 1989) are more common in the elder. Numerous drug interactions can occur with antacids, cimetidine, warfarin, and anticonvulsants (Verbeeck, 1990), and careful monitoring during therapy is warranted. Although long-term use of NSAIDs should be avoided in older patients (American Geriatrics Society Panel on Chronic Pain in Older Persons, 1998; Cleary & Carbone, 1997; Leland, 1999), some conditions associated with inflammation may necessitate their use (Ferrell, 1996; Nguyen, 1996; Schnitzer, 1998).

It is important that older adults using NSAIDs on a regular basis be carefully monitored, since side effects can be severe and even life-threatening. Evaluation of hemoglobin/hematocrit and stool guaiac sample to monitor for gastrointestinal bleeding and of blood urea nitrogen and/or serum creatinine to screen for renal insufficiency should be conducted every 3 months. New classes of

NSAIDs, such as the Cox-2 inhibitor, are becoming available; these agents might be a great benefit to older adults by minimizing the serious side effects.

Adjuvants. Medications that enhance analgesic effects are often administered as adjuvants to pain management when treating chronic pain conditions. Antidepressants, anticonvulsants, sedative/antianxiety agents, steroids, muscle relaxants, and amphetamines often are used as adjuvant analgesics. Adjuvants can contribute to primary pain control, treatment of side effects, and alleviation of psychologic distress (Cleary & Carbone, 1997; Stein & Ferrell, 1996). Unfortunately, adjuvants also can produce frequent side effects, some of which are not treatable (Ferrell, 1998; Herr & Mobily, 1997; Popp & Portenory, 1996). Older adults are particularly sensitive to the anticholinergeic effects of amitriptyline and other antidepressants, the central nervous system side effects of neuroleptics and to the delirium associated with local anesthetics (Ferrell, 1996; Hoffman et al., 1998). Thus these drugs should be used with great caution, incorporating careful drug selection, lower starting doses, cautious dose escalation, and frequent monitoring for adverse effects. Due to misperceptions related to the typical purpose of adjuvants (e.g., to treat depression), careful explanations and education are important in promoting a positive response to these agents.

Route of Administration. Because of the age-related changes mentioned earlier, guidelines should be followed when selecting the most effective route of administration. Unless contraindicated by absorption problems or swallowing ability, oral medication should be used whenever possible. Degenerated muscle related to inactivity, poor nutrition, dehydration, and decreased peripheral circulation lead to highly variable and diminished drug absorption, insufficient plasma concentrations, and delayed onset of action with intramuscular administration; therefore this route should be avoided. Other routes of administration, such as sublingual, buccal, rectal, subcutaneous, or intravenous, may be preferred. Poor compliance with oral dosing in long-term drug therapy may necessitate an alternate route (e.g., fentanyl patch). Long-term rectal administration has been successful with controlled-release morphine (Bruera, Schoeller, Fainsinger, & Kastelan, 1992), and the transdermal route (e.g., fentanyl) is now widely used. Transdermal fentanyl provides a treatment option for older adults who are unable to swallow or absorb an oral opiate and improves compliance of therapy. However, transdermal analgesia should not be used when rapid dose titration is required (Popp & Portenoy, 1996).

The use of patient-controlled analgesia (PCA) has been shown effective in elders with postoperative pain (Duggleby & Lander, 1992; Egbert, Battit, Welch, & Barlett, 1990). It is important to spend extra time with the older adult to teach use of the PCA and to evaluate her use of the PCA. Close monitoring and titration are warranted (Ferrell, Cronin-Nash, & Warfield, 1992). PCA equipment can also be adapted for those physically unable to press the button, such as patients with rheumatoid arthritis (Pasero, 1994), or a designated other, such as family member or nurse, can be responsible for dose administration (Pasero & McCaffery, 1996).

Dosing. Dosing of analgesics for older adults must be titrated and individualized in order to achieve maximum pain control. A safe recommendation for dosing of the elder is to lower the starting doses by 25% to 50% of the usual adult dose (Pasero & McCaffery, 1996) and to titrate the dose up or down based on the individual's response. Because older patients can experience a longer duration of action of opioids, less frequent dosing may be more appropriate than decreasing the dosage (Stein, 1996).

Administration of analgesics around the clock is a recommended standard of treatment that provides stable analgesic blood levels for older adults experiencing acute pain and prevents pain from becoming out of control. It also provides the individual with a sense of security that his pain is being attended to through a scheduled plan. The reader is referred to Ferrell (1991) and Popp and Portenoy (1996) for information on specific drugs and dosages for older adults.

Compliance with the pharmacologic regimen can be particularly problematic for older adults, especially with complex regimens and long-term therapy. In fact, research has shown that 50% of the elderly do not take their prescribed pain medications appropriately (Austin, Cody, Eyres, Hefferin, & Krasnow, 1986). Selecting agents (e.g., opioids and NSAIDs) that can be administered with single or twice daily dosing can increase compliance.

Medication administration schedules, calendars, and pill organizers are tools that may aid in this process (Morgan, Lindley, & Berry, 1994). Placing a schedule or reminder where it will be seen at the appropriate time, such as on the bathroom mirror or refrigerator, and incorporating medication administration into the older adult's schedule before another routine activity can also be helpful (e.g., taking medicine before meals and at bedtime).

Nonpharmacologic Interventions

Nonpharmacologic interventions can be classified into two categories: physical or cutaneous stimulation interventions and cognitive-behavioral interventions. Physical or cutaneous stimulation interventions involve stimulating the skin and underlying tissues to moderate or relieve pain. Cognitive-behavioral interventions focus on helping the individual cope with the pain being experienced by altering the interpretation of the sensation of pain and enhancing self-control.

Pharmacologic interventions in the management of pain for older adults is often complicated by age-related physiologic changes that affect pharmacokinetics and pharmacodynamics, by problems that result from polypharmacy and by idiosyncratic drug reactions. Consequently, nonpharmacologic interventions can be particularly valuable and effective. These interventions, when used in combination with pharmacologic approaches, will result in more effective pain control, less reliance on medications, fewer side effects, and less clinical impairment (American Geriatrics Society Panel on Chronic Pain in Older Persons, 1998; Ferrell, 1991; Foley, 1990; Gagliese & Melzack, 1997; McCaffery & Beebe, 1989; Middaugh, Levin, Kee, Barchiesi, & Roberts, 1988; Nguyen, 1996; Owens & Ehrenreich, 1991). Although many health care providers perceive older adults to be indifferent, unwilling, or unable to use nonpharmacologic interventions, research reveals that older patients are often very responsive to the use of these interventions (Gagliese & Melzack, 1997; Middaugh et al., 1988; Sorkin, Rudy, Hanlon, Turk, & Stieg, 1990). Not only have older adults been found to be responsive, but in comparing them to younger individuals, investigators have noted that geriatric clients often showed greater interest in these programs, were more compliant, more willing to work hard for degrees of improvement, and were generally free of work-related issues that often hinder progress for younger persons.

Cutaneous Stimulation Interventions.   Cutaneous stimulation interventions provide important noninvasive methods for managing pain in older adults. A variety of different modalities are available, including thermal agents (application of heat and cold), transcutaneous electrical nerve stimulation (TENS), and massage (simple massage and acupressure). These modalities are very effective in managing pain and are easily performed, inexpensive, and noninjurious when used properly. They can readily be taught to the client and/or significant others, enabling them to implement these interventions independently.

One of the most important, but often unused, advantages of cutaneous stimulation interventions is their applicability to multiple areas. These techniques are effective when applied directly to the site of pain. However, they also can be extremely effective when applied to a site distal to, proximal to, or contralateral to the site of pain, to trigger points, or on or around acupressure or acupuncture points. Specific activities related to the use of these interventions can be found in the NIC interventions (Iowa Intervention Project, 2000) on Cutaneous Stimulation, Heat/Cold Application, Transcutaneous Electrical Nerve Stimulation (TENS), Simple Massage, and Acupressure.

Thermal Agents.   A wide range of thermal agents is available, including hot and cold packs, hydrotherapy (i.e., tub baths or shower sprays), and paraffin baths (i.e., application of heat to a specific area by immersion in warm paraffin), as well as more sophisticated technologic devices that provide infrared therapy, short-wave diathermy, and ultrasound. Research examining the effectiveness of thermal agents in controlling pain has been relatively extensive, although few studies have included or focused specifically on older adults. The effectiveness of thermal agents for managing joint pain from osteoarthritis and rheumatoid arthritis in older adults has been demonstrated (Barr, 1993). Research on pain management for older adults with rheumatoid arthritis (Davis, Cortez, & Rubin, 1990) found that application of heat and use of a heated pool, tub, or shower was one of the most helpful methods in alleviating pain. Although older adults might be reluctant to use cold, clinical practice indicates that cold is often more effective in managing pain, especially pain related to muscle or joint pathology. Moreover, alternating heat and cold is often more effective than the use of either alone.

A number of factors associated with aging contribute to increased risk of thermal injury: (1) decreased reactivity of the thermoregulatory system; (2) decreased autonomic and vasomotor responses; (3) reduction in circulation and loss of sweat glands associated with atrophy of the skin; and (4) decreased perception of thermal changes (Kauffman, 1987). In addition, heating of large body surfaces and consequent vasodilation can place hazardous demands on cardiac output (Kauffman, 1987). Conversely, use of cold can cause a temporary increase in systolic and diastolic blood pressure, thereby posing a risk for hypertensive individuals (Michlovitz, 1990). Application of cold to extremities is contraindicated for older adults with arterial insufficiency due to peripheral vascular disease (McCaffery & Beebe, 1989). Many of these concerns can be alleviated with careful selection and precautionary use of thermal modalities. In general, operating temperatures for heating agents should be lowered for use with the elderly, while temperatures for cooling agents should be raised. Also, use of both hot and cold packs may require additional insulation with dry toweling, and treatment times may need to be shortened.

Transcutaneous Electrical Nerve Stimulation. TENS involves stimulation of cutaneous and peripheral nerves via electrodes on the surface of the skin. TENS can be very effective as an adjunctive intervention for the management of pain in older adults and has been found to be particularly effective for the relief of low back pain, diabetic neuropathies, shoulder pain or bursitis, fractured ribs, postherpetic neuralgia, myofascial pain, and advanced painful malignancies (Ferrell & Ferrell, 1991).

Although few side effects have been noted with the use of TENS, some special considerations for its use with the elder are indicated. TENS therapy is contraindicated for individuals using demand-type synchronous cardiac pacemakers. It is also suggested that electrical stimulation be avoided on the anterior chest or over the carotid sinuses of individuals with cardiac histories.

Important parameters for the most effective use of TENS are selection of the best site(s) for placement of electrodes (i.e., directly over the pain, acupuncture or acupressure points, spinal nerve roots, proximal or contralateral sites) and adjustment of the electrical current amplitude and pulse pattern. Thorough searching and adjustment may be necessary for optimum pain control, often requiring an experienced clinician or therapist to initiate therapy and train clients or caregivers.

Massage. Massage is the application of friction or pressure to skin and underlying tissues either superficially, deeply, or via vibrations. Massage is effective in managing pain in multiple ways: through stimulation of large nerve fibers that close the gate and block transmission of pain messages; by decreasing muscle spasm or tension; by increasing circulation and promoting capillary and arteriolar dilation, thereby reducing edema associated with pain; and by stimulating release of endorphins (McCaffery & Beebe, 1989; Edgar & Smith-Hanrahan, 1992). Clients generally report that massage is comforting, soothing, and relaxing. Also, massage can transmit a powerful message of acceptance and caring and enhance nurse-client communication.

Acupressure is a form of massage that uses pressure at trigger or acupuncture sites. Pressure can be applied with sustained firm pressure of 15 seconds to 5 minutes using the fingers, knuckle, or thumb, objects such as a rubber ball, or ice. It is believed that acupressure relieves pain by stimulating pressure fibers that are larger, myelinated and rapidly conducting afferent fibers. When these are stimulated, the pressure fibers close the spinal cord gating mechanism to impulses from the small unmyelinated fibers that conduct pain (McCafferey & Beebe, 1989).

The use of massage as an adjunctive therapy in pain management has several advantages. Client effort and involvement are minimal, which can be important when energy level or function is limited. Family members or significant others can be trained in the use of massage when clinician availability is limited. Contraindications to the use of massage include avoiding massage with fractures, phlebitis, skin lesions, over recent injuries or infected areas, or with patients with increased bleeding time.

Cognitive-Behavioral Interventions

Cognitive-behavioral interventions provide a variety of techniques that can be used effectively in the management of pain in the elder. Specific interventions include progressive muscle relaxation, passive muscle relaxation, autogenic training, meditation, biofeedback, and hypnosis, among others. In general, cognitive behavioral interventions promote a sense of relaxation and control. They are particularly useful in the management of chronic pain. By its very definition, chronic pain implies a chronically stressful experience that can result in autonomic and/or

muscular responses associated with painful sensations. The result is often muscle spasm, decreased blood flow to tissues, and secretion of pain-producing substances that can cause or augment existing pain. The emotional response to these occurrences can further exacerbate physical responses, contributing to a spiral of pain, anxiety, and muscle tension. Interventions that promote relaxation are effective in reducing or modulating pain by interrupting this spiral of events. Other benefits associated with these interventions include improved sleep, decreased fatigue, enhanced mood, and an increased sense of personal control over the pain (Gagliese & Melzack, 1997; Haley & Dolce, 1986; Manetto & McPherson, 1996; McCaffery & Beebe, 1989). The reader is referred to the NIC interventions Simple Relaxation Therapy, Progressive Muscle Relaxation, Autogenic Training, Simple Guided Imagery, Distraction, Meditation Facilitation, Biofeedback, and Hypnosis (Iowa Intervention Project, 2000) for specific activities related to these interventions.

Although there is increasing evidence of the efficacy of these interventions for the management of pain, particularly chronic pain, older adults are often considered poor candidates for their use and are seldom given ample opportunity to benefit from them (Gagliese & Melzack, 1997; Manetto & McPherson, 1996; Portenoy & Farkash, 1988). Clearly, there are factors that must be considered that would compromise the use of these interventions, including cognitive deficits, severe depression, and expressed mistrust of psychologic formulations inherent in some of these interventions (i.e., imagery). However, many older adults have the cognitive capacity to participate in these interventions and are willing to try them. Given the potential efficacy of these interventions in managing pain, advanced age should not preclude the use of these interventions.

Modifications can be made in the use of these interventions for older adults that make them more easily learned and used. Keefe, Beaupre, Weiner, and Siegler (1996) suggest minor changes in training procedures, including having older clients keep their eyes open while listening to relaxation tapes to minimize chances of falling asleep, reducing the length of practice sessions to reduce fatigue, and practicing at times when clients are least likely to be fatigued. Briefer training sessions can be structured for clients with shortened attention spans (Manetto & McPherson, 1996). For older individuals who have difficulty hearing the trainer or training tapes, visual aids can be developed and used. Finally, the importance of including significant others to assist the individual in learning the techniques and in providing coaching, reinforcement, motivation, or other assistance as needed cannot be overstated. Clinical experience suggests that older adults will be more accepting of these interventions when clear rationales for their use (i.e., to decrease the need for, and side effects from, medication regimens) and indications of their effectiveness are presented.

CASE STUDY

The major NIC intervention for Mr. Green, Pain Management, provides a comprehensive perspective on nursing activities to alleviate or reduce his pain. Although all of the pain-related interventions described previously in this chapter potentially could be beneficial for Mr. Green, a number of specific interventions were particularly effective: Analgesic Administration, Heat/Cold Application, Transcutaneous Electrical Nerve Stimulation (TENS), Simple Massage, Autogenic Training, and Distraction.

Since Mr. Green was taking Relafen, an NSAID, it was important that he be monitored for symptoms of gastric irrigation; complete blood count (CBC), blood urea nitrogen, serum creatinine, and liver function tests were warranted periodically. Although pharmacologic therapy is very beneficial for individuals such as Mr. Green, the potentially serious side effects make the use of other nonpharmacologic modalities for pain relief particularly important.

Incorporating nonpharmacologic interventions such as Distraction and Autogenic Training provided multiple benefits. Since Mr. Green's favorite forms of distraction were reading and watching television, these activities, as well as the autogenic training, provided periods of time when he was able to rest his hips and back. For individuals with osteoarthritic pain, a balance of rest and activity, incorporating several rest breaks during the day, is recommended. Often an hour of non-weightbearing rest in the afternoon will permit increased activity without pain later in the day. In addition, providing autogenic training for Mr. Green enabled him to more fully relax the muscles surrounding the affected joints, as well as providing general relaxation and preventing the spiral of muscle tension and pain. The muscle spasms in his back and the resultant pain were further relieved with implementation of the Simple Massage intervention and the Heat/Cold Application intervention. Alternating heat and cold has been found to be more effective in some patients than use of either modality alone. Because Mr. Green associated cold with increased pain, he was originally reluctant to try alternating these modalities. He discovered, however, that use of cold, or alternating cold with heat, was more effective in reducing both his pain and the muscle spasms he experienced. For an added sense of warmth when using cold packs, simultaneous use of a heating pad or blanket on other parts of his body was effective. TENS therapy was instituted to help control the pain that radiated to Mr. Green's leg and foot and was extremely effective.

All of the nonpharmacologic interventions were interventions that could be taught to Mr. Green and his wife, providing measures that could be used independently and thereby providing both of them with a greater sense of control over the pain he experienced. With the implementation of the interventions described, Mr. Green was able to realize a number of positive outcomes, including an improvement in Pain Level, greater use of Pain Control Behaviors, fewer disruptive effects (Pain: Disruptive Effects) and an improved Comfort Level.

SUMMARY

Management of pain in elders poses an important challenge for nurses. To ensure quality of life for older adults, careful assessment and evaluation of pain with appropriate interventions based on sound clinical judgment is essential. The myth that pain and old age go hand in hand must be dispelled. If we cannot promise our older adults that the best is, indeed, yet to be, we must strive to make their lives as pain free as possible.

REFERENCES

Acute Pain Management Guideline Panel. (1992). *Acute pain management: Operative or medical procedures and trauma. Clinical practice guideline.* AHCPR Pub. No. 92-0032. Rockville, MD: Agency for Health Care Policy and Research, Public Health Service, U.S. Department of Health and Human Services.

Ahles, T. A., Blanchard, E. B., & Ruckdeschel, J. D. (1983). The multidimensional nature of cancer-related pain. *Pain, 17,* 277-288.

American Geriatrics Society Panel on Chronic Pain in Older Persons. (1998). The management of chronic pain in older persons. *Journal of the American Geriatrics Society, 46*(5), 635-651.

American Pain Society. (1999). *Principles of analgesic use in the treatment of acute pain and cancer pain* (4th ed.). Glenview, IL: American Pain Society.

Angel, M. (1982). The quality of mercy. *New England Journal of Medicine, 306,* 98-99.

Austin, C., Cody, C., Eyres, P., Hefferin, E., & Krasnow, R. (1986). Hospice home care pain management: Four critical variables. *Cancer Nursing, 9,* 58-65.

Baker, S. P., O'Neill, B., & Karpf, R. S. (1984). *The injury fact book.* Lexington, MA: Lexington Books.

Barr, J. O. (1993). Conservative pain management for the older patient. In A. A. Guccione (Ed.), *Geriatric physical therapy: Principles and practice* (pp. 283-306). St. Louis, MO: Mosby.

Bates, M. S., Edwards, W. T., & Anderson, K. W. (1993). Ethno-cultural influences on variation in chronic pain perception. *Pain, 52,*(1), 101-112.

Beck, A. T., Ward, C., Mendelson, M., Mock, J., & Erbaugh, J. (1961). An inventory for measuring depression. *Archives of General Psychiatry, 4,* 561-571.

Bernabei, R., Gambassi, G., Lapane, K., Landi, F., Gatsonis, C., Dunlop, R., Lipsitz, L., Steel, K., & Mor, V. (1998). Management of pain in elderly patients with cancer. *Journal of the American Medical Association, 279*(23), 1877-1882.

Beyer, J. E., & Aradine, C. R. (1986). Content validity of an instrument to measure young children's perceptions of the intensity of their pain. *Journal of Pediatric Nursing, 1,* 386-395.

Bieri, D., Reeve, R., Champion, G., Addicoat, L., & Ziegler, J. (1990). The Faces Pain Scale for the self-assessment of the severity of pain experienced by children: Development, initial validation, and preliminary investigation for ratio scale properties. *Pain, 41,* 139-150.

Blazer, D., Hughes, D., & George, L. (1987). The epidemiology of depression in an elderly community population. *The Gerontologist, 27,* 281-287.

Bonica, J. J. (1990). General considerations of chronic pain. In J. J. Bonica (Ed.), *The management of pain* (2nd ed., pp. 180-196). Philadelphia: Lea & Febiger.

Brattberg, G., Mats, T., & Anders, W. (1989). The prevalence of pain in a general population: The results of a postal survey in a county of Sweden. *Pain, 37,* 215-222.

Brody, E. M., & Kleban, M. H. (1983). Day-to-day mental and physical health symptoms of older people: A report on health logs. *The Gerontologist, 23,* 75-85.

Brown, G., Nicassio, P., & Wallston, K. (1989). Pain coping strategies and depression in rheumatoid arthritis. *Journal of Consulting and Clinical Psychology, 57,* 652-657.

Browning, R. (1895). Rabbi Ben Ezra. In H. E. Scudder (Ed.), *The complete poetical work of browning.* Boston: Houghton Mifflin.

Bruera, E., Schoeller, T., Fainsinger, R. L., & Kastelan, C. (1992). Custom-made suppositories of methadone for severe cancer pain. *Journal of Pain and Symptom Management, 7,* 372-374.

Butler, R. H., & Gastel, B. (1980). Care of the aged: Perspectives of pain and discomfort. In L. E. Ng & J. J. Bonica (Eds.), *Pain, discomfort, and humanitarian care: Proceedings of the national conference.* New York: Elsevier.

Cleary, J. F., & Carbone, P. P. (1997). Palliative medicine in older patients. *Cancer, 80*(7), 1335-1347.

Cleeland, C. S., Gonin, R., Hatfield, A. K., Edmondson, J. H., Blum, R. H., Stewart, J. A., & Pandya, K. J. (1994). Pain and its treatment in outpatients with metastatic cancer. *New England Journal of Medicine, 220*(9), 592-596.

Cohen-Mansfield, J., & Marx, M. S. (1993). Pain and depression in the nursing home: Corroborating results. *Journal of Gerontology, 48*(2), 96-97.

Copp, L. A. (1990). The spectrum of suffering. *American Journal of Nursing, 90*(8), 35-39.

Corse, A. M., & Kuncl, R. W. (1991). Peripheral neuropathy. In L. R. Barker, J. R. Burton, & P. D. Zieve (Eds.), *Principles of ambulatory medicine* (4th ed., pp. 1240-1256). Baltimore: Lippincott Williams & Wilkins.

Crook, J., Rideout, E., & Brown, G. (1984). The prevalence of pain complaints among a general population. *Pain, 18,* 299-314.

Dalton, J. (1989). Nurses' perceptions of their pain assessment skills, pain management practices, and attitudes toward pain. *Oncology Nursing Forum, 16*(2), 225-231.

Davis, G., Cortez, C., & Rubin, B. (1990). Pain management in the older adult with rheumatoid arthritis or osteoarthritis. *Arthritis Care and Research, 3*(3), 127-131.

Davis, M. A. (1988). Epidemiology of osteoarthritis. *Clinical Geriatric Medicine, 4*(2), 241-255.

de Stoutz, N. D., Bruera, E. B., & Suarez-Almazor, M. (1995). Opioid rotation for toxicity reduction in terminal cancer patients. *Journal of Pain and Symptom Management, 10,* 378-384.

Doan, B., & Wadden, N. (1989). Relationships between depressive symptoms and description of chronic pain. *Pain, 36,* 75-84.

Donovan, M. (1989). Relieving pain: The current bases for practice. In S. Funk, E. Tornquist, M. Champagne, L. Copp, & R. Wiese (Eds.), *Key aspects of comfort: Management of pain, fatigue, and nausea* (pp. 25-34). New York: Springer.

Downie, W. W., Leatham, P. A., Rhind, V. M., Wright, V., Brancho, J. A., & Anderson, J. A. (1978). Studies with pain rating scales. *Annals of the Rheumatic Diseases, 37,* 378-381.

Duggleby, W., & Lander, J. (1992). Patient-controlled analgesia for older adults. *Clinical Nursing Research, 1*(1), 107-113.

Edgar, L., & Smith-Hanrahan, C. (1992). Nonpharmacologic pain management. In J. H. Watt-Watson & M. I. Donovan (Eds.), *Pain management: Nursing perspective* (pp. 162-202). St. Louis, MO: Mosby.

Egbert, L. D., Battit, G. E., Welch, C. E., & Barlett, M. K. (1990). Randomized trial of postoperative patient controlled analgesia vs intramuscular narcotics in frail elderly men. *Archives of Internal Medicine, 150,* 1897-1903.

Faherty, B. S., & Grier, M. R. (1984). Analgesic medication for elderly people post-surgery. *Nursing Research, 33*(6), 369-372.

Feldt, K. S., Ryden, M. B., & Miles, S. (1998). Treatment of pain in cognitively impaired compared with cognitively intact older patients with hip-fracture. *Journal of the American Geriatrics Society, 46*(9), 1079-1085.

Ferrell, B. A. (1991). Pain management in elderly people. *Journal of the American Geriatrics Society, 39,* 64-73.

Ferrell, B. A. (1996). Overview of aging and pain. In B. R. Ferrell & B. A. Ferrell (Eds.), *Pain in the elderly* (pp. 1-10). Seattle, WA: IASP Press.

Ferrell, B. A. (1998). The management of pain in older patients. *American Medical Directors Association 1998 Symposium Excerpts,* 7-8.

Ferrell, B. A., & Ferrell, B. R. (1991). Principles of pain management in older people. *Comprehensive Therapy, 17*(8), 53-58.

Ferrell, B. A., Ferrell, B. R., & Osterweil, D. (1990). Pain in the nursing home. *Journal of the American Geriatrics Society, 38*(4), 409-414.

Ferrell, B. A., Ferrell, B. R., & Rivera, L. (1995). Pain in cognitively impaired nursing home patients. *Journal of Pain and Symptom Management, 10,*(8), 591-598.

Ferrell, B. R., Cronin-Nash, C., & Warfield, C. (1992). The role of patient-controlled analgesia in the management of cancer pain. *Journal of Pain and Symptom Management, 7*(3), 149-154.

Foley, K. (1985). Treatment of cancer pain. *New England Journal of Medicine, 113,* 84-95.

Foley, K. M. (1987). Pain syndromes in patients with cancer. *Medical Clinics of North America, 71*(2), 169-184.

Foley, K. M. (1990). Pain management in the elderly. In W. R. Hazzards, R. Andres, & E. L Bierman (Eds.), *Principles of geriatric medicine and gerontology.* Hightstown, NJ: McGraw-Hill.

Gagliese, L., & Melzack, R. (1997). Chronic pain in older people. *Pain, 70*(1), 3-14.

Gyldenvand, T., & Tunick, P. (1989). Validation of the nursing diagnosis alteration in comfort: Chronic pain. In R. M. Carroll-Johnson (Ed.), *Classification of nursing diagnoses: Proceedings of the eighth conference* (pp. 284-290). Baltimore: Lippincott Williams & Wilkins.

Haley, W., Turner, J., & Romano, J. M. (1985). Depression and chronic pain patients: Relation to pain, activity, and sex differences. *Pain, 23,* 337-343.

Haley, W. E., & Dolce, J. J. (1986). Assessment and management of chronic pain in the elderly. *Clinical Gerontologist, 5,* 435-455.

Harkins, S. W., Kwentus, J., & Price, D. D. (1984). Pain and the elderly. In C. Benedetti, D. R. Chapiman, & G. Moricca (Eds.), *Advances in pain research and therapy* (vol. 7, pp. 103-122). New York: Raven Press.

Harkins, S. W., & Price, D. D. (1992). Assessment of pain in the elderly. In D. Turk & R. Melzack (Eds.), *Handbook of pain assessment* (pp. 315-331). New York: The Guilford Press.

Harkins, S., Price, D., & Martelli, M. (1986). Effects of age on pain perception: Thermonociception. *Journal of Gerontology, 41*,(1), 58-63.

Haythornthwaite, J., Seiber, W., & Kerns, R. (1991). Depression and the chronic pain experience. *Pain, 46*, 177-184.

Herr, K. A., & Mobily, P. R. (1997). Chronic pain in the elderly. In E. Swanson & T. Tripp-Reimer (Eds.), *Advances in gerontological nursing: Chronic illness and the older adult* (pp. 82-111). New York: Springer Publishing.

Herr, K., & Mobily, P. (1991). Complexities of pain assessment in the elderly: Clinical considerations. *Journal of Gerontological Nursing, 17*(4), 12-19.

Herr, K., & Mobily, P. (1992). Geriatric mental health: Chronic pain and depression. *Journal of Psychosocial Nursing, 30*(9), 7-12.

Herr, K., & Mobily, P. (1993). Comparison of selected pain assessment tools for use with the elderly. *Applied Nursing Research, 6*(1), 39-46.

Herr, K. A., Mobily, P. R., Kohout, F. J., & Wagenaar, D. (1998). Evaluation of the faces pain scale for use with older patients. *Clinical Journal of Pain, 14*(1), 29-38.

Herr, K., Mobily, P., Richardson, G., & Spratt, K. (1998, Oct. 25). *An evaluation of the use of selected pain scales to evaluate pain intensity using experimental pain in elder and nonelderly.* Poster presentation at the annual conference of the American Pain Society, New Orleans, LA.

Herr, K., Mobily, P., & Smith, C. (1993). Depression and the experience of chronic back pain: A study of related variables and age differences. *Clinical Journal of Pain, 9*, 104-114.

Hickey, T. (1988). Changing health perceptions of older patients and the implications for assessment. *Geriatric Medicine Today, 7*(6), 59-66.

Hofmann, M. T., Farnon, C. U., Javed, A., & Posner, J. D. (1998). Pain in elderly hospice patients. *American Journal of Hospice & Palliative Care, 15*(5), 259-265.

Hofland, S. L. (1992). Elder belief: Blocks to pain management. *Journal of Gerontological Nursing, 18*(6), 19-24, 39-40.

Hurley, A. C., Volicer, B. J., Hanrahan, P. A., Houde, S., & Volicer, L. (1992). Assessment of discomfort in advanced Alzheimer patients. *Research in Nursing & Health, 15*(5), 369-377.

International Association for the Study of Pain (IASP). (1986). Pain terms: A current list with definitions and notes on usage. *Pain, 3*, S216.

Iowa Intervention Project. J. C. McCloskey & G. M. Bulechek (Eds.). (2000). *Nursing interventions classification (NIC)* (3rd ed.). St. Louis, MO: Mosby.

Iowa Outcomes Project. M. Johnson, M. Maas, & S. Moorhead (Eds.). (2000). *Nursing outcomes classification (NOC)* (2nd ed.). St. Louis, MO: Mosby.

Jacobson, E. W. (1996). Osteoarthritis. In J. Noble (Ed.), *Primary care medicine* (2nd ed., pp. 1093-1097). St. Louis, MO: Mosby.

Jacox, A., Carr, D. B., Payne, R., et al. (1994). *Management of cancer pain. Clinical practice guideline No. 9.* AHCPR Publication No. 94-0592. Rockville, MD. Agency for Health Care Policy and Research, U. S. Department of Health and Human Services, Public Health Service.

Jay, L., & Miller, T. (1990). Chronic pain and the geriatric patient. In T. Miller (Ed.), *Chronic pain* (vol. II, pp. 821-838). Madison, WI: International Universities Press, Inc.

Jensen, M. P., Karoly, P., Riordan, E. F., Bland, F., & Burns, R. S. (1989). The subjective experience of acute pain—An assessment of the utility of 10 indices. *The Clinical Journal of Pain, 5*, 153-159.

Kaiko, R. F., Wallenstein, S. L., Rogers, A. G., Grabinski, P. Y., & Houde, R. W. (1982). Narcotics in the elderly. *Medical Clinics of North America, 66*(5), 1079-1089.

Katz, S., Ford, A. B., Moskowitz, R. W., Jackson, B. A., & Jaffe, M. W. (1963). Studies of illness in the aged. The index of activities of daily living: A standardized measure of biological and psychological function. *Journal of the American Geriatrics Association, 185*, 914-919.

Kauffman, T. (1987). Thermoregulation and use of heat and cold. In J. O. Littrup (Ed.), *Therapeutic considerations for the elderly* (pp. 69-91). New York: Churchill Livingstone.

Keefe, F. J., Beaupre, P. M., Weiner, D. K., & Siegler, I. C. (1996). Pain in older adults: A cognitive-behavioral perspective. In B. R. Ferrell & B. A. Ferrell (Eds.), *Pain in the elderly* (pp. 11-20). Seattle, WA: IASP Press.

Kerns, R., Turk, D., & Rudy, T. (1985). The West Haven–Yale Multidimensional Pain Inventory (WHYMPI). *Pain, 23*, 345-356.

Kwentus, J. A., Harkins, S. W., Lignon, N., & Silvermann, J. J. (1985). Current concepts of geriatric pain and its treatment. *Geriatrics, 40*(4), 48-57.

Lau-Ting, C., & Phoon, W. O. (1988). Aches and pains among Singapore elderly. *Singapore Medical Journal, 29*, 164-167.

Lawton, M. P., & Brody, E. M. (1969). Assessment of older people: Self-maintaining and instrumental activities of daily living. *The Gerontologist, 9*, 179-186.

Leland, J. Y. (1999). Chronic pain: Primary care treatment of the older patient, *Geriatrics, 54*(1), 23-28, 33-34, 37.

Loeser, J. D. (1990a). Peripheral nerve disorders (peripheral neuropathies). In J. J. Bonica (Ed.), *The management of pain* (2nd ed., pp. 211-219). Philadelphia: Lea & Febiger.

Loeser, J. D. (1990b). Herpes zoster and postherpetic neuralgia. In J. J. Bonica (Ed.), *The management of pain* (2nd ed., pp. 257-263). Philadelphia: Lea & Febiger.

Madison, J. L., & Wilkie, D. J. (1995). Family members' perceptions of cancer pain: Comparisons with patient sensory report and by patient psychologic status. *Nursing Clinics in North America, 30*(4), 625-645.

Mahoney, F., & Barthel, D. (1965). Functional evaluation: The Barthel Index. *MS Medical Journal, 14*(2), 61-65.

Manetto, C., & McPherson, S. E. (1996). The behavioral-cognitive model of pain. *Clinics in Geriatric Medicine, 12*(3), 461-471.

Marzinski, L. (1991). The tragedy of dementia: Clinically assessing pain in the confused, nonverbal elderly. *Journal of Gerontological Nursing, 17*(6), 25-28.

Matthews, G., Zarrow, V., & Osterholm, J. (1973). Cancer pain and its treatment. *Seminars in Drug Treatment, 3*(1), 45-72.

McCaffery, M., & Beebe, A. (1989). *Pain: Clinical manual for nursing practice.* St. Louis, MO: Mosby.

McCaffery, M., & Ferrell, B. (1991). How would you respond to these patients in pain? *Nursing, 91*(6), 34-37.

McCue, J. D. (1998). Appropriate analgesic selection in the long-term care setting. *American Medical Directors Association 1998 Symposium Excerpts:* 15-16.

McFarland, G. K., & McFarlane, E. A. (1997). *Nursing diagnosis and intervention* (3rd ed.). St. Louis, MO: Mosby.

McGrath, P. A., DeVeber, L. L., & Hearn, M. T. (1985). Multidimensional pain assessment in children. In H. L. Field, R. Dubner, & R. Cevero (Eds.), *Advances in pain research and therapy* (pp. 387-393). New York: Raven Press.

McGuire, D. B. (1992). Comprehensive and multidimensional assessment and measurement of pain. *Journal of Pain and Symptom Management, 7,*(5), 312-319.

Melding, P. (1991). Is there such a thing as geriatric pain? *Pain, 46,* 119-121.

Melzack, R. (1975). The McGill pain questionnaire: Major properties and scoring methods. *Pain, 1,* 277-299.

Melzack, R. (1987). The short-form McGill pain questionnaire. *Pain, 30,* 191-197.

Melzack, R., & Wall, P. D. (1965). Pain mechanisms: A new theory. *Science, 150,* 971-979.

Melzack, R., & Wall, P. D. (1982). *The puzzle of pain.* New York: Basic Books.

Michlovitz, S. L. (1990). *Thermal agents in rehabilitation* (2nd ed.). Philadelphia: F. A. Davis.

Middaugh, S., Levin, R., Kee, W., Barchiesi, F., & Roberts, J. (1988). Chronic pain: Its treatment in geriatric and younger patients. *Archives of Physical Medicine and Rehabilitation, 69,* 1021-1026.

Miller, J., Neelon, V., Dalton, J., Ng'andu, N., Bailey, D., Jr., Layman, E., & Hosfeld, A. (1996). The assessment of discomfort in elderly confused patients: A preliminary study. *Journal of Neuroscience Nursing, 28*(3), 175-182.

Miller, R. R., & Jick, H. (1978). Clinical effects of meperidine in hospitalized medical patients. *Journal of Clinical Pharmacology, 18,* 180-189.

Mobily, P., Herr, K., Clark, M. K., & Wallace, R. (1994). An epidemiologic analysis of pain in the elderly. *Journal of Aging and Health, 6*(2), 139-154.

Mobily, P., Herr, K., Rapp, C. G., & Ansley, T. (1999, August 27). *Prevalence and impact of pain in older adults in long term care facilities.* Paper presented at the ninth World Congress on Pain, Vienna, Austria.

Moore, A. K., Vilderman, S., Lubenskyi, W., McCans, J., & Fox, G. S. (1990). Differences in epidural morphine requirements between elderly and young patients after abdominal surgery. *Anesthesia and Analgesia, 70,* 316-320.

Morgan, A., Lindley, C., & Berry, J. (1994, Jan./Feb.). Assessment of pain and patterns of analgesic use in hospice patients. *American Journal of Hospice & Palliative Care,* 13-19, 22-25.

Murphy, D., McDonald, A., Power, A., Unwin, A., & MacSullivan, R. (1988). Measurement of pain: A comparison of the visual analogue with a nonvisual analogue scale. *The Clinical Journal of Pain, 3,* 197-219.

National Institutes of Health. (1986). The integrated approach to the management of pain. *National Institutes of Health Consensus Development Conference Statement, 6*(3). Bethesda, MD: National Institute of Health.

Nguyen, D. M. (1996). The role of physical medicine and rehabilitation in pain management. *Clinics in Geriatric Medicine, 12*(3), 517-529.

Nishikawa, S. T., & Ferrell, B. A. (1993). Pain assessment in the elderly. *Clinical Geriatrics in Long Term Care, 1,* 15-28.

North American Nursing Diagnosis Association. (1999). *Nursing diagnoses: Definitions & classification 1999-2000.* Philadelphia: Author.

Owens, M. K., & Ehrenreich, D. (1991). Literature review of non-pharmacologic methods for the treatment of chronic pain. *Holistic Nursing Practice, 6*(1), 24-31.

Parmalee, P. A., Smith, B., & Katz, I. R. (1993). Pain complaints and cognitive status among elderly institution residents. *Journal of the American Geriatrics Society, 41,* 517-522.

Pasero, C. (1994). *Acute pain management policy and procedure guideline manual.* Rolling Hills Estates, CA: Academy Medical Systems.

Pasero, C., & McCaffery, M. (1996). Postoperative pain management in the elderly. In B. R. Ferrell & B. A. Ferrell (Eds.), *Pain in the elderly* (pp. 445-468). Seattle, WA: IASP Press.

Popp, B., & Portenoy, R. (1996). Management of chronic pain in the elderly: Pharmacology of opioids and other analesic drugs. In B. R. Ferrell & B. A. Ferrell (Eds.), *Pain in the elderly* (pp. 21-34). Seattle, WA: IASP Press.

Portenoy, R. D., & Farkash, A. (1988). Practical management of non-malignant pain in the elderly. *Geriatrics, 43*(5), 29-47.

Portenoy, R. K. (1988). Drug treatment of pain syndromes. *Seminars of Neurology, 7*(2), 139-149.

Portenoy, R. K. (1994). Opioid therapy for chronic nonmalignant pain: Current status. In H. L. Fields & J. C. Liebeskind (Eds.), *Pharmacological approaches to the treatment of chronic pain: New concepts and critical issues, progress in pain research and management* (pp. 247-288). Seattle, WA: IASP Press.

Porter, F. L., Malhotra, K. M., Wolf, C. M., Morris, J. C., & Smith, M. C. (1996). Dementia and response to pain in the elderly. *Pain, 68*(2-3), 413-421.

Radloff, L. (1977). The CES-D Scale: A self-report depression scale for research in the general population. *Applied Psychological Measurement, 1*(3), 385-401.

Rankin, M., & Snider, B. (1984). Nurses' perceptions of cancer patients' pain. *Cancer Nursing, 11,* 203-209.

Riordan, M. P. (1991). Validation of the defining characteristics of the nursing diagnosis, alteration in comfort: Pain. In A. M. McLane (Ed.), *Classification of nursing diagnoses: Proceedings of the seventh conference* (pp. 221-228). St. Louis, MO: Mosby.

Roth, S. H. (1989). Merits and liabilities of NSAID therapy. *Rheumatic Diseases Clinics of North America, 15,* 470-498.

Rovner, B. W., German, P. S., Broadhead, J., Morriss, R. K., Brant, L. J., Blaustein, J., & Folstein, M. F. (1990). The prevalence and management of dementia and other psychiatric disorders in nursing homes. *International Psychogeriatrics, 2*(1), 13-24.

Roy, R., & Thomas, M. R. (1986). A survey of chronic pain in an elderly population. *Canadian Family Physician, 32,* 513-516.

Schnitzer, T. J. (1998). Non-NSAID pharmacologic treatment options for the management of chronic pain. *American Journal of Medicine, 105*(1B), 45s-52s.

Scudds, R. J., & Robertson, J. (1998). Empirical evidence of the association between the presence of musculoskeletal pain and physical disability in community-dwelling senior citizens. *Pain, 75*(2-3), 229-235.

Sengstaken, E. A., & King, S. A. (1993). The problems of pain and its detection among geriatric nursing home residents. *Journal of the American Geriatrics Association, 41*(5), 541-544.

Short, L. M., Burnett, M. S., Egbert, A. M., & Parks, L. H. (1990). Medicating the postoperative elderly: How do nurses make their decisions? *Journal of Gerontological Nursing, 16*(7), 12-17.

Silverman, M. A., & Temple, J. D. (1992). Cancer in the elderly patient: Unique aspects of prevention, management and screening. *Journal of the Florida Medical Association, 79,* 89-92.

Simon, J. M., Nolan, L., & Baumann, M. A. (1995). Validation of the nursing diagnoses acute pain and chronic pain. *Nursing Diagnosis, 6*(2), 199-203.

Simons, W., & Malabar, R. (1995). Assessing pain in the elderly patients who cannot respond verbally. *Journal of Advanced Nursing, 22*(4), 663-669.

Sorkin, B., Rudy, R., Hanlon, R., Turk, D., & Stieg, R. (1990). Chronic pain in old and young patients: Differences appear less important than similarities. *Journal of Gerontology: Psychological Sciences, 45,* 64-68.

Stein, W. M. (1996). Cancer pain in older patients. In B. R. Ferrell, & B. A. Ferrell (Eds.), *Pain in the elderly* (pp. 69-80). Seattle, WA: IASP Press.

Stein, W. M., & Ferrell, B. A. (1996). Pain in the nursing home. *Clinical Geriatric Medicine, 12*(3), 601-613.

Tait, R. C. (1993). Management of pain in the elderly. In P. A. Szwabo & G. T. Grossberg (Eds.), *Problem behaviors in long-term care: Recognition, diagnosis & treatment* (pp. 133-146). New York: Springer Publishing.

Teske, K., Daut, R., & Cleeland, C. (1983). Relationships between nurses' observations and patients' self-reports of pain. *Pain, 16,* 289-296.

Townes, A. S. (1991). Osteoarthritis. In L. R. Barker, J. R. Burton, & P. D. Zieve (Eds.), *Principles of ambulatory medicine* (4th ed., pp. 917-929). Baltimore: Lippincott Williams & Wilkins.

Tucker, M. A., Andrew, M. F., Ogle, S. J., & Davison, J. G. (1989). Age associated change in pain threshold measured by transcutaneous neuronal electrical stimulation. *Age & Ageing, 18,* 241-246.

Turk, D., & Melzack, R. (Eds.). (1992). *Handbook of pain assessment.* New York: The Guilford Press.

Turk, D. C., & Rudy, T. E. (1988). Toward an empirically derived taxonomy of chronic pain patients: Integration of psychological assessment data. *Journal of Clinical and Consulting Psychology, 56,* 233-238.

Tyler, D., Tu, A., Douthit, J., & Chapman, C. R. (1993). Toward validation of pain measurement tools for children: A pilot study. *Pain, 52,* 301-309.

Verbeeck, R. K., (1990). Pharmacokinetic drug interactions with nonsteroidal anti-inflammatory drugs. *Clinical Pharmacokinetics, 19,* 44-66.

Weiner, D., Peterson, B., & Keefe, F. (1999). Chronic pain-associated behaviors in the nursing home: Resident versus caregiver perceptions. *Pain, 80*(3), 577-588.

Weiner, D., Pieper, C., McConnell, E., Martinez, S., & Keefe, F. (1996). Pain measurement in elders with chronic low back pain: Traditional and alternative approaches. *Pain, 67*(2-3), 461-467.

Wielde, K. M. (1996). Evaluating outcomes in chronic non-malignant pain. *ASPMN Pathways, 5*(1), 9-10.

Wigley, F. M. (1991). Rheumatoid arthritis. In L. R. Barker, J. R. Burton & P. D. Zieve (Eds.), *Principles of ambulatory medicine* (4th ed., pp. 943-963). Baltimore: Lippincott Williams & Wilkins.

World Health Organization. (1990). *Cancer pain relief and palliative care.* Geneva: World Health Organization.

Yates, P., Dewar, A., & Fentiman, B. (1995). Pain: The views of elderly people living in long-term residential care settings. *Journal of Advanced Nursing, 21*(4), 667-674.

Yesavage, J., Brink, T., Rose, T., Lum, O., Huang, V., Adey, M., & Leirer, V. (1983). Development and validation of a geriatric screening scale: A preliminary report. *Journal of Psychiatric Research, 17,* 37-49.

Zaccharias, M., Pfeifer, M. V., & Herbison, P. (1990). Comparison of two methods of intravenous administration of morphine for post-operative pain relief. *Anaesthesia and Intensive Care, 18,* 205-209.

Zatzick, D. F., & Dimsdale, J. E. (1990). Cultural variations in response to painful stimuli. *Psychosomatic Medicine, 52,* 544-557.

CHAPTER 37

SENSORY/PERCEPTUAL ALTERATIONS

Elizabeth A. Swanson and Jan Drury

Perception is the process of receiving, integrating, classifying, discriminating, and assigning meaning to stimuli. This process assists human beings to receive input through sensory receptors and respond in ways that facilitate their adaptation to surroundings. Sensory receptors provide information about the outside world and serve as feedback mechanisms to tell us how well we are adjusting (Avant & Helson, 1973).

PREVALENCE

The population group most adversely affected by sensory alterations is older adults. Nearly 13% of persons over the age of 65 have some form of visual impairment that is not correctable (U.S. Department of Health and Human Services [USDHHS], 1990). In addition, 30% of adults aged 65 through 74 years and 50% of those 75 through 79 years suffer some degree of hearing loss (USDHHS, 1993). With the rate of sensory loss increasing with age and persons living longer, the rates of these losses are only expected to increase.

Loss of vision and hearing are especially prevalent among persons in nursing homes. As many as 25% of elderly nursing home residents have been found to have unrecognized significant visual impairment (Horowitz, 1994). In a study in Baltimore, black nursing home residents were found to be 50% more likely to be blind than their white counterparts (Tielsch, Javitt, Coleman, Katz, & Summer, 1995). Mahoney (1998), also assessing residents from nursing homes, found that 55% of the 104 randomly selected residents were moderately to profoundly hearing impaired. In addition, if those with mild hearing loss were included with those profoundly hearing impaired, the overall prevalence rate of residents with any hearing loss was 96%.

Untreated and uncompensated sensory losses often lead to social isolation and functional decline among elderly individuals in institutions and in their own homes (Horowitz, 1994; Kivett, 1994). Nurses who work with elderly individuals are best able to observe sensory losses and intervene to minimize the deleterious effects on the elders' functional abilities and social opportunities. Kreeger, Raulin, Grace, and Priest (1995), in assessing elderly psychiatric patients, found that when hearing deficits were corrected, improvement in cognitive and be-

havioral tests resulted. This finding confirms that failure to evaluate for hearing loss can lead to an overestimation of cognitive and behavioral problems and result in poor patient outcomes.

Other consequences result for the elderly with kinesthetic losses and the allied sense of touch. These two senses work together to maintain the individuals' body orientation in space (Burggraf & Stanley, 1989). The effects of these dysfunctions relate to gait, movement, response, and sensitivity. Thus affected persons often lean backwards when they stand and require assistance to keep from falling in that direction (Bohannon, 1996). Proprioceptive loss in diseases like stroke, peripheral vascular disease, and other sensory deficits also can be involved in falls, pedestrian accidents, and accidental drug ingestion (Kallman & Kallman, 1989).

Gustatory and olfactory senses remain remarkably intact with aging, although changes can be seen, especially when coupled with systemic disease, medication, surgery, or chemotherapy (Ship, Duffy, Jones, & Langmore, 1996). Changes in the sense of taste and smell have many implications for nutrition and the enjoyment associated with eating and drinking. When food does not smell or taste good, older adults may consume only one kind of food source to the exclusion of others.

Sensory alterations are often exacerbated by the stress of life changes that occur with aging, including retirement, death of a significant other and friends, physical changes associated with aging, and changes in self-perception. In addition, senescence or the process of aging itself is described as the progressive loss of restorative and adaptive responses that serve to maintain functional capacity.

Carnevali and Patrick (1986) suggested that older persons have a balancing act to maintain. They must equalize the activities of daily living, demands of daily living, increasingly fragile coping abilities, and support systems; this balancing act becomes more precarious over the years. Although some demands lessen with age, many demands continue. New demands also are added due to role and status changes, shifts in financial priorities and resources, and health problems. At the same time new demands are added, support systems and available resources often diminish.

A number of antecedents to sensory alteration are suggested in the literature by various authors (Burnside, 1988;

Gordon, 1987; Topf, 1994). It is crucial for nurses to be cognizant of these conditions and use relevant information to identify the appropriate nursing diagnoses. Intervention selection aims at minimizing the impact of sensory changes on older person's abilities to (1) function within the environment, (2) respond to the demands of the environment, and (3) react to the cognitive and affective implications. It also is crucial to evaluate the effectiveness of selected interventions by collecting information on nursing outcomes. The nurse needs to identify outcomes that are attainable and reasonable to expect as a result of the interventions provided (Iowa Intervention Project, 2000; Iowa Outcomes Project, 2000).

RELATED FACTORS/ETIOLOGIES

The most recent related factors/etiologies identified by NANDA (1999) are altered sensory perception; excessive environmental stimuli; psychologic stress; altered sensory reception, transmission, and/or integration; insufficient environmental stimuli; biochemical imbalances for sensory distortion (e.g., illusions, hallucinations); electrolyte imbalance; and biochemical imbalance.

Proprioception changes occur in the elderly due to many causes. Normal aging related to decreased agility and dexterity could be retarded by a well-balanced nutritional intake and remaining active. However, the impact of chronic disease often limits physical abilities for the elderly. Activities of daily living (ADL) limitations may result in an actual loss of function due to dizziness, falling, or decreased range of motion with pain and stiffness as associated with joint disease. Alternately, changes may be self-imposed, as with cumulative changes or sudden losses. Those changes may be so disconcerting that the elder chooses to self-limit activity. Other etiologies for proprioception problems can be one or a combination of any of the following; adjustment to the weight or size of an assistive device, changes in mental status, medication (vasodilators, alcohol, drug abuse, psychoactive agents, or antihypertensives), chronic illness and resultant neuromuscular or skeletal involvement such as diabetes, hypertension, cardiovascular disease, or arthritis, and vision and hearing changes. Benign positional vertigo, ampullary disequilibrium, macular disequilibrium, vestibular ataxia of aging, and Ménière's disease all can affect balance, ambulating, and self-care abilities. Often there is a decrease in reaction time and an overall loss of confidence in abilities. Of course, isolation, anxiety, sleep disorders, depression, and/or malnutrition can exacerbate any of the underlying etiologies (Forbes, 1996; Guida, 1993; Lueckenotte, 1996; Sellards, 1993).

Visual changes are well documented and are progressive but not necessarily comparable for all elderly persons. The conjunctiva thins and becomes yellow. Tear ducts are reduced in their capacity to produce tears and lubricate the eyes. Arcus senilis typically develops. The pupil decreases in size and in its ability to constrict. Similar changes occur in the iris. The lens becomes more rigid and opaque, which alters the way light is transmitted and focused. The overall effect is that visual clarity, color and light perception, and the fields of vision are reduced. In addition, pain or discomfort caused by cataracts, glaucoma, neuropathy, retinopathy, and/or blepharitis can occur (Hodges & Staab, 1996; Hogstel, 1992; Lueckenotte, 1996; Miller, 1993).

Hearing loss is not an expected result of aging and is more commonly associated with family history, past noise insults (chronic or acute), and/or underlying conductive or sensorineural disease. Presbycusis (sensorineural hearing loss) is the most common reason for hearing loss in the elderly. Age-related changes noted in the auricle are largely due to continued cartilage formation and to loss of skin elasticity. The auditory canal narrows. There is decreased vestibular sensitivity and degeneration of the ossicular joints. Higher frequency consonants such as *t, f, z, th,* and *sh* are difficult to hear or absent for the older adult. Within the ear structure, cilia in both the outer and inner auditory canal become thick and coarse and less pliable. As the cerumen glands atrophy, cerumen tends to be drier; it becomes hard and impacted and blocks passages. Drug reactions or interactions can cause distracting buzzing, ringing, or other untoward effects in the ears that decrease the ability to hear (Hogstel, 1992; Lueckenotte, 1996).

The sense of smell is often affected by the aging process. There is a rapid decline in the ability to smell and distinguish odors at age 70, in part due to decreased functioning of the olfactory nerve receptors. In the early stages of aging, this change is more apparent in men, but it has an equal presence in men and women in the late stages of aging. Other causes can be chronic illness that affect sensorineural receptors, medications (especially opiate analgesics, some antithyroid agents, some cardiovascular agents, tetracycline, and nose drops or sprays). Allergies and upper respiratory infections also greatly interfere with the sense of smell, although these changes are not specific to aging. Taste is closely related to smell in that perception of aroma is important in how a food tastes. Age-related changes in taste center on the decreasing number of nerve endings, papillae, and taste buds and the reduced ability to distinguish the four main tastes (sweet, sour, bitter, and salty). The most common underlying causes for problems in the elder's taste ability is related directly to poor dental hygiene, poor condition of teeth or ill-fitting dentures, dryness of the mouth, chronic or acute disease processes, and medication action-interaction (Forbes, 1996; Lueckenotte, 1996; Sommer, 1993; Zignego-Smith, 1993).

The last sense to be defined in terms of etiology is that of tactile-sensation. Touch is intermingled with all the other senses in that the functioning level of each of the other senses affects it. Like all the senses, chronic or acute illnesses (especially those with neurologic implications) affect the ability of the elder to distinguish temperature and pain and to pinpoint the sensation. Elders do experience a decrease in their reaction time and an overall slower response time in recognizing and reacting to stimuli. The loss of subcutaneous tissue and the loss of elasticity of the skin aids in the loss of sensory abilities regarding touch sensation. Loss or degeneration of the capillaries accelerates in the aged. Medication may cause interference with the ability to accurately feel and discern stimuli accurately (Burke, 1992; Forbes, 1996; Hodges & Staab, 1996; Zignego-Smith, 1993).

ASSESSMENT

The first step is a thorough assessment of the perceptual system during the individual's health history and physical examination. Gross inspection of the visible sensory receptors followed by testing the receptors is advocated. The interpretive, integrative, and adaptive mechanisms can be assessed at the same time by asking specific questions and implementing testing procedures. Understanding changes that occur with aging also helps to direct the assessment. For example, older adults can exhibit a longer reaction time and require an increased amount of time to take in and process information in order to respond appropriately to environmental cues. In addition, assessments should include directions for elders that are clear, concise, and timed appropriately.

It is important to include in the assessment how older adults manipulate and function within their surroundings. For optimal results, tests of functional abilities need to be conducted in quiet, uncluttered areas with natural lighting. Because these procedures may be new experiences for elders, expectations of the testing should be clearly explained and ample time is allowed for processing of information and for feedback.

Vision

In the United States, visual impairment affects 12 million people (Vader, 1992). Of utmost significance is that approximately 10% of the elders have undetected eye disease or visual impairment. Symptoms can develop quite gradually and vary among older adults. Some associated visual changes are increased time needed for accommodation; night vision and peripheral vision reduction; and more difficulty in fine detail and color discrimination. Other persons may note a halo around lights and complain about a dry, itchy feeling in their eyes (Gallman, 1995). Recent researchers are suggesting other associated visual changes with aging: scope of visual attention and speed of visual processing. In work examining whether some cognitive deficits associated with aging could be related to a restricted scope of visual attention, Kosslyn, Brown, and Dror (1999) compared 24 elderly and 24 young adults. Participants viewed two different sizes of displays. Each display contained four light-gray squares arranged as tips

of a plus sign, then black "X" marks appeared and subjects indicated when they noted the Xs. Study results indicated that the elderly had more difficulty focusing on larger areas of space when compared to younger persons and that elderly could more easily adjust their attention to smaller areas than to larger areas.

Another study of visual attention conducted by Gottlob and Madden (1998) hypothesized that older and younger persons would differ in the speed of visual processing. Adult age differences in the time course of the allocation of visual attention were examined in two different experiments that included the same 10 younger adults (M = 22 years) and 10 older adults (M = 68 years). The results of Experiment 1 demonstrated that older adults accumulated information about target identity at a slower rate than the younger subjects. To equate performance in a baseline condition in a spatial-cuing model (Gottlob & Madden, 1998), the target duration was set for each subject using the data of the first experiment. The researchers found that performance between age-groups was comparable. Thus they concluded that in this spatial-cuing paradigm, an age-related change is evident in sensory processing, not attentional allocation.

With the high percent of elders affected and the range of visual changes that do occur with aging, a significant number of older persons are at risk for injury due to their reduced visual capability. For example, they may fall or take the wrong medications. In addition, the visual cues helpful in determining appropriate behavior or responses can be misinterpreted or lost. Participation in hobbies, such as reading or other leisure-time activities, becomes more difficult. Ultimately, due to their visual impairments, elderly individuals may not be able to drive. With the loss of intrinsic enjoyment from leisure activities, and perhaps compounded by the loss of independence through not driving, elders may begin to experience some degree of social isolation, which, in turn, may further impact their sensory-perceptual abilities (Foxall, Barron, Von Dollen, Shull, & Jones, 1994).

A standard Snellen vision chart is used to determine distance vision and the Rosenbaum chart is used for near vision. A surrogate for the Rosenbaum is the newspaper, if the persons are able to read. If persons are unable to read, directional arrows or pictures may be used. Caution is required, however, in using the Snellen chart to assess older adults' vision. Watanabe (1994) noted that elders with excellent Snellen visual acuity had difficulty reading over-the-counter medication labels. Visual fields also should be checked to assess the individuals' peripheral vision and their abilities to accommodate to near and far distances. Kavanaugh and Tate (1996) suggested that indicators of visual impairment not be based in traditional assessment techniques. Nontraditional indicators might include difficulty identifying faces, difficulty getting food onto a fork, difficulty locating familiar objects, or brushes against the wall while walking. Similarly, Kelly (1995) constructed an

Inventory of Functional Visual Status to identify visual capability in older adults. The subscales of this inventory are management of medications, transportation, mobility, shopping, food preparation, and leisure activities. These assessment tools and the Snellen chart should provide nursing personnel with sufficient data to assess the visual capacity of older adults in a variety of settings. As Kelly (1996) contended, the effect of vision on functional status as opposed to visual acuity testing alone is the most critical clinical consideration when evaluating the vision of older adults.

Hearing

Hearing loss is a common problem for elders. About 40% to 50% of individuals over the age of 65 have a hearing loss (Gantz, Schindler, & Snow, 1995). Three types of disorders—presbycusis, central deafness, and conduction deafness—account for the losses. The first two may cause permanent hearing loss and may require assistive devices; conduction deafness can be reversed if it is due to a treatable condition like cerumen accumulation. Zeeger (1986) identified the defining characteristics of hearing loss as a change in the perception of hearing, tinnitus, change in the ability to detect high-frequency sounds, withdrawal, anxiety, inappropriate responses in conversational speech, and clinical evidence of impaired hearing.

Hearing loss is a very serious health problem for the elder. Pope-Spies (1995) in her work acknowledges that the sounds of music, background noise (i.e., birds singing, crickets chirping), and the human voice substantially modify people's perceptions of their experiences. Similarly, other studies have shown that social isolation, depression, acting inappropriately, and paranoia are associated with impaired hearing (Chen, 1994; Jerger, Chmiel, Wilson, & Luchi, 1995; Logan, Bess, & Lichenstein, 1990). In addition, there have also been numerous affective changes associated with hearing loss: acceptance, resignation, shyness, defensiveness, bitterness, and hate (Chen, 1994; Mahoney, 1993; Pope-Spies, 1995; Walczak, Bernstein, Senzer, & Mohr, 1993). Bess and her colleagues' (1989) work highlighted the impact of hearing deficits in this population. In a study of 153 noninstitutionalized elderly individuals, they concluded that poor hearing was associated with both functional and psychosocial impairment.

Auditory impairment has definite implications for the functioning and safety of older adults. A most serious consequence of a hearing impairment is that elders can become inappropriately labeled as confused or uncooperative when communication is misinterpreted and they respond improperly. Individuals may have difficulty with specific consonants like r and t. For example, elders may perceive the word "sing" instead of "thing" or "fine" rather than "sign." Objective data supporting this phenonomen is part of an epidemiologic study of hearing disorders in

older adults conducted by Wiley et al. (1998). Word recognition performance (NU-6 word lists in quiet and in competing messages) was examined on 3189 adults aged 48 to 59 years, 60 to 69 years, 70 to 79 years, and 80 to 94 years. Overall, scores for all measures were worse for older age groups and poorer for men when compared to women. In addition, word recognition scores in competing message were poorer than scores in quiet for all persons in all age groups. Although degree of hearing loss accounted for the largest portion of variation in the word recognition portion of variation in word recognition scores, the observed age and gender differences were still significant after adjusting for sensorineural hearing loss (Wiley et al., 1998). Thus warnings such as verbal messages or alarms may be misunderstood or missed entirely. Orientation cues like the ticking of a clock or background sounds become muffled or lost.

Assessment of the auditory receptors begins with a check of the ear canals for mechanical obstruction. If cerumen is present, a softening product is recommended to clear the canal. After this is accomplished, visualization of the canal with an ophthalmoscope should reveal healthy pink membranous lining and an eardrum that is a pearly silver-gray flat-looking disc. In screening for hearing acuity, nurses may use a tuning fork, a loud ticking clock, or verbal cues at measured distances (Meador, 1995). Gantz, Schindler, and Snow (1995) suggested a technique to differentiate between sensorineural and conductive hearing loss in the elder. Strike a tuning fork (512 cycles/second) and place it on the middle of the individuals' forehead. If the tone is louder in the impaired ear, this suggests a conductive loss. If hearing is better in the normal ear, a sensorineural loss is suggested. Ventry and Weinstein (1982) have developed the Hearing Handicap Inventory for the Elderly (Table 37-1). In a later writing, Chen (1994) suggested use of this tool or ones like it in addition to the traditional auditory assessments, since it can assist nurses to examine the functional, emotional, and social impact of hearing loss.

Kinesthetic Sense

Kinesthesia or the sense by which position, weight, and movement are perceived (Miller & Keane, 1987), is referred to in a limited manner in the literature. Other terms like position sense and proprioception are referred to more frequently (Bohannon, 1996; Carter, 1986; Kallman & Kallman, 1989; Roussel, 1995; Tideiksaar, 1989). Proprioceptive information obtained from cervical mechanoreceptors activates reflexes in the muscles of the eye, neck, and extremities to assist in maintaining an upright posture and orienting the body to its position in space. This mechanism declines with age and contributes to disequilibrium problems (Wyke, 1979). In addition, the perception of joint position sense in the lower extremities, which ensures proper foot placement while walking, also

Table 37-1 Hearing Handicap Inventory for the Elderly

INSTRUCTIONS:

The purpose of this scale is to identify the problems your hearing loss may be causing you. Answer *YES, SOMETIMES,* or *NO* for each question. *Do not skip a question if you avoid a situation because of your hearing problem.* If you use a hearing aid, please answer the way you hear *without* the aid.

	Yes (4)	Some-times (2)	No (0)
S-1. Does a hearing problem cause you to use the phone less often than you would like?	_____	_____	_____
E-2. Does a hearing problem cause you to feel embarrassed when meeting new people?	_____	_____	_____
S-3. Does a hearing problem cause you to avoid groups of people?	_____	_____	_____
E-4. Does a hearing problem make you irritable?	_____	_____	_____
E-5. Does a hearing problem cause you to feel frustrated when talking to members of your family?	_____	_____	_____
S-6. Does a hearing problem cause you difficulty when attending a party?	_____	_____	_____
E-7. Does a hearing problem cause you to feel "stupid" or "dumb"?	_____	_____	_____
S-8. Do you have difficulty hearing when someone speaks in a whisper?	_____	_____	_____
E-9. Do you feel handicapped by a hearing problem?	_____	_____	_____
S-10. Does a hearing problem cause you difficulty when visiting friends, relatives, or neighbors?	_____	_____	_____
S-11. Does a hearing problem cause you to attend religious services less often than you would like?	_____	_____	_____
E-12. Does a hearing problem cause you to be nervous?	_____	_____	_____
S-13. Does a hearing problem cause you to visit friends, relatives, or neighbors less often than you would like?	_____	_____	_____
E-14. Does a hearing problem cause you to have arguments with family members?	_____	_____	_____
S-15. Does a hearing problem cause you difficulty when listening to TV or radio?	_____	_____	_____
S-16. Does a hearing problem cause you to go shopping less often than you would like?	_____	_____	_____
E-17. Does any problem or difficulty with your hearing upset you at all?	_____	_____	_____
E-18. Does a hearing problem cause you to want to be by yourself?	_____	_____	_____
S-19. Does a hearing problem cause you to talk with family members less often than you would like?	_____	_____	_____
E-20. Do you feel that any difficulty with your hearing limits or hampers your personal or social life?	_____	_____	_____
S-21. Does a hearing problem cause you difficulty when in a restaurant with relatives or friends?	_____	_____	_____
E-22. Does a hearing problem cause you to feel depressed?	_____	_____	_____
S-23. Does a hearing problem cause you to listen to TV or radio less often than you would like?	_____	_____	_____
E-24. Does a hearing problem cause you to feel uncomfortable when talking to friends?	_____	_____	_____
E-25. Does a hearing problem cause you to feel left out when you are with a group of people?	_____	_____	_____

FOR CLINICIAN'S USE ONLY: Total Score: _____
                               Subtotal E: _____
                               Subtotal S: _____

From Ventry, I, & Weinstein, B. (1982). The hearing handicap inventory for the elderly: A new tool, *Ear Hear, 3,* 128-134.

decreases with age (Skinner, Barrack, & Cook, 1984). The identification of defining characteristics for kinesthesia are lacking, although one could use the assessment results and alterations in posture as defining characteristics of the diagnosis.

Several tests are available for identification of potential or actual difficulties in kinesthesia. The nurse must always prepare the older adult for these tests and provide safety measures in each step of the testing. One of the most common test methods is the Romberg test. The nurse asks the individual to stand with feet together and arms at sides. Once in position, the person closes her eyes. Some swaying is normal, although one should not proceed with further testing if the Romberg reflex cannot be achieved. If the person is able to do this, the test is repeated with the individual standing on one foot, then the other one. The objective of the assessment is to hold the pose for 5 seconds with a steady balance. Another tool for assessment is to have the older adult walk barefoot with eyes open and then with eyes closed. The nurse measures the pattern, stability, body position, and arm movement of the individual. If the individual can perform this successfully, the next test is to have him walk heel to toe and walk a straight line with arms at sides. Again, a small amount of swaying is normal. The nurse can test for balance, agility, and coordination by having the elder pat the knees with alternating palm and back of hand and touch each finger in sequence from index to small finger with the thumb. Persons can also be asked to run the heel of one foot down the shin of the opposite leg, starting below the knee and going toward the ankle. Other tests include having elders close their eyes and touch the index finger of one hand to the nose and then repeat with the opposite hand, gradually increasing rapidity of motion. Older adults' perception of where their bodies are in space and also where each body part is located in relation to the body is measured in these tests. It is essential for the nurse to stay close to the elder and provide stability to prevent falls and/or injury during all of the above tests (Lueckenotte, 1996).

To test older adults' perception of passive movements of the extremities, they are asked to move a finger or big toe up and down, and, while the eyes are closed, requested to indicate the direction in which the extremity is being moved. It is critical for the person being examined to have a few test runs before initiating the examination. In addition, the examiner should vary the order of the movement and must hold the digit by the sides.

Gustatory and Olfactory Senses

The gustatory and olfactory receptors work together to keep individuals hydrated and nutritionally healthy and to provide information about foods, beverages, and potentially dangerous substances (Ship et al., 1996). These processes remain remarkably intact with aging, although coupled with systemic disease, medications, surgery, and chemotherapy common with older adults, effects in these senses can be seen. Changes in the gustatory and olfactory senses have many implications in the areas of nutrition and the enjoyment associated with eating and drinking. A study conducted by Keller (1993) found that the prevalence of undernutrition in 200 long-term care persons was close to 50%. When food does not smell or taste good, the result may be the ingestion of one kind of food source to the exclusion of others. Duffy, Backstrand, and Ferris (1995) found that older women between the ages of 65 and 93 had less of a preference for strongly sour or bitter foods and ate fewer citrus fruits and vegetables. In addition, they observed that women with a decreased sense of smell and taste ate more saturated fat. Older persons with diabetes who are unable to detect a high concentration of sugar might have more difficulty controlling sugar consumption (Ship et al., 1996). Similarly, the inability to distinguish salt may interfere with hypertensive elders' compliance with a low-salt diet. Even more common is the elders' response that the food is "bland" or has no taste,

decreasing the drive to consume food (Evans, Henkin, & Leopold, 1994). Thus defining characteristics specific to Sensory/Perceptual Alterations: Gustatory are heavy use of salt, sugar, or other spices; complaints about the taste of the food; or medications that impact gustatory sensation and decrease appetite.

Generally, most of the changes that occur in aging with taste and smell are in the area of olfactory dysfunction (Yen, 1996). Ship et al. (1996) commented that taste remains robust with advancing age. Yen (1996) continued the discussion by stating that half of the populations of older adults between the ages of 65 and 80 years have lost much or all of their olfactory sensation. Gallman (1995) suggested decreased olfactory sensation as the major defining characteristic.

Dry mouth or xerostomia is a common complaint of older adults, although there is no evidence that the aging process is responsible for its occurrence (Schaid, 1993). Early studies suggested that dry mouth and aging were associated with one another, but later research in controlled situations demonstrated no change in saliva production with age (Baum, 1989). The dominant causes associated with xerostomia include Sjogren's syndrome, radiation therapy, and medications. Other causes are salivary gland diseases, hormonal dysfunction, allergies, dehydration, blood loss anemia, mouth breathing, smoking, upper respiratory tract infections, menopause, diabetes, emotional changes, and vitamin A deficiency.

Offering various common scents like coffee, garlic, vinegar, nutmeg, and cinnamon best assesses the olfactory sensation. Time should be allotted for the older adults to exhale between the different scents to ensure that the separate smells do not linger in the nasal passages.

Common tastes such as popcorn (with or without salt) and lemonade (with various amounts of sweetness) can be used to assess taste. Time and the cleaning of the palate with a neutral liquid between samples must be done so that a pure taste will be produced with each assessment.

Tactile Sense

Touch can be defined in terms of the elder's sensation related to actual tactile information received from neuron receptors. This is an orienting factor so that the older adults can respond appropriately to the environment. The response to painful stimuli or to variations in temperature can protect and orient older individuals. Touch can also refer to the more psychologic benefits of being touched by others. The latter is often regarded as caring touch that portrays positive emotional regard and a sensation of well-being. They may be held and comforted, loved, and rewarded in these ways. Loss of caring touch from family, friends, and even caregivers can cause many emotional reactions, including isolative behavior, sadness, or depression. Touching and being touched often involve similar receptors, but the message carries individual meanings based on the perception of that touch, such as pet therapy and familiar caregivers (Lueckenotte, 1996).

Generally, touch provides information about the relationship between the environment and self. If the information is incomplete, the response within the environment may be altered. For many people, touching and being touched are associated with acceptance and a sense of well-being. Specifically, tactile sensations provide individuals with information on heat, cold, and pain. Gallman (1995) suggested that decreased sensitivity to touch is the defining characteristic for this particular diagnosis.

Touching individuals on the face, arms, and legs with wisps of cotton and having them identify when and where they are being touched assesses the sensations of touch. After this initial information is gained, discrimination of touch can be determined by using a safety pin and having individuals identify if the sensation is sharp (using the pointed end) or dull (using the hinge end). In addition, assessment of individuals' ability to discriminate two pinpricks simultaneously placed at varying distances from one another is also completed. Further testing can also include the identification of various textures of fabrics or common objects by touch and temperature assessment.

The reader is referred to Jarvis (1996) or another general physical assessment text for more detailed assessment procedure information. Additionally, individuals may need to be referred to pertinent specialists for more definitive examination and treatment.

CASE STUDY

J. Solana is a 72-year-old widow living with her granddaughter. She has a younger sister who lives within 2 miles of her residence. She is of Hispanic descent and has lived in the United States for the past 30 years. She receives Social Security payments from her previous employment as a factory worker. She helps with the care of her two great grandchildren and does the cooking for the family. Mrs. Solana has the medical diagnoses obesity, kyphoscoliosis, diabetes mellitus, and iron deficiency anemia. She was recently discharged from the hospital for a *Staphylococcus*-infected wound on her right leg; the wound occurred when a car hit her. The driver stated "She just stepped right out in front of me." She was discharged while taking erythromycin and is being seen daily by a visiting nurse, who provides wound care and monitors her diabetes. Although she is heavy, Mrs. Solana has experienced a 20-pound weight loss over the last month. The family comments that Mrs. Solana has been speaking very loudly in family conversations during the past several months and sometimes responds inappropriately to questions. The family also states that she seems more stressed by her great grandchildren's behavior since she was injured.

Mrs. Solana is able to remember conversations and responds with appropriate affect, although background noise appears to interfere with her ability to concentrate.

Hearing is slightly diminished in both ears, as indicated by the whisper test. On assessing sounds via a tuning fork, Mrs. Solana perceives the sound equally in both ears. Assessment revealed a decrease in auditory acuity since it was last assessed 2 years ago. Mrs. Solana enjoys interacting with one person at a time, but describes difficulty hearing when there is background noise. She wears reading glasses that were purchased at the local drug store and states she needs to get a new pair, since newspaper print is now blurred. Mrs. Solana has bridgework in the upper left side of her mouth that fits properly. She likes all foods and truly enjoys her meals especially when her sister visits and dines with her. She is able to identify tastes and smells accurately, although she notes that she must put more flavoring and spices in the food to smell it. Family members comment that she is using many more "hot" spices than when she was younger. They also state that she is increasingly complaining of having a dry mouth. Mrs. Solana responds accurately to light touch and pain sensation on her face and upper extremities. Responses for light touch are not accurate on the lower extremities, and she is unable to distinguish between dull and sharp stimuli on her lower extremities as well. When position sense is assessed, she correctly identifies the direction of movement of her fingers bilaterally and quickly. The response to the direction of movement of her great toes is slower. She has 1+ bilateral edema in her feet and ankles. She has an unsteady gait and prefers to walk with the assistance of another person, although she can get around in the house by holding on to furniture, rails, and counters.

The following nursing diagnoses were specified for Mrs. Solana: Sensory/Perceptual Alterations: Auditory; Sensory/Perceptual Alterations: Visual; Sensory/Perceptual Alterations: Tactile; Sensory/Perceptual Alterations: Kinesthetic; Sensory/Perceptual Alterations: Gustatory; and Sensory/Perceptual Alterations: Olfactory. These diagnoses were related to impaired sensory reception and transmission, neuropathy secondary to diabetes, and edema secondary to obesity and limited mobility.

NURSING DIAGNOSIS

Nurse authors working with the content area of sensory/perceptual alterations have suggested a variety of diagnostic formats. During the seventh conference work of the North American Nursing Diagnosis Association (NANDA), two diagnostic labels in the area of sensory/perceptual dysfunction were identified: Unilateral Neglect and Sensory/Perceptual Alterations (S/PA): Visual, Auditory, Kinesthetic, Gustatory, Tactile, Olfactory (McLane, 1987). Gordon (1987) suggested three specific diagnoses: Sensory/Perceptual Alterations: Uncompensated Deficit; Sensory/Perceptual Alterations: Input Excess (or sensory overload); and Sensory/Perceptual Alterations: Input Deficit. Drury and Akins (1991) noted that the last two diagnoses both address the elder's responses to change or disruption in the quality or quantity of incoming stimuli and have similar and overlapping etiologies. It was previously felt that these two diagnoses were dissimilar enough to warrant presenting separately, but in the refinement process, it became clear that more similarities than differences exist among the different diagnostic formats. In addition, the authors support a heightened degree of specificity, which will enhance the planning of care for older adults and which has the potential to truly impact the quality of care. Thus the content of the chapter will be organized around the diagnosis Sensory/Perceptual Alterations (specify: Visual, Auditory, Kinesthetic, Gustatory, Tactile, Olfactory).

The defining characteristics for Sensory/Perceptual Alterations (Specify: Visual, Auditory, Kinesthetic, Gustatory, Tactile, Olfactory) have remained generally constant (Carroll-Johnson, 1989): disoriented in time, in place, or with persons; altered abstraction and conceptualization; changes in problem-solving abilities, behavior patterns, sensory acuity, usual response to stimuli, posture, and muscular tension (Cox et al., 1993). Anxiety, apathy, restlessness, irritability, hallucinations, and fatigue, indications of body-image alterations, and altered communication patterns also are listed as characteristic of this diagnostic label (Carroll-Johnson, 1989). The most recent revision of the diagnosis Sensory/Perceptual Alterations defines it as "a state in which an individual experiences a change in the amount or patterning of incoming stimuli accompanied by a diminished, exaggerated, distorted, or impaired response to such stimuli." This included some revision of defining characteristics. These changes include the addition of poor concentration, auditory distortions, reported or measured change in sensory acuity, irritability, change in problem-solving abilities, change in behavior pattern, altered communication patterns, and visual distortions as defining characteristics (NANDA, 1999). It is generally thought that to be most useful the defining characteristics or signs and symptoms need to be specific to the nursing diagnosis (e.g., Sensory/Perceptual Alterations: Gustatory) and distinguish that particular diagnosis from other diagnoses. Selected examples of defining characteristics that specify and distinguish across the different sensory perceptual diagnoses are presented in the following sections.

NURSING-SENSITIVE OUTCOMES

The following nursing-sensitive outcomes, classified by the Nursing Outcomes Classification (NOC) (Iowa Outcomes Project, 2000), are appropriate for the NANDA label Sensory/Perceptual Alterations (NANDA, 1999): Anxiety Control, Body Image, Cognitive Ability, Cognitive Orientation, Distorted Thought Control, and Energy Conservation. Associated outcomes include Electrolyte & Acid/Base Balance, Endurance, Fluid Balance, Neurological Status, Rest, and Sleep. The following NOC outcomes are most useful in the nursing management of an elder with sensory alterations, since they relate directly to the effectiveness of interventions to resolve or compensate for sensory losses: Self-Care, Mobility Level, Balance, Communication Ability, Social Involvement, Loneliness, Nutritional Status, and Well-Being. Other outcomes for specific sensory/perceptual alteration diagnoses (visual, auditory, kinesthetic, gustatory, tactile, olfactory) are listed in Table 37-2.

NURSING INTERVENTIONS

The selection of nursing interventions is a component of the clinical decision making of the nurse (Iowa Intervention Project, 2000). Creativity and common sense are vital in developing nursing interventions and activities for older adults with sensory/perceptual alterations. The nurse can teach older adults various techniques to compensate for sensory losses. Generally, nurses may discuss environmental strategies, encourage older adults to use multiple or alternate senses, and assist them to focus on other environmental cues to help compensate for areas of deficiency. For example, persons with compromised vision can be taught to skim the walls and articles of furniture with their hand to orient themselves to the position within the room. The nurse can call attention to a draft coming through a window in the room to orient elders spatially to the room. Or the nurse can teach them to identify smells from food preparation to orient them to the time of day.

Environmental Management Interventions

Vision Interventions.   Nursing interventions for the enhancement and compensation of visual impairment are based on altering environmental conditions or using low-vision aids (Kelly, 1995). Usually the goals of the selected interventions of environmental management are to maintain social interaction and optimize physical functioning. Thus numerous activities fall into the category of Environmental Management. The use of bright (not glaring) colors increases color contrast and helps elders identify living areas, corners, and staircases (Horowitz, 1994). According to Maguire (1996), older adults, compared to younger people, need three times the color contrast to identify patterns clearly. Colors in the red-yellow range are more easily distinguished than those in the blue-green range. Since the use of red-yellow enhances depth perception, strips of these colors along the edges of stairs or at the bottom of walls are beneficial to older individuals (Kelly, 1996).

Trent (1994) provided another perspective on the use of color with elders in nursing homes. Cool colors promote a calm, relaxed, and quiet atmosphere to serve as a retreat from the more stimulating areas of the facility. Warm colors attract attention, create excitement, and stimulate actions and can be used in the areas of the facility where stimulation is desired. It has also been suggested that light colors

Table 37-2	Suggested Nursing-Sensitive Outcomes and Nursing Interventions SENSORY/PERCEPTUAL ALTERATIONS	
Nursing Diagnoses	**Nursing-Sensitive Outcomes**	**Nursing Interventions**
Sensory/Perceptual Alterations: Auditory	Hearing	Referral
	Concentration	Communication Enhancement: Hearing Deficit
	Information Processing	Teaching: Psychomotor Skill
	Communication Ability	
	Safety Behavior: Personal	Environmental Management: Safety
	Knowledge: Personal Safety	Teaching: Personal Safety
	Body Image	Body Image Enhancement
	Social Involvement	Socialization Enhancement
	Loneliness	
	Quality of Life	
Sensory/Perceptual Alterations: Visual	Vision	Referral
	Communication Ability	Communication Enhancement: Visual Deficit
	Cognitive Orientation	Learning Facilitation
	Self-Care: Activities of Daily Living (ADL)	Teaching: Self-Care
	Self-Care: Instrumental Activities of Daily Living (IADL)	Anticipatory Guidance
	Anxiety Control	Anxiety Reduction
	Mobility Level	Exercise Promotion
	Safety Behavior: Personal	Environmental Management: Safety
	Knowledge: Personal Safety	Teaching: Personal Safety
	Quality of Life	
Sensory/Perceptual Alterations: Kinesthetic	Balance	Exercise Therapy: Balance
	Mobility Level	Exercise Promotion
	Safety Behavior: Fall Prevention	Fall Prevention
	Knowledge: Personal Safety	Teaching: Personal Safety
	Self-Care: Instrumental Activities of Daily Living (IADL)	Teaching: Self-Care
	Fear Control	Emotional Support
		Security Enhancement
Sensory/Perceptual Alterations: Tactile	Well-Being	Touch
	Safety Behavior: Personal	Environmental Management
	Knowledge: Personal Safety	Teaching: Safety
Sensory/Perceptual Alterations: Olfactory	Safety Behavior: Home Physical Environment	Environmental Management
	Safety Behavior: Personal	Teaching: Personal Safety
	Nutritional Status	Nutritional Counseling
		Nutrition Management
Sensory/Perceptual Alterations: Gustatory	Nutritional Status	Teaching: Diet Modification
	Quality of Life	Appetite Enhancement
		Fluid Management

create space and uplift, while dark colors absorb light and over time increase monotony and despair. Trent (1994) contended that residents with dementia recognize their rooms by color more than by any other variable. Kavanaugh and Tate (1996) also suggested the use of colors to label dresser drawers and other places where activities of daily living take place. Color contrast is a very important and cost-effective tool in assisting persons to orient themselves, make the most of their cognitive abilities, and maximize their functional independence.

Lighting without glare in living areas is recommended (Kelly, 1996). Reducing the number of reflective surfaces (e.g., large areas of glass, high-glossed floor finishing) can minimize glare. It is also important to acknowledge that sudden contrasts between bright sunlight and shade or indoors and outdoors compromise the vision of individuals until they can accommodate (Jarvis, 1996). Nightlights in living areas are invaluable to older adults to facilitate the transition from light to dark areas. Sunglasses, hats with broad brims, and umbrellas are recommended for use during outdoor excursions to assist elders with their compromised vision.

Other nursing interventions and activities can be instituted to manipulate the individual's environment to compensate for sensory losses. Handrails, large print or pictorial directional signs, calendars, and clocks can assist older adults in their orientation to person or place (Jubeck, 1992). Consistent placement of objects within their environment is also important, traffic patterns through rooms should be kept clear of clutter, and wide spaces should be left between furniture to facilitate movement and prevent injury (Kelly, 1995).

In a separate article, Kelly (1996) also provides guidelines for medication usage for visually impaired older adults to ensure their compliance. For example, position the medications in the person's visual field, improve signage, and periodically assess the individual's ability to take medications. All of these suggestions are useful in teaching-counseling the older adults and family who are visually impaired.

Hearing Interventions. Numerous nursing activities can be implemented to enhance hearing. In any interactions with older adults with a hearing impairment, the nurse should gain the person's attention through touch before starting the conversation, speak slowly with careful enunciation of words, and lower the pitch of the voice while not increasing the volume (Jubeck, 1992). Increased volume forces the pitch of the voice into higher frequencies and further decreases comprehension. In addition, to increase understanding of the spoken word, the nurse should use simple words and short sentences and directly face individuals when speaking to them.

Nurses have usually approached sensory impairments through the traditional recommendations of eyeglasses or hearing aids. These devices can help older adults to function independently in a variety of settings as well as enhance their ability to socialize. Mion (1992) and Jerger et al. (1995) suggested that some nontraditional sensory prosthetics, such as closed-circuit television reading devices, talking typewriters and computers, alerting devices, talking clocks, speech amplifiers, and microprocessor-based communication systems should also be considered for older adults.

Gustatory and Olfactory Interventions. Properly fitting dentures are essential and must be kept clean to enhance the taste of foods. The environment also can be controlled to enhance the taste of food. An unhurried meal that looks, smells, and tastes good and that is served in a pleasant, sociable surrounding increases the enjoyment of dining as well as the taste and appetite.

Kinesthetic Interventions. To ensure the safety of persons with kinesthetic deficits, dangerous objects need to be removed from the environment. Individuals also need to be protected from exposure to excessive heat and cold. There is also the likelihood that they may require assistance moving within the physical environment until they are able to make adaptations to their changes in position sensations (Cox et al., 1993).

Individuals with dementia are predisposed to problems maintaining spatial orientation (Liu, Gauthier, & Gauthier, 1991). To deal with spatial orientation problems during bathing, Miller (1994) promoted the use of individualized care, avoidance of rapid transportation to bathing areas without the use of cues, and enhancement of the privacy for the residents. In addition, Miller (1994) recommended environmental restructuring, remodeling bathrooms in nursing homes to resemble residential bathrooms and discouraging the use of central bathing areas for these residents. Other aspects suggested by Miller (1994) and reinforced by Danner, Beck, Heacock, and Modlin (1993) are the use of multiple sensory channels of individuals with dementia and enhancing other senses to elicit more functional responses in living. For example, residents with dementia might be consistently handed the same jacket or shoes as a cue to the event of walking.

Nurses must be aware of the impact that societal expectation of mental impairment and behavioral frailty has on the self-images of elders. The sheer fact of its existence can create the potential for it to become a self-fulfilling prophecy. As has been previously discussed, when persons no longer use the sight or hearing to gain information, alternative techniques must be developed. It is critical for nurses to accompany learning of new methods with time to ventilate feelings and time to grieve about sensory losses. In addition, elders might need some assistance identifying new coping strategies.

Counseling Interventions

Vision and Hearing Interventions. An essential part of the rehabilitation process involves educating and counseling older adults and their family members. The nurse should provide instructions in the proper care and use of adaptive devices for vision and hearing. This instruction needs to include hands-on practice, step-by-step instructions, and written clues for effective use. For example, individuals need to become familiar with replacing batteries, inserting the hearing aid, and adjusting the controls (Jerger et al., 1995); allowing time for return demonstrations is important. Due to the presentation in commercial advertisements, expectations of hearing aids are often unrealistically high. Many persons expect that hearing aids will correct to the same degree as glasses (Jerger et al., 1995). Individuals need to be informed that there is often a period of adjustment with visual and hearing aids, since people need to become used to the appliances and amplified sight and sound.

Gustatory and Olfactory Interventions. Selected instructions can be suggested to older adults as a means to enhance their taste perception. The addition of spices allowed within the confines of the therapeutic diet will enhance flavors and increase taste perception (Yen, 1996). Altering food texture, temperature, and color also helps to maintain food enjoyment (Ship et al., 1996). Foods must be in solution for the taste buds to sense flavor, so taking fluids that are salty, sweet, or carbonated with solid foods may improve taste, especially if mouths are dry.

Schaid (1993) suggested the use of hard, sugarless candies and other acid-containing substances, humidifiers, foods that require chewing (e.g., celery, carrots), and sugarless chewing gum to assist older adults with xerostomia. In addition, she suggested health promotion activities like nutritional counseling, dental hygiene and check-ups, a fluoride preparation, and avoidance of foods that increase dryness of the mouth (e.g., crackers, hot spices).

Kinesthetic and Tactile Interventions. NIC offers a number of possible nursing interventions for the nursing diagnosis Sensory/Perceptual Alterations: Tactile: Circulatory Precautions; Counseling; Environmental Management: Safety, Pressure Management, and Skin Surveillance (Iowa Intervention Project, 2000). Nurses can further assist individuals with sensory/perceptual alterations by instructing them to enhance their other senses. For example, the use of a variety of textures in the home environment increases object recognition. Nurses can also assist older adults by the conscious use of touch (Moore & Gilbert, 1995). Touch serves to orient elders to their spatial environment and also has the beneficial effect of conveying love and belonging. Touch also assists elders to experience their surroundings to the fullest. All of these approaches promote orientation to the physical environment of elders with the supplementary benefit of promoting independence.

Referral Interventions. The nurse's role in the care of older adults needs to include referrals to an appropriate specialist (e.g., audiologist, ophthalmologist, optometrist, physical therapist) for a detailed examination when warranted. Various specialized resource information centers, including the Agency on Aging (www.aoa.dhhs.gov), the American Association of the Deaf-Blind Advocacy (www/tr/wosc.osshe.edu/DBLINK/aadb.htm), the American Association of Retired Persons (www.aarp.org), the American Council of the Blind (www.acb.org), and the National Council on the Aging (www.ncoa.org), can

provide further information and suggestions for care. These websites contain information on disaster assistance for the elderly, retirement and financial planning, federal legislation, consumer tips, Social Security educational materials, and adult daycare services. Local chapters of these various organizations could help the older adult identify new approaches.

CASE STUDY

Table 37-3 contains the nursing diagnoses, interventions, and outcomes that were identified by the nurse and Mrs. Solana. Mrs. Solana and the nurse agreed that the goals for her care should include uncompromised or mildly compromised vision and hearing with the use of prostheses, consistent symptom control behavior, consistent concentration, independent mobility with an assistive device, steady or increased social involvement to at least a moderate level, improved quality of life, and a substantial level of personal safety knowledge.

Auditory and vision outcomes were selected by Mrs. Solana and the nurse because they felt that resolution of these sensory alterations would improve Mrs. Solana's communication and concentration and enable her to maintain her independence and continue contributing to her family's care. The NOC outcome Neurological Status: Cranial Sensory/Motor Function was not considered a useful outcome for Mrs. Solana, although hearing and vision are indicators for that particular outcome that can be measured. Treatment for Mrs. Solana's hearing and vision deficits will not reverse losses in sensory nerve function. Rather, treatment is compensatory to enhance sensory reception.

The NOC outcome Symptom Control was selected to monitor Mrs. Solana's management of her diabetes. To assess the extent that correction of hearing and vision improved her ability to concentrate, the NOC outcome Concentration was selected. Mobility Level also was chosen as an outcome because of its importance for Mrs. Solana's maintenance of independent function, because of the need to monitor progress following her accident, and because of the impact of mobility on circulation and the reduction of peripheral dependent edema that compromises kinesthesia. Social Involvement is an important outcome for Mrs. Solana to the extent that she is able to continue to assist her family, interact with her sister, especially during mealtimes, and possibly increase the social activities that she enjoys. The outcome of Quality of Life was selected as it relates to independence and the importance of her involvement in her family and the reestablishment of social activity. It was planned for Mrs. Solana to achieve at least a substantial level of Knowledge: Personal Safety.

The *Nursing Interventions Classification (NIC)* offers a number of nursing interventions that are appropriate for assisting Mrs. Solana: Communication Enhancement: Hearing Deficit; Communication Enhancement: Visual Deficit; Teaching: Individual; Counseling; Coping Enhancement; Environmental Management, Environmental

Table 37-3	Nursing Diagnoses, Outcomes, and Interventions for MRS. SOLANA	
Nursing Diagnoses	**Nursing-Sensitive Outcomes**	**Nursing Interventions**
SENSORY/PERCEPTUAL ALTERATIONS: AUDITORY *Defining Characteristics* Speaks loudly to converse Some responses inappropriate Distracted by noise Change in auditory acuity	**HEARING COMPENSATION BEHAVIOR** *Indicators* Responds appropriately in conversation Demonstrates voice-hearing acuity Uses hearing aid(s) correctly Concentration Responds appropriately to auditory cues Maintains attention	**REFERRAL** *Activity* Refer for auditory testing and hearing aid **COMMUNICATION ENHANCEMENT: HEARING DEFICIT** *Activities* Facilitate appointment for hearing examination, as appropriate Facilitate use of hearing aids, as appropriate Keep hearing aid clean
SENSORY/PERCEPTUAL ALTERATIONS: VISION *Defining Characteristics* Unable to read newspaper Eyeglasses ineffective Night vision decreased	**VISION COMPENSATION BEHAVIOR** *Indicators* Wears eyeglasses correctly Wears contact lens correctly Ability to see and read newsprint **SOCIAL INVOLVEMENT** *Indicators* Interaction with neighbors Interaction with family members	**REFERRAL** *Activity* Refer for visual examination and eyeglasses
SENSORY/PERCEPTUAL ALTERATIONS: TACTILE *Defining Characteristics* Altered touch of legs and feet 1+ edema of feet and ankles	**KNOWLEDGE: PERSONAL SAFETY** *Indicators* Description of skin intactness measures Description of safety risks **SYMPTOM CONTROL** *Indicators* Recognizes symptom variation Uses preventive measures Uses warning signs to seek health care **ROLE PERFORMANCE** *Indicator* Performance of family role behaviors	**TEACHING: INDIVIDUAL** *Activities* Determine the patient's learning needs Instruct about foot injuries Educate high-risk individuals and groups about environmental hazards Teach to recognize hypoglycemia and hyperglycemia **ENVIRONMENTAL MANAGEMENT: SAFETY** *Activities* Remove hazards from environment Provide adaptive devices to increase safety Increase lighting
IMPAIRED PHYSICAL MOBILITY *Defining Characteristics* Unstable gait Requires assistance to walk Lower extremity injury	**MOBILITY LEVEL** *Indicators* Balance performance Ambulation: walking Transfer performance Description of safety risks **SAFETY STATUS: FALLS OCCURRENCE** *Indicators* Number of falls while walking Number of falls while standing Number of falls while transferring	**EXERCISE THERAPY: AMBULATION** *Activities* Assist patient to establish realistic increments in distance for ambulation Encourage independent ambulation within safe limits Instruct patient-caregiver about safe transfer and ambulation techniques Assist patient to establish realistic increments in distance for ambulation Encourage independent ambulation within safe limits Instruct how to fall to minimize injury Instruct about fall risks

Continued

	Nursing Diagnoses, Outcomes, and Interventions for	
Table 37-3	**MRS. SOLANA—cont'd**	

Nursing Diagnoses	Nursing-Sensitive Outcomes	Nursing Interventions
SENSORY/PERCEPTUAL ALTERATIONS: GUSTATORY *Defining Characteristics* Complains of dry mouth Family states that she appears to be using more spices on food	**SAFETY BEHAVIOR: PERSONAL** *Indicators* Arrangement of secure living environment Preparation of food to minimize illness Correct use of assistive devices **FLUID BALANCE** *Indicators* Body weight stable Peripheral edema not present Abnormal thirst not present	**ENVIRONMENTAL MANAGEMENT** *Activities* Create a pleasant, calm eating atmosphere Provide written materials regarding medications, supplies, and assistive devices **FLUID MANAGEMENT** *Activities* Give fluids, as appropriate Consult physician if signs and symptoms of fluid volume excess persist or worsen **FLUID MONITORING** *Activity* Monitor weight
SENSORY/PERCEPTUAL ALTERATIONS: KINESTHETIC *Defining Characteristics* Altered touch of legs and feet 1+ edema of feet and ankle	**AMBULATION: WALKING** *Indicators* Walks with effective gait Walks up steps Walks at moderate pace	**EXERCISE THERAPY: AMBULATION** *Activities* Assist patient to establish realistic increments in distance for ambulation Encourage independent ambulation within safe limits Instruct patient-caregiver about safe transfer and ambulation techniques
SENSORY/PERCEPTUAL ALTERATIONS: OLFACTORY *Defining Characteristics* Complains of dry mouth Family states that she appears to be using more spices on food	**NUTRITIONAL STATUS: NUTRIENT INTAKE** *Indicators* Caloric intake Protein intake Vitamin intake **NUTRITIONAL STATUS** *Indicator* Nutrient intake	**NUTRITION MANAGEMENT** *Activities* Encourage increased intake of protein, iron, and vitamin C, as appropriate Offer herbs and spices as alternative to salt Encourage patient to wear properly fitted dentures and/or acquire dental care

Nursing Outcomes Classification (NOC) 5-point Likert measurement scales:

Hearing Compensation Behavior:	1 = Never demonstrated; 2 = Rarely demonstrated; 3 = Sometimes demonstrated; 4 = Often demonstrated; 5 = Consistently demonstrated.
Vision Compensation Behavior:	1 = Never demonstrated; 2 = Rarely demonstrated; 3 = Sometimes demonstrated; 4 = Often demonstrated; 5 = Consistently demonstrated.
Social Involvement:	1 = None; 2 = Limited; 3 = Moderate; 4 = Substantial; 5 = Extensive.
Knowledge: Personal Safety:	1 = None; 2 = Limited; 3 = Moderate; 4 = Substantial; 5 = Extensive.
Symptom Control:	1 = Never demonstrated; 2 = Rarely demonstrated; 3 = Sometimes demonstrated; 4 = Often demonstrated; 5 = Consistently demonstrated.
Role Performance:	1 = Not adequate; 2 = Slightly adequate; 3 = Moderately adequate; 4 = Substantially adequate; 5 = Totally adequate.
Mobility Level:	1 = Dependent, does not participate; 2 = Requires assistive person and device; 3 = Requires assistive person; 4 = Independent with assistive device; 5 = Completely independent.
Safety Status: Falls Occurrence:	1 = Over 9; 2 = 7-9; 3 = 4-6; 4 = 1-3; 5 = None.
Safety Behavior: Personal:	1 = Not adequate; 2 = Slightly adequate; 3 = Moderately adequate; 4 = Substantially adequate; 5 = Totally adequate.
Fluid Balance:	1 = Extremely compromised; 2 = Substantially compromised; 3 = Moderately compromised; 4 = Mildly compromised; 5 = Not compromised.
Ambulation: Walking:	1 = Dependent, does not participate; 2 = Requires assistive person and device; 3 = Requires assistive person; 4 = Independent with assistive device; 5 = Completely independent.
Nutritional Status: Nutrient Intake:	1 = Not adequate; 2 = Slightly adequate; 3 = Moderately adequate; 4 = Substantially adequate; 5 = Totally adequate.
Nutritional Status:	1 = Extremely compromised; 2 = Substantially compromised; 3 = Moderately compromised; 4 = Mildly compromised; 5 = Not compromised.

Management: Safety; Fluid Management, Fluid Monitoring, Nutrition Management; Fall Prevention; Exercise Therapy: Ambulation; and Referral (Iowa Intervention Project, 2000). The nurse selected Communication Enhancement: Hearing Deficit; Exercise Therapy: Ambulation; Teaching: Individual; Environmental Management; Environmental Management: Safety; and Referral, as illustrated in Table 37-3. The first line of intervention the nurse prescribed for Mrs. Solana was Referral for hearing and visual examinations to obtain corrective prostheses. When the hearing and/or visual prostheses were obtained, efforts were directed at teaching Mrs. Solana the proper care and use of the hearing aid and eyeglasses. The nurse also assisted Mrs. Solana to develop solutions for any problems encountered in using the prostheses. The next focus of treatment was to teach Mrs. Solana measures to be taken to enhance her personal safety, such as increased lighting and removal of environmental hazards. The nurse also helped Mrs. Solana with ambulation and exercise to maintain and enhance her mobility. All of the interventions were aimed at maintaining her independence and her useful role within the family unit and at maintaining or increasing satisfactory social relationships and experiences.

SUMMARY

Older adults experience a wide variety of sensory and perceptual alterations. Uncompensated losses can lead to functional decline, to social isolation, and to decreased quality of life. Nursing care for persons with sensory losses must be based upon a detailed assessment. Nursing can be instrumental in helping older persons to identify losses that are correctable and to seek treatment for those losses. Moreover, nurses can teach older adults creative ways to compensate for losses that are not correctable.

REFERENCES

Avant, L. L., & Helson, H. (1973). Theories of perception. In B. Wolman (Ed.), *Handbook of general psychology* (pp. 419-450). Upper Saddle River, NJ: Prentice Hall.

Baum, B. J. (1989). Salivary gland fluid secretion during aging. *Journal of the Geriatric Society, 37,* 453-458.

Bess, F., Lichtenstein, M., Logan, S., Burger, C., & Nelson, E. (1989). Hearing impairment as a determinant of function in the elderly. *Journal of the Geriatric Society, 37,* 123-128.

Bohannon, R. W. (1996). Clinical implications of neurologic changes during the aging process. In C. B. Lewis (Ed.), *Aging: The health care challenge* (pp. 177-188). Baltimore: Lippincott Williams & Wilkins.

Burggraf, V., & Stanley, M. (1989). *Nursing the elderly: A care plan approach.* Philadelphia: Lippincott, Williams & Wilkins.

Burke, M. M. (1992). Sensation. In M. M. Burke & M. B. Walsh (Eds.), *Gerontologic nursing.* (pp. 86-116). St. Louis, MO: Mosby.

Burnside, I. M. (1988). *Nursing and the aged* (3rd ed.). Hightstown, NJ: McGraw-Hill.

Carnevali, D. L., & Patrick, M. (1986). *Nursing management for the elderly* (2nd ed.). Baltimore: Lippincott Williams & Wilkins.

Carroll-Johnson, R. (1989). *Classification of nursing diagnoses: Proceedings of the eighth conference.* Baltimore: Lippincott Williams & Wilkins.

Carter, A. B. (1986). The neurological aspects of aging. In I. Rossman (Ed.), *Clinical geriatrics* (pp. 326-351). Baltimore: Lippincott Williams & Wilkins.

Chen, H. L. (1994). Hearing in the elderly: Relation of hearing loss, loneliness, and self-esteem. *Journal of Gerontological Nursing, 20*(6), 22-28.

Cox, H. C., Hinz, M. D., Lubno, M. A., Newfield, S. A., Ridenour, N. A., Slater, M. M., & Sridaromont, K. L. (1993). *Clinical applications of nursing diagnosis: Adult, child, women's psychiatric, geronic and home health considerations.* Philadelphia: F. A. Davis.

Danner, C., Beck, C., Heacock, P., & Modlin, T. (1993). Cognitively impaired elders: Using research findings to improve nursing care. *Journal of Gerontological Nursing, 19*(4), 5-11.

Drury, J., & Akins, J. (1991). Sensory/perceptual alterations. In M. Maas, K. Buckwalter, & M. A. Hardy (Eds.), *Nursing diagnoses and interventions for the elderly* (pp. 369-389). Reading, MA: Addison Wesley Longman.

Duffy, V. B., Backstrand, J., & Ferris, A. (1995). Olfactory dysfunction and related nutritional risk in free-living elderly women. *Journal of American Dietician Association, 95,* 879-884.

Evans, W. J., Henkin, R. I., & Leopold, D. A. (1994). Loss of taste or smell: A rational approach. *Patient Care, 28*(15), 40-64.

Forbes, E. (1996). Sensory functions: Hearing, vision, taste, and smell. In S. P. Hoeman (Ed.), *Rehabilitation nursing,* (pp. 307-346). St. Louis, MO: Mosby.

Foxall, M. J., Barron, C. R., Von Dollen, K., Shull, K. A., & Jones, P. A. (1994). Low-vision elders living arrangements, loneliness and social support. *Journal of Gerontological Nursing, 20*(8), 6-14.

Gallman, R. L. (1995). The sensory system and its problem in the elderly. In M. Stanley & P. G. Beare (Eds.), *Gerontological nursing* (pp. 135-147). Philadelphia: F. A. Davis.

Gantz, B. J., Schindler, R. A., & Snow, J. B. (1995). Adult hearing loss: Some tips and pearls. *Patient Care, 29*(14), 77-88.

Gioiella, E. C., & Bevil, C. W. (1985). *Nursing care of the aging client.* Norwalk, CT: Appleton & Lange.

Gordon, M. (1987). *Manual of nursing diagnosis.* Hightstown, NJ: McGraw-Hill.

Gottlob, L. A., & Madden, D. J. (1998). Time course of allocation of visual attention after equating for sensory differences: An age-related perspective. *Psychology and Aging, 13*(1), 138-149.

Guida, P. (1993). Coordination change. In T. L. Glover & P. A. Loftis (Eds.), *Decision making in gerontologic nursing* (pp. 4-5). St. Louis, MO: Mosby.

Hodges, L. C., & Staab, A. S. (1996). *Gerontological nursing.* Philadelphia: Lippincott Williams & Wilkins.

Hogstel, M. O. (1992). *Clinical manual of gerontological nursing.* St. Louis, MO: Mosby.

Horowitz, A. (1994). Vision impairment and functional disability among nursing home residents. *The Gerontologist, 34*(3), 316-323.

Iowa Intervention Project. J. C. McCloskey & G. M. Bulechek (Eds.). (2000). *Nursing interventions classification (NIC)* (3rd ed.). St. Louis, MO: Mosby.

Iowa Outcomes Project. M. Johnson, M. Maas, & S. Moorhead (Eds.). (2000). *Nursing outcomes classification (NOC)* (2nd ed.). St. Louis, MO: Mosby.

Jarvis, C. (1996). *Physical examination and health assessment* (2nd ed.). Philadelphia: W. B. Saunders.

Jerger, J., Chmiel, R., Wilson, N., & Luchi, R. (1995). Hearing impairment in older adults: New concepts. *Journal of the American Geriatrics Society, 43,* 928-935.

Jubeck, M. E. (1992). Are you sensitive to the cognitive needs of the elderly? *Home Healthcare Nurse, 10*(5), 20-25.

Kallman, H., & Kallman, S. (1989). Accidents in the elderly populations. In W. Reichel (Ed.), *Clinical aspects of aging* (pp. 547-558). Baltimore: Lippincott Williams & Wilkins.

Kavanaugh, K. M., & Tate, B. (1996). Recognizing and helping older persons with vision impairments. *Geriatric Nursing, 17*(2), 68-71.

Keller, H. H. (1993). Malnutrition and institutionalized elderly: How and why? *Journal of the American Geriatrics Society, 41,* 1212-1218.

Kelly, M. (1995). Consequences of visual impairment on leisure activities of the elderly. *Geriatric Nursing, 16*(6), 273-275.

Kelly, M. (1996). Medications and the visually impaired elderly. *Geriatric Nursing, 17*(2), 60-62.

Kivett, D. E. (1994). The importance of emotional and social isolation to loneliness among very old rural adults. *The Gerontologist, 34,* 340-346.

Kosslyn, S. M., Brown, H. D., & Dror, I. E. (1999). Aging and the scope of visual attention. *Gerontology, 45,* 102-109.

Kreeger, J. L., Raulin, M. L., Grace, J., & Priest, B. L. (1995). Effect of hearing enhancement on mental status ratings in geriatric psychiatric patients. *American Journal of Psychiatry, 152,* 629-631.

Liu, L., Gauthier, L., & Gauthier, S. (1991). Spatial disorientation in persons with early senile dementia of the Alzheimer type. *American Journal of Occupational Therapy, 45*(1), 67-74.

Logan, S. A., Bess, F. H., & Lichenstein, M. J. (1990). Hearing impairment as a major determinant of function in the elderly. *Journal of American Academy of Audiology, 1*(1), 54-61.

Lueckenotte, A. G. (1996). *Gerontologic nursing.* St. Louis, MO: Mosby.

Maguire, G. H. (1996). Activities of daily living. In C. B. Lewis (Ed.), *Aging: The health care challenge* (pp. 47-77). Baltimore: Lippincott Williams & Wilkins.

Mahoney, D. F. (1993). Cerumen impaction: Prevalence and detection in nursing homes. *Journal of Gerontological Nursing, 19*(4), 23-30.

Mahoney, D. F. (1998). Cerumen impaction and hearing impairment among nursing home residents: Nursing implications. In V. Burggraft & R. Barry (Eds.), *Gerontological nursing current practice and research* (pp. 159-168). Thorofare, NJ: Slack Incorporated.

McLane, A. M. (1987). *Classification of nursing diagnoses: Proceedings of the seventh conference.* St. Louis, MO: Mosby.

Meador, J. A. (1995). Cerumen impaction in the elderly. *Journal of Gerontological Nursing, 21*(12), 43-45.

Miller, B. F., & Keane, C. B. (1987). *Encyclopedia and dictionary of medicine, nursing, and allied health* (4th ed.). Philadelphia: W. B. Saunders.

Miller, R. I. (1994). Managing disruptive responses to bathing by elderly residents. *Journal of Gerontological Nursing, 20*(11), 35-39.

Miller, S. (1993). Decreased vision. In T. L. Glover & P. A. Loftis (Eds.), *Decision making in gerontologic nursing* (pp. 118-121). St. Louis, MO: Mosby.

Mion, L. C. (1992). Environmental structuring. In G. M. Bulchek & J. C. McCloskey (Eds.), *Nursing interventions: Essential nursing treatments* (pp. 254-264). Philadelphia: W. B. Saunders.

Moore, J. R., & Gilbert, D. A. (1995). Elderly residents: Perceptions of nurses' comforting touch. *Journal of Gerontological Nursing, 21*(1), 6-13.

North American Nursing Diagnosis Association. (1999). *Nursing diagnoses: Definitions & classification 1999-2000.* Philadelphia: Author.

Pope-Spies, D. (1995). Music, noise, and the human voice in the nurse-patient environment. *IMAGE: Journal of Nursing Scholarship, 27*(4), 291-296.

Roussel, L. (1995). The neurological system and its problems in the elderly. In M. Stanley & P. G. Beare (Eds.), *Gerontological nursing* (pp. 174-188). Philadelphia: F. A. Davis.

Schaid, E. C. (1993). Dry mouth in the elderly. *Journal of Gerontological Nursing, 19,* 42-44.

Sellards, P. C. (1993). Balance change, In T. L. Glover & P. A. Loftis (Eds.), *Decision making in gerontologic nursing.* (pp. 2-3). St. Louis, MO: Mosby.

Ship, J. A., Duffy, V., Jones, J. A., & Langmore, S. (1996). Geriatric oral health and its impact on eating. *Journal of the American Geriatrics Society, 44,* 456-464.

Skinner, H. B., Barrack, R. L., & Cook, S. D. (1984). Age-related decline in proprioception. *Clinical Orthopedic, 184,* 208-211.

Sommer, C. (1993). Decreased sense of smell. In T. L. Glover & P. A. Loftis (Eds.), *Decision making in gerontologic nursing.* (pp. 120-127). St. Louis, MO: Mosby.

Tideiksaar, R. (1989). *Falling in old age: Its prevention and treatment.* New York: Springer Publishing.

Tielsch, J. M., Javitt, J. C., Coleman, A., Katz, J., & Summer, A. (1995). The prevalence of blindness and visual impairment among nursing home residents in Baltimore. *The New England Journal of Medicine, 332,* 1205-1209.

Topf, M. (1994). Theoretical considerations for research on environmental stress and health. *IMAGE: Journal of Nursing Scholarship, 26*(4), 289-293.

Trent, L. (1994). On the importance of color. *Nursing Home, 43*(7), 48-49.

U.S. Department of Health and Human Services (USDHHS). (1990). *Healthy People 2000.* National Health Promotion and Disease Prevention Objectives. Washington, DC: Public Health Services.

U.S. Department of Health and Human Services (USDHHS). (1993). *Hearing and the elderly.* Bethesda, MD: Public Health Services.

Vader, L. A. (1992). Vision and vision loss. In W. G. Langston, J. T. Turner, & P. S. Shremp (Eds.). *Nursing Clinics of North America, 27*(3), 705-714.

Ventry, I., & Weinstein, B. (1982). The hearing handicap inventory for the elderly: A new tool. *Ear & Hearing, 3*(3), 128-134.

Walczak, M., Bernstein, A. L., Senzer, C. L., & Mohr, N. (1993). Elder hearing aids infrared listening device in a geriatric day center. *Journal of Gerontological Nursing, 19*(8), 5-9.

Watanabe, R. (1994). The ability of the geriatric population to read labels on over-the-counter medication containers. *Journal of American Optometric Association, 65,* 32-37.

Wiley, T. L., Cruickshanks, K. J., Nondahl, D. M., Tweed, T. S., Klein, R., & Klein, B. E. (1998). Aging and word recognition in competing message. *Journal of the American Academy of Optometric Audiology, 9*(3), 191-198.

Wyke, B. (1979). Cervical articular contributions to pasture and gait: Their relationship to senile disequilibrium. *Age & Ageing, 8,* 251-258.

Yen, P. K. (1996). When food doesn't taste good anymore. *Geriatric Nursing, 17*(1), 44.

Zeeger, L. (1986). The effects of sensory change in older persons. *Journal of Neuroscience Nursing, 18,* 325.

Zignego-Smith, E. (1993). Taste changes and decreased sensation. In T. L. Glover & P. A. Loftis (Eds.), *Decision making in gerontologic nursing.* (pp. 136-139). St. Louis, MO: Mosby.

CHAPTER 38

UNILATERAL NEGLECT

Elizabeth A. Weitzel

Unilateral Neglect is the state in which an individual is perceptually unaware of and inattentive to one side of the body (Carroll-Johnson, 1994). This condition results from brain injury that alters perception and can be related to other perceptual problems. The lesion is most likely to be in the right parietal lobe; estimated rates for the right lobe being affected versus the left are as low as 3:1 and as high as 16:1 (Riddoch & Humphreys, 1983; Weinstein & Friedland, 1977). Therefore Unilateral Neglect is most frequently associated with left hemiplegia related to a cerebrovascular accident (CVA) of the right hemisphere. Sometimes the symptoms are most noticeable immediately after the lesion occurs, subsiding with recovery of other functions. However, some or all of the symptoms may persist and influence rehabilitation. There is also some evidence that men are more likely to have overt symptoms, perhaps related to functions being more rigidly segregated by hemisphere in the male, with verbal functions on the left and spatial functions on the right (Greshwind & Behan, 1982; McGlone, 1978). Alzheimer's disease is also a cause of Unilateral Neglect (Bartolomeo et al., 1998; Venneri, Pentore, Cotticelli, & Della Sala, 1998).

If Unilateral Neglect is not diagnosed and treated in the elder, there is potential for injury to the affected side through trauma or neglect of hygiene. The older person might not recognize the affected side as part of her body. This means the person may be unaware of the potential for danger, the need for hygiene, and the effects of trauma to the affected side. Thus older persons can accidentally burn, bruise, or cut their affected side and be completely unaware of pain or bleeding (Siev & Freishat, 1976).

When caring for the elderly client, behaviors related to Unilateral Neglect can be misdiagnosed as another psychologic problem or mental deterioration; inappropriate or ineffective interventions would then result (Gorelick, 1986). It is important that the nurse, who is aware of hygiene and other behaviors, assesses for Unilateral Neglect when brain injury has occurred. Other sensory losses with aging will exaggerate Unilateral Neglect and compound its effect on functioning. Compensating for these losses is important and should take place before making a final determination about the extent of neglect present. Elders are at risk for developing Unilateral Neglect because both CVA and subdural hematoma occur more frequently with advanced age.

Theories of the underlying deficit that results in Unilateral Neglect include disorders of (1) sensory input; (2) internal representation of space; and (3) attention to stimuli contralateral to the lesion. Studies by Riddoch and Humphreys (1983) support disordered attention as a primary part of the deficit. Kinsella, Oliver, Ng, Packer, and Stark (1993) identified scanning of external stimuli and disrupted internal representation of space. This knowledge is important when choosing interventions.

Unilateral Neglect is complicated by a variety of deficits that can accompany or account for some of its effects: anosognosia, hemianopsia, hemispatial neglect, visual inattention, and loss of proprioception.

Anosognosia has come to mean the unawareness or denial of hemiplegia (technically it means unawareness of the disease). Elderly persons with this deficit will confabulate reasons why they are not walking or using their arm. Sometimes they will deny that the limbs belong to them. For example, an elderly man claimed that his undertaker friend had replaced his arm with one from a cadaver. If an elderly person with anosognosia is given a pair of gloves, he will typically use the affected hand to put the glove on the unaffected hand, but will not put a glove on the affected hand (Friedland & Weinstein, 1977). It is not uncommon for elderly persons with anosognosia to try to get out of bed or a chair without assistance or proper safety precautions, since they are unaware of functional limitations.

Hemianopsia (also referred to as homonomous hemianopsia) is the loss of one half of the visual field, usually to the affected side. This condition usually occurs in lesions posterior to the optic chiasm and leaves a deficit on the side of hemiplegia, if it is also present (Johnson & Cyran, 1979; Nooney, 1986). The elderly person with hemianopsia is not blind in one eye, but has lost vision to one side in each eye. Hemianopsia further complicates other deficits because the person is not receiving full visual input. Johnson and Cyran (1979) describe assessment and nursing interventions for hemianopsia in more detail.

Hemispatial Neglect is inattention to the space located to one side of the midline of a person, as well as inattention to this half of the body. Elderly persons with this deficit will ignore voices or objects on the affected side. They may also neglect half of a book or meal tray on the affected side. Persons with hemispatial neglect will draw half a flower or the unaffected side of their body normally, whereas the affected side may be omitted or drawn fainter and less distinct. If the older person also has hemianopsia, he will not be aware of the loss of vision to the affected side.

Visual Inattention, which can be part of hemispatial neglect, will cause the elderly person to fail to read words on the affected side. However, when attention is called to the omitted words, they can be read without changing the direction of gaze or moving the head. This characteristic distinguishes visual inattention from hemianopsia, in which the word is not seen unless the older person's head is turned or the gaze is changed to use the functioning half of the eyes.

Proprioception is the ability to know the position of a limb through its sensory input, without looking at it or feeling it with another extremity. Loss of proprioception compounds other deficits for the elder. When proprioception is lost, safety of the affected limb becomes a problem for the older person.

Other tactile deficits include allesthesia, the perception of stimuli to the affected side as being to the opposite limb, and the extinction phenomenon. With this deficit, elderly persons can distinguish a single stimulus to their affected side, but if a stimulus is given to both extremities simultaneously, only the unaffected side is perceived. This test is referred to as double simultaneous stimulation (DSS).

Related deficits that need to be differentiated from Unilateral Neglect and that may complicate neglect behaviors include agnosia and apraxia. Agnosia is failure of the brain to recognize input from a single sense, such as vision, hearing, proprioception, or touch. The body receives the input, but the brain does not recognize the input as familiar. For example, if a key is placed in the hand of an older person with tactile agnosia and the person is asked to identify the object without being able to see it, the older person might tell you that the hand holds something cold and hard. If the person is allowed to look at the object he can correctly identify the key. Agnosias can accompany Unilateral Neglect or be present in the absence of Unilateral Neglect. Obviously, having both agnosias and Unilateral Neglect compounds the effects of the deficits for elderly individuals.

Apraxia is the inability to carry out a learned movement voluntarily or to plan and execute movement when comprehension and motor abilities are intact. A dependent elderly person with this deficit might scratch with the affected limb unconsciously, but be unable to move the limb with precision voluntarily (e.g., pick up eating utensils, appropriately fill a spoon, and bring it to her mouth when asked to do so). This deficit can appear either with Unilateral Neglect or separate from it. Apraxia also can occur on the unaffected side, further compounding the deficit and confusing the assessment. For example, an elderly person who has both a lesion in the right hemisphere and apraxia might exhibit weakness on the left and have difficulty handling a spoon correctly with the right hand for a period of time following the injury.

Several other deficits common with right hemisphere injury exist, including lack of inhibition, social inappropriateness, and verbal outburst. Conceptual deficits such as loss of abstract thinking, loss of appreciation of subtleties, and loss of attention span also can accompany right brain injury. The elderly person's retention of normal speech can mask initial identification of many of these deficits. It is beyond the scope of this chapter to discuss all of these cognitive and psychologic deficits in detail. The classic articles written by Fowler and Fordyce (1972) and the articles by Dudas (1986), Gorelick (1986), and Tellis-Nazak (1986) are resources for more detailed information.

RELATED FACTORS/ETIOLOGIES

CVA is probably the most common cause of Unilateral Neglect in elders, but any lesion to the parietal lobe, especially in the right hemisphere, can cause Unilateral Neglect to occur. Occasionally injury to other parts of the brain will result in Unilateral Neglect, but not as consistently as injury to the right parietal lobe (Heilman & Valenstein, 1977; Ishiai, Watabiki, Lee, Kanouchi, & Odajima, 1994).

ASSESSMENT

The major indicator of Unilateral Neglect is consistent inattention to stimuli on the affected side. This is often accompanied by inadequate self-care of the affected side, lack of positioning and/or safety precautions with regard to the affected side, failure to look toward the affected side, and neglect of food or reading material on the affected side (Table 38-1). The nurse should look for signs of Unilateral Neglect following brain injury, especially injury to the right hemisphere. However, this phenomenon should not be ruled out automatically with left hemisphere injury. Assessment Guide 38-1, developed by the author, is an example of a tool that is useful for assessing Unilateral Neglect.

Other health professionals can be helpful in determining the extent of deficits. However, many nurses working with elders have limited access to these professionals and must rely on their own assessment. Even when other professionals are available, it is wise for the nurse to compare a client's behavior in a "test" environment with the behavior present in daily self-care and interactions, since abilities might not appear to be the same in both contexts.

The role of fatigue must be taken into account when assessing persons with brain injury, since most deficits will be pronounced and frustration most evident when the person is fatigued (Lezak, 1976). The older person needs to be given the best circumstances to display existing abilities. Assessing the person when rested and away from distractions will result in more accurate data on which to base diagnoses and interventions (see the section on interventions for ways to decrease distractions).

Table 38-1	Unilateral Neglect
NANDA (Carroll-Johnson, 1994)	**Weitzel**
RELATED FACTORS/ETIOLOGIES	
Effects of disturbed perceptual abilities One-sided blindness Neurologic illness or trauma	Brain injury: trauma, tumor, or cerebrovascular problems Disorders of sensory input, internal representation of space, attention to stimuli contralateral to the lesion Limited or no movement to the affected extremity Loss of one half of visual field, usually to affected side Loss of ability to know the position of a limb through its sensory input, without looking at it or touching it Perception of stimuli to the affected side as being to the opposite limb Perception of only stimulus to the unaffected side when stimulus is given to both extremities Nonrecognition of affected side as part of the body Unawareness of functional limitations Inattention to the space located to one side of the elder's midline and inattention to that half of the body
DEFINING CHARACTERISTICS	
Consistent inattention to stimuli on an affected side Inadequate self-care Positioning and/or safety precautions in regard to the affected side Does not look toward affected side Leaves food on plate on the affected side	***Denial*** Function not improved by calling attention to neglected side ***Inattention*** Failure to read words on the affected side of page; when attention is called to the omitted words, they can be read without changing the direction of gaze or moving the head ***Major Indicators*** Consistent inattention to stimuli on the affected side Inadequate self-care of the affected side Lack of positioning and/or safety precautions with regard to the affected side Not looking toward the affected side Neglect of food or reading material on the affected side

Assessment Guide 38-1

TOOL FOR UNILATERAL NEGLECT

The following questions will assist the nurse in establishing the presence of neglect:

1. Is there consistent inattention to the affected side?
2. Is there inadequate self-care to the affected side?

   Dressing
   Bathing
   Application of deodorant/cologne
   Shaving
   Application of cosmetics

3. Is there lack of positioning and/or safety precautions with regard to the affected side?
4. Is food left on the plate on the affected side?
5. Does food remain in the cheek on the affected side?
6. When asked to draw a daisy, is the drawing complete or are petals missing or faint on the affected side?
7. When asked to draw self, is the drawing complete (stick figure) or are limbs on the affected side missing, distorted, or lighter?
8. When presented with two identical drawings of a face, centered with the midline of the patient's body, can both be seen? Are they perceived as having the same expression (smiling, frowning)?

Assessing the elderly person without prejudice is also important. Tellis-Nazak (1986) discusses the effects of attitudes toward aging and stroke on the rehabilitation of older clients. Health professionals, as well as society at large, often share the belief that older persons will not benefit from rehabilitation. This belief can become a self-fulfilling prophecy.

Categories of Extent of Deficit

O'Brien and Pallett (1978) describe four degrees of deficits in Unilateral Neglect: inattention, unconcern, unawareness, and denial. Inattention is the mildest form. Persons with this deficit can use the affected side and care for it if someone else draws their attention to it. Unconcern describes persons who admit the presence of a disability, but underestimate the deficit and display an affect that is inappropriate in proportion to the amount of deficit. Unawareness is described as a transitory state soon after the injury, which clears as sensorium clears. Persons with unawareness might try activities beyond their ability because they do not recognize the extent of their disability. Denial is the most severe form of Unilateral Neglect. It includes persons described previously as having anosognosia and is often complicated with hemianopsia, apraxias, and/or agnosias. Persons in denial are not accepting of their disability. It is important to understand that this condition is not part of the normal psychologic reaction to loss in which denial is protective until the psyche is ready to accept the loss. In persons with Unilateral Neglect the brain has been injured so that it no longer acknowledges the affected side as being part of the person. It is possible, however, for the extent of this deficit to diminish as the brain heals. It is important, therefore, that the older person be reassessed at regular intervals for several months following brain injury.

NURSING DIAGNOSIS

Unilateral Neglect was added as a subdiagnosis under Sensory/Perceptual Alterations in 1987 by the seventh conference of the North American Nursing Diagnosis Association (NANDA, 1999). It is defined as "the state in which an individual is perceptually unaware of and inattentive to one side of the body" (NANDA, 1999, p. 115). Unilateral Neglect is differentiated from Sensory/Perceptual Alterations in elders (see Chapter 37) in that it is the result of pathology, not of normal aging. Unilateral Neglect results from injury to brain tissue and not from alterations in the environment. It can result in some of the same behaviors as other altered sensory perceptions, but only as related to perception of one limb on half of the body; it is usually associated with hemiplegia, hemianopsia, or other sensory deficits (Heilman & Valenstein, 1977).

When relating assessment data to the nursing diagnosis Unilateral Neglect, it is useful to group older persons with inattention, unconcern, and unawareness into category, while those exhibiting denial are considered a distinct cat-

egory. Thus two distinct diagnoses emerge: Unilateral Neglect: Inattention and Unilateral Neglect: Denial. Although individuals will need interventions specific to existing deficits, there are some definite differences between interventions for these two diagnoses. Table 38-1 summarizes the assessment data that need to be collected to determine Unilateral Neglect: Inattention or Unilateral Neglect: Denial as the appropriate diagnosis. In addition, specific deficits such as hemianopsia, apraxia, agnosia, or visual-spatial relationship problems require interventions specifically addressed to these deficits. See Assessment Guide 38-2, developed by the author, for differential diagnosis of these deficits. Table 38-1 compares Weitzel's related factors/etiologies and defining characteristics with NANDA's related factors/etiologies and defining characteristics (Carroll-Johnson, 1994; NANDA, 1994).

CASE STUDY 1

T. Snow is a 70-year-old man whose condition has just stabilized following a thrombolytic stroke affecting the right hemisphere of the brain. When approached from the left, he often does not respond until the nurse is standing in front of him. If the nurse has gained his attention and then moves to his left, he responds and can see objects to which the nurse points. Mr. Snow scratches his head with his left hand but does not wash his left side when bathing. In regard to his visual field, he can see a finger held to the left side of his head without turning his head after being told that it is there, as long as there is no visual stimulation to the right side. Based on these assessment data, the nurse diagnoses Unilateral Neglect: Inattention related to right hemisphere injury as evidenced by lack of response to stimuli from the left side, unless cued.

CASE STUDY 2

R. Brown, a 68-year-old man who had a stroke of undetermined type a year ago, has hemiparesis of the left leg and hemiplegia of the left arm. He tells the nurse he could walk if he just had new shoes. He will attempt to stand unattended, but does not place his left foot flat on the floor or use his quad cane, even though he has been instructed several times to do both. Often he will fall if staff do not intervene. Mr. Brown has no sensation of touch to his left arm, fails to bathe it, and leaves it dangling in the wheel of his wheelchair. When his gaze is directed to the left, he can see his left arm only after turning his head and using the right side of his eyes. He tells the nurse that the left arm belongs to his roommate, not to him. Based on these assessment data, the nurse diagnoses Unilateral Neglect: Denial related to right hemisphere brain injury as evidenced by failure to respond to stimuli to the left side, even when cued, and by hemianopsia.

Assessment Guide 38-2

DIFFERENTIAL DIAGNOSIS—UNILATERAL NEGLECT

The following items will assist the nurse in differentiating the extent of deficits:

1. Does the person fail to use the affected limb, even though motor ability is present?
   a. Does the person use the limb when cued? Yes = inattention. No = probable apraxia.
   b. Does the person have difficulty using hygiene articles or putting on clothes right side up, etc.? Yes = apraxia.
2. Does the person run into walls or door frames, even when there is ample room, or have difficulty walking or steering a wheelchair in a straight line? Yes = visual-spatial problems.
3. Is reading material neglected on the affected side?
   a. When attention is drawn to the missing words, can they be read without moving the gaze? Yes = inattention. No = hemianopsia and/or denial.
4. When the person is looking at a fixed point in midline, can fingers brought simultaneously from behind the head be detected at the same time? No = visual defect (See No. 5).
5. Can a finger be seen on the affected side when moved from midline outward and gaze remains fixed on midline? Yes = visual inattention. No = hemianopsia.
6. If several familiar objects are placed close to the midline of an overbed table:
   a. Can all objects be named or pointed to without turning head or gaze? No = hemianopsia or denial.
   b. When head is turned to affected side, can objects be identified? Yes = hemianopsia. No = denial.
7. When touched on the affected side, is touch perceived?
   Yes:
   a. Is it perceived accurately where touched? If perceived on the opposite side, this indicates allesthesia.
   b. Is it still perceived if the opposite side is touched at the same time (DDS)? No = extinction.
   No:
   a. Is perception increased if the person looks at being touched and/or receives verbal input about touch? Yes = inattention. No = sensory hemiplegia and/or denial.
8. Does the person have trouble finding an object in a cluttered drawer, miss the cup when pouring liquids into it, or knock things over, even with the unaffected hand? Yes = apraxia or visual-spatial relationship problems.
9. Does the person use incorrect terms referring to familiar objects, not respond correctly to familiar sounds, or fail to recognize familiar objects placed in the hand with eyes closed? Yes = agnosia (type dependent on sense not functioning).
10. Does the person have difficulty estimating time passage when a clock is visible?
    a. Can the person read the clock correctly? If no and hemianopsia is not present, may indicate a form of agraphia.
    b. If yes, may indicate time orientation problems.

NURSING-SENSITIVE OUTCOMES

Expected outcomes with the nursing diagnosis Unilateral Neglect are that the neglect behavior will decrease or be compensated for and cause fewer problems for the older person in daily activities. Evaluation will necessitate re-assessment and comparison of current behaviors against previous data and defined goals for the individual.

The following nursing outcomes are appropriate for the older person with Unilateral Neglect: Safe Environment: Physical, defined as physical surroundings that minimize harm or injury; Safety Status: Personal, defined as conditions and behaviors that minimize potential for personal injury; and Self-Care: Activities of Daily Living, defined as the ability to perform the most basic physical tasks and personal care.

Box 38-1 relates the nursing diagnosis Unilateral Neglect: Inattention with expected nursing outcomes (Iowa Outcomes Project, 2000). Box 38-2 does the same for Unilateral Neglect: Denial. Not all the indicators listed in the Nursing Outcomes Classification are appropriate for the person with Unilateral Neglect, some being more general for the person living in the community and/or for children. Those that are most appropriate appear in the previously mentioned boxes.

NURSING INTERVENTIONS

Interventions for Unilateral Neglect will be discussed in three categories: general interventions, which are appropriate with both inattention and denial; interventions specific for inattention; and interventions specific for denial. Interventions for associated deficits also will be discussed. Distinguishing inattention and denial on the basis of etiologies is not precise at this time, so the determination will be made based on assessed signs and symptoms. All of the interventions are compensatory, since the etiology of brain injury cannot be reversed by the nurse. The *Nursing Interventions Classification (NIC)* (Iowa Intervention Project, 2000) intervention Unilateral Neglect Management has been amplified into the categories described previously (see Box 38-2).

| Box 38-1 | **Nursing Diagnosis, Nursing-Sensitive Outcomes, and Nursing Intervention** **UNILATERAL NEGLECT: INATTENTION** |

Nursing Diagnosis

Unilateral Neglect: Inattention

Defining characteristics

Nonrecognition of affected side as part of the body

Unawareness of functional limitations

Inattention to the space located to one side of the elder's midline and inattention to that half of the body

Failure to read words on the affected side of page; when attention is called to the omitted words, they can be read without changing the direction of gaze or moving the head

Consistent inattention to stimuli on the affected side

Inadequate self-care of the affected side

Lack of positioning and/or safety precautions with regard to the affected side

Not looking toward the affected side

Neglect of food or reading material on the affected side

Nursing-Sensitive Outcomes

Safety Behavior: Personal

Indicators

Balance of sleep and rest with activity

Use seat belts or safety seats

Shoes that fit and are tied

Clothing appropriate for activity

Assistive devices used correctly

Correct use of equipment

Safety Behavior: Home Physical Environment

Indicators

Personal alarm system

Assistive devices

Barriers to prevent burns

Safety devices

Self-Care: Activities of Daily Living (ADL)

Indicators

As independently as possible:

- Eating
- Dressing
- Toileting
- Bathing
- Grooming
- Hygiene
- Oral hygiene
- Ambulation: walking
- Ambulation: wheelchair
- Transfer performance

Nursing Intervention

Unilateral Neglect Management

Activities

Monitor for abnormal responses to three primary types of stimuli: sensory, visual, and auditory

Evaluate baseline mental status, comprehension, motor function, sensory function, attention span, and affective responses

Provide realistic feedback about patient's perceptual deficits

Perform personal care in a consistent manner with thorough explanations

Ensure that affected extremities are properly and safely positioned

Adapt the environment to the deficit by focusing on the affected side during the acute period

Encourage phone conversation, if it improves concentration

Supervise and/or assist in transferring and ambulating

Touch affected shoulder when initiating conversation

Avoid rapid movement in the room

Gradually move personal items and activity to affected side, as patient demonstrates an ability to compensate for neglect

Position bed in room, so that individuals approach and care for patient on affected side

Keep side rails up on affected side, as appropriate

Provide range of motion and massage to affected side

Give frequent reminders to redirect the patient's attention, cueing the patient to the environment

Instruct patient to scan from left to right

Encourage patient to touch and use affected body part

Gradually focus patient's attention to the affected side, as patient demonstrates an ability to compensate for neglect

Stand on affected side when ambulating with patient, as patient demonstrates an ability to compensate for neglect

Assist patient with activities of daily living from affected side, as patient demonstrates an ability to compensate for neglect

Assist patient to bathe and groom affected side first, as patient demonstrates an ability to compensate for neglect

Focus tactile and verbal stimuli on affected side, as patient demonstrates an ability to compensate for neglect

Consult with occupational and physical therapist concerning timing and strategies to facilitate reintegration of neglected body parts and function

Instruct caregivers on the cause, mechanisms, and treatment of unilateral neglect

Include family in rehabilitation process to support the patient's efforts and assist with care, as appropriate

General Interventions

Certain nursing activities are appropriate for both Unilateral Neglect: Inattention and Unilateral Neglect: Denial: controlling sensory input, psychosocial support, safety support, and family involvement. Much of the recent research related to interventions for Unilateral Neglect has been conducted by neurologists and psychologists, based on ability of the subject to accurately bisect a line. Clinical nursing investigations of Unilateral Neglect are needed to evaluate the effectiveness of nursing interventions.

Controlling Sensory Input. To increase the elder's awareness of stimuli from the affected side, it is important to control the stimuli that may interfere with the individual's ability to concentrate following brain injury. Although there is limited research support for this approach,

Box 38-2	Nursing Diagnosis, Nursing-Sensitive Outcomes, and Nursing Intervention **UNILATERAL NEGLECT: DENIAL**

Nursing Diagnosis
Unilateral Neglect: Denial
Defining characteristics
Nonrecognition of affected side as part of the body
Unawareness of functional limitations
Inattention to the space located to one side of the elder's
  midline and inattention to that half of the body
Function not improved by calling attention to neglected side
Consistent inattention to stimuli on the affected side
Inadequate self-care of the affected side
Lack of positioning and/or safety precautions with regard to
  the affected side
Lack of positioning and/or safety precautions with regard to
  the affected side
Not looking toward the affected side
Neglect of food or reading material on the affected side

Nursing-Sensitive Outcomes
Safety Status: Personal
Indicators
Sleep/rest appropriate for activity
Seat belts used in wheelchair
Shoes that fit and are tied
Clothing appropriate for activity
Assistive devices used
Correct use of equipment

Safety Behavior: Home Physical Environment
Indicators
Lighting
Personal alarm system
Assistive devices
Barriers to prevent burns
Safety devices

Self-Care: Activities of Daily Living (ADL)
Indicators
As independently as possible
Eating
Toileting
Bathing
Grooming
Hygiene

Oral hygiene
Ambulation: walking
Ambulation: wheelchair
Transfer performance

Nursing Intervention
Unilateral Neglect Management
Activities
Monitor for abnormal responses to three primary types of
  stimuli: sensory, visual, and auditory
Evaluate baseline mental status, comprehension, motor
  function, sensory function, attention span, and affective
  responses
Provide realistic feedback about patient's perceptual deficits
Perform personal care in a consistent manner with thorough
  explanations
Ensure that affected extremities are properly and safely
  positioned
Adapt the environment to the deficit by focusing on the
  unaffected side during the acute period
Encourage phone conversation, if it improves concentration
Supervise and/or assist in transferring and ambulating
Touch unaffected shoulder when initiating conversation
Place food and beverages within field of vision and turn plate,
  as necessary
Rearrange the environment to use right or left visual field,
  such as positioning personal items, television, or reading
  materials within view on unaffected side
Avoid rapid movement in the room
Avoid moving objects in the room
Position bed in room so that individuals approach and care
  for patient on unaffected side
Keep side rails up on affected side, as appropriate
Provide range of motion and massage to affected side
Consult with occupational and physical therapist concerning
  timing and strategies to facilitate reintegration of neglected
  body parts and function
Instruct caregivers on the cause, mechanisms, and treatment
  of unilateral neglect
Include family in rehabilitation process to support the
  patient's efforts and assist with care, as appropriate

---

it is validated through anecdotal observations (Fowler & Fordyce, 1972; Tilton & Maloof, 1982; Wallhagen, 1979) and research, including DSS (Berti, Maravita, Frassinetti, & Umilta, 1995). A quiet room without excessive visual stimuli (e.g., bright patterns, movement of objects or persons) is important. The presence of hemianopsia or of visual inattention can be used to advantage by putting the elderly person's unaffected side toward a wall or partition, thus decreasing input from the remainder of the room. The nurse should move slowly around the patient and speak in concrete terms, giving one instruction at a time and breaking each task into small steps. Verbal instruction can be more effective than visual demonstration, especially if the person has any visual-spatial perception disorder. Some persons have been found to concentrate better when talking on the phone than when looking at the person speaking. If this ability is evident, phone conversations can be encouraged (Box 38-2). Written cue cards listing the sequence of steps are sometimes helpful in complex tasks such as dressing, but they must be written in simple language and be kept within field of vision. It is important to encourage the older person to slow down and to discourage impulsive movements. Consistency is crucial.

There is nonsystematic empirical evidence, as well as some research, to support selective increase of stimuli to the affected side to decrease the effects of Unilateral Neglect. Marmo (1974) found that activities such as whole-body rubdowns, especially with verbal input about the affected parts being stimulated, helped to increase awareness of the affected side. Marmo also suggests positioning the person prone with the head turned to the affected side to carry out activities of daily living (ADL) or recreation, and rolling the person over the affected side. This study did not indicate if these activities are effective if the person has Unilateral Neglect: Denial. The nurse should be cautious when using these approaches with elderly persons who are frail, who have limited joint movement, or who have respiratory or cardiac problems.

Booth (1982) questions the practice of encouraging the person to perform ADL in front of a mirror unless the nurse remains present to cue attention to the affected side. However, the older person might be taught to rotate a plate occasionally while eating to counteract the problem of seeing only half of the plate. Additional interventions are included in the discussion of inattention.

Psychosocial Support. It is critical for the nurse to accept the older person's attempts to perceive, gently correct inappropriate responses, and immediately praise correct responses. A person's ability should not be overestimated simply because of intact speech and social skills. As the older person masters one set of tasks, the nurse can gradually increase the amount and complexity of tasks. It is important to be alert to mental as well as physical fatigue. When a person who had been responding appropriately begins to respond inappropriately and/or becomes frustrated, it is time to take a break.

If the elder shows emotional lability or other forms of perseveration (repeating an action or word after its usefulness is past), the nurse should redirect, interrupting with a gentle touch to the unaffected arm, ensuring the older person's attention, and then moving on to the next activity. Sometimes it will be necessary for the nurse to complete a task (e.g., feeding, dressing) for the older person if fatigue occurs and the task needs to be finished. In this case the nurse should expect successively more of the task to be completed by the older person in future attempts. The nurse should see that the patient's needs are met, while at the same time stimulating the older person to be more independent.

It is important that elderly persons with Unilateral Neglect have a stable location and as much consistency of staff as possible. Ability to cope with change will be compromised both by the effects of age and by the effects of the perceptual deficit.

Safety Support. Providing for the safety of the older person with Unilateral Neglect is another important part of the nurse's interventions. This includes ensuring that proper hygiene measures are carried out for the affected part of the body, protecting the affected part and dealing with inadequate caution on the part of the person who does not realize the extent of the disabilities present. Providing a wide armboard on a wheelchair can help keep an affected arm out of the wheels of the chair. Using a sling is usually not advised unless the arm is completely flaccid and causes balance problems. A sling limits any use that remains in the arm and fosters formation of flexion contractures at the elbow, wrist, and fingers. A seat belt can be fastened to a wheelchair for persons who cannot remember to carry out safety precautions (e.g., lock brakes, plant affected foot firmly on floor, or await assistance from staff). The need for safety should be balanced with the need for dignity and quality of life.

Family Involvement. It is also important for the family to remain involved and to be aware of the deficits and interventions appropriate for the older person. Family can assist the staff in reorienting the older person to the affected side and implementing safety precautions. Family members also can provide valuable information about the older person's usual lifestyle.

Interventions Specific to Inattention

Cueing. When a dependent older person has Unilateral Neglect: Inattention, cueing can increase the ability to use the affected side of the body. Cueing is providing stimulus to the affected side, thus increasing sensory input and awareness. Weinberg, Diller, and Gordon (1977) improved visual scanning by putting a vertical line along the left (affected side) edge of the page and numbering the lines of print. The person with inattention learned to look for these cues to increase the ability to read the whole page and not lose the place on the page. These same researchers also found that having the person identify where a touch was located on his back or estimate the size of an object could improve awareness, especially when the person was made aware of deficits and given a means to correct the deficit with simple cues (Weinberg et al., 1977).

Recent research has separated cueing into visual stimuli and limb movement on the affected side. Use of moving or changing visual stimuli on the affected side has been found to improve performance on a variety of tests (Berti et al., 1995; Butters & Kirsch, 1992; Mattingley, Bradshaw, & Bradshaw, 1994; Mattingley, Pierson, Bradshaw, Phillips, & Bradshaw, 1993). Additionally, Butters and Kirsch (1992) found that patching the eye opposite the side of neglect helps improve test results, especially when coupled with nonstatic visual stimulation to the affected side. Hjaltason and Tegner (1992) found that reduction of background stimuli increased test performance when the room was darkened and the test was in the form of light-emitting diode (LED) stimuli.

Cueing related to movement of extremities on the affected side was found helpful in reducing visual neglect in some studies (Robertson, North, & Geggie, 1992; Robertson, Tegner, Goodrich, & Wilson, 1994; Vallar, Antonucci, Guariglia, & Pizzamiglio, 1993). Nursing studies could document how this can be developed into an effective nursing intervention and added to the NIC.

Some nurse clinicians have found that placement of flashing lights or moving objects next to the affected side increases awareness of that side (Olson & Hening, 1973). Others found that wearing a watch, a favorite ring, a bell, or a charm bracelet on the affected arm helped to draw attention to it (Fowler & Fordyce, 1972; Olson & Hening, 1973). Placing the bedside table to the affected side might also increase awareness. It is important to approach the older person with Unilateral Neglect: Inattention from the affected side to increase awareness. It is also important to minimize stimulation to the unaffected side when trying to increase awareness.

CASE STUDY 1

Mr. Snow, previously given the diagnosis Unilateral Neglect: Inattention, will probably benefit from a variety of cueing activities to improve input from the affected side. He should have his room arranged so that people approach him from the affected side. Also, his bedside table should be placed to that side. With morning and evening care, he should be asked to identify where he is being touched on his back in a variety of spots. A mobile of favorite objects could be hung within eyesight on his affected side, perhaps having a chime or some other noise associated with it. A radio or TV could also be placed next to his affected side to increase auditory input. A patch could be placed over Mr. Snow's right eye while he is doing self-care and other activities requiring reduced stimulus from the unaffected side. It is anticipated that these activities would increase independence and awareness of the affected side. After a few weeks Mr. Snow should be reassessed to determine the amount of stimuli he perceives to the affected side without cueing.

Interventions Appropriate for Denial

Although the older person's Unilateral Neglect: Denial persists, there is little that can be done to increase awareness of the affected side. Thus interventions become focused on allowing persons to function as fully as possible within their limitations and to maintain safety. If the denial is so great that the older person fails to recognize any limitations, the nurse might need to become creative in developing ways to protect the person without undo constraint.

The elderly person with denial should have objects arranged on the unaffected side to allow the objects to be seen and used. This includes the bedside table, call light, and any other essential objects. Persons with denial should be approached from the unaffected side to avoid startling them or having them reject voices on the affected side. These persons will need a great deal of simplification of tasks and verbal input throughout. The meal tray should be placed on the unaffected side or turned during the meal. Sometimes the visual loss can be used to advantage by placing part of the food out of the field of vision. This strategy decreases the amount of food seen, which can simplify the task of eating.

Interventions for Associated Deficits

Apraxia.   The older person with apraxia should be helped to guide her hand through the correct movement. If the individual has problems with eating, food is put in the spoon, the spoon placed in her hand, and the movement to the mouth guided without verbal direction. This might need to be repeated several times before it can be carried out independently. Practicing putting an object in a desired place can help the older person's apraxia (Lord & Hall, 1986). The nurse could empty a bag of soft wrapped candy on the over-bed table and have the older person with apraxia pick up the candy, one piece at a time, and place each piece in a wide-mouthed cup. When all the candy is in the cup, one piece can be eaten as a reward, if the diet allows. Repeating this activity two or three times a day can increase the older person's ability to use the hand purposefully. If apraxia causes the older person to confuse top and bottom of clothing, sewing colored labels in the top can increase independence in dressing.

Agnosia.   The older person can be helped to learn to compensate for agnosia. For example, an older person with tactile agnosia can be taught to look at objects rather than depend on feel for recognition.

Visual-Spatial Relationships.   Having an uncluttered environment with essential items in easy view will help the older person locate needed items. The older person can be taught to stay toward the unaffected side in hallways and doorways to avoid hitting the affected side. Sometimes exercising to increase sitting and standing balance and keeping the head in midline will improve these problems. Robertson et al. (1994) found that persons with left Unilateral Neglect without hemiplegia could walk through a door closer to center if they moved their left arm as they approached the doorway.

Hemianopsia.   Older persons can be taught to scan with their eyes and turn their head. Elders with denial might not be able to compensate for hemianopsia. The older person should be approached from the unaffected side and asked to turn his head to follow movement toward the affected side. When taking older persons with hemianopsia out of their rooms, landmarks or color cues in the hallway can be pointed out. Loss of vision to the affected side will mean that the side visualized going down the hall will not be visible to the older person on the way back to the room.

CASE STUDY 2

Mr. Brown will probably be frustrated by any attempts at cueing that require him to learn a behavior. Selected stimuli can be given to the affected side, but this might not change his ability to function. He will need to have his room arranged with articles to his unaffected side. A wide armrest on his wheelchair could increase safety for his affected arm. If Mr. Brown continues to attempt to stand and walk unaided, a seat belt might be necessary. Landmarks close to his door that he will see when returning to his room should be pointed out. Because of the denial, Mr. Brown will require close monitoring by staff. However, with time, he might begin to respond to more stimuli on the affected side. If reassessment should confirm this improvement in status, the diagnosis should be changed to Unilateral Neglect: Inattention and the interventions altered appropriately.

SUMMARY

Unilateral Neglect can affect older persons following brain injury. It can be displayed as either inattention or denial. Nurses can treat both diagnoses best by structuring the environment. Inattention is most amenable to the intervention environmental cueing. Denial as a result of brain injury is not the same as denial following loss. Denial that results from brain injury is an inability of the brain to function correctly. The person having denial usually is not aware of any deficit or of the extent of the deficit. Denial requires the nurse to compensate for the deficit as long as the denial persists; ensuring safety and maintaining the elderly person's dignity are major nursing concerns.

REFERENCES

Bartolomeo, P., Dalla Barba, G., Boisse, M. F., Backoud-Levi, A. C., Degos, J. D., & Boller, F. (1998). Right-side neglect in Alzheimer's disease. *Neurology, 51*(4), 1207-1209.

Berti, A., Maravita, A., Frassinetti, F., & Umilta, C. (1995). Unilateral neglect and neglected field stimuli. *Cortex, 31,* 331-343.

Booth, K. (1982). The neglect syndrome. *Journal of Neurosurgical Nursing, 14*(1), 38-43.

Butters, C. M., & Kirsch, N. (1992). Combined and separate effects of eye patching and visual stimulation on unilateral neglect following stroke. *Archives of Physical Medicine and Rehabilitation, 73,* 1133-1139.

Carroll-Johnson, R. M. (Ed.). (1994). *Classification of nursing diagnoses: Proceedings of the tenth conference.* Baltimore: Lippincott Williams & Wilkins.

Dudas, S. (1986). Nursing diagnoses and intervention for rehabilitation of the stroke patient. *Nursing Clinics of North America, 23*(2), 345-357.

Fowler, R., & Fordyce, W. (1972). Adapting care for the brain injured patient. *American Journal of Nursing, 72*(10), 1832-1835.

Friedland, R. P., & Weinstein, E. A. (1977). Hemi-inattention and hemisphere specialization: Introduction and historical review. In E. A. Weinstein & R. P. Friedland (Eds.), *Advances in neurology* (vol. 1, pp. 1-31). New York: Raven Press.

Gorelick, P. B. (1986). Cerebrovascular disease: Pathology, physiology and diagnosis. *Nursing Clinics of North America, 21,* 275-288.

Greshwind, N., & Behan, N. (1982). Left-handedness: Association with immune disease, migraine and development of learning disorders. *Proceedings of the National Academy of Science, 79,* 5097-5100.

Heilman, K. M., & Valenstein, E. (1977). Mechanisms and underlying hemispatial neglect. In E. A. Weinstein & R. P. Friedland (Eds.), *Advances in neurology* (vol. 1, pp. 166-170). New York: Raven Press.

Hjaltason, H., & Tegner, R. (1992). Darkness improves line bisection in unilateral spatial neglect. *Cortex, 28*(3), 353-358.

Iowa Intervention Project. J. C. McCloskey & G. M. Bulechek (Eds.). (2000). *Nursing interventions classification (NIC)* (3rd ed.). St. Louis, MO: Mosby.

Iowa Outcomes Project. M. Johnson, M. Maas, & S. Moorhead (Eds.). (2000). *Nursing outcomes classification (NOC)* (2nd ed.). St. Louis, MO: Mosby.

Ishiai, S., Watabiki, S., Lee, E., Kanouchi, T., & Odajima, M. (1994). Preserved leftward movement in left unilateral spatial neglect due to frontal lesions. *Journal of Neurology, Neurosurgery, and Psychiatry, 57*(9), 1085-1090.

Johnson, J. H., & Cyran, M. (1979). Homonymous hemianopsia: Assessment and management. *American Journal of Nursing, 79,* 2131-2134.

Kinsella, G., Oliver, J., Ng, K., Packer, S., & Stark, R. (1993). Analysis of the syndrome of unilateral neglect. *Cortex, 29*(1), 135-140.

Lezak, M. D. (1976). *Neuropsychological assessment.* Cary, NC: Oxford University Press.

Lord, J. P., & Hall, K. (1986). Neuromuscular reeducation vs. traditional programs for stroke rehabilitation. *Archives of Physical Medicine and Rehabilitation, 67*(2), 88-91.

Marmo, N. A. (1974). A new look at the brain injured adult. *American Journal of Occupational Therapy, 28*(4), 199-200.

Mattingley, J. B., Bradshaw, J. L., & Bradshaw, J. A. (1994). Horizontal visual motion modulates focal attention in left unilateral spatial neglect. *Journal of Neurology, Neurosurgery and Psychiatry, 57*(10), 1228-1235.

Mattingley, J. B., Pierson, J. M., Bradshaw, J. L., Phillips, J. G., & Bradshaw, J. A. (1993). The effects of visible and invisible cues on line bisection. *Neuropsychologica, 31*(11), 1201-1215.

McGlone, J. (1978). Sex differences in functional brain asymmetry. *Cortex, 14,* 122-128.

Nooney, T. W. (1986). Partial visual rehabilitation of hemianopia patients. *American Journal of Optometry and Physiologic Optics, 639*(5), 382-386.

North American Nursing Diagnosis Association. (1999). *Nursing diagnoses: Definitions & classification 1999-2000.* Philadelphia: Author.

O'Brien, M. T., & Pallett, P. T. (1978). *Total care of the stroke patient.* Boston: Little, Brown.

Olson, D. O., & Hening, E. (1973). *A manual of behavior management strategies for traumatically brain-injured adults.* Chicago: Rehabilitation Institute.

Riddoch, M. J., & Humphreys, G. (1983). The effect of cueing on unilateral neglect. *Neuropsychologica, 21*(16), 589-599.

Robertson, I. H., North, N. T., & Geggie, C. (1992). Spatiomotor cueing in unilateral left neglect: Three case studies of its therapeutic effects. *Journal of Neurology, Neurosurgery and Psychiatry, 55*(9), 799-805.

Robertson, I. H., Tegner, T., Goodrich, S. J., & Wilson, C. (1994). Walking trajectory and hand movements in unilateral left neglect: A vestibular hypothesis. *Neuropsychologica, 32*(12), 1495-1502.

Siev, E., & Freishat, B. (1976). *Perceptual dysfunction in adult stroke patient.* Thorofare, NJ: Slack.

Tellis-Nazak, M. (1986). The challenge of the nursing role in rehabilitation of elderly stroke patients. *Nursing Clinics of North America, 21*(2), 399-343.

Tilton, C. N., & Maloof, M. (1982). Diagnosing the problem in stroke. *American Journal of Nursing, 82*(4), 569-601.

Vallar, G., Antonucci, G., Guariglia, C., & Pizzamiglio, L. (1993). Deficits of position sense, unilateral neglect and optokinetic stimulation. *Neuropsychologica, 31*(11), 1191-1200.

Venneri, A., Pentore, R., Cotticelli, B., & Della Sala, S. (1998). Unilateral spatial neglect in the late stage of Alzheimer's disease. *Cortex, 34*(5), 743-752.

Wallhagen, M. (1979). The split brain: Implications for care and rehabilitation. *American Journal of Nursing, 79*(12), 2118-2125.

Weinberg, J., Diller, L., & Gordon, W. A. (1977). Visual scanning training effect on reading-related tasks in acquired right brain injury. *Archives of Physical Medicine and Rehabilitation, 58*(4), 479-486.

Weinstein, E. A., & Friedland, R. P. (Eds.). (1977). *Advances in neurology* (vol. 1). New York: Raven Press.

CHAPTER 39

KNOWLEDGE DEFICIT

Vicki S. Conn, Jane M. Armer, and Karen S. Hayes

Knowledge Deficit is one of the most commonly used nursing diagnoses for adults of all ages, and client teaching is one of the most common nursing activities (Levin, Krainovitch, Bahrenburg, & Mitchell, 1989). A knowledge deficit is present when individuals possess inadequate or insufficient cognitive information or psychomotor skills concerning a specific topic such as a particular condition or treatment plan (Carpenito, 1995; Kim, McFarland, & McLane, 1995). Knowledge Deficit diagnoses and related interventions are appropriate for caregivers of impaired older adults as well as for older adults themselves. Teaching, the predominant intervention for Knowledge Deficit, is an interpersonal process using deliberately structured and sequenced communication to promote learning (Redman, 1993). The desired outcome of teaching for knowledge deficits is the acquisition of knowledge by the older adult (Figure 39-1).

Teaching older patients or their caregivers can be a challenging aspect of nursing practice. The potential rewarding benefits for older adults make teaching one of the most important nursing interventions for this vulnerable population.

Knowledge deficits occur when individuals experience a lack of information or a difficulty in applying information that leads to compromises in health (Cox et al., 1993). Lack of knowledge can lead to lack of primary prevention behaviors such as inadequate activity, lack of secondary prevention such as mammography participation, and lack of tertiary prevention such as prevention of skin breakdown in older adults with diabetes. Lack of knowledge can contribute to uninformed decision making or to anxiety in older adults who are unprepared for health care experiences (Fogarty, Curbow, Wingard, McDonnell, & Somerfield, 1999). Lack of knowledge can prevent caregivers from providing optimal home care to frail older adults resulting in unnecessary hospitalization or unwanted long-term care placement.

The purpose of nursing interventions for knowledge deficits among older adults is generally to increase knowledge. Increased knowledge, in turn, can contribute to increased self-care and self-management skills, improved decision-making, and decreased fears (Martin & Fitzsimons, 1989). For example, adequate knowledge can minimize stress during hospital discharge (Rendon, Davis, Gioiella, & Tranzillo, 1986). Effective teaching regarding effective self-management of chronic illnesses can contribute to reduced subsequent health care expenditures (Trautner, Richter, & Berger, 1993).

Patients and nurses both describe teaching as an important activity (Agre, Bookbinder, Cirrincione, & Keating, 1990; Cohen, Hausner, & Johnson, 1994). Older adults are the most commonly taught patients in hospitals (McGoldrick, Jablonski, & Wolf, 1994). Knowledge deficit is also common as a related factor for other diagnoses (Jenny, 1987). Knowledge deficits can be contributing factors to diagnoses such as Noncompliance, Anxiety, or Self-Care Deficit where the desired outcome is a behavior beyond acquisition of knowledge (Wetsch, Macklebust, Neil, & Chase, 1995). Although Knowledge Deficit is not always the appropriate primary diagnosis, teaching can be an appropriate activity for several diagnoses affected by lack of knowledge (Carpenito, 1995; Coenen et al., 1995; Jenny, 1987).

RELATED FACTORS/ETIOLOGIES

Several factors are related to the development of Knowledge Deficit (Cox et al., 1993; Kim, et al., 1995; McDougall, 1999):

1. Newly diagnosed health problems such as diabetes
2. Newly prescribed therapies, such as fluid restrictions associated with heart failure
3. Inexperience with psychomotor skills, such as manipulation of home glucose monitoring equipment
4. Lack of exposure to information or lack of recall of information
5. Misinterpretation of information
6. Lack of familiarity with information resources
7. Inability to use resources such as when literacy problems prevent reading information
8. Cognitive limitations that affect learning, such as those related to dementia or mental retardation
9. Lack of interest in learning

Depression, which is common among older adults, also can decrease motivation to learn, contributing to Knowledge Deficit. Previous teaching does not preclude the possibility of a knowledge deficit (Copeland-Owen et al., 1987).

Other diagnoses can be related to Knowledge Deficit, including Altered Health Maintenance and Noncompliance.

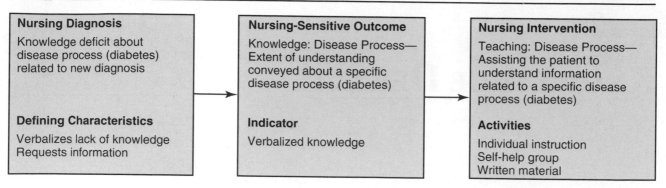

FIGURE **39-1**   Typical nursing diagnosis, outcome, and intervention for older adults.

Noncompliance can be differentiated from Knowledge Deficit in that Noncompliance reflects an informed decision, not a lack of knowledge. Powerlessness is differentiated from Knowledge Deficit by the presence of apathy. Altered Health Maintenance and Ineffective Management of Therapeutic Regimen can include knowledge deficit but are broader in scope (Cox et al., 1993; Kim et al., 1995).

ASSESSMENT

Assessment of the older adult with a knowledge deficit should address what the client already knows. The nature of the nursing assessment will vary dramatically, since the assessment will be consistent with the knowledge required for any particular patient. For example, demonstration of psychomotor skills needed to change a dressing may be assessed for one older adult, while another situation may necessitate the client verbalize signs of infection that would lead to contact with a health care provider. Developed instruments to measure knowledge have been developed for some common chronic illnesses, such as diabetes. Most often assessment uses observation of client skill and verbal questioning of client knowledge.

Assessment should also address readiness to learn (Figure 39-2). Readiness to learn is influenced by a complex constellation of factors, including intellectual capacity, development, prior life and learning experiences, illness characteristics, setting characteristics, and personal, social, and cultural characteristics (Stanton, 1985). For example, older adults with diabetes learn more when glycemic control is improved (Gradman, Laws, Thompson, & Reaven, 1993). Some settings may make learning more difficult. For example, there is some evidence that older patients have difficulty learning about medications during hospitalization (Brown, 1995). Management of anxiety might be necessary to enhance readiness to learn (Beatty & Wolf, 1996). The nurse preparing teaching strategies will need assessment information about both motivation and ability to learn (Rakel & Bulechek, 1990). Health beliefs, values, goals, and past experience influence motivation to learn (Rakel & Bulechek, 1990). Ability to learn can be affected by unmet needs such as pain, by psychologic or physiologic changes associated with attention

deficits, by problems with memory or conceptualization, or by learning disabilities (Rakel & Bulechek, 1990). Diverse memory-related impairments are common among older adults, although self-reported memory problems are not well correlated with documented difficulties (Best, Hamlett, & Davis, 1992; Durkin, Prescott, Furchtgott, Cantor, & Powell, 1995; McDougall, 1999).

Previous experiences learning health-related material should be assessed. Methods clients found particularly effective, such as involvement of the spouse or a self-help group, can then be incorporated into the current plan to both increase confidence in learning and actual learning. One especially important aspect of assessment is reading level. Almost one fifth of older adults do not read at even the fifth grade level (Doak, Doak, & Root, 1996). Tests are available to measure reading level, including the wide-range achievement test and the rapid estimate of adult literacy in medicine (REALM). Although formal tests such as these generally are not used in nursing practice, some assessment of reading ability is essential if written material will be a component of the planned teaching.

Assessment should provide the foundation for culturally appropriate care. Cultures are characterized by definitions of health, illness, and care that provide important contexts within which clients receive teaching. For example, Old Order Amish definitions of health strongly incorporate the ability to carry out work-related responsibilities (Armer & Tripp-Reimer, 1997). Teaching for Old Order Amish diagnosed with diabetes or hypertension should acknowledge the importance of work capacity as a value contributing to health decisions regarding lifestyle measures to prevent complications of these chronic illnesses.

CASE STUDY

A. Petersen is a 79-year-old woman who has lived her entire life in a small farming community where most of the residents' ancestors came from Denmark. Mrs. Petersen completed ninth grade and has raised three sons and farmed with her husband throughout her life. Mrs. Petersen's husband died several years ago, and Mrs. Petersen has remained in the family farm home. Her son,

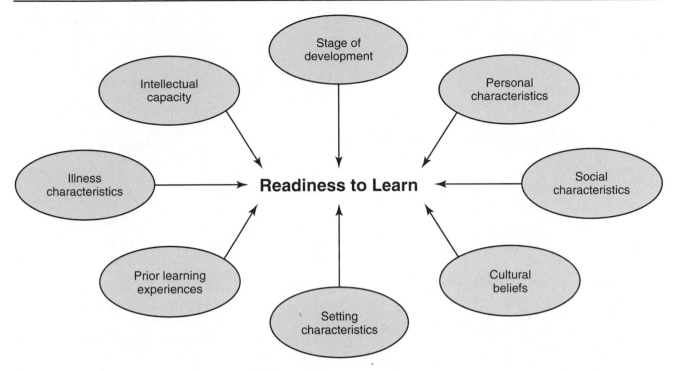

FIGURE **39-2**   Factors influencing readiness to learn.

Jens, and daughter-in-law, Marie, now run the farm and live less than one mile from Mrs. Petersen. Jens eats lunch at Mrs. Petersen's house on weekdays and picks her up for church on Sunday. Mrs. Petersen often babysits Jens' children. Mrs. Petersen has a history of mild hypertension controlled with medication, moderate knee and hip arthritis, and hearing loss partially corrected with a hearing aid. After much prompting from Jens, Mrs. Petersen visited her primary health care provider for a persisting wound on her heel. The wound began as a blister from new shoes, but has not healed over several weeks. Mrs. Petersen was diagnosed with diabetes during her care for the foot wound.

At the first visit, the nurse found that Mrs. Petersen communicated easily and had begun reading some pamphlets her primary care provider had given her. The nurse believed Mrs. Petersen was able to read, since she asked the nurse questions about how to check the bottom of her feet with her arthritic hips and knees and whether she could change the allocation of food so that her largest meal would be the lunch with Jens. Mrs. Petersen said her goals were to heal the wound, to continue to cook lunches for her son, and to continue occasional babysitting for her grandchildren. Mrs. Petersen's main concern was that diabetes not interfere with her current pattern of living.

NURSING DIAGNOSIS

Verbalized statements reflecting a lack of knowledge are the most commonly documented characteristics of the North American Nursing Diagnosis Association (NANDA) diag-

nosis Knowledge Deficit (Copeland-Owen et al., 1987; McKeighen, Mehmert, & Dickel, 1989; Pokorny, 1985; Woodtli, 1988). NANDA (1999, p. 118) has specified the following major defining characteristics for Knowledge Deficit:

1. Verbalization of the problem
2. Inaccurate performance of test
3. Inappropriate or exaggerated behaviors
4. Inaccurate follow-through of instruction

Behavioral cues, which require nursing inference to identify knowledge deficits, have infrequently been found in nursing documentation.

Knowledge Deficit diagnoses are used inappropriately when the optimal outcome is something other than an increase in level of knowledge. Martin and Fitzsimons (1989) found that hospital-based nurses often used Knowledge Deficit as a diagnosis when the desired outcome was something other than knowledge (e.g., compliance). In these cases, knowledge deficit could be identified as a related factor to legitimize teaching, while a different diagnosis (e.g., noncompliance) was linked with an appropriate nonknowledge-related outcome.

NURSING-SENSITIVE OUTCOMES

Nursing outcomes represent the client's states, actions, or behaviors (Iowa Outcomes Project, 2000; McCloskey & Bulechek, 1994). Although outcomes can be influenced by other disciplines, knowledge deficit outcomes are strongly influenced by nursing (Iowa Intervention Project, 2000).

Important knowledge outcomes identified by the Iowa Nursing Outcomes Classification (NOC) project include the following (Iowa Outcomes Project, 2000):

- Knowledge: Diet—Extent of understanding conveyed about diet (p. 260)
- Knowledge: Disease Process—Extent of understanding conveyed about a specific disease process (p. 262)
- Knowledge: Energy Conservation—Extent of understanding conveyed about energy conservation techniques (p. 264)
- Knowledge: Health Behaviors—Extent of understanding conveyed about the promotion and protection of health (p. 268)
- Knowledge: Health Resources—Extent of understanding conveyed about health care resources (p. 271)
- Knowledge: Infection Control—Extent of understanding conveyed about prevention and control of infection (p. 275)
- Knowledge: Medication—Extent of understanding conveyed about safe use of medication (p. 279)
- Knowledge: Personal Safety—Extent of understanding conveyed about preventing unintentional injuries (p. 281)
- Knowledge: Prescribed Activity—Extent of understanding conveyed about prescribed activity and exercise (p. 289)
- Knowledge: Treatment Procedure(s)—Extent of understanding conveyed about procedure(s) required as part of a treatment regimen (p. 293)
- Knowledge: Treatment Regimen—Extent of understanding conveyed about a specific treatment regimen (p. 294)

Measurement of knowledge outcomes usually is based on client verbalization of knowledge (McGoldrick et al.,

1994; McKeighen et al., 1989; Pokorny, 1985). The nurse can assess spontaneous verbalizations from patients to determine the extent to which the outcomes have been achieved. More often, the nurse asks the patient questions that elicit responses which can be evaluated for attainment of knowledge outcomes. Often the nurse can observe the patient perform a skill, such as performing exercises for diseased joint and surrounding muscles, to infer that knowledge has been obtained. Having the patient verbalize while performing the skill provides more complete information about knowledge outcomes. Although tests are rarely used in nursing practice to determine patient knowledge level, some well-developed tests are available for selected common conditions such as diabetes (Pokorny, 1985). NOC has developed a scale for measuring extent of understanding that ranges from "none" to "exhaustive" (Table 39-1).

The timing of outcomes measurement is important. Patient outcomes of interventions for Knowledge Deficit should be measured at the time that the knowledge is needed by the patient to make an appropriate decision or perform a health care behavior. While it is more convenient to assess knowledge outcomes immediately after teaching, the retention of the knowledge until the patient needs the knowledge is more important.

NURSING INTERVENTIONS

Teaching patients is the predominant intervention for Knowledge Deficit. The purpose of teaching is to increase knowledge; often nurses teach to increase knowledge so that knowledge will lead to more effective behaviors (Lorig, 1996). Teaching is a behavioral domain intervention selected from *Nursing Interventions Classification (NIC)* (Iowa Intervention Project, 2000). Teaching supports psychosocial functioning, facilitates lifestyle behav-

Table 39-1	NOC Indicators of Extent of Understanding Conveyed About a Specific Treatment Regimen				
Indicators	**None**	**Limited**	**Moderate**	**Substantial**	**Exhaustive**
Description of rationale for treatment regimen	1	2	3	4	5
Description of self-care responsibilities for ongoing treatment	1	2	3	4	5
Description of self-care responsibilities for emergency situations	1	2	3	4	5
Description of expected effects of treatment	1	2	3	4	5
Description of prescribed diet	1	2	3	4	5
Description of prescribed medication	1	2	3	4	5
Description of prescribed activity	1	2	3	4	5
Description of prescribed exercise	1	2	3	4	5
Description of prescribed procedures	1	2	3	4	5
Performance of self-monitoring techniques	1	2	3	4	5
Performance of treatment procedure	1	2	3	4	5
Selection of foods recommended in diet	1	2	3	4	5
Other: _____ (Specify)	1	2	3	4	5

ior changes, and is initiated in response to the nursing diagnosis Knowledge Deficit. Myriad research studies, including several meta-analyses, have consistently documented the effectiveness of teaching in increasing knowledge, changing health-related behaviors, and improving physiologic outcomes such as glycemic control among those with diabetes, postoperative complications, functional ability among those with arthritis, and symptom severity and interference with activities among those with Parkinson's disease (Cargill, 1992; Devine, 1992; Glasgow et al., 1992; Hawe & Higgins, 1990; Lorig & Holman, 1993; Montgomery, Lieberman, Singh, & Fries, 1994; Mullen, Mains, & Velez, 1992). Teaching also can be an appropriate strategy for other diagnoses such as ineffective management of a therapeutic regimen related to knowledge deficit (Fujita & Dungan, 1994). According to the Iowa NIC researchers, teaching is one of the most common and most frequently used nursing interventions in diverse settings (Bulechek, McCloskey, Titler, & Denehey, 1994).

Principles of Teaching and Learning

Principles of effective teaching and learning will be briefly reviewed. The interested reader is referred to recent texts for more detailed descriptions (e.g., Doak et al. [1996] for teaching those with low literacy and Rankin and Stallings [1996], Lorig [1996] or Redman [1993] for general information about teaching). Several strategies can be used to enhance the learning process (Table 39-2). Many of these strategies, including feedback, rehearsal, reinforcement, individualization, relevance, and multiple educational

Table 39-2	Selected Principles of Teaching and Learning Appropriate for Older Adults
Principle	**Strategies**
Meet unmet patient needs.	Address comfort and safety needs before teaching.
	Address anxiety if interfering with learning.
	Ensure fatigue does not prevent learning.
Create a learning-conducive environment.	Ensure a comfortable, well-lighted space.
	Minimize distractions and noise.
Pace materials.	Slow the pace of instruction for older adults.
	Match the older adult's verbal pace.
Structure teaching.	Prepare materials in an organized format.
	Plan deliberate teaching sessions.
Provide repetition leading to learning.	Provide repetition in varied formats.
	Repeat material within sessions.
	Repeat most important information most often.
Develop associating cues.	Identify current behaviors that can be linked with new behaviors.
Associate new knowledge with existing knowledge.	Ask the learner if the new information reminds him of anything he already knows.
	Use examples from the learner's own life.
	Use analogies the learner understands.
Provide essential information only.	Determine the absolutely essential information that must be learned.
	Avoid providing interesting information that will not affect learner behavior.
Teach most important information first.	Structure teaching sessions to address the most important information at the beginning.
Teach from simple to complex.	Plan the flow of teaching material to cover easier material first.
	Provide foundational information before expecting problem-solving skills.
Summarize previous learning.	Frequently summarize the previously covered essential information during sessions, at the end of sessions, and at the beginning of subsequent sessions.
Provide feedback.	Tell the learners how they are progressing toward gaining adequate knowledge.
	Help the learner assess his own progress.
Give positive reinforcement.	Praise efforts to learn.
	Praise successful learning often.
	Encourage the learner to recognize success.
Enhance transfer of learning.	Increase the similarity of the learning and application environments.
	Teach a variety of contexts so learning is not context dependent.
Use multisensory learning.	Provide instruction in multiple senses (vision + hearing).
Use multiple educational channels.	Use varied teaching strategies (lecture + discussion + role playing).
	Provide repetition by varying educational strategies.
Encourage learner interaction with material.	Ask adjunct questions to involve the learner.
	Use discussion.
	Have the learner write something addressing the material.

channels, have been documented to enhance learning in multiple studies, include meta-analytic work (Mullen, Green, & Persinger, 1985; Mullen et al., 1992; Simons-Morton, Mullen, Mains, Tabak, & Green, 1992; Weinrich, Boyd, & Nussbaum, 1989).

Many principles of patient teaching are appropriate for older adults (Cox et al., 1993; Higgins & Ambrose, 1995; Oldaker, 1992; Redman, 1993; Rendon et al., 1986). Meeting any unmet client needs prior to initiating teaching activities is important. Attention to teaching will not occur if the client experiences unmet needs, such as pain or constipation, that dominate the client's attention. During the teaching episode the nurse should be alert for evidence of fatigue that could interfere with concentration and learning. High anxiety levels may have to be managed by relaxation or other interventions to allow learning to occur. A learning-conducive environment that is quiet, well-lighted, temperature appropriate, and free of distractions allows the learner to attend to the material. Material should be paced appropriately for the individual client to increase comprehension and learning. Studies have generally found that structured teaching is more effective than unstructured teaching (Opdycke, Ascione, Shimp, & Rosen, 1992).

Repetition is a very important teaching principle. Repetition can be accomplished by providing appropriate written material to follow up personal instruction. Repetition in different formats can also be effective (Young, Aram, Seif, McManus, & Williams, 1999). Rehearsing behavior can provide a realistic repetition experience. Decreasing the time between learning and applying the learning increases the likelihood of recall and provides a reinforcing opportunity. Feedback about learning provides learners with information about their learning. Positive reinforcement should be used liberally to reinforce learning, enhance learning self-confidence, and contribute to a positive attitude toward learning.

Moving information into long-term memory requires that the new information be associated with some old knowledge and integrated into memory. Associating the new information with previous knowledge, such as by asking the learner if the new material reminds her of anything, can enhance learning. Teaching examples that are related to the individual's own life is helpful because they add realism to the learning and enhance long-term memory. Recall may also be increased by helping the learner develop a system of *associated cues,* such as taking medications with meals.

Presenting only crucial information is the best strategy to prevent overwhelming the learner. Older adults learn more when provided small amounts of specific information than when provided with larger amounts of information (Ascione & Shimp, 1984). Teaching should focus on client behaviors that are necessary to promote health and well-being. The first-taught information is best remembered. Teaching sessions should begin and end with the

most crucial information. Generally teaching should proceed from simple to complex. Confidence gained from learning simple material can increase attention to more complex information. Summarizing previous learning is an important strategy to reinforce what is known, to build on previous knowledge, and to help the client organize the knowledge in long-term memory.

Transfer of learning is most likely to occur when the application context is similar to the learning context. Transfer can also be enhanced by practicing the material in a variety of contexts so the information is not stored in long-term memory in close association with just one context. Multi-sensory teaching, that which stimulates as many senses as possible (e.g., both hearing and vision), enhances learning. Multiple educational channels, such as individual instruction plus a small group experience, also enhance learning (Champion, 1995). Common useful channels of education include didactic presentations to individuals or groups (lecture style), demonstrations, discussions, simulations or games, case studies-problems, and role-playing. The interaction of the learner with the material enhances learning. Some strategies for learner interaction include having the learner rephrase the information, having the learner solve problems, having the learner fill in the blanks with the information, and engaging the learner in a discussion about the information. Adjunct questions to the learner, such as asking clients to restate information in their own words, provides repetition, personalizes the information, and allows the teacher to evaluate learning.

Nursing Interventions for Learning Challenges Encountered by Older Adults

Teaching older adults requires individualizing the teaching process to compensate for any impairments the older adult might experience. As with all teaching situations, the interpersonal relationship between nurse and older client should be characterized by respect, acceptance, and patience. Nursing interventions related to teaching older adults should be conveyed with an optimistic attitude, expecting the older client to learn (Rendon et al., 1986). Individualization is important, since standardized programs might not be as effective for older adults as for younger adults (Brown, 1992).

Sensory changes typically require some modification of teaching efforts and materials (Kline & Scialfa, 1996) (Table 39-3). Presenting material to multiple senses has been found to be well received by older adults and can compensate for some sensory deficits (Theis & Merritt, 1994). An often overlooked intervention is to clean the older adult's glasses to improve vision. Large fonts and high-contrast materials should be used. Soft light will reduce glare; high wattage will help compensate for pupil size changes. When color-coding materials for older adults, blues and greens should be avoided, since yellow-

Table 39-3	Strategies to Promote Learning Among Older Adults With Vision and Hearing Problems
Sensory Problem	**Teaching Strategies**
Vision changes including: • Reduced acuity • Increased glare • Decreased pupil size • Yellowing of lens	Ensure glasses are clean. Use large, simple font type. Use high-contrast materials (avoid pastels). Use soft light with high wattage. Avoid blues and greens for color-coding. Present material in multiple sensory modes.
Hearing changes from presbycusis	Speak slowly and clearly. Face the older adult. Do not raise the pitch of your voice. Eliminate background noise. Provide visual cues such as gestures. Ensure that assistive device is operating.

Table 39-4	Tactics to Enhance Learning Among Older Adults With Cognitive Changes or Problems
Cognitive Problem	**Strategies**
Limited attention to learning activity	Vary the format within sessions. Ask questions often. Actively involve the learner in any manner.
Memory problems	Repetition, repetition, repetition. Design cues to stimulate recall. Ask questions frequently. Provide an organizational scheme for material. Integrate new information with previous knowledge. Encourage the use of mental pictures along with words. Use understandable analogies.
Concrete thinking tendencies	Use specifics instead of generalizations. Explain the characteristics of any concepts that must be used. Provide diverse examples of concepts.
Slowed processing of information	Reduce pace of teaching. Allow more time for responses.

ing of the lens with advanced age alters perception of these colors (Ekstrom, 1993). Speaking slowly and clearly can enhance communication with the hearing impaired. Facing the older adult allows for lipreading. Raising voice volume generally is contraindicated. Most people raise the pitch of their voice when they speak more loudly, making hearing even more difficult for older adults. Ensuring a quiet environment is essential if hearing problems are present. Visual aids can be helpful to reinforce verbal teaching. The teacher can write key words while presenting material to assist the hearing-impaired older adult.

Culture significantly influences the teaching of the older adult. Cultures set expectations of how people will perform with increasing age. These cultural expectations can influence the elder's readiness to learn new skills and information, and will likely influence the role of the family in supporting the acquisition of the new knowledge and concomitant life changes. Understanding these behavioral influences is a first step in appropriate education for the aged client. Therefore cultural assessment is an integral part of patient assessment and patient education (Tripp-Reimer & Afifi, 1989; Tripp-Reimer, Brink, & Saunders, 1984; Tripp-Reimer, Johnson, & Rios, 1995). It is important to maintain elders' cultural heritage and beliefs while maximizing their health and independence. This is particularly crucial in planning elder care because ethnic elders often are the stronghold of traditional values, beliefs, and practices. Consider the older person's folk beliefs and behaviors throughout the nursing process. Although the potential exists for conflict between folk medicines and scientific health care, research shows that folk remedies can

be pharmacologically appropriate (Tripp-Reimer & Martin, 1983) and complementary to scientific treatment in providing holistic health care (Bomar, 1989). Cultural differences should be acknowledged for the richness and diversity they provide (Bomar, 1989). Noninterference in clients' non-harmful health behaviors is crucial (Wenger, 1991). Family members should be included as strong actual or potential resources in the educational process.

Cognitive changes of multiple varieties and extents, especially memory problems, are not universal, but are common among older adults. Several principles of learning and specific strategies for those with cognitive changes can help these older adults learn (Table 39-4). Attention deficit can be addressed by asking questions, by varying the format of the teaching session, and by shifting the focus between learner and teacher. Participatory activities enhance attention (Keller, 1987). Repetition can overcome many memory problems. Repetition is especially valuable, since older adults can require more exposures to information for learning to occur (Durkin et al., 1995). Older adults often cannot remember the five to seven items that typical younger adults can remember. The nurse can compensate for short-term memory deficits by having older adults learn and pass into long-term memory fewer pieces of information before proceeding to the next content. Providing visual or written cues can assist with recall. For example, placing a note on the bathroom mirror might help an older man remember to take medication while shaving.

If the older adult exhibits memory problems, questions should be asked frequently during the teaching process to determine the extent and nature of learning (McDougall, 1999). Older adults with memory problems might need organizers supplied by the teacher to enhance the likelihood of recall. The organization of material for older adults is crucial, since age-associated decreases in the capacity to use strategies for organizing material are common (Beatty & Wolf, 1996). Older adults do prefer well-organized and structured learning experiences (Theis & Merritt, 1994). Integrating new content with previous knowledge improves retention, perhaps because it takes advantage of the stronger crystallized intelligence of older adults (Theis, 1991). Older adults have been found to learn more if the teaching is based on previous knowledge (Theis & Merritt, 1994). Using analogies in teaching can also take advantage of older adults' previous knowledge.

Older adults tend to be concrete thinkers and have some difficulty forming concepts. The teacher can explicitly label constructs and provide diverse examples to help these persons grasp conceptual material. Careful pacing of material can be helpful if slowed processing of information is apparent. A good strategy is to observe the individual's own pace of speaking and attempt to match that pace.

Encouraging older adults to form mental images can improve learning. The mental images provide more potential features for retrieval purposes when the individual needs to remember the information.

Motivation can be enhanced by contracting with clients (Figure 39-3). Contracts or mutually established goals increase the probability that the learning is meeting the learner's needs and fully incorporating the learner into the learning process (Cox et al., 1993; Rendon et al., 1986). Explicitly identifying the meaning of the material to that individual increases motivation to learn. Older adults process more deeply information that is meaningful and relevant. Motivation is also enhanced if the teaching focuses clearly on behaviors that will increase quality of life and meet the individual's goals (Rausch & Turkoski, 1999). For example, if the older adult with arthritis highly values time with extended family, teaching could be framed as contributing to maintaining mobility to visit family. Providing meaningful choices in the learning process will also enhance motivation (Keller, 1987). Of course, the nurse should model enthusiasm about learning.

Lack of confidence in the older adult who believes he is experiencing significant memory problems can hamper attempts to learn. Confidence can be enhanced by promoting success. Initial teaching should focus on the most easily learned material with frequent and explicit observations about the older adult's success in learning material. Breaking a large mass of information into more manageable pieces can also increase the belief that one can learn the material. Confidence will also be enhanced by the learner observing others who have learned successfully. The nurse's attitude toward the older adult as a competent learner can also enhance confidence (Keller, 1987).

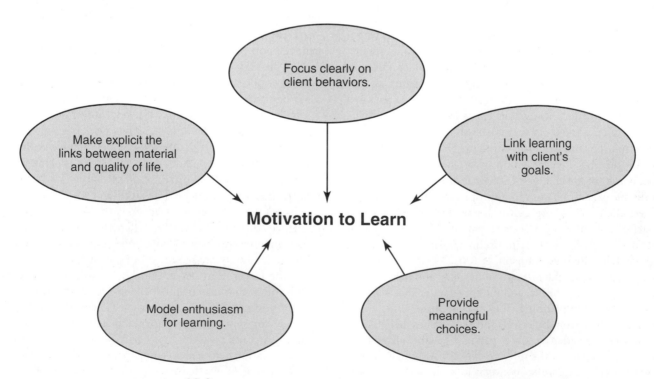

FIGURE 39-3   Strategies to enhance motivation to learn among older adults.

Problem-solving strategies among older adults tend to be based on previous experience solving problems. Older adults rely on experiential knowledge and previously practiced problem-solving procedures to solve new problems (Willis, 1996). This requires careful questioning of the learner to understand his problem-solving tactics and, ideally, teaching the new material such that it can be used with these previously learned problem-solving strategies.

Due to slowed processing of information and response time, nurses might need to spend more time conducting teaching with older adults (Clarkin, 1991; Smith, 1996). Self-paced or slowly paced information has been associated with greater learning (Kim & Grier, 1981).

Life events can interfere with learning. The older adult grieving the loss of a companion may require special or delayed teaching (Clarkin, 1991).

Fatigue can interfere with learning. Older adults experiencing sleep disturbances can develop fatigue during teaching. Teaching episodes might need to be spaced to manage fatigue.

Low literacy levels are a common problem in teaching older adults. Diverse studies reveal that many patients do not understand health care terms (Reid et al., 1994; Spees, 1991; Streiff, 1986). For example, Reid et al. (1995) found that patients with previously diagnosed chronic health problems such as diabetes recalled less than 10% of the ideas presented in a pamphlet. Another study found that 10% of pamphlets given to older adults with diabetes were as difficult to read as the *British Medical Journal* (Petterson, Dornan, Albert, & Lee, 1994). Even the material accompanying common over-the-counter medications is typically above the reading level of most older adults (Redman, 1993). Older adults who struggle to read a sentence might not be able to remember the beginning of the sentence by the time they read the end. The following strategies are appropriate for teaching older adults with low literacy (Doak et al., 1996; Hussey, 1994):

1. Use visual materials that do not require reading. For example, Hussey (1994) found medication compliance increased among low-literacy older adults when a color-coded medication schedule was used.
2. Use the most common words possible.
3. Use short sentences.
4. Use examples liberally.
5. Involve significant others in learning experiences.

Low literacy is associated with several learning difficulties besides the obvious problem of reading (Doak et al., 1996):

1. Difficulty processing images and symbols
2. Tendency to take instructions literally without being able to interpret them differently in new situations
3. Tendency to think in terms of specifics and difficulty thinking in terms of concepts
4. Limited vocabulary

5. Hesitancy about asking questions for fear of appearing unintelligent
6. Difficulty understanding graphs

Older adults with low literacy represent major teaching challenges for nurses. Well-planned and carefully executed teaching interventions can be successful in most of these challenging situations.

Diverse Strategies to Enhance Learning Among Older Adults

Advancing technologic developments provide attractive alternatives for teaching some older adults. Rippey et al. (1987) found that older adults acquired information about osteoarthritis successfully using a computer-based course, changed their health behaviors appropriately, and reported decreased pain. Computers can be tireless and patient teachers. They make possible work at an individual pace, user privacy, and unlimited review of material. They can use graphics to enhance visual stimulation, stimulate learning through questions, and provide feedback to learner and teacher (Bensen et al., 1999; Luker & Caress, 1992). Programs can incorporate age-appropriate pacing, timing, color, and animations (Rippey et al., 1987). Although not all older patients are good candidates for computer-based teaching, this alternative will be appropriate for some older adults. Even inexpensive mail-delivered educational interventions have been found effective in improving important health outcomes (Montgomery et al., 1994). Video materials can be useful for older adults. Video material should include slowly paced speech, full-face view of speakers to allow lip-reading, lack of background noise such as music, and use of realistic models of older adults. Teaching programs developed by nurses can sometimes effectively be delivered by indigenous or lay worker (Lorig & Holman, 1993). Since older adults are a very heterogeneous group, modes of delivery of teaching interventions must be individually evaluated for potential effectiveness based on the characteristics of individual learners.

Selecting and Preparing Written Materials for Teaching Older Adults

The provision of written materials can enhance learning. The selection or creation of these materials determines their potential effectiveness for older adults. There are several attributes the nurse should examine when selecting materials (Doak et al., 1996; Ekstrom, 1993; Estey, Musseau, & Keehn, 1994; Higgins & Ambrose, 1995; Petterson et al., 1994; Redman, 1993; Weinrich & Boyd, 1992):

1. Are the materials legible? Many prepared educational materials are not legible for older adults because the font size is too small. A font size of 12 to 16 points is

minimal. Photocopy-enlarging small type might not result in readable material, since some letters appear distorted when enlarged. Plain font faces should be used, since more decorative fonts (e.g., Script) are more difficult to read. Both capital and lowercase letters should be used, since all caps are difficult to read. The paper should be good quality, low-gloss paper, and the text should be in high contrast to the background.

2. Are pictures age appropriate and in high contrast? Line drawings might be more helpful, since superfluous detail can be removed.

3. Is the text readable? The grade level should not be higher than fifth grade, as even at this level significant numbers of older adults will not be able to read the material. Sentences should be short. Lists should be used instead of long sentences with clauses. The author should use an active voice. Vertical type should not be used.

4. Is the content understandable to most older adults? The material should be literal with as few concepts as possible. Specifics should predominate over generalizations. Visual cues, such as bolding or bullets, should help the older adult understand the material.

5. Is the content appropriate to the cultural context? Be aware of cultural beliefs, practices, and behaviors in lifestyle areas related to the teaching focus. Use familiar language and props to support teaching.

6. Does the material follow the principles of good teaching? Look for organization, simple-to-complex flow, repetition, etc.

Other Interventions for Knowledge Deficit

Some other interventions identified in NIC can be helpful for the older adult with knowledge deficits. For example, counseling has been combined effectively with teaching to deal jointly with information and support needs and to promote rehabilitation (Banks, 1992). Common counseling strategies identified in NIC such as active listening, questioning, providing information or feedback, and clarifying can be combined with teaching (Banks, 1992; Iowa Intervention Project, 2000). Another intervention strategy identified by NIC that could be useful is Support Group (Iowa Intervention Project, 2000). Support Group can be an appropriate intervention to deal with emotional issues that must be addressed to enhance readiness to learn (Kinney, Mannetter, & Carpenter, 1992). Support groups also can provide a setting for repetition and reinforcement of learning. Reminiscence can be a useful adjunct to help the older client deal with crisis or loss so that readiness to learn is enhanced (Hamilton, 1992). Interventions to address anxiety might be necessary to promote an optimal emotional state for teaching and learning to occur. NIC-identified anxiety reduction activities include using a calm and reassuring approach, encouraging verbalization of feelings and perceptions, or helping the older adult iden-

tify situations that precipitate anxiety (Iowa Intervention Project, 2000). Values Clarification (Wilberding, 1992) can help older adults set goals that include learning. Values Clarification, as described by NIC, helps clients see more clearly their values and the consequences of their actions, which is sometimes necessary to effect behavior change or readiness to learn (Craven & Hirnle, 1992).

CASE STUDY

The nursing diagnosis specified for Mrs. Petersen was Knowledge Deficit related to a newly diagnosed health problem. The newly diagnosed health problem was accompanied by newly prescribed therapies and inexperience with psychomotor skills (wound management and home glucose monitoring).

The nurse planned a multiple approach teaching program for Mrs. Petersen. Mrs. Petersen and the nurse agreed that a major goal would be to plan meals that would continue to foster the daily lunches between Mrs. Petersen and Jens, her son. Mrs. Petersen received several home visits from a nurse, spaced about every 3 days, to provide basic teaching about diabetes and wound management. At each visit the nurse inquired about the functioning of the patient's hearing aid and turned off the radio prior to initiating teaching. The nurse sat across the kitchen table from Mrs. Petersen in the well-lighted and comfortable kitchen with visual materials on the table. These teaching sessions included nurse-provided content using a book of pictures about diabetes and its management, demonstrations by the nurse (wound dressing, home glucose monitoring, etc.), and repeat demonstrations by Mrs. Petersen. The nurse asked frequent questions to maintain attention, involved Mrs. Petersen in active learning, assessed progress, and provided feedback. The nurse left large print material that repeated the material covered. At each return visit the nurse summarized the most crucial information from previous sessions before proceeding with new material. After the first visit the nurse observed Mrs. Petersen performing the wound care. The nurse had Mrs. Petersen prepare daily meal plans to apply her knowledge of appropriate diet. The nurse suggested that Mrs. Petersen consider joining a self-help group about 50 miles from her home. However, Mrs. Petersen did not drive after dark and declined the suggestion. The nurse convinced Mrs. Petersen to ask Jens about driving her to the meetings. Jens was able to take Mrs. Petersen to the meetings once a month, where she had the opportunity to reinforce previous learning and learn new problem-solving strategies.

Outcomes were assessed constantly as the visits occurred. The nurse asked Mrs. Petersen many questions and presented her with problem situations (such as eating at a friend's house with particular foods served) to assess her knowledge level. At her last visit the nurse watched Mrs. Petersen perform wound care, complete a blood glucose reading, and plan a week's menu. The nurse measured the knowledge outcome by observing the behavior while asking Mrs. Petersen to explain her thinking, thereby validating the knowledge acquisition. The nurse encountered Mrs. Petersen a couple years later at a church bazaar in a nearby town. Mrs. Petersen reported no subsequent wounds, continued lunches with her son, and had "good blood sugars" when checked about once a week.

SUMMARY

Knowledge deficits among older adults can hamper independence, interfere with the effectiveness of prescribed therapies, or contribute to premature long-term care placement. Teaching older adults can be one of the most challenging and rewarding nursing interventions. Carefully planned and executed teaching can enhance the quality and quantity of life for older adults.

The NIC descriptions of teaching emphasize teaching different types of content (e.g., disease process or medication) and include some teaching strategies under teaching groups, teaching individuals, and teaching psychomotor skills (Iowa Intervention Project, 2000). Many of the specific activities listed in NIC for teaching individuals are especially important for teaching older adults, such as appraising the patient's educational level, selecting appropriate teaching methods or strategies, and selecting appropriate educational materials. Teaching is an extremely complex activity, as evidenced by the many books on patient teaching. When the learner is an older adult, the level of complexity is further enhanced. While the NIC activities lack specificity for teaching older adults, that specificity is probably beyond the scope of a parsimonious classification scheme. The knowledge outcomes specified by NOC address the major dimensions of nursing-sensitive outcomes that would be expected for teaching (Iowa Outcomes Project, 2000). The congruence between the diagnosis, the NIC interventions, and the NOC outcomes provides clear evidence of the goal-directed nature of nursing care for older adults experiencing Knowledge Deficit.

REFERENCES

Agre, P., Bookbinder, M., Cirrincione, C., & Keating, E. (1990). How much time do nurses spend teaching cancer patients. *Patient Education & Counseling, 16*, 29-38.

Armer, J., & Tripp-Reimer, T. (1997). Definition of health and health promotional behaviors among midwestern Amish families. Paper presentation. Gerontological Society of America Annual Conference.

Ascione, F., & Shimp, L. (1984). The effectiveness of four education strategies in the elderly. *Geriatrics & Gerontology, 18*, 926-931.

Banks, L. (1992). Counseling. In G. Bulechek & J. McCloskey (Eds.), *Nursing interventions: Essential nursing treatments* (2nd ed., pp. 279-290). Philadelphia: W. B. Saunders.

Beatty, P., & Wolf, M. (1996). *Connecting with older adults: Educational responses and approaches*. Malabar, FL: Krieger Publishing.

Bensen, C., Stern, J., Skinner, E., Beutner, K., Conant, M., Tyring, S., Reitano, M., Davis, G., & Wald, A. (1999). An interactive, computer-based program to educate patients about genital herpes. *Sexually Transmitted Diseases, 26*(6), 364-368.

Best, D., Hamlett, K., & Davis, S. (1992). Memory complaint and memory performance in the elderly: The effects of memory-skills training and expectancy change. *Applied Cognitive Psychology, 6*, 405-416.

Bomar, P. (1989). *Nurse and family health promotion: Concepts, assessment, and interventions*. Philadelphia: W. B. Saunders.

Brown, D. (1995). Hospital discharge preparation for homeward bound elderly. *Clinical Nursing Research, 4*, 181-194.

Brown, S. (1992). Meta-analysis of diabetes patient education research: Variations in intervention effects across studies. *Research in Nursing & Health, 15*, 409-419.

Bulechek, G., McCloskey, J., Titler, M., & Denehey, J. (1994, October). Nursing interventions used in practice. *American Journal of Nursing*, 59-64.

Cargill, J. (1992). Medication compliance in elderly people: Influencing variables and interventions. *Journal of Advanced Nursing, 17*, 422-426.

Carpenito, L. (1995). *Nursing diagnosis: Application to clinical practice* (6th ed.). Baltimore: Lippincott Williams & Wilkins.

Champion, V. (1995). Results of a nurse-delivered intervention on proficiency and nodule detection with breast self-examination. *Oncology Nursing Forum, 22*(5), 819-824.

Clarkin, C. (1991). Knowledge deficit. In F. F. Rogers-Seidl (Ed.), *Geriatric nursing care plans* (pp. 48-50). St. Louis, MO: Mosby.

Coenen, A., Ryan, P., Devine, E., Werley, H., Sutton, J., & Kelber, S. (1995). Use of the nursing minimum data set to describe nursing interventions for select nursing diagnoses in an acute care setting. In M. Rantz & P. LeMone (Eds.), *Classification of nursing diagnoses: Proceedings of the eleventh conference* (pp. 131-132). Glendale, CA: Cinahl Information Systems.

Cohen, M., Hausner, J., & Johnson, M. (1994). Knowledge and presence: Accountability as described by nurses and surgical patients. *Journal of Professional Nursing, 10*, 177-185.

Copeland-Owen, S., diBenedetto, T., Furney, G., Gosnell, D., Horst, M., Keely-Knox, S., Marcello, M., Morgenstern-Stanovich, M., & Pontius, C. (1987). Validation of the nursing diagnosis knowledge deficit: Restorative measures. In A. McLane (Ed.), *Classification of nursing diagnosis: Proceedings of the seventh national conference*. St. Louis, MO: Mosby.

Cox, H., Hinz, M., Lubno, M., Newfield, S., Ridenour, N., McCarthy-Slater, M., & Sridaromont, K. (1993). *Clinical applications of nursing diagnosis*. Philadelphia: F. A. Davis.

Craven, R., & Hirnle, C. (1992). *Fundamentals of nursing: Human health and function*. Baltimore: Lippincott Williams & Wilkins.

Devine, E. (1992). Effects of psychoeducational care for adult surgical patients: A meta-analysis of 191 studies. *Patient Education & Counseling, 19*, 129-142.

Doak, C., Doak, L., & Root, J. (1996). *Teaching patients with low literacy skills* (2nd ed.). Baltimore: Lippincott Williams & Wilkins.

Durkin, M., Prescott, L., Furchtgott, E., Cantor, J., & Powell, D. (1995). Performance but not acquisition of skill learning is severely impaired in the elderly. *Archives of Gerontology & Geriatrics, 20*, 167-183.

Ekstrom, I. (1993). Printed materials for an aging population; Design considerations. *Journal of Biocommunication, 20*, 25-30.

Estey, A., Musseau, A., & Keehn, L. (1994). Patient's understanding of health information: A multihospital comparison. *Patient Education & Counseling, 24*, 73-78.

Fogarty, L. A., Curbow, B. A., Wingard, J. R., McDonnell, K., & Somerfield, M. R. (1999). Can 40 seconds of compassion reduce patient anxiety? *Journal of Clinical Oncology, 17*(1), 371-379.

Fujita, L., & Dungan, J. (1994). High risk for ineffective management of therapeutic regimen: A protocol study. *Rehabilitation Nursing, 19,* 75-79.

Glasgow, R., Toobert, D., Hampson, S., Brown, J., Lewinsohn, P., & Donnelly, J. (1992). Improving self-care among older patients with type II diabetes: The "sixty something . . ." study. *Patient Education & Counseling, 19,* 61-74.

Gradman, T., Laws, A., Thompson, L., & Reaven, G. (1993). Verbal learning and/or memory improves with glycemic control in older subjects with non-insulin-dependent diabetes mellitus. *Journal of Geriatric Psychiatry & Neurology, 41,* 1305-1312.

Hamilton, D. (1992). Reminiscence therapy. In G. Bulechek & J. McCloskey (Eds.), *Nursing interventions: Essential nursing treatments* (2nd ed., pp. 292-303). Philadelphia: W. B. Saunders.

Hawe, P., & Higgins, G. (1990). Can medication education improve the drug compliance of the elderly? Evaluation of an in hospital program. *Patient Education & Counseling, 16,* 151-160.

Higgins, L., & Ambrose, P. (1995). The effect of adjunct questions on older adults' recall of information from a patient education booklet. *Patient Education & Counseling, 23,* 41-47.

Hussey, L. (1994). Minimizing effects of low literacy on medication knowledge and compliance among the elderly. *Clinical Nursing Research, 3,* 132-145.

Iowa Intervention Project. J. C. McCloskey & G. M. Bulechek (Eds.). (2000). *Nursing interventions classification (NIC)* (3rd ed.). St. Louis, MO: Mosby.

Iowa Outcomes Project. M. Johnson, M. Maas, & S. Moorhead (Eds.). (2000). *Nursing outcomes classification (NOC)* (2nd ed.). St. Louis, MO: Mosby.

Jenny, J. (1987). Knowledge deficit: Not a nursing diagnosis. *IMAGE: Journal of Nursing Scholarship, 19,* 184-185.

Keller, J. (1987). Development and use of the ARCS model of instructional design. *Journal of Instructional Development, 10*(3), 2-10.

Kim, K., & Grier, M. (1981). Pacing effects of medication instruction for the elderly. *Journal of Gerontological Nursing, 7,* 464-468.

Kim, M., McFarland, G., & McLane, A. (Eds.). (1995). *Pocket guide to nursing diagnoses* (6th ed.). St Louis, MO: Mosby.

Kinney, C., Mannetter, R., & Carpenter, M. (1992). Support groups. In G. Bulechek & J. McCloskey (Eds.), *Nursing interventions: Essential nursing treatments* (2nd ed., pp. 326-339). Philadelphia: W. B. Saunders.

Kline, D., & Scialfa, C. (1996). Visual and auditory aging. In J. Birren & K. Schaie (Eds.), *Handbook of the psychology of aging* (4th ed., pp. 181-202). San Diego, CA: Academic Press.

Levin, R. F., Krainovitch, B. C., Bahrenburg, E., & Mitchell, C. A. (1989). Diagnostic content validity of nursing diagnoses. *IMAGE: The Journal of Nursing Scholarship, 21,* 40-44.

Lorig, K. (1996). *Patient education: A practice approach* (2nd ed.). Thousand Oaks, CA: Sage.

Lorig, K., & Holman, H. (1993). Arthritis self-management studies: A twelve year review. *Health Education Quarterly, 20,* 17-28.

Luker, K., & Caress, A. (1992). Evaluating computer assisted learning for renal patients. *International Journal of Nursing Studies, 29,* 237-250.

Martin, P., & Fitzsimons, P. (1989). The use of knowledge deficit as a nursing diagnosis made by RNs. In R. Carroll-Johnson (Ed.), *Classification of nursing diagnosis: Proceedings of the eighth conference* (pp. 364-367). Baltimore: Lippincott Williams & Wilkins.

McCloskey, J., & Bulechek, G. (1994). Classification of nursing interventions: Implications for nursing diagnosis. In R. Carroll-Johnson & M. Paquette (Eds.). *Classification of nursing diagnosis: Proceedings of the tenth conference* (pp. 113-125). Baltimore: Lippincott Williams & Wilkins.

McDougall, G. J. (1999). Cognitive interventions among older adults. *Annual Review of Nursing Research, 17,* 219-240.

McGoldrick, T., Jablonski, R., & Wolf, Z. (1994). Needs assessment for a patient education program in a nursing department. A delphi approach. *Journal of Nursing Staff Development, 10,* 123-130.

McKeighen, R., Mehmert, P., & Dickel, C. (1989). Validation of nursing diagnosis knowledge deficit. In R. Carroll-Johnson (Ed.), *Classification of nursing diagnosis: Proceedings of the eighth conference* (pp. 359-363). Baltimore: Lippincott Williams & Wilkins.

Montgomery, E., Lieberman, A., Singh, G., & Fries, J. (1994). Patient education and health promotion can be effective in Parkinson's disease: A randomized controlled trial. Propath Advisory Board. *American Journal of Medicine, 97,* 429-435.

Mullen, P., Green, L., & Persinger, G. (1985). Clinical trials of patient education for chronic conditions: A comparative meta-analysis of intervention types. *Preventive Medicine, 14,* 753-781.

Mullen, P., Mains, D., & Velez, R. (1992). A meta-analysis of controlled trials of cardiac patient education. *Patient Education & Counseling, 19,* 143-162.

North American Nursing Diagnosis Association. (1999). *Nursing diagnoses: Definitions & classification 1999-2000.* Philadelphia: Author.

Oldaker, S. (1992). Live and learn: Patient education for the elderly orthopedic client. *Orthopedic Nursing, 11,* 51-56.

Opdycke, R., Ascione, F., Shimp, L., & Rosen, R. (1992). A systematic approach to educating elderly patients about their medications. *Patient Education & Counseling, 19,* 43-60.

Petterson, T., Dornan, T., Albert, T., & Lee, P. (1994). Are information leaflets given to elderly people with diabetes easy to read? *Diabetic Medicine, 11,* 111-113.

Pokorny, B. (1985). Validating a diagnostic label: Knowledge deficits. *Nursing Clinics of North America, 20,* 641-655.

Rakel, B., & Bulechek, G. (1990). Development of alterations in learning: Situational learning disabilities. *Nursing Diagnosis, 1,* 134-146.

Rankin, S., & Stallings, K. (1996). *Patient education: Issues, principles, practices.* Baltimore: Lippincott Williams & Wilkins.

Rausch, M., & Turkoski, B. (1999). Developing realistic treatment standards in today's economic climate: Stroke survivor education. *Journal of Advanced Nursing, 30,* 329-334.

Redman, B. (1993). *The process of patient education* (7th ed.). St. Louis, MO: Mosby.

Reid, J., Klachko, D., Kardash, C., Robinson, R., Scholes, R., & Howard, D. (1995). Why people don't learn from diabetes literature: Influence of text and reader characteristics. *Patient Education & Counseling, 25,* 31-38.

Reid, J., Ringenberg, Q., Kardash, C., Robinson, R., Scholes, R., & Kunz, C. (1994). Why are some pamphlets hard for patients to read? *Missouri Medicine, 91,* 589-592.

Rendon, D., Davis, K., Gioiella, E., & Tranzillo, M. (1986). The right to know: The right to be taught . . . the elderly client. *Journal of Gerontological Nursing, 12,* 33-38.

Rippey, R., Bill, D., Abeles, M., Day, J., Downing, D., Pfeiffer, C., Thal, S., & Wetsone, S. (1987). Computer-based patient education for older persons with osteoarthritis. *Arthritis and Rheumatism,* 932-935.

Simons-Morton, D., Mullen, P., Mains, D., Tabak, E., & Green, L. (1992). Characteristics of controlled studies of patient education and counseling for preventive health behaviors. *Patient Education & Counseling, 19,* 175-204.

Smith, A. (1996). Memory. In J. Birren & K. Schaie (Eds.), *Handbook of the psychology of aging* (4th ed., pp. 236-250). San Diego, CA: Academic Press.

Spees, C. (1991). Knowledge of medical terminology among clients and families. *IMAGE: Journal of Nursing Scholarship, 23,* 225-229.

Stanton, M. (1985). Teaching patients: Some basic lessons for nurse educators. *Nursing Management, 16,* 59-62.

Streiff, L. (1986). Can clients understand our instructions? . . . in an ambulatory care setting. *IMAGE: Journal of Nursing Scholarship, 18,* 48-52.

Theis, S., & Merritt, S. (1994). Model of learner-in-context. *Nursing & Health Care, 15,* 465-468.

Theis, S. (1991). Using previous knowledge to teach elderly clients. *Journal of Gerontological Nursing, 17,* 34-38.

Trautner, C., Richter, B., & Berger, M. (1993). Cost-effectiveness of a structured treatment and teaching program on asthma. *European Respiratory Journal, 0903,* 1485-1491.

Tripp-Reimer, T., & Afifi, L. (1989). Cross-cultural perspectives on patient teaching. *Nursing Clinics of North America, 24*(3), 613-619.

Tripp-Reimer, T., Brink, P., & Saunders, J. (1984). Cultural assessment: Content and process. *Nursing Outlook, 32*(2), 78-81.

Tripp-Reimer, T., Johnson, R., & Rios, H. (1995). Cultural dimensions in gerontological nursing. In M. Stanley & J. Baer (Eds.), *Gerontological nursing.* Philadelphia: F. A. Davis.

Tripp-Reimer, T., & Martin, M. (1983). Knowledge and use of folk remedies among ethnic aged. In G. Felton & M. Albert (Eds.), *Nursing research: A monograph for non-nurse researchers* (pp. 100-113). Iowa City, IA: The University of Iowa.

Weinrich, S., Boyd, M., & Nussbaum, J. (1989). Continuing education: Adapting strategies to teach the elderly. *Journal of Gerontological Nursing, 15,* 17-21.

Weinrich, S., & Boyd, M. (1992). Education in the elderly: Adapting and evaluating teaching tools. *Journal of Gerontological Nursing, 18,* 15-20.

Wenger, A. (1991). Culture-specific care and the old order Amish. *IMPRINT, 38,* 80-82, 84, 87.

Wetsch, P., Macklebust, J., Neil, J., & Chase, S. (1995). Knowledge deficit. In M. Rantz & P. LeMone (Eds.), *Classification of nursing diagnoses: Proceedings of the eleventh conference* (pp. 411-412). Glendale, CA: Cinahl Information Systems.

Wilberding, J. (1992). Values clarification. In G. Bulechek & J. McCloskey (Eds.), *Nursing interventions: Essential nursing treatments* (pp. 315-325). Philadelphia: W. B. Saunders.

Willis, S. (1996). Everyday problem solving. In J. Birren & K. Schaie (Eds.), *Handbook of the psychology of aging* (4th ed., pp. 287-306). San Diego, CA: Academic Press.

Woodtli, A. (1988). Identification of nursing diagnoses and defining characteristics: Two research models. *Research in Nursing & Health, 11,* 399-406.

Young, B., Aram, J., Seif, A., McManus, B., & Williams, I. P. (1999). Managing osteoporosis in older people with fracture. Patients should be given written advice about lifestyle. *British Medical Journal, 319,* 383.

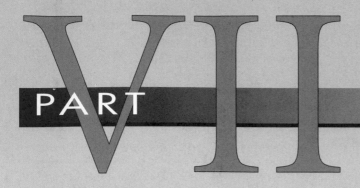

PART VII

Self-Perception–Self-Concept Pattern

OVERVIEW

In Chapter 40 Bunten discusses the multidimensional phenomenon of self-concept, which includes a person's image of his social roles and positions, body image, personality, and self-esteem. She points out that although inconsistency of research definitions and measures makes it difficult to determine conclusively whether one's self-concept is stable or changes with advancing age, the nurse may anticipate changes in the various dimensions of self-concept. She describes these changes and their impact on the older person's feelings and behavior, with special emphasis on the importance of, and difficulty in maintaining, positive self-esteem.

Depression is the most prevalent and most treatable psychiatric disorder among elders. In Chapter 41, Depression, Piven and Buckwalter provide a theoretical overview of depression in later life and suggest that nurses are in a key position to identify and treat depression based on their knowledge of mental health, physical health, and drugs used to treat illness in elders. The authors offer valuable suggestions for development of nursing diagnoses that capture the breadth of characteristics and factors associated with depression more adequately than do diagnoses in the current NANDA classification, and they emphasize the importance of nursing knowledge of biologic guidelines, psychiatric guidelines, recent clinical practice guidelines, and theories of aging for diagnosis and intervention. They advocate the development of specific nursing diagnoses based on the *DSM-IV* (APA) diagnostic criteria to improve their conceptual adequacy and, more practically, to enable nurse reimbursement. The authors describe the characteristics of depression unique to elderly individuals and review defining characteristics of the types of depression most frequently observed in older adults

using the DSM-IV: major depression, mood disorder caused by a general medical condition, adjustment disorder with depressed mood, and dysthymia. Assessment tools are presented with a recommendation for a combination of tools and multiple trials to ensure a definitive diagnosis. Using a case study, NIC interventions including cognitive, social support, and group interventions are highlighted, and somatic therapies about which the nurse must know (e.g., psychopharmacologic and electroconvulsant) are discussed. Patient goals and nursing-sensitive patient outcomes are identified from the NOC.

In Chapter 42, Body Image Disturbance, Glick discusses disruptions in the way elderly persons perceive or experience their bodies. The author views body image as a developmental process, and the chapter differentiates various aspects of that process, including body schema, body self, body fantasy, and body concept. The author presents the history of NANDA diagnoses associated with body image. Glick contrasts the broad categories of 1996 related factors with a list of specific conditions affecting older adults that may alter body image and discusses research findings and questions with respect to critical defining characteristics. Assessment is presented in terms of history-taking approaches useful with elders, and several standardized body image assessment tools are discussed. The author emphasizes the difficulty of differential diagnosis and the need to consider context, as well as the biopsychosocial aspects of body image. Using a case study, Glick discusses NIC interventions and NOC outcomes appropriate for disturbances in body image with elders.

Because of the accoutrements of aging, elderly persons are vulnerable to losses of resources and thus loss of power and control. In Chapter 43 Davidhizar and Giger examine the problem of Powerlessness in elders, reviewing defining

516

characteristics and factors related to control, grief and loss, and disability. The relationships between health behavior, powerlessness, health status, and mortality among elders are also explored. The authors identify outcomes appropriate for elders with the problem of Powerlessness, as well as common interventions and the ways in which they are likely to promote well-being, personal empowerment, and ultimately quality of life.

In Chapter 44, Anxiety and Fear, Moorhead and Brighton discuss the current state of these two historically intertwined nursing diagnoses and review their prevalence among and significance for older adults. The authors review the literature for both concepts and distinguish them from one another primarily on the basis of the person's knowledge or ignorance of the source stimulating the reaction. Fear is a reaction to a known agent, whereas anxiety is a reaction to something the person is unable to identify. Anxiety and fear assessment tools are reviewed, noting the increase in the availability and nursing use of anxiety assessment instruments since the publication of *Nursing Diagnoses and Interventions for the Elderly* (Maas, Buckwalter, & Hardy, 1991)* and the limited use of fear assessment instruments in nursing. Defining characteristics and etiologies of Anxiety and Fear that are appropriate across the life span and specific to advanced aging are presented in separate sections of the chapter, including research findings concerning the validation of defining characteristics. Many fears have been shown to concern the dependent elder. Common ones, such as fear of pain and suffering resulting from incapacitating illness; fear of

dependence; fear of loss of control; fear of abandonment, loneliness, and meaninglessness; fear of crime and victimization; fear of falling; and fear of transportation are explicated in Chapter 44. Nursing interventions aimed at anxiety and fear reduction and increased coping abilities are identified and illustrated with case studies in which the use and linkages between NANDA, NOC, and NIC are demonstrated.

In Chapter 45 Groh and Whall focus on the diagnosis Self-Esteem Disturbance. The authors analyze the concept of self-esteem and discuss research that has related self-esteem to other variables such as physical and social activity, social support, religiosity, depression, and age, concluding that depression is the variable most strongly correlated with self-esteem in older adults. Based on the literature, the authors recommend that the NANDA diagnosis Self-Esteem Disturbance be expanded to reflect a more global and comprehensive definition. Using the theoretical perspective of Roy, Groh and Whall review assessment of the critical data from which the diagnoses and probable etiologies can be inferred. Nursing interventions that restore, maintain, or promote self-esteem are described along with evaluation of desired outcomes.

In Chapter 46, Hopelessness, Farran analyzes the concept of hopelessness and explicates the NANDA diagnosis by integrating it with the four theoretical attributes of experiential process, transcendent or spiritual process, rational process, and relational process. The author suggests several instruments useful for the measurement of hopelessness, hope, depression, and suicidal intent in elders and summarizes interventions for the treatment of hopelessness associated with depression. Nursing-sensitive outcomes and nursing interventions relevant to the four attributes of hopelessness are identified and illustrated using a case study.

---

*Maas, M., Buckwalter, K. C., & Hardy, M. (Eds.) (1991). *Nursing diagnoses and interventions for the elderly*. Redwood City, CA: Addison-Wesley.

CHAPTER 40

NORMAL CHANGES WITH AGING

Donna Bunten

Human needs can be categorized as either biologic, such as hunger and thirst, or acquired through interaction with others, such as the needs for affiliation and a sense of self-worth. These needs were classified hierarchically by Maslow (1954). According to Maslow's hierarchy, physiologic needs and safety needs form a base on which other needs rest and should be met before the more complex needs for love and belonging, self-esteem, and self-actualization are addressed. These varying needs overlap, with high-level needs emerging as lower-level needs are being addressed. As nurses provide care, they are better able to understand their clients' feelings and behaviors when they consider the full spectrum of challenges to their basic needs. One of these basic needs, that of a positive self-concept, is a critical factor in maintaining physical and psychosocial well-being. The sense of self plays an important role in shaping health behaviors and outcomes and, as such, should be of primary importance to nurses (Stein, 1995).

SELF-CONCEPT

Self-concept has been defined in general terms as "the totality of the individual's thoughts and feelings that have reference to himself as an object" (*Webster's,* 1985, p. 1065). Rosenberg (1979) was more explicit, defining self-concept as the total picture or image an individual has of herself including the social roles and positions that form a part of the person's identity, body image, personality traits, and the evaluation of self known as self-esteem. Historically the terms *self-concept* and *self-esteem* have been confused and used interchangeably in much of the literature. Self-esteem is only one dimension of self-concept. Stein (1995) urges nurses to consider other dimensions of self-concept that are thought to be powerful determinants of behavior, "such as one's belief's about who one is today and expectations, fears, and wishes about what one will become in the future" (p. 187).

There is broad consensus that self-concept is multidimensional in nature, that it is a dynamic process of interaction between the individual and the environment, and that its various dimensions can be separated only for study (Bengston, Reedy, & Gordon, 1985; Binsock & George, 1990; Breytspraak, 1984). The dimensions of self-concept are thought to remain constant across age groups (Monge, 1975). In other words, the same elements compose the self for people of all ages.

The question of whether the self-concept of individuals changes with age is debatable. After conducting an extensive literature search, Bengston et al. (1985) concluded that stability and change in self-concept have both been recorded; inconsistencies in both the definition of the construct and methods of measurement have contributed to these different findings. Definition consistency of the construct of self-concept plus longitudinal and sequential data are needed before the question of whether change or stability of the concept in its totality occurs during advancing age can be answered.

It is reasonable, however, to expect some changes in the various dimensions of self-concept with aging. Kaufman (1986) noted that "the self-concept grows and changes as one continues to interpret one's environment and interactions throughout life" (p. 6). As people grow older, their interpersonal networks change, the lifelong series of entrances and exits in social groups continues, and the importance of associations changes. Separation from work or home, for example, can disrupt the older person's sense of belonging and self-concept. Elders are also presented with fewer opportunities for success and more opportunities for losses (family, friends, income), with subsequent negative consequences for their self-concepts (Freund & Smith, 1999; Hogstel, 1992). A person's image of the body is an integral part of one's concept of self. As the aging process changes the body, the image of the body can change as well. Adjustment in body image is a challenge for the older person in a society that emphasizes youth and beauty. Personality, which is also a dimension of self-concept, shows no basic change in the healthy older person (McCrae & Costa, 1982). Some characteristics of the personality may in fact become more pronounced with advancing age (Brody, 1985). A cantankerous young man may be an even more cantankerous old man; a sweet girl may be an even sweeter old woman.

The older person with a positive sense of self will feel secure throughout a wide range of experiences. The person with a positive self-concept also recognizes that he has strengths and limitations and will find it acceptable to work within the framework of those limitations (Freund & Smith, 1999). Challenges can be met as they occur and are dealt with appropriately. When a person is consistently faced with repeated failures, a negative self-concept develops. A poor self-concept leads a person to experience high anxiety, a sense of powerlessness, or inability to bring about change; maladaptive coping measures and behaviors can result (Pasquali, Arnold, DeBasie, & Alesi, 1985).

SELF-ESTEEM

Self-esteem is the evaluative dimension of self-concept or the judgment that individuals make about themselves based on feelings of being valued, useful, and competent. The self-esteem of the elderly person is challenged by ageist patterns in our society (Butler, 1975). Elders are frequently stereotyped as being universally sick, isolated, and deprived, as well as being socially inept, dependent, and nonproductive members of our society. Internalizing any or all of these negative stereotypes can erode an elder's self-esteem. Bengston et al. (1985) speculate, on the other hand, that self-esteem does not decrease for older persons who choose to emphasize positive stereotypes or for whom chronologic age is less central to their self-concept than other characteristics. Ward (1977) asked 323 noninstitutionalized volunteers aged 60 to 92 to select what age they felt themselves to be and simultaneously gathered data on self-reported feelings of self-esteem and feelings about the aged in general. He found that older persons who displayed negative attitudes toward aging and identified themselves as elders also displayed low levels of self-esteem. Positive levels of self-esteem were found in persons who still considered themselves as being middle-aged and held positive regard for the aged. Denial of old age can insulate some older persons from society's stereotypical attitudes toward the aged. It is important for nurses to understand the elderly client's perception about her age to make accurate assessments and plan interventions that will be personally acceptable and clinically appropriate for each individual. It is also important for nurses to examine their own attitudes about the aged. If they accept society's negative and illness-oriented perception of older adults, they may in turn unwittingly initiate a self-fulfilling prophecy of dependency among their older clients (Terpstra, Terpstra, Plawecki, & Struter, 1989).

The self-concept of the older person is impacted not only by changes in outward appearance, but also by diminishing vitality, increasing vulnerability for losses in physical and mental health, and the possible corresponding loss of independence. Chen (1994), for example, hypothesized that hearing loss, which is frequently associated with aging, would contribute to loneliness and a reduction in self-esteem in older adults. She found a significant correlation between hearing handicaps, loneliness, and low self-esteem. This study demonstrates that loneliness may occur even in the presence of others if communication is impaired. As elders develop increasing deficits, caregivers may take control and dignity away from them and impose their own expectations on them as well.

Ebersole and Hess (1998) noted that it must be quite difficult for the aged person to watch his self-image dissolve through the loss of independence, which is frequently associated with disabilities known to occur more frequently in the elder. If the privacy and dignity of the elder is invaded by caregivers (e.g., not using privacy curtains, entering the room without permission, treating the elder as if she was a child, or calling the elder "Dearie" instead of using a proper name), a sense of worthlessness is be reinforced. Dignity and self-esteem complement each other. Diminishment in self-esteem can lead to depression, and the elderly person can experience the feeling of having lost control over his life in these instances. Lack of control over one's life decreases self-esteem, and a perceived lack of control results in poorer adjustment, lower activity levels, and diminished physical health for older persons (Beckingham & Watt, 1995; Tallis, Fillit, & Brocklehurst, 1998). Nurses must empower older persons to discover their strengths, talents, and solutions and enhance the possibilities to meet their identified needs. Older persons must be empowered to exert control over their own lives. Collaborative decision making between clients and professionals can diminish the feeling of loss of control and increase self-esteem.

SUMMARY

Elderly persons are vulnerable to losing valued relationships. The loss of a spouse, a long-term friend or neighbor, or any relationship valued by the older person can affect that person's self-esteem. Incorporated in the concept of self-esteem is how we see ourselves as valued by others. Individuals learn about themselves from others through both verbal and nonverbal communication.

If elderly persons have been happiest when involved in many social interactions during their lifetime or happiest when retiring and inactive, these patterns will direct their expectations, their sense of satisfaction with life, and their self-esteem as they age (Birren & Schaie, 1990; Steffl, 1984). When assessing a client's needs for interaction, it is appropriate to ask about that person's interaction level at other stages of her life. The most salient level of interaction for the elderly person is highly individualized.

The factors associated with self-concept and self-esteem in older persons center around the cumulative losses experienced while aging. Multiple mental and physical assaults can lower self-esteem, which is central to the integrity of the human personality. Emotional factors and stress can precipitate physical illness, and, conversely, physical illness can trigger negative psychologic and emotional reactions. Consequently, the importance of evaluating potential problems in both spheres simultaneously is underscored. "The durability of self-esteem in later years will depend somewhat on personality, the successful negotiation of adult tasks and social integration" (Ebersole & Hess, 1998). Nurses are charged with the responsibility of recognizing the status of their elderly clients' feelings about self. They must then attempt to identify the factors that contribute to both positive and negative self-concepts and plan and initiate interventions to assist those clients whose self-concepts need enhancement.

REFERENCES

Beckingham, A. C., & Watt, S. (1995). Daring to grow old: Lessons in healthy aging and empowerment. *Educational Gerontology, 21,* 479-495.

Bengston, V., Reedy, M., & Gordon, C. (1985). Aging and self-conception: Personality processes and social context. In J. E. Birren & K. W. Schaie (Eds.), *Handbook of the psychology of aging* (2nd ed., pp. 1282-1292). New York: Van Nostrand Reinhold.

Binsock, R. H., & George, L. K. (1990). *Handbook of aging and the social sciences* (3rd ed.). San Diego, CA: Academic Press.

Birren, J. E., & Schaie, K. W. (1990). *Handbook of the psychology of aging.* San Diego, CA: Academic Press.

Breytspraak, L. M. (1984). *The development of self in later life.* Boston: Little, Brown.

Brody, E. M. (1985). *Mental and physical health practices of older people.* New York: Springer.

Butler, R. M. (1975). *Why survive? Being old in America.* New York: Harper & Row.

Chen, H. L. (1994). Hearing in the elderly: Relation of hearing loss, loneliness and self-esteem. *Journal of Gerontological Nursing, 20*(6), 22-28.

Ebersole, P., & Hess, P. (1998). *Toward healthy aging: Human needs and nursing response* (5th ed.). St. Louis, MO: Mosby.

Freund, A. M., & Smith, J. (1999). Content and function of the self-definition in old and very old age. *Journals of Gerontology. Series B, Psychological Sciences & Social Sciences, 54*(1), P55-P67.

Hogstel, M. O. (1992). *Clinical manual of gerontological nursing.* St. Louis, MO: Mosby.

Kaufman, S. R. (1986). *The ageless self.* New York: Meridian.

Maslow, A. H. (1954). *Motivation and personality.* New York: Harper & Row.

McCrae, R. R., & Costa, Jr., P. T. (1982). Self-concept and the stability of personality: Cross-sectional comparisons of self-reports and ratings. *Journal of Personality and Social Psychology, 43,* 1282-1292.

Monge, R. H. (1975). Structure of the self-concept from adolescence through old age. *Experimental Aging Research, 1,* 281-291.

Pasquali, E. A., Arnold, H. M., DeBasie, N., & Alesi, E. G. (1985). *Mental health nursing: A holistic approach* (2nd ed.). St. Louis, MO: Mosby.

Rosenberg, M. (1979). *Conceiving the self.* New York: Basic Books.

Steffl, B. M. (Ed.). (1984). *Handbook of gerontological nursing.* New York: Van Nostrand Reinhold.

Stein, K. F. (1995). Schema model of the self-concept. *IMAGE: Journal of Nursing Scholarship, 27*(3), 187-193.

Tallis, R., Fillit, H., & Brocklehurst, J. C. (Eds.). (1998). *Brocklehurst's testbook of geriatric medicine and gerontology* (5th ed.). New York: Churchill Livingstone.

Terpstra, T. L., Terpstra, T. L., Plawecki, H. M., & Struter, J. (1989). As young as you feel: Age identification among the elderly. *Journal of Gerontological Nursing, 15*(12), 4-10.

Webster's Ninth New Collegiate Dictionary. (1985). Springfield, MA: Merriam Webster.

Ward, R. (1977). The impact of subjective age and stigma on older persons. *Journal of Gerontology, 32,* 227-232.

DEPRESSION

Mary Lynn Piven and Kathleen C. Buckwalter

Depression is the most prevalent and most treatable mental disorder of later life, but often it is undiagnosed and untreated (Depression Guideline Panel, 1993). Biologic, psychologic, and social changes place older adults at high risk for the development or recurrence of depression. The consequences of unrecognized and untreated depression in elders include increased use of health care services, longer hospitalization stays, poor treatment compliance, and increased morbidity and mortality from medical illness and from suicide (Schneider & Olin, 1995). Depression has been implicated in two-thirds of all geriatric suicides (Allen & Blazer, 1991), and it is estimated that major depression costs the American economy $16 billion per year in direct costs of treatment and indirect costs from lost productivity (Depression Guideline Panel, 1993). Depressive disorder in the elder adult is associated with increased health care services (across care settings and cross culturally), increased mortality (Parmelee, Katz, & Lawton, 1992), increased pain, decreased physical, social, and role functioning, slower recovery from hip fracture (Mossey, Knott, & Craik, 1990), and increased risk for suicide (Manton, Blazer, & Woodbury, 1987) compared to those who are not depressed. The increasing population of individuals 65 and over demands improved detection and subsequent treatment in the context of scientifically based collaborative efforts by multiple disciplines.

Health care professionals, lay persons, and elders themselves often equate growing old with growing sad, disengaged, and apathetic. It is not normal to be old and sad. However, symptoms of depression are often indistinguishable from certain "expected" behaviors of growing old; therefore persistent, sensitive, and skilled observation and assessment are required to uncover masked depressive states that mimic, precede, or exist concomitantly with other organic pathologies. Depression in elders poses a significant personal and public health problem that requires skilled attention and aggressive intervention. Nurses in a variety of settings (e.g., medical hospital, long-term care, community health, psychiatric facilities) are in a critical position to identify and treat depressive conditions among elders. The nurse who understands the complex interrelationships among mental health, physical health, and the consequences of drugs commonly used to treat medical illness in elders is in a unique position to make a differential diagnosis of clinically significant depression and assist elderly clients in improving their affective state (mood). Nurses can employ a variety of interpersonal and group strategies to help alleviate depression. They also assume an important function in monitoring psychotropic and other medications that may precipitate adverse side effects or cause depression.

RELATED FACTORS/ETIOLOGIES

Current understanding of the etiology of depression suggests that there may be numerous independent or interacting psychologic and biologic factors. There is no single theory that best characterizes the occurrence of depression in late life. It is likely that, throughout life, depression represents a class of disorders with multiple causal pathways.

Psychologic Theories

Cognitive Theory. Beck et al. (1979) hypothesized that cognitive styles and distortions contribute to the development of depression. This cognitive model suggests that early life experiences create the foundation for the development of negative thought patterns and that depression is the consequence of viewing the self, the world, and the future in a negative manner (cognitive triad). The three main concepts in this theory of depression include (1) the cognitive triad, as mentioned earlier; (2) rigid and unrealistically high basic assumptions/expectations that affect the way an individual organizes information about their experiences; and (3) errors in thinking, including dichotomous (black and white, all or nothing) thinking, selective abstraction, overgeneralization, arbitrary inference, magnification, and minimization.

Learned Helplessness. Based on elements of attributional theory, this model of depression argues that cognitive and motivational deficits and emotional changes occur when an individual learns that his behavior and outcomes are independent (Seligman, 1975). Depression can occur when individuals learn that they cannot control events, when they expect a negative outcome, and when they believe that they are powerless to affect the outcome.

Biologic Theories

Genetic and Neurobiologic Factors.   The 1980s introduced exciting scientific advances in the following areas: development of brain imaging techniques; explication of the role of neurotransmitters and neuronal receptors in the formation of behavior; correction of erroneous beliefs of the brain being unchangeable after birth or unresponsive to the environment (brain plasticity); and the molecular genetics of psychobiologic diseases such as major depression (Pardes, 1986). Some aspects of the psychobiology of aging parallel those that occur in depression, including declines in growth hormone regulation, central nervous system (CNS) sertonin function and thyroid-releasing hormone (TRH) sensitivity. However, Veith and Raskind (1988) reported that there is insufficient scientific evidence to suggest that the neurobiologic changes of aging predispose the older adult to depression.

Twin and family studies have provided substantial evidence of a possible genetic etiology in depressive disorders, with the risk of affective disorder being almost four times greater among relatives with affective illness than among the general population (Blazer, 1993).

Substantial literature has detailed the search for a sensitive and specific biologic marker to aid the diagnosis of major depression. Three potential markers are discussed here: dexamethasone suppression test, sleep electroencephalogram (EEG), and serotonin or 3H-imipramine binding.

Dexamethasone Suppression Test.   The most widely established neuroendocrine change in depression is overactivity or hyperarousal of the hypothalamic pituitary adrenal (HPA) axis. The dexamethasone suppression test was originally introduced as a screening procedure for Cushing's disease, but Carroll (1982) and Carroll et al. (1976a, 1976b) established the dexamethasone suppression test (DST) as a possible marker for depression. During times of stress, adrenocorticotropic hormone is secreted from the pituitary in bursts or pulses, which stimulates the adrenal cortex to produce plasma cortisol. In many cases of major depression, the body does not shut down its own production in response to exogenous cortisol, resulting in hypercortisolemia. The procedure includes the following steps: (1) Dexamethasone 1 mg orally at 11 PM and (2) blood drawing at 8 AM, 4 PM and 11 PM the next day. Any plasma cortisol level above 5 μg/dt obtained between 9 and 24 hours after the dose of dexamethasone indicates failure of the normal suppression of cortisol levels and signifies a positive test. The DST is confounded by a variety of diseases and conditions, including Alzheimer's disease, bulimia nervosa, acute fasting, withdrawal from antidepressant drug treatment, and acute ingestion of caffeine (APA, 1994). Phenytoin and phenobarbital can accelerate the metabolism of dexamethasone,

leading to decreased sensitivity and spurious suppression response (Brown, 1989).

Sleep Electroencephalogram.   Sleep complaints are common among older adults. Unfortunately, even many health care providers believe that poor sleep is an inevitable part of growing old. In fact, stress is the most frequent cause of acute insomnia, and depression is the most frequent cause of chronic insomnia (Billiard, Partinen, Roth, & Shapiro, 1994). Scientific literature over the last three decades posits a strong relationship between sleep and psychiatric disorders. An electroencephalogram (EEG) is as unique as a fingerprint, yet it changes with age and is quite sensitive to medications. Approximately 90% of depressed inpatients show some form of EEG-verified sleep disturbance (Reynolds et al., 1988). Short rapid eye movement (REM) latency remains one of the most consistent findings in symptomatic depressed patients. However, the specificity of this finding to depression is under debate because it is also found in obsessive-compulsive disorders and schizophrenia (Armitage, 1995). A second robust feature of sleep in acutely ill depressed patients, when compared with age-matched controls, is a consistently longer first REM period (Reynolds et al., 1988). This finding appears to be greater in middle-age and elder adults than in young adults with depression.

Serotonin/3H-Imipramine Binding.   Numerous hypotheses concerning the biology of depression have focused on altered function of one or more of the monoamines that serve as synaptic neurotransmitters in the CNS (norepinephrine [NE], dopamine [DA], serotonin [5-hydroxytrytamine, 5-HT]). Each of these neurotransmitters is synthesized and mobilized in specific brain pathways that project to various parts of the brain and control a wide range of functions, including sleep, arousal, appetite, and pleasure (Hagerty, 1995). Some investigators propose that a deficiency of one or more of these monoamines might account for depression, while others claim that increased activity of the same monoamine leads to depression. Siever and Davis (1985) reformulated the catecholamine hypotheses to clarify the inconsistencies of previous studies. Within the resulting "dysregulation hypothesis of depression," depression is conceptualized not as resulting from a shortage or oversupply of catecholamines, but rather as a relative failure in the regulation of the neurotransmitters (Siever & Davis, 1985).

One of the monoamines investigated as a potential biologic marker is serotonin (5-HT), which regulates temperature, sleep, appetite, and sexual behavior (Dinan, 1996). There is good evidence that 3H-imipramine binding is intimately associated functionally and structurally with the 5-HT uptake site. These binding sites are present on human platelets, and the binding characteristics of 3H-imipramine are similar in both human brain cell and platelet membranes. The platelet receptors mimic human central nervous system receptors. Therefore changes in platelet 3H-imipramine binding may reflect changes in neuronal transport mechanism. Low platelet 3H-imipramine binding is found in patients with affective disorders, obsessive-compulsive disorder, anorexia nervosa, and panic disorder.

ASSESSMENT

No biologic marker has sufficient specificity for use in the clinical detection of major depression in the older medical patient. Consequently, the clinical interview remains the most effective method for detecting depression. The variety of theories on depression and aging illustrate the need for an individualized, multidimensional, comprehensive assessment. Burnside (1980) suggested that the interviewer attempt to make the interview pleasant for the elderly patient, conveying a sense of empathy, respect, and caring. The interviewer should be positioned close to the patient, use touch when appropriate to diminish the patient's anxiety, and be clear in stating the purpose of the interview and the length of time it will take (allow more time than for other age groups). A skilled diagnostician attends to verbal, nonverbal, and environmental cues as well as to cognitive and behavioral aspects of the client (Kneisl & Wilson, 1984). Sensory loss, confusion, communication disorders, cultural influences, shame, and fear of stigmatization can inhibit expression of feelings by elderly persons. Frequently, depressed elders are unaware of their apathetic and withdrawn behavior or assume it is part of getting old. When the client's history is lacking or withheld, the clinician must be persistent and perceptive in uncovering clues to validate a masked depressive state. Collateral history from family and staff members is valuable to corroborate clinical impressions and/or provide additional pertinent clinical history. The interview should take into account the following factors that play a role in treatment planning:

- Diagnosed medical problems, medications, functional status, nutritional status, personal and family psychiatric history, alcohol or drug usage, and thorough physical and neurologic examination
- Cognitive functioning mental status examination, including changes in cognition over time and educational level
- Psychologic strengths and symptomatology, coping skills, spirituality, sexuality, suicidal ideation, or past attempts at suicide
- Quality and quantity of social support, financial status, legal history, and potential for elder abuse
- Time course/duration and severity of depressive symptoms to differentiate the type of depression

One of the most challenging clinical problems concerns the accurate detection of depression in elders by nurses in nonpsychiatric care facilities (e.g., inpatient/out-

patient medical settings, nursing care facilities). Rehabilitation care settings appear to be more sensitive to functional impairment that is strongly associated with clinically significant depression (Berkman et al., 1986; Oxman, Berkman, Kasl, Freeman, & Barrett, 1990). Issues of poor detection have been well documented in the medical literature (Callahan et al., 1994; German et al., 1987; Rapp & Davis, 1989), but only recently have the assessment and referral patterns of nurses been described. A survey of 149 nurses from the American Nurses Association reported that respondents recognized the signs and symptoms of depression but, regardless of years of experience or level of education, a majority of respondents (52%) reported that they did not assess older patients for depression (Profitt, Augspurger, & Byrne, 1996). Further evidence of this knowledge/practice gap was found in research by Badger, Duman, and Kwan (1996). Prior to an educational intervention, 52% of 363 participants did not refer their depressed clients. Only 10% of participants routinely referred depressed clients. Badger et al. (1996) stated "assessment skills may be the more critical skill, particularly for nurses who work in acute care settings with shortened lengths of stay. Assessment and case finding may be the only intervention possible" (p. 104). However, preliminary findings by Piven et al. (1996) provides evidence that nine of 16 older patients in an acute care setting who scored as depressed on the Geriatric Depression Scale were not detected and/or referred to psychiatric nursing consultation staff. This is of concern, since there is evidence that early treatment is essential to reduce subsequent morbidity and mortality associated with depression (Depression Guideline Panel, 1993).

Assessment Tools

Various tools are available that can facilitate the assessment of an elderly patient and allow systematic data collection. Any tool used to assess elders must have established reliability and validity for use with elderly populations. Tools designed for and tested on other age groups are not likely to provide accurate findings when applied to elders. Caution must be used even with tools designed for elders because multiple extraneous variables can influence the results. For example, sensory loss, time of day, lack of patient cooperation, environmental stimuli, cultural influences, medication, and other factors can affect scores. Therefore the use of a combination of tools and multiple trials is recommended before establishing a definitive diagnosis.

Geriatric Depression Scale. The Geriatric Depression Scale (GDS) was developed as a screening tool to measure depression in elders. The GDS purposely excludes somatic symptoms that can confound detection of depression in the elderly (Brink et al., 1982; Yesavage et al., 1983). The GDS is a 30-item tool with a simple yes/no response self-report format. It can also be read to an elderly person who has visual difficulty. The GDS has been validated using both normal elders and elders undergoing treatment for depression in a variety of settings. Using a cut-off score of 11 yields a sensitivity of 0.84% and a specificity of 0.95%, whereas a more stringent cut-off score of 14 results in a sensitivity of 0.80% and a 100% specificity rate. Importantly, the GDS successfully discriminates depressed from nondepressed elders in both the physically ill elderly and in those who are receiving treatment for cognitive impairments (Yesavage et al., 1983). Concurrent validity has been established for the GDS against the other most commonly used measures of depression: Zung's Self-Rating Scale for Depression (SDS), the Hamilton Rating Scale for Depression (HamD), and Research Diagnostic Criteria (RDC).

A shorter version of the GDS, the SGDS, consists of 15 self-administered yes or no items. A correlation coefficient of 0.84 between the GDS and SGDS indicates successful differentiation of depressed and nondepressed elders (Sheikh & Yesavage, 1986).

The Center for Epidemiological Studies Depression Scale.   The Center for Epidemiological Studies Depression Scale (CES-D) consists of 20 items representing the symptoms of depressive disorder (Radloff, 1977). Response categories range from "rarely or none of the time," which is scored as 0, to "most of the time," which receives a 3. The total score is derived by summing all items, with a possible score ranging from 0 to 60. The most commonly used cut-off score to indicate depression is 16.

NURSING DIAGNOSIS

Although it is the most common psychiatric condition among older adults, the diagnosis Depression has not yet been accepted by the North American Nursing Diagnosis Association (NANDA) (1999). The authors believe this is an unfortunate oversight given the prevalence of this condition, the sequelae associated with untreated depression (suicide), and the negative impact of mood disorders on elders' quality of life. Gordon (1982) formulated a diagnosis Reactive Depression (Situational), defined as the "acute decrease in self-esteem or worth related to a threat to self-competency" (p. 166); characteristics of this diagnosis are provided in Box 41-1. In our view this diagnosis is too narrow in its acute perspective and etiologic base (powerlessness). Work continues to validate a nursing diagnosis that captures the syndrome of depressive illness (Thomas, Sanger, & Whitney, 1986; Zauszniewski, 1994). Three current NANDA nursing diagnoses have been associated with depression in clinical practice: Chronic Low Self-Esteem, which is the "long standing negative self evaluation/feelings about self or self capabilities" (NANDA, 1999, p. 113), Powerlessness, defined as the "perception that one's own actions will not significantly affect an

outcome; a perceived lack of control over a current situation or immediate happening" (p. 116), and Hopelessness, which is "a subjective state in which an individual sees limited or no alternatives or personal choices available and is unable to mobilize energy on own behalf" (p. 116) (see Box 41-1).

These diagnoses developed in a period when psychosocial/behavioral theories dominated the conceptualization of depression; consequently, they have limited ability to capture the breadth of characteristics and factors associated with depressive illness. More recently, an explosion of exciting research findings in the area of psychobiology has threatened to outpace the usefulness of current NANDA diagnostic classifications pertinent to psychiatric nursing diagnoses. To evaluate depression as an illness or disorder, and not simply a reaction to circumstances or to being old, the nurse must have some knowledge of the biologic theories of depression, the psychiatric diagnostic manual (the *Diagnostic and Statistical Manual IV*), and the clinical practice guidelines concerning the detection, diagnosis, and treatment of depression in primary care set forth by the Agency for Health Care Policy and Research (AHCPR). Theories of aging can also be useful in providing a conceptual context to assist the nurse with integrating psychosocial interventions into the treatment of depression.

Defining Characteristics

Despite variations in terminology and etiology, overall the signs and symptoms of depressive disorders remain fairly consistent throughout the life span. Individuals who are depressed may look sad, tired, and forlorn. Compared to the detection of traditional medical conditions (e.g., glucose levels in diabetes, blood urea nitrogen in kidney disease), the recognition of psychiatric disorders is largely dependent on the observation of behavior. For example, behavioral changes in depression are often episodic; in the older adult, this pattern can be difficult to recognize because of the frequent overlay of physical and emotional symptoms common in medical illness. Often, attention to grooming, hygiene, and self-presentation is neglected because of a lack of motivation. Depressed individuals are frequently tearful and sometimes are hostile, irritable, and aggressive. The feelings most often reported by depressed individuals include guilt, hopelessness, disinterest in life, isolation, loneliness, lack of pleasure, anxiety, emptiness, decreased energy, libido, and appetite, feelings of failure, inability to concentrate, self-devaluation and reproach, recurrent thoughts of death, and suicidal rumination. Signs and symptoms can include anorexia and weight loss or overeating and weight gain, sleep pattern disturbances (insomnia or hypersomnia), brooding about the past, pessimism, and social withdrawal. A markedly depressed elder may be mute and unresponsive to the assessment interview.

Box 41-1   Diagnoses Associated With Depression

Gordon Diagnosis (1982)
Reactive Depression (Situational)
Defining characteristics

Expression of hopelessness, despair

Inability to concentrate, making reading, writing, conversation difficult

Change, usually decrease in physical activities, eating, sleeping (early morning awakening), sexual activity

Continual questioning of self-worth (self-esteem)

Feeling of failure (real or imagined)

Withdrawal from others to avoid possible rejection, real or imagined

Threats or attempts to commit suicide

Suspicion or sensitivity to words and actions of others related to general lack of trust in others

Misdirected anger (toward self)

General irritability

Guilt feelings

Extreme dependency on others with related feelings of helplessness and anger

Related factor/etiology

Perceived powerlessness

NANDA Diagnoses (1999)
Chronic Low Self-Esteem (1988)
Defining characteristics

Long-standing or chronic: Self-negating verbalization; expressions of shame/guilt; evaluates self as unable to deal with events; rationalizes away/rejects positive feedback and exaggerates negative feedback about self; hesitant to try new things/situations; Minor: Frequent lack of success in work or other life events; overly conforming, dependent on others' opinions; lack of eye contact; nonassertive/passive; indecisive; excessively seeks reassurance

Related factors/etiologies

To be developed

Powerlessness (1982)
Defining characteristics

Severe: Verbal expressions of having no control or influence over situation; verbal expressions of having no control or influence over outcome; verbal expressions of having no control or influence over self-care; depression over physical deterioration that occurs despite patient compliance with regimens; apathy; Moderate: Nonparticipation in care or decision making when opportunities are provided; expressions of dissatisfaction and frustration over inability to perform previous tasks and/or activities; does not monitor progress; expression of doubt regarding role performance; reluctance to express true feelings; fearing alienation from caregivers; passivity; inability to seek information regarding care; dependence on others that may result in irritability, resentment, anger, and guilt; does not defend self-care practices when challenged; Low: Expressions of uncertainty about fluctuating energy levels; passivity

Related factors/etiologies

Health care environment; interpersonal interaction; illness-related regimen; lifestyle of helplessness

Hopelessness (1986)
Defining characteristics

Passivity, decreased verbalization; decreased affect; verbal cues (despondent content, "I can't," sighing); lack of initiative; decreased response to stimuli; decreased affect; turning away from speaker; closing eyes; shrugging in response to speaker; decreased appetite; increased/decreased sleep; lack of involvement in care/passively allowing care

Related factors/etiologies

Prolonged activity restriction creating isolation; failing or deteriorating physiologic condition; long-term stress; abandonment; lost belief in transcendent values/God

Additional NANDA Diagnoses Related to Depression
Diversional Activity Deficit
Anxiety
Impaired Verbal Communication
Constipation
Ineffective Individual Coping
Self-Esteem Disturbance
Social Isolation
Altered Nutrition: Less Than Body Requirements
Self-Care Deficit
Dysfunctional Grieving

DSM-IV Diagnoses (APA, 1994)
Major Depressive Episode

A. Five (or more) of the following symptoms have been present during the same 2-week period and represent a change from previous functioning; at least one of the symptoms is either (1) depressed mood or (2) loss of interest or pleasure (anhedonia). Do not include symptoms that are clearly due to a general medical condition, or mood-incongruent delusions or hallucinations.

1. Depressed mood most of the day, nearly every day, as indicated by either subjective report (e.g., feels sad or empty) or observation made by others (e.g., appears tearful).
2. Markedly diminished interest or pleasure in all, or almost all, activities most of the day, nearly every day (as indicated by either subjective account or observation made by others).
3. Significant weight loss when not dieting or weight gain (e.g., more than 5% of body weight in a month), or increase in appetite nearly every day (in children, consider failure to make expected weight gains).
4. Insomnia or hypersomnia nearly every day.
5. Psychomotor agitation or retardation nearly every day (observable by others, not merely subjective feelings of restlessness or being slowed down).
6. Fatigue or loss of energy nearly every day.
7. Feelings of worthlessness or excessive or inappropriate guilt (which may be delusional) nearly every day (not merely self-reproach or guilt about being sick).
8. Diminished ability to think or concentrate, or indecisiveness, nearly every day (either by subjective account or observed by others).

Continued

Box 41-1   Diagnoses Associated With Depression—cont'd

9. Recurrent thoughts of death (not just fear of dying), recurrent suicidal ideation without a specific plan, or a suicide attempt or a specific plan for committing suicide.

B. Symptoms do not meet criteria for a Mixed Episode.

C. Symptoms cause clinically significant distress or impairment in social, occupational, or other important area of functioning.

D. Symptoms are not due to the direct physiologic effects of a substance (e.g., a drug of abuse, a medication) or a general medical condition (e.g., hypothyroidism).

E. The symptoms are not better accounted for by Bereavement, i.e., after the loss of a loved one, the symptoms persist for longer than 2 months or are characterized by marked functional impairment, morbid preoccupation with worthlessness, suicidal ideation, psychotic symptoms, or psychomotor retardation.

Mood Disorder Due to a General Medical Condition

A. A prominent and persistent disturbance in mood predominates in the clinical picture and is characterized by either (or both) of the following:
   1. Depressed mood or markedly diminished interest or pleasure in all, or almost all, activities.
   2. Elevated, expansive, or irritable mood.

B. There is evidence from the history, physical examination, or laboratory findings that the disturbance is the direct physiologic consequence of a general medical condition.

C. The disturbance is not better accounted for by another mental disorder (e.g., Adjustment Disorder with Depressed Mood in response to the stress of having a general medical condition).

D. The disturbance does not occur exclusively during the course of a delirium.

E. The symptoms cause clinically significant distress or impairment in social, occupational, or other important areas of functioning.

Adjustment Disorder With Depressed Mood

Predominate manifestations are symptoms such as depressed mood, tearfulness, or feelings of hopelessness. In addition, the presence of the following:

A. The development of emotional or behavioral symptoms in response to an identifiable stressor(s) occurring within 3 months of the onset of the stressor(s).

B. These symptoms or behaviors are clinically significant as evidenced by either of the following:
   1. Marked distress that is in excess of what would be expected from exposure to the stressor.
   2. Significant impairment in social or occupational (academic) functioning.

The stress-related disturbance does not meet the criteria for another specific Axis I disorder and is not merely an exacerbation of a pre-existing Axis I or Axis II disorder.

C. The symptoms do not represent Bereavement.

D. Once the stressor (or its consequences) has terminated, the symptoms do not persist for more than an additional 6 months.

Dysthymic Disorder

A. Depressed mood for most of the day, for more days than not, as indicated either by subjective account or observation by others, for at least 2 years.

B. Presence, while depressed, of two (or more) of the following:
   1. Poor appetite or overeating.
   2. Insomnia or hypersomnia.
   3. Low energy or fatigue.
   4. Low self-esteem.
   5. Poor concentration or difficulty.
   6. Feelings of hopelessness.

C. During the 2-year period of the disturbance, the person has never been without the symptoms in Criteria A and B for more than 2 months at a time.

D. No Major Depressive Episode has been present during the first 2 years of the disturbance; i.e., the disturbance is not better accounted for by chronic Major Depressive Disorder or Major Depressive Disorder in partial remission.

E. There has never been a Manic Episode, a Mixed Episode, or a Hypomanic Episode, and criteria have never been met for Cyclothymic Disorder.

F. The disturbance does not occur exclusively during the course of a chronic Psychotic Disorder, such as Schizophrenia or Delusional Disorder.

G. The symptoms are not due to the direct physiologic effects of a substance (e.g., a drug of abuse, a medication) or a general medical condition (e.g., hypothyroidism).

H. The symptoms cause clinically significant distress or impairment in social, occupational, or other important areas of functioning.

From American Psychiatric Association. (1994). *Diagnostic and statistical manual of mental disorders* (4th ed.). Washington, DC: APA; Gordon, M. (1982). *Manual of nursing diagnosis* (p. 166). Hightstown, NJ: McGraw-Hill; North American Nursing Diagnosis Association. (1999). *Nursing diagnoses: Definitions & classification 1999-2000.* Philadelphia: The Association.

The authors recommend that NANDA develop the nursing diagnosis Depression based on the DSM-IV (APA) criteria, etiologies, and defining characteristics for major depressive episode and mood disorder caused by general medical condition. One important reason for this recommendation is that currently nurses can only be reimbursed for psychiatric services delivered in response to a DSM-IV-based diagnosis. Furthermore, the authors suggest that NANDA consider adapting the diagnosis Chronic Low Self-Esteem to incorporate more of the diagnostic criteria set forth in the DSM-IV diagnosis Dysthymic Disorder (see Box 41-1). Finally, we advise consideration of merging elements of Gordon's diagnostic category Reactive Depression (Situational) with those of the DSM-IV criteria for Adjustment Disorder with Depressed Mood (see Box 41-1).

Unique Characteristics of Depression in Elders

There are characteristics of depression specific to the elders that are not explicitly identified in the DSM-IV. It is crucial for clinicians to be aware that depressive illness in the elder, which is amenable to treatment, can mimic other organically based irreversible disorders. Many elderly patients who are thought to be demented may actually have a depressive disorder with misleading cognitive symptoms. The term *pseudodementia* refers to depression associated with and often misinterpreted as dementia. Generally, depressive illness manifests itself suddenly, whereas the organic brain syndromes appear more slowly

or, in the case of multi-infarct (vascular) dementia, in a graduated stepwise fashion (Lazarus, Davis, & Dysken, 1985). Signs of confabulation suggest there may be an organic component such as that seen in Alzheimer's disease. Demented patients often become angry and attempt to cover up the cognitive impairment when their memory is tested, whereas depressed elders may not answer questions or simply acknowledge that they do not remember (Table 41-1).

Organic disorders can also exist concomitantly with depression, and the cognitive impairment may be worsened by the depressive overlay, a situation described as "excessive disability." The elderly patient's condition is compromised beyond what would be expected by the dementing process alone. Judicious use of antidepressant medications, together with brief psychotherapy in the early stages of dementia, has been shown to alleviate

Table 41-1 Differentiating Dementia From Depression	
Dementia	**Depression**
AFFECT	
Labile, fluctuating from tears to laughter, not consistent or sustained. May show apathy, irritability, euphoria, or inappropriate affect. Normal control impaired, suggestible.	Depressed, feelings of despair that are pervasive, persistent. Anxious hypomanic. Not influenced by suggestions. May be flat, withdrawn, sad, tearful.
MEMORY	
Decreased attention for recent events; confabulation; perseveration. Irritability when memory tested.	Difficulty in concentration. Impaired learning of new knowledge. Decreased attention with secondary decrease in recent memory. May not respond when tested or will admit can't remember.
INTELLECT	
Impaired, decreased as tested by serial 7s, similarities, recent events.	Impaired but can perform serial 7s and can usually remember recent events.
ORIENTATION	
Fluctuating with varying levels of awareness. Disoriented for time, place.	May have some confusion, not as profound as in dementia.
JUDGMENT	
Poor judgment with inappropriate behavior, dress. Deterioration of personal habits and hygiene. Loss of bowel and bladder control.	May be poor, especially if suicidal, e.g., poor grooming. May be careless with medication. May risk personal safety.
SOMATIC COMPLAINTS	
Fatigue, failing health complaints with vague complaints of pain in head, neck, back.	Typical complaints include: decreased sleep, appetite, weight, libido, energy, and constipation.
NEUROLOGIC SYMPTOMS	
Dysphasia, apraxia, agnosia.	Not present.

Adapted from Zung, W. W. K. (1980). Affective disorders. In Busse, E. W., Blazer, D. G. (Eds.), *Handbook of geriatric psychiatry* (p. 357). New York: Van Nostrand Reinhold.

excess disability. Although depressive symptoms can be successfully treated in this manner, the course of the irreversible dementia remains inexorably progressive despite treatment.

Another sign of depression, especially in older persons, is excessive preoccupation with physical symptoms (somatization). Indeed, hypochondriacal symptoms seem to increase among depressed elders, whereas phobic and obsessional symptoms are diminished. Expressing bodily discomfort is often more familiar to older persons than is bringing forth symptoms of psychic pain. In a study by Koenig, Ford, and Blazer (1993), only 43% of older patients with major depressive disorder did not endorse feeling "downhearted and blue" on self-report, pointing up the unreliability of self-report and the value of coupling careful observation and queries about other symptoms associated with depressive disorder. Clinicians have noted that, because of the stigma associated with mental illness, depressed elderly patients will sometimes "cover up" depression when interacting with others by maintaining meticulous grooming and feigning a cheerful attitude. Furthermore, elderly depressed persons most often approach their family physician with somatic complaints related to depression rather than going to a psychiatrist or other mental health professional. The nurse should be alert for other signs of depressive illness in an elderly patient who consistently focuses on physical problems. Palpitations, shortness of breath, burning with urination, stomach cramps, heavy feelings in the abdomen, and dry mouth were symptoms found to be helpful in differentiating depressed from nondepressed elders (Koenig et al., 1993).

Diagnostic and Statistical Manual IV Criteria

The term *depression* is used to describe many things, including a mood, a symptom, a disease, or a syndrome (Buschmann & Rossen, 1993). Symptoms of sadness or demoralization are common in elders faced with challenges to physical and social integrity. Loss of a spouse, diagnosis of a medical illness, and adjustment to a long-term care facility can cause stress and even periods of demoralization in an older person. Moods fluctuate as one adjusts to the vicissitudes of life. Distinguishing normal adjustments to life changes from depressive symptoms is critical to the accurate detection and assessment of clinically relevant depression in the older adult. The *Diagnostic and Statistical Manual IV,* (DSM-IV), published by the American Psychiatric Association (1994), provides a categorical approach to the diagnosis of mental disorders that is largely atheoretical. The current manual includes several categories of depression differentiated by onset, precipitating factors, symptoms, severity, and duration. Familiarity with the following diagnostic categories will assist the nurse in categorizing the severity of depressive symptoms in order to plan appropriate intervention(s) for optimal outcome(s).

Older adults may suffer from different types of depression. There is growing evidence that a significant minority of elders suffer from depressive symptoms that do not meet DSM-IV criteria for major depression as outlined in Box 41-1 but that nonetheless affect their quality of life and may lead to a more severe mood disorder (Meyers, 1994). In a 1-year longitudinal study examining the incidence and persistence of depression among nursing home residents, Parmelee, Katz, and Lawton (1992) found that on initial evaluation, 15% of the 868 subjects displayed possible major depression and another 16.5% exhibited minor depressive symptoms. Follow-up of 448 residents 1 year later revealed that 40% of those with major depression had experienced no remission in symptoms, and a significant percentage (16.2%) of those categorized as "minor depressives" had developed major depression. This suggests that minor or sub-syndromal depression cannot necessarily be considered a transitory or easily managed disorder among frail elders. Space limitations prevent an exhaustive examination of each of the mood disorders detailed in the DSM-IV, therefore only those most commonly observed in older adults will be detailed here.

Major Depressive Disorder.   The diagnostic criteria for Major Depressive Episode as listed in the DSM-IV are provided in Box 41-1. The accurate detection and diagnosis of major depression in elders with concurrent medical problems is probably the greatest clinical challenge because of the difficulty of distinguishing symptoms of physical illness from those of depressive disorder. Controlling for alcohol use, severity of medical illness, and functional status, Koenig et al. (1993) found that the following observer-rated depressive symptoms most strongly differentiated depressed from nondepressed male patients: loss of interest and pleasure (anhedonia), middle insomnia (awakening too early and unable to return to sleep), suicidal thoughts, and hypochondriasis (excessive concern with health problems). In a self-report of depressive symptoms, a positive response to feeling "restless and fidgety" was the self-rated item most strongly related to having major depressive disorder, followed by "often bored" and depressed mood. Loss of interest in work or usual activities, when observed by the clinician or reported by the patient, is a particularly important sign that a major depressive disorder may be present. Loss of pleasure (anhedonia), sleep disturbance, and intense feelings of despair and discouragement may be useful in separating major depression from dysthymia.

Mood Disorder Resulting From a General Medical Condition.   The primary feature of this mood category is persistent mood disturbance judged to be the direct physiologic effect of a general medical condition. Numerous medical conditions that are common in the elderly can cause mood symptoms, including, for example, neurologic disease (e.g., Huntington's disease, Parkinson's disease), endocrine disease (e.g., hyperthyroidism and hypothyroidism), cerebrovascular disease (e.g., stroke), metabolic disorders (e.g., vitamin B deficiency), autoimmune disorders (e.g., systemic lupus erythematosus), and cancer (e.g., pancreatic cancer) (see Box 41-1). Therefore Mood Disorder Due to a General Medical Condition should always be considered as the basis of affective changes in physically compromised elders.

Adjustment Disorder With Depressed Mood. The hallmark of an Adjustment Disorder is the appearance of significant emotional or behavioral symptoms within 3 months of an identifiable stressor, with the amount of distress judged to be in excess of what would be expected given the quality of the stressor and/or causing significant social or occupational (academic) functional impairment (see Box 41-1). Given the often numerous and unremitting stressors many elders are subjected to, this diagnosis is also quite viable in older populations.

Dysthymia. Dysthymia is characterized by at least 2 years of chronically depressed mood, associated with other depressive symptoms that are less severe than those present in major depressive disorder (see Box 41-1). It should be considered in those elders who describe themselves as "always sad, low, or down in the dumps."

In the following case study particular attention has been given to aspects of assessment, patient strengths, and adaptive behaviors. To ensure that these often overlooked aspects of the elder are included, the authors recommend that a specific, regularly updated section of the care plan be devoted to "signs of growth/strengths," and that these crucial aspects of the patient (no matter how minimal they may seem) be stressed in every form of communication related to the geriatric patient's status (e.g., shift report, progress notes, physician rounds, reports given to family members, interactions with the patient). Shifting the focus away from problems will ensure that the strengths of the patient are fortified and encouraged to progress by all who have contact with the elder.

CASE STUDY

K. Ray is an 85-year old male residing on the health-related floor in a long-term care facility. His wife is on the skilled nursing care unit in the same facility. Mr. and Mrs. Ray lived independently up until about a year ago, when Mrs. Ray suffered a massive stroke, leaving her comatose. She was described as a doting wife and a meticulous housekeeper. Mr. Ray was a mason for 40 years, with an eighth grade education. They had two children. One son is married and living out of state; another son died at age 28 from cancer over 20 years ago. Over the last 2 months, staff in the facility have noted that Mr. Ray has refused to visit his wife, has become progressively more focused on bodily aches and pains, and has required prodding to attend to personal hygiene. Although Mr. Ray currently appears of normal weight, records from admission indicate a 15-pound weight loss and poor appetite. Night shift staff have reported that over the last 3 weeks Mr. Ray has asked for sleeping medication for problems with awakening too early in the morning and then returning to sleep. Although Mr. Ray has been pleasant and cooperative with nursing staff in the past, he has begun to make negative statements about the residents and nursing staff and recently threatened to hit another resident. The staff obtained permission to consult with a geropsychiatric nurse clinician, who then came to the facility to assess the patient.

Medical records revealed that Mr. Ray had been essentially healthy during his adult years. With the patient's permission, a phone call was placed to his son, who corroborated Mr. Ray's report that there was no personal or family history of alcohol abuse or depression. He has no physical limitations and had been physically active gardening and taking daily walks with the family dog prior to admission.

Mr. Ray appeared gaunt, disheveled, and tired. His hair was uncombed, and he had several days' worth of stubble on his face. When addressed, he emitted a pervasive feeling of despair with an undercurrent of anger and despondency. The nurse used a Mini Mental Status Exam (MMSE) as a guide to assess Mr. Ray's cognitive status. He was reluctant to converse, but became less anxious when the nurse touched his arm and asked him to share a cup of coffee with her. Mr. Ray was oriented in all spheres, with judgment, remote memory, and recent memory intact. His thoughts flowed logically and he did not demonstrate any perceptual difficulty. His gait was obviously slow though steady. He spoke hesitantly of the many losses he had encountered in his life, both past and recent. When asked what things he did to get through difficult times in the past he looked puzzled, then explained he never considered his needs since his wife's were more important. He indicated that his wife grieved quite openly and demonstratively, and he often felt the need to console her rather than himself. When the nurse broached the subject of his wife's condition it became apparent that Mr. Ray felt irrationally guilty, blaming himself for not having insisted that she see a doctor when she complained of feeling dizzy. "I was always complaining about money, so she didn't want to spend the money on a doctor." Highlights of the nurse's assessment of Mr. Ray are presented below, illustrating principles of therapeutic communication and examples of the kinds of questions the nurse might ask, always allowing adequate time for patient response between questions.

NURSE: Mr. Ray, do you think about dying or killing yourself? How often? How long? (If yes, do you have a plan to kill yourself? How? Do you have the means?) *Assessment of suicidal ideation*

PATIENT: (withdrawing, angrily) You think I'm crazy, don't you? *Fear of stigmatization*

NURSE: (touching his arm, emphasizing her response with direct eye contact) Mr. Ray, you are not crazy. Everything you have said makes perfect sense to me. You are thinking very clearly and logically. (pause)	*Expression of caring touch, contact*
NURSE: The staff and I are concerned about you because you seem blue and down in the dumps most of the time. How would you describe your mood? Do you feel this depressed nearly every day? For how long?	*Establishes subjective description of mood, severity, and duration*
NURSE: Do you enjoy things as much as you used to? Have you stopped doing things you used to do? For how long? What stopped you from doing those things?	*Assess for anhedonia, severity, and duration and of physical, social, occupational, and functional impairment*
NURSE: I understand you have lost 15 pounds; have you tried to lose weight? How long has your appetite been less? Have you noticed the loss?	*Assess for increase or decrease in appetite* *Validation*
NURSE: The night staff have noticed that you are having some trouble sleeping. Some people have difficulty falling asleep, staying asleep, or awakening early. Do you have any of these? How often?	*Assess for insomnia or hypersomnia, duration, and severity*
NURSE: Do you feel on edge and nervous? Slowed down? How's your energy level? Do you feel tired a lot? For how long? Are you able to get done the things you want to do?	*Assess psychomotor retardation or agitation* *Assess energy and fatigue level, duration, and severity*
NURSE: Do you feel you are a worthwhile individual?	*Assess self-image, self-esteem*
NURSE: Is your mind still as clear as it used to be? How's your concentration?	*Assess concentration, decisiveness*
NURSE: You aren't eating or sleeping well. You've lost weight, and these things suggest to me that you are feeling depressed. I can understand fully why you are feeling blue. It seems very normal that you feel sad. (Pause.) I would like to help you to feel better and maybe even be happy again. (Pause, nurse takes his hand.) Sometimes when people have suffered great losses they are able to feel better if they can	*Seeking patient input, collaboration*
share their feelings with another person. You have been holding your sadness inside for a long time now and it's affecting your health. (Pause.) I would like to help you. You don't have to suffer alone. I think together we can work this out. Would you be willing to share your feelings with me? (Long silence.) Only you can tell us how you feel.	*Reinforcing patient's control*
PATIENT: (withdraws his hand and wipes away a tear) If I could sleep better I'd feel better.	*Shifting focus from feelings to somatic complaints*
NURSE: That's probably very true. Maybe a goal we could work on would be to help you sleep longer at night. (Pause.) Do you think if you shared your upsetting feelings with me during the day you might feel more restful at night? (Long silence, no answer.)	*Validation Collaboration, mutual goal setting Redirecting*
NURSE: I imagine it feels uncomfortable to you to think about sharing your sadness with me. You don't know me very well. (Pause.) Maybe we could start by talking about some of the good times you've had in your life? Would that feel more comfortable to you?	*Validation, empathy Establishing trust by refocusing temporarily on less painful issues, being direct, refocusing on feelings*
PATIENT: (Pause.) Will you come every day?	*Seeking clarification suggests acceptance*

Based on the assessment interview historical data, a GDS score of 14, and collateral information obtained from a phone call to Mr. Ray's son, the geropsychiatric nurse clinician suspected that Mr. Ray was suffering from Major Depression. She contacted the attending staff physician and discussed her clinical impressions. Subsequent to the telephone discussion, the physician started Mr. Ray on an antidepressant. The geropsychiatric nurse clinician assisted the nursing staff in care planning for Mr. Ray by identifying relevant nursing diagnoses. In Mr. Ray's case, NANDA diagnosis Self-Esteem Disturbance was more appropriate than Chronic Low Self-Esteem because of the time-limited nature of his depressive illness and associated impaired self-esteem (see Chapter 45, Self-Esteem Disturbance).

The nurse also identified Mr. Ray's strengths, which are as follows:

- Is in excellent physical condition; has absence of chronic illness; is completely mobile; is agile and fully ambulatory
- Possesses adaptive strengths; has endured significant losses in his life
- Had a solid marriage and good relationships with his neighbors in the community and belonged to a pater-

nal organization much of his life, indicating the ability to maintain meaningful relationships
- Derived much satisfaction from caring for the family dog
- Has strong religious beliefs
- Is physically attractive
- Used to make his own wine
- Agreed to meet with the geropsychiatric clinician
- Scored 26 on MMSE, indicative of intact intellectual functioning
- Is nonsuicidal
- Resides on the health-related unit among many other highly functional peers
- Is financially secure
- Has been assisting his roommate to the dining room recently
- Is knowledgeable about gardening

This list of strengths was made a permanent part of Mr. Ray's record, along with the nursing and psychiatric diagnoses; it was reviewed and updated at biweekly multidisciplinary care conferences.

NURSING-SENSITIVE OUTCOMES

Several outcomes identified in the *Nursing Outcomes Classification (NOC)* (Iowa Outcomes Project, 2000) are relevant to late-life depression: Suicide Self-Restraint, Mood Equilibrium, Hope, and Coping. These outcomes and their NOC definitions and indicators are listed and briefly discussed below. The outcomes Knowledge: Disease Process and Knowledge: Medication, which are not discussed further, also are important for cognitively intact elders, who can benefit from understanding their illness and the pharmacologic interventions that are part of the treatment plan. The outcome Grief Resolution can be relevant for elders who are experiencing depression related to grief; Grief Resolution is discussed in some detail in Chapter 49, Grieving.

Suicide Self-Restraint is defined as the "ability to refrain from gestures and attempts at killing self" (Iowa Outcomes Project, 2000, p. 410). Indicators for Suicide Self-Restraint are shown in Table 41-2. Although Mr. Ray was not actively suicidal, the fact that elders are a high risk group for suicide (rate for all ages is 12.2 per 100,000, whereas elders commit suicide at almost twice this rate, or 20.1 per 100,000), makes this outcome relevant for the diagnosis Depression in older adults.

Mood Equilibrium, a key outcome for depressed elders, is defined as "appropriate adjustment of prevailing emotional tone in response to circumstances" (Iowa Outcomes Project, 2000, p. 306). Indicators of mood equilibrium are listed in Table 41-2. These indicators cover both depression and mania as might be found in bipolar disorder (e.g., speech at moderate pace, exhibits absence of flight of ideas, grandiosity, and euphoria). Several of the indicators (e.g., exhibits concentration, wears appropriate clothing) could be compromised in cognitively impaired elders

Table 41-2 Outcome Indicators: SUICIDE SELF-RESTRAINT, MOOD EQUILIBRIUM, HOPE, AND COPING

Outcomes	Indicators
SUICIDE SELF-RESTRAINT	Expresses feelings; maintains connectedness in relationships; seeks help when feeling self-destructive; verbalizes suicidal ideas if present; verbalizes control of impulses; refrains from gathering means for suicide; does not give away possessions; does not require treatment for suicide gestures or attempts; refrains from using mood-altering substance(s); discloses plan for suicide; upholds suicide contract; maintains self-control without supervision; does not attempt suicide
MOOD EQUILIBRIUM	Exhibits appropriate affect; exhibits nonlabile mood; exhibits impulse control; reports adequate sleep (at least 5 hr/24 hr); exhibits concentration; exhibits appropriate grooming and hygiene; wears appropriate clothing for situation and weather; maintains stable weight; reports normal appetite; reports compliance with medication and therapeutic regimen; speech at moderate pace; exhibits absence of flight of ideas; exhibits absence of grandiosity; exhibits absence of euphoria; shows interest in surroundings; absence of suicide ideation; reports appropriate energy level; reports ability to accomplish daily task
HOPE	Expression of a positive future orientation; expression of faith; expression of belief in self; expression of belief in others; expression of will to live; expression of reasons to live; expression of meaning in life; expression of optimism; expression of inner peace; expression of sense of self-control; demonstration of zest for life; setting of goals
COPING	Identifies effective coping patterns; identifies ineffective coping patterns; verbalizes sense of control; reports decrease in stress; verbalizes acceptance of situation; seeks information concerning illness and treatment; modifies lifestyle as needed; adapts to developmental changes; uses available social support; employs behaviors to reduce stress; identifies multiple coping strategies; uses effective coping strategies; avoids unduly stressful situations; verbalizes need for assistance; seeks professional help as appropriate; reports decrease in physical symptoms of stress; reports decrease in negative feelings; reports increase in psychologic comfort

Table 41-3	Nursing Diagnoses, Nursing-Sensitive Outcomes, and Nursing Interventions MAJOR DEPRESSION	

Nursing Diagnoses	Nursing-Sensitive Outcomes	Nursing Interventions
HOPELESSNESS		
Defining Characteristics	Hope	Develop a plan of care that involves
Passivity, decreased verbalization; decreased affect; verbal cues (e.g., despondent content, "I can't," sighing); lack of initiative; decreased appetite; increased/decreased sleep; lack of involvement in care/passively allowing care	Mood Equilibrium (all Self-Care outcomes; Social Support)	degree of goal attainment, moving from simple to more complex goals (Teaching: Prescribed Medication; Teaching: Disease Process; Counseling)
Related Factors/Etiologies		Involve patient actively in own care; encourage relationship with
Prolonged activity restriction creating isolation; long-term stress		significant others (Self-Care Deficit; Socialization Enhancement)
POWERLESSNESS		
Defining Characteristics	Health Beliefs: Perceived Control; Health Beliefs: Perceived Resources	Encourage patient to identify strengths; explore previous successes; praise
SEVERE: Verbal expressions of having no control or influence over situation		progress toward goals (Counseling; Hope Instillation; Coping
MODERATE: Guilt		Enhancement)
CHRONIC LOW SELF-ESTEEM		
Self-negating verbalization; expression of shame/guilt; indecisive	Role Performance Social Interaction Skills	Monitor lack of follow-through in goal attainment; reinforce strengths that patient identifies (Decision-Making Support; Self-Esteem Enhancement)

without depression. In addition, indicators may be misleading in terms of differential diagnosis, as discussed earlier in connection with pseudodementia, although dementia and depression can and do coexist in some elders. Mood Equilibrium is perhaps the most important outcome in the case of Mr. Ray, and weekly evaluation was instituted.

Hope is an outcome indicative of resolution of depression. According to the NOC system, Hope is defined as "presence of internal state of optimism that is personally satisfying and life-supporting" (Iowa Outcomes Project, 2000, p. 235). In many respects, Hope is closely related to the outcome Psychosocial Adjustment: Life Change, which is especially relevant to elders suffering from Adjustment Disorder with Depressed Mood (Table 41-3). It is noteworthy that some of the indicators of this outcome (i.e., demonstration of zest for life) may be more appropriate for younger rather than older adults, especially nondepressed but physically frail elders, and those who reside in institutional settings. Indicators of Hope are shown in Table 41-2. In the case of Mr. Ray, the significant life stressor that might have precipitated his depression was his wife's massive stroke; there was no hope for her recovery. This outcome was to be evaluated with Mr. Ray on a quarterly basis.

Coping is defined as "actions to manage stressors that tax an individual's resources" (Iowa Outcomes Project, 2000, p. 192). In many cases elders must learn to cope with

great losses, such as the death or impairment of loved ones, that can lead to depression. Achievement of the NOC indicators of Coping constitutes a real nursing challenge; progress toward achieving this outcome should be evaluated on a monthly basis with depressed elders. Indicators for Coping are shown in Table 41-2.

Since the primary treatment for depression in all age groups is antidepressant medication, it might be useful to have an outcome related to "Medication Response." Response to antidepressants typically occurs within 4 to 6 weeks of initiation of treatment. Relevant nursing activities would include, for example, close monitoring of appetite, sleep, and activity level along with subjective and objective evaluations of mood. Outcome indicators would then reflect re-establishment of normal patterns of sleep, eating, and levels of activity and mood, in the absence of adverse side effects such as dry mouth, confusion, sweating, orthostatic hypotension, blurry vision, urinary retention, cardiotoxicity, and hepatotoxicity.

CASE STUDY

The geropsychiatric nurse clinician, together with Mr. Ray, his physician, and his son, established the following initial goals of treatment: (1) to reduce and eventually remove all signs and symptoms of the depressive syndrome; (2) to restore psychosocial functioning to that of the asymptomatic state; and (3) to reduce the likelihood of relapse and recurrence (Depression Guideline Panel, 1993). In addition to these broad treatment goals, the nurse identified specific short- and long-term goals she would use to evaluate the success of the nursing interventions. Short-term goals included the following:

1. Express feelings by identifying one feeling from his feeling list daily
2. Reduce pacing and combative behaviors
3. Engage in one daily group activity of choice
4. Express feeling in one-to-one interactions daily with primary care nurse
5. Accurately appraise coping behaviors
6. Become more assertive by practicing one assertive interaction every day
7. Assist in all self-care activities daily (i.e., shave self, dress self)
8. Interact with peers informally in activity room
9. Identify and appraise past adaptive coping mechanisms

Long-term goals included the following:

1. Resume former sleep patterns (sleeping past 0500 daily)
2. Visit wife, read to her, assist in her care once a week to daily
3. Attend and participate in "griever's group" weekly meeting
4. Be prepared for wife's inevitable death by talking about it and expressing feelings

NURSING INTERVENTIONS

Several nursing interventions can be appropriate in the treatment of older adults with depression: Caregiver Support, Hope Instillation, Presence, Security Enhancement, Crisis Intervention, Anticipatory Guidance, Decision-Making Support, Body Image Enhancement, Self-Esteem Enhancement, Socialization Enhancement, Support System Enhancement, Coping Enhancement, and Cognitive Restructuring. However, the following five nursing interventions defined by the *Nursing Interventions Classification (NIC)* (Iowa Intervention Project, 2000) address the key signs and symptoms of depression in the older adult: Suicide Prevention, Teaching: Disease Process, Teaching: Prescribed Medication, Emotional Support, and Counseling. Ideally, given the breadth and complexity of depressive illness, some or all of the above interventions will be used in combination, based on individualized assessment of the cause(s) and presentation of depressive symptoms in the older adult.

Suicide Prevention

The intervention Suicide Prevention is defined as "reducing risk of self-inflicted harm for a patient in crisis or severe depression" (Iowa Intervention Project, 2000, p. 620). Activities included in this intervention are as follows:

- Determine whether patient has specific suicide plan identified
- Determine history of suicide attempts
- Place patient in least restrictive environment that allows for necessary level of observation
- Refrain from negatively criticizing
- Place patient in room with protective window coverings, as appropriate
- Instruct patient and significant other in signs, symptoms, and basic physiology of depression
- Facilitate discussion of factors or events that precipitated the suicidal thoughts
- Provide psychiatric counseling, as appropriate
- Instruct family on possible warning signs or pleas for help patient may use
- Encourage the person to make a verbal no-suicide contract
- Protect patient from harming self
- Demonstrate concern about patient's welfare
- Remove dangerous items from the patient's environment
- Observe closely during suicidal crisis
- Instruct family that suicidal risk increases for severely depressed patients as they begin to feel better
- Escort patient during off-ward activities, as appropriate
- Facilitate support of patient by family and friends
- Refer patient to psychiatrist, as needed

Accurate assessment of the older patient for suicidal ideation includes direct questions regarding presence of recurrent thoughts of death (not just the fear of dying) and recurrent suicidal ideas. Second, the absence or presence of a suicidal plan can provide some clues as to the seriousness of the individual's depressive illness. Information about whether the patient has access to a mechanism to commit suicide (owns or knows how to access a gun) and the formation of a plan (leaving a note, etc.) can provide clues as to the severity of the depression and the seriousness of self-harm threat. The nurse can use such behavioral interventions as establishing a verbal or written contract promising no self-harm. Patients unwilling to contract not to hurt themselves require expedient evaluation by a physician and constant surveillance until the physician's evaluation is complete.

Teaching: Prescribed Medication

The NIC intervention label Teaching: Prescribed Medication is defined as "preparing a patient to safely take prescribed medications and monitor for their effects" (Iowa Intervention Project, 2000, p. 650). Activities included under this intervention are as follows:

- Instruct the patient to recognize distinctive characteristics of the medications(s), as appropriate

- Instruct the patient on the purpose and action of each medication
- Instruct the patient on the proper administration/application of each medication
- Instruct the patient to perform needed procedures before taking a medication, as appropriate
- Instruct the patient on which criteria to use when deciding to alter when taking medication dosage/schedule, as appropriate
- Instruct the patient on specific precautions to observe when taking medications, as appropriate
- Instruct the patient on how to relieve and/or prevent certain side effects, as appropriate
- Instruct the patient on the signs and symptoms of over- and under-dosage
- Instruct the patient on the proper care of devices used for administration
- Provide the patient with written information about the action, purpose, side effects, and so on of medications
- Instruct the patient to carry documentation of prescribed medication regimen
- Inform the patient of possible changes in appearance and/or dosage when filling generic medication prescriptions
- Caution the patient against giving prescribed medications to others
- Provide information on medication reimbursement, as appropriate
- Inform the patient of both the generic and brand names of each medication
- Instruct the patient on the dosage, route, and duration of each medication
- Evaluate the patient's ability to self-administer medications
- Inform the patient what to do if a dose of medication is missed
- Inform the patient of consequences of not taking or abruptly discontinuing medications, as appropriate
- Instruct the patient on possible adverse side effects of each medication
- Instruct the patient on appropriate actions to take if side effects occur
- Inform the patient of possible drug-food interactions, as appropriate
- Instruct the patient on proper disposal of needles and syringes at home, as appropriate, and where to dispose of the sharps container in his community
- Assist the patient to develop a written medication schedule
- Instruct the patient on how to fill prescriptions, as appropriate
- Warn the patient of the risks associated with taking expired medications
- Determine the patient's ability to obtain required medications

- Provide information on cost savings programs/organizations to obtain medications and devices, as appropriate

Antidepressant medication may be prescribed to treat moderate to severe depression. Education of the older patient regarding the appearance, dosage, and side effects of antidepressant medication, as well as the expected duration of treatment, is essential to optimal patient care. Inclusion of a significant other or spouse in this teaching can help to reinforce the elder's learning and help to ease the learning burden of beginning a new medication.

Teaching: Disease Process

The NIC intervention Teaching: Disease Process is defined as "assisting the patient to understand information related to a specific disease process" (Iowa Intervention Project, 2000, p. 640), in this case, the disease process of depression. A number of activities, listed here, are subsumed under this intervention, all of which can be appropriate for the depressed elder.

- Appraise the patient's current level of knowledge related to specific disease process
- Describe the common signs and symptoms of the disease, as appropriate
- Identify possible etiologies, as appropriate
- Avoid empty reassurances
- Provide information about available diagnostic measures, as appropriate
- Discuss therapy/treatment options
- Encourage the patient to explore options/get a second opinion, as appropriate or indicated
- Instruct the patient on measures to control/minimize side effects of the disease, as appropriate
- Refer the patient to local community agencies/support groups, as appropriate
- Provide the phone number(s) to call if complications occur
- Explain the pathophysiology of the disease and how it relates to the anatomy and physiology, as appropriate
- Describe the disease process, as appropriate
- Provide information to the patient about condition, as appropriate
- Provide the family/significant other(s) with information about the patient's progress, as appropriate
- Discuss lifestyle changes that may be required to prevent future complications and/or control the disease process
- Describe rationale behind management/therapy/treatment recommendations
- Describe possible chronic complications, as appropriate
- Explore possible resources/support, as appropriate
- Instruct the patient on which signs and symptoms to report to health care provider, as appropriate

- Reinforce information provided by other health care team members, as appropriate

Education of the older adult regarding the normal ebb and flow of human emotions and how normal sadness can be distinguished from depressive disorder is integral to patient teaching. The nurse might confront generational differences in attitudes toward low mood. For instance, older adults might have been reared with the life view that depression is a character weakness or that it can be solved by "pulling oneself up by one's bootstraps." Information should be provided regarding "marker symptoms," e.g., what one may expect to improve with treatment. For example, if early morning awakening has been a symptom of depression, the nurse would educate the patient that decrease and cessation of this symptom should occur with successful treatment of depression. When appropriate, spouses and/or family members should also be educated about the nature of depression, its course, and the relative costs and benefits of treatment options (Depression Guideline Panel, 1993).

Emotional Support

The NIC intervention Emotional Support, defined as "provision of reassurance, acceptance, and encouragement during times of stress" (Iowa Intervention Project, 2000, p. 300), is another strategy for treatment of depression in older adults. Most of the activities listed under the Emotional Support intervention are appropriate for management of depression. However, the interested reader is referred to Chapter 49 (Grieving) for an alternative view to the linear, stage-specific view of the grieving process, as assumed under the activity "Provide support during denial, anger, bargaining and acceptance phases of grieving." Other activities under the intervention Emotional Support are listed here:

- Discuss with the patient the emotional experience(s)
- Assist patient in recognizing feelings of anxiety, anger, or sadness
- Discuss consequences of not dealing with guilt and shame
- Facilitate patient's identification of usual response pattern in coping with fears
- Identify the function that anger, frustration, and rage serve for the patient
- Stay with the patient and provide assurance of safety and security during periods of anxiety
- Reduce demand for cognitive functioning when patient is ill or fatigued
- Support the use of appropriate defense mechanisms
- Encourage the patient to express feelings of anxiety, anger, or sadness
- Listen to expressions of feelings and beliefs
- Provide support during denial, anger, bargaining, and acceptance phases of grieving

- Encourage talking or crying as means to decrease the emotional response
- Provide assistance in decision making
- Refer for counseling, as appropriate

When successfully applied, this intervention provides elders with a sense of hope and decreases their sense of isolation and alienation. An important aspect of any intervention for depressed elders is involvement of family via education and interpretation of depressive symptoms whenever possible.

Counseling

The NIC intervention Counseling is defined as "use of an interactive helping process focusing on the needs, problems, or feelings of the patient and significant others to enhance or support coping, problem-solving, and interpersonal relationships" (Iowa Intervention Project, 2000, p. 238). Virtually all of the activities listed under this intervention are appropriate for use with depressed older adults:

- Establish a therapeutic relationship based on trust and respect
- Demonstrate empathy, warmth, and genuineness
- Establish the length of the counseling relationship
- Establish goals
- Provide privacy and ensure confidentiality
- Provide factual information, as necessary and appropriate
- Encourage expression of feelings
- Assist patient to identify the problem or situation that is causing the distress
- Use techniques of reflection and clarification to facilitate expression of concerns
- Ask patient/significant others to identify what they can/cannot do about what is happening
- Assist patient to list and prioritize all possible alternatives to a problem
- Identify any differences between the patient's view of the situation and the view of the health care team
- Determine how family behavior affects patient
- Verbalize the discrepancy between the patient's feelings and behaviors
- Use assessment tools (e.g., paper and pencil measures, audiotape, videotape, or interactional exercises with other people) to help increase patient's self-awareness and counselor's knowledge of situation, as appropriate
- Reveal selected aspects of one's own experiences or personality to foster genuineness and trust, as appropriate
- Assist patient to identify strengths and reinforce these
- Encourage new skill development, as appropriate
- Encourage substitution of undesirable habits with desirable habits
- Reinforce new skills
- Discourage decision making when the patient is under severe stress

There is scientific evidence that psychotherapy (counseling) alone can be used successfully as a first-line treatment for mild to moderate major depression; there also is minimal evidence that psychotherapy alone is effective in severe or psychotic forms of depression (Depression Guideline Panel, 1993). There is a notable lack of outcome studies that compare the effects of different psychotherapeutic interventions in the over-65 population. A few studies have demonstrated that the combination of psychotherapy and medication has been more efficacious in relieving depression than either intervention alone (Rush & Beck, 1978; Thompson & Gallagher, 1986). As for medication, monitoring for symptom response is imperative. If therapy is ineffective after 6 weeks, or if therapy "does not result in nearly a full symptomatic remission within 12 weeks, a switch to medication may well be appropriate since there is clear evidence of its specific efficacy" (Depression Guideline Panel, 1993, p. 73).

Behavioral Therapy

Therapy based on social learning theory (Bandura, 1987) and functional analysis of behavior (Ferster, 1973) includes such interventions as setting up a daily schedule, practicing assertiveness, or problem solving. A meta-analysis of psychotherapy trials in outpatients with major depressive disorder suggests that the overall efficacy of behavioral therapy was 55.3%. Behavioral therapy was 9.1% more effective than other forms of psychotherapy and 23.9% more effective than medication alone (Depression Guidelines Panel, 1993). There is some evidence that behavior therapy is more effective than relaxation training on improved mood at follow-up (McLean & Hakstian, 1990), but this approach needs additional research in older populations.

Cognitive Therapy

Beck (1967) focused on the cognitive processes of depression. His contribution is based primarily on the theory that depressive signs stem from the negative "self-talk" characteristic of depressed individuals. This negative triad or cognitive set consists of attitudes and beliefs regarding the self, the world, and the future. Beck characterized depressed individuals as creating their own depression by distorting interpretations of reality, focusing on and reinforcing the negative. The therapeutic approach consistent with Beck's theory (cognitive therapy) involves the conscious restructuring of the negative thought processes of depressed individuals, using a time-limited (thus efficient) approach. Modification of conscious thoughts, feelings, and behaviors identified as promoting the depressive state is the primary goal of this therapy. The therapist and patient collaborate, through mutual goal setting, to achieve the desired cognitive and affective changes. For adult outpatients suffering from depression, efficacy for cognitive therapy was 46.6% for all persons evaluated and

51.3% for geriatric outpatients (Depression Guideline Panel, 1993).

Vague and "mysterious" approaches to therapy, in which the objectives are not clear and the therapist remains disengaged, are poorly tolerated by most elderly persons. A combination of cognitive and behavioral interventions is promoted by therapists who work with elders because of the time efficiency, the reinforcement of self-control, and the relative ease with which the technique can be learned by caregivers (Chaisson, Beutler, Yost, & Tallendes, 1984). Elders have been found to be more accepting and responsive to cognitive/behavioral approaches because of the collaborative stance of the therapist and the explicitness and practicality of stating specific cognitive and behavioral outcomes, which are easily recognized (reinforced) in the course of therapy.

Interpersonal Therapy

The theoretical basis of this type of therapy suggests that interpersonal problems serve to cause, exacerbate, or maintain depression. Interpersonal therapy is focused on the patient's relationship to significant others rather than on the intrapsychic focus of brief dynamic therapy. Interpersonal therapy targets patients' relationships as the focus of intervention and is designed to assist patients to modify either their relationships or their expectations about those relationships. In addition to patient education regarding the nature and course of depressive illness, the therapist provides a corrective or healthy relationship with the patient to supply a model of a satisfying interpersonal relationship. In so doing, the therapist actively converses, empathizes, and validates the patient's thoughts and feelings (Peplau, 1952; Sullivan, 1954).

There is some evidence from a 12-week period of acute-phase randomized trials in outpatients with nonpsychotic major depression that interpersonal therapy was as effective as amitriptyline in decreasing depressive symptoms. Interestingly, the amitriptyline seemed to target the vegetative symptoms earlier, while the interpersonal therapy treatment group reported earlier improvement of suicidal ideation, work, interest, and mood (DiMascio et al., 1979a, 1979b). The efficacy of interpersonal therapy has exceeded that of cognitive therapy by 13.2%, that of placebo plus clinical management by 22.6%, and that of imipramine by 12.3% (Depression Guideline Panel, 1993). However, the value of interpersonal therapy for depressed elders warrants further investigation.

Brief Dynamic Therapy

The theoretical underpinnings of this therapy are based on the idea that emotional distress (depression) is derived from unresolved, intrapsychic conflicts from early life. Therefore the therapeutic approach to treatment involves resolution of intrapsychic conflicts and restructuring of the personality. To be suitable for psychodynamically oriented psychotherapy, older adults must be motivated, capable of introspection and psychologic insight, show evidence of good adaptation earlier in life, and be able to tolerate strong emotions (Davanloo, 1980).

Meta-analysis of six randomized controlled trials using brief dynamic therapy suggested an efficacy of 34.8%, although the target population was not elders. Overall, this therapy might have a weaker effect, compared to the directive, more structured therapies (interpersonal, behavioral, and cognitive), especially for older adults (Depression Guideline Panel, 1993).

Supportive Therapy

Whereas the aforementioned therapies are tied to theories of psychopathology, supportive therapy techniques are not theory-driven. Instead, they are based on what works and what seems to make the patient feel and function better. Supportive therapy involves evaluating the patient's psychologic strengths and weaknesses and helping the individual to make choices that increase her functional capacity. The therapist often strives to reduce the patient's anxiety, which might be interfering with the adequate use of typical coping devices. The therapist supports the patient's healthy defenses and assists the patient in finding ways of coping with stress when the individual's own defenses are inadequate. Appropriate elderly candidates for supportive psychotherapy include healthy, high-functioning patients undergoing extreme stress as well as frail elders with limited capacity for insight and poor verbal skills (Winston, Pinsker, & McCullough, 1986).

Special Focus of Group Work With Elders

A geriatric group can be designed for a variety of purposes. Severely depressed and cognitively impaired elders will benefit from sensory stimulation, reality orientation, and remotivation activities. Persons with a variety of affects can be beneficial in stimulating withdrawn patients and calming anxious members. A cohort group that focuses on reminiscing and life review can facilitate these processes for persons reluctant to engage in reminiscing on a one-to-one basis. Movement, music, art, and psychodrama tend to bring forth creativity and expression of feelings (catharsis) that might not surface without stimulation. The curative factors of "universality" and "instillation of hope" can be especially beneficial for members of a "grievers" or widow's group, since the members can share their loss experiences (Table 41-4).

Group work, when applied with sensitivity, caring, planning, organization, skill, and self-investment, can be fun and rewarding. Anecdoctal evidence supports the effectiveness of this intervention with the elderly; however, there are few outcome studies comparing the effectiveness of different types of geriatric group work. Nurses, both in the community and in long-term care settings, are in prime positions to explore this cost-effective, therapeutic intervention through ongoing research efforts. For complete guides to group work with elders, the reader is referred to Burnside (1984).

Milieu Therapy

Behavioral principles and group process theory form the major foundations for constructing a therapeutic milieu. Perhaps no other psychotherapeutic intervention has such strong implications for nursing in long-term care settings. The scientific structuring of the environment to promote health, foster individual strengths, and affect personal growth in patients is clearly the nurse's domain. Milieu therapy has preventive as well as therapeutic value and must be a major consideration in all long-term care settings.

To best meet the needs of each unique elder within a diverse and changeable patient-staff community, the geriatric milieu must be dynamic and evolving. Staff-related factors (nurse/patient ratio, interpersonal variables,

Table 41-4	Curative Factors in Group Work With the Elderly
Socialization	Provides replacement of meaningful relationships and stimulation of social skills. Allows for celebration of holidays and social events and reminiscing among cohorts. Provides opportunities to resume former roles (chairman, secretary, president, etc.).
Group cohesiveness	Refers to the "stick-togetherness" characterized by group membership. Provides for a sense of belonging (e.g., an old cohort group may begin to view themselves as the "biologic elite" within a facility). Reaffirms ability to be liked and make friends. Provides for expression of affection and physical contact, esteem, and validation.
Universality	Provides a sense of "We're all in this together." Enables members to see themselves in others and to share experiences, successes, and losses.
Instillation of hope	Complements universality. Enables members to see that others have suffered and survived similar situations. Members can share adaptive strengths and coping skills.
Altruism	Very important. Members are provided opportunities to feel needed and to help others. Reinforces self-esteem. Often the support and advice received from peers is integrated more readily than "professional advice."

Adapted from Yost, E. B., & Corbishley, M. A. (1985). Group therapy. In Chaisson-Stewart, G. M. (Ed.), *Depression in the elderly: An interdisciplinary approach.* New York: John Wiley & Sons.

attitudes and interactions, staffing patterns and composition, and level of skill) have a profound influence on the prevailing atmosphere and must be included in the milieu assessment and structuring. Box 41-2 provides a useful framework for organizing the complex concept of milieu into a workable format. Examples illustrate how to categorize elements in the environment. Once the elements in each long-term care facility have been categorized, the staff and residents, if at all possible (we recommend an ongoing "milieu committee"), can determine which elements should be manipulated or altered to promote health, foster growth, and prevent deterioration based on individual strengths and needs.

Pharmacologic Interventions

Antidepressant medication has been effective in alleviating moderate to severe depression in elders; however, caution must be exercised because of the following:

- The risk of death from suicide by overdose
- Poor adherence, due to greater sensitivity to side effects
- Medically significant side effects
- The need for education of the patient and family about depression and its treatment
- Intercurrent medical disease that interferes with proper antidepressant dosing
- Occult self-medication with drugs such as alcohol
- Inadequate family support to continue taking medication properly (Depression Guideline Panel, 1993)

Biologic and pharmacokinetic changes that accompany aging influence the absorption, distribution, metabolism, and excretion of most medications. Additionally, the anticholinergic, cardiovascular, and neurologic side effects of many of the commonly used antidepressants can be pronounced in elders. Patients with significant cardiac disease will require particularly judicious use of medication and careful monitoring. The previous good response of a patient or family member indicates that the same medication should be considered.

Generally, the drugs in the antidepressant class known as the secondary amines (e.g., nortriptyline and desipramine) are as efficacious as the tertiary amines (e.g., imipramine and amitryptyline) in relieving depression in late life and have the advantage of fewer anticholinergic and sedative side effects. However, for agitated, depressed elders, more sedating antidepressants might be warranted. The recommended geriatric dosage is always lower than the recommended dosages found in drug handbooks for the general population (usually one-third to one-half lower). It is also generally recommended that the daily dosage be divided into two or three doses to avoid the sudden rise in blood levels that may accentuate side effects. Table 41-5 lists characteristics of the most commonly used antidepressants.

A newer generation of antidepressants, known as selective serotonin reuptake inhibitors (SSRIs), are comparable to the tricylics in terms of efficacy, but have a more promising side effect profile. Among the advantages of the SSRIs in elderly patients are a decreased potential for fatal

---

Box 41-2 Milieu Components	
Structure	**Support**
Regular mealtimes	Nourishment
Scheduled activities	Medication
Predictability and routine consistency	Social support
Bowel/bladder program	Reassurance
Shift change	Visitors
Medication time	Physical therapy, occupational therapy
Vital signs	Spiritual expression, consistent, positive
Regular physician visits	Staff attitudes
Bedtime	Handrails
Primary nursing	Mutual goal setting
Care planning	Exercise
Evaluation	
	Validation
Containment	Reality orientation, feedback, acceptance
Physical aspects of the facility: interior design, safety features, atmosphere, space, privacy, lighting, location, temperature, noise, odors, colors, infection control, restraints, confinement, isolation, "homey"	Interaction, contact with world
	Music, touch, warmth, creative expression, sensory stimulation
	Focus on positive aspects of behavior, "downplay" negative
Atmosphere of rooms, roommates	Newspaper, TV, one to one relationships
Access to public transportation, "Knock before entering"	Patient autonomy and decision making
	Excursions outside

Adapted from Gunderson, J. G., Will, O. A., Mosher, L. R. (1983). *Principles and practice of milieu therapy,* New York: Aronson.

Table 41-5 Characteristics of Selected Antidepressant Drugs

Drug	Level of Sedation	Anticholinergic Activity	Degree of Orthostatic Hypotension	Recommended Geriatric Dosage (mg/day)
Tricyclic tertiary amines				
• Amitryptyline	Very high	Very high	High	25-150
• Doxepin	High	High	Middle	25-150
• Imipramine	Middle	Middle	High	25-150
Tricyclic secondary amines				
• Despramine	None	Low	Low	25-150
• Protriptyline	None	Middle	Low	5-30
• Nortriptyline	Low	Middle	Low	10-35
Tricyclic dibenzoxazepine				
• Amoxapine	Middle	Middle	Low	25-150
Tetracyclic				
• Maprotiline	Middle	Middle	Low	25-150
Other				
• Trazodone	Middle	Very low	Low	50-200

Drug/Class	Trade Name	Dosage (mg/day)	Common Side Effects
Monocyclic			Increased restlessness, anxiety, insomnia
• Bupropion	Wellbutrin	300-450	
SSRIs			For all SSRIs listed: anxiety, insomnia, nausea, diarrhea, headache, decreased appetite, delayed orgasm, decreased libido
• Fluoxetine	Prozac	20-60	
• Sertraline	Zoloft	50-200	
• Paroxetine	Paxil	20-50	
• Fluvoxamine	Luvox	50-300	
Serotonin-norepinephrine reuptake inhibitor			Nausea, dose-related hypertension
• Venlafaxine	Effexor	75-300	
Phenylpiperazine antidepressants			Hypotension, lightheadedness, bradycardia, confusion, vision changes, dry mouth, nausea, constipation, diarrhea, urinary retention, rash
• Nefazodone	Serzone	50-600	

Data from Ouslander, J. G., Small, G. W. (1984, October). Management of depression in the elderly patient with physical illness, *Geriatric Medicine Today, 3*(10), 94.

overdose and fewer anticholinergic side effects. However, even though effective in alleviating depression, the SSRIs should be used with caution. Some, like fluoxetine, can result in weight loss, agitation, sexual dysfunction, and sleep difficulty in elders. Therefore the SSRIs sertraline and paroxetine are usually recommended for older patients, as they tend to produce less agitation. New drugs such as venlafaxine (Effexor), which is both a serotonin and norepinephrine reuptake inhibitor, and nefazodone (Serzone) show great promise in treating late life depression safely as well.

Agitated depressed elders not responsive to the tricyclic class of antidepressants may benefit from a monoamine oxidase inhibitor (MAOI) such as tranylcypromine

(Parnate) or phenelzine (Nardil). Tyramine must be eliminated from the diet and sympathomimetic medications must be discontinued to prevent hypertensive crisis associated with these drugs. For clinical trials of MAOI, lithium, or other psychotropic medications that are particularly challenging to administer and regulate in elders, we recommend obtaining geropsychiatric consultation.

Electroconvulsant Therapy

The 2- to 3-week lag time between onset of antidepressant drug therapy and symptom relief is a significant liability for severely depressed elders whose health is in danger. When suicide or starvation is a real threat or when antidepressants are ineffective or contraindicated, electroconvulsive therapy (ECT) should be considered. The main criteria for selecting ECT as the treatment of choice are the severity of depression and the necessity for immediate results (Zung, 1980).

Because of advances in the use of muscle relaxants and anesthesia, ECT is rapidly effective and safe with judicious screening. The unilateral method has been shown to decrease the confusion and recent memory loss associated with this intervention. Essentially, ECT can serve as a life-saving measure in the elderly and is especially effective in the relief of delusional depression. Ignorance and negative emotions associated with early, less sophisticated use of ECT should not enter into decisions regarding the appropriateness of this intervention.

earlier in his plan of care. Initially she worked toward developing trust and establishing a therapeutic alliance (Counseling) to enable him to work through the grief process associated with his wife's condition (Emotional Support) and to develop more effective coping patterns (Coping Enhancement). She also taught Mr. Ray about the antidepressant nortriptyline, which had been prescribed for him (Patient Teaching: Prescribed Medication) and about depression itself (Teaching: Disease Process). The nurse consultant scheduled meetings with Mr. Ray's primary nurse, dietitian, social worker, and activity specialist, so that the interventions could be consistently applied and reinforced.

Based on Mr. Ray's strengths and the assessment data obtained earlier, Mr. Ray was invited to join an assertiveness class. Applying behavioral principles, the nursing home staff consistently identified, praised, and reinforced positive changes in his behavior, assertive interactions, and expression of feelings (Suicide Prevention).

The nurse also worked individually with Mr. Ray on cognitive restructuring (Cognitive Restructuring) in an effort to reduce his guilt; the nurse encouraged expression of feelings by using a "feelings list." This approach eventually helped Mr. Ray to recognize his own grieving behavior. He was invited to join a "griever's group" at the nursing home but he initially refused. Despite his reluctance to join the group, nursing staff continued to support Mr. Ray in the grieving process (see Chapter 49, Grieving) and to listen to his concerns actively and empathetically (Emotional Support).

CASE STUDY

The geropsychiatric nurse clinician determined that Mr. Ray was not actively suicidal, that he had no history of previous attempts, and that he could remain on the health-related floor of the facility. She advised the nursing staff to refrain from criticizing Mr. Ray's appearance and behavior, educated them about the warning signs of suicide, and conducted an environmental assessment of Mr. Ray's room for dangerous objects.

The geropsychiatric nurse clinician, together with Mr. Ray's physician, decided to combine both counseling and pharmacotherapy. After the nurse educated Mr. Ray about antidepressant medications and their effects, he agreed to this plan of care. The geropsychiatric nurse consultant spent a great deal of time helping Mr. Ray understand the antidepressant medication the doctor had prescribed for him, as Mr. Ray was initially reluctant to take "mind pills" and "uppers." She also met with the staff of the long-term care facility to discuss the medication and the observation of possible side effects. When he visited, Mr. Ray's son actively participated in the educational process. The nurse also sent him information regarding late life depression and its treatment. The nurse kept Mr. Ray's son involved through monthly phone consultations.

The nurse met with Mr. Ray twice a week and used several of the NIC interventions discussed or identified

SUMMARY

The diagnosis Depression is multifaceted and characterized by a varied constellation of behaviors, feelings, and signs. Rarely does depression exist as an isolated clinical entity. Rather, biochemical, social, physical, psychologic, and environmental factors present in a complex interplay that makes diagnosis difficult and easy to miss. A series of assessment tools and tips can aid in this task.

Since no NANDA diagnosis currently exists for depression per se, it is difficult to link NIC interventions and NOC outcomes with this diagnosis. However, Table 41-2 illustrates related diagnoses, interventions, and outcomes that can assist the nurse in addressing this major health concern among older adults. Due to the prevalence of depression in the elderly and its consequences when undiagnosed and untreated, it is recommended that NANDA develop the nursing diagnosis Depression based on the DSM-IV (APA) criteria, etiologies, and defining characteristics for major depressive episode and mood disorder due to general medical condition.

Gerontologic nurses in acute care, community, and long-term care settings have a broad armamentarium of psychiatric and nursing interventions to employ. Cognitive and behavioral strategies are particularly effective with depressed elders. Group and milieu approaches can be very helpful in preventing and alleviating depression. The nurse must also be knowledgeable of somatic treatments (e.g., medications and ECT), which are often employed as adjunctive treatments with elders. Appropriate and timely intervention can foster improved mood, lessening of depressive symptoms, improved coping, and increased hope. These outcomes represent critical components of well-being in the elderly.

REFERENCES

Allen, A., & Blazer, D. G. (1991). Mood disorders. In J. Sadavoy, L. Lazarus, & L. Jarvik (Eds.), *Comprehensive review of geriatric psychiatry* (pp. 337-351). Washington, DC: American Psychiatric Press.

American Psychiatric Association. (1994). *Diagnostic and statistical manual of mental disorders* (4th ed.). Washington, DC: Author.

Armitage, R. (1995). Microarchitectural findings in sleep EEG in depression: Diagnostic implications. *Biological Psychiatry, 37,* 72-84.

Badger, T. A., Duman, R., & Kwan, T. (1996). Knowledge of depression and application to practice: A program evaluation. *Issues in Mental Health Nursing, 17,* 93-109.

Bandura, A. (1987). *Social learning theory.* Englewood Cliffs, NJ: Prentice Hall.

Beck, A. T. (1967). *Depression, clinical, experimental and theoretical aspects.* New York: Harper & Row.

Beck, A. T., Rush, A. J., Shaw, B. F., & Emery, G. (1979). *Cognitive therapy of depression.* New York: Guilford Press.

Berkman, L. F., Berkman, C. S., Kasl, S., Freeman, D. H., Leo, L., Ostfeld, A. M., Cornoni-Huntley, J., & Brody, J. A. (1986). Depressive symptoms in relation to physical health and functioning in the elderly. *American Journal of Epidemiology, 124*(3), 372-388.

Billiard, M., Partinen, M., Roth, R., & Shapiro, C. (1994). Sleep and psychiatric disorders. *Journal of Psychosomatic Research, 38,* 1-2.

Blazer, D. (1993). *Depression in late life* (2nd ed.). St. Louis, MO: Mosby.

Brink, T. L., Yesavage, J. A., Lum, O., Heersema, P. H., Adey, M., & Rose, T. L. (1982). Screening tests for geriatric depression. *Clinical Gerontologist, 1*(1), 37-43.

Brown, G. M. (1989). Neuroendocrine probes as biological marker of affective disorders: New directions. *Canadian Journal of Psychiatry, 34,* 819-823.

Burnside, I. M. (1980). *Psychosocial nursing care of the aged* (2nd ed.). Hightstown, NJ: McGraw-Hill.

Burnside, I. M. (1984). *Working with the elderly: Group process and techniques.* Sudbury, MA: Jones & Bartlett.

Buschmann, M., & Rossen, E. (1993). Depression in older women. *Journal of Women's Health, 2,* 317-322.

Callahan, C. M., Hendrie, H. C., Dittus, R. S., Brater, D. C., Hui, S. L., & Tierney, W. M. (1994). Improving treatment of late life depression in primary care: A randomized clinical trial. *Journal of the American Geriatrics Society, 42,* 839-846.

Carroll, B. J. (1982). The dexamethasone test for melancholia. *British Journal of Psychiatry, 140,* 292-304.

Carroll, B. J., Curtis, G. C., & Mendels, J. (1976a). Neuroendocrine regulation in depression I: Limbic system-adrenocortical dysfunction. *Archives of General Psychiatry, 33,* 1039-1044.

Carroll, B. J., Curtis, G. C., & Mendels, J. (1976b). Neuroendocrine regulation in depression II: Discrimination of depressed from nondepressed patients. *Archives of General Psychiatry, 33,* 1051-1058.

Chaisson, G. M., Beutler, L., Yost, E., & Tallendes, J. (1984). Treating depressed elderly. *Journal of Psychosocial Nursing & Mental Health Services, 22*(5), 25-30.

Chaisson-Stewart, G. M. (1985). An integrated theory of depression. In G. M. Chaisson-Stewart (Ed.), *Depression in the elderly: An interdisciplinary approach.* New York: John Wiley & Sons.

Davanloo, H. (1980). A method of short-term psychotherapy. In H. Davanloo (Ed.), *Short term dynamic psychotherapy* (pp. 43-71). New York: Aronson.

Depression Guideline Panel. (1993, April). *Depression in primary care: Volume 1. Detection and diagnosis. Clinical practice guideline, Number 5.* Rockville, MD. U.S. Department of Health and Human Services, Public Health Service, Agency for Health Care Policy and Research. AHCRP Publication No. 93-0550.

DiMascio, A., Klerman, G. L., Weissman, M. M., Prusoff, B. A., Neu, C., & Moore, P. (1979a). A control group for psychotherapy research in acute depression: One solution to ethical and methodological issues. *Journal of Psychiatric Research, 15,* 189-197.

DiMascio, A., Weissman, M. M., Prusoff, B. A., Neu, C., Zwilling, M., & Klerman, G. L. (1979b). Differential symptoms reduction by drugs and psychotherapy in acute depression. *Archives of General Psychiatry, 36,* 1450-1456.

Dinan, T. G. (1996). Noradrenergic and serotonergic abnormalities in depression: Stress-induced dysfunction: *Journal of Clinical Psychiatry, 57* (Suppl. 4), 14-18.

Ferster, C. B. (1973). A functional analysis of depression. *American Psychologist, 28,* 857-870.

German, P. S., Shapiro, S., Skinner, E. A., Von Korff, M., Klein, L. E., Turner, R. W., Teitelbaum, M. L., Burke, J., & Burns, B. J. (1987). Detection and management of mental health problems of older patients by primary care providers. *Journal of the American Medical Association, 257*(4), 480-493.

Gordon, M. (1982). *Manual of nursing diagnosis.* Hightstown, NJ: McGraw-Hill.

Gunderson, J. G., Will, O. A., & Mosher, L. R. (1983). *Principles and practice of milieu therapy.* New York: Aronson.

Hagerty, B. M. (1995). Advances in understanding major depressive disorder. *Journal of Psychosocial Nursing, 33,* 27-34.

Iowa Intervention Project. J. C. McCloskey & G. M. Bulechek (Eds.). (2000). *Nursing interventions classification (NIC)* (3rd ed.). St. Louis, MO: Mosby.

Iowa Outcomes Project. M. Johnson, M. Maas, & S. Moorhead (Eds.). (2000). *Nursing outcomes classification (NOC)* (2nd ed.). St. Louis, MO: Mosby.

Kneisl, C. R., & Wilson, H. S. (1984). *Handbook of psychosocial nursing care.* Reading, MA: Addison Wesley Longman.

Koenig, H. G., Ford, S. M., & Blazer, B. G. (1993). Should physicians screen for depression in elderly medical patients?: Results of a decision analysis. *International Journal of Psychiatry in Medicine, 23,* 239-263.

Lazarus, L. W., Davis, J. M., & Dysken, M. W. (1985). Geriatric depression: A guide to successful therapy. *Geriatrics, 40*(6), 43-53.

Manton, K. G., Blazer, D. G., & Woodbury, M. A. (1987). Suicide in middle age and later life: Sex and race specific life table and cohort analyses. *Journal of Gerontology, 42,* 219-227.

McLean, P. D., & Hakstian, A. R. (1990). Relative endurance of unipolar depression treatment effects: Longitudinal follow-up. *Journal of Consultation in Clinical Psychology, 58,* 482-488.

Meyers, B. (1994). Epidemiology and clinical meaning of "significant" depressive symptoms in later life: The question of sub-syndromal depression. *The American Journal of Geriatric Psychiatry, 2,* 188-193.

Mossey, J. M., Knott, K., & Craik, R. (1990). The effects of persistent depressive symptoms on hip fracture recovery. *Journal of Gerontology, 45,* 163-168.

North American Nursing Diagnosis Association. (1999). *Nursing diagnoses: Definitions & classification 1999-2000.* Philadelphia: Author.

Oxman, T. E., Berkman, L. F., Kasl, S., Freeman, D. H., & Barrett, J. (1990). Social support and depressive symptoms in the elderly. *American Journal of Epidemiology, 135,* 356-368.

Pardes, H. (1986). Neuroscience and psychiatry: Marriage or co-existence. *American Journal of Psychiatry, 143,* 1205-1212.

Parmelee, P. A., Katz, I. R., & Lawton, M. P. (1992). Depression and mortality among institutionalized aged. *Journal of Gerontology, 47,* 3-10.

Peplau, H. E. (1952). *Interpersonal relations in nursing.* New York: G. P. Putnam's Sons.

Piven, M. L. S., Schacht, E., Brems, C. S., Hradek, E., Hegamin-Younger, C. Keen, P., & Buckwalter, K. (1996). *Multidimensional functional assessment of elders in the general hospital.* Unpublished manuscript.

Profitt, C., Augspurger, P., & Byrne, M. (1996). Geriatric depression: A survey of nurses' knowledge and assessment practices. *Issues in Mental Health Nursing, 17,* 123-130.

Radloff, L. S. (1977). A self-report depression scale for research in the general population. *Applied Psychological Measurement, 1,* 385-401.

Rapp, S. R., & Davis, K. M. (1989). Geriatric depression: Physicians knowledge, perceptions, and diagnostic practices. *The Gerontologist, 29,* 252-257.

Reynolds, C. F., Kupfer, D. J., Houck, P. R., Hoch, C. C., Stack, J. A., Berman, S. R., & Zimmer, B. (1988). Reliable discrimination of elderly depressed and demented patients by electroen-cephalographic sleep data. *Archives of General Psychiatry, 45,* 258-264.

Rush, A. J., & Beck, A. T. (1978). Cognitive therapy of depression and suicide. *American Journal of Psychiatry, 32*(2), 201-219.

Schneider, L. S., & Olin, J. T. (1995). Efficacy of acute treatment for geriatric depression. *International Psychogeriatrics, 7,* 7-25.

Seligman, M. (1975). *Helplessness: On depression, development and death.* San Francisco: W. H. Freeman.

Sheikh, J. I., & Yesavage, J. A. (1986). Geriatric Depression Scale (GDS): Recent evidence and development of a shorter version. *Clinical Gerontologist, 5*(1/2), 165-173.

Siever, L. J., & Davis, K. L. (1985). Overview: Toward a dysregulation hypothesis of depression. *American Journal of Psychiatry, 142,* 1017-1031.

Sullivan, H. S. (1954). *The psychiatric interview.* New York: W. W. Norton.

Thomas, M. D., Sanger, E., & Whitney, J. D. (1986). Nursing diagnosis of depression. *Journal of Psychosocial Nursing, 24,* 6-12.

Thompson, L. W., & Gallagher, D. (1986, Spring). Psychotherapy for late life depression. *Generations,* 38-41.

Veith, R. C., & Raskind, M. A. (1988). The neurology of aging: Does it predispose to depression? *Neurobiology of Aging, 9,* 101-117.

Winston, A., Pinsker, H., & McCullough, L. (1986). A review of supportive psychotherapy. *Hospital and Community Psychiatry, 37,* 1105-1114.

Yesavage, J., Brink, T., Rose, T., Lum, O., Huang, V., Adey, M., & Otto Leirer, V. (1983). Development and validation of a geriatric depression screening scale: A preliminary report. *Journal of Psychiatric Research, 17,* 37-49.

Yost, E. B., & Corbishley, M. A. (1985). Group therapy. In G. M. Chaisson-Stewart (Ed.), *Depression in the elderly: An interdisciplinary approach.* New York: John Wiley & Sons.

Zauszniewski, J. A. (1994). Nursing diagnosis and depressive illness. *Nursing Diagnosis, 5,* 106-114.

Zung, W. W. K. (1980). Affective disorders. In E. W. Busse & D. G. Blazer (Eds.), *Handbook of geriatric psychiatry.* New York: Van Nostrand Reinhold.

CHAPTER 42

BODY IMAGE DISTURBANCE

Orpha J. Glick

Body image is a multidimensional construct that reflects an individual's total body experience over time. It represents the cognitive and affective integration of sensory, intrapersonal, and interpersonal information one receives from or about the body. Nurses (Bille, 1977; Drench, 1994; Fawcett & Frye, 1980; Liviskie, 1973; Popkess-Vawter, 1989; Stein, 1995; Wilson, 1981), neurologists, psychiatrists, and psychologists (Gorman, 1969; Helman, 1995; Henker, 1979; Lipowski, 1977) have hypothesized that body image is a critical factor in health and illness.

A disturbance in body image is an impairment in the way an individual perceives or conceives of his body. The disturbance may be related to a disorder that affects any level of body experience, it represents a discrepancy between the individual's perception and reality, and it can be accompanied by negative judgments and attitudes toward the body or body function (Gordon, 1994).

Nurses have written about the importance of body image and disturbance of body image in health promotion and in care during illness. One of the earliest studies of body image disturbance was reported by Rubin (1967), who studied body image as a factor in maternal role taking. More recently, the nursing diagnosis Altered Body Image was included in the list of diagnoses generated at the First National Conference on Classification of Nursing Diagnosis in 1973. Since then, the wording of the diagnosis has been changed to Body Image Disturbance (Carroll-Johnson, 1989). According to Metzger and Hiltunen (1987), Body Image Disturbance is among the 10 most frequently reported diagnoses.

This chapter focuses on the nursing diagnosis and management of Body Image Disturbance in older adults who have or are at risk for developing impairments or alterations in perception or conception of their bodies. The conceptual structure for discussing body image is grounded in the complex interplay of neurobiologic and psychosocial phenomena of body experience. The concept of body image is examined as a foundation for understanding the clinical manifestations and related factors of Body Image Disturbance as well as to establish the relevance of the diagnosis for elderly populations.

BODY IMAGE: A DEVELOPMENTAL PROCESS

Body image as a phenomenon of human experience is difficult to describe because it is a theoretical abstraction of an individual's sensory-perceptual, cognitive, affective, and social experiences with the body. When viewed as a developmental process, body image is fluid and dynamic and changes throughout the life span. Some of these changes are very profound and occur rapidly, whereas others evolve more slowly. For example, during childhood and adolescence there are rapid changes in physical and mental growth as the central nervous system matures and the individual develops physically, emotionally, and socially. As the individual ages, body changes are subtler and occur gradually through daily life experiences such as body movement, hunger (or satiation), positive (or negative) interpersonal interactions, and intrapersonal reflection. The impact of any of these experiences on the construction of body image may or may not be a part of conscious awareness.

Most definitions of body image presented in the literature have incorporated perceptual, cognitive, and affective (feelings, attitudes) dimensions. Gorman (1969), however, has differentiated "precept" (perception) of body from "concept" (conception) of body. He noted, for example, that "body image is the conception of the body rather than a perception" (p. 17). This suggests that it is more a construction of the mind than a sensory image with spatial characteristics that is developed by the visual apparatus. This view is consistent with the schema model of self-concept described by Stein (1995). According to Stein, schemas are knowledge structures that are derived from experience, that are stored in long-term memory, and that subsequently operate as frameworks for processing information.

Shontz (1975) believed that individuals experience their bodies at different levels of perception. He described four integrated yet distinguishable levels: (1) body schema; (2) body self (boundary); (3) body fantasy; and (4) body concept. These levels are hierarchical in that they become more abstract as they move further from sensory experience. Moreover, each level of body experience incorporates phenomena from previous levels. The four levels are described here to provide a conceptual structure for studying and comprehending the complex nature of body image phenomena.

Body Schema

The most fundamental type of body experience is body schema. According to Shontz (1975), body schema has a neurobiologic basis and is "preprogrammed" in the infant's nervous system. It is further developed through physical maturation and processing information received during motor activity and learning (Gorman, 1969; Shontz, 1975).

Body schema incorporates sensory-perceptual information about body structures and functions. It provides the psychobiologic foundation for the development of certain basic psychomotor skills. For example, body schema integrates the wide range of postures for physical activity that are mediated by proprioception. Recall that proprioceptive feedback enables individuals to locate body parts in space and makes it possible for them to assume postures and to sequence movements required for motor function. Body schema also includes a topographic representation of the body. Topographic body schema operates to locate stimuli on or from the surface of the body. This safety mechanism warns the individual about potential injury and confirms the body boundary. Although body schemata influence awareness, they usually are not the focus of an individual's awareness. Shontz (1975) compared the role of body schema in awareness as the role of "ground" in the view of perception held by Gestalt psychology. He noted that "a body schema is the ground against which stimulation to the body is perceived as the figure" (p. 64).

The significance of body schema in human function was established in the early 1900s by neurologists who observed severe distortions in body perception in patients with brain damage. Gorman (1969) credited Henry Head, a neurologist, with developing the idea of body schema from extensive study of kinesthetic perception and the role of body posture and movement in the evaluation of body schema. The observation that distortion was most common when brain lesions occurred in the parietal lobe led to the assumption that brain localization for body image functions was the parietal lobe, particularly the posterior zone of the nondominant hemisphere (Fisher & Cleveland, 1968; Shontz, 1969). This notion is consistent with the knowledge that somatic sensory information is received and processed by regions of the parietal lobe and that it is integrated with sensory and motor signals from other cortical and subcortical brain regions and memory (past experience) in the association cortex (Kupfermann, 1991).

Body Self

The second level of body experience is "self." This level reflects the individual's experiences and perception with the body boundary and the differentiation between the "self" and the "nonself" (Shontz, 1975). Body boundaries are usually described in terms of strength or definiteness in contrast to weakness or indefiniteness (Vinck & Pierloot, 1977). Fisher and Cleveland (1968) are credited with some

of the most extensive work on the relationship among body boundary perception and somatic function, psychic function, and personality characteristics. These investigators used projective methods (Rorschach Ink Blot Test) to develop measures of high barrier (strong) versus high penetration (weak) body boundary perceptions. According to Vinck and Pierloot (1977), individuals with definite, clearly articulated body boundaries (high barrier scores) have a "clearer awareness" of body surface and demonstrate more intense reactions to injury of boundary regions (e.g., skin or muscle) and less reaction to injury of dysfunction in internal regions of the body. Conversely, persons with less definite, weak body boundary perceptions (higher penetration scores) are more sensitive to internal body regions (e.g., cardiac, gastrointestinal) and tend to react more intensely to injury or dysfunction in the internal regions.

The perception of body boundary also influences the definition and use of personal space. This extends the perception of the body boundary beyond the body itself. For example, the differentiation of self from the nonself serves as a reference for perceiving spatial direction such as in front of, behind, and above, as well as distance from the body (Shontz, 1975). These perceptions determine how one relates to other objects in space as well as to individuals in social interaction (Helman, 1995). Moreover, Gorman (1969) and others (Bleeker & Mulderij, 1992) have maintained that not only does body image extend beyond the body boundary (when defined as external surface) to external space and prostheses, it also extends to tools or vehicles that are intimately associated with the body (e.g., leg brace, cane, or wheelchair). Helman (1995) characterized this extension of body boundary as "symbolic skins."

In addition to the biologic and psychologic significance of body boundary, the differentiated self involves the social dimension of body image. Schilder (1950), a psychiatrist whose work focused on the influence of visual sensation on the development of body image, is viewed as the first person to address the role of social sanctions and responses in the development of body image (Drench, 1994). The impact of social responses on individuals' attitudes and beliefs about the appearance and function of their bodies is well known. The differentiated self is accompanied by self-evaluations and judgments (e.g., good vs. bad) depending on the individual's perception of others' reactions. These self-evaluations may or may not be accurate representations of reality.

Although individuals often are not consciously aware of the profound emotional and social significance of body boundary perception, accurate perception and self-differentiation contribute to one's sense of body integrity and safety as well as to self-hood (Helman, 1995). As previously noted, perceptions of body boundaries can be assessed by projective techniques such as the Rorschach Ink

Blot Test. The Draw-a-Person test has also been used and will be described in a later section of this chapter.

Body Fantasy

The fantasy level, the third level of body experience, contains the symbolic content of one's body experience (Shontz, 1975). Fantasies may encompass idealized body appearance or function. For example, elderly individuals with or without compromised health may fantasize their bodies as youthful and healthy. Mabry (1979) postulated that older adults often perceive their bodies as younger.

The stimuli for fantasy perceptions can originate from internal responses or from external input from social sources. Shontz (1975) believed that this dimension of body experience embodies the emotional and psychologic content of body image and most likely results from social sanctions throughout life. The fantasy level of body image can also be measured by projective techniques such as the Rorschach and Draw-a-Person tests. Because body fantasy is subjective and represents a more abstract level of body experience, results of projective tests may simultaneously have multiple meanings and be very difficult to interpret (Shontz, 1975).

Body Concept

Body concept, the fourth and most abstract level of body experience, incorporates one's knowledge about body structure and function that is accumulated through learning and life experiences. Although this dimension may be related to health and health practices, it is not essential to the function of body schemata (Shontz, 1975). This level of body experience is frequently used by health professionals to increase clients' comprehension and knowledge of their body functions and the way in which these functions may be altered by pathology and treatment. Hypothesized outcomes of educating individuals about their bodies are increased compliance and self-care, as well as disease prevention and health protection (Helman, 1995). However, the extent to which knowledge of one's anatomy and physiology actually influences behavior in health or illness has not been consistently documented in the health education literature.

The preceding description represents body image as both stable and dynamic in that it is situationally responsive to life changes (Hooker, 1992) and involves the integration or reintegration of basic levels of sensory experiences and perception (schema, body boundary), and cognitive levels of imagination, information processing, and knowledge (fantasy, concept). This results in a unified "gestalt" in the individual's conception of body appearance, structure, and function and the use of the body as an instrument for physical and psychosocial action. Although individuals may have a high level of knowledge about their bodies, it is clear that many of the body experiences described usually are not a part of awareness until body appearance or function is disturbed by developmental changes or by illness, injury, or disability (Drench, 1994; Morse, Bottorff, & Hutchinson, 1995).

The complexity of body image phenomena is further compounded by the interface of the concept with three closely related psychosocial constructs: self-esteem, personal identity, and role performance (Drench, 1994; Matteson, McConnell, & Linton, 1996; Stein, 1995). Self-esteem is the personal judgment of value or worth that individuals have about their body, person, intellect, or performance. Self-esteem is expressed in the attitudes that individuals have toward themselves (Coopersmith, 1967). The significance of self-esteem in human function in health and illness throughout life is well documented. Personal identity is defined as the individual's composite view of her own physical, intellectual, and emotional attributes, as well as achievements and aspirations. Personal identity is closely related to social role performance (Matteson et al., 1996; Murray, 1972). Conversely, the roles one assumes become a part of personal identity. For example, the role of grandparent incorporates certain personal and social characteristics and expectations. An individual's perception of self-worth and identification with "grandparenting" is intricately related to success and satisfaction in performing that role. Similarly, the perception of adequacy in body function is also linked to the performance of the role (Matteson et al., 1996).

The constructs of body image, self-esteem, personal identity, and role performance just described and their interrelationships are illustrated as overlapping circles by the North American Nursing Diagnosis Association (NANDA). The size of each component varies with the importance placed on it by an individual at a given time (Kim & Moritz, 1982). During the Fourth National Conference (1980), the concepts self-esteem, personal identity, and role performance, previously labeled as individual diagnoses, were added to body image as dimensions of self-concept. The nursing diagnosis label became "Self-Concept, Disturbance in: Body Image, Self-Esteem, Role Performance, Personal Identity" (Kim & Moritz, 1982). However, after the Eighth Conference, NANDA again labeled each of these dimensions as separate diagnoses (Carroll-Johnson, 1989).

PREVALENCE

Although it is commonly believed that elderly individuals are at high risk for disturbances in body image, little research documents the prevalence of these disturbances in this population. Moreover, there is little systematic exploration of their responses to alterations in body image. In a 1986 review, Janelli reported only six studies that included older adults in the sample. She also noted that the most frequently used instrument was human figure drawings and that many of the studies compared college and grade school children with psychiatric patients and institutionalized older adults. Janelli (1986) concluded that "overall, the studies indicated there are differences in body image perception among older adults and young persons as indicated in human figure drawings." The cause of these differences, however, is not clear. Janelli (1986) suggested that more research is needed to determine the effects of variables such as age, health status, and personality on older adults' perceptions of their bodies.

Hoffman (1983) examined perception of body image in adults age 65 to 83 and the effect of stress-related life events on their responses. Contrary to common belief, the subjects demonstrated moderately high (positive) body image scores. However, when the subjects were divided into two groups (stressed versus nonstressed), group differences were found, with "stressed" subjects being five times more likely to score low on the questionnaire than "nonstressed" subjects. The term *stressed* was operationalized as persons who had experienced severe illness, surgery, or widowhood within the last 5 years. Hoffman (1983) concluded that stress negatively affects body image in that stressed individuals think less positively about their body structure and function. These results, however, are difficult to interpret because sample size and the content of the questionnaire were not included in the report. Issues of validity and reliability also were not addressed.

Norris (1978), who conducted pioneering work in concept development of body image phenomena, suggested that threats to body image integrity induced by "normal" aging might be attenuated by an individual's inner psychologic and intellectual resources. This notion is supported by several researchers who found that age per se is not a risk factor for the development of body image disturbances (Bille, 1977; Hoffman, 1983; Lakin, 1960; Plutchik, Weiner, & Conte, 1971). More recent study of developmental processes and coping have shown similar results (Coward, 1996; Hansell & Mechanic, 1991).

RELATED FACTORS/ETIOLOGIES

Disturbance of body image in elderly adults can be caused by or associated with a wide range of organic and functional pathology, trauma, treatment modalities, and intrapsychic and interpersonal responses (Box 42-1). Studies have shown that lack of sensation in a body part, as well as perceptual changes due to visual disturbance or loss of position sense, can alter one's body image (Shontz, 1969). Organic brain lesions such as a hemispheric cerebrovascular accident (CVA) can generate alterations in body schema, particularly when the lesion occurs in the parietal lobe. These disturbances are manifested by inattention to the affected side (unilateral neglect) as well as to the environment (Mesulam, 1985). Other organic brain lesions are those causing dementia (e.g.,

Alzheimer's disease) and loss of motor control (Parkinson's disease).

Body image can be altered by musculoskeletal disorders, in particular by deformities and the constant presence of pain. Body image can be altered by pain alone. For example, an elderly person who has painful joints caused by arthritis might perceive the joint as being huge and overpowering other body parts or functions. Although the individual might be cognitively aware that other people do not perceive the joint in the same way, the presence of pain focuses the joint(s) as the center of his world (Eastman, 1983). Moreover, individuals who are experiencing discomfort often feel, behave, or appear differently than their usual pattern (Driscoll, 1985).

Psychopathology can be a source of body image disturbance. For example, individuals with schizophrenia have described feelings of changed body size or shape, of having lost a portion of their body, or of their body being "permeated" with poison. Depression, on the other hand, can be characterized by expressions of body "deterioration" and "disintegration" (Fisher & Cleveland, 1968).

Treatment modalities for acute or chronic diseases can alter body image. For example, surgical treatments such as enterostomy, mastectomy, radical neck resections, and extremity amputation result in visible changes in structure or function. Although less visible, treatments such as hysterectomy, coronary artery bypass, and organ transplants also require a reintegration of how the body looks and feels.

Some authors believe that lifesaving technologic advances have allowed more body image problems to surface than previously encountered (Henker, 1979). Similarly, advances in health care have made it possible for the population to age in the absence of epidemics and infections that raised mortality rates in previous generations. Increased longevity and changes in lifestyle patterns have increased the incidence and prevalence of chronic degenerative diseases, which, in turn, reduce functional capacity. Although elderly persons are becoming more valued as a result of growing social awareness, the American ideal of the independent individual functioning on her own remains (Hansell & Mechanic, 1991). This bias affects elders in a fundamental way, since interpersonal feedback is one of the factors involved in the formation and maintenance of one's body image. If the feedback given elders is negative and society continues to place greater value on youth and beauty than on life experience and wisdom, it is logical to predict that some individuals will be at risk for negative self-perceptions and attitudes regarding their capacity to function.

In addition to negative societal responses and increased susceptibility to chronic disease, older adults experience many losses (Drench, 1994): loss of occupation, loss of role function(s), loss of support systems, and loss of personal items (e.g., home, household items, automobile). Retirement brings about a loss of work role as well as social roles and expectations associated with occupational

Box 42-1	Pathophysiologic and Psychopathologic Conditions and Therapeutic Measures That Can Potentiate Body Image Disturbance

Surgical excision/alteration of body parts

- Enterostomy
- Mastectomy
- Hysterectomy
- Cardiovascular surgery
- Radical neck surgery
- Laryngectomy

Surgical or traumatic amputation
Burn injury
Facial trauma

Eating disorders

- Anorexia nervosa
- Bulimia

Obesity
Musculoskeletal alteration

- Arthritis

Alteration in integument

- Psoriasis
- Scars secondary to trauma/surgery

Brain lesions

- Cerebrovascular accidents
- Dementia
- Parkinson's disease

Affective disorders

- Depression
- Schizophrenia

Disfiguring endocrine disorder

- Acromegaly
- Cushing's syndrome

Chemical substance abuse
Diagnostic procedures
Loss or diminution of function

- Impotence
- Movement/control
- Sensory/perception
- Memory

Treatment modalities

- High technology (e.g., defibrillator implants, joint prostheses, dialysis)
- Chemotherapy

Pain
Psychosocial changes/losses

- Voluntary or forced changes in work or social roles
- Significant other support
- Divorce
- Personal possessions (home, household items, finances)
- Translocation/relocation

Societal responses to aging (ageism)

- Negative interpersonal feedback
- Emphasis on productivity

Knowledge deficit(s) (personal, caregiver, or societal)

identity and success (Mor-Barak, Scharlach, Birba, & Sokolov, 1992). In addition to social roles, occupation is deeply integrated into an individual's body image. For example, farmers are often viewed as strong, vigorous, and independent. Murray (1972) stated that "one's very essence may be felt to be a farmer, miner, musician or nurse." Consequently, retirement or injury requiring the cessation or alteration in work role can result in uncertainty about one's identity. Theriault (1994) maintained that retirement is a major life event that requires an internal reorganization of perceptions and expectations.

Actual loss or diminution of physical and mental function(s) can threaten body image wholeness for older adults. These losses can be induced by normal aging or by illness (Drench, 1994; Glick & Tripp-Reimer, 1996; Matteson et al., 1996). Norris (1978) noted that the body "communicates aging." When an individual perceives an aspect of his body as inferior, the inferiority is often generalized

to the total concept of self (Fisher & Cleveland, 1968). Norris (1978) maintained that feelings and perceptions about one's self or body image define and limit the capacity for function. This suggests that if older adults are assisted in developing a body image that is consistent with reality and maintaining a body appearance that is consistent with the internalized concept of the body, immobilizing impairments in body image can be reduced or prevented.

Loss of physical or mental functions frequently alters one's ability to control body functions. Developing control of body parts (e.g., hands, legs) and functions (e.g., dressing, grooming, locomotion) is accomplished through movement and exploration throughout early development. Once the neurobiologic, affective, and cognitive capacity for control is achieved, however, it becomes integrated into one's body image and identity. Only when one is threatened with a potential or actual loss of control of function does it enter conscious awareness and engender a profound effect on body image (Morse et al., 1995). Rubin (1968) stated, "To lose or be threatened with the loss of a complex coordinated and controlled functional activity which has been achieved and integrated into the personal system is to lose or be threatened with the loss of self." When this occurs, the mobilization of coping resources is compounded by feelings of inadequacy, shame, and grief. Consequently, efforts to realign body image depend on successful resolution of these and other affective responses (Drench, 1994; Matteson et al., 1996).

Another major loss experienced by elderly adults is the loss of their informal support system(s) (Murray, 1972). Informal support systems for elders include spouses, children or other family members, neighbors, and friends or peers (Stoller & Earl, 1983). In a sample of 753 noninstitutionalized elderly adults, Stoller and Earl found that a spouse provided the major support for elderly married individuals who were physically impaired. On the other hand, unmarried individuals with few family members relied more heavily on their friends for assistance and support. In a more recent study of 81 noninstitutionalized adults, Burbank (1992) found that relationships were a primary source of "meaning" in their lives and that the spouse relationship was most frequently listed as the "most meaningful."

The impact on individuals of losing part or all of their support system is less clear than that associated with illness and disability. However, one might hypothesize an indirect effect based on the belief that stress levels increase one's susceptibility to disease and illness and that social support is a resource for stress management. Thomas, Goodwin, and Goodwin (1985) maintained that social support is becoming accepted as an important determinant of health status in elders. They found, for example, that healthy older adults in their sample ($n = 256$) who had "good" social support systems tended to show lower serum cholesterol and uric acid levels and higher indices of immune function. These findings were independent of age, body mass, tobacco use, alcohol intake, and degree of perceived psychologic distress. These findings suggest that a support system not only ameliorates existing dysfunction from disturbances in body image related to chronic illness or disability, but also serves to decrease the risk of illness and concomitant disturbances in body experiences.

Disturbance in body image can be caused by inadequate knowledge or inaccurate perceptions about capacity for function. For example, elderly clients can perceive themselves as weaker or more dependent than objective tests indicate. Conversely, they can perceive themselves as stronger and more vigorous than they actually are and overextend themselves physically or socially. The inaccuracy of perception can result either from cultural factors such as the current emphasis on being young and slender or from American beliefs about health and illness

(Helman, 1995). Similarly, there can be illusions or delusions associated with illness and toxicity of medications. Physical factors such as the loss of a body function or part or prolonged dependency on a machine (e.g., dialysis) can result in inaccurate perceptions. When physical changes occur suddenly, as in traumatic injury, CVA, or surgical excision, time is required to reintegrate sensory experiences as well as the psychosocial impact of change. The extent to which changes in body appearance, structure, and function cause body image disturbance(s) depends on the rate of onset, the severity, the visibility, and the meaning of the change to the individual (Driscoll, 1985; Lubkin, 1986; Shontz, 1975).

The related factors of body image disturbances accepted and listed by NANDA can be grouped into the following categories: (1) biophysical; (2) cognitive/perceptual; (3) psychosocial; (4) cultural or spiritual; (5) developmental changes; (6) illness; (7) trauma or injury; (8) surgery; and (9) illness treatment (NANDA, 1999, p. 112). Note that these are broad categories of related factors that do not elaborate specific conditions in which disturbance in body image may occur. Although not exhaustive, an expanded list of pathologic, treatment, and psychosocial conditions that affect older adults and that may alter body image was generated from the literature and is presented in Box 42-1. Clearly, not all clients in these circumstances experience disturbances in body image; however, all of these conditions should be assessed to rule out a diagnosis of actual or risk for Body Image Disturbance.

ASSESSMENT

The assessment of clients for evidence of disturbance in body image includes a search for the presence of behavior patterns that indicate actual or risk for body image disturbance. This can be done by interview and clinical observation or by obtaining more formal measurements of body image.

Clinical Interview and Observations

Assessment of body image perception and attitudes includes the collection of subjective and objective data. Subjective data include clients' verbal statements about their body structure or function as well as their attitudes toward their bodies. For example, statements such as "It feels like my body is separated from me" reflect a distortion in body perception. Labels for body function or appearance, such as "dirty," "fat," or "small," can reflect negative feelings about the body. Subjective data are obtained during history-taking interviews or during subsequent interactions with the client. Carpenito (1987) suggested several open-ended questions for assessing the various aspects of body image. For example, individuals' attitudes toward their bodies can be assessed by asking "How do you feel about the changes in your body?" Perception of body image can be determined by asking "How would you describe your body?" and "How has getting older changed the way you feel about your body?" Other questions that can be used to assess body image include the following:

- "Before you were sick (came to the nursing home, and so on) how did you feel about people who were sick (in a nursing home, and so on)?"
- "How do you feel about not being able to move as well?" (or some other limitation)
- "What do you think caused the changes?"
- "Do you think your family understands what is happening to you?"
- "What kind of help is available to you?"

Objective data are composed of the caregiver's observations of behavior, such as the refusal to touch or look at a body part, refusal to discuss or use prosthetic devices, and failure to participate in self-care. Objective data can be obtained during verbal interactions as well as during other care activities with the client.

Assessment Tools

A number of assessment tools can be used to obtain more formal measurements of body image. Several of these tools can be applied to clinical assessment, whereas others may be more useful when conducting research. A summary of the characteristics of the most widely used instruments follows.

The Body-Cathexis Scale, developed by Secord and Jourard (1953), is a five-point Likert scale that measures the "degree of feeling of satisfaction or dissatisfaction with the various parts or processes of the body" (Secord & Jourard, 1953). Individuals are asked to rate their feelings toward 46 body parts (e.g., hair, lips, nose, fingers, wrists, legs) and functions (e.g., appetite, breathing, elimination, sexual activity). In addition, characteristics such as height, body build, profile, and gender are included. A score of five signifies a strongly positive attitude toward a body part or function, a score of one indicates a strongly negative attitude, and a score of three reflects a neutral attitude. Overall scores that are high indicate a more positive body attitude or image than lower scores.

Although the Body-Cathexis Scale frequently is used in body image research, the validity of the instrument continues to be an issue. Several researchers reasoned that, because body image cannot be precisely defined, one cannot know whether the instrument is measuring what it is supposed to measure. However, concurrent validity has been found with other measures of body image such as the Draw-a-Person test and perception of body space (Fawcett & Frye, 1980).

The Draw-a-Person Test is one of the most widely used body image assessment tools. Schilder (cited in Gorman, 1969) has been credited with the development of the technique. Several approaches to figure drawing tasks have been used. First, clients have been asked to draw a picture of themselves on a blank piece of paper or within a line frame. This is sometimes referred to as the "self-portrait" and has been used to assess perception of body schema (Bach, Tracy, & Huston, 1971), perception of body boundary (Fawcett, 1978), and body concept (Silberfarb, Phelps, Hauri, & Solow, 1978). In other instances, subjects have been asked to draw a person (Lakin, 1960) or, more specifically, to draw a "figure of a nude male and a nude female" (Plutchik, Conte, Weiner, & Teresi, 1978).

In using the Draw-a-Person test, the assumption is made that what a person draws actually represents an image of the person who produced it. This assumption has been challenged by several researchers. In reviewing a series of studies using figure drawing, Fisher and Cleveland (1968) concluded that there has been little success in differentiating characteristics of the drawings that are linked with body image from those that reflect skill in drawing or the testing method (i.e., the kind of instructions given to the client or subject). Gorman (1969) noted that, in contrast to the criticism of several researchers, clinicians believe that human figure drawings are valuable for diagnosing certain psychologic phenomena. For example, several characteristics of figure drawings suggest disorders of the central nervous system: (1) sketchy, broken, scribbled lines; (2) distortions of "true" anatomic pattern, including loss of symmetry; and (3) the "footing" of the figure appears tentative and insecure. Gorman (1969) maintained that, when used with other types of assessment such as interviews, physical and laboratory examination, and medical history, human figure drawings can add useful information about body image, particularly in estimating outlines of the body concept.

The interpretation of figure drawings as a measure of body image disturbances is also compounded by sensory-perceptual disorders such as hemianopsia or some other perceptual-motor dysfunction. Plutchik et al. (1978) noted that drawings of normal elders might be easily confused with those of psychiatric patients regardless of the age of the patient. These investigators compared figure drawings of four groups of subjects: (1) normal adults, (2) adult psychiatric inpatients, (3) senior citizens, and (4) elderly psychiatric patients. They found few differences among normal elders (senior citizens) and hospitalized elderly psychiatric patients. The drawings of normal elders and young adult psychiatric patients also showed similar characteristics. These investigators suggested that "norms based upon figure drawings of children or adults may not apply to the elders and that, therefore, figure drawings may be a less useful diagnostic tool for elders than they are for children or adults." Although figure drawings might reflect actual perceptions of body image, it would be difficult to determine whether or not the etiology of the disturbance was related to body schema or a higher level of body experience, such as body boundary and personal space.

The Baird Body Image Assessment Tool (BBIAT) is an 11-item Likert scale (1 = strongly disagree, 5 = strongly agree) that is designed to be used at the bedside. Seven of the 11 items are questions directed to the client, including, "Do you perceive yourself differently as a result of this surgical procedure or illness?" The remaining four items are observations regarding the presence of "prominent body feature(s)," "evidence or complaint of pain," "major change in affect," and "equipment present" (Baird, 1985). The items for the tool were developed from the literature and the investigator's experience. Ten patients immobilized with orthopedic problems were used for preliminary testing. Although this is a short tool and may be more useful in clinical practice than other measures of body image, further testing and refinement are required to establish the validity and reliability of the measure.

The Tennessee Self-Concept Scale (TSCS) was developed in 1965 by Fitts and has been used extensively to study self-concept. The TSCS consists of 100 self-descriptive statements. Self-perceptions are ranked on a five-point scale, with one indicating an item is completely false as a descriptor and five indicating an item is completely true as a descriptor of self. The items represent three subsets of self-concept: (1) identity, which represents what the individual is; (2) self-satisfaction, which reflects how a person feels about herself; and (3) behavior, which is what an individual does or how he acts. Individuals who score high tend to see themselves as valuable people, whereas those with low scores tend to see themselves as less than desirable (Fitts, 1965).

The TSCS is divided into five scales: (1) physical self, (2) moral-ethical self, (3) personal self, (4) family self, and (5) social self. The physical self measures the perception that one has of one's body, its function and appearance, and state of health and sexuality. The moral-ethical self deals with the moral, ethical, and religious aspects of the self. The personal self describes perceptions regarding individuals' personal adequacy, self-respect, and self-confidence apart from their body and social relationships. The family self describes how individuals see their relationships and role within their group of family and close friends and their sense of adequacy as a member of that group. The social self deals with one's sense of worth in relation to other people in general (Fitts, 1965).

Although the TSCS was developed to study self-concept, it has been used to target body image phenomena in a group of people who had rheumatoid arthritis. Eastman (1983) found that the only scale on which the sample consistently scored lower than the norm was on the physical self scale. The mean of her sample fell at the fourth percentile. In addition, results of the physical self scale and scores on the Body-Cathexis Scale were highly correlated in this sample.

Noting a lack of sensitivity in standardized measures of body image, Mock (1993) used a Body Image Visual Analog Scale (BIVAS) as a measure of intensity of body satisfaction. The 100-millimeter scale had anchor points ranging from complete dissatisfaction to complete satisfaction. Mock described the instrument as rapid, convenient, easy to use, and more sensitive than standardized measures. The major disadvantage identified was that the BIVAS only measures the one dimension of satisfaction.

NURSING DIAGNOSIS

NANDA (1999) has defined Body Image Disturbance as "confusion in mental picture of one's physical self" (p. 111). The range in manifestations of body image disturbance varies widely and is consistent with the levels of body experience and the wide range of related factors. Table 42-1 lists the defining characteristics identified and accepted by NANDA (1999). Note that the defining characteristics encompass sensory-perceptual, attitudinal, emotional, and behavioral attributes that might be present. In addition to listing relevant behavioral manifestations, the NANDA work specifies that in order to justify making the diagnosis Body Image Disturbance, the client must have a verbal or nonverbal response to actual or perceived changes in structure or function (NANDA, 1999). These are referred to as "critical" defining characteristics.

Although the NANDA (1999) list of defining characteristics is consistent with descriptions of responses associated with disturbances in body image reported in the literature, systematic validation has only begun. Metzger and Hiltunen (1987) conducted a retrospective nurse identification study to examine the content validity of the 10 most frequently reported nursing diagnoses. Fehring's (1986) model for obtaining content validity estimates was used. Five "critical" and 12 "supporting" cues (defining characteristics) were identified for the diagnosis Body Image Disturbance. Critical cues included those items (from the NANDA list) with a validity ratio of 0.75 or higher. Supporting cues were defined as items with ratios between 0.50 and 0.75. Items with ratios less than 0.50 were not included in the report.

The findings of this study are congruent with the NANDA position that verbal or nonverbal responses to actual or perceived change in structure and/or function are critical defining characteristics that need to be present to make the diagnosis Body Image Disturbance. However, validity ratios of 0.75 and above were also obtained for the items "negative feelings about body," "verbalization of: fear of rejection or of reaction by others," and "preoccupation with change or loss." This suggests that there might be additional critical defining characteristics that should be considered requisite for making the diagnosis. Metzger and Hiltunen (1987) suggested that research using large randomly selected national samples be conducted to seek

Table 42-1	Nursing Diagnosis, Outcomes, and Interventions for MRS. VICK

NURSING DIAGNOSIS

BODY IMAGE DISTURBANCE

Defining Characteristics

Refusal to participate in self-care
Refusal to leave her room
Discontinued use of cosmetics and personal clothing
Refusal to use walker
Verbalized feelings of worthlessness
Exaggerated dependence
Reduction in social activity

Nursing-Sensitive Outcomes	Nursing Interventions
BODY IMAGE *Indicators* Willingness to touch affected body part Willingness to use strategies to enhance appearance and function Adjustment to changes in body function Adjustment to changes in physical appearance Congruence between body reality, body ideal, and body presentation Description of affected part	**BODY IMAGE ENHANCEMENT** *Activities* Determine patient's and family's perceptions of alteration in body image versus reality Assist patient to use personal item Assist patient to discuss changes caused by illness or surgery, as appropriate Facilitate discussion of actual changes Monitor positive/negative self statements **ENVIRONMENTAL MANAGEMENT** *Activity* Assist to personalize living space
GRIEF RESOLUTION *Indicators* Expresses feelings about loss Verbalizes reality of loss Verbalizes acceptance of loss Reports a decrease in preoccupation with loss Maintains grooming and hygiene Shares loss with significant others Reports involvement in social activities	**GRIEF WORK FACILITATION** *Activities* Assist patient to identify initial reaction to the loss Encourage identification of greatest fears concerning the loss Encourage discussion of previous loss experiences Support progression through personal grieving stages Assist to identify personal coping strategies Assist in identifying modifications process **COGNITIVE RESTRUCTURING** *Activities* Help the patient accept the fact that self-statements mediate emotional arousal Point out styles of dysfunctional thinking Assist patient in labeling the painful emotion Assist patient to analyze own interpretation of situation Assist patient to replace faulty interpretations with more reality-based interpretations of stressful situations, events, interactions

Nursing Outcomes Classification (NOC) 5-point Likert measurement scales:

Body Image: 1 = Never positive; 2 = Rarely positive; 3 = Sometimes positive; 4 = Often positive; 5 = Consistently positive.
Grief Resolution: 1 = Not at all; 2 = To a slight extent; 3 = To a moderate extent; 4 = To a great extent; 5 = To a very great extent.

confirmation of the findings. In addition, prospective clinical studies with randomized samples of clients are needed to document the presence of these and presently unknown defining characteristics and etiologies. For example, Driscoll (1985) noted that refusing to wear a prosthesis or use an assistive device might indicate a disturbance in body image. Clinical validation of body image disturbances in elderly clients is critical, since there is little systematic study of body image experiences in this segment of the population.

C A S E   S T U D Y

L. Vick is a 72-year-old woman who cared for her home and husband with quiet precision for 50 years. One day while in her home, she was hurrying and suddenly tripped, fell, and broke her hip. She was taken to a nearby hospital where her hip was pinned. Her postoperative course progressed well until the third day when she developed a deep vein thrombosis. The thrombosis eventually resulted in a below-the-knee (BK) amputation of the right leg. In a few weeks, Mrs. Vick went from complete independence to dependence by the loss of her lower extremity.

Mrs. Vick was transferred to a nursing home, where she rarely spoke, made no attempt to learn to use the walker, and refused to go to the dining room to eat or participate in activities. Her husband usually joined her for the noon and evening meal; she ate well at those meals and chatted with him in her room. She refused to participate in her personal care, including the care of her long hair, which she had worn in a bun for 58 years. Her hair was cut short by the staff to facilitate care. She had no personal items from her home in her room. When staff approached Mrs. Vick about her apathy and dependency, she responded by saying, "I'm no good without my leg."

A nursing student who asked to care for Mrs. Vick noted the lack of personal items in her possession, both toiletries and clothing. Mr. Vick said that his wife did not want to use cosmetics anymore since her surgery, so he took them home. He attributed the lack of personal clothing to weight loss. He explained that Mrs. Vick had once been a large woman, weighing around 170 lbs. Now because she wouldn't eat unless he was there, she weighed closer to 130 lbs. and "nothing fits her." He also shared with the student the pride Mrs. Vick had felt in her long hair and the lovely combs with which she held it in place.

NURSING-SENSITIVE OUTCOMES

The primary desired outcome for a client with Body Image Disturbance is Body Image, defined as "positive perception of own appearance and body function" (Iowa Outcomes Project, 2000, p. 123). Table 42-2 lists suggested indicators for this outcome. Indicators for assessing the degree of outcome achievement focus on the frequency with which the client manifests positive descriptions of his body and self, as well as statements of satisfaction with body appearance and function. Adjustments to changes in structure or function and health status are indicators of having reconstructed or realigned his body image consistent with changes in form and function. Reconstruction of body image is accomplished through sensorimotor as well as cognitive and social processes. This is consistent with the interplay between biologic and psychosocial processes that occurs with normal development and maintenance of body image.

Finally, willingness to use strategies that enhance appearance and function of the body are behavioral manifestations that support judgments about successful integration of changes. This includes the ability to maintain or achieve body control in performing personal and social role functions. The significance of body control in facilitating independent function and self-care is self-evident. It is particularly relevant when autonomy in function is or will be compromised by chronic illness and disability. Lubkin (1986) stated that "when clients can understand, determine, and participate in self-care, they gain a sense of control over chronic illness and resultant bodily changes."

Grief Resolution can be considered as an intermediate outcome for body image disturbance intervention. Although emotions such as shock, anger, fear, and depressed mood are viewed as "normal" responses to threatened or actual loss of body integrity or function, there is agreement that persistent negative emotional states impede the cognitive processing required for accurate or realistic perceptions of the body's appearance or capacity for function. Grief Resolution is defined as "adjustment to actual or impending loss" (Iowa Outcomes Project, 2000, p. 223). Relevant indicators assessing the degree of grief resolution in body image disturbance include the extent to which the client (1) expresses feelings about the loss, (2) verbalizes the reality and acceptance of the loss, (3) discusses the meaning of the loss, (4) reports or manifests less preoccupation with the loss, and (5) expresses positive expectations for the future.

Individual success in attaining successful reintegration of body image depends on the etiology of the body image disturbance and, more important, on the value the individual places on the body part or function that is altered (Henker, 1979). Lubkin (1986) also suggested that the visibility of the change can affect the outcome.

In addition to characteristics of the body image insult, the client's coping resources will affect the outcomes of intervention. Resources such as a supportive spouse or other significant person(s), personality, and previous experience are key factors in success or failure in the coping process (Wilson, 1981). For example, in discussing stress responses in elderly clients with changes in body image, Motta (1981) stated that persons who have lived into old age "have probably been successful in developing strategies to deal with anxiety" and thus have established coping patterns. This is not to say that body image disturbances in older adults are less profound. Rather, it is possible that longevity is related to the use of successful adaptation to life changes. Finally, it should be noted that, in addition to the physical assistance given by professional health caregivers, their unbiased sensitivity to the aged client's body image experiences is a coping resource that contributes to the development of positive feelings, attitudes, and perceptions about his body.

| Table 42-2 | Suggested Nursing-Sensitive Outcomes and Nursing Interventions BODY IMAGE DISTURBANCE |

NURSING DIAGNOSIS

BODY IMAGE DISTURBANCE

Defining Characteristics

Critical:

- Verbal response to actual or perceived change in structure/ function
- Nonverbal response to actual or perceived change in structure and/or function

Objective:

- Not looking at body part
- Not touching body part
- Hiding or overexposing body part
- Change in social involvement
- Change in ability to estimate spatial relationship of body to environment

Subjective:

- Verbalization of change in lifestyle
- Fear of rejection or of reaction by others
- Focus on past strength, function, or appearance
- Negative feelings about body (helplessness, hopelessness, or powerlessness)
- Preoccupation with change or loss
- Emphasis on remaining strengths, heightened achievement
- Extension of body boundary to incorporate environment

Nursing-Sensitive Outcomes

BODY IMAGE

Indicators

Internal picture of self
Congruence between body reality, body ideal, and body presentation
Description of affected body part
Willingness to touch affected body part
Satisfaction with body appearance
Satisfaction with body function
Adjustment to changes in physical appearance
Adjustment to changes in body function
Adjustment to changes in health status
Willingness to use strategies to enhance appearance and function

Nursing Interventions

BODY IMAGE ENHANCEMENT

Activities

Use anticipatory guidance to prepare patient for changes in body image that are predictable
Determine patient's body image expectations based on developmental stage
Assist patient to discuss changes caused by illness or surgery, as appropriate
Facilitate discussion of actual change
Assist patient to separate physical appearance from feelings of personal worth, as appropriate
Assist patient to discuss changes caused by aging, as appropriate
Identify the significance of the patient's culture, religion, race, sex, and age on body image
Monitor positive/negative self statements
Monitor patient's ability to look at and touch body
Determine whether or not body perception induced social isolation
Determine if a change in body image has contributed to increased social isolation
Assist patient in identifying parts of her body that have positive perceptions associated with them
Identify means of reducing the impact of any disfigurement through clothing, wigs, or cosmetics, as appropriate

GRIEF RESOLUTION

Indicators

Expresses feelings about loss
Verbalizes reality of loss
Verbalizes acceptance of loss
Describes meaning of the loss or death
Discusses unresolved conflicts
Reports decreased preoccupation with loss
Maintains grooming and hygiene
Seeks social support

GRIEF WORK FACILITATION

Activities

Assist the patient to identify the nature of the attachment to the lost object or person
Encourage expression of feelings about the loss
Encourage discussion of previous loss experiences
Encourage identification of greatest fears concerning the loss
Include significant others in discussions and decisions, as appropriate

Continued

Suggested Nursing-Sensitive Outcomes and Nursing Interventions—cont'd	
Table 42-2 BODY IMAGE DISTURBANCE—cont'd	
Nursing-Sensitive Outcomes	**Nursing Interventions**
Shares loss with significant others Expresses positive expectations for the future	Assist to identify personal coping strategies Communicate acceptance of discussing loss Identify sources of community support
BODY IMAGE *Indicators* Congruence between body reality, body ideal, and body presentation Willingness to use strategies to enhance appearance and function Willingness to use body (part) in daily function	**COGNITIVE RESTRUCTURING** *Activities* Help the patient accept the fact that self-statements mediate emotional arousal Help patient understand the inability to attain desirable behaviors frequently results from irrational self-statements Point out styles of dysfunctional thinking Assist patient in labeling the painful emotion Assist patient to replace faulty interpretations with more reality-based interpretations of stressful situations, events, and interactions
KNOWLEDGE: DISEASE PROCESS *Indicators* Description of disease process Description of risk factors Description of effects of disease Description of usual disease course Description of precautions to prevent complications **KNOWLEDGE: TREATMENT REGIMEN** *Indicators* Description of self-care responsibilities for ongoing treatment Description of expected effects of treatment Performance of self-monitoring techniques Performance of self-care	**TEACHING: DISEASE PROCESS** *Activities* Appraise the patient's current level of knowledge related to specific disease process Explain pathophysiology of the disease and how it relates to the anatomy and physiology, as appropriate Describe common signs and symptoms of the disease, as appropriate Provide the family/significant other(s) with information about the patient's progress Discuss lifestyle changes that may be required to prevent future complications and/or control the disease process Discuss therapy/treatment options Describe rationale behind management/therapy/treatment recommendations Instruct the patient on measures to control/minimize symptoms, as appropriate Instruct the patient on which signs and symptoms to report to health care provider, as appropriate Reinforce information provided by other health care team members, as appropriate
MUSCLE FUNCTION *Indicators* Flexibility of movement (agility) Muscle tone Strength of muscle contraction Speed of movement Sustained muscle movement Steadiness of movement Control of movement Expressions of confidence in physical capacity	**EXERCISE PROMOTION** *Activities* Appraise patient's health beliefs about physical exercise Encourage verbalization of feelings about exercise or need for exercise Instruct patient about desired frequency, duration, and intensity of the exercise program Assist patient to prepare and maintain a progress graph/chart to motivate adherence with the exercise program Instruct the patient in techniques to avoid injury while exercising Assist patient to schedule regular periods for the exercise program into weekly routine Assist to identify and schedule reinforcement (rewards)

NURSING INTERVENTIONS

Recovery from a body image disturbance requires a reintegration of feelings and body experiences to develop a revised image consistent with reality (Drench, 1994). Reintegration is a process of recognition, acceptance, and resolution (Carpenito, 1987). The individual must first recognize that a change in body structure, function, or perception has taken place, then these changes must be internalized to resolve the conflict successfully. Matteson et al. (1996) noted that the previously developed body image must be discarded and that new perceptions and abilities must be acquired and incorporated. Drench (1994) suggested that persons whose body image is not central to the self-concept might be more able to realistically assess their situation and make necessary modifications in perception or function.

Although there is agreement that body image disturbances and the attendant emotional responses can impede recovery from the illness or injury and its treatment, nursing research investigating specific interventions to facilitate reintegration of body image has been very limited. Consequently, there are few tested guidelines for intervention. The majority of body image literature addressing measures to promote reintegration is based on clinical anecdotes and case studies. These interventions have generally been grounded in the reasoning used to explain the development of body image (i.e., touch, vision, and kinesthesia). Others address the need for the client to resolve affective responses to conflicts arising from discrepancies experienced between the internalized model of the body form and the adjustment necessitated by changes in the body or one's control of the body. Table 42-2 lists the primary interventions that are appropriate for Body Image Disturbance.

Body Image Enhancement

Body Image Enhancement is defined as "improving a patient's conscious and unconscious perceptions and attitudes toward his/her body" and encompasses activities that are done to assist clients to confront and adjust their conscious and unconscious perceptions and attitudes toward their body (Iowa Intervention Project, 2000, pp. 182-183). This intervention is largely an interpersonal process, in which interactions are designed to assist the individual to move toward the integration or reintegration of changes that have occurred or are anticipated to occur.

One of the Body Image Enhancement activities is to assist the client to prepare for alterations in body structure or function (anticipatory guidance). Preparation for alterations in body structure, function, or appearance is a preventive measure designed to desensitize individuals to the shock that frequently accompanies sudden changes (Henker, 1979). Another major component of the intervention is facilitating discussion of the extent of actual change and whether change is precipitated by pathology,

by its treatment, or by normative aging-related changes or life events. Realistically examining the extent and nature of the change can assist the client to separate physical changes from her perception of personal worth (self-esteem). Misperceptions and inaccurate attributions or overgeneralization can lead to overwhelming anxiety and depression (Henker, 1979; Pender, 1996). It should be made clear that threatening body changes do not signal an end to the self (Pender, 1996). Ersek (1992) has cautioned, however, that there can be too much (or conversely, too little) reality orientation. She described a hypothesized curvilinear relationship between reality negotiation and adaptive outcomes, but concluded that, given a supportive environment, persons can redefine their own reality.

In addition to helping clients explore the reality of their body image disturbance, Body Image Enhancement includes providing opportunity and assistance in looking at, touching, dressing, and using altered body parts as a mechanism for incorporating sensory information into the thought processes regarding the change (McDowell, 1983; Wilson, 1981). Similarly, assisting the client to engage in body movement and exercise can assist in re-establishing confidence in her abilities to again control and use her body. This activity can be accompanied by emphasizing the unaltered parts of the body and building on the body resources that have not been directly affected (Drench, 1994).

Another component of Body Image Enhancement is identifying social support resources. The importance of engaging the client's network is grounded in the belief that involvement and acceptance of significant others is a major factor in the reintegration process: one's own acceptance of and adjustment to change is often reflected in the sanctions of significant others. Drench (1994) suggested that family and friends can help a person to discover and accept a new body image. Formal caregivers and significant others are cautioned to ensure that there is congruence between verbal and behavioral messages in order to facilitate trust and to communicate that the worth of the person has been retained.

Engaging social support resources can also include referrals to support groups. It has been clinically and scientifically demonstrated that associations with persons in similar circumstances who have made successful adjustments constitute positive role model assistance in making transitions to a new satisfactory body image or self-image. Finally, it is suggested that the caregiver monitor the client throughout the adaptive process for evidence of social isolation. Henker (1979) suggested that resocialization should be encouraged early in the recovery process because a prolonged pattern of social isolation is very difficult to break.

Grief Work Facilitation

A second and related intervention for body image disturbance is Grief Work Facilitation. Research has shown that many clients experience changes in the appearance or function of the body as a major loss that is accompanied by profound emotional responses (Henker, 1979). Grief Work Facilitation is defined as "assistance with the resolution of a significant loss" (Iowa Intervention Project, 2000, p. 358). Activities focus on exploring the nature of the loss with the client and assisting him to describe feelings about the loss. Facilitating the client's grief work ameliorates emotional responses such as anger, fear, and depression (Drench, 1994; Henker, 1979). Henker noted that addressing the feeling states of the client lowers tension so that the cognitive elements of information processing can be engaged and adaptive responses can be mobilized.

Caregiver and self-monitoring of emotion over time is essential. Wilson (1981) noted that a satisfactory physical outcome is not necessarily an indication of successful resolution of the affective responses. Again, engaging the client's significant others can facilitate the client's progress through the grieving process. According to Drench (1994), mourning is a necessary phase of adjustment to loss of body image. It is important for formal and informal care systems to allow the time required to resolve the grief because emotional adjustment is contingent on resolution.

Cognitive Restructuring

A third intervention for body image disturbance is Cognitive Restructuring, which addresses the importance of engaging in positive thought patterns. Cognitive Restructuring is defined as "challenging the patient to alter distorted thought patterns and view self and the world more realistically" (Iowa Intervention Project, 2000, p. 219). The activities are directed toward assisting the client to understand that self-statements mediate emotional arousal and that dysfunctional beliefs can sabotage attempts to alter behavior and achieve reality-based interpretations and goals (Pender, 1996). Cognitive Restructuring also incorporates assisting clients to identify, clarify, and label feelings and to identify and analyze their own interpretations and sources of negative feelings. Finally, the client is assisted in constructing and rehearsing positive, reality-based self-statements as a mechanism for redirecting thought patterns. Thus this intervention focuses on the client's thinking, imagery, and attitudes toward the self (Pender, 1996).

The theoretical underpinning of Cognitive Restructuring focuses on the centrality of cognition in generating adaptive behavioral and affective responses. Because the individual's view of self and her personal world is central to how she acts, change processes are entered through thoughts and images (Pender, 1996; Scandrett-Hibdon, 1992). Information processing is directed toward teaching clients to think logically and create positive rather than negative self-statements and images.

Cognitive Restructuring also can include the construction of "possible selves." Possible selves are "conceptions of the self in the future" and can be positive (hoped for) or negative (feared self) (Hooker, 1992, p. 86). Possible selves can operate as a stimulus or incentive to engage in actions that move a person toward achievement of a desired or possible state of being (Ryff, 1993). Cross and Markus (1991) characterized possible selves as "blueprints for personal change and growth" (p. 232). These investigators also suggested that difficult or painful states can be endured in the present if they are directly relevant to a desired self at some future time.

Teaching: Disease Process

It has been suggested that knowledge about body structure and function (body concept) as well as attitudes toward one's body and self (cathexis) are basic to self-care practices (Smit & Kee, 1992). Patient education has been viewed as one method of informing individuals about their bodies and health care needs. Drench (1994) noted that reintegration or reconstruction of body image can be facilitated by knowledge of structure and function. Although there is widespread use of patient education as a nursing intervention, only two early studies were found that explored relationships between patient education and body image phenomena.

Mabry (1979) studied the effects of planned instruction on body image and the use of ambulatory aids by 70 elderly adults (age 60 and above) living independently. Body image was measured with the Body-Cathexis Scale developed by Secord and Jourard. A structured interview was used to identify the need for and verbal acceptance (or rejection) of ambulatory aids. The planned instruction was composed of a 20- to 30-minute health information class about the correct use of ambulatory aids. Teaching methods included demonstration, lecture-discussion, and modeling. Content of the instruction included body changes accompanying aging, the effect of body changes on locomotion, and the value of supportive devices (canes and walkers) on safety in movement. Results of the study showed that subjects' attitudes toward their body improved (as measured by the Body-Cathexis Scale) in the treatment and control groups, with no gain in the placebo group. There was, however, no significant difference in acceptance of ambulatory aids as indicated by responses to the interview questions. These findings suggest that learning about their body improved subjects' attitudes toward their body but did not facilitate resolution of emotional responses to the use of ambulatory aids. It is also likely that the emotional impact of requiring the use of assistive devices such as a cane or walker is very profound and thus requires interventions that go beyond giving information and incorporate activities that address the affective and cognitive dimensions of body.

Bille (1977) also used the Body-Cathexis Scale to investigate the relationship between body image and learning self-care and subsequent compliance with treatment protocols for myocardial infarction. He reasoned that one way of reducing anxiety generated by an illness such as myocardial infarction is to learn about the disease or illness. He noted, however, that clients frequently experience a time lag in revising their body image and that failure to internalize body injury (e.g., damaged heart) into the body image may impede the learning process. Subjects for the study included 24 male patients age 32 to 75 who were admitted to the hospital with a clinical diagnosis of acute or probable myocardial infarction. Compliance was measured 1 month after discharge by a telephone interview. First, patients were asked for their perception of the self-care information given by physicians in eight areas of content (medications, diet, physical activity, stressful situations, work, weight loss, smoking, and use of alcohol). Second, they were asked to estimate the extent to which they followed the advice given in each area during the month following hospitalization. The third part of the interview addressed areas of difficulty that were encountered in following the advice given. No attempt was made to validate patients' perceptions with physicians' perceptions of the instruction. Compliance score ranges based on the interview responses were reported as percentages of the 32 items. Thus scores could range from 0% to 100% compliance. In addition to compliance scores, 40 items (multiple-choice, true-false, and completion) tested knowledge of the self-care information given for the eight areas.

Results of the study showed no significant correlation between body image as measured by the Body-Cathexis Scale and knowledge scores. Furthermore, there were no significant relationships between amount of learning and ratio of reported compliance. There was, however, a significant correlation between body image scores and compliance. Patients who reported a more positive body image also reported higher compliance with posthospitalization prescriptions. These findings are consistent with the finding that self-concept is significantly related to self-care (Smit & Kee, 1992). Bille (1977) suggested that these patients might place a higher value on caring for their bodies, whereas individuals who feel more negative might place less value. When body image scores and compliance ratio were analyzed by age, there was no significant relationship between age and satisfaction with body parts and functions (body-cathexis). Similarly, there was no relationship between age and knowledge. On the other hand, age did have a positive effect on compliance behavior. It is not known whether this is a function of value or of more time to carry out the prescribed self-care.

Exercise Therapy and Promotion

The role of exercise and movement therapy in maintaining function and well-being of older adults has been documented by research since the early 1980s (Bassett, McClamrock, & Schmelzerm, 1982; Bortz, 1980; Fuller, 1982; Goldberg & Fitzpatrick, 1980). Fuller (1982) concluded that the "functional losses attributed to aging alone may, in reality, represent the combined effect of true aging changes, unrecognized incipient disease processes and an increasingly sedentary life style." In a review of literature on exercise in elderly persons, Wagner, LaCroix, Buchner, and Larson (1992) also spoke to relationships between use of the body and the vitality of body functions and suggested that efforts to increase physical activity can reverse the effects of deconditioning from inactivity.

Although no research was found that tested exercise and movement as interventions for body image disturbance in older adults, recent research has consistently shown that there are general health benefits of exercise as well as positive relationships to physical and psychologic function (Stewart, King, & Haskell, 1993). It is suggested here that if body function is maintained or improved even in the presence of chronic disease, the risk of body image disturbance and ensuing crippling affective responses that may accompany chronic illness or loss of function could be minimized. Fuller (1982) noted that, although exercise doesn't "erase wrinkles," it can improve physical appearance by maintaining muscle tone and decreasing body fat. Moreover, maintaining or improving physical fitness and function has been associated with more positive perceptions of health (Elward & Larson, 1992) and with improvements in functional status (Wagner et al., 1992).

In addition to examining the effects of exercise and physical activity, researchers have addressed major issues in exercise promotion for older adults. Barriers to engaging in systematic, planned physical activity include ageism views held by clinicians and society, prevalence of affective status such as depression, lack of transportation and finances, weather conditions, lack of knowledge and/or experience, and safety issues (Hogue & McConnell, 1996). Bokovoy and Blair (1994) and others have noted that some older adults are put off by regimented protocols and complicated instructions that frequently are used in traditional exercise prescriptions. Blair, Kohl, and Gordon (1992) have advocated using a "lifestyle exercise" approach, in which older adults are assisted to integrate more physical activity into their daily lives and to look for ways they could expend more energy. Blair et al. (1992) also encouraged clinicians to attend to physical activity patterns of their older adult clients on a routine basis and to use behavioral principles in assisting clients to engage in exercise. Recommendations include teaching self-monitoring, engaging social support networks, setting goals in terms of small incremental changes, and assisting clients in identifying and eliminating barriers. Older clients can also be shown how to plan for their own reinforcement.

The recommendations just described are consistent with the activities that are included in the *Nursing Interventions Classification (NIC)* intervention Exercise Promotion, defined as "facilitation of regular physical exercise to maintain or advance to a higher level of fitness and health" (Iowa Intervention Project, 2000, p. 316). Exercise Promotion is an intervention that can be used to prevent body image disturbances in "well" elderly adults. It can also be used in conjunction with therapeutic exercise interventions such as Exercise Therapy: Balance, Exercise Therapy: Joint Mobility, or Exercise Therapy: Muscle Control (Iowa Intervention Project, 2000) to treat body image disturbances that arise from acute pathology and/or its treatment or from trauma.

The feasibility and efficacy of specific exercise interventions to enhance self-perception and function of elderly adults are well documented. There is evidence that function can be safely improved with exercise in older adults who have chronic musculoskeletal disease, and the pain they experience can be decreased (Ettinger et al., 1997). Furthermore, improved function can bring about positive change in the way older adults perceive and feel about themselves. However, because few researchers have used body image as a dependent variable, the specific effect of movement or exercise therapy and promotion on body image, per se, remains undetermined.

The nursing interventions discussed are directed toward biologic, emotional, cognitive, and social dimensions of disturbed body image in elderly clients. Body Image Enhancement, Grief Work Facilitation, and Cognitive Restructuring address emotional responses and perceptual inaccuracies or distortions that may occur with actual or perceived changes in body structure or function. Movement and Exercise Promotion or therapy assist in developing muscle strength, joint flexibility, motor control, and endurance required to use the body effectively for independent function in everyday living. When physical exercise is conducted in a group, it also offers social stimulation and emotional support. Movement and exercise also provide sensory input and reinforce sensorimotor feedback systems. Finally, client education is used to provide and clarify information about body changes and functions as well as ways the body, even though modified, can be used for self-care and daily activity.

It should be noted that the interventions for Body Image Disturbance discussed in this section are not viewed as being comprehensive. Rather, they represent examples of interventions that could be used and tested with elderly clients who have or are at risk for body image disturbances. Shontz (1974) suggested that treatment decisions for body image disturbances should be based on the causes or sources of the disturbance, the level of body image experience that is affected, and the personal or social functions that are altered. He states, "There is no apriori reason to assume that basic sensorimotor capacities need to be enhanced or that intensive psychotherapy is needed; each patient must be understood and treated as an individual" (Shontz, 1974, p. 469).

CASE STUDY

The nursing student recognized the following defining characteristics of Body Image Disturbance in Mrs. Vick's behavior:

- Refusal to participate in self-care
- Refusal to leave her room
- Discontinued use of cosmetics and personal clothing
- Signs of grief, anger, despair
- Preoccupation with disability
- Refusal to use walker
- Verbalized feelings of worthlessness
- Exaggeration of dependence
- Change in social activity patterns

The following tentative nursing diagnoses were identified for Mrs. Vick:

1. Body Image Disturbance related to her below-the-knee amputation
2. Depression related to (a) decreased mobility, (b) disturbance in body image
3. Ineffective Coping related to depression and sensory perceptual alteration
4. Altered Nutrition, Less Than Body Requirements related to ineffective coping or depression
5. Risk for Dysfunctional Grieving related to depression

The following nursing intervention activities were undertaken for Mrs. Vick (Table 42-2):

1. Consulting with the family regarding Mrs. Vick's past patterns of grooming and dress (Body Image Enhancement)
2. Engaging Mr. Vick's assistance in obtaining and encouraging the use of personal items (e.g., clothing, makeup, pictures) (Body Image Enhancement and Grief Work Facilitation)
3. Engaging in therapeutic (1:1) interpersonal interaction with a focus on clarifying and shaping a realistic image of body form and capacity for function (Cognitive Restructuring)
4. Esthetically enhancing and personalizing the present living environment to increase sensory experience and to reestablish Mrs. Vick's personal identity (Environmental Management)
5. Encouraging physical exercise to retain joint mobility and proprioceptive stimulation (Exercise Therapy: Range of Motion [ROM], Exercise Therapy: Motor Control)

With the help of Mr. Vick, several new dresses in Mrs. Vick's favorite color were obtained, and her cosmetics were returned to the nursing home. At the same time, the student began to assist Mrs. Vick to modify the image she had developed since her amputation and its concomitant losses. Their daily interactions focused on her feelings about the losses she had experienced, including the loss of her leg. They also discussed ways to view and strengthen the dimensions of her body structure and function that weren't changed by the illness and surgery as well as options for a prosthesis and ambulatory aids. The student assisted Mrs. Vick with passive and active knee and hip exercises to maintain joint mobility. In addition to purchasing new clothes, Mr. Vick brought pictures to hang on the walls of her room and provided new jeweled barrettes to replace the combs in her hair. In the course of several weeks, Mrs. Vick began to participate in her care, combing her hair, applying makeup, and choosing the clothing she preferred to wear that day. She began to ask for a mirror to check her appearance before she left the room. She still preferred to eat in her own room with her husband, but no longer protested going to the dining room for activities.

SUMMARY

Body image phenomena are of concern to nurses because they have been identified as having a major (although frequently unconscious) impact on health and illness behavior. Yet there is little concrete knowledge about the nature of body image experiences, particularly in elderly persons. The abstract and multidimensional characteristics as well as the psychologic fusion of body experiences with other dimensions of an individual's self-concept render it very difficult to isolate, define, and test clinically. Differential diagnosis is also compounded by obscure clinical manifestations as well as by potential or actual coexisting nursing diagnoses that may be manifested by similar defining characteristics. In Mrs. Vick's case, for example, coexisting diagnoses may be Reactive Depression, Ineffective Individual Coping, Self-Esteem Disturbance, or Sensory/Perceptual Alterations.

Clearly, the knowledge and clinical expertise required to diagnose and treat actual or risk for body image disturbances in older adults are more complex and comprehensive than can be illustrated in a simplified case study. In addition to theoretical and clinical knowledge of body image phenomena, knowledge about aging is required to appreciate and become sensitive to the diversity in experiences and needs of elderly individuals. Although there is limited research documenting the nature of body image experiences in elders, there is some evidence that aging per se does not induce body image disturbances (Bille, 1977; Lipowski, 1977; Plutchik et al., 1978). What is suggested, however, is that elderly clients who are at risk for or have disturbances in body image related to pathologic or social events are individuals who, at the same time, may be coping with body and social changes that occur with "normal aging" (Driscoll, 1985; Lubkin, 1986; McDowell, 1983). These changes are often experienced as losses and may compound the responses to and treatment of loss of body image integrity (Lubkin, 1986). It should also be emphasized that disturbances in body image may range from transient short-term alterations to very profound and chronic changes in perception. Similarly, pathologic and social conditions that cause or contribute to body image disturbance may occur gradually or be very sudden. Wilson (1981), for example, noted that 30% of patients with rectal cancer are admitted to hospitals as emergencies. When this occurs, the individual must cope with the emotional impact as well as with the reality of a stoma while in a "crisis situation." This means that nursing diagnosis and treatment of body image disturbance(s) must consider the context of the disturbance as well as the biopsychosocial composition of body image phenomena.

REFERENCES

Bach, P., Tracy, H. W., & Huston, J. (1971). The use of self-portrait method in evaluation of hemiplegia. *Southern Medical Journal, 64,* 1475-1484.

Baird, S. (1985). Development of a nursing assessment tool to diagnose altered body image in immobilized patients. *Orthopedic Nursing, 4,* 47-54.

Bassett, C., McClamrock, E., & Schmelzerm, O. (1982). A 10-week exercise program for senior citizens. *Geriatric Nursing, 3,* 103-105.

Bille, D. A. (1977). The role of body image in patient compliance and education. *Heart & Lung, 6,* 143-148.

Blair, S., Kohl, H., & Gordon, N. (1992). Physical activity and health: A lifestyle approach. *Medicine Exercise Nutrition and Health, 1,* 54-57.

Bleeker, H., & Mulderij, K. (1992). The experience of motor disability. *Phenomenology & Pedagogy, 10,* 1-18.

Bokovoy, J., & Blair, S. (1994). Aging and exercise: A health perspective. *Journal of Aging and Physical Activity, 2,* 243-260.

Bortz, W. M. (1980). Effect of exercise on aging—effect of aging on exercise. *Journal of the American Geriatrics Society, 28,* 49-51.

Burbank, P. (1992). An exploratory study: Assessing the meaning of life among older adult clients. *Journal of Gerontological Nursing, 18*(9), 19-28.

Carpenito, L. J. (1987). Self-concept, disturbance. In *Nursing diagnosis: Application to clinical practice* (2nd ed.). Baltimore: Lippincott Williams & Wilkins.

Carroll-Johnson, R. (Ed.). (1989). *Classification of nursing diagnoses: Proceedings of the eighth conference.* Baltimore: Lippincott Williams & Wilkins.

Coopersmith, S. (1967). *The antecedents of self-esteem.* New York: Freeman.

Coward, D. (1996). Self-transcendence and correlates of a healthy population. *Nursing Research, 45* (2), 116-121.

Cross, S., & Markus, H. (1991). Possible selves across the life span. *Human Development, 34,* 230-255.

Drench, M. E. (1994). Changes in body image secondary to disease and injury. *Rehabilitation Nursing, 19*(1), 31-36.

Driscoll, P. (1985). Change in body image. In J. Pigg, P. W. Driscoll, & R. Caniff (Eds.), *Rheumatology nursing: A problem oriented approach* (pp. 283-293). New York: John Wiley & Sons.

Eastman, L. (1983). *Self-concept, body image and the performance of activities of daily living in individuals with rheumatoid arthritis.* Unpublished master's thesis, The University of Iowa, Iowa City, IA.

Elward, K., & Larson, E. (1992). Benefits of exercise for older adults. *Clinics in Geriatric Medicine, 8*(1), 35-50.

Ersek, M. (1992). Examining the process and dilemmas of reality negotiation. *IMAGE: Journal of Nursing Scholarship, 24*(1), 19-25.

Ettinger, W. H., Burns, R., Messier, S. P., Applegate, W., Resjeski, W. J., Morgan, T., Shumaker, S., Berry, M. J., O'Toole, M., Monu, J., & Craven, T. (1997). A randomized trial comparing aerobic exercise and resistance exercise with a health education program in older adults with knee osteoarthritis. The fitness arthritis and seniors trial (FAST). *Journal of the American Medical Association, 227*(1), 25-31.

Fawcett, J. (1978). Body image and the pregnant couple. *American Journal of Maternal Child Nursing, 3,* 227-233.

Fawcett, J., & Frye, S. (1980). An exploratory study of body image dimensionality. *Nursing Research, 29,* 324-327.

Fehring, R. (1986). Validating diagnostic labels: Standardized methodology. In M. E. Hurley (Ed.), *Classification of nursing diagnosis: Proceedings of the sixth conference* (pp. 183-190). St. Louis, MO: Mosby.

Fisher, S., & Cleveland, S. E. (1968). *Body image and personality* (2nd ed.). St. Louis, MO: Warren H. Green.

Fitts, W. H. (1965). *Tennessee self-concept scale: Manual and test booklet.* Nashville, TN: Department of Mental Health.

Fuller, E. (1982). Exercise: Getting the elderly going. *Patient Care, 16,* 67-110.

Glick, O. J., & Tripp-Reimer, T. (1996). The Iowa conceptual model of gerontological nursing. In E. Swanson & T. Tripp-Reimer (Eds.), *Series on issues in gerontological nursing* (pp. 11-55). New York: Springer.

Goldberg, W. G., & Fitzpatrick, J. J. (1980). Movement therapy with the aged. *Nursing Research, 29,* 339-345.

Gordon, M. (1994). *Nursing diagnosis: Process and application* (2nd ed.). Hightstown, NJ: McGraw-Hill.

Gorman, W. (1969). *Body image and image of the brain.* St. Louis, MO: Warren H. Green.

Hansell, S., & Mechanic, D. (1991). Body awareness and self-assessed health among older adults. *Journal of Aging and Health, 3*(4), 473-492.

Helman, C. G. (1995). The body image in health and disease: Exploring patients' maps of body and self. *Patient Education and Counseling, 26,* 169-175.

Henker, F. (1979). Body-image conflict following trauma and surgery. *Psychosomatics, 20,* 812-820.

Hoffman, R. (1983). Manifestations of body image changes in the elderly due to stress and a model for nursing treatment. *New Mexico Nurse, 28,* 4-8.

Hogue, C., & McConnell, E. (1996). *Exercise and the elderly.* Paper presented at the Gerontological Nursing Interventions Conference, Iowa City, Iowa.

Hooker, K. (1992). Possible selves and perceived health in older adults and college students. *Journal of Gerontology, 42,* 85-95.

Iowa Intervention Project. J. C. McCloskey & G. M. Bulechek (Eds.). (2000). *Nursing interventions classification (NIC)* (3rd ed.). St. Louis, MO: Mosby.

Iowa Outcomes Project. M. Johnson, M. Maas, & S. Moorhead (Eds.). (2000). *Nursing outcomes classification (NOC)* (2nd ed.). St. Louis, MO: Mosby.

Janelli, L. M. (1986). Body image in older adults: A review of the literature. *Rehabilitation Nursing, 11,* 6-8.

Kim, M. J., & Moritz, D. A. (Eds.). (1982). *Classification of nursing diagnoses: Proceedings of the third and fourth national conferences.* St. Louis, MO: Mosby.

Kupfermann, I. (1991). Localization of higher cognitive and affective functions: The association cortices. In E. Kandel, J. H. Schwartz, & T. M. Jessell (Eds.), *Principles of neuroscience* (3rd ed., pp. 823-838). New York: Elsevier.

Lakin, M. (1960). Formal characteristics of human figure drawings by institutionalized and noninstitutionalized aged. *Journal of Gerontology, 15,* 76-78.

Lipowski, Z. J. (1977). The importance of body experience for psychiatry. *Comprehensive Psychiatry, 18,* 473-479.

Liviskie, S. (1973). Definition of boundaries after burn injury. *Maternal Child Nursing Journal, 2,* 101-109.

Lubkin, I. (1986). Body image. In *Chronic illness impact and intervention* (pp. 167-179). Sudbury, MA: Jones & Bartlett.

Mabry, E. R. (1979). *Effects of planned instruction on body image and the use of ambulatory aids by well-elderly clients.* University Microfilm International.

Matteson, M., McConnell, E., & Linton, A. (1996). *Gerontological nursing* (2nd ed., pp. 711-718). Philadelphia: W. B. Saunders.

McDowell, D. (1983). The special needs of the older colostomy patient. *Journal of Gerontological Nursing, 9,* 294-296.

Mesulam, M. M. (1985). Attention, confusional states and neglect. In M. M. Mesulam (Ed.), *Principles of behavioral neurology* (pp. 125-168). Worcester, MA: F. A. Davis.

Metzger, K. L., & Hiltunen, E. F. (1987). Diagnostic content validation of ten frequently reported nursing diagnoses. In A. McLane (Ed.), *Classification of nursing diagnoses: Proceedings of the seventh conference* (pp. 144-153). St. Louis, MO: Mosby.

Mock, V. (1993). Body image in women treated for breast cancer. *Nursing Research, 42*(3), 153-157.

Mor-Barak, M. E., Scharlach, A. E., Birba, L., & Sokolov, J. (1992). Employment, social networks and health in retirement years. *International Journal of Aging and Human Development, 35*(2), 145-159.

Morse, J. M., Bottorff, J. L., & Hutchinson, S. (1995). The paradox of comfort. *Nursing Research, 44*(1), 14-19.

Motta, G. (1981). Stress and the elderly: Coping with a change in body image. *Journal of Enterostomal Therapy, 8,* 21-22.

Murray, R. (1972). Body image development in adulthood. *Nursing Clinics of North America, 7,* 617-629.

Norris, C. (1978). Body image: Its relevance to professional nursing. In C. Carlson & B. Blackwell (Eds.), *Behavioral concepts and nursing intervention* (2nd ed., pp. 5-36). Baltimore: Lippincott Williams & Wilkins.

North American Nursing Diagnosis Association. (1999). *Nursing diagnoses: Definitions & classification 1999-2000.* Philadelphia: Author.

Pender, N. (1996). *Health promotion in nursing practice* (3rd ed., pp. 171-172). Norwalk, CT: Appleton & Lange.

Plutchik, R., Conte, H. R., Weiner, M. B., & Teresi, J. (1978). Studies of body image, IV. Figure drawing in normal and abnormal geriatric and nongeriatric groups. *Journal of Gerontology, 33*(1), 68-75.

Plutchik, R., Weiner, M. B., & Conte, H. (1971). Studies of body image, I. Body worries and discomfort. *Journal of Gerontology, 26,* 344-380.

Popkess-Vawter, S. (1989). Assessment of positive and negative body image in normal weight and overweight females. In R. Carroll-Johnson (Ed.), *Classification of nursing diagnoses: Proceedings of the eighth conference* (pp. 313-319). Baltimore: Lippincott Williams & Wilkins.

Rubin, R. (1967). Attainment of the maternal role. *Nursing Research, 16,* 237-245.

Rubin, R. (1968). Body image and self-esteem. *Nursing Outlook, 16,* 20-23.

Ryff, C. (1993, March). *The self in later life. Gerontology News.* Washington, DC: The Gerontological Society of America.

Scandrett-Hibdon, S. (1992). Cognitive appraisal. In G. Bulechek & J. McCloskey (Eds.), *Nursing interventions essential nursing treatments* (2nd ed., pp. 462-471). Philadelphia: W. B. Saunders.

Schilder, P. (1950). *Image and appearance of the human body.* New York: Universities Press.

Secord, P., & Jourard, S. (1953). The appraisal of body-cathexis: Body-cathexis and the self. *Journal of Consulting Psychology, 17,* 343-347.

Shontz, F. C. (1969). *Perceptual and cognitive aspects of body experience.* San Diego, CA: Academic Press.

Shontz, F. C. (1974). Body image and its disorders. *International Journal of Psychiatry Medicine, 5,* 461-472.

Shontz, F. C. (1975). *Psychological aspects of physical illness and disability.* Indianapolis, IN: MacMillan.

Silberfarb, P. M., Phelps, P. J., Hauri, P., & Solow, C. (1978). Effects of intestinal bypass surgery on body concept. *Journal of Consulting Clinical Psychology, 46*(6), 1415-1418.

Smit, M., & Kee, C. (1992). Correlates of self-care among the independent elderly. *Journal of Gerontological Nursing, 18*(9), 13-18.

Stein, K. (1995). Schema model of self-concept. *IMAGE: Journal of Nursing Scholarship, 27*(3), 187-193.

Stewart, A. L., King, A. C., & Haskell, W. L. (1993). Endurance exercise and health-related quality of life in 50-65 year old adults. *The Gerontologist, 33*(6), 782-789.

Stoller, E., & Earl, L. (1983). Help with activities of daily life: Sources of support for the noninstitutionalized elderly. *The Gerontologist, 23*(1), 64-70.

Theriault, J. (1994). Retirement as a psychosocial transition: Process of adaptation to change. *International Journal of Aging and Human Development, 38*(2), 153-170.

Thomas, P., Goodwin, H., & Goodwin, J. (1985). Effect of social support on stress-related changes in cholesterol level, uric acid level and immune function in an elderly sample. *American Journal of Psychiatry, 142*(6), 735-737.

Vinck, J., & Pierloot, R. (1977). Body image boundary definiteness and psychopathology. *Acta Psychiatrica Belgica, 77,* 348-359.

Wagner, E., LaCroix, A., Buchner, D., & Larson, E. (1992). Effects of physical activity on health status in older adults. *Annual Review of Public Health, 13,* 451-468.

Wilson, D. (1981). Changing the body's image. *Nursing Mirror, 152,* 38-40.

CHAPTER 43

POWERLESSNESS

Ruth E. Davidhizar and Joyce Newman Giger

Power plays a significant role in human encounters. Power is defined as a combination of authority and influence derived from a variety of sources including position, expertise, and personal qualities (Prescott & Dennis, 1985). A position may give power when an office or role gives authority to the individual in that office or role. Power derived from personal knowledge and education may give power that accompanies expertise. Power from personal qualities occurs when personal characteristics increase personal feelings of attractiveness. A perception of powerlessness can happen to all people regardless of age. However, the problems associated with powerlessness can be greatly exacerbated among elderly persons, who tend to have fewer resources and [illegible] rely upon for suppo[illegible] lessness among eld[illegible] without an in-dept[illegible] powerlessness.

Bacharach and La[illegible] dimensions of the p[illegible] ence. Authority invol[illegible] ated with an adminis[illegible] formal and relates to [illegible] convince others of [illegible] 1980). These dimensi[illegible] appear to be relativel[illegible] the power to hire an[illegible] position or expertise [illegible] phenomenon that is created by personal feelings. An individual who subjectively feels powerful has more power than another person in a similar position or circumstance who feels powerless. Both authority and influence are dimensions that are under personal control and that can be personally altered by changing one's personal mental state. Thus, although authority and influence arise in part from external sources, they are also internally generated and in part are under personal control (Mirowsky, 1997).

Empowerment occurs when feelings of power are internalized to oneself or facilitated in someone else. Feelings of empowerment are basic and essential for optimal self-actualization. In fact, for elders, personal feelings of empowerment are a tool that results in positive attitudes for self and others and in feelings of control over the environment. Lack of feelings of power leads to insecurity, emotional distress, and depression and can hinder effective relationships with significant others and health care professionals.

Feelings of power do not automatically come with being born into a position of social status or with educational accomplishment. For some, regardless of position and status, lack of feelings of power are pervasive throughout life. For other people, feelings of personal power seem to have come naturally and seem embedded in the individual's personality even from birth. For still others, the ability to feel personal power seems to develop over time and results from great effort. Nevertheless, regardless of the security and feeling of personal power with which an adult may enter the ranks of elders, feelings of power [illegible]ress, grief, [illegible]g process, [illegible] to feelings [illegible]

[illegible]quences for [illegible] associated [illegible]ors among [illegible]983) con-[illegible]ler persons [illegible]ntly associ-[illegible]

[illegible]lving total [illegible]

The clear association between feelings of powerlessness and preventive health care behaviors was established in the early work of Rodin and Langer (1977), who noted that there was a positive health effect of a control-relevant intervention among the institutionalized aged population they studied. Seeman and Lewis (1995) conducted a similar study on older men (ages 45 to 59) and mature women (ages 30 to 44) in which data were collected periodically over a 10-year period. Findings from this study suggested that there is a direct correlation between declining health and increased powerlessness. Further findings from this study also indicated that an increased sense of mastery is related to a decreased sense of powerlessness. Older men and mature women were more likely to score comparably on predictors of powerlessness and declining health status.

Powerlessness remains an excellent predictor of mortality, especially when an individual's initial level of activity is severely limited and when psychologic symptoms and satisfaction with health status are factored into the overall equation. While powerlessness was an excellent predictor of mortality among both older men and mature women, the best predictor of mortality, among those happy and unhappy with their health status, was age. Seemingly, findings from this extremely important study suggested that in each year, among both older men and mature women, powerlessness was significantly associated with greater activity limitations and increased psychologic symptoms. In addition, further analysis of their data suggested that change in health status was significantly associated with change in the sense of powerlessness. In fact, increased powerlessness accompanied deterioration in health status and was predictive of increased health problems. While mortality is more frequently seen among elders who have feelings of powerlessness, particularly men, Seeman and Lewis (1995) concluded that such is the case only in individuals who were initially unhappy with their health.

Not only does lack of feelings of control affect the morale of elderly clients, but family and caregiver morale and self-esteem are affected as well (Davidhizar, 1994). Reactions to the chronically ill person vary among significant others, but feelings of powerlessness frequently are cyclic so that as clients feel increasingly powerless, so do caregivers.

Thus power, empowerment, and powerlessness are important concepts for elders and for the health care professionals with whom they interact. The diagnosis of powerlessness can be critical to the holistic assessment of the elderly person; subsequent interventions by the health care professional can be critical to facilitating feelings of well-being.

RELATED FACTORS/ETIOLOGIES

The classic work of Johnson (1967) noted that certain experiences such as hospitalization could possibly contribute to the sense of powerlessness. Some of the etiologies originally identified by Johnson, e.g., internal locus of control, institutional and health care environments, are as relevant now as they were more than 30 years ago. The introduction of the concept of powerlessness into nursing care and the nursing literature by Carpenito (1983) also viewed powerlessness derived from hospitalization as a state in which an individual experiences or perceives an inability to control certain events. Powerlessness is a result of the impinging, multiplural stressors of the stressor occurring. While the effects of hospitalization can produce a sense of powerlessness among all individuals, it can be especially enhanced in elderly individuals. For elders who are hospitalized or in long-term care facilities, segregation

from others, failure to receive personalized care, and aged stereotyping can lead to strong and negative feelings of powerlessness (Koch & Webb, 1996). The resolution of feelings of loss and grief is very complex and varies from individual to individual and from situation to situation. Among elders, feelings of powerlessness frequently play a significant role, since American society relates feelings of power to the young and tends to withdraw attribution of power as individuals age (Meis, 1985). Johnson further noted that health and the recovery in many instances are factors which cannot be totally controlled by the individual. Thus, for many individuals who perceive themselves as "powerless," the concepts of fate and chance are strongly embedded in health, illness, and wellness behaviors.

Carpenito (1983) identified three categories of etiologic and contributing factors related to powerlessness: (1) pathophysiologic factors, which result from any disease process; (2) situational factors, which involve a lack of information, personal characteristics that highly value control, or hospital or institutional limitations; and (3) maturational factors, processes that are evolving across the life span. The North American Nursing Diagnosis Association (NANDA) also has identified several etiologies of powerlessness: the health care environment, interpersonal interactions, illness-related regimens, and a lifestyle of helplessness (NANDA, 1999, p. 117).

RELATED FACTORS/RISK FACTORS

Numerous factors and related concepts affect feelings of powerlessness in older adults. Primary among these are perceived control, grief and loss, and disability.

Perceived Control

A number of researchers have studied the effects of giving power and perceived control to an individual and the resulting changes in feelings of self-worth. Elderly persons, in a study by Langer and Rodin (1976), who were given responsibility for their own care in a nursing home setting, took a more active responsibility, i.e., took responsibility for the care of plants and were allowed to make choices as to activities. The elderly residents of a long-term care facility, particularly those who perceived greater choice and responsibility and were more involved in social interactions, reported higher levels of morale. Rodin also correlated choice with well-being.

Locus of control has also been evaluated in elderly persons in relation to feelings of well-being. Reid, Haas, and Hawkings (1977) related external locus of control with powerlessness and external locus of control with negative feelings of depression. Ziegler and Reid (1979) noted that feelings of control in a group of community elders were positively correlated with health, knowledge of service, and use of services. In a second study, Ziegler and Reid (1979) noted that for elderly persons on a chronic care hospital unit, control was correlated with life satisfaction, tranquility, self-concept, and subject senescence.

Menec and Chipperfield (1997) compared perceived control in relation to age groups. The analysis suggested that perceived control interacted with functional status for old-old (80+) adults, but not for young-old (65 to 79 years old) adults in terms of perception of health, hospitalization, and mortality. Thus it appears there may be a buffering effect of perceived control in relation to different age groups in the elderly. However, other researchers have reported no difference between age and stress and coping. For example, Aldwin, Sutton, Chiara, and Spiro (1996) found no age difference in perceived stressfulness of the problem, appraisals of harm or loss, and coping efficacy when middle-aged, young-old, and old-old men were interviewed.

Nystrom and Segesten (1995) reported that peace of mind was promoted in elderly nursing home patients by instructional activities, by genuine encounters, and through empowering supportive interventions. Health education that supported a realistic picture of the situation and supported methods to deal with situations at hand was noted to have an empowering effect. Tollett and Thomas (1995) used Miller's Model of Patient Power Resources to study the effect of nursing interventions on feelings of hope, self-efficacy, self-esteem, and decreased depression among homeless veterans. Those who received the nursing intervention were less depressed and had increased levels of hope and self-esteem.

Locus of control is a significant concept in relation to powerlessness. Rotter (1975) recognized the need for situation-specific measures related to a variety of situations when the goal is the prediction of behavior in specific situations. According to Rotter's (1966) social learning theory, locus of control is an expectancy, as opposed to a motivational construct, and should therefore only be measured by expectancy items. Consequently, information-seeking behavior might be a function of the value an individual attaches to a healthy life, such as the belief that seeking preventive health care information will help maintain health. Typically, individuals with an internal health-related locus of control place high value on health and the actions that can be taken to promote health. Powerlessness is related to external locus of control, and consequently individuals who feel powerless take few actions that can promote health. Johnson (1967), who first introduced the concept of powerlessness to nursing, noted that an understanding of powerlessness might provide insight into understanding the health-related behavior of individuals. Johnson utilized Seeman's (1959) definition of powerlessness as "the expectancy or probability held by the individual that his own behavior cannot determine outcomes or reinforcements he seeks" (p. 785) and related it to Rotter's (1954) theory of social learning. Johnson (1967) concluded that, for individuals "who do not always behave as

expected," the concept of powerlessness offers an explanation to behavior.

Grief and Loss

Grief and loss are also related to feelings of powerlessness. Authors have outlined the stages of grief as a process that individuals go through in reacting to loss. Kubler-Ross (1978) proposed five stages of grief. She related the stages to the experience of dying individuals and those bereaved at a loss. Although not supported by scientific quantitative research, many individuals believe these stages accurately represent the experience of grieving: (1) denial and isolation, (2) anger, (3) bargaining, (4) depression, and (5) acceptance. Initially, feelings of shock, disbelief, and denial are experienced and serve as buffers that enable the individual to mobilize alternative defenses. Sadness and crying follow as awareness develops. Acceptance evolves to gradual relinquishing of the lost object or person, investing in new interests and people, and adjusting, in the case of the death of a spouse, to living alone. If the acceptance stage of grief is completed, the individual no longer feels emotional pain and the struggle to adjust is eliminated. However, for many individuals the loss triggers feelings of powerlessness that are not resolved and continue over time. Dysfunctional grief occurs when feelings of grief are present for more than a year and are accompanied by extreme guilt, hopelessness, suicidal ideation, and powerlessness (McMahon, 1992).

Disability

As the number of elders increases, more suffer from chronic disability. Chronic disability refers to a disabling condition including illness, injury, or physical handicap that causes a limitation or incapacity (*Webster's New World Dictionary*, 1991). While each chronic disability presents unique demands on the individual and significant others, Miller (1992) makes two generalizations that can be applied to most chronic situations: (1) the client experiences impaired functioning in more than one, and usually in multiple, body-mind-spirit systems, and (2) the demands on the client related to the disability can never be completely eliminated (Tuck, Sobel, Follick, & Youkilis, 1990). Thus chronic disability is a condition that requires multiple adjustments throughout the life span and is accompanied for many individuals by feelings of powerlessness.

Chronic disability has also been defined by Lubkin (1986) as "the irreversible presence, accumulation, or latency of disease states or impairments that involve the total human environment for supportive care and self-care, maintenance of function and prevention of further disability" (p. 6). Many demands are made on the individual and significant others. Reif (1975) noted that individuals with chronic disabilities have symptoms that interfere with many normal activities and routines, have medical regimens that are limited in effectiveness, and have symptoms that disrupt patterns of living. Thus not only are the symptoms and the disability limiting, but the treatment regimen may be limiting as well. For many elders, adjustment is not just a single occurrence, but must be ongoing if substantial changes are to be made in health status. Coping with feelings of powerlessness is often ongoing as well.

NURSING DIAGNOSIS

Powerlessness has been defined by Miller (1992) as the perception of the individual that one's own actions will not significantly affect an outcome. In other words, powerlessness is the feeling one has no control over events. Feelings of powerlessness can result from a situation that an individual believes is unalterable. When a change or loss has occurred, personal factors, factors in the environment, and factors related to the situation contribute to feelings of powerlessness. Powerlessness is a potential problem when one or more of the power resources of physical strength, psychologic stamina, self-concept, energy, knowledge, motivation, and belief system are in any way compromised (O'Heath, 1991).

NANDA (1999) defines Powerlessness as the "perception that one's own action will not significantly affect an outcome; a perceived lack of control over a current situation of immediate happening" (p. 116). NANDA further classifies characteristics of powerlessness as "severe," "moderate," and "low." In many ways these characteristics are similar to the early work of Miller (1992) and are primarily operational by definition.

As early as 1967, Johnson indicated that there was a need to identify powerlessness as operative when considering or postulating a determinant of behavior. According to Johnson, there are several problems inherent in the use of powerlessness as an operative definition. These problems are found in the assessment area, and consequently there is no norm beyond which an individual could say with absolute certainty that powerlessness manifested in the form of probability values could be established.

Defining characteristics of powerlessness include (1) expressed dissatisfaction over inability to control a given situation and (2) refusal or hesitancy to participate in health care decision making (Carpenito, 1983). Associated characteristics include apathy, aggression, violent behaviors, anxiety, uneasiness, resignation, acting-out behaviors, and depression. These characteristics, however, are not mutually exclusive to the single diagnosis of powerlessness and could be indicative of a number of other nursing diagnoses as well.

By simple definition, powerlessness is a feeling of loss of control. Patients, and particularly elders, experience two reactions to the loss of control. For many individuals, regardless of age, there is tremendous guilt associated with

loss of control. These feelings are often manifested through such behaviors as hostility, anger, withdrawal, and depression. When such behaviors are manifested, it is often difficult for the individual to recognize that people in the environment are concerned with his personal well-being and consequently the restoration of power.

Zerwekh (1983) identified several defining characteristics related to Powerlessness: body language, minimal verbalization, anxiety, and swings between retreat and antagonism. Relevant body languages that might have a direct correlation with Powerlessness include shifting eyes, crossed legs and arms, or restlessness movements. While the patient may have minimal verbalization, it is essential to consider behaviors that are in opposition to this, including constant complaints or excessive demands. When an individual has a perception of powerlessness, there can be a profound alteration in thought processes. It is also interesting to note that individuals most vulnerable to powerlessness are those whose development and situational experiences increase their susceptibility to stressful events (Zerwekh, 1983).

While differential diagnosis for Powerlessness is often not possible because of its lack of refinement or development as a nursing diagnosis, several nursing diagnoses can lead to a diagnosis of Powerlessness (e.g., impaired mobility).

CASE STUDY

C. Smith is a 79-year-old African American female who was admitted to the hospital for uncontrolled insulin-dependent diabetes mellitus (type 1). In addition to diabetes, Mrs. Smith also has hypertension, for which she takes triamterene (Dyazide) once daily, and a history of coronary artery disease and arthritis affecting her knee and elbow joints. Mrs. Smith weighs 245 lbs and is 5 feet 2 inches tall. Mrs. Smith's weight has been a source of concern for her because, coupled with her arthritis, diabetes, and coronary heart disease, it has severely curtailed her overall activity level. Mrs. Smith has 4 children (ages 40, 45, 55, and 56), all of whom reside more than 500 miles away. Until this hospitalization, Mrs. Smith, a widow of some 15 years, had been caring for herself unaided. Although Mrs. Smith had been seen by her physician for the control of her diabetes, she had not been compliant with her dietary or treatment regimen. In addition to her other disability conditions, Mrs. Smith also has a vision and hearing impairment.

Upon admission, Mrs. Smith's random blood glucose level was 391 mg/dl. The nurse asked her about her dietary and exercise patterns. Mrs. Smith told the nurse she mostly eats cereal, canned soups, and lunchmeat sandwiches because it is too hard to cook just for herself. She had tried numerous diets in the past, but had never had even short-lasting success losing weight. She knows she is supposed to exercise, but her arthritis makes it difficult for her to take even a short walk. She usually checks her blood sugar each morning, but hesitates to vary her insulin dose very much because she fears insulin reactions. She told the nurse she didn't think it mattered much anyway what she ate or how much insulin she took. Her sugars simply always ran high.

Mrs. Smith also expressed a lack of satisfaction in her life. Each day is the same, with few opportunities for enjoyment. She usually sees her children only once a year. Someone will call her every couple of weeks, but she does not understand why they cannot keep in closer contact. She had to give up driving due to her deteriorating vision, so now transportation is a major problem. She spends most days watching TV and sees little more to hope for.

NURSING-SENSITIVE OUTCOMES

Just as powerlessness tends to increase feelings of depression and inadequacy, increasing feelings of power can have an empowering and positively uplifting effect. Empowerment of elders can increase quality of life and feelings of well-being. Nurses working with elders need both feelings of empowerment and the skills to empower clients. Facilitating effective self-care in patients requires a style that nurtures others to develop themselves. Manz and Sims (1989) call this style "super leadership" or the ability to lead others to lead themselves. Professionals have the responsibility to bring out the best in those they serve (Gunden & Crissman, 1992). When a patient is empowered to take self-directed actions for self-care, it is a high level of patient care. Nursing Outcomes Classification (NOC) outcomes that are most important for the nurse to monitor are Quality of Life, defined as "an individual's expressed satisfaction with current life circumstances" (Iowa Outcomes Project, 2000, p. 347); Well-Being, "an individual's expressed satisfaction with health status" (p. 443); Self-Esteem, the "personal judgment of self-worth" (p. 391); and Decision Making, defined as the "ability to choose between two or more alternatives" (p. 194). The nurse also may choose some NOC Knowledge outcomes. Outcomes and selected indicators most relevant for measurement and documentation are in Box 43-1.

A nurse can facilitate these outcomes for elders by endowing them with the knowledge needed to improve their personal care (e.g., using the intervention Teaching: Individual) and with an understanding that the outcome Self-Esteem makes a difference in future health care decisions and behaviors. Positive recognition and praise for self-care are powerful motivators and can enhance adherence to a self-care plan in the future.

NURSING INTERVENTIONS

Empowerment can be defined many ways. Empowerment, according to *Webster's New World Dictionary* (1991), is "the process of enabling oneself to use one's power or of giving ability of power to another." Empowerment posi-

tively influences change. Change and power have a positive interactive influence. When change is successfully implemented, it empowers individuals. If change is not successfully implemented, empowerment dissipates. When individuals are empowered, change is more likely to occur, whereas change is less likely to occur without empowerment. Nursing treatments must therefore assist persons with developing the resources needed to increase their abilities to effect needed changes or to enhance behaviors that are effective in meeting goals.

A number of nursing interventions in the Nursing Interventions Classification (NIC) (Iowa Intervention Project, 2000) are useful for the treatment of Powerlessness: Assertiveness Training, Behavior Modifications: Social Skills, Mutual Goal Setting, Patient Contracting, Decision-Making Support, Cognitive Restructuring, Socialization Enhancement, Self-Esteem Enhancement, and Teaching: Individual. Other NIC interventions are useful for nurses to use depending on the individual circumstances for a person with a diagnosis of Powerlessness. The reader is encouraged to review other NIC interventions for their potential in the treatment of Powerlessness. Box 43-1 contains the NANDA diagnosis, signs and symptoms of Powerlessness, selected NIC Interventions and indicators that will most likely be selected by nurses to treat Powerlessness in elderly clients and to effect positive changes in outcomes.

Empowerment may come from external and internal forces. For example, it can be externally motivated through positive relationships with other persons including significant others and health care professionals. For the institutionalized elder, empowerment can come through being given decisions to make regarding patient care. For the elderly client in home care, empowerment can be actualized through the opportunity to make decisions for oneself. NIC interventions Mutual Goal Setting, Patient Contracting, and Decision-Making Support maximize the elder's participation in decisions about care. For example, when the nurse gives the elderly client a decision-making opportunity to decide when the nurse should return and what procedures the client would like assistance with, the client is empowered to make decisions that can affect the outcome of care. Empowerment can also come as a result of praise from others for persistence with a medical regimen or for maintaining a positive attitude in the midst of negative circumstances.

When empowerment is internally induced, it comes from personal feelings and thoughts and is closely related to self-concept or self-image. It can come from self-examination or from the self-confidence that results when a personal goal is accomplished. It is facilitated by receiving positive feedback from significant others (including nurses) for accomplishments, from nurses and others reinforcing personal strengths, and from receiving unconditional love from caregivers regardless of attitude or actions.

Suggested Nursing-Sensitive Outcomes and Nursing Interventions	
Box **43-1** **POWERLESSNESS**	

Nursing Diagnosis
Powerlessness
Defining characteristics
Verbal expression of having no control over self-care
Verbal expressions of having no control or influence over
    situation
Verbal expressions of having no control or influence over
    outcome
Resentment, anger, guilt
Withdrawal
Depression
Loss
Grief
Refusal or hesitancy to participate in health care decisions
Minimal verbalization
Anxiety
Swings between retreat and antagonism

Nursing-Sensitive Outcomes
Quality of Life
Indicators
Satisfaction with health status
Satisfaction with social circumstances
Satisfaction with self-concept

Well-Being
Indicator
Satisfaction with ability to cope

Self-Esteem
Indicators
Confidence level
Feelings about self-worth
Description of self

Decision Making
Indicators
Identifies alternatives
Weighs alternatives
Chooses among alternatives

Nursing Interventions
Socialization Enhancement
Activities
Encourage patience in developing relationships
Give positive feedback when patient reaches out to others

Assertiveness Training
Activities
Differentiate between assertive, aggressive, and passive-aggres-
    sive behaviors
Instruct patient in the different ways to act assertively

Cognitive Restructuring
Activities
Point out styles of dysfunctional thinking
Assist patient to replace faulty interpretations with more
    reality-based interpretations of stressful situations, events,
    and interactions

Self-Esteem Enhancement
Activities
Encourage patient to identify strengths
Reinforce the personal strengths that patient identifies
Assist patient to identify positive responses from others

Mutual Goal Setting
Activities
Assist patient in identifying realistic, attainable goals
Encourage patient to state goals clearly, avoiding the use of
    alternatives
Assist patient in developing a plan to meet goals

Decision-Making Support
Activities
Help patient identify the advantages and disadvantages of each
    alternative
Provide information requested by patient

Patient Contracting
Activities
Encourage patient to identify own goals, not those she believes the
    health care provider expects
Assist the patient in setting realistic time limits
Encourage the patient to identify appropriate, meaningful
    reinforcers or rewards

Teaching: Individual
Activities
Inform of importance of adhering to medication prescribed
Inform of purpose and benefits of activity or exercise
Inform of importance of balanced diet

Self-Awareness Enhancement
Activities
Assist patient to identify the values that contribute to self-concept
Assist patient to identify guilty feelings
Assist patient to identify positive attributes of self

Italics: Refers to interventions and outcomes for case study.
Nursing Outcomes Classification (NOC) 5-point Likert measurement scales:
Quality of Life, Well-Being, and Self-Esteem: 1 = Extremely compromised; 2 = Substantially compromised;
                                  3 = Moderately compromised; 4 = Mildly compromised; 5 = Not compromised.
Decision Making: 1 = Never demonstrated; 2 = Rarely demonstrated; 3 = Sometimes demonstrated;
                                    4 = Often demonstrated; 5 = Consistently demonstrated.

The ability to feel power and to empower others may be derived from referent power. By definition, referent power is the ability to influence others. Referent power accompanies certain personality characteristics. Here again, Self-Esteem Enhancement and Socialization Enhancement include activities that help individuals appreciate and use power in relationships. For example, personal charm and enthusiasm can empower an individual to have influence over others. Such things as having good manners, being empathetic with a focused manner, having good listening skills, and exhibiting charisma and enthusiasm can enhance an elderly individual's personal empowerment and ability to develop positive relationships.

Personal power is derived from knowledge and competency. Self-confidence is developed when an elder gains specific education and experience. Personal expertise elicits respect from others. There are a number of NIC Teaching interventions that nurses can use to educate elderly patients about Activity Exercise, Medication, Diet, or Disease Process and Treatment.

Empowerment is achieved best by dynamic, charismatic, and far-sighted individuals with a vision. The art of empowering elders is a process that involves "building, developing and increasing power through cooperating, sharing, and working together" (Rothstein, 1995).

To empower others it is first necessary for the nurse to have personal feelings of power. Empowered individuals have a positive self-concept. Personal needs to feel important and to feel useful are met. Nurses who are themselves empowered in their work settings feel that they are part of a worthwhile enterprise and experience positive accomplishments. In health care settings, nurse empowerment is facilitated by structures that enable nurses to handle uncertainties as they try out new behaviors. Empowering structures establish clear role expectations and authority to carry out the expectations. There must be clear expectations for each person's responsibilities. Role expectations are reaffirmed when individuals are affirmed and supported for doing their work well (Rothstein, 1995).

The personal management of self is critical to feeling empowered. Personal empowerment means having self-awareness, comfort with self, and self-confidence. For an insecure and dependent individual, feelings of empowerment may involve a radical departure from past behaviors.

Empowerment also requires a certain mindset. To feel empowered, productive thinking needs to be present. There must be feelings of personal control over personal perceptions. Empowered individuals know they have power that is not dependent on external forces. While external forces can reaffirm and expedite feelings of power, true empowerment comes from within.

The empowered individual must also set realistic expectations. Having realistic, rather than unrealistic or unattainable expectations helps to eliminate the disappointment of not being able to reach goals. Realistic expectations also help the individual to think productively. Personal feelings of empowerment provide the power to change situations and the way situations are perceived. The empowered individual has a sense of perspective, for example, to find the humor in an incongruous situation. The empowered individual may even look for situations that represent personal comedy in order to share humor and a feeling of fun with others.

Empowerment also requires an adequate level of trust in self. The intervention Self-Awareness Enhancement assists an elder to explore and understand feelings, motivations, and behavior in order to let go of guilt and feelings of "not doing enough." Self-awareness can help elders stay calm in a crisis and maintain positive self-esteem and self-image when things are going badly.

For elders to have feelings of personal power, they need to be assisted to enhance self-awareness. Teaching: Individual is an intervention used with varied specific content so that elderly persons understand the importance of adequate rest, breaks in the day, taking time out for fun, looking at things with humor, and looking out for oneself to achieve a healthy state. Self-awareness and knowledge can enable the elder to say "no" to involvement that awakens feelings that are too personal.

Self-nurture involves using strategies that support self-esteem. These strategies can include positive thought, such as "I've done this many times before and it has always gone well. This will go well too." Self-nurturing thoughts can also involve celebrating accomplishments, trying new things, and learning more about self.

Self-Responsibility Facilitation also facilitates the maintenance of a sense of empowerment. Novice professionals often find themselves feeling responsible for everything. Once responsibilities are clearly delineated and understood, then the amount of work expected to meet these responsibilities can be clearly identified. The question "How important will my doing this work right now be 5 years from now?" can help keep things in perspective.

CASE STUDY

Mrs. Smith's nurse made the diagnosis of Powerlessness related to chronic illness, lack of control over weight and blood sugar, and lack of social involvement. The nurse talked with Mrs. Smith about her willingness to participate in a long-term plan to increase her feelings of control over her circumstances. Mrs. Smith was initially reluctant to participate in any new plan. The nurse took time to explain both the approaches that she thought would be helpful and the outcomes she thought Mrs. Smith might be able to accomplish. Mrs. Smith agreed that it would be wonderful if she could accomplish the outcomes Quality of Life, Well-Being, Self-Esteem, and Decision Making. Because these outcomes were highly desirable, Mrs. Smith agreed to try a new plan.

The nurse incorporated several nursing interventions into Mrs. Smith's plan of care. The most important intervention during Mrs. Smith's hospitalization was Teaching: Individual. The nurse held daily teaching sessions with Mrs. Smith regarding insulin administration, diet, and exercise. During these sessions the nurse helped Mrs. Smith to plan simple meals that she could make without great effort. A dietitian also participated in these teaching sessions to help Mrs. Smith understand how to promote a steady, slow weight loss. The nurse recommended that Mrs. Smith try attending a congregate meal site in her community, in hopes that she would get more varied meals. The nurse did review foods that might be on the congregate meals menu that Mrs. Smith should avoid or consume sparingly.

The congregate meal piece contributed to a second nursing intervention, Socialization Enhancement. The nurse hoped that Mrs. Smith would experience positive social interactions at the meal site that would give her increased confidence in her personal relationships. The nurse also gave Mrs. Smith the phone number for the local elderly transportation service, so that she could arrange rides to the congregate meal site.

Other important interventions were Mutual Goal Setting, Patient Contracting, and Self-Esteem Enhancement. The nurse and the dietitian both helped Mrs. Smith to identify specific, realistic goals for both her blood sugar level and her weight. Mrs. Smith was given a written copy of these goals for easy reference. The nurse observed Mrs. Smith perform each blood sugar check and had her state her rationale for choosing a particular dose of insulin. The nurse used good decisions and successful outcomes as opportunities to convey confidence in Mrs. Smith's abilities. Poor decisions and unsuccessful outcomes were used as opportunities for additional teaching. The nurse helped Mrs. Smith to identify personal strengths she could use in meeting her goals. These included having a history of enjoying cooking, being physically able to prepare meals, and still having sufficient vision to check her blood sugar levels and accurately draw up her insulin.

Finally, the nurse anticipated that Mrs. Smith would need support upon returning home. She obtained Mrs. Smith's consent for a home care referral and, in making the referral, informed the home care agency of Mrs. Smith's need for ongoing reinforcement of her abilities and of the goals she had set.

SUMMARY

An important dimension of personal power is the ability to feel empowered and to empower others. Careful assessment of position power, of expertise power, and of the personal characteristics that add or detract from personal power can increase self-awareness and assist a person to maximize strengths and develop weak areas.

Each individual has power that is recognized and power that is not recognized. When the nurse makes an effort to evaluate feelings of personal empowerment among the elder and family members of the elder, deficiencies can be identified. When the nurse plans and uses treatments that foster and promote feelings of empowerment, personal growth, and positive attitudes, the elderly client is more likely to adhere to a health care regimen that promotes optimal functioning.

REFERENCES

Aldwin, C. M., Sutton, K. J., Chiara, G., & Spiro, A., III. (1996). Age differences in stress, coping, and appraisal: Findings from the Normative Aging Study. *Journals of Gerontology. Series B, Psychological Sciences & Social Sciences, 51*(4), P179-P188.

Bacharach, S., & Lawyer, E. (1980). *Power and politics in organizations.* San Francisco: Jossey-Bass.

Carpenito, L. J. (1983). *Nursing diagnosis: Application to clinical practice.* Baltimore: Lippincott Williams & Wilkins.

Davidhizar, R. (1994). Powerlessness of caregivers in home care. *Journal of Clinical Nursing, 3*(3), 155-158.

Fuller, S. (1978). Inhibiting helplessness in the elderly. *Journal of Gerontological Nursing, 4,* 18-23.

Gunden, E., & Crissman, S. (1992). Leadership skills for empowerment. *Nursing Administration Quarterly, 16*(3), 6-10.

Hanes, C., & Wild, B. (1977). Locus of control and depression among noninstitutionalized elderly persons. *Psychological Reports, 41,* 581-585.

Iowa Interventions Project. J. C. McCloskey & G. M. Bulechek (Eds.). (2000). *Nursing interventions classification (NIC)* (3rd ed.). St. Louis, MO: Mosby.

Iowa Outcomes Project. M. Johnson, M. Maas, S. Moorhead (Eds.). (2000). *Nursing outcomes classification (NOC)* (2nd ed.). St. Louis, MO: Mosby.

Johnson, D. (1967). Powerlessness: A significant determinant of patient behavior. *Journal of Nursing Education, 6*(2), 39-44.

Koch, T., & Webb, C. (1996). The biomedical construction of aging: Implications for nursing care of older people. *Journal of Advanced Nursing, 23*(5), 954-959.

Kubler-Ross, E. (1978). *To live until we say good-bye.* Englewood Cliffs, NJ: Prentice Hall.

Langer, E., & Rodin, J. (1976). The effects of choice and enhanced personal responsibility for the aged: A field experiment in an institutional setting. *Journal of Personality Social Psychology, 34,* 191-203.

Lubkin, I. (1986). *Chronic illness: Impact and interventions.* Boston: Jones & Bartlett.

Manz, C., & Sims, H. (1989). *Super leadership.* Englewood Cliffs, NJ: Prentice Hall.

McMahon, A. (1992). The mentally ill elderly. In J. Haber, A. McMahon, P. Price-Hoskins, & B. Sideleau (Eds.), *Comprehensive psychiatric nursing* (pp. 729-750). St. Louis, MO: Mosby.

Meis, M. (1985). Loneliness and the elderly. *Orthopedic Nursing, 6,* 17-19.

Menec, V. H., & Chipperfield, J. G. (1997). The interactive effect of perceived control and functional status on health and mortality among young-old and old-old adults. *Journals of Gerontology. Series B, Psychological Sciences & Social Sciences, 52*(3), P118-P126.

Miller, J. (1992). *Coping with chronic illness* (2nd ed.). Philadelphia: F. A. Davis.

Mirowsky, J. (1997). Age, subjective life expectancy, and the sense of control: The Horizon hypothesis. *Journals of Gerontology.*

Series B, Psychological Sciences & Social Sciences, 52(3), S125-S134.

North American Nursing Diagnosis Association. (1999). *Nursing diagnoses: Definitions & classification 1999-2000.* Philadelphia: Author.

Nystrom, A., & Segesten, K. (1995). Support of the experience of health in lucid elderly nursing home patients; registered nurses perceptions. *Scandinavian Journal of Caring Sciences, 9*(3), 145-152.

O'Heath, K. (1991). Powerlessness. In M. Maas, K. Buckwalter, & M. Hardy (Eds.), *Nursing diagnoses and interventions for the elderly* (pp. 449-459). Reading, MA: Addison Wesley Longman.

Prescott, P., & Dennis, K. (1985). Power and powerlessness in hospital nursing departments. *The Journal of Professional Nursing,* 348-355.

Reid, D., Haas, G., & Hawkings, D. (1977). Locus of desired control and positive self-concept of the elderly. *Journal of Gerontology, 32,* 441-448.

Reif, L. (1975). Beyond medical intervention strategies for managing life in face of chronic illness. In M. Davis, M. Kramer, & A. Strauss (Eds.), *Nurses in practice: A perspective on work environment* (pp. 261-273). St. Louis, MO: Mosby.

Rodin, J., & Langer, E. J. (1977). Long term effects of a controlled-relevant intervention with the institutionalized aged. *Journal of Personality & Social Psychology, 35,* 897.

Rothstein, L. (1995). The empowerment effort that came undone. *Harvard Business Review,* 20-26.

Rotter, J. (1954). *Social learning and clinical psychology.* Englewood Cliffs, NJ: Prentice Hall.

Rotter, J. (1966). Generalized expectancies for internal versus external control of reinforcements. *Psychological Monographs, 80,* 1-8.

Rotter, J. (1975). Some problems and misconceptions related to the construct of internal versus external control of reinforcement. *Journal of Consulting Clinical Psychology, 43,* 56-63.

Seeman, M. (1959). The meaning of alienation. *American Sociological Review, 24,* 783-791.

Seeman, M., & Lewis, S. (1995). Powerlessness, health and mortality of longitudinal stress of older men and mature women. *Social Science & Medicine, 41*(4), 517-528.

Seeman, M., & Seeman, T. E. (1983). Health behavior and personal autonomy. *Journal of Health and Social Behavior, 24,* 144.

Tollett, J., & Thomas, S. (1995). A theory based nursing intervention to instill hope in homeless veterans. *Advances in Nursing Science, 18*(2), 76-90.

Tuck, D., Sobel, H., Follick, M., & Youkilis, H. (1990). A sequential criterion analysis for assessing coping with chronic illness. *Journal of Human Stress, 6,* 35-40.

Webster's New World Dictionary. (1991). Englewood Cliffs, NJ: Prentice Hall.

Zerwekh, J. (1983, Summer/Autumn). Empowering the no longer patient. *Washington State Journal Nursing,* 12-17.

Ziegler, M., & Reid, D. (1979). Correlates of locus of control of desired control in two samples of elderly persons: Community residences and hospitalized persons. *Journal of Consulting Psychology, 47,* 977-981.

CHAPTER 44

ANXIETY AND FEAR

Sue A. Moorhead and Veronica A. Brighton

The nursing diagnoses Anxiety and Fear have been included in nursing literature since the first National Conference on the Classification of Nursing Diagnoses was convened in St. Louis in 1973. Over the last 25 years the status of these two nursing diagnoses has been invariably intertwined. At one point Anxiety was removed from the list of approved nursing diagnoses, an action that intensified efforts to clarify the differences between these two feeling states. Despite many attempts to differentiate Anxiety from Fear, the major difference continues to be definitional in nature. This chapter will discuss the current status of these two diagnoses, identify relevant assessment tools available, and discuss nursing interventions and patient outcomes for these diagnoses.

ANXIETY

Anxiety is a commonly discussed concept in the nursing and health care literature and is frequently encountered with patients regardless of setting. A computerized literature search identified over 5000 published articles containing "anxiety" in the abstract since 1993. An examination of this literature quickly reveals that anxiety affects individuals experiencing a wide variety of events (Table 44-1). Nurses often assist patients in these situations.

Prevalence

Anxiety disorders are the most prevalent of all the mental disorders in the United States (Blair & Ramones, 1996). Substantial advances have been made in the identification and treatment of panic disorder, social phobia, generalized anxiety disorders, and posttraumatic stress disorder (Lydiard, Brawman-Mintzer, & Ballenger, 1996). Anxious behavior can result from a treatable physiologic medical illness, a psychiatric illness, or an exaggerated or normal response to life events. Table 44-2 contains a listing of the anxiety disorders in the *Diagnostic and Statistical Manual of Mental Disorders* (4th edition) (DSM IV).

From the psychiatric viewpoint, several authors suggest that anxiety disorders, as a group, are the most common condition in the elderly. The prevalence of anxiety in the elderly is lower when compared to younger age groups (Blazer, George, & Hughes, 1991; Sheikh & Salzman, 1995), but it tends to be clinically significant (Markovitz,

1993). Hocking and Koenig (1995) estimated that between 10% and 20% of patients over 65 experience clinically significant symptoms of anxiety. Fernandez, Levy, Lachar, and Small (1995) reported that depression and anxiety in later life are second in frequency only to dementia. Most of the elderly residing in nursing homes and residential care facilities have mental disorders, with up to 75% having dementia (Snowdon, 1993).

Weiss (1994) found that older adults are susceptible to mood disruptions from a variety of sources, including primary anxiety or mood disorders, medical illnesses and treatments, and psychosocial stressors; the most common disturbance is mixed anxiety and depression. Liebowitz (1993) discussed the pros and cons of adding mixed anxiety and depression to the DSM-IV as a new category. Today mixed anxiety and depression increasingly is identified as a separate diagnosis (Kuzel, 1996). In a study of community-dwelling elders, Smith, Colenda, and Espeland (1994) identified that anxiety and depression are highly correlated even in the elderly who report low levels of anxiety and depression. Martin, Flemming, and Evans (1995) stated that the development of depression in the geriatric population is associated with a higher risk of suicide than with any other age group. Heidrich (1993), in a study of elderly women, found that poor health, regardless of age, was associated with more depression and anxiety and that these women also had lower levels of autonomy and positive relationships with others.

An extensive review of the literature by Smith, Sherrill, and Colenda (1995) identified that, although anxiety disorders appear to be less prevalent in the elder, anxiety associated with medical and psychiatric disorders and subsyndromal anxiety are significant sources of morbidity in this age group. Steinberg (1994) found that anxiety disorders in the elderly cause considerable morbidity and dysfunction and increase mortality rates. The initial onset of primary generalized anxiety and other anxiety disorders in the elderly may be rare, but these problems tend to be chronic in nature and may persist into old age.

With the increasing numbers of elderly individuals in society, anxiety is a problem of significant dimension. Few systematic studies of the course, severity, and treatment of anxiety disorders have been performed despite an increased interest in anxiety in younger groups (Steinberg,

Table 44-1	Literature Review Associating Anxiety to Life Events
Event	**Literature**
Preoperative Periods	Allen, Knight, Falk, & Strang, 1992; Augustin & Hains, 1996; Friedman, Badere, & Fitzpatrick, 1992; Gaberson, 1991; Markland & Hardy, 1993; Salmon, 1993; Shafer, Fish, Gregg, Seavello, & Kosek, 1996; Steelman, 1990; Winter, Paskin, & Baker, 1994
Invasive or threatening health-related tests or examinations	Foxwell & Alder, 1993; Ludwick-Rosenthal & Neufeld, 1993; Nugent, Tamlyn-Leaman, Isa, Reardon, & Crumley, 1993; Palakanis, DeNobile, Sweeney, & Blankenship, 1994; Peterson, 1991; Weller & Hener, 1993; Zlotogorski, Tadmor, Duniec, Rabinowitz, & Diamant, 1995
Aging	Lasher & Faulkender, 1993
Stress	Robinson, 1990
Retirement	MacEwen, Barling, Kelloway, & Higginbottom, 1995; Theriault, 1994
Severe burns	Franulic, Gonzalez, Trucco, & Vallejos, 1996
Acquired immunodeficiency syndrome (AIDS)	Evans, Kassof, Beckham, & Handel-Kindred, 1990
Abuse	Trimpey, 1989
Heart attacks	Conn, Taylor, & Wiman, 1991; Webb & Riggin, 1994
Cancer	Carroll, Kathol, Noyes, Wald, & Clamon, 1993; Gram & Slenker, 1992; Hurt, McQuellon, Barrett, 1994; Lampic, von Essen, Peterson, Larsson, & Sjoden, 1996
Illness of a family member	Daly, Kleinpell, Lawinger, & Casey, 1994; Halm, 1990; Higginson & Priest, 1996; Johnson & Frank, 1995; Leske, 1996; Mintz, van Horn, & Levine, 1996; O'Connell, 1989; Potinkara & Paunonen, 1996; Rukholm, Bailey, Coutu-Wakulczyk, & Bailey, 1991; Snelling, 1994
Family caregivers	Anderson, Linto, & Steward-Wynne, 1995; Neundorfer, 1991
Pain	Ferrell-Torry & Glick, 1993; Heath, 1992; McCracken & Gross, 1993; Wald, 1991
Alcohol use	Kranzier, 1996; Weissman, 1988a
Educational testing	Summers, Hoffman, Neff, Hanson, & Pierce, 1990
Computer technology	Negron, 1995
Loss and grief	Zisook, Schneider, & Schuchter, 1990

1994). Blair and Ramones (1996) described their view that anxiety is undertreated:

> Anxiety, perhaps more than other psychiatric symptoms, is also victim of stigma and bias, not only from a cultural perspective, but in the professional communities as well. This contributes to a poor understanding of anxiety, difficulty in diagnosis, inadequate assessment, mismanagement of treatment, and can lead to confusion and splitting concerning appropriate pharmacological intervention. The results are that anxiety is severely undertreated in psychiatric settings (p. 9).

The National Institute of Mental Health reports that only 1 in 5 persons suffering from an anxiety disorder will ever seek medical attention, and that only 25% of all patients with general anxiety disorder will receive any treatment at all (Weissman, 1988a, 1988b). The majority of anxious individuals often see physicians repeatedly, describe a variety of diffuse complaints, or self-medicate with over-the-counter medications, alcohol, or other substances (Blair & Hildreth, 1991; Blair & Ramones, 1994). Hyman and Cassem (1989) estimate that the suicide rate among untreated patients suffering from anxiety disorders is about 15%.

Related Factors/Etiologies

The etiologies of Anxiety are varied and occur across an individual's life span. It is important to identify the etiol-

ogy of Anxiety so that an appropriate nursing intervention can be selected. Box 44-1 summarizes the etiologies found in the nursing literature. NANDA (1999) identified 17 possible etiologies of Anxiety. Whitley (1992a) reduced related factors into the broad categories "perception of threat" and "impending change." Tueth (1993) suggested that anxiety in the elder is more often a symptom of an underlying mental or physical disorder than a primary diagnosis. Anxiety is easy to recognize in patients, but difficult to diagnose because it spans a continuum ranging from a normal state, to distress, to a disabling, fully developed disorder (Fernandez et al., 1995). Box 44-2 lists the organic factors associated with anxiety symptoms that should be considered and ruled out when making a diagnosis related to anxiety.

Assessment

Many types of assessment tools have been developed to measure the concept of anxiety for research and clinical purposes. A distinction frequently is made between anxiety as an emotional state and the personality trait that leads individuals to demonstrate habitual anxiousness (Vogel, 1991). State anxiety is characterized by the feelings of apprehension, tension, and increased autonomic nervous system activity. Nurses in all specialty areas encounter this type of anxiety in patients because of its situational and/or transient nature that surfaces because of

Table 44-2	DSM-IV Anxiety Disorders	
Anxiety Disorder	**Definition**	**DSM-IV Code**
Panic attack	A discrete period in which there is the sudden onset of intense apprehension, fearfulness, or terror, often associated with feelings of impending doom	Code with disorder in which panic attack occurs
Agoraphobia	Anxiety about, or avoidance of, places or situations from which escape might be difficult (or embarrassing) or in which help may not be available in the event of having a panic attack or paniclike symptoms	Code with disorder in which agoraphobia occurs
Panic disorder without agoraphobia	Characterized by recurrent unexpected panic attacks about which there is persistent concern	300.01
Panic disorder with agoraphobia	Characterized by both recurrent unexpected panic attacks and agoraphobia	300.21
Agoraphobia without history of panic disorder	Characterized by the presence of agoraphobia and paniclike symptoms without a history of unexpected panic attacks	300.22
Specific phobia	Characterized by clinically significant anxiety provoked by exposure to a specific feared object or situation, often leading to avoidance behavior	300.29
Social phobia	Characterized by clinically significant anxiety provoked by exposure to certain types of social or performance situations, often leading to avoidance behavior	300.23
Obsessive-compulsive disorder	Characterized by obsessions (which cause marked anxiety or distress) and/or compulsions (which serve to neutralize anxiety)	300.3
Posttraumatic stress disorder	Characterized by the reexperiencing of an extremely traumatic event accompanied by symptoms of increased arousal and by avoidance of stimuli associated with the trauma	309.81
Acute stress disorder	Characterized by symptoms similar to those of posttraumatic stress disorder that occur immediately in the aftermath of an extremely traumatic event	308.3
Generalized anxiety disorder	Characterized by at least 6 months of persistent and excessive anxiety and worry	300.02
Anxiety disorder caused by a general medical condition	Characterized by prominent symptoms of anxiety that are judged to be a direct physiologic consequence of a general medical condition	293.89
Substance-induced anxiety disorder	Characterized by prominent symptoms of anxiety that are judged to be a direct physiologic consequence of drug abuse, medication, or toxin exposure	Code by specific substance of abuse
Anxiety disorder not otherwise specified	Included for coding disorders with prominent anxiety or phobic avoidance that do not meet criteria for any specific anxiety disorder (or anxiety symptoms about which there is inadequate or contradictory information)	300.00

Data from American Psychiatric Association. (1994). *Diagnostic and statistical manual of mental disorders (4th ed.).* Washington, DC: Author.

environmental or personal stress. In contrast, trait anxiety is thought to be a personality characteristic that is more firmly entrenched in socioeconomic status. Trait anxiety occurs when the self-concept of the individual is challenged or threatened in some way. This type of anxiety is usually a long-standing personality trait and is expressed by a fairly specific behavior pattern (Spielberger, 1975). Patients with trait anxiety are more likely to be treated by psychiatric and mental health nurses. The distinctions made between state and trait anxiety are widely accepted and used across disciplines and are clearly clinically useful.

Table 44-3 lists 13 assessment tools and relevant research studies found in the literature. This table clearly depicts the popularity of the State-Trait Anxiety Inventory

(STAI) (Spielberger, Gorsuch, Lushene, Vagg, & Jacobs, 1983) as an assessment tool. Almost 30 studies, many from nursing, have used these instruments to measure anxiety in adult patients. Stanley, Beck, and Zebb (1996) conducted a study of older adults with and without generalized anxiety disorder to evaluate the psychometrics of four different instruments. The State-Trait Anxiety Inventory was found to be a reliable measure of anxiety in older populations, although scores were lower for the elderly than for younger groups. The researchers concluded that this might indicate that older individuals would be more likely to report certain types of symptoms. Gender differences on measures of anxiety were not found to be significant in older anxious and nonanxious adults in this study.

Box 44-1	Related Factors/Etiologies ANXIETY

Vogel (1991)
Loss of objects
Loss of external supplies
Loss of support systems
Loss of sensory function
Loss of social control
Fear of losses due to the aging process
Maladaptive coping strategies
Declining mental abilities
Declining physical abilities
Cognitive impairment

NANDA (1999)
Unconscious conflict about essential values/goals of life
Threat to self-concept
Threat of death
Threat to or change in health status
Threat to or change in environment
Threat to or change in role functioning

Threat to or change in interaction patterns
Situational/maturational crisis
Interpersonal transmission/contagion
Unmet needs

Whitley (1992a)
Threat to self-concept
Unmet needs
Situational crisis
Maturational crisis
Threat to or change in role functioning
Threat to or change in role status
Threat to or change in environment
Threat to or change in socioeconomic status
Unconscious conflict about essential values/goals in life
Interpersonal transmission and contagion
Threat to or change in interaction patterns
Threat of death

Box 44-2	Organic Factors Associated With Symptoms of Anxiety

Pharmacologic Agents
Stimulants, including caffeine
Thyroid replacement
Nicotine and alcohol withdrawal
Cannabis or other hallucinogen
Neuroleptics
Corticosteroids
Sedative-hypnotic withdrawal or paradoxical reactions
Aspirin
Sulfonamides
Bronchodilators and decongestants

Endocrine Disorders
Hyperthyroidism and hypothyroidism
Cushing's disease
Hyperparathyroidism
Carcinoid syndrome
Hypoglycemia
Pheochromocytoma
Hypercortisolism

Neurologic Disorders
Epilepsy
Migraine
Demyelinating diseases

Delirium
Dementia

Other
Heavy metal intoxication
Vitamin B_{12} deficiency
Mitral valve prolapse
Physical exertion
Lactic acidosis
Hypoxemia and chronic obstructive pulmonary disease (COPD)
Pulmonary embolism
Porphyria
Collagen-vascular disease
Brucellosis
Renal dysfunction

Data from Fernandez, F., Levy, J. K., Lachar, B., & Smith, G. W. (1995). The management of depression and anxiety in the elderly. *Journal of Clinical Psychiatry, 56*(Suppl 2), 20-29.

Table **44-3**	Measurement Instruments for Anxiety		
Tool	**Focus**	**Items**	**Studies**
State-Trait Anxiety Inventory (STAI Form Y) (Spielberger, Gorsuch, Lushene, Vagg, & Jacobs, 1983)	Designed to elicit feelings of anxiousness Contains subscales for state and trait anxiety	20 items 4-point Likert scale Range of scores: 20-80 Low anxiety = 20-39 Medium = 40-59 High = 60-80	Allen et al. (1992) Augustin & Hains (1996) Barnason, Zimmerman, & Nieveen (1995) Bokinskie (1992) Daly, Kleinpell, Lawinger, & Casey (1994) Elliot (1993) Ferrell-Torry & Glick (1993) Fraser & Ross-Kerr (1993) Friedman, Badere, & Fitzpatrick (1992) Gift, Moore, & Soeken (1992) Halm (1990) Markland & Hardy (1993) O'Connell (1989) Okun, Stein, Bauman, & Silver (1996) Olson & Sneed (1995) Palakanis, DeNobile, Sweeney, & Blankenship (1994) Rankin, Gfeller, & Gilner (1993) Rose, Conn, & Rodeman (1994) Rukholm et al. (1991) Shuldham, Cunningham, Hiscock, & Luscombe (1995)
Jackson Personality Research Inventory (JPI) (Jackson, 1977, 1979)	Developed and tested on community samples rather than psychiatric populations	20-item anxiety subscale 6-point Likert scale	Heidrich (1993)
Hospital Anxiety and Depression Scale (HAD) (Zigmond & Snaith, 1983)	Brief questionnaire designed to indicate the presence of a depressive anxiety disorder in medically ill patients	Contains 14 items (7 anxiety, 7 depression) Potential range of scores 0-21 Each response is weighted with a score from 1 to 3	Carroll, Kathol, Noyes, Wald, & Clamon (1993) Elliot (1993) Lampic, von Essen, Peterson, Larsson, & Sjoden (1996) Shuldham et al. (1995) Silverstone (1994)
Anxiety Defining Characteristics Tool (ADCT) (Young, 1986)	Developed to measure the defining characteristics of the nursing diagnosis Anxiety	52 items 4-point Likert scale	Lampic et al. (1996) Shuldham et al. (1995) Young (1986)
Anxiety about Aging Scale (AAS) (Lasher & Faulkender, 1993)	Assesses four dimensions of aging and three types of fears	84 items	No studies found
Brief Symptom Inventory (BSI) Derogatis & Spencer (1982)	Contains a subscale for anxiety	5 items 5-point Likert scale	No studies found
Panic and Agoraphobia Scale (Bandelow, 1995)	Developed to assess the severity of panic disorders and agoraphobia Intended for use in clinical trials Measures factors that impair the quality of life	Both observer and self-rating forms are available with matching items Observer form takes about 10 minutes to complete	No studies found
Social Phobia and Anxiety Inventory (SPAI) (Turner, Beidel, Dancu, & Stanley, 1989)	Developed to measure social phobias Includes cognitive, somatic, and behavioral dimensions of social fear	32-item scale 7-point Likert scale Separate score for agoraphobia and social phobia	Osman, Barrios, Aukes, & Osman (1995)

Continued

Table 44-3	Measurement Instruments for Anxiety—cont'd		
Tool	**Focus**	**Items**	**Studies**
Symptom Questionnaire (Kellner, 1987)	Designed to measure changes in psychologic distress in effectiveness research	92 items Contains a 23-item anxiety subscale Short form contains anxiety and depression subscales	Bull, Luo, & Maruyama (1994)
Profile of Mood States (POMS) (McNair, Lorr, & Droppleman, 1971)	Anxiety subscale focuses on musculoskeletal and somatic tension and psychomotor manifestations	Has been used with older adults	Conn, Taylor, & Wiman (1991) Giese & Schomer (1986) Oldridge, Streiner, Hoffmann & Guyatt (1995) Olson & Sneed (1995)

The Beck Anxiety Inventory (BAI) (Beck, Epstein, Brown, & Steer, 1988) was developed to create a clinical measure of anxiety appropriate for use with psychiatric patients. A second purpose for the development of this tool was to ensure that the items used would be independent of symptoms of depression. Cox, Cohen, Direnfeld, and Swinson (1996), in a recent evaluation of this inventory, questioned whether this instrument measures panic attacks rather than anxiety. Further tests of this instrument are warranted. Elliott (1993) compared three instruments—the STAI, the Hospital Anxiety and Depression Scale (HADS), and the Linear Analogue Anxiety Scale (LAAS); all three instruments were found to be valid measures of clinical anxiety.

See Table 44-3 for several relatively new scales that focus on specific types of anxiety, perhaps reflecting a trend to develop tools that measure specific aspects or types of anxiety. The Anxiety Defining Characteristic Tool is based on the work of NANDA. Few studies were found that have used this instrument. Future work needs to be done on the reliability and validity of the scales presented in Table 44-3.

Nursing Diagnosis

Many studies have validated the importance of Anxiety as a nursing diagnosis. Jones and Jacob (1981) found Anxiety as the third most frequently identified nursing diagnosis, occurring in patients of all ages and levels of health status and associated with all categories of medical diagnoses. Kim et al. (1984) found anxiety to be one of the top ten diagnoses identified by nurses working with cardiovascular patients. Gordon (1982) reported Anxiety as one of 10 most frequently identified nursing diagnoses from 1980 to 1984. Metzger and Hiltunen (1987) included Anxiety because of its frequent use by nurses in its validation study. Coenen et al. (1995), in a study using the Nursing Minimum Data Set, found Anxiety to be one of the top six nursing diagnoses in an acute care setting.

Anxiety was developed as a nursing diagnosis in 1973 based on the work of Peplau. The early diagnosis specified four levels of intensity: mild, moderate, severe, and panic (Gebbie & Lavin, 1995). In 1980 a controversy surfaced as to whether anxiety should be considered a diagnosis or be used only as a defining characteristic of Ineffective Coping, Knowledge Deficit, or Fear. In 1980 the North American Nursing Diagnosis Association (NANDA) eliminated Anxiety as a nursing diagnosis and made it a defining characteristic of the diagnosis Fear (Kim & Moritz, 1982).

Three early studies (Burke, 1982; Jones & Jacob, 1981; Yocum, 1984) focused on differentiating Anxiety from Fear. These studies demonstrated that nurses discriminate between the two concepts and treat patients differently. More recently, Bay and Algase (1999) developed a process model that reflects distinct characteristics of fear and anxiety. It is clear that anxiety is frequently observed by nurses in practice (Whitley, 1989). In 1982 Anxiety was again recommended for inclusion in the NANDA classification. Anxiety was defined as "a vague, uneasy feeling whose source is often nonspecific or unknown to the individual" (NANDA, 1994, p. 86). The most recent definition of Anxiety is "a vague uneasy feeling of discomfort or dread accompanied by an autonomic response; the source is often nonspecific or unknown to the individual; a feeling of apprehension caused by anticipation of danger. It is an altering signal that warns of impending danger and enables the individual to take measures to deal with threat" (NANDA, 1999, p. 134).

NANDA accepted a total of 29 defining characteristics for anxiety (17 subjective symptoms and 12 objective symptoms) when it was added back to the classification in 1982 (Kim, McFarland, & McLane, 1997; NANDA, 1994, p. 86). Defining characteristics subsequently have been defined and refined by several authors. There are presently 73 defining characteristics, with 9 behavioral symptoms, 16 affective symptoms, 2 objective symptoms, 3 subjective symptoms, 30 physiologic symptoms, and 13 cognitive symptoms. These patient behaviors provide the signs and symptoms for diagnosing this problem.

Several nurse validation studies were conducted in the 1980s. Aukamp (1986) conducted a validation study using both clients (30 pregnant women) and maternity nurses. Both groups agreed on two defining characteristics: "verbalized feelings about being anxious" and "apprehension." Whitley (1986), using Fehring's (1986, 1987, 1994) Diagnostic Content Validity Model in a study of nurse NANDA members, found the following five defining characteristics as critical indicators of anxiety: "anxious," "worried," "increased tension," "apprehension," and "regretful." In another study that used the Fehring model, Metzger and Hiltunen (1987) identified "fear of unspecific consequences" and "distress" as additional indicators of Anxiety. Kinney and Guzetta (1989), in a nurse validation study using magnitude estimation scaling, identified the following five defining characteristics of Anxiety: "expressed anxiety," "verbal complaints of anxiety," "motor activity," "nervous habits," and "apprehension." Lopez and Risey (1988), using the Fehring technique, identified the following nine defining characteristics of anxiety as critical: "anxious," "apprehension," "worried," "restlessness," "focus on self," "fear of unspecific consequences," "extraneous movement," "facial tension," and "difficulty in cognitive functioning." "Regretful" was rejected as a defining characteristic in this study.

Wake, Fehring, and Fadden (1994) conducted a multinational diagnostic content validation study that included anxiety. This study identified three critical defining characteristics across subjects from Belgium, Canada, Columbia, England, France, and the United States: "anxious," "panic," and "nervous." Variations by country were found for "distressed" and "sympathetic stimulation." The authors concluded that "country variations in these ratings may be the result of limitations of translation, language differences, or cultural differences" (p. 235).

Only two studies in the 1980s were found that used clinical validation methods to identify the defining characteristics of Anxiety. In a study using cardiovascular patients, Kim et al. (1984) found that psychosocial indicators of stress such as feeling "anxious, tense, or restless" and behaviors such as "tranquilizer use, nervous mannerisms, questioning, and depression" were frequently identified as defining characteristics of anxiety. This study also identified concern about life events (illness, future, family, finances) as a defining characteristic of anxiety. In a second clinical validation study by Fadden, Fehring, and Rossi (1987), most of the NANDA defining characteristics of anxiety were observed by clinical nurse specialists in the 49 medical-surgical patients studied; however, none reached a significant clinical diagnostic validity level using Fehring's technique. The studies conducted in the 1980s were primarily based on expert nurse opinion. More studies validating the defining characteristics with patient data are needed.

Four lists of defining characteristics for Anxiety from different sources are highlighted in Box 44-3. Three of the lists (NANDA, 1999; Vogel, 1991; Whitley, 1992a) reflect a nursing viewpoint. The list of signs and symptoms from Zisook, Schneider, and Schuchter (1990) arose from a study of anxiety and bereavement conducted in San Diego. This study followed widows and widowers over the first 2 years after the death of a spouse. The attributes identified in this bereavement study are consistent with the characteristics identified in the nursing studies. Whitley (1992a) divided the signs and symptoms of Anxiety into four areas: Physiologic: Sympathetic; Physiologic: Parasympathetic; Psychological/Behavioral; and Cognitive. Whitley's (1992a) discussion provides the most extensive list of defining characteristics found in the literature.

Nursing-Sensitive Outcomes

The general goals of nursing care for patients with the nursing diagnosis of Anxiety are to (1) prevent severe anxiety or panic from developing; (2) eliminate or reduce incapacitating anxiety states; (3) identify sources of anxiety; and (4) increase effective coping skills (McFarland & McFarlane, 1993). The Nursing Outcomes Classification (NOC) links a total of 11 outcomes with the diagnosis Anxiety. Primary outcomes include Aggression Control, Anxiety Control, Coping, Impulse Control, Self-Mutilation Restraint, and Social Interaction Skills. Additional outcomes associated with Anxiety are Acceptance: Health Status, Grief Resolution, Parent-Infant Attachment, Psychosocial Adjustment: Life Change, and Symptom Control (Iowa Outcomes Project, 2000, p. 467).

Nursing Interventions

It is important to treat anxiety because these disorders contribute to excess disability and further compromise quality of life for older individuals (Fernandez et al., 1995; Schweizer & Rickels, 1996). Management of anxiety in the elderly often involves the use of psychotropic drugs. It is very important to carefully monitor these types of medications in the elderly because of their increased sensitivity to toxic side effects, their decreased physical resiliency, and the risk of dependency and withdrawal (Gomez & Gomez, 1994). When these types of medications are needed, the choice of drugs must be individualized (Markovitz, 1993). Weiss (1996) identified that the general principles of treating the elderly with anti-anxiety drugs should include relief of symptoms with minimal sedation effects, improvement in sleep, freedom from autonomic and cognitive toxicity, and no physical dependence or drug interactions. The best pharmaceutical options for most elderly patients are short half-life benzodiazepines in low doses (Gomez & Gomez, 1994). The benefits and the risks of managing anxiety with medication must be considered.

Box 44-3	Defining Characteristics ANXIETY

Vogel (1991)
Pacing
Hand wringing
Tics or tremors
Repetitive actions such as twisting or rubbing
Elevated blood pressure
Elevated pulse rate
Muscle tension
Headache
Sleeplessness
Facial flushing
Subjective statements ("I feel nervous")
Aggressiveness
Disturbing dreams
Crying
Avoidance of decision-making situations
Inability to make decisions
Memory impairment
Inability to focus on content
Obsession with physical complaints

NANDA (1999)
Behavioral
Diminished productivity
Scanning and vigilance
Poor eye contact
Restlessness
Glancing about
Extraneous movement
Expressed concerns due to change in life events
Insomnia
Fidgeting

Affective
Regretful
Irritability
Anguish
Scared
Jittery
Overexcited
Painful and persistent increased helplessness
Rattled
Uncertainty
Increased wariness
Focus on self
Feelings of inadequacy
Fearful
Distressed
Apprehension
Anxious

Objective
Trembling/hand tremors
Insomnia

Subjective
Shakiness
Worried
Regretful

Physiologic
Voice quivering
Increased respiration
Urinary urgency
Increased pulse
Pupil dilation
Increased reflexes
Abdominal pain
Sleep disturbance
Tingling in extremities
Increased tension
Cardiovascular excitation
Increased perspiration
Facial tension
Anorexia
Heart pounding
Diarrhea
Urinary hesitancy
Fatigue
Dry mouth
Weakness
Decreased pulse
Facial flushing
Superficial vasoconstriction
Twitching
Decreased blood pressure
Nausea
Urinary frequency
Faintness
Respiratory difficulties
Increased blood pressure

Cognitive
Blocking of thought
Confusion
Preoccupation
Forgetfulness
Rumination
Impaired attention
Decreased perceptual field
Fear of nonspecific consequences
Tendency to blame others
Difficulty concentrating
Diminished ability to problem solve
Diminished learning ability
Awareness of physiologic symptoms

Zisook, Schneider, & Schucter (1990)
Nervousness
Suddenly scared
Fearful
Tense, keyed up
Terror, panic
Restlessness
Faintness, dizziness
Pains in chest
Nausea, upset stomach
Trouble getting breath

Box 44-3	Defining Characteristics ANXIETY

Hot or cold spells
Numbness, tingling
Weakness
Feelings easily hurt
Feeling people unfriendly
Feeling inferior to others
Feeling self-conscious
Trouble remembering things
Blocked in getting things done
Having to check/double-check what you do
Difficulty making decisions
Mind going blank
Trouble concentrating
Afraid in open spaces
Afraid to travel on bus, train
Avoid things due to fear
Feeling uneasy in crowds
Nervous when left alone

Whitley (1992a)
Physiologic: Sympathetic
Increased pulse
Increased blood pressure
Increased respirations
Face flushed
Respiratory difficulties
Increased reflexes
Twitching
Trembling
Tremors
Restlessness
Extraneous movements
Insomnia
Weakness
Pupil dilatation
Anorexia
Dry mouth
Increased perspiration
Facial tension
Voice quivering

Physiologic: Parasympathetic
Decreased pulse
Decreased blood pressure
Faintness/fainting
Abdominal pain
Nausea
Diarrhea
Urinary urgency
Urinary frequency

Psychologic
Increased tension
Apprehension
Worried
Distressed
Focus on self
Uncertainty
Fearful
Scared
Fear of unspecific consequences
Jittery
Poor eye contact
Glancing about
Feelings of inadequacy
Rattled
Increased helplessness
Increased wariness
Expressed concerns about changes in life events

Cognitive
Difficulty concentrating
Diminished learning ability
Diminished ability to problem solve
Blocking of thoughts
Decreased perceptual field
Forgetfulness
Impaired attention
Diminished productivity
Preoccupation
Confusion

Because of the many problems associated with anti-anxiety medications, nondrug strategies might be preferred (Hocking & Koenig, 1995), especially for patients with mild to moderate anxiety levels (Danton, Altrocchi, Antonuccio, & Basta, 1994). Snowdon (1993) maintained that, for older persons in nursing homes, attention should be given to improving their living environment before commencing psychotropic medications. Nurses who prescribe for patients in these types of settings must observe the Omnibus Budget Reconciliation Act (OBRA) regulations that dictate a preference for psychosocial treatments over drug therapy, avoidance of chemical or physical restraints, and minimal use of psychotropic medications (Weiss, 1994).

A wide variety of types of nursing interventions have been recommended for the treatment of anxiety (Table 44-4). The nurse should consider situational and patient characteristics as well as the degree and duration of anxiety symptoms when choosing an intervention. Nursing interventions for anxiety may focus on (1) providing information to increase a patient's sense of control and decrease uncertainty, (2) meeting basic needs, (3) assisting the patient to relax, or (4) helping patients to reconceptualize their thoughts about the threat or situation (McFarland & McFarlane, 1997).

The extensiveness of available interventions for the nursing diagnosis Anxiety is further demonstrated by the extensive list of nursing interventions linked to this

Table 44-4	Suggested Interventions Literature for Anxiety
Intervention	**Literature**
THERAPEUTIC TOUCH	Heidt, 1981; Olson & Sneed, 1995; Olson, Sneed, Bondonna, Ratliff, & Dias, 1992; Simington & Laing, 1993
TEACHING: PREOPERATIVE	Allen et al., 1992; Anderson & Masur, 1989; Peterson, 1991
INFORMATION GIVING	Dodds, 1993; Foxwell & Alder, 1993; Ludwick-Rosenthal & Neufeld, 1993; Nugent et al., 1993
HUMOROUS DISTRACTION	Gaberson, 1991
MUSIC THERAPY	Augustin & Hains, 1996; Barnason et al., 1995; Henry, 1995; Kaempf & Amodei, 1989; Moss, 1987; Palakanis et al., 1994; Standley, 1986; Steelman, 1990; Summers et al., 1990
RELAXATION	Gift et al., 1992; Mandle, Jacobs, Arcari, & Domar, 1996; Markland & Hardy, 1993; Mynchenberg & Dungan, 1995; Renfroe, 1988; Rickard, Scogin, & Keith, 1994; Weber, 1996
BIBLIOTHERAPY	Lidren et al., 1994; Marrs, 1995
BACK MASSAGE	Fraser & Ross-Kerr, 1993
ANXIETY MANAGEMENT	Childs-Clarke, Whitfield, & Cadbury, 1989
SUPPORT GROUPS	Halm, 1990
GUIDED IMAGERY	Heath, 1992; Thompson & Coppens, 1994
DIVERSIONAL ACTIVITIES	Friedman et al., 1992
COGNITIVE REFRAMING	Chambless & Gillis, 1993; Teasdale, 1993
INFORMATION GIVING TO FAMILY MEMBERS	Bokinskie, 1992; Johnson & Frank, 1995; Leske, 1996; O'Connell, 1989; Silva, 1979

patient problem by the Iowa Intervention Project (2000). A total of 46 unique interventions are identified from the Nursing Interventions Classification (NIC). Seven of these interventions are on the suggested list and include Anxiety Reduction, Calming Technique, Coping Enhancement, Dementia Management, Examination Assistance, Presence, and Telephone Consultation. The remaining 40 interventions are suggested as "additional optional interventions" the nurse might choose. Those not mentioned previously in this chapter are Allergy Management, Anger Control Assistance, Animal-Assisted Therapy, Anticipatory Guidance, Art Therapy, Autogenic Training, Biofeedback, Childbirth Preparation, Counseling, Crisis Intervention, Distraction, Elopement Precautions, Energy Management, Environmental Management, Exercise Promotion: Stretching, Genetic Counseling, Grief Work Facilitation: Perinatal Death, High-Risk Pregnancy Care, Humor, Hypnosis, Labor Induction, Labor Suppression, Medication Prescribing, Meditation Facilitation, Music Therapy, Progressive Muscle Relaxation, Reminiscence Therapy, Reproductive Technology Management, Security Enhancement, Simple Guided Imagery, Simple Relaxation Therapy, Support Group, Teaching: Individual, Teaching: Preoperative, Teaching: Prescribed Medication, Teaching: Procedure/Treatment, Urinary Incontinence Care: Enuresis, Visitation Facilitation, and Vital Signs Monitoring (Iowa Intervention Project, 2000, p. 715). This linkage list provides an even broader view of possible nursing interventions to treat anxiety than found in the literature review of research studies.

When planning interventions for the treatment of anxiety in the elderly it is important to be cognizant of the great variation among older adults. The nurse must be willing to tailor the use of cognitive-behavioral interventions and/or medications to meet the individual needs of each patient (Sheikh & Salzman, 1995). Both of these types of interventions can be effective (Steinberg, 1994). Impressive advances in the treatment of anxiety have been demonstrated in past decades. Much of the focus, however, has been on short-term, symptom-focused treatment that has not been sufficient for many individuals. Additional psychotherapy-type treatments might be needed to provide long-term benefits (Shear, 1995). Multisite investigations are now underway that combine proven psychosocial interventions with effective drug treatments; these research efforts might provide insight and have synergistic effects for the treatment of anxiety in the future (Barlow & Lehman, 1996).

CASE STUDY 1

D. Nance was a 78-year-old woman who continued to live alone in her two-bedroom home in the same neighborhood where she had lived with her husband for 40 years. Mr. Nance died 10 years ago, and Mrs. Nance's married children, who no longer lived in the community, spoke with pride of their mother's independence and involvement in church and senior citizen activities. The city, determined to build a new recreation facility in the block where Mrs. Nance lived, offered to purchase her home for a good price. Her children were pleased because they felt this would give their mother an opportunity to live in an apartment, which would be easier to care for. Mrs. Nance showed little reaction to the offer, although she stopped going to church and was rarely seen outside. She stopped calling her children and, when they called, spoke in a soft voice and talked about moving. Finally, when she did not answer her phone, her children came to see her. They found her unkempt, visibly agitated, walking with a shuffling gait, and with marked hand tremors. They took her to a physician who found that her pulse and blood pressure were alarmingly elevated. The physician recognized her anxiety and prescribed an anti-anxiety agent. The physician warned the family that medication was a temporary measure and that more long-lasting solutions for their mother's anxiety would have to be found.

As Box 44-4 depicts, Mrs. Nance had multiple etiologies for Anxiety and experienced many of the defining characteristics of this diagnosis. Box 44-4 also identifies the patient outcomes and nursing interventions selected for Mrs. Nance. The outcome, Anxiety Control, defined as the "personal actions to eliminate or reduce feelings of apprehension and tension from an unidentified source" (Iowa Outcomes Project, 2000, p. 116) was selected to monitor Mrs. Nance's ability to reduce her anxious feelings. Six specific indicators from this outcome were selected to determine if her anxiety was decreasing, staying the same, or increasing after intervention by a nurse. The nursing intervention selected was Anxiety Reduction, defined as "minimizing apprehension, dread, foreboding, or uneasiness related to an unidentifiable source of anticipated danger" (Iowa Intervention Project, 2000, p. 146).

CASE STUDY 2

T. and F. Rose have been married for 56 years. Mr. Rose is 78 years old and Mrs. Rose is 74 years old. Two months ago, Mrs. Rose developed incapacitating physical problems that resulted in her being admitted to a local nursing home. Mr. Rose tried to visit her regularly, but because he refused to use public transportation, he had to rely on his son to take him for visits. Just recently his son made a job change that required him to move to another part of the country. Because he would no longer be available to assist his elderly father, the son had Mr. Rose admitted to the same nursing home in which Mrs. Rose resided.

Though usually pleasant, Mr. Rose seemed upset and apprehensive after moving to the long-term care facility. He continuously expressed worry about his wife's condition and once confided to a nurse his own concern about becoming physically or mentally disabled. His son did not contact him after his admission, and whenever asked about his son, Mr. Rose became quite agitated and replied, "Him? Oh, he's the one who forgot about me." A niece called and visited him frequently, but Mr. Rose stated, "She's a nice girl, but I don't want to count on her too much. You know, you just can't tell when she'll lose interest in an old man." Although Mr. Rose appeared to be adjusting to life in the facility, he complained to a

---

Box **44-4**	Nursing Diagnosis, Outcome, and Intervention for **MRS. NANCE**

Nursing Diagnosis	Reports increased length of time between episodes
Anxiety	Maintains concentration
Defining characteristics	Reports absence of physical manifestations of anxiety
Shakiness	Behavioral manifestations of anxiety absent
Apprehension	Reports adequate sleep
Increased tension	
Jittery	Nursing Intervention
Restlessness	**Anxiety Reduction**
Trembling/hand tremors	*Activities*
Distresses	Seek to understand the patient's perspective of a stressful situation
Overexcited	Listen attentively
	Reinforce behavior, as appropriate
Related factors/etiologies	Encourage verbalization of feelings, perceptions, and fears
Threat to self-concept	Identify when level of anxiety changes
Threat to or change in health status	Support the use of appropriate defense mechanisms
Threat to or change in environment	Determine patient's decision-making ability
Threat to or change in role functioning	Administer medications to reduce anxiety, as appropriate
Threat to interaction patterns	Clearly state expectations for patient's behavior
Situational/maturational crisis	
Nursing-Sensitive Outcome	
Anxiety Control	
Indicators	
Uses effective coping strategies	
Reports decreased duration of episodes	

Nursing Outcomes Classification (NOC) 5-point Likert measurement scale:
Anxiety Control: 1 = Never demonstrated; 2 = Rarely demonstrated; 3 = Sometimes demonstrated;
              4 = Often demonstrated; 5 = Consistently demonstrated.

coresident, "It's so different living here from at home. I don't think I'll ever get used to it here. And living here costs so much. I'm scared I'll run out of money. How do you keep paying?"

Though Mr. Rose was physically stable, alert, oriented, and nearly totally independent in all activities of daily living, he appeared fearful and tense and had spells of heart palpitations that the physician said had no physiologic cause.

Box 44-5 identifies the patient outcome and nursing intervention selected for Mr. Rose. The outcome, Coping, defined as "actions to manage stressors that tax an individual's resources" (Iowa Outcomes Project, 1997, p. 136), was selected to measure the degree to which Mr. Rose was able to cope and adjust to his new living situation. The NIC intervention, Coping Enhancement, defined as "assisting a patient to adapt to perceived stressors, changes, or threats that interfere with meeting life demands and roles" (Iowa Intervention Project, 2000, p. 234), was the logical intervention. Mr. Rose had many life changes occurring in rapid succession and help by the nurse with coping strategies was anticipated to reduce his feelings of anxiety.

FEAR

It is necessary to distinguish fear from anxiety. Jones and Jacob (1981) summarized the understandings of fear and anxiety represented in the literature into three major clusters. First, fear and anxiety are used as synonymous, interchangeable concepts. Second, fear and anxiety are distinctly different experiences. Finally, fear and anxiety are not well-differentiated. Danesh (1977) described fear and anxiety as similar, but different experiences. Yocum (1984) reviewed the literature defining fear and anxiety and emphasized that both fear and anxiety are separate nursing diagnoses and, furthermore, are not symptoms of other diagnoses. Her report supported the notion of fear as a quick and often short-lived response to specific, identifiable danger. Taylor-Loughran (1989) described the relationship between fear and anxiety and suggested the possibility of a fear-anxiety syndrome. The common distinction made between fear and anxiety in both nursing and nonnursing literature is the ability to identify the etiologic agent of a fearful response and the inability to specify the cause of anxiety (Barry, 1984; Danesh, 1977; Jones &

Box 44-5	Nursing Diagnosis, Outcome, and Intervention for **MR. ROSE**

Nursing Diagnosis **Anxiety** *Defining characteristics* Uncertainty Cardiovascular excitation Apprehension Increased tension Worried Distressed Expressed concerns due to change in life events *Related factors/etiologies* Threat to or change in environment Threat to or change in role functioning Threat to or change in interaction patterns Threat to self-concept Unmet needs Nursing-Sensitive Outcome **Coping** *Indicators* Verbalizes sense of control Reports decrease in stress Verbalizes acceptance of situation Modifies lifestyle as needed Uses available social support Employs behaviors to reduce stress	Uses effective coping strategies Verbalizes need for assistance Reports decrease in physical symptoms of stress Adapts to developmental changes Nursing Intervention **Coping Enhancement** *Activities* Appraise the impact of the patient's life situation on roles and relationships Help the patient to identify the information he is most interested in obtaining Encourage an attitude of realistic hope as a way of dealing with feelings of helplessness Introduce patient to persons (or groups) that have successfully undergone the same experience Support the use of appropriate defense mechanisms Encourage verbalizations of feeling, perceptions, and fears Appraise patient's needs/desires for social support Determine the risk of patient's inflicting self-harm Encourage family involvement Assist the patient to identify positive strategies to deal with limitations and manage needed lifestyle or role changes Assist the patient to clarify misconceptions Assist the patient to identify available support systems

Nursing Outcomes Classification (NOC) 5-point Likert measurement scale:
Coping: 1 = Never demonstrated; 2 = Rarely demonstrated; 3 = Sometimes demonstrated; 4 = Often demonstrated;
          5 = Consistently demonstrated.

Jacob, 1981; Whitley, 1992b; Yocum, 1984). Stuart (1995) provided a useful separation of these two concepts:

Fear is an individual ideation with a specific source or object that the person can identify and describe. Fear involves the intellectual appraisal of a threatening stimulus; anxiety involves the emotional response to that appraisal. A person generally fears a set of circumstances that may occur at some point in the future. A fear is caused by physical or psychological exposure to a threatening situation. Fear produces anxiety. The two emotions are differentiated in speech; we speak of "having" a fear, but of "being" anxious (p. 328).

Just as fear must be distinguished from anxiety, it must also be differentiated from phobia. True phobias are recognized as psychopathologic conditions. The *Diagnostic and Statistical Manual of Mental Disorders (DSM-IV)* (American Psychiatric Association, 1994, p. 405) described the essential feature of specific phobic disorders as a "marked and persistent fear of clearly discernible, circumscribed objects or situations." The phobic adult realizes that the fearful response is disproportionately unreasonable in relation to the actual danger of the threat. In a normal fear response the degree of response is consistent with the actual threat. "Insight into the excessive or unreasonable nature of the fear tends to increase with age and is not required to make the diagnosis in children" (p. 406). Anxiety sensitivity is the "fear of anxiety-related sensations, which arises from beliefs that these sensations have harmful somatic, psychological or social consequences" (Taylor, 1993, p. 289). Anxiety sensitivity is thought to play an important role in causing panic attacks.

Related Factors/Etiologies

The origins of fear are potentially limitless. However, a review of the literature on fears of the elderly reveals a small body of information. Cesarone's (1991) literature review suggested that the sources of fear in the elderly can be loosely clustered into five major categories. Fears related to the physical body included fears of pain, suffering, and incapacitating illness (Copp, 1981; Eyde & Rich, 1983). Fears related to the psyche included fears of dependence, loss of control, and becoming burdensome on family and loved ones (Brodie, 1978; Carter & Galliano, 1981; Castles & Murray, 1979; Copp, 1981; Eyde & Rich, 1983). Several authors have described a fear of dying or fears related to dying (Castles & Murray, 1979; Nolan, 1984; Spencer & Dorr, 1975; Williams, 1976). However, most often these fears of dying can be identified more realistically as fear of pain and suffering, fear of loneliness, fear of meaninglessness, fear of the unknown, and/or fear of abandonment. Using a medical model orientation, Roth (1978) suggested that "the psychopathology of old age appears to center ultimately on the fear of dying" (p. 557). Wass and Myers (1982) asserted that the aged are no more fearful of death than any other group of individuals

and that often the elderly seem to be less fearful of death than younger persons. Brodie (1978) stated that "Contrary to the findings of other investigators, the 'most feared' items of retirees did not include death, which was noted as one of the 'least feared' items" (p. 70).

Another category of fears of the elderly are those fears related to social interaction and/or significant others. Fear of loss through death or injuries of a loved one were disclosed, as was fear of speaking before a group. Fears related to crime and victimization among the elderly have been widely documented and form the final category of fears (Ebersole & Hess, 1998; Jeffords, 1983; Kennedy & Silverman, 1985; Lebowitz, 1975; Norton & Courlander, 1982; Pollack & Patterson, 1980; Sundeen & Mathieu, 1976). These fears have been studied in elderly who reside in urban communities and most often have been shown to be related to the community. It also has been shown that fears of crime and victimization can be reduced when proactive steps are taken to increase the elderly individual's sense of security.

Closely related to the fear of victimization is the fear of transportation. Commuting (by any modality) places the elderly individual at increased risk for physical mishap and injury or crime (Ebersole & Hess, 1998). Teri and Lewinsohn (1986) suggested that elderly people may experience a fear of change or disruption of regular routines. Fear of diagnostic tests, especially mental status examinations, was also cited. This fear perhaps might more accurately be labeled as a fear of being unhealthy or mentally incompetent. Copp (1981) suggested that financial fears can be a serious concern for the elder. Ebersole and Hess (1998) suggested that the institutionalized elder can be fearful of invasive touching by nurses and other caregivers.

Fear of falling has been commonly identified in older adults; the result can be a restriction in activity (Arfken, Lach, Birge, & Miller, 1994; Burker et al., 1995). Arfken et al. (1994) also suggested that "the prevalence of fear of falling is greater in women and that it is associated with increased frailty and recent experience with falls" (p. 565). Whitley (1992b) identified eight related factors for fear, which are summarized in Box 44-6. To date, 14 related factors for the diagnosis of fear have been developed by NANDA.

Assessment

To complete a comprehensive assessment of a client's fear, the nurse must both inquire about subjective experiences and observe the physiologic and behavioral manifestations of the affective state. Rachman's (1994) literature review suggested that many people exaggerate the intensity of a fear-provoking situation and that those persons who are most fearful are the individuals who are most likely to overpredict their fear response. The assessment also must seek to identify the source of the fear. Assessment of fear may be successfully accomplished by direct observation and questioning, by indirect measurement of

---

Box 44-6   Related Factors/Etiologies
FEAR

Cesarone (1991)

Fears related to the physical body

- Fear of disease or illness
- Fear of pain
- Fear of prolonged suffering

Fears related to the psyche

- Fear of abandonment
- Fear of attachment
- Fear of becoming a burden
- Fear of dependence
- Fear of failure to adapt
- Fear of incompetence
- Fear of loss
- Fear of "loss of control"
- Fear of mental illness

Fears related to dying

- Fear of death
- Fear of loneliness
- Fear of meaninglessness
- Fear of punishment

Fear related to social interaction and significant others

- Fear of illness or injury to loved one
- Fear of death of loved one
- Fear of speaking in front of a group

Other miscellaneous fears

- Fear of change
- Fear of crime and victimization
- Fear of financial insecurities
- Fear of medical/psychiatric tests
- Fear of transportation
- Fear of touch

Whitley (1992b)

Natural or innate origins

- Sudden noise
- Heights
- Pain
- Loss of physical support

Learned response

- Conditioning
- Modeling from or identification with others

Separation from support system in a potentially threatening way

- Hospitalization
- Treatments

Knowledge deficit or unfamiliarity
Sensory impairment
Phobic stimulus or phobia
Environmental stimuli

---

changing physiologic states, and/or through the use of formal assessment tools.

Table 44-5 identifies the assessment tools found in the literature dealing with the concept of fear. Most of these tools seek to identify and assess the level and types of fear the individual is experiencing. The Fear Questionnaire (Marks & Mathews, 1979) and the Fear Survey Schedule (Wolpe & Lang, 1964) deal with fears from a global perspective but have not been used much by nurses. The other two instruments address specific types of fears: fear of pain and fear of spiders.

Nursing Diagnosis

Fear was initially identified as a nursing diagnosis at the first National Conference on the Classification of Nursing Diagnoses in 1973. Eight subcategories were also generated. Four of the subcategories represented what was called "functional fear," and four reflected "nonfunctional fear." Each of the eight fear subcategories were also qualified by degree as mild, moderate, severe, or panic (Gebbie & Lavin, 1995). This diagnostic formulation of Fear persisted for 7 years.

At the 1980 National Conference the general assembly accepted the diagnosis of Fear and the label was changed to a single category with one defining characteristic, the "ability to identify the object of fear" (Kim & Moritz, 1982, p. 290). The NANDA definition of Fear is "anxiety caused by consciously recognized and realistic danger. It is a perceived threat, real or imagined. Operationally, fear is the presence of an immediate feeling of apprehension and fright; source known and specific; subjective responses that act as energizers but cannot be observed; and objective signs that are the result of the transformation of energy into relief behaviors and responses" (NANDA, 1999, p. 137).

It is possible for an elderly individual to be frightened of almost any object or experience that potentially poses a threat. To identify the existence of Fear, the nurse must know the signs and symptoms that represent it. NANDA (1999) has identified 28 defining characteristics of Fear. Whitley's study (1992b) identified subjective and objective defining characteristics of Fear (Box 44-7). Subjective defining characteristics include increased tension, being apprehensive and scared, and impulsiveness. The individual also states or demonstrates that the source of the fear is

Table 44-5	Measurement Instruments for Fear		
Tool	**Focus**	**Items**	**Studies**
Fear Questionnaire (Marks & Mathews, 1979)	Contains three subscales to assess clinical phobias: agoraphobia, social, blood, and injury	15 items 0-8 scale 40 top score	Chisholm & Hurley (1994) Cox, Parker, & Swinson (1996) Osman, Barrios, Osman, & Markway (1993) Stanley, Beck, & Zebb (1996)
Fear Survey Schedule (Wolpe, 1983; Wolpe & Lange, 1964)	Contains the following anxiety-evoking stimuli: animal; social or interpersonal; tissue damage, illness, and death; noises; classical phobias; and a miscellaneous category (e.g., falling, strange places, failure, imaginary creatures)	72 items 5-point Likert scale	Berggren, Carlsson, Gustafsson, & Hakeberg (1995) Chisholm & Hurley (1994) Davey, Burgess, & Rashes (1995) Stravynski, Basoglu, Marks, Sengun & Marks (1995)
Fear of Spiders Questionnaire (Syzmanski & O'Donohue, 1995)	Assesses fear of spiders Covers the following domains: cognitive, behavioral, physiologic, negative attitudes, and fear of harm by spiders	228 items 7-point Likert scale Self-report	No studies found
Fear of Pain Questionnaire (McNeil, Rainwater, & Aljazireh, 1986)	Assesses fear of painful stimuli Includes three subscales for minor pain, severe pain, and medical pain	Scale 1-5 30 items Self-report	McCracken, Gross, Aikens, & Carnrike (1996)

known. Objective defining characteristics include increased heart rate, blood pressure and respiratory rate, pallor, pupil dilatation, concentration on the source of the fear, increased alertness, and fight/flight behaviors (Whitley, 1992b). In a later study, Whitley identified five critical defining characteristics of Fear: fearfulness, fright, cardiovascular excitation, apprehension, and being scared. Two of these, apprehension and cardiovascular excitation, are also identified as defining characteristics of Anxiety (Whitley, 1994).

Nursing-Sensitive Outcomes

According to NOC, the only suggested outcome for the nursing diagnosis Fear is Fear Control, defined as the "personal actions to eliminate or reduce disabling feelings of alarm aroused by an identifiable source" (Iowa Outcomes Project, 2000, p. 216). Additional associated outcomes suggested are Anxiety Control, Comfort Level, and Coping.

Anxiety Control, the "personal actions to eliminate or reduce feelings of apprehension and tension from an unidentifiable source" (Iowa Outcomes Project, 2000, p. 116), seems by definition to be an incorrect outcome for fear, although it might possibly be used to deal with anxiety associated with fear. Comfort Level, defined as "extent of physical and psychological ease" (Iowa Outcomes Project, 2000, p. 173), and Coping, "actions to manage stressors that tax an individual's resources" (Iowa

Outcomes Project, 2000, p. 192), would be appropriate outcomes if Fear Control were not selected.

Nursing Interventions

Three NIC interventions are primary for the NANDA diagnosis of Fear: Anxiety Reduction, "minimizing apprehension, dread, foreboding or uneasiness related to an unidentified source of anticipated danger" (Iowa Intervention Project, 2000, p. 146); Coping Enhancement, "assisting a patient to adapt to perceived stressors, changes or threats which interfere with meeting life demands and roles" (p. 187); and Security Enhancement, "intensifying a patient's sense of physical and psychological safety" (p. 483).

NIC offers many other interventions that might be relevant for the nursing diagnosis of Fear: Cognitive Restructuring, Counseling, Crisis Intervention, Decision-Making Support, Environmental Management, Examination Assistance, Preparatory Sensory Information, Presence, Support System Enhancement, and Telephone Consultation. In addition, 24 additional optional interventions are suggested, including Anger Control Assistance, Biofeedback, Communication Enhancement: Visual Deficit, Meditation Facilitation, Self-Esteem Enhancement, Teaching: Preoperative, and Vital Signs Monitoring. Also, some interventions listed for the nursing diagnosis of Anxiety may be appropriate for treating the anxiety that can accompany Fear (Iowa Intervention Project, 2000, p. 736).

Box 44-7

Defining Characteristics
FEAR

NANDA (1999)
Feeling of dread related to an identifiable source

Cesarone (1991)
Subjective
Affective responses
Cognitive responses
Apprehension
Decreased self-assurance
Dread
Expectation of danger to self
Fright
Impulsiveness
Inability to concentrate
Intense focus on the threat
Nervousness
Panic
Tension
Terror

Physical Sensations
Palpitation
Sinking feeling in the pit of stomach
Tightness in throat

Physiologic Responses
Decreased gastrointestinal activity
Diaphoresis
Dry mouth
Increased blood pressure
Increased heart rate
Increased muscle tension
Increased respirations
Pupil dilation
Superficial vasoconstriction
Urinary frequency

Behavioral Manifestations
Avoidance or attack behavior
Disorganization of speech
Hand tremors
Impairment of performance
Increased alertness
Increased quantity of verbalizations
Increased questioning/information seeking
Increased rate of verbalizations
Motor incoordination

Narrowed or fixed focus of attention
Physical flight
Possible immobilization
Restlessness
Voice tremors/pitch changes

Whitley (1992b)
Subjective
Apprehensive
Frightened
Increased tension
Decreased self-assurance
Afraid
Scared
Terrified
Panicky
Jittery
Dread
Alarm
Impulsiveness

Objective
Identifies object of fear
Immediate response to object of fear
Increased alertness
Concentration on the source
Wide-eyed
Attach behavior
Focus on "it" out there
Fight behavior/aggression
Flight behavior/withdrawal
Increased heart rate
Increased blood pressure
Shunting of blood from skin and gastrointestinal tract to the
    heart, central nervous system, and skeletal muscles
Anorexia
Nausea
Vomiting
Diarrhea
Muscle tightness and fatigue
Urinary frequency
Increased respiratory rate
Shortness of breath
Pallor
Diaphoresis
Pupil dilation

Systematic desensitization has been used successfully for the treatment of phobias. The patient develops a hierarchy of feared situations from those that are less feared to those that are intensely feared. Deep muscle relaxation is taught to the patient, and the hierarchy of feared images is presented to the client while he is in the deep relaxation state (Stuart, 1995). This is an intervention that might be used by advanced nurse practitioners and possibly should be developed for future editions of NIC.

CASE STUDY 3

S. Jackson is 68 years of age and has been widowed for 5 years. Although Mrs. Jackson has no children, several other widows about her age, including her sister-in-law, live in the same inner-city apartment building and keep an eye on one another. During the past year, however, two widows have died and the apartment building has fallen into the hands of a landlord who is letting the

Box 44-8	Nursing Diagnosis, Outcome, and Intervention for **MRS. JACKSON**

Nursing Diagnosis
Fear
Defining characteristics
Ability to identify object of fear
Frightened
Scared
Stays home
Expectation of danger to self

Related factors/etiologies
Fear of crime and victimization
Loss of friends and husband
Deteriorating living environment

Nursing-Sensitive Outcome
Fear Control
Indicators
Monitors intensity of fear
Plans coping strategies for fearful situations

Uses effective coping strategies
Reports increased length of time between episodes
Maintains social relationships
Maintains physical functioning

Nursing Intervention
Security Enhancement
Activities
Discuss specific situations or individuals that threaten the
    patient or family
Help the patient/family identify what factors increase sense of
    security
Assist patient to identify usual coping responses
Assist patient to use coping responses that have been
    successful in the past

Nursing Outcomes Classification (NOC) 5-point Likert measurement scale:
Fear Control: 1 = Never demonstrated; 2 = Rarely demonstrated; 3 = Sometimes demonstrated; 4 = Often demonstrated;
              5 = Consistently demonstrated.

building get very rundown (e.g., broken windows and mice). The deaths of her friends and husband and the decline of her home are daily reminders of her own imminent death and the powerlessness she feels to do anything about the apartment building. Mrs. Jackson has always been active and tries to walk regularly. She used to go out and visit her friends, attend church, and attend social events at the senior center, but more and more she watches TV at night in place of other activities. Mrs. Jackson watches lots of news and also crime shows, despite the fact she finds these "upsetting and scary because there's so much crime going on now." She worries she will be mugged someday.

Mrs. Jackson has had diabetes and hypertension for 10 years, sees a nurse practitioner in an outpatient clinic in a large health care facility regularly, and has been able to control both chronic diseases successfully with diet, exercise, and medication. Lately, however, both her walking and her visits to the nurse practitioner have been greatly curtailed, since she has become very frightened about leaving her apartment and does not feel safe in the neighborhood.

The nursing diagnosis Fear and the selected nursing-sensitive outcome and nursing intervention for Mrs. Jackson are summarized in Box 44-8. The NOC outcome Fear Control is defined as the "personal actions to eliminate or reduce disabling feelings of alarm aroused by an identifiable source" (Iowa Outcomes Project, 2000, p. 216). Six indicators were selected to follow her progress. The intervention, Security Enhancement, defined as "intensifying a patient's sense of physical and psychological safety" (Iowa Intervention Project, 2000, p. 571), was

chosen to address Mrs. Jackson's fear directly. Four nursing activities were selected from this nursing intervention. These activities focused on identifying situations that were threatening to her and those that made her feel safe, as well as on coping skills.

SUMMARY

The nursing diagnoses Anxiety and Fear have clinical relevance to nurses from many specialties. Their long history of inclusion in the NANDA classification speaks to their importance. Future work to identify distinct and different defining characteristics and etiologies for the two diagnoses is critical. Otherwise the nurse is caught in a circular diagnostic cycle: once the source of anxiety is identified, anxiety must be redefined as fear. Of equal importance is the use of DSM-IV diagnoses by nurses as more advanced practitioners are prepared in the future. To date, nursing diagnoses have ignored important concepts related to anxiety such as depression and phobias. This makes the use of standardized language for some nurses difficult at best. The diagnosis of Anxiety needs to address patients with trait anxiety as well as it does patients with state anxiety. The chronic nature of personality anxiety disorders makes this critical. It is important that Anxiety and Fear be refined and validated with additional studies by nurses. Only then can linkages between classifications such as NANDA, NIC, and NOC be used to improve the care of patients experiencing anxiety and fear.

REFERENCES

Allen, M., Knight, C., Falk, C., & Strang, V. (1992). Effectiveness of a preoperative teaching program for cataract patients. *Journal of Advanced Nursing, 17,* 303-309.

American Psychiatric Association. (1994). *Diagnostic and statistical manual of mental disorders* (4th ed.). Washington, DC: Author.

Anderson, C. S., Linto, J., Steward-Wynne, E. G. (1995). A population-based assessment of the impact and burden of caregiving for long-term stroke survivors. *Stroke, 26*(5), 843-849.

Anderson, K. O., & Masur, F. T. (1989). Psychologic preparation for cardiac catheterization. *Heart & Lung, 18*(2), 154-163.

Arfken, C. L., Lach, H. W., Birge, S. J., & Miller, J. P. (1994). The prevalence and correlates of fear of falling in elderly persons living in the community. *American Journal of Public Health, 84*(4), 565-570.

Augustin, P., & Hains, A. A. (1996). Effect of music on ambulatory surgery patients' preoperative anxiety. *AORN Journal, 63*(4), 750, 753-758.

Aukamp, V. (1986). Knowledge deficit and anxiety as nursing diagnoses in third trimester of pregnancy: An exploratory study to identify the defining characteristics and contributing factors. Unpublished doctoral dissertation. University of Texas, Austin.

Bandelow, B. (1995). Assessing the efficacy of treatments for panic disorder and agoraphobia. *International Clinical Psychopharmacology, 10*(2), 73-81.

Barlow, D. H., & Lehman, C. L. (1996). Advances in the psychosocial treatment of anxiety disorders. Implications for national health care. *Archives of General Psychiatry, 53*(8), 727-735.

Barnason, S., Zimmerman, L., & Nieveen, J. (1995). The effects of music interventions on anxiety in the patient after coronary bypass grafting. *Heart & Lung, 24*(2), 124-132.

Barry, P. D. (1984). *Psychosocial nursing: Assessment and intervention.* Baltimore: Lippincott Williams & Wilkins.

Bay, E. S., & Algase, D. L. (1999). Fear and anxiety: A simultaneous concept analysis. *Nursing Diagnosis, 10*(3), 103-111.

Beck, A. T., Epstein, N., Brown, G., & Steer, R. A. (1988). An inventory for measuring clinical anxiety: Psychometric properties. *Journal of Consulting and Clinical Psychology, 56,* 893-897.

Berggren, U., Carlsson, S. G., Gustafsson, J. E., & Hakeberg, M. (1995). Factor analysis and reduction of a Fear Survey Schedule among dental phobic patients. *European Journal of Oral Sciences, 103*(5), 331-338.

Blair, D. T., & Hildreth, N. A. (1991). PTSD and the Vietnam veteran: The battle for treatment. *Journal of Psychosocial Nursing and Health Services, 29,* 15-20.

Blair, D. T., & Ramones, V. A. (1994). Psychopharmacologic treatment of anxiety. *Journal of Psychosocial Nursing and Health Services, 32,* 49-53.

Blair, D. T., & Ramones, V. A. (1996). The undertreatment of anxiety: Overcoming confusion and stigma. *Journal of Psychosocial Nursing and Health Services, 34*(6), 9-18, 41-42.

Blazer, D., George, L. K., & Hughes, D. (1991). The epidemiology of anxiety disorders: An age comparison. In C. Salzman & B. D. Lebowitz (Eds.), *Anxiety in the elderly* (pp. 17-30). New York: Springer.

Bokinskie, J. C. (1992). Family conferences: A method to diminish transfer anxiety. *Journal of Neuroscience Nursing, 24*(2), 129-133.

Brodie, J. N. (1978). Social behavior of the elderly: Effects of fearfulness and perceived locus of control. *Issues in Mental Health Nursing, 1*(1), 64-75.

Bull, M. J., Luo, D., & Maruyama, G. (1994). Symptom questionnaire anxiety and depression scales: Reliability and validity. *Journal of Nursing Measurement, 2*(1), 25-36.

Burke, S. O. (1982). A developmental perspective on the nursing diagnoses fear and anxiety. *Nursing papers: Perspectives in nursing* (pp. 59-64). Montreal, Canada: School of Nursing, McGill University.

Burker, E. J., Wong, H., Sloane, P. D., Mattingly, D., Preisser, J., & Mitchell, C. M. (1995). Predictors of fear of falling in dizzy and non-dizzy elderly. *Psychology & Aging, 10*(1), 104-110.

Carroll, B. T., Kathol, R. G., Noyes, R., Wald, T. G., & Clamon, G. H. (1993). Screening for depression and anxiety in cancer patients using the Hospital Anxiety and Depression Scale. *General Hospital Psychiatry, 15*(2), 69-74.

Carter, C., & Galliano, D. (1981). Fear and loss of attachments: A major dynamic in the social isolation of the institutionalized elderly. *Journal of Gerontological Nursing, 7,* 342-349.

Castles, M. R., & Murray, R. B. (1979). *Dying in an institution: Nurse/patient perspectives.* Norwalk, CT: Appleton & Lange.

Cesarone, D. (1991). Fear. In M. Mass, K. Buckwalter, & M. Hardy (Eds.), *Nursing diagnoses and interventions for the elderly* (pp. 460-468). Reading, MA: Addison Wesley Longman.

Chambless, D. L., & Gillis, M. M. (1993). Cognitive therapy of anxiety disorders. *Journal of Consulting & Clinical Psychology, 61*(2), 248-260.

Childs-Clarke, A., Whitfield, W., & Cadbury, S. (1989). Anxiety management groups in clinical practice. *Nursing Times, 85*(30), 49-52.

Chisholm, D. C., & Hurley, J. D. (1994). Personality traits associated with fear. *Psychological Reports, 74*(3 Pt 1), 847-850.

Coenen, A., Ryan, P., Sutton, J., Devine, E. C., Werley, H. H., & Kelber, S. (1995). Use of the Nursing Minimum Data Set for select nursing diagnoses and related factors in an acute care setting. *Nursing Diagnosis, 6*(3), 108-114.

Conn, V. S., Taylor, S. G., & Wiman, P. (1991). Anxiety, depression, quality of life, and self-care among survivors of myocardial infarction. *Issues in Mental Health Nursing, 12,* 321-331.

Copp, L. A. (1981). *Care of the aging.* New York: Churchill Livingstone.

Cox, B. J., Cohen, E., Direnfeld, D. M., & Swinson, R. P. (1996). Does the Beck Anxiety Inventory measure anything beyond panic attack symptoms? *Behavior Research & Therapy, 34*(11-12), 949-961.

Cox, B. J., Parker, J. D., & Swinson, R. P. (1996). Confirmatory factor analysis of the Fear Questionnaire with social phobia patients. *British Journal of Psychiatry, 168*(4), 497-499.

Daly, K., Kleinpell, R. M., Lawinger, S., & Casey, G. (1994). The effect of two nursing interventions on families of ICU patients. *Clinical Nursing Research, 3*(4), 414-422.

Danesh, H. B. (1977). Anger and fear. *American Journal of Psychiatry, 134,* 1109-1112.

Danton, W. G., Altrocchi, J., Antonuccio, D., & Basta, R. (1994). Nondrug treatment of anxiety. *American Family Physician, 49*(1), 161-166.

Davey, G. C., Burgess, I., & Rashes, R. (1995). Coping strategies and phobias: The relationship between fears, phobias and methods of coping with stressors. *British Journal of Clinical Psychology, 34*(Pt 3), 423-434.

Derogatis, L. R., & Spencer, P. M. (1982). *BSI: Administration and procedures. Manual I.* Baltimore: Clinical Psychometric Research.

Dodds, P. (1993). Access to the coping strategies: Managing anxiety in elective surgical patients. *Professional Nurse, 9*(1), 45-52.

Ebersole, P., & Hess, P. (1998). *Toward healthy aging: Human needs and nursing response* (5th ed.). St. Louis, MO: Mosby.

Elliot, D. (1993). Comparison of three instruments for measuring patient anxiety in a coronary care unit. *Intensive & Critical Care Nursing, 9*(3), 195-200.

Evans, C. L. S., Kassof, M., Beckham, E., & Handel-Kindred, J. (1990). Reducing AIDS anxiety on the unit with preventive infection control. *Journal of Psychosocial Nursing, 28*(1), 36-39.

Eyde, D. R., & Rich, J. A. (1983). *Psychological distress in aging.* Rockville, MD: Aspen.

Fadden, T., Fehring, R., & Rossi, E. K. (1987). Validation studies: Paper presentations. In A. M. McLane (Eds.), *Classification of nursing diagnoses: Proceedings of the seventh conference* (pp. 113-120). St. Louis, MO: Mosby.

Fehring, R. J. (1986). Validating diagnostic labels: Standardized methodology. In M. E. Hurley (Ed.), *Classification of nursing diagnoses: Proceedings of the sixth conference* (pp. 183-190). St. Louis, MO: Mosby.

Fehring, R. J. (1987). Methods to validate nursing diagnoses. *Heart & Lung, 16*(6), 625-629.

Fehring, R. J. (1994). The Fehring model. In R. M. Carroll-Johnson & M. P. Paquette (Eds.), *Classification of nursing diagnoses: Proceedings of the tenth conference* (pp. 55-62). Baltimore: Lippincott Williams & Wilkins.

Fernandez, F., Levy, J. K., Lachar, B., & Small, G. W. (1995). The management of depression and anxiety in the elderly. *Journal of Clinical Psychiatry, 56*(Suppl 2), 20-29.

Ferrell-Torry, A. T., & Glick, O. J. (1993). The use of therapeutic massage to modify anxiety and the perception of cancer pain. *Cancer Nursing, 16*(2), 93-101.

Foxwell, M., & Alder, E. (1993). More information equates with less anxiety: Reducing anxiety in cervical screening. *Professional Nurse, 9*(1), 32-36.

Franulic, A., Gonzalez, X., Trucco, M., & Vallejos, F. (1996). Emotional and psychosocial factors in burn patients during hospitalization. *Burns, 22*(8), 618-622.

Fraser, J., & Ross-Kerr, J. (1993). Psychophysiological effects of back massage on elderly institutionalized patients. *Journal of Advanced Nursing, 18*(2), 238-245.

Friedman, S. B., Badere, B., & Fitzpatrick, S. (1992). The effect of television viewing on preoperative anxiety. *Journal of Post Anesthesia Nursing, 7*(4), 243-250.

Gaberson, K. (1991). The effect of humorous distraction on preoperative anxiety: A pilot study. *AORN Journal, 54*(6), 1258-1263.

Gebbie, K. M., & Lavin, M. E. (1995). *Classification of nursing diagnoses: Proceedings of the first national conference.* St. Louis, MO: Mosby.

Giese, H., & Schomer, H. (1986). Life-style changer and mood profile of cardiac patients after an exercise rehabilitation program. *Journal of Cardiopulmonary Rehabilitation, 6*, 30-37.

Gift, A. G., Moore, T., & Soeken, K. (1992). Relaxation to reduce dyspnea and anxiety in COPD patients. *Nursing Research, 41*(4), 242-246.

Gomez, G. E., & Gomez, E. A. (1994). The use of psychotropic drugs to treat the elderly. *Journal of Psychosocial Nursing & Mental Health Services, 32*(12), 30-34.

Gordon, M. (1982). *Manual of nursing diagnosis.* New York: McGraw-Hill.

Gram, I. T., & Slenker, S. E. (1992). Cancer anxiety and attitudes toward mammography among screening attenders, nonattenders, and women never invited. *American Journal of Public Health, 82*(2), 249-251.

Halm, M. A. (1990). Effects of support groups on anxiety of family members during critical illness. *Heart & Lung, 19*(1), 62-71.

Heath, A. H. (1992). Imagery: Helping ICU patients control pain and anxiety. *Dimensions of Critical Care, 11*(1), 57-62.

Heidrich, S. M. (1993). The relationship between physical health and psychological well-being in elderly women: A developmental perspective. *Research in Nursing and Health, 16*, 123-130.

Heidt, P. (1981). Effect of therapeutic touch on anxiety level of hospitalized patients. *Nursing Research, 30*(1), 32-37.

Henry, L. L. (1995). Music therapy: A nursing intervention for the control of pain and anxiety in the ICU: A review of the literature. *Dimensions of Critical Care Nursing, 14*(6), 295-304.

Higginson, I., & Priest, P. (1996). Predictors of family anxiety in the weeks before bereavement. *Social Science & Medicine, 43*(11), 1621-1625.

Hocking, L. B., & Koenig, H. G. (1995). Anxiety in medically ill older patients: A review and update. *International Journal of Psychiatry in Medicine, 25*(3), 221-238.

Hurt, G. J., McQuellon, R. P., & Barrett, R. J. (1994). After treatment ends: Neutral time. *Cancer Practice, 2*(6), 417-420.

Hyman, S. E., & Cassem, N. H. (1989). Managing the person with psychiatric illness. In E. Rubenstein & D. D. Federmann (Eds.), *Science American Medicine, 13*, 1-18.

Iowa Intervention Project. (2000). In J. C. McCloskey & G. M. Bulechek (Eds.). *Nursing interventions classification (NIC)* (3rd ed.). St. Louis, MO: Mosby.

Iowa Outcomes Project. (2000). In M. Johnson, M. Maas, & S. Moorhead (Eds.). *Nursing outcomes classification (NOC)* (2nd ed.). St. Louis, MO: Mosby.

Jackson, D. N. (1977). Reliability of the Jackson Personality Research Inventory. *Psychological Reports, 40*, 613-614.

Jackson, D. N. (1979). *Jackson Personality Inventory Manual.* Goshen, NY: Research Psychologists Press.

Jeffords, C. R. (1983). The situational relationship between age and fear of crime. *International Journal of Aging & Human Development, 17*, 103-111.

Johnson, M. J., & Frank, D. I. (1995). Effectiveness of a telephone intervention in reducing anxiety in families of patients in an intensive care unit. *Applied Nursing Research, 8*(1), 42-43.

Jones, P., & Jacob, D. F. (1981). Nursing diagnosis: Differentiating fear and anxiety. *Nursing Papers, 13*(4), 20-29.

Kaempf, G., & Amodei, M. E. (1989). The effect of music on anxiety. *AORN Journal, 50*(1), 112-118.

Kellner, R. (1987). *Manual of the Symptom Questionnaire.* Albuquerque, NM: University of New Mexico.

Kennedy, L. W., & Silverman, R. A. (1985). Significant others and fear of crime among the elderly. *International Journal of Aging & Human Development, 20,* 241-256.

Kim, M. J., Amoroso-Seritella, R., Gulanick, M., Moyer, K., Parsons, E., Scherbel, J., Stafford, M. J., Suhayda, R., & Yocum, C. (1984). Clinical validation of cardiovascular nursing diagnoses. *Classification of nursing diagnoses: Proceedings of the fifth national conference* (pp. 128-138). St. Louis, MO: Mosby.

Kim, M. J., McFarland, G. K., & McLane, A. M. (1997). *Pocket guide to nursing diagnoses* (7th ed.). St. Louis, MO: Mosby.

Kim, M. J., & Moritz, D. A. (1982). *Classification of nursing diagnoses: Proceedings of the third and fourth conference.* New York: McGraw-Hill.

Kim, M. J., Seritella, R. A., & Gulanick, M. (1984). Clinical validation of cardiovascular nursing diagnoses. In M. J. Kim, G. K. McFarland, & A. M. McLane (Eds.), *Classification of nursing diagnoses: Proceedings of the fifth national conference.* St. Louis, MO: Mosby.

Kinney, M., & Guzetta, C. (1989). Testing a measuring technique to study nursing diagnoses. In R. M. Carroll-Johnson (Ed.), *Classification of nursing diagnoses: Proceedings of the eighth national conference* (pp. 419-420). Baltimore: Lippincott Williams & Wilkins.

Kranzier, H. R. (1996). Evaluation and treatment of anxiety symptoms and disorders in alcoholics. *Journal of Clinical Psychiatry, 57*(Suppl 7), 15-21, discussion 22-24.

Kuzel, R. J. (1996). Treating comorbid depression and anxiety. *Journal of Family Practice, 43*(6 Suppl), 45-53.

Lampic, C., von Essen, L., Peterson, V. W., Larsson, G., & Sjoden, P. O. (1996). Anxiety and depression in hospitalized patients with cancer: Agreement in patient-staff dyads. *Cancer Nursing, 19*(6), 419-428.

Lasher, K. P., & Faulkender, P. J. (1993). Measurement of aging anxiety: Development of the Anxiety about Aging Scale. *International Journal of Aging & Human Development, 37*(4), 247-259.

Lebowitz, B. D. (1975). Age and fearfulness: Personal and situational factors. *Journal of Gerontology, 30,* 696-700.

Leske, J. S. (1996). Intraoperative progress reports decrease family member's anxiety. *AORN Journal, 64*(3), 424-425, 428-436.

Lidren, D. M., Watkins, P. L., Gould, R. A., Clum, G. A., Asterio, M., & Tulloch, H. L. (1994). A comparison of bibliotherapy and group therapy in the treatment of panic disorder. *Journal of Consulting & Clinical Psychology, 62*(4), 865-869.

Liebowitz, M. R. (1993). Mixed anxiety and depression: Should it be included in DSM-IV? *Journal of Clinical Psychiatry, 54*(Suppl), 4-7, 17-20.

Lopez, A., & Risey, B. (1988). *Anxiety: Validation of a nursing diagnosis.* Unpublished manuscript, Louisiana University Medical Center, New Orleans, LA.

Ludwick-Rosenthal, R., & Neufeld, R. W. (1993). Preparation for undergoing an invasive medical procedure: Interacting effects of information and coping style. *Journal of Consulting & Clinical Psychology, 61*(1), 156-164.

Lydiard, R. B., Brawman-Mintzer, O., & Ballenger, J. C. (1996). Recent developments in the psychopharmacology of anxiety disorder. *Journal of Consulting & Clinical Psychology, 64*(4), 660-668.

MacEwen, K. E., Barling, J., Kelloway, E. K., & Higginbottom, S. F. (1995). Predicting retirement anxiety: The roles of parental

socialization and personal planning. *Journal of Social Psychology, 135*(2), 203-213.

Mandle, C. L., Jacobs, S. C., Arcari, P. M., & Domar, A. D. (1996). The efficacy of relaxation response interventions with adult patients: A review of the literature. *Journal of Cardiovascular Nursing, 10*(3), 4-26.

Markland, D., & Hardy, L. (1993). Anxiety, relaxation and anesthesia for day-case surgery. *British Journal of Clinical Psychology, 32*(Part 4), 493-504.

Markovitz, P. J. (1993). Treatment of anxiety in the elderly. *Journal of Clinical Psychiatry, 54*(Suppl), 64-68.

Marks, I. M., & Mathews, A. M. (1979). Brief standard self-rating for phobic patients. *Behavioral Research Therapy, 17,* 263-267.

Marrs, R. W. (1995). A meta-analysis of bibliotherapy studies. *American Journal of Community Psychology, 23*(6), 843-870.

Martin, L. M., Flemming, K. C., & Evans, J. M. (1995). Recognition and management of anxiety and depression in elderly patients. *Mayo Clinic Proceedings, 70*(10), 999-1006.

McCracken, L. M., & Gross, R. T. (1993). Does anxiety affect coping with pain? *Clinical Journal of Pain, 9*(4), 253-259.

McCracken, L. M., Gross, R. T., Aikens, J., & Carnrike, C. L., Jr. (1996). The assessment of anxiety and fear in persons with chronic pain: A comparison of instruments. *Behaviour Research & Therapy, 34*(11-12), 927-933.

McFarland, G. K., & McFarlane, E. A. (1997). *Nursing diagnosis & intervention* (3rd ed.). St. Louis, MO: Mosby.

McNair, D., Lorr, M., & Droppleman, L. (1971). *Educational and industrial testing service manual of the profile of mood states.* San Diego, CA: Educational and Testing Service.

McNeil, D. W., Rainwater, A. J., & Aljazireh, L. (1986). *Development of a methodology to measure fear of pain.* Paper presented at the annual meeting of the Association of Advancement of Behavior Therapy, Chicago.

Metzger, K. L., & Hiltunen, E. F. (1987). Diagnostic validation of 10 frequently reported nursing diagnoses. In A. M. McLane (Ed.), *Classification of nursing diagnoses: Proceedings of the seventh conference* (pp. 144-53). St. Louis, MO: Mosby.

Mintz, M. C., van Horn, K. R., & Levine, M. J. (1996). Developmental models of social cognition in assessing the role of family stress in relatives' predictions following brain injury. *Brain Injury, 9*(2), 173-186.

Moss, V. A. (1987). The effect of music on anxiety in the surgical patient. *Perioperative Nursing Quarterly, 3*(3), 9-12.

Mynchenberg, T. L., & Dungan, J. M. (1995). A relaxation protocol to reduce patient anxiety. *Dimensions of Critical Care Nursing, 14*(2), 78-85.

Negron, J. A. (1995). The impact of computer anxiety and computer resistance on the use of computer technology by nurses. *Journal of Nursing Staff Development, 11*(3), 172-175.

Neundorfer, M. M. (1991). Coping and health outcomes in spouse caregivers of persons with dementia. *Nursing Research, 40*(6), 260-265.

Nolan, T. F. (1984). Thanatological counseling of adults and their families. In S. Lego (Ed.), *The American handbook of psychiatric nursing.* Baltimore: Lippincott Williams & Wilkins.

North American Nursing Diagnosis Association. (1994). *Nursing diagnoses: Definitions and classification 1995-1996.* Philadelphia: Author.

North American Nursing Diagnosis Association. (1999). *Nursing diagnoses: Definitions & classification 1999-2000.* Philadelphia: Author.

Norton, L., & Courlander, M. (1982). Fear of crime among the elderly: The role of crime prevention programs. *The Gerontologist, 22,* 388-393.

Nugent, L. S., Tamlyn-Leaman, K., Isa, N., Reardon, E., & Crumley, J. (1993). Anxiety and the colposcopy experience. *Clinical Nursing Research, 2*(3), 267-277.

O'Connell, M. (1989). Anxiety reduction in family members of patients in surgery and postanesthesia care: A pilot study. *Journal of Post Anesthesia Nursing, 4*(1), 7-16.

Okun, A., Stein, R. E., Bauman, L. J., & Silver, E. J. (1996). Content validity of the Psychiatric Symptom Index, CES-Depression Scale, and State-Trait Anxiety Inventory from the perspective of DSM-IV. *Psychological Reports, 79*(3 Pt 1), 1059-1069.

Oldridge, N., Streiner D., Hoffmann, R., & Guyatt, G. (1995). Profile of moods states and cardiac rehabilitation after acute myocardial infarction. *Medicine & Science in Sports & Exercise, 27*(6), 900-905.

Olson, M., & Sneed, N. (1995). Anxiety and therapeutic touch. *Issues in Mental Health Nursing, 16*(2), 97-108.

Olson, M., Sneed, N., Bondonna, R., Ratliff, J., & Dias, J. (1992). Therapeutic touch and post-Hurricane Hugo stress. *Journal of Holistic Nursing, 10*(2), 120-136.

Osman, A., Barrios, F. X., Aukes, D., & Osman, J. R. (1995). Psychometric evaluation of the Social Phobia and Anxiety Inventory in college students. *Journal of Clinical Psychology, 51*(2), 235-243.

Osman, A., Barrios, F. X., Osman, J. R., & Markway, K. (1993). Further psychometric of the Fear Questionnaire: Responses of college students. *Psychological Reports, 73*(3 Pt 2), 1259-1266.

Palakanis, K. C., DeNobile, J. W., Sweeney, W. B., & Blankenship, C. L. (1994). Effect of music therapy on state anxiety in patients undergoing flexible sigmoidoscopy. *Diseases of the Colon & Rectum, 37*(5), 478-481.

Peterson, M. (1991). Patient anxiety before cardiac catheterization: An intervention study. *Heart & Lung, 20*(6), 643-647.

Pollack, L. M., & Patterson, A. H. (1980). Territoriality and fear of crime in elderly and nonelderly homeowners. *Journal of Social Psychology, 111,* 119-129.

Potinkara, H., & Paunonen, M. (1996). Alleviating anxiety in nursing patients' significant others. *Intensive & Critical Care Nursing, 12*(6), 327-334.

Rachman, S. (1994). The overprediction of fear: A review. *Behavior Research & Therapy, 32*(7), 683-690.

Rankin, E. J., Gfeller, J. D., & Gilner, F. H. (1993). Measuring anxiety states in the elderly using the State-Trait Anxiety Inventory for Children. *Journal of Psychiatric Research, 37*(1), 111-117.

Renfroe, K. L. (1988). Effect of progressive relaxation on dyspnea and anxiety in patients with chronic obstructive pulmonary disease. *Heart & Lung, 17,* 408-413.

Rickard, H. C., Scogin, F., & Keith, S. (1994). A one year follow-up of relaxation training for elders with subjective anxiety. *The Gerontologist, 34*(1), 121-122.

Robinson, L. (1990). Stress and anxiety. *Nursing Clinics of North America, 25*(4), 935-943.

Rose, S. K., Conn, V. S., & Rodeman, B. J. (1994). Anxiety and self-care following myocardial infarction. *Issues in Mental Health Nursing, 15*(4), 433-444.

Roth, N. (1978). Fear of death in the aging. *American Journal of Psychotherapy, 32,* 552-560.

Rukholm, E., Bailey, P., Coutu-Wakulczyk, G., & Bailey, W. B. (1991). Needs and anxiety levels in relatives of intensive care unit patients. *Journal of Advanced Nursing, 16,* 920-928.

Salmon, P. (1993). The reduction of anxiety in surgical patients: An important nursing task or the medicalization of preparatory worry. *International Journal of Nursing Studies, 30*(4), 323-330.

Schweizer, E., & Rickels, K. (1996). The long term management of generalized anxiety disorders: Issues and dilemmas. *Journal of Clinical Psychiatry, 57*(Suppl 7), 9-12.

Shafer, A., Fish, M. P., Gregg, K. M., Seavello, J., & Kosek, P. (1996). Preoperative anxiety and fear: A comparison of assessments by patients and anesthesia and surgery residents. *Anesthesia & Analgesia, 83*(6), 1285-1291.

Shear, M. K. (1995). Psychotherapeutic issues in long term treatment of anxiety disorder patients. *Psychiatric Clinics of North America, 18*(4), 885-894.

Sheikh, J. I., & Salzman, C. (1995). Anxiety in the elderly: Course and treatment. *Psychiatric Clinics of North America, 18*(4), 871-883.

Shuldham, C. M., Cunningham, G., Hiscock, M., & Luscombe, P. (1995). Assessment of anxiety in hospital patients. *Journal of Advanced Nursing, 22*(1), 87-93.

Silva, M. (1979). Effects of orientation information on spouses' anxieties and attitudes towards hospitalization and surgery. *Research in Nursing & Health, 2,* 127-136.

Silverstone, P. H. (1994). Poor efficacy of the Hospital Anxiety and Depression Scale in the diagnosis of major depressive disorder in both medical and psychiatric patients. *Journal of Psychosomatic Research, 38*(5), 441-450.

Simington, J. A., & Laing, G. P. (1993). Effects of therapeutic touch on anxiety in the institutionalized elderly. *Clinical Nursing Research, 2*(4), 438-450.

Smith, S. L., Colenda, C. C., & Espeland, M. A. (1994). Factors determining the level of anxiety in geriatric primary care patients in a community dwelling. *Psychosomatics, 35*(1), 50-58.

Smith, S. L., Sherrill, K. A., & Colenda, C. C. (1995). Assessing and treating anxiety in elderly persons. *Psychiatric Services, 46,* 36-42.

Snelling, J. (1994). The effect of chronic pain on the family unit. *Journal of Advanced Nursing, 19*(3), 543-551.

Snowdon, J. (1993). Mental health in nursing homes: Perspectives on the use of medications. *Drugs & Aging, 3*(2), 122-130.

Spencer, M. G., & Dorr, C. J. (1975). *Understanding aging: A multidisciplinary approach.* Norwalk, CT: Appleton & Lange.

Spielberger, C. D. (1975). Stress and anxiety. In I. G. Garason & C. D. Spielberger (Eds.), *Stress and anxiety.* Philadelphia: Hemisphere.

Spielberger, C. D., Gorsuch, R. L., Lushene, P., Vagg, P. R., & Jacobs, G. A. (1983). *Manual for the State-Trait Anxiety Inventory.* Palo Alto, CA: Consulting Psychologists, Press.

Standley, J. M. (1986). Music research in medical/dental treatment: Meta-analysis and clinical applications. *Journal of Music Therapy, 23,* 55-122.

Stanley, M. A., Beck, J. G., & Zebb, B. J. (1996). Psychometric properties of four anxiety measures in older adults. *Behavior Research & Therapy, 34*(10), 827-838.

Steelman, V. M. (1990). Intraoperative music therapy: Effects on anxiety, blood pressure. *AORN Journal, 52*(5), 1026-1034.

Steinberg, J. R. (1994). Anxiety in elderly patients: A comparison of azapirones and benzodiazepines. *Drugs & Aging, 5*(5), 335-345.

Stravynski, A., Basoglu, M., Marks, M., Sengun, S., & Marks, I. M. (1995). Social sensitivity: A shared feature of all phobias. *British Journal of Clinical Psychology, 34*(Pt 3), 343-351.

Stuart, G. W. (1995). Anxiety responses & anxiety disorders. In G. W. Stuart & S. J. Sundeen (Eds.), *Principles & practices of psychiatric nursing* (5th ed., pp. 327-353). St. Louis, MO: Mosby.

Summers, S., Hoffman, J., Neff, J. A., Hanson, S., & Pierce, K. (1990). The effects of 60 beats per minute music on test taking anxiety among nursing students. *Journal of Nursing Education, 29*(2), 66-70.

Sundeen, R. A., & Mathieu, J. T. (1976). The fear of crime and its consequences among the elderly in three urban communities. *The Gerontologist, 16*, 211-291.

Szymanski, J., & O'Donohue, W. (1995). Fear of spiders questionnaire. *Journal of Behavior Therapy & Experimental Psychiatry, 26*(1), 31-34.

Taylor, S. (1993). The structure of fundamental fears. *Journal of Behavioral Therapy and Experimental Psychiatry, 24*(4), 289-299.

Taylor-Loughran, S. (1989). Defining characteristics of the nursing diagnoses fear and anxiety: A validation study. *Applied Nursing Research, 2*(4), 178-186.

Teasdale, K. (1993). Information and anxiety: A critical reappraisal. *Journal of Advanced Nursing, 18*, 1125-1132.

Teri, L., & Lewinsohn, P. M. (1986). *Geropsychological assessment and treatment.* New York: Springer.

Theriault, J. (1994). Retirement as a psychosocial transition: Process of adaptation and change. *International Journal of Aging & Human Development, 38*(2), 153-170.

Thompson, M. B., & Coppens, N. M. (1994). The effects of guided imagery on anxiety levels and movement of clients undergoing magnetic resonance imaging. *Holistic Nursing Practice, 8*(2), 59-69.

Trimpey, M. L. (1989). Self-esteem and anxiety: Key issues in an abused women's support group. *Issues in Mental Health Nursing, 10*, 297-308.

Tueth, M. J. (1993). Anxiety in the older patient: Differential diagnosis and treatment. *Geriatrics, 48*(2), 51-54.

Turner, S. M., Beidel, C., Dancu, V., & Stanley, M. A. (1989). An empirically derived inventory to measure social fears and anxiety: The social phobia and anxiety inventory. *Psychological assessment. Journal of Consulting and Clinical Psychology, 1*(1), 35-40.

Vogel, C. H. (1991). Anxiety. In M. Mass, K. Buckwalter & M. Hardy (Eds.), *Nursing diagnoses and interventions for the elderly* (pp. 469-479). Reading, MA: Addison Wesley Longman.

Wake, M. M., Fehring, R. J., & Fadden, T. C. (1994). Multinational diagnostic content validation of anxiety, hopelessness, and ineffective airway clearance. *Classification of nursing diagnoses: Proceedings of the tenth conference.* Baltimore: Lippincott Williams & Wilkins.

Wald, M. F. (1991). Pain anxiety and powerlessness. *Journal of Advanced Nursing, 16*, 388-397.

Wass, H., & Myers, J. E. (1982). Psychosocial aspects of death among the elderly: A review of the literature. *Personnel Guidance Journal, 61*, 131-137.

Webb, M. S., & Riggin, O. Z. (1994). A comparison of anxiety levels of female and male patients with myocardial infarction. *Critical Care Nurse, 14*(1), 118-124.

Weber, S. (1996). The effects of exercises on anxiety levels in psychiatric inpatients. *Journal of Holistic Nursing, 14*(3), 196-205.

Weiss, K. J. (1994). Management of anxiety and depression syndromes in the elderly. *Journal of Clinical Psychiatry, 55*(Suppl 5), 5-12.

Weiss, K. J. (1996). Optimal management of anxiety in older patients. *Drugs & Aging, 9*(3), 191-201.

Weissman, M. M. (1988a). Anxiety and alcoholism. *Journal of Clinical Psychiatry, 49*(Suppl 10), 17-19.

Weissman, M. M. (1988b). The epidemiology of anxiety disorders: Rates, risks, and familial patterns. *Journal of Psychiatric Research, 22*(Suppl 1), 99-114.

Weller, A., & Hener, T. (1993). Invasiveness of medical procedures and state anxiety in women. *Behavioral Medicine, 19*(2), 60-65.

Whitley, G. G. (1986). *Validation of the nursing diagnosis anxiety: A nurse consensus survey.* Unpublished doctoral dissertation, Northern Illinois University, DeKalb, IL.

Whitley, G. G. (1989). Anxiety: Defining the diagnosis. *Journal of Psychosocial Nursing, 27*(10), 7-12.

Whitley, G. G. (1992a). Concept analysis of anxiety. *Nursing Diagnosis, 3*(3), 107-116.

Whitley, G. G. (1992b). Concept analysis of fear. *Nursing Diagnosis, 3*(4), 155-161.

Whitley, G. G. (1994). Expert validation and differentiation of the nursing diagnoses anxiety and fear. *Nursing Diagnosis, 5*(4), 143-150.

Williams, J. C. (1976). Allaying common fears. In P. S. Chaney (Ed.), *Dealing with death and dying.* Jenkintown, PA: Nursing Skillbook. Intermed Communications.

Winter, M. J., Paskin, S., & Baker, T. (1994). Music reduces stress and anxiety in the surgical holding area. *Journal of Post Anesthesia Nursing, 9*(6), 340-343.

Wolpe, J. (1983). *The practice of behavior therapy* (3rd ed.). New York: Pergamon Press.

Wolpe, J., & Lang, P. J. (1964). A fear survey schedule for use in behavior therapy. *Behavior, Research & Therapy, 2*, 27-30.

Yocum, C. J. (1984). The differentiation of fear and anxiety. In M. J. Kim, G. K. McFarland, & A. M. McLane (Eds.), *Classification of nursing diagnoses: Proceedings of the 5th national conference* (pp. 352-355). St. Louis, MO: Mosby.

Young, L. (1986). *A validation study of the nursing diagnosis anxiety in hospital patients.* Unpublished master's thesis. Marquette University, Milwaukee, WI.

Zigmond, A. S., & Snaith, R. P. (1983). The hospital anxiety and depression scale. *Acta Psychiatrica Scandinavica, 67*(6), 361-370.

Zisook, S., Schneider, D., & Schuchter, S. R. (1990). Anxiety and bereavement. *Psychiatric Medicine, 8*(2), 83-95.

Zlotogorski, Z., Tadmor, O., Duniec, E., Rabinowitz, R., & Diamant, Y. (1995). Anxiety levels of pregnant women during ultrasound examination: Coping styles, amount of feedback and learned resourcefulness. *Ultrasound in Obstetrics & Gynecology, 6*(6), 425-429.

CHAPTER 45

SELF-ESTEEM DISTURBANCE

Carla J. Groh and Ann L. Whall

Self-esteem refers primarily to the self-worth individuals place on themselves. Self-esteem is a dynamic process of interaction between the individual and the environment (George, 1990). It is an individual's self-evaluation that expresses an attitude of approval or disapproval and indicates the extent to which the individual believes himself to be capable, significant, successful, and worthy (Coopersmith, 1967). A person's self-esteem is thought to be multidimensional (Binsock & George, 1990; Rosenberg, 1979) and related to life satisfaction (Coopersmith, 1967). Recent nursing literature postulates that self-esteem is one of many components of the self and is derived from the array of cognitions included in self-concept (Stein, 1995). Self-esteem is hard to isolate and identify (Brandon, 1969), but it affects thinking processes, desires, values, and goals and is the single most significant factor in behavior. The centrality of self-esteem in maintaining physical and psychosocial well-being is widely recognized in nursing. Despite its importance, self-esteem is remarkably neglected in nursing research and often overlooked in clinical practice (Stein, 1995).

The degree to which self-esteem changes with age remains uncertain (George & Bearon, 1980). In an extensive review of the literature on stability and change in self-perceptions during later life, Bengston, Reedy, and Gordon (1985) found documentation supporting both perspectives. Rosenberg (1979) argued that individuals have a tendency to maintain pre-existing self-conceptions even in the face of threatening evidence. More current research has supported his argument. Research findings of Baltes and Schmid (1987), McCrae and Costa (1988), and Kaufman (1986) found that self-concept, personality traits, and self-esteem change remarkably little with advanced age.

It also has been proposed that the older person's sense of self-worth might actually increase as greater self-acceptance develops. A study conducted by Gove, Ortega, and Briggs Style (1989) found support for this "maturational effect" on self-esteem in a probability sample of adults in the contiguous United States. The investigators concluded that self-esteem increases somewhat with age, more strongly for males than females. Other social scientists, however, have argued that self-conceptions are expected to be responsive to changes in the social environment and that self-esteem might be a more situationally

reactive phenomenon than a direct result of aging (Goldberg & Fitzpatrick, 1980). Research will need to use consistent definitions and gather longitudinal and sequential data to investigate whether self-esteem changes or is stable during the later years of life (Bunten, 1997).

Research has indicated that self-esteem is a key coping resource and an important correlate of psychologic well-being in later life (Dietz, 1996; Krause, 1987, 1999). Coopersmith (1967) found that persons with high self-esteem are generally happier, more independent, more self-confident, less anxious, and more effective in meeting environmental demands than those with low self-esteem. Persons with high self-esteem do not pretend to be perfect, they recognize their limitations, and they expect to grow and improve (Frey & Carolock, 1989). Persons with low self-esteem are likely to be alienated and to feel incapable of controlling their lives. Low self-esteem can make a person prone to illness, whereas high self-esteem might contribute to the prevention of illness. It is important, therefore, that nurses understand self-esteem and be able to identify the factors that facilitate and maintain positive self-esteem in older adults from diverse cultural and ethnic backgrounds.

Maintenance and/or restoration of self-esteem in older adults is a significant social and health care issue. The U.S. Bureau of the Census (Day, 1992) predicts a "gerontologic explosion" as the baby boom generation reaches old age. The Bureau projects that there will be more than 70 million people older than age 65 by 2030. Although the great majority of older adults negotiate late life changes with grace, good humor, and equanimity, gerontologists suggest that older adults are at high risk for self-esteem disturbance due to age-related events and stresses experienced in late life (Binstock & George, 1990; Silverstone, 1996; Taft, 1985).

RELATED FACTORS/ETIOLOGIES

Several research studies have investigated the relationship between either physical health, mental health, or perception of well-being and self-esteem. Studies have shown that hearing loss has a significant effect on self-esteem (Chen, 1994; Loeb & Sarigiani, 1986; Yachnik, 1986) as well as on loneliness (Chen, 1994). Other studies have shown that poor health, regardless of age, is associated with more depression and anxiety and lower levels of positive relationships and autonomy (Heidrich, 1993). In a subsequent study, Heidrich (1994) found that worse physical health was related to higher levels of depression and that depression was a significant predictor of self-concept. Worse physical health, however, was not a direct predictor of self-concept.

In a related study, Parent and Whall (1984) investigated the relationship between physical activity, self-esteem, and depression. They found a strong relationship between certain physical activities and self-esteem. The physical activities that were most significant and had the greatest impact on the older adult's self-esteem were those activities that involved social interaction and contact with others.

Other studies have investigated the relationship between either social support, religiosity, or social roles and self-esteem. The research findings related to social support and self-esteem are inconclusive. Two studies of community-dwelling older adults found a strong correlation between social support and self-esteem. Frazier (1982), in a study of 126 community-dwelling older adults, found that perceived social support was positively correlated with depression and self-esteem: participants who perceived greater support were less depressed and had higher self-esteem than those who did not. Although Heidrich (1994) did not examine the concept of social support per se, the results of her study found that positive relations with others and a sense of purpose in life were the strongest predictors of self-concept. In contrast, Nelson (1989), in a sample of 26 institutionalized elderly individuals, found only a moderate correlation between social support and self-esteem that did not reach statistical significance. It may be that social support is not sufficient to mitigate the effects of institutionalization on feelings of self-worth and self-capability.

Only a few studies have investigated the relationship between self-esteem and religiosity. Krause (1995), in a sample of 1005 community-dwelling adults 65 years of age or older, found that religiosity was related to feelings of self-worth. More specifically, self-esteem was highest among older adults who exhibited either the least or the most religious involvement. Nelson (1989) found similar results. Although she did not examine the relationship between self-esteem and religiosity per se, Nelson did find that religious participation was significantly correlated with depression, in that subjects who frequently participated in some type of religious activity were less depressed than those who did not. If the inverse relationship between self-esteem and depression holds true, then one could postulate that those subjects who frequently participated in religious activities were less depressed and had higher self-esteem than those who did not.

The relationship between self-esteem and salient life roles is a recent area of inquiry. Theorists have proposed that stressors arising in highly valued roles exert a more noxious effect on health and well-being than events emerging in roles that are less important to older adults (Burke, 1991; Thoits, 1991). Thoits (1995) speculated that some older adults try to cope with salient role stressors by devaluing the importance of the role in which the life event emerged. However, the notion that people try to confront stressors by devaluing the importance of that role has not been empirically tested (Krause, 1999), nor is this devaluation theory endorsed by others.

In a recent study by Krause (1999) the role of self-esteem was examined as a potentially important variable in how older adults cope with stress in social roles they value highly. A nationally representative sample of older adults was interviewed at two points in time: 1992-1993 and 1996-1997. Completed data were compiled for 589 older adults. Global feelings of self-worth were measured with three indicators taken from the scale developed by Rosenberg (1979). The reliability of this brief composite was 0.749. The mean score for this brief composite was 14.061 (SD = 1.5; range = 4 to 15). The results suggested that a strong sense of role-specific self-esteem is associated with a lower probability of role devaluation, regardless of the amount of stress present. Thus feelings of self-worth associated with a particular role influence whether that role is devalued over time (Krause, 1999). Krause concluded that it is not sufficient merely to obtain an inventory of all the roles occupied by an older adult, but that we also must assess feelings of self-worth associated with each role.

The relationship between self-esteem and depression merits special consideration. Many of the studies cited in this chapter investigated the relationship between self-esteem and depression, in addition to the other variables already discussed. All of the studies found a strong and significant negative relationship between these two variables: as depression increased, self-esteem decreased. Indeed, depression is the variable most strongly correlated with self-esteem in older Euro-American adults (Heidrich, 1993, 1994; Nelson, 1989; Parent & Whall, 1984). This is especially relevant, since high rates of depression are correlated with physical disability. Yet older adults are not prevalent users of mental health and rehabilitation services (Silverstone, 1996). Thus depression often goes untreated and can result in lower self-esteem. However, most of the research that supports the statistically significant negative relationship between depression and self-esteem has focused predominantly on middle-class Euro-Americans and lower socioeconomic African American women. Findings of research with middle-class African American women have not supported the relationship between self-esteem and depression. Both Stokes (1999) and Warren (1997) suggested that the Rosenberg Self-Esteem Scale might not be a valid measure of self-esteem in middle-class African American women. Furthermore, Warren (1997), citing past research on self-esteem in African Americans, suggested that these individuals do not universally have low self-esteem when comparisons are made between their peers and not other groups. Thus future research should continue to examine the variable of self-esteem in the development of depression in different classes of African Americans (Warren, 1997) as well as in other ethnic and cultural groups.

RISK FACTORS

Gerontologic research has identified several risk factors for self-esteem disturbances in older adults. Institutionalization, which becomes more likely the longer a person lives, can increase the risk for self-esteem disturbances. High self-esteem or the continued belief in self-adequacy and capability is counterproductive to life in many institutional settings, where not speaking out and conforming are valued. Feelings of worthiness can be shattered as people are infantilized by such phrases as "my baby" or "be a good girl." For the older adult, adjustment to institutionalization is related to loss of one's rights, initiatives, feelings, wishes, and desires. In these situations the patient is "adjusted" when many of the features of low self-esteem are manifested. Thus institutionalization can be counterproductive to high levels of self-esteem, even if the institutional objectives and philosophy indicate otherwise. In addition, a major depressive disorder is diagnosed in 12% of persons in institutions providing long-term or short-term care. Moreover, 23% to 31% of persons living in these settings have significant depressive symptoms even though they do not meet the criteria for a major depressive disorder as identified in the fourth edition of the *Diagnostic and Statistical Manual of Mental Disorders (DSM-IV)* (Alexopoulos, 1995).

Gender can be a risk factor for self-esteem disturbances. The majority of the aging population are women. Older women experience a myriad of health problems and social issues that can result in low self-esteem. Women have greater morbidity due to chronic conditions (e.g., arthritis, osteoporosis, heart disease, diabetes, cancer and its sequelae, incontinence, and depression) and more limitations in self-care than do men (Dimond, 1996). Threats to self-competence can cause individuals to view themselves as useless and unable to change or control their life situations. The result can be loss of self-esteem and feelings of inferiority. Growing older in a society that has few respected roles for older women can bring a multiplicity of stressful experiences: sexism, ageism, loss of work and social roles, loss of support systems, and the death of a spouse, siblings, and/or parents. Furthermore, great proportions of older women live in poverty. Minkler and Stone (1985) observed that to be old, poor, and female is to experience "triple jeopardy." The consequences of "triple jeopardy" are further heightened by ethnicity. Hispanic and African American women are at particularly high risk of living in poverty and poor health as they age (Dimond, 1993).

ASSESSMENT

Gerontologic research investigating the relationship between self-esteem and aging have identified many of the above as risk factors for self-esteem disturbances in older adults. Roy's (1976, 1984) adaptation model views humans as biopsychosocial beings. The person is in constant interaction with a changing environment, confronting physical, social, and psychologic changes. Roy's model offers nursing a framework on which to base the assessment of older adults' capabilities and abilities to adapt to the numerous changes that confront them. Roy postulated that a person learns or acquires mechanisms that are used to cope with impinging environmental changes. Responding positively to these changes requires adaptation and brings about health. Illness or maladaptation occurs when the person is unable to respond positively to the stimuli in the environment.

The stimulus most immediately confronting the person is called the focal stimulus and is the one to which the older adult must make an adaptive response. This is the cause of the behavior. An example of a focal stimulus might be an environmental change such as a move to less independent living or loss of a friend through death or relocation. Focal stimuli can have a profound impact on the critical attributes of self-esteem. Contextual stimuli are all other stimuli present that contribute to the behavior caused by the focal stimuli. Contextual stimuli can be either external or internal, such as developmental age or stresses of illness. Stimuli whose effects on the given situation are unclear are called residual stimuli. These stimuli are based on general knowledge and/or intuitive impressions such as beliefs, attitudes, experiences, or traits that cannot be validated by the older adult (Andrews & Roy, 1991).

Roy's adaptation model discusses the assessment of the stimuli and the notion that the nurse must also assess four adaptive modes: self-concept, role function, physiologic changes, and interdependence changes. The integration of the nursing diagnosis approach and Roy's adaptation model includes assessing the defining characteristics of self-esteem and the older adult's adaptive capabilities. The data obtained from the assessment helps the nurse determine the most effective way to change the course of events toward the desired adaptation. The nurse's mode of intervention is to increase, decrease, or maintain stimulation.

To assess the defining characteristics of self-esteem disturbance, the nurse could observe the older adult's behavior and ask questions. Box 45-1 presents some areas the nurse might want to observe and possible questions to ask. These questions, in addition to others, can help relate a disturbance in self-esteem to its causes.

Assessment Instruments

The Rosenberg Self-Esteem Scale has been used in several studies to measure self-esteem level. It is unidimensional

Box 45-1	Nursing Observations and Questions

Nursing Observations

Does he appear comfortable around others?

Does he initiate conversation with others, or does he tend to isolate himself?

Does he express his opinions/needs/wants to the appropriate people? Or does he negate his needs?

Does he maintain eye contact when talking with others?

Does he use hand gestures or other nonverbal movements when talking?

Does he speak in low tones, or does he speak to be heard?

Does he appear neat and clean or disheveled and unkempt?

Interview Questions

How would you describe yourself?

Do you feel good about your abilities, or do you feel saddened or depressed? If so, about what?

Are there changes or losses that have become problematic?

Are the changes in your capabilities, the things you cannot do, a problem for you?

How do you feel about the changes related to your body?

What things annoy or bother you or make you fearful, anxious, or depressed?

in nature and is designed to measure attitudes toward the self along a favorable-to-unfavorable dimension. Rosenberg (1979) defined self-esteem as self-acceptance or a basic feeling of self-worth. The Self-Esteem Scale consists of 10 items of the Likert type, allowing one of four responses: strongly agree, agree, disagree, and strongly disagree. Integral values are assigned to each scale point, and the total score is obtained by simple summation. The Self-Esteem Scale has been administered to large and diverse samples of all ages. Many of the studies cited in this chapter used this instrument to measure self-esteem (Krause, 1995; Nelson, 1989; Parent & Whall, 1984). However, other instruments that measure self-esteem are also available, including the Coopersmith (1967) Self-Esteem Inventory and the Tennessee Self-Concept Scale (Fitts, 1964).

It is generally recommended to assess a concept using an instrument developed to measure that specific concept. However, instruments not designed specifically to measure self-esteem can be used to assess for self-esteem disturbances. In convergent validity efforts, Rosenberg (cited in George & Bearon, 1980) and Parent and Whall (1984) have suggested the use of the Beck Depression Inventory (BDI). Other depression instruments include the Geriatric Depression Rating Scale, the Center for Epidemiologic Studies (CES-D) scale, the Hamilton Depression Rating Scale (Ham-D), and the Zung Depression Rating Scale. Research findings have supported the inverse relationship between self-esteem and depression in older adults. Therefore it is feasible that one could assess depression as an indirect way to assess self-esteem.

There is one caution in using any standardized instrument to assess self-esteem disturbances. A nursing assessment includes the exercise of clinical judgment and the drawing of inferences based on an entire body of knowledge. Therefore although the instruments may be of value and assistance, a comprehensive assessment using more than one method to measure self-esteem is required.

In summary, assessment includes the following activities:

1. Observe the older adult's behavior and her interactions with others

2. Interview the older adult using the questions suggested in Box 45-1 and other appropriate questions to address the defining characteristics of self-esteem

3. Use the Rosenberg Self-Esteem Scale and/or Beck Depression Inventory to confirm the assessment

CASE STUDY

K. Case, age 73, had been married for 49 years. Her husband died last year, and since then she has experienced an exacerbation of arthritis and diabetes. Physically Mrs. Case is having increased difficulty getting around and is frequently in pain. She was diagnosed with diabetes 10 years ago. Her blood sugar levels were fairly well managed with an oral agent until a year ago. Since that time, her blood sugar level consistently has been greater than 170 mg/100 ml, but she refuses insulin injections. Mrs. Case is not sleeping well at night and feels anxious "for no reason." Since she does not feel well, she has stopped going to the senior citizen center, where she used to go three times a week.

Mrs. Case admits to feeling sad and lonely since her husband died, but also admits that she and her husband did not have a good relationship. She describes Mr. Case as mentally abusive and frequently critical and demeaning toward her. She cries intermittently and is not eating because she says she's "no longer worth anything." On occasion, Mrs. Case has alluded to blaming herself for her husband's death. She recalls hearing a thud during the night that he died, but did not get up to investigate because she thought the cat had knocked a book off the shelf. Mrs. Case says "If only I had gotten up to see what the noise had been . . . when I found Jack in the morning, he was cold and stiff . . . I don't know how long he laid there."

Mrs. Case has two children, a son and a daughter. Mrs. Case states that her relationship with the daughter is strained and that the daughter doesn't visit very often: "she's really busy, you know." Mrs. Case's son is struggling with chronic alcoholism and is not able to be supportive at this time. Mrs. Case expresses anger at her husband for dying and leaving her to deal with their son, but also blames the son for contributing to his father's death. Mrs. Case's best friend recently moved out of state.

The nursing staff at the health clinic where Mrs. Case receives her care were stunned to see several changes in Mrs. Case since her last visit 6 weeks ago. Her appearance was disheveled, and her clothes were wrinkled and slightly stained. When the nurse practitioner asked Mrs. Case how things were going, she responded "I'm tired . . . nobody cares about me." Sensing a disturbance in self-esteem and feelings of depression, the nurse practitioner began an assessment.

The nurse asked the following questions to assess the defining characteristics of self-esteem. These questions assisted the nurse in identifying the related factors that the interventions will address.

- How would you describe yourself?
- How do you feel about your abilities?
- Do you feel saddened or depressed? If so, about what?
- Are there losses you are concerned about?
- Are there changes in your capabilities? Are the things you cannot do, a problem for you?
- How do you feel about changes related to your body and not being able to get around as well as you used to?
- What things annoy or bother you or make you feel fearful, anxious, or depressed?

Mrs. Case identified that because she was having difficulty walking, she missed working in her garden and being outside. What she feared most was the possibility that she would eventually be confined to a wheelchair and would need to move to an extended care facility. Mrs. Case stated she was restless and anxious and would cry for no apparent reason. She stated "I feel like I don't belong . . . my husband's gone, my children don't pay much attention to me, and my best friend moved away . . . nobody really cares if I live or die." Because self-esteem disturbance was evident, but the extent uncertain, the BDI was administered. Mrs. Case was not suicidal, but was moderately depressed.

Next the three types of stimuli were identified. The focal stimulus—the stimulus most immediately confronting the person and the one to which the older adult must make an adaptive response—was Mrs. Case's decreased ability to get around and her pain. The contextual stimuli—those stimuli that contributed to the behavior caused by the focal stimuli—were identified as feelings of depression, hopelessness, worthlessness, and guilt. The residual stimuli, including beliefs, attitudes, experiences, or traits that cannot be validated, were identified as Mrs. Case's fears that this was the end of her life and that she was worthless.

Roy's (1976) four adaptive modes (self-concept, physiologic integrity, role function, and interdependence) were also assessed to further determine Self-Esteem Disturbance. Physiologically it was uncertain to what extent Mrs. Case's mobility would improve. It was thought that if Mrs. Case required a wheelchair in the future, her home could be evaluated for environmental modifications that would allow her a sense of independence and greater mobility. It was felt that Mrs. Case's joint pain could be more effectively managed. In assessing interdependence it was noted that Mrs. Case was feeling increasingly incapable of being self-sufficient. Mrs. Case also viewed her role function as

being greatly compromised in that she no longer had a husband or children to care for and about. In reality, Mrs. Case felt that she no longer had a role or function in life.

NURSING DIAGNOSIS

Gordon (1992) identified the "self-perception–self-concept" pattern as one of the 11 functional health patterns found within the nursing diagnosis system. She further listed the diagnosis of Self-Esteem Disturbance as an accepted diagnosis within the self-perception–self-concept pattern. The North American Nursing Diagnosis Association (NANDA) defines Self-Esteem Disturbance as the "negative self-evaluation/feelings about self or self-capabilities, which may be directly or indirectly expressed" (NANDA, 1999, 112), and its defining characteristics are presented in Box 45-2. A majority of the defining characteristics must be present for the diagnosis of Self-Esteem Disturbance to be made. It is not necessary that all defining characteristics be present because everyone does not express disturbances in self-esteem in the same way.

NANDA has developed two additional nursing diagnoses related to self-esteem that are relevant to older adults: Chronic Low Self-Esteem and Situational Low Self-Esteem. Chronic Low Self-Esteem is defined as "long-standing negative self-evaluation/feelings about self or self-capabilities" (NANDA, 1999, p. 113), which may be directly or indirectly expressed; Situational Low Self-Esteem is defined as "negative self-evaluation/feelings about self that develop in response to a loss or change in an individual who previously had a positive self evaluation" (NANDA, 1999, p. 113). While it is quite feasible that an older adult may have experienced a negative self-evaluation most of her life, it is more likely that changes in self-esteem are situationally related for the majority of older adults. As previously noted, older adults are at risk for self-esteem changes caused by age-related events and stresses experienced in late life (Binstock & George, 1990; Silverstone, 1996; Taft, 1985). Although Self-Esteem Disturbance and Situational Low Self-Esteem are most relevant for older adults, the nurse will need to conduct a comprehensive assessment in order to differentiate between these nursing diagnoses and to implement appropriate interventions.

The research literature has defined self-esteem as an individual's self-evaluation of his worth but has not described how a person with a negative self-evaluation might feel, what he might say about himself, or how he might behave. NANDA's defining characteristics, on the other hand, do identify specific behaviors, verbalizations, and feelings that can be used as a starting point when assessing self-esteem. However, the NANDA definition of Self-Esteem Disturbance is narrow in scope and does not acknowledge the various factors that affect self-esteem in the older adult. For example, the current definition states

| Box 45-2 | Suggested Nursing-Sensitive Outcome and Nursing Intervention SELF-ESTEEM DISTURBANCE |

Nursing Diagnosis
Self-Esteem Disturbance
Defining characteristics
Diagnostic cues (supported by evidence)
Self-negating verbalizations and one or more of the following:

- Lack of eye contact
- Head flexion
- Shoulder flexion

Supporting cues
- Expressions of shame/guilt
- Rationalizes away/rejects positive feedback and exaggerates negative feedback about self
- Hesitant to try new things/situations
- Hypersensitivity to slight or criticism

Compensations

- Grandiosity
- Denial of problem obvious to others
- Projection of blame/responsibility for problems
- Rationalizing personal failures

Related factors/etiologies
To be developed

Nursing-Sensitive Outcome
Self-Esteem
Indicators
Verbalization of self-acceptance
Lower levels of depression, anxiety
Acceptance of compliments from others
Increased socialization and involvement
Improved physical appearance and hygiene
Increased willingness to try new activities

Nursing Intervention
Self-Esteem Enhancement
Activities
Therapeutic communication
Participation in group therapy
Assist the older adult to reframe current situation
Assist the older adult to identify strengths and limitations

---

that Self-Esteem Disturbance is a negative self-evaluation/feelings about self or self-capabilities with no reference to why an older adult might feel that way. Theoretical writings and empirical findings suggest that a more global and comprehensive definition of Self-Esteem Disturbance might be more relevant. There is growing evidence to support that self-esteem is influenced by environmental (George, 1990), social (Frazier, 1982; Heidrich, 1994), physical (Chene, 1991), religious (Krause, 1995; Nelson, 1989) and emotional (Heidrich, 1993, 1994; Nelson, 1989; Parent & Whall, 1984) factors. The inclusion of these contributing factors in the NANDA definition of Self-Esteem Disturbance might assist nurses in the assessment of self-esteem and facilitate more appropriate interventions and realistic outcomes.

NURSING-SENSITIVE OUTCOMES

The outcome Self-Esteem is the "personal judgment of self-worth" (Iowa Outcomes Project, 2000, p. 391). This could be evaluated objectively using the indicators and measurement procedures noted in Box 45-2.

NURSING INTERVENTIONS

Nurses need to recognize the diversity of older adults. As we work with older adults from varying religious and cultural backgrounds, we need to grow more sensitive to varying values, attitudes, and beliefs as we develop and implement nursing interventions. The interventions de-

scribed in this chapter are based on the NIC interventions for Self-Esteem Disturbance (Iowa Intervention Project, 2000) and on Roy's (1976, 1984) adaptive model, but with the above caveats in mind. One suggested intervention, Self-Esteem Enhancement, is defined by NIC as "assisting a patient to increase his/her personal judgment of self worth" (Iowa Intervention Project, 2000, p. 580). The interventions involve both the adaptation level of the older adult in the four modes and the stimuli. To promote adaptation, other stimuli may need to be managed. According to Andrews and Roy (1986), management of stimuli involves altering, increasing, decreasing, removing, or maintaining the stimuli. The nursing intervention involves selection of which stimuli to change (e.g., focal or contextual) and the approach with the highest probability of bringing about adaptation. Whenever possible, the focal stimulus is the focus of the nursing intervention, but when this is not possible, contextual stimuli can be managed in order to broaden the possible adaptation level. The steps in the nursing intervention, therefore, must increase the older adult's personal judgment of self-worth. This can be accomplished by increasing, decreasing, or maintaining the stimuli.

Several activities can be implemented by nurses to increase an older adult's perception of self-worth. First, the nurse could help the older adult see the focal stimuli as having a positive valuing influence rather than being another negative devaluing experience (Roy, 1976). Second, therapeutic communication might be helpful. The nurse could help the older adult reframe her view of the situation. The older adult might be able to understand that feelings of sadness, loss, anger, and unhappiness are normal responses to life changes. Through therapeutic communication the nurse can help older adults understand what maturational or situational crisis they are experiencing, what is expected of them, and what they expect of themselves. Third, older adults need to understand, define, accept, and try out control of the environment that they identify as comfortable. The older adult's self-evaluation needs to be satisfying and to include a view of self as competent with opportunities to achieve feedback to continue that view. With this kind of positive picture of self, the older adult will be able to change self-views, yet maintain self-esteem and adapt through self-concept.

CASE STUDY

Based on the data obtained in the assessment, the following diagnosis was specified for Mrs. Case: Low Self-Esteem related to decreased ability to ambulate and increased joint pain (focal stimuli). Mrs. Case validated that not being able to walk as well and the possible consequences of such were the most upsetting factors immediately present in her life.

The interventions identified as appropriate for Mrs. Case focused on increasing her personal judgment of self-worth. This was accomplished initially by addressing Mrs. Case's decreased ability to ambulate and increased joint pain (focal stimuli). The nurse practitioner arranged for Mrs. Case to be evaluated by the physical therapy department to assess her functional potential. It was found that Mrs. Case had peripheral neuropathy secondary to the diabetes. Physical therapy was recommended three times a week for muscle strengthening. Mrs. Case agreed to insulin once she understood that the insulin might help in decreasing some of her physical symptoms. In addition, a comprehensive assessment of Mrs. Case's pain was conducted, and her analgesic schedule was adjusted.

Other activities related to the contextual and residual stimuli were implemented to increase Mrs. Case's personal judgment of self-worth. Mrs. Case was encouraged to participate in group therapy and discuss some of the losses she was experiencing (e.g., death of her husband and her related guilt, strained relations with children, relocation of her best friend, and decline in physical health). Mrs. Case began to feel that people did care about her and that she was worth caring about. Mrs. Case continued to exhibit symptoms of depression and was evaluated by a geropsychiatrist, who prescribed an antidepressant.

Mrs. Case was also connected to the local transportation system for senior citizens, which increased her mobility potential tremendously. Although Mrs. Case needed frequent encouragement and support, she participated in the treatment plan and experienced a greater sense of control and self-esteem.

Although the outcomes of the physical therapy were still in doubt after 5 months, Mrs. Case was able to use a walker for short distances in her house. When she went out, Mrs. Case used a wheelchair because she tired easily and was slow. Being able to use a walker at home and a wheelchair when out was a compromise that Mrs. Case could live with.

Mrs. Case's joint pain and blood glucose levels were better controlled, and she reported feeling physically better. This progress had a direct impact on Mrs. Case's self-esteem. The questions that had initially been asked of Mrs. Case were again used to assess Mrs. Case's current level of self-esteem. This assessment noted that Mrs. Case was beginning to exhibit some of the critical attributes of high self-esteem; that is, she felt less depressed and had a positive view of her progress. She continued to have some disbelief in her ability to follow through on the group therapy because it was emotionally painful, but she became convinced that change was both possible and evident. Reassessment with the BDI demonstrated a lesser degree of depression at this time.

SUMMARY

It is imperative that nurses in all realms of the health care system be able to recognize disturbances in self-esteem and know how to treat it. The nursing diagnosis Self-Esteem Disturbance is particularly significant for older adults because it often is associated with depression, anxiety, and other age-related stressors. Because of the multiplicity of factors that can be associated, assessment can be difficult. However, a comprehensive assessment is necessary to establish parameters for what can be expected from that person. The Rosenberg Self-Esteem Scale and Beck's Depression Inventory are examples of standard assessment tools that nurses can use to develop a definitive diagnosis. Nursing interventions are aimed at assisting the older adult to increase his personal judgment of self-worth. The desired outcome is for the older adult to have a perception of self-worth. Nurses are often in a strategic position to intervene with older adults who suffer from a disturbance in self-esteem.

REFERENCES

Alexopoulos, G. (1995). Mood disorders. In H. Kaplan & B. Sadock (Eds.), *Comprehensive textbook of psychiatry/VI* (pp. 2566-2568). Baltimore: Lippincott Williams & Wilkins.

Andrews, H., & Roy, C. (1986). *Essentials of the Roy adaptation model.* Norwalk, CT: Appleton & Lange.

Andrews, H., & Roy, C. (1991). Essentials of the Roy Adaptation model. In C. Roy & H. A. Andrews (Eds.), *The Roy adaptation model: The definitive statement.* Norwalk, CT: Appleton & Lange.

Baltes, M. M., & Schmid, U. (1987). Psychological gerontology. *German Journal of Psychology, 11,* 87-123.

Bengston, V., Reedy, M., & Gordon, C. (1985). Aging and self-conception: Personality processes and social context. In J. E. Birren & K. W. Schaie (Eds.), *Handbook of the psychology of aging* (2nd ed., pp. 1282-1292). New York: Van Nostrand Reinhold.

Binstock, R., & George, L. (1990). *Handbook of aging and the social sciences* (3rd ed.). San Diego, CA: Academic Press.

Brandon, N. (1969). *The psychology of self-esteem: A new concept of man's psychological nature.* Los Angeles: Nash.

Bunten, D. (1997). Self perception/self concept pattern: Normal changes with aging. In M. Maas, K. Buckwalter, M. Hardy, T. Tripp-Reimer, & M. Titler (Eds.), *Nursing diagnoses, interventions, and nursing-sensitive outcomes for the elders: Epidemiologic rationale.* Thousand Oaks, CA: Sage.

Burke, P. J. (1991). Identity process and social stress. *American Sociological Review, 56,* 836-849.

Chen, H. L. (1994). Hearing in the elderly: Relation of hearing loss, loneliness and self-esteem. *Journal of Gerontological Nursing, 20*(6), 22-28.

Chene, A. (1991). Self-esteem of the elderly and education. *Educational Gerontology, 17,* 343-353.

Coopersmith, S. (1967). *The antecedents of self-esteem.* Boston: Freeman Cooper.

Day, J. C. (1992). Population projections of the United States by age, sex, race, and Hispanic origin: 1992 to 2050. *Current Population Reports* (Series P25, No. 1092). Washington, DC: U.S. Government Printing Office.

Dietz, B. E. (1996). The relationship of aging to self-esteem: The relative effects of maturation and role accumulation. *International Journal of Aging and Human Development, 43*(3), 249-266.

Dimond, M. (1993). Older women: Social policies and health care. *Journal of Gerontological Nursing, 19,* 5-6.

Dimond, M. (1996). Older women: Social policies and health care. In V. Burggraf & R. Barry (Eds.), *Gerontological nursing: Current practice and research* (pp. 9-15). Thorofare, NJ: Slack Inc.

Fitts, W. H. (1964). *Tennessee self-concept manual* (3rd ed.). Los Angeles: Western Psychological Services.

Frazier, C. (1982). Depression, self-esteem, and physical health as a function of social support in the elderly. *Dissertation Abstracts International, 306,* DA831-1282.

Frey, D., & Carolock, C. J. (1989). *Enhancing self esteem* (2nd ed.). Bristol, PA: Accelerated Development.

George, L. (1990). Social structure, social processes, and social-psychological states. In R. Binstock & L. George (Eds.), *Handbook of aging and the social sciences* (3rd ed., pp. 186-204). San Diego, CA: Academic Press.

George, L., & Bearon, L. (1980). *Quality of life in older persons: Meaning and measurement.* New York: Human Sciences Press.

Goldberg, W., & Fitzpatrick, J. (1980). Movement therapy with the aged. *Nursing Research, 29*(6), 339-346.

Gordon, M. (1992). *Nursing diagnosis: Process and application.* Hightstown, NJ: McGraw-Hill.

Gove, W. R., Ortega, S. T., & Briggs Style, C. (1989). The maturational and role perspectives on aging and self through the adult years: An empirical evaluation. *American Journal of Sociology, 95*(5), 1117-1145.

Heidrich, S. (1993). The relationship between physical health and psychological well-being in elderly women: A developmental perspective. *Research in Nursing and Health, 16,* 123-130.

Heidrich, S. (1994). The self, health, and depression in elderly women. *Western Journal of Nursing Research, 16*(5), 544-555.

Iowa Intervention Project. J. C. McCloskey & G. M. Bulechek (Eds.). (2000). *Nursing interventions classification (NIC)* (3rd ed.). St. Louis, MO: Mosby.

Iowa Outcomes Project. M. Johnson, M. Maas, & S. Moorhead (Eds.). (2000). *Nursing outcomes classification (NOC)* (2nd ed.). St. Louis, MO: Mosby.

Kaufman, S. R. (1986). *The ageless self: Sources of meaning in late life.* Madison, WI: University of Wisconsin Press.

Krause, N. (1987). Life stress, social support, and self-esteem in an elderly population. *Psychology and Aging, 2,* 349-356.

Krause, N. (1995). Religiosity and self-esteem among older adults. *Journal of Gerontology: Psychological Sciences, 50B*(5), 236-246.

Krause, N. (1999). Stress and the devaluation of highly salient roles in late life. *Journal of Gerontology: Social Sciences, 54B*(2), S99-S108.

Loeb, R. C., & Sarigiani, P. (1986). The impact of hearing impairment on self-perceptions of children. *Volta Review, 88*(2), 89-100.

McCrae, R. R., & Costa, P. T. (1988). Age personality and the spontaneous self-concept. *Journal of Gerontology: Social Sciences, 43,* S177-S185.

Minkler, M., & Stone, R. (1985). The feminization of poverty. *The Gerontologist, 25,* 351-357.

Nelson, P. (1989). Social support, self-esteem, and depression in the institutionalized elderly. *Issues in Mental Health Nursing, 10,* 55-68.

North American Nursing Diagnosis Association. (1999). *Nursing diagnoses: Definitions & classification 1999-2000.* Philadelphia: Author.

Parent, C., & Whall, A. (1984). Are physical activity, self-esteem and depression related? *Journal of Gerontological Nursing, 10,* 8-11.

Rosenberg, M. (1979). *Conceiving the self.* New York: Basic Books.

Roy, C. (1976). *Introduction to nursing: An adaptation model.* Englewood Cliffs, NJ: Prentice Hall.

Roy, C. (1984). *Introduction to nursing: An adaptation model* (2nd ed.). Englewood Cliffs, NJ: Prentice Hall.

Silverstone, B. (1996). Older people of tomorrow: A psychosocial profile. *The Gerontologist, 36*(1), 27-32.

Stein, K. (1995). Schema model of the self-concept. *IMAGE: Journal of Nursing Scholarship, 27*(3), 187-193.

Stokes, C. A. (1999). *The relationship between self-esteem and health promoting behaviors in African American women.* Unpublished master's thesis. University of Detroit Mercy, Detroit, MI.

Taft, L. (1985). Self-esteem in later life: A nursing perspective. *Advances in Nursing Science, 8,* 77-84.

Thoits, P. A. (1991). On merging identity and stress research. *Social Psychology Quarterly, 54,* 101-112.

Thoits, P. A. (1995). Identity-relevant events and psychological symptoms: A cautionary tale. *Journal of Health and Social Behavior, 36,* 72-82.

Warren, B. J. (1997). Depression, stressful life events, social support, and self-esteem in middle class African American women. *Archives of Psychiatric Nursing, XI*(3), 107-117.

Yachnik, M. (1986). Self-esteem in deaf adolescents. *American Annals of the Deaf, 131*(4), 305-310.

CHAPTER 46

HOPELESSNESS

Carol J. Farran

Feelings of hopelessness may be associated with the numerous losses experienced during this life stage—loss of physical health and function, loss of family and friends by death, and changes in work, leisure patterns, and residence (Farran & Popovich, 1990). Consequently, the concept of hopelessness is of major importance in the care of elderly persons. Ironically, most studies of elders have examined hope instead of hopelessness (Farran, Herth, & Popovich, 1995). In many ways, hope and hopelessness are opposite sides of the same coin. One cannot be understood without understanding the other; they create a necessary dialectic (Lynch, 1965). Studies of hope and hopelessness in elders have included grieving widows and widowers, persons with cancer, and persons in community-based care, long-term care, senior citizen centers, and inpatient geropsychiatric units (Farran et al., 1995).

Other terms that are closely related to hopelessness include helplessness, powerlessness, depression, and suicidal behaviors. Seligman's (1975) theoretical work and research on learned helplessness/hopelessness suggest a sequence to these behaviors. Persons are initially confronted with multiple events that are outside their own control. They attempt to respond or change their situation, but whatever they do is not adequate to bring about the desired changes. They become discouraged, and their motivation to take action or initiate responses to the situation is undermined. They begin believing that their success or failure is independent of their own actions, and they begin doing less and less. Feelings of helplessness lead them to try even less to change their situation. These feelings of helplessness and powerlessness can lead to hopelessness, depression, and in some cases even death (Schulz, 1980; Solomon, 1982; Uncapher, Gallagher-Thompson, Osgood, & Bongar, 1998).

Hopelessness must also be understood in the context of depression and suicidal behaviors. Beck's cognitive approach to depression suggests that negative feelings and moods such as depression and hopelessness are associated with irrational and distorted thoughts (Beck, 1963, 1967). Treatment involves changing these irrational and distorted thoughts to more rational and appropriate thought patterns. Research with elderly psychiatric patients has further noted that hopelessness is the strongest predictor of suicidal intent (Beck, Kovacs, & Weissman, 1975; Beck, Steer, Kovacs, & Garrison, 1985; Uncapher et al., 1998).

Existing research on hope and hopelessness and the theoretical formulations that support our understanding of helplessness, powerlessness, depression, and suicidal behaviors are vital to understanding hopelessness in the care of elders. Elders are particularly prone to feelings of hopelessness and depression because of the multiple changes and losses that occur in their lives, and these changes occur when they have less energy and fewer resources than they had earlier in their lives.

ASSESSMENT

The occurrence of hopelessness in older persons can be evident in many aspects of their lives. When persons feel hopeless they may have difficulty articulating their goals for the future, they may hold onto goals that are rigid, inflexible, unattainable, or unrealistic, or they may have negative expectations about achieving these goals (Averill, Catlin, & Chon, 1990; Farran et al., 1995; Moltmann, 1975; Stotland, 1969).

Hopelessness can occur when intrapersonal, interpersonal, and environmental/sociologic resources are limited, or when a person does not have the necessary cognitive, affective, or behavioral resources (Farran et al., 1995). The description of hopelessness given by the North American Nursing Diagnosis Association (NANDA) incorporates the intrapersonal, interpersonal, and environmental aspects of hopelessness through the following phrases: unable to mobilize energy, decreased decision-making capabilities, giving up, abandonment/separation from others, and isolation due to disease (Carpenito, 1995). Particular attention also needs to be given to the larger environmental/sociologic issues that can affect elderly persons' feelings of hopelessness, including their earlier war-related experiences, deprivations, poverty, violence, and abuse.

Hopelessness may be characterized by the absence of action (Engel, 1968), by appropriate action toward an inappropriate goal (Kastenbaum & Kastenbaum, 1971), or by misguided action away from one's situation (rather than directly facing it) (LeShan, 1989; Lynch, 1965). NANDA addresses the action component of hopelessness in references to the following symptoms: passivity, decreased verbalization; decreased affect; despondent verbal cues; lack of initiative; decreased response to stimuli; and lack of involvement in care (Carpenito, 1995; NANDA, 1999).

Hopelessness involves an inhibition of one's motivational system (Korner, 1970) and may involve alterations in either internal or external feelings of control (Rotter, 1966). Both "too high" or "too low" expressions of internal or external control can be associated with hopelessness. Persons with "too high" feelings of internal control in uncontrollable external situations (illness, stress) can feel hopeless because they may have inadequate resources to attain their goal, or their goals may be inappropriate for their external situation. Likewise, persons with "too low" internal feelings of control can have a depreciated sense of self and feel as though they never get a break or as though things never work out for them (Farran et al., 1995). Persons with "too high" levels of external control can be unrealistic about help that they anticipate from others to resolve a problem and thus assume no personal control. Other persons can have "too low" a sense of external control because others have so frequently failed them (Engel, 1968). NANDA's references to the relationship between control and hopelessness speak to the individual seeing limited alternatives or personal choices (Carpenito, 1995).

Hopelessness also is related to an individual's perspective of time. Hopelessness generally involves an inability to think about or imagine a tolerable future, as seen in persons who are experiencing current traumatic losses, change, or grief (Frank, 1968; Kastenbaum & Kastenbaum, 1971; Lynch, 1965; Melges & Bowlby, 1969). Other time alterations associated with hopelessness include (Farran et al., 1995) persons who have always felt hopeless (such as those persons with a personality disorder); persons who are chronically mentally ill or criminals (LeShan, 1989; Melges & Bowlby, 1969; Stotland, 1969); persons who express a past and future hopelessness and live mainly for the present (including those with character disorders, alcoholism, or drug addiction) (Melges & Bowlby, 1969); and persons who are clinically depressed or suicidal and who may have hopeless feelings about both the present and the future. NANDA descriptions suggest that hopelessness involves a view of the limited present alternatives, as well as a pattern of dealing with the past and future, but not with the here and now (Carpenito, 1995).

NANDA suggests that hopelessness can be associated with abandonment or separation from others, loss of significant others by death or divorce, prolonged caretaking of others, or impaired relationships (Carpenito, 1995). Understanding the relational roots of hopelessness is necessary for targeting of specific interventions and outcomes. The close association between hopelessness and the relational process very likely forms the basis for effective nurse-patient interactions. Persons who are hopeless can have difficulty trusting others (Erikson, 1982; Melges & Bowlby, 1969), they can have difficulty imagining that others can provide any assistance to them (Engel, 1968;

Isani, 1963; Lynch, 1965; Schmale & Iker, 1971), or they can have no one who can provide them love and support.

A number of relational patterns can contribute toward hopelessness. For some persons, supportive relationships have never been present, resulting in perpetual feelings of hopelessness (parental deprivation). For other persons, relationships have been the cause of particular pain and contribute toward the person's hopelessness (physical/sexual abuse). Still other persons experience more transitory feelings of hopelessness because of changes brought about in their relationships through death, divorce, or illness (Farran et al., 1995).

Measures of Hopelessness

Two measures of hopelessness have been used in elders (Farran et al., 1995). The Beck Hopelessness Scale has been used to quantify hopelessness associated with psychologic conditions and has been found to be one of the best predictors of suicide (Beck, Brown, Berchick, Stewart, & Steer, 1990; Beck et al., 1985; Beck, Weissman, Lester, & Trexler, 1974). It has been the only reliable instrument measuring hopelessness in old, frail, multiply impaired nursing home residents (Abraham, 1991). This 20-item measure includes three dimensions of hopelessness: affective, motivational, and cognitive.

The Geriatric Hopelessness Scale was developed to quantify hopelessness in nonpsychiatric elderly populations and reliably measures hopelessness in situations of high and low depression (Fry, 1984). This measure examines specific and generalized cognitions of pessimism and futility concerning oneself and the future. The measure's four factors focus on hopelessness associated with the following situations: loss of physical and cognitive abilities; loss of personal/interpersonal worth and attractiveness; recovering spiritual faith and receiving spiritual grace; and receiving nurturance, recovering respect, and remembrance in the present and after death.

An abbreviated clinical assessment of hopelessness is summarized in Assessment Guide 46-1 and is based upon a more extensive assessment of hope and hopelessness published previously (Farran et al., 1995). These four attributes of hopelessness are included in this clinical assessment: experiential, transcedent spiritual, rational, and relational.

Measures of Hope

A wide variety of hope measures have been used successfully with elders (Farran et al., 1995): the Hopefulness Scale (Mercier, Fawcett, & Clark, 1984); the Stoner Hope Scale (Stoner, 1988); the State-Trait Hope Scale (Grimm, 1984); the Miller Hope Scale (Miller & Powers, 1988); the Hope Index (Staats, 1987); the Nowotny Hope Scale (Nowotny, 1989); the Herth Hope Scale (Herth, 1991); the Herth Hope Index (Herth, 1992); and the Snyder Hope

HOPELESSNESS

I. Experiential Attributes
   A. What current situations are contributing to this person's feelings of hopelessness?
   B. On a scale of 1 to 10, with 1 being least hopeless and 10 being most hopeless, how hopeless is the individual?
   C. Is this person clinically depressed?
   D. Does this person express any suicidal thoughts or behaviors?

II. Spiritual/Transcendent Process
   A. What religious/spiritual practices or rituals have sustained this person in the past?
   B. Is the individual able to "give voice" to the deeper issues being raised by her situation?
   C. How does this person find meaning or purpose in life?
   D. Is this person able to "rise above" her particular situation on an individual or spiritual level?

III. Rational/Irrational Thought Process
   A. Goals
      1. Does this person have goals for the future?
      2. Are these goals general/specific, rigid/flexible, or attainable?
      3. Are the individual's goals consistent with family member goals?
   B. Resources
      1. Does the individual have internal resources to meet his goals (determination, courage, optimism)?

2. Does the individual have physical energy to meet her goal?
3. Does the individual have family and/or community resources to support his desired goals?
   C. Action
      1. Is the individual taking appropriate and/or realistic action to meet goals?
      2. Are others acting in behalf of the patient?
      3. Are these actions congruent with the patient's actions?
   D. Control
      1. What is the source of the individual's sense of control—internal or external?
      2. Are feelings of being in control consistent with available resources?
   E. Time
      1. What past and present experiences of hopelessness has the individual had?
      2. What are the individual's feelings concerning the future?

IV. Relational Process
   A. How connected is the patient to other persons?
   B. Are other persons available for the patient?
   C. Are these relationships supportive or confrontational?

Scale (Snyder et al., 1991). Several related measures on Hope and Will to Live have also been developed by the Nursing Outcomes Classification (NOC) (Iowa Outcomes Project, 2000).

Measures of Depression

If an individual experiences hopelessness, a careful assessment of depression must also be made. This assessment is better made using the DSM III-R criteria (American Psychiatric Association, 1987), as opposed to more general criteria established by NANDA. Hopelessness is one symptom in a complex of other depression symptoms such as feeling sad, blue, low, or down in the dumps, and possibly irritability. Classification as a psychiatric disorder requires that depressive symptoms be prominent and persistent, with at least four out of seven symptom complexes needing to be present almost every day for at least 2 weeks. Pertinent symptoms include the following: changes in ap-

petite, weight, and sleep patterns; psychomotor agitation or retardation; loss of interest or pleasure in activities; loss of energy or fatigue; feelings of worthlessness, self-reproach, or guilt; difficulty thinking, slowed thinking, or indecisiveness; and recurrent thoughts or wishes of death, suicidal ideation, or suicidal attempts (Table 46-1). A number of quantitative depression measures, successfully used with elderly persons, could also be used, including the Beck Depression Scale (Beck et al., 1974) and the Geriatric Depression Scale (Yesavage, 1988).

Measures of Suicidal Intent/Behaviors

In the event of suicidal thoughts and/or behaviors, a thorough assessment of suicidal risk and potential must be made. The risk of elder suicide is greater for persons with the following characteristics: male; Protestant; white; widowed or divorced; low-paying job; retired or unemployed; poor physical health; having recently seen a

Suggested Nursing-Sensitive Outcomes and Nursing Interventions

Table 46-1   HOPELESSNESS

Nursing Diagnosis	Nursing-Sensitive Outcomes	Nursing Interventions
HOPELESSNESS *Related Factors/Etiologies* Experiential process • Prolonged activity restriction creating isolation • Failing or deteriorating physiologic condition • Long -term stress	ACCEPTANCE: HEALTH STATUS ENDURANCE GRIEF RESOLUTION HOPE PSYCHOSOCIAL ADJUSTMENT: LIFE CHANGE QUALITY OF LIFE REST SYMPTOM CONTROL WELL-BEING WILL TO LIVE	ACTIVE LISTENING ANXIETY REDUCTION BEHAVIOR MODIFICATION CALMING TECHNIQUE COUNSELING CRISIS INTERVENTION DYING CARE EMOTIONAL SUPPORT GRIEF WORK FACILITATION GUILT WORK FACILITATION HOPE INSTILLATION LIMIT SETTING PAIN MANAGEMENT SELF-AWARENESS ENHANCEMENT SELF-CARE ASSISTANCE THERAPEUTIC TOUCH TOUCH
Defining Characteristics Depression • Lack of initiative • Passivity decreased verbalization • Decreased affect • Decreased appetite • Increased/decreased sleep • Psychomotor agitation/retardation • Feelings of worthlessness, self-reproach • Guilt • Thinking/indecisiveness	ACCEPTANCE: HEALTH STATUS DISTORTED THOUGHT CONTROL HOPE MOOD EQUILIBRIUM PSYCHOSOCIAL ADJUSTMENT: LIFE CHANGE QUALITY OF LIFE SELF-ESTEEM SLEEP WILL TO LIVE	**HOPELESSNESS WITH DEPRESSION** ANGER CONTROL ASSISTANCE HEALTH SCREENING BEHAVIOR MANAGEMENT: SELF-HARM COGNITIVE RESTRUCTURING MEDICATION ADMINISTRATION MEDICATION MANAGEMENT MOOD MANAGEMENT SLEEP ENHANCEMENT
Suicidal thoughts/behaviors • Suicidal ideation • Previous suicidal attempts • Suicidal plan	IMPULSE CONTROL SELF-MUTILATION RESTRAINT SUICIDE SELF-RESTRAINT	**HOPELESSNESS WITH SUICIDAL IDEATION/ BEHAVIORS** SUICIDE PREVENTION SURVEILLANCE
	COPING SPIRITUAL WELL-BEING	**HOPELESSNESS/SUICIDAL BEHAVIORS/INPATIENT HOSPITALIZATION** ELOPEMENT PRECAUTIONS MILIEU THERAPY SECLUSION
Spiritual or transcendent process • Decreased verbalization • Lost belief in transcendent values/God • Inability to personally transcend situation	DECISION MAKING INFORMATION PROCESSING	COPING ENHANCEMENT SPIRITUAL SUPPORT VALUES CLARIFICATION

Rational or irrational thought process
   Goals
 	
  • Difficulty establishing goals
		DECISION-MAKING SUPPORT
		MUTUAL GOAL SETTING
		PATIENT CONTRACTING
		SELF-MODIFICATION ASSISTANCE

Table 46-1	Suggested Nursing-Sensitive Outcomes and Nursing Interventions—cont'd	
	HOPELESSNESS—cont'd	

Nursing Diagnosis	Nursing-Sensitive Outcomes	Nursing Interventions
• Rigid, inflexible, unattainable, unrealistic goals • Negative expectation concerning goals		

Resources
• Intrapersonal
  • Apathy/lack of energy
  • Decreased decision-making capabilities
  • Giving up
	ENERGY CONSERVATION
	REST
	ROLE PERFORMANCE
		ANTICIPATORY GUIDANCE
		ASSERTIVENESS TRAINING
		BIBLIOTHERAPY
		COGNITIVE STIMULATION
		COPING ENHANCEMENT
		ENERGY MANAGEMENT
		HUMOR
		SELF-ESTEEM ENHANCEMENT

• Interpersonal
  • Abandonment/separation from others
• Environmental/sociologic
  • Isolation due to disease
  • War/poverty/violence/abuse
	LONELINESS
	SOCIAL INVOLVEMENT
	SOCIAL SUPPORT
	KNOWLEDGE: HEALTH BEHAVIORS
	KNOWLEDGE: HEALTH RESOURCES
	REST
		SIMPLE GUIDED IMAGERY
		SIMPLE RELAXATION THERAPY
		FAMILY INVOLVEMENT PROMOTION
		FAMILY MOBILIZATION
		MULTIDISCIPLINARY CARE CONFERENCE
		SUPPORT GROUP
		SUPPORT SYSTEM ENHANCEMENT
		PRESENCE
		ABUSE PROTECTION SUPPORT

Action • Passivity/lack of initiative • Appropriate action toward inappropriate goal • Misguided action • Decreased verbalization/affect	DECISION MAKING LEISURE PARTICIPATION DISTORTED THOUGHT CONTROL HEALTH BELIEFS: PERCEIVED CONTROL	RECREATION THERAPY SELF-RESPONSIBILITY FACILITATION HEALTH EDUCATION LEARNING FACILITATION TEACHING: INDIVIDUAL REMINISCENCE THERAPY
Control • Altered internal control • Altered external control • Sees limited alternatives		
Time • Altered feelings about past, present, and future • Limited present alternatives		
Relational • Distrust in others • Inability to imagine that others can/will help • Abandonment/separation from others • Loss of significant relationships • Prolonged caretaking of others • Impaired relationships	CAREGIVER EMOTIONAL HEALTH CAREGIVER-PATIENT RELATIONSHIP CAREGIVER STRESSORS CAREGIVER WELL-BEING COMMUNICATION: EXPRESSIVE ABILITY HEALTH BELIEFS: PERCEIVED RESOURCES LONELINESS SOCIAL INTERACTION SKILLS SOCIAL INVOLVEMENT	ANIMAL-ASSISTED THERAPY CAREGIVER SUPPORT BEHAVIOR MODIFICATIONS: SOCIAL SKILLS COMPLEX RELATIONSHIP BUILDING FAMILY INTEGRITY PROMOTION FAMILY PROCESS MAINTENANCE FAMILY SUPPORT FAMILY THERAPY ROLE ENHANCEMENT THERAPY GROUP

physician for health-related concerns; presence of depression, alcoholism, low self-concept, or loneliness; prior history of poor relationships; history of mental illness in the family; and rigid, tunnel vision and circular reasoning (Horton-Deutsch, Clark, & Farran, 1992; Osgood, 1992). The Beck Scale of Suicide Ideation is designed to measure the presence, intensity, and severity of suicidal ideation (Beck, Steer, & Ranieri, 1988).

NURSING DIAGNOSIS

NANDA (1999) defines Hopelessness as "a subjective state in which an individual sees limited or no alternatives or personal choices available and is unable to mobilize energy on own behalf" (p. 76). A second definition, offered by Farran et al. (1995), suggests that Hopelessness is "an essential experience of the human condition. It functions as a feeling of despair and discouragement; a thought process that expects nothing; and a behavioral process in which the person attempts little or takes inappropriate action."

While both definitions have similarities, the second definition of Hopelessness has several qualities that are not immediately evident in the NANDA definition. The phrase, "hopelessness is an essential experience of the human condition," immediately links hopelessness with the following existential theoretical perspective: certain things happen to us as humans, and although these experiences are not always pleasant, they have the potential to help us grow and become better persons (Nauman, 1971; Yalom, 1980). Another strength of the Farran et al. definition lies in its specific references to "feelings, thoughts, and behaviors." By specifying what constitutes the subjective state of Hopelessness, a framework is created for assessing these components, for identifying related outcomes, and for targeting specific interventions to meet these outcomes.

Relationship Between Hopelessness and Hope

An appreciation of the close relationship between hope and hopelessness is vital to preventing hopelessness and maintaining hopefulness. A model depicting these constructs is presented in detail in Farran et al. (1995). The model suggests that hopelessness and hope share the following aspects: their roots of development both lie in intrapersonal, interpersonal, and environmental/sociologic perspectives (Erikson, 1982; Fromm, 1968); they share situational determinants and can both be influenced by life stage, by stages or symptoms of a particular illness, and by treatment settings (Herth, 1990a); they both involve experiential, transcendent, rational, and relational processes; and neither of them is absolute in their range—they may be fluid, transient, or intermittent (Engel, 1968; Lynch, 1965).

Levels of Hopelessness

Hopelessness can be experienced on at least two levels. At the most basic level, hopelessness is experienced in the face of difficult life experiences such as the death of a spouse, the diagnosis of cancer, or living with a debilitating chronic illness (Farran et al., 1995). At this level, feelings of hopelessness are more transitory and can be dealt with once persons mobilize their resources. When dealt with at this level, feelings of hopelessness can even result in enhanced mental, physical, and spiritual functioning or quality of life. At a more pathologic level hopelessness has a more pervasive hold on a person, is manifest along with depression and suicidal ideation (Beck et al., 1975; Uncapher et al., 1998), and is characterized by diminished physical, mental, and spiritual health. At this level hopelessness is particularly relevant to elderly individuals, as research suggests that suicide rates are higher among the elderly population than among any other age-group (McIntosh, 1995).

Attributes of Hopelessness

Four theoretical attributes are vital to understanding hopelessness: experiential process, transcendent/spiritual process, rational process, and relational process (Farran et al., 1995). These four attributes are integrated with the definition, defining characteristics, and related factors of Hopelessness proposed by NANDA, as noted in Table 46-1.

Experiential Process. Hopelessness has been described as an experiential process—it affects one's feelings, thoughts, and behaviors (Farran et al., 1995). Etiologically, hopelessness has often been described in relation to such painful and inescapable situations as concentration camp or prisoner of war experiences (Frankl, 1963; Nardini, 1952) and as involving a sense of "trial, captivity or suffering" (Fromm, 1968; Marcel, 1962; Moltmann, 1975). The experience of hopelessness also involves feelings of powerlessness concerning one's ability to change these external circumstances (Frankl, 1978).

Hopelessness, powerlessness, and depression are particularly relevant to elderly persons and are reflected in NANDA's definition, defining characteristics, and related factors. While occurring at a different level than actual concentration camp or prisoner of war experiences, hopelessness that is associated with such etiologies as "prolonged activity restriction, failing or deteriorating physiological condition, and long-term stress" creates its own feelings of being trapped and personalizes one's experiences with "trial, captivity, and suffering." The feelings of powerlessness and depression associated with hopelessness are reflected in such terms as "sees no alternatives or personal choices and is unable to mobilize energy on own behalf." Powerlessness and depression are further characterized by major defining characteristics such as passivity, decreased verbalization, decreased affect, and verbal cues such as "I can't" and by minor characteristics such as lack of initiative, decreased response to stimuli, decreased appetite, changes in sleep patterns, and lack of involvement in care or passive allowing of care (Carpenito, 1995).

Suicidal thoughts and behaviors associated with hopelessness exist when the "individual is at risk for inflicting direct harm" (Carpenito, 1995, p. 832). An individual may just think about suicide (ideation), may have an actual plan, and/or may make an actual suicide attempt.

Transcendent or Spiritual Process. Persons who feel hopeless misperceive their own spiritual or transcendent potential (Farran et al., 1995). They might talk about the "black cloud" that hovers over them or declare that "God has withdrawn himself from me" (Marcel, 1962, p. 47). A characteristic of hopelessness is a particular muteness or inability to cry out to a "Higher Power" or other persons (Soelle, 1975). Questions such as "Why?," "Why me?," or "What do I make of this experience?" may be identified, but not articulated. NANDA has attempted to capture this impaired transcendent process by including in specified signs and symptoms decreased verbalization or verbal cues; including as a related factor lost belief in transcendent values/God also reflects an impaired transcendent process (Carpenito, 1995). Transcendence or the ability to "rise above" one's current situation may also occur on a more individual/personal level.

Rational or Irrational Thought Process. Hopelessness has been described as an irrational thought process that may involve alterations in at least five areas: goals, resources, action, control, and time perspective (Farran et al., 1995). Hopelessness, as an irrational thought process, is further compared and contrasted with NANDA's definition, defining characteristics, and related factors (Table 46-1).

CASE STUDY

D. Martin was a 65-year-old widowed female who lived in her own home. She was oriented to person, place, and time. Her physical problems began about 2 years previously when she fell after leaving an Al Anon meeting. She broke her ankle and at the same time was diagnosed with Parkinson's disease. For the next year she managed well in her own home. One year later she suffered a stroke that resulted in right hemiplegia. She spent many months in a rehabilitation center and was eventually discharged to her home with assistance. One person stayed with her during days, and another came for the night. The Parkinson's disease continued to progress, making ambulation and activities of daily living more difficult, but not impossible. She was admitted to a community-based mental health

program for older adults and treated for depression over an 8-month period.

Three days after her stroke, her husband went on a drinking spree, had a massive heart attack, and died in the intensive care unit. Mrs. Martin described his death as a "suicide." Mrs. Martin was unable to see her husband or attend his funeral. The two of them had a pact in which they agreed, "that she would go first because he was more of a loner and could do without other people." Mrs. Martin felt betrayed and abandoned after his death.

Mrs. Martin's mother had died 4 years previously. Mrs. Martin's family had a history of caring for their elders, including Mrs. Martin's grandmother, an aunt, Mr. Martin's father, and Mrs. Martin's mother. Mrs. Martin's only daughter died at the age of 7 from rheumatic heart disease. The daughter would have been 36 years old at the time of Mrs. Martin's stroke. Mrs. Martin felt that, in spite of having been a caregiver all of her life, she now had no family members to care for her.

Mrs. Martin's diagnosis of hopelessness was etiologically related to her numerous long-term stressors, including changes in her own physical health and loss of significant relationships (experiential attributes of hopelessness). She had spiritual distress as evidenced by her feelings of abandonment and her difficulty understanding why a loving God would have let her suffer so (Transcendent/Spiritual attribute of hopelessness). Mrs. Martin's hopelessness was further evidenced in her discouragement about her current situation and concerns about what would become of her in the future (rational aspects of hopelessness). Her goal was to stay in her own home as long as possible. She had adequate financial resources for the time being. Her personal energy fluctuated day to day, and her prolonged activity restriction made it difficult at times to take appropriate action or to mobilize energy on her own behalf. She felt a sense of powerlessness in that many events in the past had been out of her control, but she possessed a sense of personal fortitude and stick-to-itiveness. She had faced difficult life experiences in the past, she was discouraged about her present situation, and she longed for a time in the future where things might be better. Mrs. Martin had a history of strong family caring relationships, although she felt abandoned by her husband and young daughter. She enjoyed the workers who were placed in her home. She often talked with and was consoled by her cocker spaniel, Chi Chi.

NURSING-SENSITIVE OUTCOMES

The four attributes of hopelessness provide a basis for identifying outcomes (Iowa Outcomes Project, 2000). Outcomes may be relevant to several attributes of hopelessness, but are not always duplicated for brevity. Table 46-1 summarizes these outcomes by attribute.

The major outcome of interest relevant to the experiential process attribute of Hopelessness is Hope. Other supporting outcomes might include Acceptance: Health

Status, Psychosocial Adjustment: Life Change, Endurance, Grief Resolution, Quality of Life, Rest, Symptom Control, Well-Being, and Will to Live (Iowa Outcomes Project, 2000). In the event that depression accompanies the individual's feelings of hopelessness, appropriate outcomes would include Acceptance: Health Status, Distorted Thought Control, Hope, Mood Equilibrium, Psychosocial Adjustment: Life Change, Quality of Life, Self-Esteem, Sleep, and Will to Live (Iowa Outcomes Project, 2000). Outcomes associated with suicidal thoughts/behaviors would include Impulse Control, Self-Mutilation Restraint, and Suicide Self-Restraint (Iowa Outcomes Project, 2000).

Outcomes relevant to the transcendent/spiritual process attribute of Hopelessness include improved Coping, Spiritual Well-Being (Iowa Outcomes Project, 2000), and increased meaning and purpose-in-life.

Outcomes pertinent to the rational/irrational attributes of Hopelessness might include the following: goals—Decision Making and Information Processing; intrapersonal resources—Energy Conservation, Rest, and Role Performance; interpersonal resources—Loneliness, Social Involvement, and Social Support; environmental resources—Knowledge: Health Behaviors, Knowledge: Health Resources, and Rest; action—Decision Making and Improved Leisure Participation; control—Distorted Thought Control and Health Beliefs: Perceived Control (Iowa Outcomes Project, 2000).

Outcomes associated with the relational attribute of hopelessness could include Caregiver Emotional Health, Caregiver-Patient Relationship, Caregiver Stressors, Caregiver Well-Being, Communication: Expressive Ability, Health Beliefs: Perceived Resources, Loneliness, Social Interaction Skills, and Social Involvement (Iowa Outcomes Project, 2000).

NURSING INTERVENTIONS

Nursing interventions can be categorized by the four attributes of Hopelessness identified earlier. Table 46-1 identifies Nursing Interventions Classification (NIC) intervention labels that can be used in response to these attributes of hopelessness (Iowa Intervention Project, 2000). Intervention labels can be used in response to several attributes, but are listed just once for brevity.

Experiential Process Interventions

Interventions that respond to the experiential attribute of hopelessness acknowledge the physical, psychologic, and spiritual pain that can precipitate hopelessness. The major intervention is that of Hope Instillation, which can be further supported by a broad range of interventions (Table 46-1). Interventions for persons who are experiencing depression and suicidal ideation/behaviors in both outpatient and inpatient psychiatric settings also are summarized in Table 46-1. The major intervention for depres-

sion is Mood Management, although this would be supported by a variety of other interventions (Table 46-1). For suicidal thoughts/behaviors, the main interventions would include Suicide Prevention and Surveillance.

Transcendent or Spiritual Process

The primary interventions in this category are Spiritual Support and Values Clarification (Table 46-1). These interventions are further supported by a thorough assessment of "the individual's source of love and relatedness, means of forgiveness, meaning and purpose-in-life and hopes" (Farran et al., 1995, pp. 112-113). Persons with a prior spiritual practice can be assisted to maintain or reconnect with the spiritual/religious base or rituals that have provided comfort in the past. If the individual does not espouse a prior or current spiritual/religious tradition, more general interventions can focus on enhancing the person's coping skills and ability to transcend the situation on a personal level. In any case, interventions should acknowledge the individual's muteness or inability to "give voice" to the questions and concerns raised by his particular situation. Interventions also should work toward assisting the individual to "make sense" or find meaning in his current situation, since having meaning and purpose in life is vital to resolving hopelessness (Korner, 1970).

Rational or Irrational Thought Process

Existing research has consistently noted the importance of cognitive strategies for maintaining hope and diminishing hopelessness (Herth, 1990a, 1990b; Hull, 1989; Miller, 1985, 1991; Wright, 1983).

Since Hopelessness is often marked by difficulties in establishing realistic goals, a major focus of interventions is on Mutual Goal Setting (Table 46-1). Interventions may be directed further toward assisting individuals to be flexible in modifying their goals as their situation worsens, to be realistic in assessing their progress in meeting their goals (Wright, 1983), and to define progress in "the twitch of a toe rather than in the steps of the dance."

Effective interventions also are aimed toward bolstering the individual's intrapersonal, interpersonal, and environmental/sociologic resources. Intrapersonal attributes such as determination, courage, and optimism are vital to regaining Hope (Herth, 1990a, 1990b; Miller, 1991). Interventions for Hopelessness might include Assertiveness Training, Bibliotherapy, Simple Guided Imagery, and to listen to uplifting music (Herth, 1990a, 1990b; Miller, 1991). Humor has frequently been cited as another intrapersonal means of dispelling Hopelessness (Herth, 1990a, 1993; Miller, 1991). Energy Management is essential for the mobilization of hope and prevention of Hopelessness (Herth, 1990a, 1990b). Other interventions are summarized in Table 46-1.

Interventions directed toward bolstering interpersonal resources involve the mobilization of the individual's informal and formal social support network, including support groups, assistance with meals and shopping, assistance with personal care, and respite care. Environmental/sociologic resources that diminish hopelessness might involve simply "being with" the individual and initiating abuse protection, if necessary.

Persons who feel hopeless often take no action, appropriate action toward an inappropriate goal, or misguided action. Persons may need to be taught reality surveillance skills so that they can assume greater self-responsibility and ground their hope in reality (Wright & Shontz, 1968). Increasing the number of pleasurable events through increased activity and/or recreation also can decrease levels of hopelessness and depression (Teri & Gallagher-Thompson, 1991).

Persons who feel hopeless often perceive that their lives are out of control. Thorough assessment needs to be directed toward determining what perceptions of control are distorted (internal/external control) and what events or responses can realistically be controlled. Appropriate interventions include Health Education, Learning Facilitation, and Teaching: Individual (Table 46-1). Cognitive-behavioral interventions can assist persons to gain a more realistic picture of which events can be controlled (Beck, 1967). Creative but simple methods of facilitating control also might be needed. A nursing home study found that residents who were given a plant to care for and allowed increased choice and control reported lower levels of hopelessness and depression.

The continuity between one's past, present, and future can be disrupted in persons who feel hopeless. Persons who are seriously ill have often reported that their feelings about the future are quantified not in calendar time, but rather through family and through meaning attached to life events (Herth, 1990a). Reminiscence Therapy has been an effective intervention for dealing with past, present, and future events and has been associated with decreased levels of depression.

Relationships are crucial to the mobilization, support, or maintenance of Hope and to the prevention of Hopelessness in elders (Farran et al., 1995; Herth, 1990a, 1990b, 1993). Enhancement of a sense of connectedness within a caring environment has consistently been identified as critical to fostering Hope in persons, regardless of their age or health condition (Haase, Britt, Coward, Leidy, & Penn, 1992). Hope-fostering strategies are summarized in the following paragraphs and in Table 46-1.

Complex relationship building, including being present, available, and actively listening to clients and their family, is an important Hope-fostering strategy (Farran et al., 1995). Research suggests that Hope and Hopelessness are "contagious," that what one person does affects another, and that positive interpersonal relationships between nurse, patient, and family are vital to maintaining

Hope and preventing Hopelessness (Wake & Miller, 1992). Nurses serve as catalysts to create internal and external conditions that assist patients and families to share and pass on their feelings.

Other Hope-fostering strategies involve competent care and comfort directed toward the patient, family teaching concerning what should be anticipated, and allowing family members to be physically present with a loved one (Family Integrity Promotion, Family Process Maintenance, and Family Support) (Hull, 1989; Miller, 1991). Attachment ideation (Miller, 1985) encourages patients to talk about the persons most significant to them, to focus on their loved one's attributes, and to reminisce about happy experiences that have been shared. Even if the person is confused or unresponsive, the nurse can use attachment ideation through statements like the following: "Hazel was here; it sounds as though you two had great fun at your cottage."

To instill and maintain hope in others requires that the nurse must have hope, love, and confidence in herself (Farran et al., 1995; Herth, 1989; Miller, 1991; Watson, 1985). "Being with" the patient, the "therapeutic use of self" and belief in the nurse-patient relationship as a partnership rather than an expert relationship are keys to fostering Hope (O'Malley & Menke, 1988).

CASE STUDY

Outcomes established with Mrs. Martin included Psychosocial Adjustment: Life Change and Grief Resolution. She did not agree to the outcomes Acceptance: Health Status or Grief Resolution, stating, "I can acknowledge the death of my young daughter, but accept it . . . no, never."

The nurse went to Mrs. Martin's home once weekly for 8 months. To assist Mrs. Martin in dealing with her changes in physical health and loss of significant relationships, the nurse focused on first establishing a trusting relationship (Erikson, 1982). Interventions included Active Listening, Anxiety Reduction, Calming Technique, Counseling, Emotional Support, Grief Work Facilitation, Guilt Work Facilitation, Hope Instillation, Self-Awareness Enhancement, and Self-Care Assistance. Since her symptoms of depression were evident primarily in mood changes, interventions were directed toward mood management. Mrs. Martin evidenced no suicidal thoughts or behaviors.

In response to her questions about God and suffering, interventions were directed toward spiritual support. Mrs. Martin had been active in a local congregation, and her pastor regularly came to see her and provide communion. Mrs. Martin's prior association with Al Anon further supported her transcendent/spiritual attributes. She maintained regular contact with her sponsor, regularly practiced cognitive-restructuring techniques such as "Let go and let God," and often recited the Serenity Prayer.

Mrs. Martin's goal to remain in her own home was realistic, considering her financial resources. Her primary area of difficulty was that she had such negative expectations concerning her goals. Decision-Making Support and

Mutual Goal Setting were the primary interventions used by the nurse.

Mrs. Martin's intrapersonal resources included a strong sense of personhood, courage, and humor in spite of multiple life changes; however, her energy fluctuated, given her Parkinson's disease and residual stroke damage. Her assertiveness skills, self-esteem, and sense of humor were supported; her coping skills were enhanced; and her limited energy was managed.

Although she felt abandoned by the deaths of her husband and daughter, she established an affectionate relationship with her daytime in-home worker. Interventions were directed toward Grief Work Facilitation and Anger Control Assistance. Support was provided to both of her caregivers. At one point it became apparent that the nighttime care worker was emotionally abusing Mrs. Martin. Elder Abuse Protection Support interventions were initiated, and that caregiver was removed from the home.

Mrs. Martin's primary area of difficulty was with passivity. Behavioral modification approaches were useful, as was Self-Responsibility Facilitation.

Mrs. Martin desired high levels of internal control in the face of uncontrollable external events such as her own health, but experienced low feelings of external control pertaining to events such as her husband's "suicidal" death. Techniques of reality Surveillance were used (Wright & Shontz, 1968), as were Grief Work Facilitation, Guilt Work Facilitation, and Anger Control Assistance.

Mrs. Martin's feelings primarily focused on present feelings of hopelessness. She was encouraged to ventilate her feelings of anger and to reminisce about her past positive experiences.

In addition to interventions noted for interpersonal resources, Animal-Assisted Therapy was initiated. Mrs. Martin's dog generally sat on the floor right next to her during home visits. If Mrs. Martin cried, her dog cocked his head and seemed to understand. In some cases, both the nurse and Mrs. Martin used the dog as an intermediary. Mrs. Martin would tell the dog things that she was not quite ready to incorporate within her own personhood, and the nurse would make suggestions to the dog that Mrs. Martin was not quite ready to hear.

Mrs. Martin's depressive symptoms became more controlled over time as she coped with her stressors. Her limited energy was managed, and her mood and self-esteem improved. Mrs. Martin exhibited higher levels of hopefulness in terms of personal satisfaction; she maintained her spiritual connectedness with herself, Al Anon friends, others, and God. Mrs. Martin eventually made the decision to sell her own home and move to another state with her daytime worker, Rose, and her husband. Upon her dismissal from the mental health program, she was processing information concerning her care, participating in leisure activities such as watching TV, and acknowledging an increase in perceived control and will to live. The relationship between Mrs. Martin and her caregiver was based on positive interactions and connections. Rose, in a sense, became Mrs. Martin's daughter. Mrs. Martin worked with her attorney to ensure that her assets were protected, while at the same time providing remuneration to Rose for her care. Upon her dismissal from the mental health program, her social environment was safe and she continued to have social involvement and support from others.

SUMMARY

The prevention of Hopelessness and maintenance of Hope in elderly persons are of vital importance. Often feelings of hopelessness are accompanied by depression and possibly even suicidal thoughts and behaviors. It is vital for clinicians to understand that hopelessness, depression, and suicidal behaviors are treatable maladies.

Treatment involves an acknowledgment of the experiential aspects of the elderly person's situation that causes feelings of hopelessness. Acknowledgement of the individual's lament and underlying feelings is vital. Interventions also necessitate a "calling forth" of the individual's transcendent/spiritual attributes. While not everyone owns a spiritual heritage, each elderly person owns a history of having already "made it through" multiple difficult life experiences. These existing qualities need to be called forth in a rational way. Elderly persons can be assisted to examine their goals, resources, actions, feelings of control, and perspective of time. Relationships are vital and provide an anchor and a way out of Hopelessness. Expected outcomes include adjustment to life circumstances, improved coping abilities, improved mood and self-esteem, and improved relationships. The outcomes most desired are decreased hopelessness, increased hope, and will to live.

REFERENCES

Abraham, I. (1991). The geriatric depression scale and hopelessness index: Longitudinal psychometric data on frail nursing home residents. *Perceptual and Motor Skills 72*, 875-878.

American Psychiatric Association. (1987). *Diagnostic and statistical manual of mental disorders (DSM-III-R)* (3rd ed., rev.). Washington, DC: Author.

Averill, J. R., Catlin, G., & Chon, K. K. (1990). *Rules of hope.* New York: Springer.

Beck, A. T. (1963). Thinking and depression. *Archives of General Psychiatry, 9*, 324-333.

Beck, A. T. (1967). *Depression: Clinical, experimental, and theoretical aspects.* New York: Harper & Row.

Beck, A. T., Brown, G., Berchick, R. J., Stewart, B. L., & Steer, R. A. (1990). Relationships between hopelessness and ultimate suicide: A replication with psychiatric outpatients. *American Journal of Psychiatry, 147*(2), 190-195.

Beck, A. T., Kovacs, M., & Weissman, A. (1975). Hopelessness and suicidal behavior. *Journal of American Medical Association, 234*(11), 1146-1149.

Beck, A. T., Steer, R. A., Kovacs, M., & Garrison, B. (1985). Hopelessness and eventual suicide: A 10-year prospective study of patients hospitalized with suicidal ideation. *American Journal of Psychiatry, 142*, 559-563.

Beck, A. J., Steer, R. A., & Ranieri, W. F. (1988). Scale for suicide ideation: Psychometric properties of a self-report version. *Journal of Clinical Psychology, 44*, 499-505.

Beck, A. T., Weissman, A., Lester, D., & Trexler, L. (1974). The measurement of pessimism: The hopelessness scale. *Journal of Consulting and Clinical Psychology, 42*(6), 861-865.

Carpenito, L. J. (1995). *Nursing diagnosis: Application to clinical practice.* Baltimore: Lippincott Williams & Wilkins.

Engel, G. L. (1968). A life setting conducive to illness: The giving up–given up complex. *Annals of Internal Medicine, 69,* 293-300.

Erikson, E. H. (1982). *The life cycle completed: A review.* New York: W. W. Norton.

Farran, C. J., Herth, K. A., & Popovich, J. M. (1995). *Hope and hopelessness: Critical clinical constructs.* Thousand Oaks, CA: Sage.

Farran, C. J., & Popovich, J. (1990). Hope: A relevant concept for geriatric psychiatry. *Archives in Psychiatric Nursing, 4,* 127-130.

Frank, J. (1968). The role of hope in psychotherapy. *International Journal of Psychiatry, 5*(5), 383-395.

Frankl, V. E. (1963). *Man's search for meaning.* New York: Washington Square Press.

Frankl, V. E. (1978). *The unheard cry for meaning.* New York: Washington Square Press.

Fromm, E. (1968). *The revolution of hope: Toward a humanized technology.* New York: Harper & Row.

Fry, P. (1984). Development of a geriatric scale of hopelessness. *Journal of Counseling Psychology, 31*(3), 322-331.

Grimm, P. (1984). *The state-trait hope inventory: A measurement project.* Unpublished manuscript, University of Maryland School of Nursing.

Haase, J., Britt, T., Coward, D., Leidy, N., & Penn, P. (1992). Simultaneous concept analysis of spiritual perspective, hope, acceptance and self-transcendence. *IMAGE: Journal of Nursing Scholarship, 24*(2), 141-147.

Herth, K. A. (1989). The relationship between level of hope and level of coping response and other variables in patients with cancer. *Oncology Nursing Forum, 16*(1), 67-72.

Herth, K. A. (1990a). Fostering hope in terminally ill people. *Journal of Advanced Nursing, 15,* 1250-1259.

Herth, K. A. (1990b). The relationship between hope, coping styles, concurrent losses, and setting to grief resolution in elderly widow(er)s. *Research in Nursing and Health, 13,* 109-117.

Herth, K. A. (1991). Development and refinement of an instrument to measure hope. *Scholarly Inquiry for Nursing Practice: An International Journal, 5*(1), 39-51.

Herth, K. A. (1992). An abbreviated instrument to measure hope: Development and psychometric evaluation. *Journal of Advanced Nursing, 17,* 1251-1259.

Herth, K. A. (1993). Hope in older adults in community and institutional settings. *Issues in Mental Health Nursing, 14*(2), 139-156.

Horton-Deutsch, S., Clark, D. C., & Farran, C. J. (1992). Chronic dyspnea and suicide in elderly men. *Hospital and Community Psychiatry, 43*(12), 1198-1203.

Hull, M. (1989). Family needs and supportive nursing behavior during terminal cancer: A review. *Oncology Nursing Forum, 16,* 787-792.

Iowa Intervention Project. J. C. McCloskey & G. M. Bulechek (Eds.). (2000). *Nursing Interventions Classification (NIC)* (3rd ed.). St. Louis, MO: Mosby.

Iowa Outcomes Project. M. Johnson, M. Maas, & S. Moorhead (Eds.). (2000). *Nursing Outcomes Classification (NOC)* (2nd ed.). St. Louis, MO: Mosby.

Isani, R. (1963). From hopelessness to hope. *Perspectives in Psychiatric Care, 1*(2), 15-17.

Kastenbaum, R., & Kastenbaum, B. S. (1971). Hope, survival, and the caring environment. In E. Palmare & F. D. Jeffers (Eds.), *Prediction of life span* (pp. 249-271). Lexington, MA: Heath Lexington Books.

Korner, J. N. (1970). Hope as a method of coping. *Journal of Consulting and Clinical Psychology, 34*(2), 134-139.

LeShan, L. (1989). *Cancer as a turning point.* New York: E. P. Dutton.

Lynch, W. F. (1965). *Images of hope: Imagination as healer of the hopeless.* Baltimore: Helicon Press.

Marcel, G. (1962). *Homo viator: Introduction to a metaphysics of hope* (E. Crawford Trans.). New York: Harper & Row.

McIntosh, J. (1995). Suicide prevention in the elderly (age 65-99). *Suicide and Life-Threatening Behaviors, 25*(1), 22-35.

Melges, F. T., & Bowlby, J. (1969). Types of hopelessness in psycho-pathological process. *Archives of General Psychiatry, 20,* 690-699.

Mercier, M., Fawcett, J., & Clark, D. (1984). *Hopefulness: A preliminary examination.* Unpublished manuscript, Rush-Presbyterian-St. Luke's Medical Center, Chicago.

Miller, J. F. (1985, Jan.). Inspiring hope. *American Journal of Nursing,* 22-25.

Miller, J. F. (1991). Developing and maintaining hope in families of the critically ill. *AACN Clinical Issues, 2*(2), 307-315.

Miller, J. F., & Powers, M. (1988). Development of an instrument to measure hope. *Nursing Research, 37*(1), 6-10.

Moltmann, J. (1975). *The experiment hope.* Philadelphia: Fortress Press.

Nardini, J. E. (1952). Survival factors in American prisoners of war of the Japanese. *American Journal of Psychiatry, 109,* 241-248.

Nauman, S. E. (1971). *The new dictionary of existentialism.* New York: Philosophical Library.

North American Nursing Diagnosis Association. (1999). *Nursing diagnoses: Definitions & classification 1999-2000.* Philadelphia: Author.

Nowotny, M. (1989). Assessment of hope in patients with cancer: Development of an instrument. *Oncology Nursing Forum, 16*(1), 75-79.

O'Malley, P., & Menke, E. (1988). Relationship of hope and stress after M.I. *Heart & Lung, 17*(2), 184-190.

Osgood, N. J. (1992). *Recognizing the warning signs.* New York: Lexington Books.

Rotter, J. B. (1966). Generalized expectations for internal versus external control of reinforcement. *Psychological Monographs: General and Applied, 80*(1), Whole No. 609, 1-18.

Schmale, A. H., & Iker, H. P. (1971). Hopelessness as a predictor of cervical cancer. *Social Science and Medicine, 5,* 95-100.

Schulz, R. (1980). Aging and control. In J. Garber & M. E. P. Seligman (Eds.), *Human helplessness theory and applications* (pp. 261-277). San Diego, CA: Academic Press.

Seligman, M. E. P. (1975). *Helplessness: On depression, development, and death.* San Francisco, CA: W. H. Freeman.

Snyder, C., Harris, C., Anderson, J., Holleran, S., Irving, L., Sigmon, S., Yoshinobu, L., Gibb, J., Langelle, C., & Harney, P. (1991). The will and the ways: Development and validation of an individual-differences measure of hope. *Journal of Personality and Social Psychology, 60*(4), 570-585.

Soelle, D. (1975). *Suffering* (E. R. Kalin, Trans.). Philadelphia: Fortress Press. (Original work published 1973.)

Solomon, K. (1982). Social antecedents of learned helplessness in the health care setting. *The Gerontologist, 22*(3), 282-287.

Staats, S. (1987). Hope: Expected positive affect in an adult sample. *Journal of Genetic Psychology, 148*(3), 357-364.

Stoner, M. (1988). Measuring hope. In M. Stromborg (Ed.), *Instruments for clinical nursing practice* (pp. 133-140). Norwalk, CT: Appleton & Lange.

Stotland, E. (1969). *The psychology of hope.* San Francisco: Jossey-Bass.

Teri, L., & Gallagher-Thompson, D. (1991). Cognitive-behavioral interventions for treatment of depression in Alzheimer's patients. *The Gerontologist, 31*(3), 413-416.

Uncapher, H., Gallagher-Thompson, D., Osgood, N. J., & Bongar, B. (1998). Hopelessness and suicidal ideation in older adults. *The Gerontologist, 38*(1), 62-70.

Wake, M., & Miller, J. (1992). Treating hopelessness; Nursing strategies from six countries. *Clinical Nursing Research, 1*(4), 347-365.

Watson, J. (1985). *Nursing: the philosophy and science of caring.* Denver, CO: Associated University Press.

Wright, B. (1983). Coping, succumbing, and hoping. In *Physical disability: A psychosocial approach* (2nd ed., pp. 193-216). New York: Harper & Row.

Wright, B., & Shontz, F. (1968). Process and tasks in hoping. *Rehabilitation Literature, 29*(11), 322-331.

Yalom, I. D. (1980). *Existential psychotherapy.* New York: Basic Books.

Yesavage, J. A. (1988). Geriatric depression scale. *Psychopharmacology Bulletin, 24*(4), 709-711.

VIII

Role-Relationship Pattern

OVERVIEW

In Chapter 47 Bunten reviews the normal changes in roles and relationships across the life span and observes that most changes in aging are associated with individuals exiting formal roles. She discusses factors believed to ease role transitions, including the assumption of new roles for the elder, and the importance of social support.

In Chapter 48, Relocation Stress Syndrome, Johnson explores the significance of the diagnosis for nursing practice and for the well-being of institutionalized elders. The author reviews the extensive research documenting the primarily negative effects of relocation on elders and suggests objective assessment tools to evaluate for these effects. NIC interventions are discussed in the context of the major general interventions found in the literature, preparation for relocation, and facilitating decision-making control. Finally, the author identifies outcomes sensitive to nursing intervention, including the broad outcome Psychosocial Adjustment: Life Change and several more specific outcomes and measures. She suggests revisions in NIC and NOC that would facilitate the use of these classifications in nursing practice and research relevant to this diagnosis.

In Chapter 49 Whiting and Buckwalter offer a conceptualization of Grieving that takes issue with the traditional view. The concept is reframed from the point of view of the elderly person who is experiencing grief. The authors argue that a dysfunctional, problem-oriented perspective promotes labeling on the part of caregivers, tends to negate the highly individualized nature of the grief experience, and discourages the use of nursing interventions that provide support and facilitate coping throughout the normal process of grieving. Nursing assessment is described in depth. The nursing intervention ENUF (empathy, nonjudgment, unconditional positive regard, feeling focus) is recommended as an approach to assist the grieving individual. Outcomes useful for evaluating

nursing interventions are identified, including the NOC outcome Coping and other coping-related perceptions specific to the grieving process.

In Chapter 50 on Social Isolation, Waterman, Blegen, Clinton, and Specht define the diagnosis as the quantity and quality of social contact below that required to sustain an individual's well-being. The authors discuss etiology in terms of barriers to social contact and suggest combining two NANDA diagnoses, Social Isolation and Impaired Social Interaction, into a single diagnosis using the label of the former. Authors also identify defining characteristics for the proposed diagnosis, nursing-sensitive outcomes, and interventions to overcome barriers to social contact and to support the patient until barriers are overcome.

Elders experience a high incidence of cerebral vascular accidents, as well as other conditions that result in impaired communication. Impaired communication often disrupts role behaviors and relationships for elders. In Chapter 51 Emick-Herring discusses the physiology of communication problems and focuses on communication diagnoses, including Impaired Verbal Communication: Aphasia and Impaired Verbal Communication: Dysarthria. The author recommends augmenting these diagnostic labels to include nonverbal communication. She discusses several types of aphasia, including expressive, receptive, and global. The important role of the nurse and the interdisciplinary team in providing interventions in the categories of environmental management, support behaviors, behavior to enhance communication, and education is addressed. The importance of an appropriate environment for language retraining and for reinforcement and assistance with prescribed speech therapy is emphasized. The author offers suggestions for changes in NIC and NOC to enhance their usefulness for clinical practice with this diagnosis.

Family members today are responsible for a good share of the care dependent elders receive. In Chapter 52 Given, Kozachik, Collins, DeVoss, and Given discuss the role strain that accompanies informal care and suggest diagnostic-specific interventions and outcomes using the standardized nursing language classifications.

In Chapter 53, Risk for Violence: Self-Directed or Directed at Others, Ingram deals with the phenomenon of violent behavior that is a common concern for health care professionals who work with institutionalized elders. Using a model of prediction of violence developed by Stokman, the author describes the diagnosis and its assessment in three spheres: long-term vulnerabilities; short-term stressors; and contextual triggers. Selection of the most appropriate NIC interventions and NOC outcomes is also discussed.

In Chapter 54 on Self-Determination, Weiler and Moorhead discuss the right of elderly persons to make personal health care decisions. This diagnosis is particularly important because changes in physical and/or mental

capacity can subject elders to imbalanced power relationships with loss of autonomy when they enter the health care delivery system. Advanced directives, such as the living will and durable power of attorney, are discussed along with the need for nurses to understand the wishes and preferences of elderly persons. The use of NIC interventions and NOC outcomes is demonstrated using four case studies, and suggestions are made for future work on the diagnosis Self-Determination and related interventions and outcomes.

In Chapter 55, Altered Family Processes, Davis examines the role of nursing diagnosis and intervention within the context of the family in the community. Family assessment tools are presented and evaluated. The author uses a case study to illustrate assessment, diagnosis, interventions, and outcomes related to both family process and family caregiving skills.

CHAPTER 47

NORMAL CHANGES WITH AGING

Donna Bunten

Role and relationship pattern describes an individual's perception of his major roles and associated responsibilities in his current situation, including whether interactions and relationships are satisfying. Interaction requires that the elderly person have the ability and desire to communicate and available opportunities for socialization. Role and relationship entrances and exits, threats of change or loss, and transitions between roles present major challenges for aging adults. Aging successfully requires continual adaptation to change within the individual, the family, and the broader environment.

ROLE CHANGES

Most role changes in early life are entrances involving voluntary assumptions of increasing responsibility. Role changes in later life are more often exits, which may be involuntary and/or result in the loss of responsibility (Aiken, 1995; Atchley, 1994; Binstock & George, 1994; Dugan & Kivett, 1994; Pearlin & Skaff, 1996). The mental, emotional, and physical health of people of all ages is related to their ability to cope with and adapt to the changes in their lives. Adaptation to changes in roles and relationships may be facilitated in several ways. During the life course, events such as the transition from worker to retiree or from active parent to grandparent are examples of normative events associated with advancing age (Atchley, 1994). Many adults prepare for expected changes, and this preparation assists in smoothing out transitions (Atchley, 1994; Solomon, 1996). Solomon (1996) points out that, "Life changes per se do not create stress, rather, adverse effects result from events that are considered unexpected or for which people are unprepared" (p. 48).

Other factors can ease transitions between roles and relationships: being aware of the problem, having a supportive milieu, having a positive attitude, feeling a sense of control over the situation, and having the knowledge to satisfactorily adjust to whatever change(s) might be involved (Ebersole & Hess, 1998). The importance of roles in assisting elders to adapt to change comes from the affiliations, prestige, status, wealth, and influence associated with them (Atchley, 1994). Having at least one major role sustained during loss or transition is helpful when adapting to change (Carter & Cook, 1995). For example, an elderly woman who is involved in a supportive relationship with her children will find the role of mother helping her through the transition from wife to widow. Relationships offer a means of support for individuals by acting as a buffer against stress and stressful events (Carter & Cook, 1995). All associations, whether with family, friends, work groups, religious groups, or other social groups, give people information about the appropriateness of their behavior and act to reinforce their identity and self-esteem (Binstock & George, 1994).

Roles and relationships can change in many ways across the life span. Some roles cease to exist. People retire or lose their spouses. New roles can emerge. The grandparent role presents itself to many as a new and satisfying role. Some roles and relationships continue through late maturity, but change in nature. Markus and Herzog (1991) describe, for example, the change that occurs in the parent and child relationship through the years. The parent of a young child provides large amounts of physical and emotional care. Being the parent of a middle-aged or older adult can involve a reversal in the nature of the relationship, with the parent accepting guidance or even physical support from the mature child.

Elders have generally been identified as being able to adapt successfully to change and to any associated stress during transitions between roles and/or relationships. Individual differences, especially in the older person's desire and ability to make or enhance new roles and supportive relationships, will affect successful adaptation to change (Hansson & Carpenter, 1994). For many elderly individuals the period of transition between roles and relationships is a time to develop new and enriching relationships and activities (Ebersole & Hess, 1998; Hansson & Carpenter, 1994).

Many elderly persons find that retirement and widowhood affect established patterns of behavior and relationships. Successful adaptation to these role changes primarily depends on the self-reported importance of the role lost to the person's identity and on the availability of new roles to substitute for the old ones (Carter & Cook, 1995).

Some of today's cohort of older persons are victims of mandatory retirement. Forced retirement left them without the functional role of worker that had contributed to their positive sense of self and justified their social future. Newer generations of elderly people working in most public and private positions find legislation protecting them from mandatory retirement. Workers today may choose to take early retirement offered by many organizations. The person who chooses to retire is still faced with the adjustments associated with becoming a retired person. Carter and Cook (1995) found that having good health and an adequate income are of paramount importance in the decision to retire and in finding satisfaction after that event. The presence of a strong social network, other roles, and activities and relationships that continue after retirement have a positive effect on the retired person's sense of well-being (Carter & Cook, 1995; Floyd et al., 1992; Freund & Smith, 1999).

Many older persons find retirement to be a period of increased fulfillment and participate in volunteer and other leisure activities. Binstock (1996) found that 63% of African-American elders and 53% of Caucasian elders surveyed were volunteers. Volunteering provides the rewards of enhancing self-esteem and feeling useful and offers a means for social and psychologic stimulation. Volunteer service done by elderly persons frequently fills gaps in social service programs, many of which assist other older persons (Ebersole & Hess, 1998).

Floyd et al. (1992) found that life satisfaction in retirement is associated with replacing rewards gained from work activities with rewarding leisure activities. Unfortunately, retirement planning seminars available to many adults today frequently ignore activity-oriented planning.

The elderly person who becomes widowed is also presented with many demands and opportunities. The older woman is more than three times as likely as the elderly man to be widowed (Taeuber, 1993). In 1990 nearly half of all women 65 years old or older were widowed, compared with only 14% of elderly men (American Association of Retired Persons, 1994). Elderly widows frequently found past fulfillment in activities centered around home and family, and many never worked outside of the home. Upon becoming widows these women find themselves faced with the loss not only of their companion, confidant, and sex partner, but also of their financial provider, business manager, household repairman, car mechanic, etc. Some elderly widows must seek employment to remain financially solvent, only to find that their lack of experience in the job market, lack of skills, and age itself make them less desirable in today's competitive job arena. They must negotiate responsibilities of these new and often uncomfortable roles in addition to working through the grief process itself. The need to learn new skills and develop new relationships can be viewed as a hardship, but it can also have a positive dimension (Anderson & Diamond, 1995). Elderly widows can develop a new and pleasing sense of self-reliance as they succeed in developing new skills and relationships.

Men who are widowed do not have an easier road than women in adjusting to life without their spouse. Common challenges faced by widowers focus around household chores such as cooking, meal planning, and initiating and planning social activities (Anderson & Diamond, 1995; Atchley, 1994; Campbell & Silverman, 1987). In three of four marriages the male dies first. Thus men don't expect to be left alone and are reported to be psychologically less prepared to be alone (Campbell & Silverman, 1987). Unlike widows, who are frequently found attending bereavement support groups or engaging in social activities together, older men have not formed groups based on their widowhood (Atchley, 1994). Older men are less likely to have a confidant other than their spouse. The Campbell and Silverman (1987) study reported that having a male confidant was most beneficial during adjustment to bereavement. These authors found that even when many male respondents were lacking such a friendship, they were reluctant to seek help or to accept help when it was offered. Field (1999), in reporting the results of the Berkeley Older Generation Longitudinal study, noted, "Men declined in number of new friends, in their desire for close friendships, in the less intimate nature of their interactions with friends, and in involvement in beyond-family activities, while women did not change" (p. 325).

ROLE ADAPTATIONS

Both widows and widowers have been found to benefit from social support, which can provide a link between traumatic life events and adjustment to a successful new life. Having someone to reach out to during bereavement has been found to result in less depression (Anderson & Diamond, 1995; Kanacki, Jones, & Galbraith, 1996) and decreased mortality rates (Ryan & Austin, 1989). Social support can act directly on health by serving as a buffer against the harmful physical and mental consequences of traumatic events (Mor-Barak, Miller, & Syme, 1991).

The loss of a spouse has been identified as the most important risk factor contributing to loneliness in later life. However, the loss or absence of any attachment figure (friend, relative, pet, etc.) contributes to feelings of emotional isolation, emptiness, and loneliness in elders (Austin, 1989; Dugan & Kivett, 1994; Weiss, 1973). Effective relationships are a necessary part of human function and lead to better health and the feeling of well-being for persons of all ages (Martire, Schulz, Mittelmark, & Newsom, 1999).

Studies of the benefits of relationships most often focus on the issue of social support, which typically is defined as the presence of a supportive network or support actions, attitudes, and emotional climate provided by others (Hansson & Carpenter, 1994). Three types of social support can be distinguished, with each providing a different type of benefit. Instrumental support provides tangible benefits such as money, housing, transportation, or shopping. Informational support provides new information, opinions, and other resources helpful with decision making and problem solving. Emotional support provides the sense of belonging and the benefit of feeling that someone cares and will give of themselves for you. Relationships can provide one or all of these benefits (Hansson & Carpenter, 1994). Support systems are also characterized as providing either formal or informal support. Informal support is traditionally defined as help provided by family and friends, while formal support is help provided by professionals (Fulks & Molinari, 1995).

Today, families continue to provide the bulk of instrumental and emotional support for older and/or chronically impaired relatives (van Tilburg, 1998). Increased life expectancies mean that more of today's elders will likely be in need of assistance. Consequently, adult caregivers can spend a longer period of years giving parent care than they did caring for their children (Hansson & Carpenter, 1994). However, future cohorts of elderly persons are more likely to enjoy better health in old age and need less assistance for shorter periods of time than previous cohorts (Silverstone, 1996).

Spouses are the major providers of help to persons under age 75 in the 1990s and in need of personal care, meal preparation, housework, or shopping. While these spouses may experience significant strain if they are also having health problems, they may find that caregiving provides them with a sense of purpose and competence.

If the older person cannot receive care from a spouse, the care is usually provided by one or more adult children. Adult daughters give the greatest proportion of care to widowed mothers. Women, particularly daughters, have been found to assume more responsibility for personal care than sons, who are more likely to provide supervision, transportation, and financial assistance (Atchley, 1994; Horowitz, 1985). Uhlenberg (1993) points out that most caregivers cite both positive and negative aspects of parent care and that many do not describe their caregiving as a burden. He postulates that other roles (spouse, parent, worker) may in fact have a positive influence on caregivers by producing buffering effects.

Several demographic and societal trends affect the family's participation in providing elder care: increases in the numbers of multigenerational families; increases in divorce; reconstructed and single-parent families; geographic mobility within families; fewer siblings found in younger generations to provide support; and a growing number of elderly individuals who are childless (Choi, 1994; Hansson & Carpenter, 1994). Ethnic background and the timing of family role transitions also affect the nature and availability of caregiving by families (Burton, 1996; Talamantes, Cornell, Espino, Lichtenstein, & Hazuda, 1996).

There is great variability in today's definition of family. The family might consist of married or unmarried couples, extended family members, same gender couples, or persons who are not actual kin of the elderly person but who have assumed family roles and responsibilities (Ebersole & Hess, 1998). All of a client's possible supportive relationships should be identified when addressing and attempting to meet the diverse needs of elderly individuals. Because of geographic remoteness and occupational obligations, families may play a decreasing role in providing direct care services needed by older people in the future. However, they likely will assume an increasingly important role in mediating between older persons and social and medical services. Caregivers will need education about available resources and the manipulation of bureaucratic procedures to help them support dependent elders. Potential caregivers must also be reminded that unasked-for support may be regarded as unpleasant by persons of all ages because of its implied incompetence (Smith & Goodnow, 1999).

Ryan and Austin (1989) remind nurses that available social support is salient to both physical and mental health in elders. The loss of physical, mental, social, and/or economic resources can change the position of the elderly person's place in the social world. The loss of productive roles, of significant others, of self-esteem, and perhaps of home and possessions put some older persons at risk for anxiety and fear associated with a world that is unfamiliar to them. These critical transitions are a hallmark of aging and require continual adaptation.

SUMMARY

The provision of opportunities to take advantage of an environment that offers new roles with defined responsibilities and new relationships will likely enhance the older person's feeling of well-being. Recognition of elderly individuals who are at risk for experiencing role and relationship changes and their possible detrimental effects can help health care professionals identify those who are likely to benefit most from various interventions.

REFERENCES

Aiken, L. R. (1995). *Aging: An introduction to gerontology.* Thousand Oaks, CA: Sage.

American Association of Retired Persons. (1994). *A profile of older Americans* (PF3049/1294/f996). Washington, DC: Program Resources Department.

Anderson, K. L., & Diamond, M. F. (1995). The experience of bereavement in older adults. *Journal of Advanced Nursing, 22,* 308-315.

Atchley, R. C. (1994). *Social forces and aging: An introduction to social gerontology* (17th ed., pp. 160-173). Belmont, CA: Wadsworth.

Austin, A. G. (1989). Becoming immune to loneliness: Helping the elderly fill the void. *Journal of Gerontology, 15*(9), 25-28.

Binstock, R. H. (1996). Our social selves grow older. *The Gerontologist, 36*(1), 124-128.

Binstock, R. H., & George, L. K. (1994). *Handbook of aging and the social sciences* (3rd ed.). San Diego, CA: Academic Press.

Burton, L. M. (1996). Age norms, the timing of family role transitions, and intergenerational caregiving among aging African American women. *The Gerontologist, 36*(2), 199-208.

Campbell, S., & Silverman, P. R. (1987). *Widower: When men are left alone.* New York: Prentice Hall Press.

Carter, M. A. T., & Cook, K. (1995, Sept.). Adaptation to retirement: Role changes and psychological resources. *The Career Development Quarterly, 44,* 67-82.

Choi, N. G. (1994). Patterns and determinants of social service utilization: Comparison of childless elderly and elderly parents living with or apart from their children. *The Gerontologist, 34*(3), 353-362.

Dugan, E., & Kivett, V. R. (1994). *Relationships in old age: Coping with the challenge of transition.* New York: Guilford Press.

Ebersole, P., & Hess, P. (1998). *Toward healthy aging: Human needs and nursing response* (5th ed.). St. Louis, MO: Mosby.

Field, D. (1999). Continuity and change in friendships in advanced old age: Findings from the Berkeley Older Generation Study. *International Journal of Aging and Human Development, 48*(4), 325-346.

Floyd, F. J., Haynes, S. N., Doner, W., Winemiller, D., Lemsky, C., Burgy, T. M., Werle, M., & Heilman, N. (1992). Assessing retirement satisfaction and perception of retirement experiences. *Psychology and Aging, 7*(4), 609-621.

Freund, A. M., & Smith, J. (1999). Content and function of the self-definition in old and very old age. *Journals of Gerontology. Series B, Psychological Sciences & Social Sciences, 54*(1), P55-P67.

Fulks, J. S., & Molinari, V. (1995). The young-old and the old-old: Issues of well-being, family, and social support. *Journal of Geriatric Psychiatry, 28*(2), 197-215.

Hansson, R. O., & Carpenter, B. N. (1994). *Relationships in old age: Coping with the challenge of transition.* New York: Guilford Press.

Horowitz, A. (1985). Sons and daughters as caregivers to older parents: Differences in role performance and consequences. *The Gerontologist, 25*(6), 613-617.

Kanacki, L. S., Jones, P. S., & Galbraith, M. E. (1996). Social support and depression in widows and widowers. *Journal of Gerontological Nursing, 22*(2), 39-45.

Markus, H. R., & Herzog, A. R. (1991). The role of self-concept in aging. In K. W. Schaie & M. P. Lawton (Eds.), *Annual review of gerontology* (pp. 123-126). New York: Springer.

Martire, L. M., Schulz, R., Mittelmark, M. B., & Newsom, J. T. (1999). Stability and change in older adults' social contact and social support: The Cardiovascular Health Study. *Journals of Gerontology: Series B, Psychological Sciences & Social Sciences, 54*(5), S302-S311.

Mor-Barak, M. E., Miller, L. S., & Syme, L. S. (1991). Social networks, life events, and health of the poor, frail elderly: A longitudinal study of the buffering versus the direct effect. *Family Community Health, 14*(2), 1-13.

Pearlin, L. I., & Skaff, M. M. (1996). Stress and the life course: A paradigmatic alliance. *The Gerontologist, 32*(2), 239-247.

Ryan, M. C., & Austin, A. G. (1989). Social support and social networks in the aged. *IMAGE: Journal of Nursing Scholarship, 23*(3), 176-180.

Silverstone, B. (1996). Older people of tomorrow: A psychosocial profile. *The Gerontologist, 36*(1), 27-32.

Smith, J., & Goodnow, J. J. (1999). Unasked-for support and unsolicited advice: Age and the quality of social experience. *Psychology & Aging, 14*(1), 108-121.

Solomon, R. (1996). Coping with stress: A physician's guide to mental health in aging. *Geriatrics, 51*(7), 46-52.

Taeuber, C. M. (1993). *Sixty-five plus in America/Current population reports.* (Special Studies/P23-178RV/Bureau of Census). Washington, DC: United States Government Printing Office.

Talamantes, M. A., Cornell, J., Espino, D. V., Lichtenstein, M. J., & Hazuda, H. P. (1996). SES and ethnic differences in perceived caregiver availability among young-old Mexican Americans and non-Hispanic Whites. *The Gerontologist, 36*(1), 88-99.

Uhlenberg, P. (1993). Demographic changes and kin relationships in later life. In G. L. Maddox & M. P. Lawton (Eds.), *Annual review of gerontology and geriatrics* (Vol. 3, pp. 219-238). New York: Springer.

van Tilburg, T. (1998). Losing and gaining in old age: Changes in personal network size and social support in a four-year longitudinal study. *Journals of Gerontology. Series B, Psychological Sciences & Social Sciences, 53*(6), S313-S323.

Weiss, R. S. (1973). *Loneliness, the experience of emotional and social isolation.* Cambridge, MA: MIT Press.

CHAPTER 48

RELOCATION STRESS SYNDROME

Rebecca A. Johnson

Relocation has been defined as the change in environment that takes place when people move their primary living space from one location to another. The process of relocation includes changes in the life situation that stimulate the move, decision making and preparing for the move, the actual physical move, and adjustment to the new surroundings (Remer & Buckwalter, 1990).

Litwak and Longino (1987) have identified three moves that older adults undertake. The first move usually occurs shortly after retirement and is based on the desire to live amidst particular amenities in a desirable climate. This relocation, commonly called migration, may involve traveling long distances. In response to health changes the second move is usually to a location that is closer to identified support networks such as adult children, family members, or long-time friends. For many older adults this may be the final move. However, for others a third move occurs when it becomes necessary for them to live in more supportive housing because of declining functional ability and/or health.

Additional moves may take place as older adults require increasingly more complex levels of assistance with daily living or actual nursing care. Finally, older adults may move because of situational changes in their supportive housing facilities or nursing homes or because their care requirements necessitate that they move to different locations within the facilities or nursing homes.

Nurses are especially appropriate health care professionals to assist older adults who relocate. Nurses have identified a consistency in patients' responses to relocation, developed a nursing diagnosis of Relocation Stress Syndrome (Barnhouse, Brugler, & Harkulich, 1992), and validated patients' responses through empirical study. Relocation Stress Syndrome (RSS) has been defined by the North American Nursing Diagnosis Association (NANDA) as "physiologic and/or psychological disturbances as a result of transfer from one environment to another" (Carpenito, 1995, p. 728; NANDA, 1999, p. 107). Relocation Stress and Risk for Relocation Stress are two other related nursing diagnoses identified by NANDA.

Application of the diagnosis RSS permits professionals to recognize as a constellation what have been described in most of the literature as the effects of relocation. The diagnostic label by its entirely negative orientation, like most of the empirical literature, assumes that these effects are negative. However, some research has found that relocation is not necessarily a negative event for older adults (Haddad, 1981; Harwood & Ebrahim, 1992; Johnson, 1996; Middleton, 1985; Rajacich & Faux, 1988; Storandt & Wittels, 1975). Therefore it is necessary to recognize that, much like any other nursing diagnosis, RSS may occur in varying degrees and is not an inevitable consequence of relocation.

NURSING DIAGNOSIS

Risk Factors

Risk factors for RSS include the following: previous relocation experiences, length of time spent in previous residence (Deane, 1990), extent of environmental change in the current relocation, willingness to relocate (Ferraro, 1981), inadequate preparation for relocation, losses of loved ones (Freedman, 1996; Freedman, Berkman, Rapp, & Ostfeld, 1994), resources (Collins, King, & Kokinakis, 1994), physical and/or mental health (Colsher & Wallace, 1990; Rowles, 1983), functional ability (Miller, Longino, Anderson, James, & Worley, 1999; Wolinsky, Callahan, Fitzgerald, & Johnson, 1993), feelings of powerlessness, and lack of an adequate support system (Glazebrook, Rockwood, Stolee, Fisk, & Gray, 1994; Montgomery & Kosloski, 1994). The more risk factors that are present, the more likely that the problems will develop.

Table 48-1 shows the high degree of similarity between the related factors that have been articulated by NANDA and those that have been empirically derived. However, the NANDA characteristics for RSS include a much greater degree of detail, identifying that each related factor may occur secondary to numerous situations or conditions. For example, moderate to high degree of environmental change in the new environment is listed as occurring secondary to decreased control of individual care, decrease or change in available caregivers, change in patient monitoring equipment, physical differences between the two environments, increased noise/activities in the new environment, inconsistencies in care, or decreased privacy and changes in lifestyle. While none of these factors has been the focus of research, they have been discussed as incidental to the related factors themselves.

Table 48-1	NANDA and Empirically Derived Related Factors/Etiologies RELOCATION STRESS SYNDROME	
NANDA Related Factors/Etiologies	**Empirically Derived Related Factors/Etiologies**
PATHOPHYSIOLOGIC	
Decreased physical health status Increased stress before relocation Depression Decreased self-esteem	Physical and/or mental health Functional ability Feelings of powerlessness Willingness to relocate Incontinence
SITUATIONAL	
Moderate to high degree of environmental change History and types of previous transfers Past, concurrent, and recent losses Little or no preparation for the impending move	Extent of environmental change in the current relocation Previous relocation experiences Length of time spent in previous residence Losses (of loved ones or resources) Inadequate preparation for relocation Lack of an adequate support system

ASSESSMENT

The most commonly studied characteristics of RSS include depression, anxiety (Thomasma, Yeaworth, & McCabe, 1990), deterioration in mental status, decreased life satisfaction (Wells & MacDonald, 1981), decreased self-perceived social support (Tesch, Nehrke, & Whitbourne, 1989), behavior changes (Lander, Brazil, & Ladrigan, 1997; Thomas et al., 1990; Young, Forbes, & Hirdes, 1994), and morbidity (Ferraro, 1982). Additionally, there exists a considerable body of research conducted primarily during the 1970s, with contradictory findings on mortality related to relocation (Aldrich & Mendkoff, 1963; Borup & Gallego, 1981; Bourestom & Tars, 1974; Coffman, 1983; Markus, Blenkner, Bloom, & Downs, 1971; Pablo, 1977).

Depression and Anxiety

Depression, which may or may not be accompanied by anxiety, has been identified by researchers studying the effects of relocation in older adults (Johnson, 1992; Liebowitz, 1974), particularly in older women (Dimond, McCance, & King, 1987). Onset of depression was found to occur shortly after the older adult became aware of impending relocation (Brody, Kleban, & Moss, 1974; Liebowitz, 1974) and to persist during relocation and for up to 4 months after relocation (Anthony, Procter, Silverman, & Murphy, 1987).

Sad affect, verbalizations of sadness, withdrawal, changes in sleeping or eating habits, weight change, gastrointestinal disturbances, or worsening of chronic conditions such as pain and limited mobility may be indicative of depression in older adults. Additionally, persons might seek more assistance from the nurse or be more dependent in doing things previously done with less assistance (Lander et al., 1997).

Deterioration in Mental Status, Life Satisfaction, and Social Support

Deterioration in mental functioning (Dube, 1982; Wells & MacDonald, 1981) and increased aggression among older adults with psychiatric disorders (Thomas et al., 1990) have been identified as consequences of relocation. In particular, mental functioning can be negatively influenced when extreme degrees of change in the environment occur and environmental cues are lost.

Declines in life satisfaction (Pino, Rosica, & Carter, 1978; Wells & MacDonald, 1981) have been found among older adults who relocate. Life satisfaction appears to be particularly vulnerable when the degree of change in the environment in relocation is extreme (i.e., from community to nursing home), when the relocation is involuntary, or when the older adult is not prepared for relocation. However, a primarily positive interpretation of the meaning of relocation has also been identified in elderly religious sisters experiencing involuntary, intrainstitutional relocation (Johnson, 1996).

Additionally, Tesch, Nehrke, and Whitbourne (1989) found that relocation resulted in a decrease in social support. Other researchers have found a decline in social involvement (Anthony et al., 1987; Bourestom & Tars, 1974; Lander et al., 1997). On the other hand, Armer (1996) reported that, as might be expected, social support was critical in promoting adjustment to relocation.

Morbidity

Findings regarding the effect of relocation on health and morbidity are not definitive. Ferraro (1982) reported a decline in health and functioning even associated with voluntary relocation. Other researchers have also found health to decline after relocation (Johnson, 1992), the

Box 48-1

NANDA and Empirically Derived Defining Characteristics
RELOCATION STRESS SYNDROME

NANDA Defining Characteristics	
Major	Verbalization of insecurity in new living situation
Loneliness	Vigilance
Apprehension	Weight change
Depression	Withdrawal
Anxiety	
	Empirically Derived Defining Characteristics
Minor	Deterioration in mental status
Change in eating habits	Decline in life satisfaction
Sleep disturbance	Decrease in social support
Dependency	Decrease in social involvement
Insecurity	Behavior changes
Lack of trust	Increased need for PRN pain medications
Gastrointestinal disturbances	Decline in health and functioning
Increased verbalization of needs	Mortality
Need for excessive reassurance	Falls
Restlessness	Weight loss
Sad affect	Increase in medical visits
Unfavorable comparison of post- or pre-transfer staff	Decline in self-care
Verbalization of being concerned/upset about transfer	

number of medical visits to increase (Lander et al., 1997), and the need for PRN pain medications to increase (Gallagher & Walker, 1990). However, improvements in emotional health (Eckert & Haug, 1984), physical health (Borup, Gallego, & Heffernan, 1979; Engle & Graney, 1993) and physical function have also been documented (Harwood & Ebrahim, 1992; Pablo, 1977). Further investigation is needed for conclusions to be drawn. As is shown in Box 48-1, most of the NANDA-derived defining characteristics of RSS have not been validated through research. Investigation of the prevalence of these characteristics would be a very helpful line of investigation.

Assessment Tools

Objective assessment tools can facilitate proper diagnosis and treatment of elders experiencing relocation. Ideally, assessment should occur both prior to and following relocation. However, as relocation decisions can be made precipitously in response to catastrophic health events, assessment at both times might not be feasible. At a minimum, assessment needs to occur during the period shortly following relocation. Reassessment weekly for 4 to 6 weeks can be particularly informative. Comparison of sequential assessment findings can help in planning long-term interventions.

Geriatric Depression Scale.   Brink et al. (1982) developed the Geriatric Depression Scale (GDS) in response to a need for an instrument well suited to older patients. The long form of this screening tool consists of 30 phrases with yes/no responses and takes approximately 10 to 15 minutes to administer. A shortened, 15-item version is

also available. The GDS has been tested and found to be effective with populations of older patients (Norris, Gallagher, Wilson, & Winograd, 1987; Yesavage et al., 1983). A score of 10 or higher suggests depression and should trigger a referral for more comprehensive evaluation of mood state (Norris et al., 1987). This instrument is easily administered either in person or over the phone; in addition, persons can complete the instrument as a self-report test. The instrument can be found by accessing the original Brink et al. reference. For additional information on assessment of depression, the reader is referred to Chapter 41.

Profile of Mood States.   The Profile of Mood States (POMS) (McNair, Lorr, & Droppleman, 1981) is a 65-item closed-ended instrument that assesses the following subscales: Tension, Depression, Anger, Vigor, Fatigue, and Confusion. It takes 15 to 20 minutes to administer and has been used effectively with older people (Kaye et al., 1988). Scoring is more complex for this tool than for the GDS and requires a published manual. Subscale scores can be considered individually, and a Total Mood Disturbance Score can be obtained by summing the scores of five of the subscales. The POMS and the scoring manual are available commercially from EDITS, Inc., San Diego, CA, 92167.

Mini-Mental Status Exam.   This instrument is a screening tool for cognitive intactness but is not diagnostic for dementia (Folstein, Folstein, & McHugh, 1975). It consists of 11 items that measure orientation, memory, and attention. The Mini-Mental Status Exam (MMSE) takes approximately 10 to 15 minutes to administer and has been found to be reliable and valid with elderly patients. Oral responses are required in Part One (maximum score of 21). Part Two assesses subjects' abilities to follow simple verbal and written commands in writing a sentence, folding paper, and copying a design (maximum score of 9). The overall maximum possible score on the MMSE is 30 (higher score equals better cognitive function). A score of 24 or lower suggests cognitive impairment.

Self-Perceived Health Questions.   Self-perceived health can be assessed by asking older adults to rate the following: their current health overall, their current health compared with their health 1 year ago, and their current health compared with the health of others their age. A 4-point scale (excellent, good, fair, or poor) is used (Kaplan & Camacho, 1983). A study of 6928 adults over a 9-year period found that self-perceived health was significantly related to mortality when age, gender, health practices, social network participation, income, education, health relative to age peers, morale, depression, and happiness were controlled. Similarly, Ferraro (1982) found that self-ratings of health were significantly related to an objective measure of health status (disability scale) among 3402 elderly subjects. Self-rated health also was predictive of mortality in a study conducted by Mossey and Shapiro (1982), who controlled for age, gender, life satisfaction, income, and urban or rural residence in their sample of 3128 elders.

Iowa Self Assessment Inventory.   The Iowa Self Assessment Inventory (ISAI) assesses most of the signs and symptoms of RSS. This 56-item instrument, scored on a 4-point Likert-type scale, takes approximately 15 minutes to administer to well elderly persons. The ISAI aims to identify their resources, status, and abilities in the following seven components: economic resources, emotional balance, physical health status, trusting others, mobility, cognitive status, and social support. Scores on the ISAI range from 8 to 32, with higher scores indicating more of a particular resource or ability. The ISAI was developed for use with community-dwelling elders and has been found to be an effective assessment tool with this population (Gilmer et al., 1991; Morris et al., 1990). The ISAI has most commonly been used with well elders and should be tested with more infirm elders. In addition, it has been translated into several different languages and tested cross-culturally on elderly subjects in France, Scandinavia, Belgium, and Canada as well as in the United States.

CASE STUDY

K. Brendan, an 85-year-old woman who has been a resident of The Family Retirement Home for the past 12 years, was forced to move 2 weeks ago because of a renovation project aimed at creating a special area for residents who required more than intermediate nursing care. Staff prepared residents for the relocation by informing them of the progress of the building renovation, discussing their new rooms and common spaces, and allowing them to express their concerns and ask questions. When the renovation was complete, the residents who were to relocate were given a tour of the new wing, and those who were able to do so chose their new rooms. Residents' belongings were packed by nursing staff, and relocation was completed in 1 day.

Mrs. Brendan has one daughter who lives a great distance away. She herself has lived in the area for the past 5 years. Spinal degeneration resulting from osteoporosis gives Mrs. Brendan chronic pain. Since moving, she has required up to four scheduled and two PRN analgesic doses per day. Before moving, she took no PRN analgesics. She now spends 1 day each week in bed because of pain and shortness of breath due to worsened congestive heart failure. She also has poor vision and moderate short-term memory impairment. Since moving to the new wing, Mrs. Brendan mostly sits alone in her room with the door closed. She frequently calls for staff to put her to bed because she has "nervous legs." She refuses to join in the nightly sing-alongs, previously a favorite activity, because she doesn't know anyone in the new wing of the home. Staff members note that Mrs. Brendan is less able than before the move to recall the time for meals.

As a follow-up, all residents who moved were assessed by the Assistant Director of Nursing. Mrs. Brendan was determined to be suffering from RSS based on her score of 18 on the Geriatric Depression Scale, her worsened health status, decreased social involvement, and worsened mental status. During the assessment, Mrs. Brendan stated that she thought she was "going downhill fast." In addition to relocating, her history also contained the following related factors for RSS: poor health, loss of some of her personal belongings because of smaller space allocations in the new wing of the building, and lack of social support due to the distance from her daughter and not having any friends in the facility or the surrounding area.

NURSING-SENSITIVE OUTCOMES

The desired outcomes of nursing interventions to prevent or minimize RSS are listed in Box 48-2. The *Nursing Outcomes Classification (NOC)* (Iowa Outcomes Project, 2000) presents several nursing outcomes expected when RSS is resolved. Clearly the most salient and inclusive NOC outcome is the resident's psychosocial adjustment to this significant life change. This is, however, a very broad outcome. Adjustment can include any of the following outcomes: Anxiety Control, Coping, Decision Making, Family Participation in Professional Care, Hope, Social Interaction Skills, Social Involvement, or Social Support. Some outcomes not recognized by NOC result from the older adult exerting control over relocation: Mood Equilibrium, Quality of Life, Self-Esteem, Spiritual Well-Being, and Well-Being. However, of these outcomes, only Social Support, Coping, and Quality of Life are included in the NANDA, NOC, and NIC linkages specifically for demonstrating resolution of RSS (Johnson et al., 2000).

Additional associated NOC outcomes for RSS include Grief Resolution, Caregiver Home Care Readiness, and Caregiver Adaptation to Patient Institutionalization (Johnson et al., 2000). Grief Resolution, in particular, is a very useful outcome for RSS, since loss of home, personal belongings, social network, and support might be inevitable results of relocation. Testing some of the *Nursing Interventions Classification (NIC)* (Iowa Intervention Project, 2000) interventions aimed at Grief Resolution would be a very fruitful area of research. It is curious, however, that Caregiver Home Care Readiness is included in the linkages for RSS. For this outcome to be applicable, relocation of the older adult to the caregiver's home would need to take place. Most outcomes are not specific enough to be only applicable under such narrow circumstances. Caregiver readiness for home care might not be a meaningful outcome given the wide range of other NOC outcomes related to caregivers.

The NOC outcomes linked with RSS by Johnson et al. (2000) are surprisingly brief, given the considerable number of dependent variables that have been found to be influenced by interventions for RSS. Moreover, many outcomes have not been systematically tested (see Box 48-2).

Assessing for outcomes might involve administering the same assessment tools used to diagnose RSS (for depression —GDS; other mood disturbances & well-being—POMS; cognitive status—MMSE; social and economic resources and functional ability—ISAI; and self-perceived health). Life satisfaction might be assessed as an indicator of overall well-being using the Life Satisfaction Index (LSI) (Neugarten, Havighurst, & Tobin, 1961). Self-esteem can be evaluated using the Rosenberg Self-Esteem Scale (Rosenberg, 1962), and hope can be measured using the Herth Hope Index (Herth, 1992). These outcome measures are briefly discussed below.

Life Satisfaction Index

The Life Satisfaction Index (LSI) uses an agree/disagree format that is very easy to administer to older adults and that has been used successfully with this population. Form A consists of 20 self-report statements about well-being. Form B consists of 12 statements that assess the following characteristics: zest versus apathy, resolution and fortitude, congruence between desired and achieved goals, positive self-concept, and mood tone. The higher the score, the more satisfied the individual is with his current life situation.

Herth Hope Index

The Herth Hope Index (HHI) (Herth, 1992) is a 12-item scale with a 4-point Likert-type format designed for use in clinical settings. It has been used successfully with elderly persons and features enlarged print for readability. Scores range from 12 to 48, with higher scores indicating better outcomes. The HHI measures cognitive, affective, and affiliative dimensions of hope and is aimed at assessing changes in hope in response to interventions. The HHI has been found to have an internal consistency of 0.88 to 0.97 and a test-retest reliability coefficient of 0.87 to 0.91 when tested over a 2-week period with acute, chronic, and terminally ill adult patients (mixed age groups) and their family caregivers (Farran, Herth, & Popovich, 1995).

Rosenberg Self-Esteem Scale

The Rosenberg Self-Esteem Scale (Rosenberg, 1962) is a 10-item tool that measures a basic feeling of self-worth. It is a unidimensional scale and uses a 4-point Likert format. Reliability coefficients reportedly range from 0.85 to 0.92, and validity correlations range from 0.56 to 0.83 (Lewis, 1982). These reliability and validity findings are based on a population of mixed ages.

NURSING INTERVENTIONS

Once a diagnosis of RSS is established, the nurse must identify and implement appropriate nursing interventions. Box 48-3 shows a list of NIC (Iowa Intervention Project, 2000) interventions for RSS that have been subjected to empirical testing with older adults. Also listed are some interventions that logically address the defining characteristics of RSS, but that have not been specifically tested by research. The interventions Admission Care, Coping Enhancement, Decision-Making Support, and

Box 48-2	NOC Outcomes Expected for Resolution of Relocation Stress Syndrome
Systematically Tested Outcomes Psychosocial Adjustment: Life Change Coping Quality of Life Social Support Mood Equilibrium Depression Amelioration Anxiety Reduction Improved Self-Perceived Health Positive Meaning	Decreased Morbidity Life Satisfaction **Non–Systematically Tested Outcomes** Caregiver Adaptation to Patient Institutionalization Caregiver Home Care Readiness Grief Resolution Self-Esteem (although a NOC outcome, it is not specified for RSS) Hope (although a NOC outcome, it is not specified for RSS)

Box 48-3	NIC Interventions Appropriate for Relocation Stress Syndrome

Empirically Tested Interventions	Animal-Assisted Therapy
Preparation for Relocation	Anxiety Reduction
Admission Care	Art Therapy
Anticipatory Guidance	Bibliotherapy
Coping Enhancement	Calming Techniques
Counseling	Environmental Management
Emotional Support	Family Integrity Promotion
Health Care Information Exchange	Guided Imagery
Reminiscence Therapy	Hope Instillation
Socialization Enhancement	Humor
Support System Enhancement	Medication
Values Clarification	Music Therapy
	Simple Massage
Facilitating Control	Simple Relaxation Therapy
Counseling	Support Groups
Emotional Support	Therapeutic Touch
Mutual Goal Setting	Touch
Non–Empirically Tested Interventions	
Active Listening	
Anger Control	

Values Clarification have been evaluated not as separate interventions but as inherent components of the two main interventions discussed in the literature: preparation for relocation (enhancing predictability of relocation and new surroundings) and facilitating the older adult's control in decisions about relocation.

Preparing for Relocation

Preparation has been almost exclusively tested in an institutional context where relocation became necessary because of changing care needs of the older adult or changing organization or structure of the facility. Particularly in the current health care environment, relocation can occur precipitously, decreasing opportunities for comprehensive preparation (Everard, Rowles, & High, 1994).

Degree of preparation ranges from simply telling older adults that relocation is necessary and imminent (Thomas et al., 1990) to seeking their involvement in the relocation process (known in the NIC language as Mutual Goal Setting) (Kowalski, 1981). Preparation may include a variety of activities: conducting site visits (known in the NIC language as Health Care Information Exchange, Admission Care, or Anticipatory Guidance) (Amenta, Weiner, & Amenta, 1984; Grant, Skinkle, & Lipps, 1992); enhancing their social support network (known in the NIC language as Support System Enhancement); directing their focus away from the relocation (Johnson & Hlava, 1994); and creating and adhering to a schedule for relocation activities given to relocating elders at least a month in advance (Thomasma et al., 1990).

Two preparation interventions are not directly identified in the NIC taxonomy. Creating and adhering to a schedule for relocation activities, because of its level of specificity, may be more appropriately included as an activity under the NIC intervention of Security Enhancement. If older adults know in advance what is to happen during their relocation process, their security can be enhanced throughout the process. Directing older adults' focus away from the relocation may be included as an activity under the NIC intervention of Coping Enhancement. If they are able to refocus from relocation onto other events, they might be better able to cope with the relocation process. However, the difficulty of listing these interventions as activities, subsumed under NIC interventions, increases the likelihood that they will get lost when nurses are seeking interventions for RSS. This can result in an incomplete approach to preventing or resolving RSS.

Walker and Gallagher (1990) found that physical and emotional health indices improved in older adults who were temporarily moved out of their care facility. Preparation for the move included informing the residents several months prior to the move (known in the NIC taxonomy as Anticipatory Guidance), sending letters describing the move to their close family members (known in the NIC as Support System Enhancement or Family Mobilization), having informational meetings with residents and family members (known in the NIC as Anticipatory Guidance, Family Involvement Promotion, or Support System Enhancement), and conducting individual sessions with each resident in order to discuss the move, encourage expression of concerns, and answer questions (known in the NIC as Counseling, Coping Enhancement, Emotional Support, or Hope Instillation). The importance of scheduling the relocation well in advance and adhering to the schedule was emphasized by Thomasma et al. (1990), who found that anxiety worsened when relocation was announced only 1 week in advance and when older adults were unsure of the date on which they would relocate.

Grant, Skinkle, and Lipps (1992) found that elderly nursing home residents who were relocated to a new facility expressed a need for more information about the new nursing home, the quality of care, the general layout of the facility, the layout of their new rooms, and other residents of the facility (known in the NIC as Anticipatory Guidance). Residents expressed most concern about losing their personal belongings, getting lost in the new facility, and having staff be less responsive. Latino elders might fear that discrimination and language barriers will result in poor care (Johnson, Schwiebert, Alvarado-Rosenmann, Pecka, & Shirk, 1997).

Relocation stress can be minimized through careful screening and selection of residents so that the most mentally and physically impaired individuals experience the least extreme degree of relocation (for example, to areas within the same facility versus to another facility) (Powell, Walker, Christie, Mitchell-Pederson, & Rauscher, 1990; Pruchno & Resch, 1988; Rantz & Egan, 1987). This intervention is not addressed in the NIC taxonomy. Additionally, maintaining continuity in caregivers has been empirically found to be beneficial (Powell et al., 1990) but not addressed in the NIC taxonomy. A multidisciplinary approach to planning relocation (Pino et al., 1978; Pruchno & Resch, 1988) was also viewed as beneficial. This intervention is related most closely to Discharge Planning in the NIC taxonomy.

Close interpersonal relationships with friends living in the nursing home (Tesch et al., 1989), with family and friends outside of the facility (Armer, 1996), or with care staff within the facility (Wells & MacDonald, 1981) have been related to stability of life satisfaction, physical and mental health, and psychosocial adaptation of older relocating adults. These factors may be most closely related to the NIC interventions of Socialization Enhancement, Family Mobilization, Visitation Facilitation, and Family Support. The most beneficial approach to preparation appears to be a multifaceted strategy combining individual and group preparation with information sharing, counseling, fostering social relationships, and promoting control of the older adult over the relocation.

Facilitating Older Adults' Control in Relocation

A sense of control over relocation is linked to elders' definitions of "home." Several psychosocial processes forge the link between older adults and their homes. A working knowledge of the physical environment helps link older adults to their home. In addition, possessions that have meaning to older individuals and that represent their life course personalize the home. Some belongings were found to have such strong attachment for the older adults that they were perceived as direct representations, extensions, or embodiments of self (Rubinstein, 1990).

Older adults "fine-tune" their home environments to enhance their physical comfort and facilitate their daily routines and activities; they gradually centralize their operating environment as their physical capabilities change (Rubinstein, 1990). Thus even older adults who are bedridden, if cognitively capable, create an environmental milieu that is comfortable to them (i.e., via placement of tissues, reading materials, a drinking glass). This milieu may be increasingly scaled down and become more sterile and less "homelike" as disability increases.

Clearly the process of identifying a place as "home" implies that individuals have control over their surroundings. This control is often minimized or nonexistent for older adults who must relocate and eliminate personal possessions because of space limitations in the new environment. This is one of the reasons that the assisted living movement is growing so fast in this country.

These activities aimed at creating "home" are specific enough to be subsumed under the NIC interventions. However, doing this may result in their "loss" for RSS. In contrast, considering these activities to be separate interventions that are more specific to RSS may result in a more complete plan of care for relocating older adults.

Johnson, Schwiebert, and Alvarado Rosenmann (1994) found that, although community-dwelling older adults intended to make their own decision to relocate to a nursing home, most nursing home residents in fact did not make the decision to relocate. Although most older adults studied by Reinardy (1992) did not have total control in making the decision to move to a nursing home, those who did make the decision were found to have better physical, social, and psychologic functioning, social interaction, activity, and satisfaction with services. Likewise, Smith and Brand (1975) found that older adults who relocated voluntarily had better life satisfaction than those who were forced to relocate.

Control, as described in the literature, pertains to a wide range of issues: where to move, when to move, what to move, the layout and organization of the new environment, and what personal belongings will be moved. While it is clear from a review of extant research that control by older adults over relocation needs further investigation, it is possible to identify some aspects of control that may prevent or minimize RSS.

When the older adult relocates voluntarily with greater control over the process and environment, outcomes are more positive (Ferraro, 1981; Armer, 1996; Danermark & Ekstrom, 1990; Mirotznik & Ruskin, 1985; Schulz & Brenner, 1977; Wells & MacDonald, 1981). However, control beyond basic decisions also is important (Rutman & Freedman, 1988). Walker and Gallagher (1990) found that it was important for older adults to be consulted regarding orchestration of the move and characteristics of the new surroundings.

Choosing room location; room color and furnishings, supervising packing of belongings; participating in a residence's council (a means of communicating opinions and concerns to administration); and selecting menus for daily meals have been found to enhance adjustment to relocation (Grant Skinkle and Lipps, 1992; Harwood & Ebrahim, 1992; Amenta, Weiner, & Amenta, 1984).

More than a decade ago, Everard, Rowles, and High (1994) recognized that facility or institutional needs and policies can conflict with the needs and desires of older adults, as well as with their need to exert control over the relocation process. Older adults who relocate due to declining functional ability might experience even greater limits on their opportunities to exert control (Wolinsky et al., 1993). However, research findings consistently identify that control is important in minimizing relocation stress, no matter what the precipitating circumstances. Thus it is critical that nurses intervene in order to advocate for as much control as possible by older adults over their process of relocation. The NIC interventions that most closely approximate the notion of control are Patient Rights Protection, Self-Responsibility Facilitation, and Mutual Goal Setting. Even in situations where there may be little overall control, making smaller decisions can enhance control and promote psychologic well-being (Housely, 1992).

Lacking in the NIC list are interventions related to decision-making support. Clearly, according to the research findings, this is a needed addition. Older adults may need decision-making support on multiple levels, as has been discussed. Decision-making support may not be limited to the older adult. Families may need this type of support, as research has shown that most commonly they are key participants in the relocation decision-making process (Johnson et al., 1994).

Interventions Tested Empirically But Not in Relocation Contexts

A number of interventions are reported in the literature, which might be beneficial in preventing or minimizing the symptoms of RSS. These interventions are aimed at specific symptoms of RSS and warrant testing in a relocation context. Reminiscence Therapy, either in group or individual formats, may be of benefit following relocation in terms of ameliorating depression (Youssef, 1990) and yielding positive effects (Johnson, 1992). This intervention is included in the NIC taxonomy for RSS.

Pet ownership can buffer the effects of stressful life events among elders (Siegel, 1990), and Animal-Assisted Therapy has been found to positively influence social behaviors among institutionalized older adults (Kongable, Buckwalter, & Stolley, 1989). Use of religious beliefs and practices as well as social support have also been found to be beneficial in alleviating depression (Buschmann & Hollinger, 1994; Dean, Kolody, & Wood, 1990; Koening et al., 1992; Mullins & Dugan, 1991; Palinkas, Wingard, &

Barret-Connor, 1990; Pressman, Lyons, Larson, & Strain, 1990). These interventions are addressed through the NIC interventions Spiritual Support, Socialization Enhancement, Emotional Support, and Support System Enhancement.

The use of humor to produce a statistically significant decrease in agitation (Tennant, 1995) and an improvement in morale has been demonstrated in nursing home residents. Humor is included in the NIC taxonomy for RSS. Relaxation Therapy can positively influence the self-esteem of older adults (Bensink, Godbey, Marshall, & Yarandi, 1992) and also alleviate depression (Arean et al., 1993); however, it is not included in the NANDA, NOC, and NIC linkages for RSS. Related interventions such as Activity Therapy, Recreation Therapy, Art Therapy, and Music Therapy are included in the NIC. These interventions can be beneficial in the context of relocation of older adults, but need to be more clearly designed for and empirically tested in a relocation context. Other interventions worthy of testing are listed in Box 48-3. Johnson (1999) has compiled recommended interventions to assist relocating elders.

CASE STUDY

The Family Retirement Home houses 325 older adults in either condominiums, independent living apartments with meal service, assisted living apartments, intermediate care, or skilled nursing beds. The gerontologic nurse practitioner employed by the center identified RSS as a problem when Mrs. Brendan moved from the assisted living apartments into the intermediate nursing unit. There were no programs in place to ease resident transitions between levels of care.

The gerontologic nurse practitioner created a task force consisting of one resident from each level of the facility (a total of five), the social worker, and the activity coordinator. The task force was charged with development of a Relocation Assistance Plan. The Relocation Assistance Plan was initiated by the nurse coordinator, who is responsible for all resident transfers.

The resident task force members starred in a brief videotape, describing their relocation experience, providing tips about what personal belongings are especially needed, and describing the advantages of their level of care. Other residents also gave testimonials about the positive attributes of their care setting. The videotape of the intermediate unit, included as part of the Relocation Assistance Plan, was loaned to Mrs. Brendan, together with a videocassette recorder to view it.

The resident task force members also formed a "buddy network," a group of residents willing to advise and shepherd new residents or ones relocating within the facility. Mrs. Brendan's buddy served as a resource person, making frequent contact with her before relocation and during the first month following relocation.

A biweekly support group was formed for residents in the process of relocating or recently relocated to the Intermediate Care Unit and skilled nursing facility (SNF) units.

This group had access to counseling, information sharing, and periodic social events. Mrs. Brendan's family members were encouraged to attend one or more group sessions at her invitation. Additionally, the gerontologic nurse practitioner made regular contact with Mrs. Brendan during the first 3 months following her relocation on an as-needed basis. The purpose of these contacts was to assess Mrs. Brendan for RSS, to answer questions, and to provide individual counseling to facilitate her adaptation to the new environment.

Information folders were created for distribution to each resident anticipating relocation. The folders included information about the level of accommodation to which the resident was moving (meal service, housekeeping, transportation, assistance with settling personal belongings, and care activities), a pictorial directory of staff members, a map of the unit to which they were relocating, rules of conduct, and rights and privileges of residents. The packet also included a questionnaire that asked about present concerns, assistance needed, and first, second, and third preferences for rooms. Through this material, Mrs. Brendan was able to gain a familiarity with her new home on the Intermediate Care Unit, to recognize key staff members readily, to specify her room preference, and to plan for how her new room would look.

The nursing coordinator also met with Mrs. Brendan to provide her with the information packet and the videotape depicting the Intermediate Care Unit and to discuss these materials. The nursing coordinator also gave Mrs. Brendan a tour of the unit, explained the "buddy network" and assigned Mrs. Brendan a buddy, and described the activities of the support groups. The nursing coordinator helped her complete the preference questionnaire and discussed her responses with her.

Approximately 2 weeks after relocation the gerontologic nurse practitioner conducted an assessment of Mrs. Brendan using the Geriatric Depression Scale, self-perceived health questions, and the Iowa Self-Assessment Inventory. Prescriptions for her treatment were based on which signs and symptoms of RSS were most problematic for Mrs. Brendan. The gerontologic nurse practitioner gave a Relocation Assistance Plan evaluation tool to her, which she completed and returned to the members of the resident task force. Reassessment every 2 weeks using the Geriatric Depression Scale, self-perceived questions, and the Iowa Self Assessment Inventory was planned.

SUMMARY

Box 48-4 links the signs and symptoms of RSS with the appropriate NIC nursing interventions and anticipated NOC nursing outcomes. There is logical flow between each of these three areas. Research has shown that preparation of relocating older adults and maximization of their control in the relocation process enhances adjustment (insofar as they want and are capable of control). However, applying the individual nursing interventions as they are precisely worded in the NIC presents some difficulty. For example, while "Active Listening" is specified as a separate nursing intervention in the NIC, in most of the literature on relocation, this activity is assumed as part of preparation for relocation. It could be argued that active listening is a necessary but assumed component of any patient teaching or counseling. If this is the case, then it is unclear why specifying this intervention is beneficial.

The same argument may hold for other NIC interventions, such as Anticipatory Guidance, Calming Technique, Emotional Support, Values Clarification, Coping Enhancement, or Socialization Enhancement. Each of these interventions may be inherent components of a comprehensive process of preparing older

---

Box 48-4	Suggested Nursing-Sensitive Outcomes and Nursing Interventions **RELOCATION STRESS SYNDROME**

Nursing Diagnosis	**Quality of Life**
Relocation Stress Syndrome	**Self-Esteem**
Defining characteristics	**Social Interaction Skills**
Depression	**Social Involvement**
Anxiety	**Social Support**
Mental status decline	**Spiritual Well-Being**
Decreased life satisfaction	**Well-Being**
Behavior changes	
Social support decline	Nursing Interventions
Morbidity	**Active Listening**
	Admission Care
Nursing-Sensitive Outcomes	**Anticipatory Guidance**
Anxiety Control	**Coping Enhancement**
Coping	**Counseling**
Decision Making	**Emotional Support**
Family Participation	**Family Involvement Promotion**
Hope	**Mutual Goal Setting**
Mood Equilibrium	**Socialization Enhancement**
Psychosocial Adjustment: Life Change	**Values Clarification**

adults for relocation. If these interventions are not separate, but combine to form the amalgam of preparation for relocation, then empirically testing them as discrete variables may be impractical and/or unproductive.

Application of NOC nursing outcomes is less problematic in terms of the existing literature on relocation. However, given the considerable literature demonstrating appropriate outcomes for RSS, it is clear that the NOC linkage list for RSS needs to be expanded (Johnson et al., 2000). Several NOC outcomes are missing, which can be expected in light of the NIC interventions that are used. Those that are glaringly absent include Anxiety Control, Mood Equilibrium, Social Interaction Skills, Social Involvement, Well-Being, Hope, Family Participation in Professional Care, and Spiritual Well-Being.

There seems to be a rather direct fit of the NIC interventions to the NANDA related factors and defining characteristics for RSS (Johnson et al., 2000). However, the relationship between the NIC interventions and NOC outcomes for RSS is more difficult to ascertain given the brevity and broadness of the current NOC linkage list for RSS. Some NOC outcomes for RSS (Coping, Quality of Life, and Social Support) directly reflect the obverse of the defining characteristics of RSS (Johnson et al., 2000). Others (Caregiver Adaptation to Patient Institutionalization, Caregiver Home Care Readiness, and Grief Resolution) do not directly correspond to either the identified defining characteristics of RSS or the NIC interventions delineated for RSS. For the NIC and NOC taxonomies to be completely beneficial in planning care for older adults suffering from RSS, revision of the linkages is needed so that the NIC interventions flow from the NANDA defining characteristics, which in turn flow seamlessly into the NOC outcomes. This revision will not only facilitate effective use of the NIC and NOC with RSS, but it will form a logical framework for the much needed empirical testing of interventions and validation of outcomes.

REFERENCES

Aldrich, C., & Mendkoff, E. (1963). Relocation of the aged and disabled: A mortality study. *Journal of the American Geriatrics Society, 11*(3), 185-194.

Amenta, M., Weiner, A., & Amenta, D. (1984). Successful relocation of elderly residents. *Geriatric Nursing, 5*(8), 356-360.

Anthony, K., Procter, A., Silverman, A., & Murphy, E. (1987). Mood and behavior problems following the relocation of elderly patients with mental illness. *Age & Ageing, 16*, 355-365.

Arean, P., Perri, M., Nezu, A., Schein, R., Christopher, F., & Joseph, T. (1993). Comparative effectiveness of social problem-solving therapy and reminiscence therapy as treatments for depression in older adults. *Journal of Consulting and Clinical Psychology, 61*(6), 1003-1010.

Armer, J. (1996). An exploration of factors influencing adjustment among relocating rural elders. *IMAGE: Journal of Nursing Scholarship, 28*(1), 35-40.

Barnhouse, A., Brugler, C., & Harkulich, J. (1992). Relocation stress syndrome. *Nursing Diagnosis, 3*(4), 166-167.

Bensink, G., Godbey, K., Marshall, M., & Yarandi, H. (1992). Institutionalized elderly, relaxation, locus of control, self-esteem. *Journal of Gerontological Nursing, 13*(4), 30-36.

Borup, J., & Gallego, D. (1981). Mortality as affected by interinstitutional relocation: Update and assessment. *The Gerontologist, 21*(1), 4-7.

Borup, J., Gallego, D., & Heffernan, P. (1979). Relocation: Its effect on health, functioning and mortality. *The Gerontologist, 20*(4), 468-479.

Bourestom, M., & Tars, S. (1974). Alterations in life patterns following nursing home relocation. *The Gerontologist, 14*, 506-510.

Brink, T., Yesavage, J., Lum, O., Hiersema, P., Adey, M., & Rose, T. (1982). Screening tests for geriatric depression. *Clinical Gerontologist, 1*, 37-43.

Brody, E., Kleban, M., & Moss, M. (1974). Measuring the impact of change. *The Gerontologist, 14*, 299-307.

Buschmann, M., & Hollinger, L. (1994). Influence of social support and control on depression in the elderly. *Clinical Gerontologist, 14*(4), 13-28.

Carpenito, L. (1995). *Nursing diagnosis: Application to clinical practice* (6th ed.). Baltimore: Lippincott Williams & Wilkins.

Coffman, T. (1983). Toward an understanding of geriatric relocation. *The Gerontologist, 23*(5), 297-304.

Collins, C., King, S., & Kokinakis, C. (1994). Community service issues before nursing home placement of persons with dementia. *Western Journal of Nursing Research, 16*(1), 40-56.

Colsher, P. L., & Wallace R. B. (1990). Health and social antecedents of relocation in rural elderly persons. *Journal of Gerontology, 45*(1), S32-38.

Danermark, B., & Ekstrom, M. (1990). Relocation and health effects on the elderly: A commented research review. *Journal of Sociology & Social Welfare, 17*(1), 25-49.

Dean, A., Kolody, B., & Wood, P. (1990). Effects of social support from various sources on depression in elderly persons. *Journal of Health and Social Behavior, 31*, 148-161.

Deane, G. (1990). Mobility and adjustments: Paths to the resolution of residential stress. *Demography, 27*(1), 65-79.

Dimond, M., McCance, K., & King, K. (1987). Forced residential relocation: Its impact on the well-being of older adults. *Western Journal of Nursing Research, 9*(4), 445-464.

Dube, A. (1982). The impact of moving a geriatric population: Mortality and emotional aspects. *Journal of Chronic Disease, 35*(1), 61-64.

Eckert, J., & Haug, M. (1984). The impact of forced residential relocation on the health of the elderly hotel dweller. *Journal of Gerontology, 39*(6), 753-755.

Engle, V., & Graney, M. (1993). Stability and improvement of health after nursing home admission. *Journal of Gerontology, 48*(1), S17-23.

Everard, K., Rowles, G., & High, D. (1994). Nursing home room changes: Toward a decision-making model. *The Gerontologist, 34*(4), 520-527.

Farran, C., Herth, K., & Popovich, J. (1995). *Hope and hopelessness: Critical clinical constructs.* Thousand Oaks, CA: Sage.

Ferraro, K. (1981). Relocation desires and outcomes among the elderly: A longitudinal analysis. *Research on Aging, 3*(2), 166-181.

Ferraro, K. (1982). The health consequences of relocation among the aged in the community. *Journal of Gerontology, 38*(1), 90-96.

Folstein, M., Folstein, S., & McHugh, P. (1975). Mini-mental state: A practical method for grading the cognitive state of patients for the clinician. *Journal of Psychiatric Research, 12*, 189-198.

Freedman, V. (1996). Family structure and the risk of nursing home admission. *Journal of Gerontology, 51B*(2), S61-69.

Freedman, V. A., Berkman, L. F., Rapp, S. R., & Ostfeld, A. M. (1994). Family networks: Predictors of nursing home entry. *American Journal of Public Health, 84*(5), 843-845.

Gallagher, E. M., & Walker, G. (1990). Vulnerability of nursing home residents during relocations and renovations. *Journal of Aging Studies, 4*(1), 31-46.

Gilmer, J., Cleary, T., Lu, D., Morris, W., Buckwalter, K., Andrews, P., Boutelle, S., & Hatz, D. (1991). The factor structure of the Iowa Self-Assessment Inventory. *Educational and Psychological Measurement, 51*(2), 365-375.

Glazebrook, K., Rockwood, K., Stolee, P., Fisk, J., & Gray, J. (1994). A case control study of the risks for institutionalization of elderly people in Nova Scotia. *Canadian Journal on Aging, 13*(1), 104-117.

Grant, P., Skinkle, R., & Lipps, G. (1992). The impact of an interinstitutional relocation of nursing home residents requiring a high level of care. *The Gerontologist, 32*(6), 834-842.

Haddad, B. (1981). Intra-institutional relocation: Measured impact upon geriatric patients. *Journal of the American Geriatrics Society, 29,* 86-88.

Harwood, R., & Ebrahim, S. (1992). Is relocation harmful to institutionalized elderly people? *Age & Ageing, 21*(1), 61-66.

Herth, K. (1992). An abbreviated instrument to measure hope: Development and psychometric evaluation. *Journal of Advanced Nursing, 17,* 1251-1259.

Housely, W. F. (1992). Psychoeducation for personal control: A key to psychological well-being of the elderly. *Educational Gerontology, 18,* 785-794.

Iowa Intervention Project. J. C. McCloskey & G. M. Bulechek (Eds.). (2000). *Nursing interventions classification (NIC)* (3rd ed.). St. Louis, MO: Mosby.

Iowa Outcomes Project. M. Johnson, M. Maas, & S. Moorhead (Eds.). (2000). *Nursing outcomes classification (NOC)* (2nd ed.). St. Louis, MO: Mosby.

Johnson, R. A. (1992). *Account-making and the meaning of translocation for elders.* Unpublished doctoral dissertation. Iowa City, IA: University of Iowa.

Johnson, R. A. (1996). The meaning of relocation among elderly religious sisters. *Western Journal of Nursing, 18*(2), 172-185.

Johnson, R. A. (1999). Helping older adults adjust to relocation: Nursing interventions and issues. In L. Swanson & T. Tripp-Reimer (Eds.), *Life transitions in the older adult: Issues for nurses and other health professionals* (pp. 52-72). New York: Springer.

Johnson, M., Bulechek, G., Dochterman, J., Maas, M., & Moorhead, S. (2000). *Nursing diagnoses, outcomes, & interventions: NANDA, NOC, and NIC linkages.* St. Louis: Mosby.

Johnson, R. A., & Hlava, C. (1994). Translocation of elders: Maintaining the spirit. *Geriatric Nursing, 15*(4), 209-212.

Johnson, R. A., Schwiebert, V. B., & Alvarado Rosenmann, P. (1994). Factors influencing nursing home placement decisions. *Clinical Nursing Research, 3*(3), 269-281.

Johnson, R. A., Schwiebert, V. B., Alvarado-Rosenman, P., Pecka, G., & Shirk, N. (1997). Residential preferences and elder care views of Hispanic elders. *Journal of Cross Cultural Gerontology, 12*(1), 91-107.

Kaplan, G., & Camacho, T. (1983). Perceived health and mortality: A nine-year follow-up of the human population laboratory cohort. *American Journal of Epidemiology, 117*(3), 292-303.

Kaye, J., Lawton, M. P., Gitlin, L., Kleban, M., Windsor, L., & Kaye, D. (1988). Older peoples performance on the profile of mood state (POMS). *Clinical Gerontologist, 7*(3/4), 35-56.

Koening, H., Cohen, J., Blazer, D., Pieper, C., Meador, I., Shelp, F., Goli, V., DiPasquale, B. (1992). Religious coping and depression among elderly, hospitalized medically ill men. *American Journal of Psychiatry, 149*(12), 1693-1700.

Kongable, L., Buckwalter, K., & Stolley, J. (1989). The effects of pet therapy on the social behavior of institutionalized Alzheimer's clients. *Archives of Psychiatric Nursing, 3*(4), 191-198.

Kowalski, N. (1981). Institutional relocation: Current programs and applied approaches. *The Gerontologist, 21*(5), 512-519.

Lander, S., Brazil, A., & Ladrigan, P. (1997). Intrainstitutional relocation. Effects on residents' behavior and psychosocial functioning. *Journal of Gerontological Nursing, 23*(4), 35-41.

Lewis, F. (1982). Experienced personal control and quality of life in late-stage cancer patients. *Nursing Research, 31*(2), 113-119.

Liebowitz, B. (1974). Impact of intra-institutional relocation. Special report from the Philadelphia geriatric center. Background and the planning process. *The Gerontologist, 14*(4), 293-294.

Litwak, E., & Longino, C. (1987). Migration patterns among the elderly: A developmental perspective. *The Gerontologist, 27*(3), 266-272.

Markus, E., Blenkner, M., Bloom, M., & Downs, R. (1971). The impact of relocation upon mortality rates of institutionalized aged persons. *Journal of Gerontology, 26*(4), 537-541.

McNair, D., Lorr, M., & Droppleman, L. (1981). *Profile of mood states. EDITS manual.* San Diego, CA: Educational and Industrial Testing Service.

Middleton, G. (1985, April/May/June). Study of the impact of an environmental change on the elderly. *Psychiatric Nursing.* 11-13.

Miller, M., Longino, C., Anderson, R., James, M., & Worley, A. (1999). Functional status, assistance, and the risk of a community-based move. *The Gerontologist, 39*(2), 187-200.

Mirotznik, J., & Ruskin, A. (1985). Interinstitutional relocation and the elderly. *Journal of Long Term Care Administration, 13*(4), 127-131.

Montgomery, R. J., & Kosloski, K. (1994). A longitudinal analysis of nursing home placement for dependent elders cared for by spouses vs. adult children. *Journal of Gerontology, 49*(2), S62-74.

Morris, W., Buckwalter, K., Cleary, T., Gilmer, J., Hatz, D., & Studer, M. (1990). Refinement of the Iowa Self-Assessment Inventory. *The Gerontologist, 30*(2), 243-248.

Mossey, J., & Shapiro, E. (1982). Self-rated health: A predictor of mortality among the elderly. *American Journal of Public Health, 72*(8), 800-808.

Mullins, L., & Dugan, E. (1991). Elderly social relationships with adult children and close friends and depression. *Journal of Social Behavior and Personality, 6*(2), 315-328.

Neugarten, B., Havighurst, R., & Tobin, S. (1961). The measurement of life satisfaction. *Journal of Gerontology, 16,* 134-143.

Norris, J., Gallagher, D., Wilson, A., & Winograd, C. (1987). Assessment of depression in geriatric medical outpatients: The validity of two screening measures. *Journal of the American Geriatrics Society, 35*(11), 989-995.

North American Nursing Diagnosis Association. (1999). *Nursing diagnoses: Definitions & classification 1999-2000*. Philadelphia: Author.

Pablo, R. Y. (1977). Intra-institutional relocation: Its impact on long-term care patients. *The Gerontologist, 17*(5), 426-435.

Palinkas, L., Wingard, D., & Barret-Connor, E. (1990). The biocultural context of social networks and depression among the elderly. *Social Science Medicine, 30*(4), 441-447.

Pino, C. J., Rosica, L. M., & Carter, T. J. (1978). The differential effects of relocation on nursing home patients. *The Gerontologist, 18*(2), 167-171.

Powell, C., Walker, J., Christie, M., Mitchell-Pederson, L., & Rauscher, C. (1990). The unexpected relocation of elderly inpatients in response to a threatened strike. *Journal of Advanced Nursing, 15*, 423-429.

Pressman, P., Lyons, J., Larson, D., & Strain, J. (1990). Religious belief, depression, and ambulating status in elderly women with broken hips. *American Journal of Psychiatry, 147*(6), 758-760.

Pruchno, R., & Resch, N. (1988). Intrainstitutional relocation: Mortality effects. *The Gerontologist, 28*(3), 311-317.

Rajacich, D., & Faux, S. (1988). The relationship between relocation and alterations in mental status among elderly hospitalized patients. *The Canadian Journal of Nursing Research, 20*(4), 31-42.

Rantz, M., & Egan, K. (1987, October). Reducing death from translocation syndrome. *American Journal of Nursing*, 1351-1352.

Reinardy, J. (1992). Decisional control in moving to a nursing home: Post admission adjustment and well-being. *The Gerontologist, 32*(1), 96-103.

Remer, D., & Buckwalter, K. (1990). Decreasing relocation stress. *Continuing Care, Sept.*, 26-27, 42 & 50.

Rosenberg, M. (1962). Self esteem and concern with public affairs. *Public Opinion Quarterly, 26*, 201-211.

Rowles, G. (1983). Between worlds: A relocation dilemma for the appalachian elderly. *International Journal of Aging and Human Development, 17*(4), 301-314.

Rubinstein, R. (1990). Personal identify and environmental meaning in later life. *Journal of Aging Studies, 4*(2), 131-147.

Rutman, D., & Freedman, J. (1988). Anticipating relocation: Coping strategies and the meaning of home for older people. *Canadian Journal on Aging, 7*(1), 17-30.

Schulz, R., & Brenner, G. (1977). Relocation of the aged: A review and theoretical analysis. *Journal of Gerontology, 32*(3), 323-333.

Siegel, J. (1990). Stressful life events and use of physician services among the elderly: The moderating role of pet ownership. *Journal of Personality and Social Psychology, 58*(6), 1081-1086.

Smith, R., & Brand, F. (1975). Effects of enforced relocation on life adjustment in a nursing home. *International Journal of Aging and Human Development, 6*(3), 249-259.

Storandt, M., & Wittels, I. (1975). Maintenance of function in relocation of community-dwelling older adults. *Journal of Gerontology, 30*(5), 608-612.

Tennant, I. (1995). Laugh it off: The effect of humor on the well-being of the older adult. *Journal of Gerontological Nursing, 16*(12), 11-17.

Tesch, S., Nehrke, M., & Whitbourne, S. (1989). Social relationships, psychosocial adaptation and intrainstitutional relocation of elderly men. *The Gerontologist, 29*(4), 517-523.

Thomas, M., Ekland, E., Griffin, M., Hagerott, R., Leichman, S., Murphy, H., & Osborne, O. (1990). Intrahospital relocation of psychiatric patients and effects on aggression. *Archives of Psychiatric Nursing, 4*(3), 154-160.

Thomasma, M., Yeaworth, R., & McCabe, B. (1990). Moving day: Relocation and anxiety in institutionalized elderly. *Journal of Gerontological Nursing, 16*(7), 18-24.

Walker, S., & Gallagher, E. (1990). Environmental change and disruption in an extended care setting: Implications for the nursing role. *Perspectives, Spring*, 6-12.

Wells, L., & MacDonald, G. (1981). Interpersonal networks and pros-relocation adjustment of the institutionalized elderly. *The Gerontologist, 21*(2), 177-183.

Wolinsky, F. D., Callahan, C. M., Fitzgerald, J. F., & Johnson, R. J. (1993). Changes in functional status and the risks of subsequent nursing home placement and death. *Journal of Gerontology, 48*(3), S93-101.

Yesavage, J., Brink, T., Rose, T., Lum, O., Huang, V., Adey, M., & Leirer, V. (1983). Development and validation of a geriatric depression screening scale: A preliminary report. *Journal of Psychiatric Research, 17*(1), 37-49.

Young, J. E., Forbes, W. F., & Hirdes, J. P. (1994). The association of disability with long-term care institutionalization of the elderly. *Canadian Journal on Aging, 13*(1), 24-29.

Youssef, F. (1990). The impact of group reminiscence counseling on a depressed elderly population. *Nurse Practitioner, 15*(4), 32-37.

CHAPTER 49

GRIEVING

Gwen Whiting and Kathleen C. Buckwalter

Death and bereavement are unfortunate facts of life for older adults and the persons who care for them. Grief is a universal phenomenon that has been conceptualized in many different ways (Bowlby, 1961; Engel, 1960a; Freud, 1973; Lindemann, 1974; Parkes, 1972), and yet it rarely has been studied systematically. Little is known about the time course associated with grief (Parkes, 1997), about the importance, frequency, or manifestations of unresolved grief, or about the morbidity and mortality associated with bereavement (Zisook, Shuchter, & Schuckit, 1985). Nor is the natural history of grief in older adults understood well (Dimond, 1981).

Nurses who work with older adults must understand the process of grieving to provide effective support and to promote adjustment to loss. Appropriate nursing interventions and guidance during the grieving process are important to prevent grief-related psychiatric disorders, medical illnesses, and social incapacitation (Parkes, 1965, 1997; Zisook, DeVaul, & Click, 1982).

Theories of grief, loss, and dying have been developed largely to describe a logical sequence or stages of events (Kübler-Ross, 1969). These theories are helpful unless they are used to impose upon others some preconceived timeline or hypothesized "proper" or "appropriate" way in which to grieve (Solari-Twadell, Bunkers, Wang, & Snyder, 1995). Many studies of grief and bereavement are based on crisis theory, a theory that is too narrow to adequately conceptualize the multidimensional experience of grief among elders. Crisis theory implies resolution of a grief reaction in a very short period of time, whereas empirical evidence suggests that grieving requires both time and resources (Dimond, 1981).

Understanding the grieving process can be facilitated by using a four-part "feel/think/act/believe" paradigm of change and growth (Figure 49-1). According to this paradigm, successful change is accomplished when feeling, thinking, and acting are balanced and congruent with a core set of beliefs and values generated throughout the individual's life (Kearney, 1986; Moses & Kearney, 1995). However, when persons think without feeling or act without thinking, or think, act, or feel in a manner incongruent with their inner set of values or beliefs, they may have difficulty coping with change and loss.

Many changes precipitate a grieving process. The changes inherent in growing older, especially in the pres-

ence of chronic illness or disability, impact the dreams, hopes, illusions, and fantasies of aging persons. One context within which to view grieving is that of a cycle that begins with attachment, goes through loss, and returns to renewed attachment. With this cycle in mind, the many and cumulative losses that often accompany old age can be seen as "shattering" attachment dreams. The process of separating from such "lost" dreams prepares the way for emotion-driven reexamination of core values. As bereaved older adults go through a process of reevaluation and active grieving, they prepare themselves to attach anew (Patterson, 1996). This cycle, from attachment to renewed attachment, is embedded in the larger cycle of human development, an intrinsic part of human existence (Moses & Kearney, 1995) shaped by personal history and mutual interaction with others and the environment (Solari-Twadell et al., 1995).

As individuals move through life, they generate many important dreams (Moses, 1985; Moses & Kearney, 1995), including dreams about their later years. Yearnings for completion, peace and contentment, fulfilled responsibilities, financial and material comfort and security, time to be with a partner, and enjoyment of children and grandchildren are only a few of the many dreams and fantasies attached to the later years of life. At the core of these dreams are intense feelings emanating from the elderly individual's unique perception and experience of self and the world.

When core-level dreams are threatened a grieving process begins (Moses, 1983). Death of a spouse, for example, destroys the surviving partner's dreams that depend on the spouse's presence. Degenerative or debilitating illnesses that affect an individual's ability to function physically and/or mentally affect both the impaired individual and family members. The loss of core-level dreams is often so personal that nurses and other health care professionals might not be aware of what is happening. Even the affected elderly individual is frequently confused by the grieving process and the feelings generated.

Through grieving an individual separates from a significant lost dream or projection into the future. The individual struggles with social, emotional, and philosophical issues and reevaluates core-level attitudes and values (Moses, 1977). The process supports personal growth and enables the older individual to create new, more attainable dreams, even in the face of lost ones.

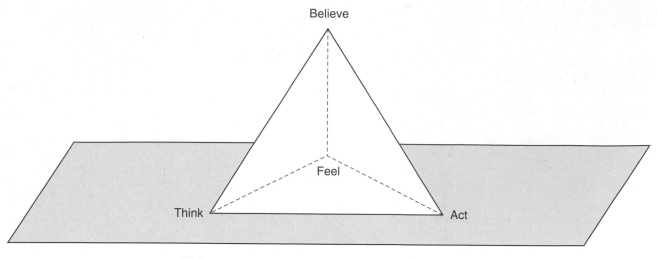

FIGURE **49-1**   Feel/think/act/believe paradigm. (Copyright © Dr. Kenneth Moses.)

Grieving is spontaneous, unlearned, and lifelong (Moses, 1977; Moses & Van Heck-Wulatin, 1981), and the feelings that result appear to be intrinsic and cross-cultural (Lewis & Rosenblum, 1974). Persons who are grieving experience a variety of feeling states, most notably denial, anxiety, guilt, depression, anger, and fear. Although these feeling states are often devalued and denigrated, both by elders themselves and by health care professionals, they are necessary for successful readjustment in the face of change. In addition, feeling-level interactions with a significant other are necessary for the successful evolution of the grieving process (Moses, 1977); in other words, we can't and don't grieve in isolation. The feeling states of denial, anger, anxiety, depression, guilt, and fear occur in no specific order, one is not a prerequisite for another, and they can be felt simultaneously.

Denial is a normal, natural, and necessary part of healthy grieving. Elderly individuals encountering loss situations can deny the existence of the loss or change, the extent and permanence of the loss, the impact of the loss, or the feelings associated with the loss (Aspinwall & Brunhart, 1996; Moses & Van Heck-Wulatin, 1981). Each form of denial serves the same purpose, namely, to keep the grieving person from having to deal with feelings associated with the loss experience too abruptly and from being overwhelmed by the experience (Morley, 1997). Viewing denial as an impediment to early and effective intervention and treatment devalues the grieving individual's felt experience. Denial provides time to build both internal strength and external supports that facilitate successful coping. An enormous amount of energy is necessary to accomplish the building of internal and external supports. Nurses who attempt to "break through" the denial and convince elderly persons of the fact, permanence, and impact of their loss or to persuade them to follow through on all medical recommendations will often be frustrated and disappointed (Collins et al., 1995).

Regaining and maintaining balance in the face of the loss or change requires many personal and internal adjustments (Moses, 1983, 1985) and often vast changes in knowledge, attitudes, beliefs, and behaviors. These adjustments require enormous energy and skill. Anxiety both mobilizes these energies and focuses them on the important task of reestablishing the balance of thoughts/beliefs, feelings, and actions (Moses, 1983; Prigerson et al, 1996).

Guilt is the most difficult and disconcerting of all the grief states. It is difficult for both elderly persons and health professionals to view guilt as acceptable and facilitating growth. Yet guilt allows grieving individuals to reevaluate their beliefs about how they affect the world, the validity of their morals, and the usefulness of their ethical structures (Moses, 1983). How and why one defines certain elements as either their fault or an occurrence of fate is a personal, internal struggle. The goal of this struggle is to develop a system that allows the older adult to deal effectively with the vicissitudes of life. A healthy stance avoids both the absurdity of assuming full responsibility for all life events and the equally absurd position of disclaiming responsibility for anything (Moses, 1983; Moses & Van Heck-Wulatin, 1981).

Although Western culture generally views depression as pathologic, this feeling state can be a normal, necessary, and healthy part of the grieving process. Everyone has a need to be competent, yet definitions of competency change as individuals age. Depression helps older individuals confront their definition of competence both within their current life experience and in the context of loss and change.

Within our culture, strong feelings and expressions of anger are considered immature and inappropriate in the context of "responsible behavior," and we work hard to expunge angry expression in all age groups. At the same time, we have an internalized sense of justice and injustice (Moses, 1977, 1983; Moses & Van Heck-Wulatin, 1981). If we treat others fairly, we expect them to reciprocate in kind. Chronic illness and disability violate this sense of justice and fairness in older persons who have worked, saved, and planned for retirement or travel.

Fear confronts issues of abandonment, vulnerability, and risk in the face of change and loss. New attitudes, beliefs, and definitions concerning the individual's ability to reattach must be formed, knowing the risk inherent in building a new dream (Moses, 1977, 1983; Moses & Van Heck-Wulatin, 1981). Our society has fostered an even greater sense of vulnerability among older adults. The changes and losses experienced by older persons put them in even closer touch with their mortality, sometimes precipitously and often painfully. Helping older persons face their fears enables them to struggle with reattachment, even in the midst of vulnerability and risk (see Chapter 44, Anxiety and Fear).

RELATED FACTORS/ETIOLOGIES

Four variables influence the duration and course of the grieving process: the nature of the elder's support system; the elder's past history with transforming experiences; the elder's emotional maturity; and how pivotal or central the loss is to the elder's life.

Support System

The cultural milieu in which one is raised defines what is acceptable and unacceptable. Persons raised to believe that denial, anxiety, depression, anger, guilt, or fear are wrong to experience and inappropriate to express will subjugate those feelings, and the grieving process will arrest in response to those negative cultural injunctions. The significant others who surround and attempt to support the older person experiencing loss also affect the grieving process. Grieving is facilitated in the context of a relationship with a person who is willing and able to be authentically present. Friends, family, and health care professionals who communicate disapproving subcultural messages, who are too distracted by their own grief to be fully present, or who are unwilling or unable to tolerate the older adult's expression of feelings associated with grieving will discourage grieving or offer "help" instead of support. Common ways that people offer such discouraging "help" include the following exhortations: "Face reality; . . . it's not as bad as you think; . . . be strong; . . . it's not your fault; . . . these things happen; . . . it will turn out for the best; . . . calm down; . . . you can handle this; . . . pull yourself together; . . . don't cry; . . . there's nothing to be afraid of." The clear and common message that underlies all of these expressions is: "Don't feel what you're feeling; if you do, don't express it!" These inhibitory messages from others can reinforce inner voices of the grieving elder that impugn the feelings of grief as a sign of weakness, dependency, self-indulgence,

stupidity, lack of discipline, cowardice, a character flaw, or even insanity. Together these internal and external voices function as powerful environmental restraints on the grieving process.

History of Loss

The time and course of grieving is also impacted by the older individual's history of loss. When a person experiences a core-level loss for the first time, the feelings that emerge are both overwhelming and confusing. If one successfully works through the bereavement process, one experiences a growing, life-changing transformation. When subsequent losses occur the individual is more able to recognize the experience and to acknowledge and trust the path she needs to follow. Although this does not make the experience of loss any less painful, it does reduce the added pain and misspent time that result from resisting the grieving process. Those who are unsuccessful in dealing with loss tend to recall only the distress and bewilderment, not the release.

Emotional Maturity

The third variable that influences the time and course of grieving is emotional maturity. Constraints originate from childhood traumas and unresolved developmental crises that directly affect psychosocial growth and emotional maturity. A person who has achieved emotional maturity, by definition, has successfully traversed the territory of grieving core-level losses in the past. That person is more apt to use the skills and insights that grew out of those past experiences.

Centrality of the Loss

The last variable that affects the grief process is how central the loss is to one's life. Losing a spouse is a painful loss, but for the older adult who loses a spouse after 50 years of marriage and who has no children or other relatives in his life, the grieving process might be even harder. Peripheral losses, that is, losses where the attachment is not deep, are painful, but usually do not result in life-changing transformations. Only core-level losses do that.

Individuals who have many attachments will more likely have an intact support system to assist them in grieving after the loss. For the elder who has a single, meaningful relationship in her life and that relationship is lost, the grieving process will be more difficult and lengthy. In the latter circumstance, older adults suffer not only the loss of a loved one, but also the loss of their whole support system when it is needed most. In this situation an older person might be heard to say, "She's the only one I ever loved, the only one who could help me at a time like this, and now she's gone" (Moses & Kearney, 1995).

ASSESSMENT

In assessing grief in older adults the nurse should explore several key questions: How central to the older adult's life was the attachment; that is, how many of his life dreams were shattered by the loss? How exclusive was the attachment; that is, was this one of many deep attachments or the older adult's only or primary attachment?

A number of instruments have been developed to capture the concept of grief and loss among older adults and among those who care for them. In the latter category, for example, researchers have used the Impact of Patient Death Questionnaire (Adams, Hershatter, & Moritz, 1991) to evaluate the effects of patient death on the nursing staff in a long-term care setting (O'Hara, Harper, Chartrand, & Johnston, 1996). Several other tools purport to measure the impact of grief on family caregivers and non–health care professionals, including the Texas Revised Inventory of Grief (Faschingbauer, 1981) and the Grief Experience Inventory. The Grief Experience Inventory (Sanders, Mauger, & Strong, 1979) comprises nine subscales: despair, anger-hostility, guilt, social isolation, loss of control, rumination, depersonalization, somatization, and death anxiety.

A psychiatrically based assessment tool, the Inventory of Grief, was initially developed (Faschingbauer, DeVaul, & Zisook, 1977) as a 14-item self-report scale with two distinct factors: "present feelings" and "past behavior and feelings immediately following the object loss." The instrument was expanded to 58 items in an effort to measure frequency and time course of grief-related behaviors and feelings (Zisook et al., 1982). Research using the expanded tool demonstrated that grief did not end at any circumscribed time interval, although most "symptoms" peaked between 1 and 2 years after loss of a loved one. Many behaviors and symptoms appeared to persist indefinitely, and certain preoccupations and painful memories continued to affect bereaved respondents strongly after 10 years.

Zisook and DeVaul (1983) extracted three items from the expanded inventory to create the Unresolved Grief Index. Nine items on the Zung Depression Scale were significantly correlated with items on this new index, suggesting a stable (over time) relationship between depression and unresolved grief. However, the research was carried out with middle-aged rather than elderly respondents.

Dimond, Caserta, & Lund (1994) combined qualitative and quantitative approaches, using interview data and standardized measures of depression. These investigators cautioned against using measures of depression as the sole indicator of post-bereavement depression to the exclusion of the life context of the elder in the interpretation of scores. They argued that a comprehensive nursing assessment includes determination of concurrent life experiences that might exacerbate grief. They suggested that the following questions can be useful in providing a more complete picture of the life experience of the older adult after death of a spouse (Dimond et al., 1994, p. 266):

1. Can you tell me about how your spouse died?
2. How have others treated you since the death? What have they said to you, and how has this made you feel?
3. How have your children and other members of your family handled the death? Have they been helpful to you?
4. Can you tell me about other things that have happened to you, or are happening to you now, that are making things harder for you?
5. Have you made any big changes in your life since your spouse died, such as moving or selling your home?

McFarland and Wasli (1986, p. 79) outlined a 10-point nursing assessment for the nursing diagnosis of Dysfunctional Grieving that also evaluates some of the critical elements recommended by the authors: the elder's support system, past history and emotional maturity, and the centrality of the loss is to the elder's life:

1. Are defining characteristics of dysfunctional grieving present?
2. What is the nature of the loss? When did it occur?
3. How did the patient perceive the loss? Did it have special meaning or value? What is the significance of the loss in relation to the patient's perceived and real abilities to meet his own needs?
4. What stage of grieving and behavioral manifestations does the patient currently show?
5. What is the patient's behavior between actual occurrence of loss and the present?
6. How has the patient coped with loss in the past? What strengths were demonstrated in coping with loss?
7. Is the patient at high risk for dysfunctional grieving? Examples of such patients are those with:
   a. Poor relationship with person prior to death
   b. Social isolation or poor social network
   c. History of multiple past losses and use of maladaptive coping strategies.
   d. Presentation of a brave, stoic front
8. What is the nature of the social network present?
9. What is the degree of depression? Are there suicidal tendencies?
10. What are significant others' reactions to the patient's response to loss?

Finally, any assessment of grieving must include an in-depth examination of the grief-related feeling states denial, anxiety, guilt, depression, anger, and fear. Elderly individuals who are experiencing denial might appear to reject what the health care professional has to offer or to be engaging in "doctor shopping," looking for an acceptable diagnosis and rejecting those with catastrophic implications (Collins et al., 1995). These older individuals often become vulnerable to "quackery" as they search for and involve themselves in unusual and unorthodox treatments (Moses, 1983). Some elders who deny the impact of a change may appear to have all the necessary resources, knowledge, and attitudes to deal with the loss with no outward manifestation or acknowledgment of stress. Many health care professionals encourage this behavior in an effort to minimize the difficulty of implementing necessary treatments. Other elderly individuals who deny feelings may acknowledge that a difficult, permanent change has occurred, but claim that "it doesn't matter; it just doesn't upset me," or "I don't know what you're all so upset about." These individuals can exhibit incongruencies, such as thinking without feeling or acting without thinking, and have trouble coping with whatever change or loss has occurred. Unfortunately, elderly persons with any form of denial will not perceive the need to alter their current attitudes, behaviors, values, or feelings regarding the loss or diagnosis (Moses, 1983) and may appear defensive and agitated or rigid and affectless (Moses, 1983, 1985).

Older individuals who encounter loss and change, especially those in long-term care settings, can exhibit generalized anxiety. Sometimes anxiety can be so great that it immobilizes the individual (see Chapter 44).

Guilt can be experienced in one of three ways. Older individuals often believe that they caused their own loss experience through poor health habits, smoking, alcohol or drug abuse, contraction of an avoidable disease, or other occurrences that they felt were within their control. This is the most logical manifestation of guilt and therefore is the easiest to accept. Guilt also can be demonstrated in a belief that the loss is fair or just punishment for wrongdoing in the past, even in the absence of any direct connections. This type of guilt has a less logical basis and is easier to counter. Finally, guilt can be evidenced in the philosophical stance that "good things happen to good people; bad things happen to bad people." Thus the grieving individual feels guilt simply because the loss occurred (Moses & Van Heck-Wulatin, 1981).

Older adults can express depression through judgments of themselves as weak (impotent), useless (incapable), and worthless (valueless). They see themselves as having no influence or impact in important areas of life. Expressing feelings of "anger turned inward," a sense of impotence and valuelessness, enables the elder to let go of old definitions of competence and see themselves as competent, adequate, potent, and valuable once again (Moses, 1983).

Older adults who experience anger while grieving often project their anger onto persons that they perceive as the cause of their loss or change. The "targets" for their anger can include physicians, family members, nurses, and others who seem to be the source and/or reminder of the loss and the injustice. Ironically, the very people on whom the anger is displaced often are those most needed by the older person suffering from loss or change. In some cases, older persons direct their anger at science, at God, or at life in general. This displacement keeps them from confronting internal values, beliefs, and attitudes regarding fairness and justice and from restructuring core level issues to generate a more reality-based internal sense of fairness (Moses, 1983).

Fear often can be detected in grieving persons, especially institutionalized elders who have lost control of their environment, their bodily functions, the expression of their individuality, or the autonomy and intimacy of their relationships with others. These individuals can express painful awareness of their vulnerability, which they might be experiencing for the first time and which they are likely to be experiencing in a new and unacceptable way. They also might express doubts regarding the wisdom of trying to reattach and reconnect themselves to the world, only to be hurt again (Moses, 1983).

CASE STUDY 1

D. Fox, age 66, was suddenly and unexpectedly widowed 6 months ago. She seemed to handle the death of her husband well, living alone in the family home, working part-time, and caring for herself. However, her daughter reportedly noticed piles of unpaid bills for the mortgage and insurance, as well as Social Security forms that had not been filled out. When a friendly visitor from the local Council on Aging asked about the papers, Mrs. Fox looked "blank," then responded, "Oh, they'll be taken care of. Everything will be fine." When pressed further, Mrs. Fox changed the subject or walked out of the room.

When Mrs. Fox's uncharacteristic and nonchalant behavior continued and her insurance policy was canceled for nonpayment, her daughter took her to a geriatric assessment clinic. The daughter informed the nurse that Mr. Fox had always handled the couple's finances. Mrs. Fox used her own paycheck only for "pin money and little extras." Otherwise, Mr. Fox had taken care of all financial matters during the marriage. Next the nurse obtained a brief history from Mrs. Fox concerning her husband's death. The dialogue revealed that Mrs. Fox felt her daughter was a "worrywart" and that she didn't need to be talking to anyone. Mrs. Fox advised the nurse that she was not really sure why her daughter seemed concerned about her financial security, noting that in all her years she had never worried about finances before and that everything had been just fine.

CASE STUDY 2

C. Lloyd, age 73, had been widowed for 10 years. She had one married daughter living in another state and a 40-year-old mentally retarded daughter living with her. Mrs. Lloyd initially called her local community mental health center (CMHC) asking for some medication to help her sleep and for assistance with her retarded daughter's "difficult" behavior. Early sessions with both mother and daughter were for evaluation purposes. The daughter was referred for evaluation of her medication and current medical needs and assigned a nurse therapist to assist her with her feeling-level issues regarding (1) her retardation, (2) having her elderly mother as her only companion, and (3) the unresolved loss of her father. Because Mrs. Lloyd complained of persistent insomnia and anorexia and had lost 15 pounds over the past 2 months, the therapist also evaluated the need for her to have assistance in dealing with her own issues regarding her husband, her daughter, and her own anticipated death. Mrs. Lloyd had a great deal of difficulty accepting help initially. She tearfully explained that she wanted the nurse-therapist to come, but kept saying, "We should be talking about my daughter, not me. I'll be okay if I just get some sleep and start eating."

CASE STUDY 3

P. Smythe, age 70, was released from the hospital after recovery from a myocardial infarction. The extent of the damage was relatively minor, and his physicians gave him permission and encouragement to engage in light activity, especially walking. Before his infarction Mr. Smythe was an active businessman. He ran a large corporation, was on the boards of several other large companies, played golf, swam, and traveled a great deal with his wife. His heart attack occurred on the golf course. After his return home, however, Mr. Smythe remained virtually housebound, refusing even to walk around his home. Every time his wife encouraged him or reminded him that the doctor said he should walk he would become angry and say "What does he know?" or "I will when I'm ready. Now leave me alone." Then she'd tell him he shouldn't feel angry because the doctors were just doing their job. The doctor made a referral to a geriatric nurse practitioner to monitor Mr. Smythe's blood pressure and, more importantly, to try to assist Mrs. Smythe in dealing with diet and exercise issues. The nurse spent initial sessions listening to Mr. Smythe angrily talk about doctors and "those hospital people" who tell him what to do and "run his life." He snapped at his wife several times when she tried to explain why the doctors were telling him to exercise.

NURSING DIAGNOSIS

Medical and psychiatric models most often have viewed grief along a continuum, with "normal grief" at one end and "pathologic grief reactions" (e.g., neurotic and psychosomatic symptoms) at the other end (Volkan, 1970). However, even "normal" grief has been considered an illness by some because it is a discrete syndrome with predictable symptomatology (Engel, 1960b). In keeping with the illness perspective of the grieving process, four related nursing diagnoses were set forth in 1973: arrested grieving;

arrested grieving, potential; delayed onset of grieving; and delayed onset of grieving, potential (Kim & Moritz, 1982). In 1980 these diagnoses became synthesized under the diagnostic label "Dysfunctional Grieving," which the North American Nursing Diagnoses Association (NANDA) currently defines as "Extended, unsuccessful use of intellectual and emotional responses by which individuals, families, communities attempt to work through the process of modifying self-concept based upon the perception of loss" (NANDA, 1999, p. 124).

The term *dysfunctional* has been used to describe any experience that inhibits persons from going on with their lives (Gordon, 1982). Dysfunctional grieving implies being "stuck in one phase of grieving, demonstrating excessive emotional reactions or excessive length of time in a phase" (McFarland & Wasli, 1986, p. 77). The literature suggests that potential outcomes of dysfunctional grieving include failure to attain acceptance and successful adaptation, engagement in prolonged, excessive denial, and the development of mental illness, especially depression. The terms *complicated, unresolved, morbid, neurotic, pathologic, abnormal, deviant, chronic, delayed, exaggerated, atypical,* and *distorted* also refer to this same "dysfunctional" element in the grieving process.

The following defining characteristics of Dysfunctional Grieving have been outlined by NANDA: verbal expression of distress at loss; denial of loss; expression of guilt; expression of unresolved issues; anger; sadness; crying; difficulty expressing loss; alterations in eating habits, sleep patterns, dream patterns, activity level, libido, concentration, and/or pursuits of tasks; idealization of lost object; reliving of past experiences with little or no reduction (diminishment) of intensity of the grief; interference with life functioning; developmental regression; labile affect; alterations in concentration and/or pursuits of tasks (NANDA, 1999, pp. 124-125). These characteristics are difficult to differentiate from depressive symptomatology and other psychiatric conditions (see Chapter 41).

Related factors identified by NANDA include actual or perceived object loss, with the term *object loss* being used in the broadest sense. Thus, as noted in Table 49-1, object loss includes people, possessions, a job, status, home, ideals, and parts and processes of the body (NANDA, 1999, p. 125).

Bell (1995, p. 236) has called NANDA's "dysfunctional" approach to the grieving process a "lens of pathology." This dysfunctional perspective judges depression, anger, fear, guilt, anxiety, and denial to be inappropriate when they extend beyond some arbitrarily proscribed time period or level of intensity. Thus older adults who do not conform to a stereotyped set of psychologic and physiologic reactions or whose period of recovery deviates from some predetermined norm (Dimond, 1981) are labeled "dysfunctional grievers."

Moreover, the nursing interventions that flow from this dysfunctional framework are often ineffective because they focus predominantly on "doing something for" the bereaved rather than recognizing and honoring their suffering (Solari-Twadell, Bunkers, Wang, & Snyder, 1995). This approach devalues their core-level feelings, sacrificing insight and understanding of the grief experience (Frank, 1991; Solari-Twadell et al., 1995). In so doing, outcomes for bereaved older adults are often less than optimal.

Indeed, compelling research evidence suggests that the grieving process is a highly individualized and unique experience. Grief and loss are affected by a variety of social and situational factors, sex roles, and cultural values and practices (Clayton, Halikas, & Maurice, 1971; Faschingbauer, 1981; Glick, Weiss, & Parkes, 1974; Lowenthal & Haven, 1968; Maddison & Viola, 1968; Rees & Lufkins, 1967; Vachon, 1976). Furthermore, systematic assessment efforts confirm that bereavement is characterized by a wide constellation of behaviors, feelings, and symptoms (Zisook et al., 1982), the meaning of which cannot be defined by an observer.

In taking issue with NANDA's diagnostic perspective and dysfunctional view of grieving, this chapter reframes the concept of grieving from the vantage point of the elderly bereaved person and argues that grieving is usually a functional process. From the authors' perspective, grieving—even prolonged grieving—is part of the process of living, rather than an impediment to life. Thus we reject the indiscriminate application of labels (e.g., "inappropriate," "negative," "dysfunctional") traditionally used to describe the emotions experienced as elderly persons struggle to redefine, reevaluate, and reattach (cope) in the context of their loss(es). Although grieving can be superimposed upon premorbid psychiatric/psychologic problems, most elderly persons experience grieving as a normal, though individually defined, dynamic process. Indeed, the term *dysfunctional* trivializes and minimizes problems, perpetuates a sense of powerlessness and hopelessness about the future, and limits both practitioners and elders who are labeled as dysfunctional from proposing other distinctions about themselves (Bell, 1995). Consequently, it is proposed that consideration be given to developing a nursing diagnosis labeled Grieving, defined as "a normal, spontaneous, unlearned, lifelong, functional process that is part of living and is uniquely defined by the person experiencing the loss." Table 49-1 contrasts NANDA's definition, related factors, and defining characteristics for Dysfunctional Grieving with those for Grieving set forth by the authors.

Table 49-1	Dysfunctional Grieving and Grieving: Comparison of Definitions, Defining Characteristics, and Related Factors/Etiologies
Dysfunctional Grieving (NANDA, 1999)	**Grieving (Whiting and Buckwalter)**
DEFINITION	
Extended, unsuccessful use of intellectual and emotional responses by which individuals, families, communities attempt to work through the process of modifying self-concept based upon the perception of loss	A normal, spontaneous, unlearned, lifelong, functional process that is part of living and is uniquely defined by the person experiencing the loss
DEFINING CHARACTERISTICS	
Verbal expression of distress at loss; denial of loss; expression of unresolved issues; anger; sadness; crying; difficulty in expressing loss; alterations in: eating habits, sleep patterns, dream patterns, activity level, libido; idealization of lost object; reliving of past experiences; interference with life functioning; developmental regression; labile affect; alterations in concentration and/or pursuits of tasks	Redefinition, reevaluation, and reattachment in the context of loss Depression Anger Fear Guilt Anxiety Denial Reassessment of attitudes and values Struggle with social, emotional, and philosophic structures
RELATED FACTORS/ETIOLOGIES	
Actual or perceived object loss; objects may include people, possessions, a job, status, home, ideals, parts, and processes of the body	Feel/think/act/believe paradigm out of sync Inability to fulfill dreams, illusions, fantasies, and projections into the future Profound impact on existential issues related to attachment, meaning, vitality, values, choice, and ownership

NURSING-SENSITIVE OUTCOMES

Outcomes traditionally associated with resolution of the NANDA diagnosis Dysfunctional Grieving are embedded in a time-constrained, linear conceptualization of the grieving process (McFarland and Wasli, 1986, p. 82), in which the individual:

1. Engages in normal grief work, that is, works through the phases of normal grieving (e.g., denial, anger, bargaining, realization of loss, and acceptance and reintegration)
2. Demonstrates a reasonable amount of time in phases of grieving
3. Demonstrates nonexcessive and nonprolonged emotional reactions
4. Restructures and reorders life constructively

The *Nursing Outcomes Classification (NOC)* (Iowa Outcomes Project, 2000) has identified a number of outcomes relevant to the grieving process: Comfort Level; Endurance; Hope; Will to Live; Psychosocial Adjustment: Life Change; Anxiety Control; Caregiver Emotional Health; Self-Esteem; Quality of Life; Social Involvement; Spiritual Well-Being; Loneliness; and Mood Equilibrium. However, none of these outcomes are specific to grieving. Will to Live, for example, refers to one's own illness/treatment; similarly, all of the citations underlying the outcome Psychosocial Adjustment: Life Change come from the retirement literature rather than from the bereavement literature.

The two NOC outcomes most pertinent to the nursing diagnosis of grieving are Grief Resolution and Coping. Grief Resolution is defined as "adjustment to actual or impending loss" (Iowa Outcomes Project, 2000, p. 223) (Box 49-1). The NOC indicator "progresses through stages of grief" seems predicated on a staging conceptualization of the bereavement process that stands in contrast to a nonlinear movement through the various feeling (grieving) states of denial, anxiety, fear, guilt, depression, and anger. But importantly, the NOC indicator places no time constraints on the process (e.g., resolution achieved by 12 months after loss). One might argue that the elder who is in a feeling state of denial or depression, for example, would be unable to achieve several of the NOC indicators such as participating in funeral planning or seeking social support. Furthermore, the older adult whose life-long partner has been lost might not report "normal sexual desire."

Coping is the behavioral (or functional) enactment of attitudinal and philosophic changes that grow out of the grieving process. Although grieving is a prerequisite of coping, both are evident shortly after the onset of a loss. Indicators for the NOC outcome Coping are listed in Box 49-2 (Iowa Outcomes Project, 2000).

Wright (1960) and Moses (1983, 1985) have described four keys to coping with grief: containing the impact of the loss, devaluing "normal" standards, enlarging scope of values, and shifting from comparative to asset values. These concepts can be used to measure the success of an individual's grief journey.

Successful grieving requires containing the impact of the loss. A core-level loss affects an individual's entire life. The impact of the loss is generalized, creating the feeling that "everything" is lost, ruined, or meaningless. Coping with loss requires a careful and accurate assessment of what is actually affected (lost), what is salvageable, and what aspects of life have been unscathed by the loss. Such a sorting process helps the individual contain the impact of the loss so that it does not feel ever-present. Persons who are containing the impact of their loss can identify aspects of their lives that remain unchanged. They also will report an increase in psychologic comfort and positive expectations about the future.

Successful grieving depends on devaluing "normal" standards. Loss is not valued as "normal." Society treats loss as a low-incidence occurrence that only affects certain people. It is not considered "normal" to have an impaired child, to be wheelchair bound, to struggle with a manic-depressive disorder, or to suffer with a terminal illness. Indeed, loss can create feelings of inferiority in grieving

Box 49-1	**Nursing-Sensitive Outcome Indicators** **GRIEF RESOLUTION**
Expresses feelings about loss	Expresses spiritual beliefs about death
Verbalizes reality of loss	Verbalizes acceptance of loss
Describes meaning of the loss or death	Participates in planning funeral
Maintains current will	Maintains advance directives
Discusses unresolved conflict(s)	Reports absence of somatic distress
Reports decreased preoccupation with loss	Maintains living environment
Maintains grooming and hygiene	Reports absence of sleep disturbance
Reports adequate nutritional intake	Reports normal sexual desire
Seeks social support	Shares loss with significant others
Reports involvement in social activities	Progresses through stages of grief
Expresses positive expectations about the future	

Box 49-2	Nursing-Sensitive Outcome Indicators COPING	
Identifies effective coping patterns	Identifies ineffective coping patterns
Verbalizes sense of control	Reports decrease in stress
Verbalizes acceptance of situation	Seeks information concerning illness and treatment
Modifies lifestyle as needed	Adapts to developmental changes
Uses available social support	Employs behaviors to reduce stress
Identifies multiple coping strategies	Uses effective coping strategies
Avoids unduly stressful situations	Verbalizes need for assistance
Seeks professional help as appropriate	Reports decrease in physical symptoms of stress
Reports decrease in negative feelings	Reports increase in psychologic comfort

older persons and inhibit social integration. Coping requires rejection of the "normal" standards that devalue bereaved or afflicted people. Persons who have devalued the normal standards verbalize their disbelief in the normal standards of society and see themselves as normal. They accept responsibility for making their needs known and verbalize a sense of control. They seek social support and work with other responsible individuals to meet those needs.

Successful grieving incorporates enlarging one's scope of values. Ironically, as people grow and develop, the values they hold often become narrow and constricted. When a substantive loss fundamentally shakes an individual's value system, it can enlarge the scope of that person's values. This process of enlarging the scope of values facilitates coping. Persons who are enlarging the scope of their values will be able to see themselves as valuable and potentially link their sense of value to a variety of abilities, activities, and relationships. They will report involvement in social activities and use of behaviors that reduce stress and enhance coping.

Successful grieving entails shifting from comparative values to asset values. Some people appear more concerned about how they compare to others than about their own assets. Older adults who value themselves only when they "measure up" to others will judge themselves as inferior after a loss. As a result, losses become devastating. Elders who concentrate on their own abilities, accomplishments, knowledge, and experiences can more quickly and easily make use of these assets to assist in creating new dreams. Therefore coping with loss includes shifting from comparative values to asset values. Persons who are successfully shifting their values can describe their unique and individual experiences and gifts and will report sharing those experiences and gifts with others. They also will report involvement in social activities and using behaviors to reduce stress and promote coping.

It is proposed here that the indicators described by Wright (1960) and Moses (1983, 1985) be incorporated as outcomes in a new Grieving/Coping Model. As shown in Figure 49-2, elderly persons who have successfully

coped with loss and change will be able to reenter the world and undertake the developmental tasks of older age with new skills, perspectives, insights, and attitudes. The "hallmark of the resolution of grief is the ability of the bereaved to recognize that they have grieved and can now return to work, re-experience pleasure, and respond to the companionship of love of others" (Zisook et al., 1985, p. 497).

NURSING INTERVENTIONS

There is a dearth of nursing investigations evaluating interventions to facilitate the grieving process in elders. Rather, most articles identify needs of the bereaved or set forth anecdotally based suggestions for providing support. In reality, health care professionals tend to offer bereaved older adults an array of treatments aimed at ameliorating the pain or "curing" the affliction of grieving (Moses, 1993). These include, for example, the use of medications, hypnosis, and/or relaxation exercises.

More recently, attention has turned to ways in which nursing homes can assist staff, families, and other residents in the grieving process, including using hospice organizations as a source for information and grief counseling, pastoral counseling, holding memorial services, and sending out personalized sympathy cards or other direct expressions of sympathy (Kavanaugh, 1995).

A number of interventions identified in the third edition of the *Nursing Interventions Classification (NIC)* (Iowa Intervention Project, 2000) are important to the concept of grieving in older adults, but most have not been empirically validated for this purpose. These include, for example, Active Listening; Anger Control Assistance; Anxiety Reduction; Cognitive Restructuring; Coping Enhancement; Counseling; Crisis Intervention; Emotional Support; Family Support; Mood Management; Presence; and Spiritual Support. However, the most relevant NIC intervention is Grief Work Facilitation, defined as "assistance with the resolution of a significant loss" (Iowa Intervention Project, 2000, p. 358). This intervention incorporates a number of activities, as listed in Box 49-3.

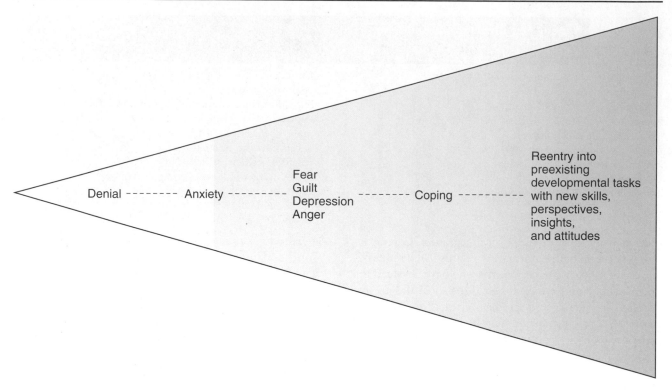

FIGURE **49-2**   Grieving-coping model.

While most of the NIC activities used to implement the Grief Work Facilitation intervention are in keeping with the authors' conceptualization of the grieving process, there is an underlying implication in certain of the intervention activities that grieving is a series of steps to be followed and that grieving is done in discrete stages that must be followed to be successfully completed. That is, the two NIC activities italicized in Box 49-3 seem to suggest that the grieving process is linear and sequential rather than a cyclical, fluid, and dynamic process impelled by feeling states. Seeing grieving in such a stepwise progression can view persons who have "skipped" some of the steps as having a pathologic disorder. It also increases the likelihood that interventions will be formula-like recipes (i.e., a specific set of instructions to be followed precisely) for working through losses rather than like maps that can be used to guide, support, and orient the elder through the unfamiliar and sometimes terrifying terrain of personal transformation following loss(es) (Moses, 1993).

ENUF

Successful intervention with the grieving process is based on the belief that people are best helped by creating an environment in which they can better experience and help themselves. These interventions require that the "helper" have the willingness and ability to be authentically present. The environment must reflect very specific attitudes toward and values for the older adult, succinctly captured in the acronym ENUF (Moses, 1983; Moses & Kearney, 1995), which is defined as follows:

*E*mpathy is the concerted effort to gain an accurate perception of another's experience and then to congruently share that perception in one's own unique style and personal manner.

*N*onjudgment is an attitude of acceptance, free of evaluation, regardless of content shared.

*U*nconditional positive regard is a philosophy about the nature of human beings that affirms the value of all people, as they are, simply because they exist.

*F*eeling focus is the act of emphasizing feelings instead of content in interactions of an emotional nature.

Empathizing, the first component of ENUF, is the concerted effort to gain an accurate perception of another's experience and to congruently share that perception in one's own words, unique style, and personal manner. Empathizing requires a concerted effort. In this context the nurse focuses full attention, training, skill, knowledge, history, sensitivity, and awareness in the moment. There is no one and nothing more important than the grieving elder and that which she is sharing. This sense of being present is best captured when the nurse is both willing and able to act on the words, "There is no place in the world I would rather be, no one with whom I would rather be, and nothing I would rather be doing, than being me, sitting here with you, now" (Rosenthal, 1994, p. 214).

Box 49-3	Nursing Intervention Activities **GRIEF WORK FACILITATION**

Identify the loss

Encourage expression of feelings about the loss

Encourage discussion of previous loss experiences

Encourage identification of greatest fears concerning the loss

Support progression through personal grieving stages

Assist to identify personal coping strategies

Communicate acceptance of discussing the loss

Use clear words, such as dead or died, rather than euphemisms

Encourage expression of feelings in ways comfortable to the child, such as writing, drawing, or playing*

Identify sources of community support

Reinforce progress made in the grieving process

Assist the patient to identify the nature of the attachment to the lost object or person

Assist the patient to identify the initial reaction to the loss

Encourage the patient to verbalize memories of the loss, both past and current

Instruct in phases of the grieving process, as appropriate

Include significant others in discussions and decisions, as appropriate

Encourage patient to implement cultural, religious, and social customs associated with the loss

Answer children's questions associated with the loss*

Encourage children to discuss feelings*

Assist the child to clarify misconceptions

Support efforts to resolve previous conflict, as appropriate

Assist in identifying modifications needed in lifestyle

*Identifies activities more relevant to children than older adults.

To empathize the nurse must be actively engaged in the relationship, working right along with the grieving elder. This is more than a process of simply listening to words and following along, then parroting back the words heard. Neither is it a technique to be followed with textbook perfection. Empathy hinges on the nurse's efforts to gain an accurate perception of that which the grieving person is sharing. The facilitative power of empathizing grows not simply from gaining an accurate perception of the elder's experience; rather, it emerges from the process of making the effort. The potential to facilitate the grief work is created by the nurse's interest and concern. Involvement, intimacy, and trust cannot be assumed to exist simply because one person is experiencing pain and the other is offering help. Rather, it is demonstrated through the concerted effort of the nurse to understand the elder's experience. The consistency and reliability of this effort, as perceived by the elder, supports the growth of trust and rapport out of which the grief work develops (Moses & Kearney, 1995).

Empathizing is the concerted effort to gain an accurate perception of another's experience. The key element in rapport is the trust that one will be understood. Trust makes it possible for the elderly person to risk talking about feelings that he fears might be misunderstood. The accuracy of the nurse's perceptions is continually validated and improved by verifying with the elder. The only way to know that one's perception matches another's experience is to ask. Nurses practicing ENUF regularly confirm their perceptions with their patients. They typically follow simple declarative statements about what they are perceiving with straightforward inquiries about the accuracy of those perceptions. By sharing their perceptions and then asking simple questions such as, "Is that what it's like for you?" nurses simultaneously verify their accuracy and

express their intention to understand. The purpose is not just to get confirmation that the nurse's perception is accurate, but, as importantly, to demonstrate the nurse's involvement with the patient in the process. Empathizing works in a relationship because the effort of the nurse is a match for the work of the bereaved older adult (Moses & Kearney, 1995).

When helpers simply announce that they understand or make declarations without checking their accuracy, rapport is often negatively affected. Rather than facilitating the grieving process, such declarations often bring it to an impasse. Even if the nurse is accurate, elders may perceive the words as an intrusion into their process. Sometimes patients react to this intrusion by seeing the helper as brilliant, clairvoyant, or even magical. Other times they see the helper as an arrogant know-it-all. When that happens, authenticity is lost and a negative experience ensues (Moses & Kearney, 1995).

Nurses who use ENUF have to deal with their own feelings and thoughts about what their older patients are relating. Grief work often involves processing intense pain, and if nurses are fully present in this process, it is impossible for them to avoid having their own feelings stirred. The key is to remember that the focus is on what the elder is feeling. To the extent that nurses use their own feelings to provide them with clues as to what patients might be feeling and then reflect this in their questions, they can assist in the task of empathizing. Rather than sharing their reactions as interpretations about the elder, nurses practicing ENUF express their reactions as statements about their experiences, thus expanding the interaction rather than restricting the process (Moses & Kearney, 1995).

It is important for nurses practicing ENUF to respond in their own words, style, and manner. In so doing, they bring themselves into the interaction rather than mirroring back the patient's own words. This is one way that empathizing differs from "active listening." The point is not to show that one heard the elder's words, but to demonstrate one's intention to accurately perceive what those words mean and to be fully present (Moses & Kearney, 1995).

Being nonjudgmental, the second component of ENUF, is an attitude, not a technique. It is based on the belief that growth takes place when an individual takes a risk. In the grieving process, it is important to risk letting go of lost, shattered dreams. Taking this risk permits the creation of new, more attainable dreams. However, for this to happen the elder must feel safe enough to take risks. It is necessary for the nurse to establish rapport and engage the elder in the work of the grieving process. Empathizing nonjudgmentally is essential to this trust-building process. Creating an environment free from the threats created by criticism, punishment, or blame makes risk-taking possible. The nurse helps establish a facilitative environment by avoiding all judgments about the elder's feelings, thoughts, actions, or beliefs. In this way the nurse provides a model that elders can use to suspend their own internal judgments.

The intention to be nonjudgmental is not limited to simply being nice or sympathetic. The "shoulds" and "shouldn'ts" that arise in the bereaved are driving forces in their internal belief systems. Any critical or judgmental response from helpers that elicits this dynamic can derail the helping process. Most helpers find it easy to understand how negative judgments can evoke an elder's negative experience of herself. It is somewhat more difficult, however, to see how positive judgments and sympathetic support can also have negative outcomes.

When an older adult asks, "Is it wrong for me to be angry about this?" a common response might well be to say, "Why no, that's perfectly natural." If the elder appears reassured, it is even more difficult to understand the potential disservice done to the process. One of the pitfalls of this response, however, is that the elder and the helper have colluded to put the helper in the judgment seat. That feeling was natural, but what about others? When will the elder come to an "unnatural" feeling, and what will happen then?

Feelings arise spontaneously in the grieving process. It is simply not the case that some are justified and some are not. A patient's feelings may or may not be expressed congruently, but the sense of how they fit into the client's feel/think/act/believe system can only be assessed in the experience of the older patient. Clarity about the elder's experience cannot be established through judgments based on external observation alone, but can only be gained by empathetic feedback. Forming an accurate perception of such experiences is the basic task of the nurse, and expressing those perceptions nonjudgmentally is the only way to continue that experience for the elder (Moses & Kearney, 1995).

The third component of ENUF is unconditional positive regard. This philosophy, set forth by Carl Rogers (1965), affirms the value of all people simply because they exist. In order for nurses to facilitate the grieving process of the elder, they must empathize in an unconditional manner. Unconditional regard communicates the message, "I value, care for and respect you without ifs, ands, or buts. You can neither earn nor lose your right to that respect, caring, or valuing. It is part of the birthright to which all human beings are entitled." This attitude is not conveyed simply by verbalizing the sentiment. Rather, the behavior and the effort to demonstrate caring, valuing, and respect, applied consistently, far outweigh the words.

Qualified acceptance of the older patient deters successful engagement in the relationship to do the work of grieving. Being aware of and respecting the distinction between acceptance of the person and approval of their behavior or lifestyle is a fundamental prerequisite for offering genuine unconditional acceptance. Within such a context, all sorts of difficult, even repugnant or frightening behavior on the part of the older patient can be responded to with this unconditional acceptance.

To understand the meaning of unconditional acceptance one must understand the value and place of acceptance in the work of grieving. Acceptance, in this context, refers to the belief that core-level or existential issues are part of the human experience and worthy of respect. Neither the nature of these issues nor the feeling states generated by the shattering of the attachment dreams invalidates one's right to love and be loved. An individual's right to be accepted can neither be guaranteed by socially approved deportment nor lost by the failure to live up to the expectations of others. Such conditions violate both the boundaries and the feel/think/act/believe integrity of all parties involved (Moses & Kearney, 1995).

With many elders it is easy for helpers to almost reflexively express their concern: "Of course I'm not upset with you. This is a very difficult time. Most people, men included, would be weeping as you are." It may be harder to express this concern when an older patient is manifesting a form of grieving that is more difficult for the nurse to tolerate: an anxious elder who cannot sit still and is too distracted to finish a thought or complete a sentence; a guilty elder whose self-blame defies all logic; a fearful elder whose sense of dread is articulated in paranoid ways; a suicidal, hostile, or violent elder; or a self-abusive or denying older adult. Unconditional acceptance sends the same message of respect, valuing, and caring to troublesome older patients and to pleasant, cooperative ones (Moses & Kearney, 1995).

The attitude of acceptance on the part of the nurse is not a guarantee that the nurse and the older patient will work together. Sometimes no match can be found between what the nurse has to offer and what the elder is willing and able to receive. In that case, arrangements for another health care professional to work with the elder or a referral for more intensive services may be appropriate.

Grieving is a spontaneous, unlearned, feeling process. The feelings must be shared with a significant other in order for their functions to be served. For this reason the maintenance of a focus on feelings, the fourth component of ENUF, is a critical element in practice. Maintaining this focus helps elders discover the issues impacted by their loss and the coping mechanisms that are no longer useful in responding to the loss (Moses & Kearney, 1995). The feeling states of grieving are neither simple nor static. Nurses using ENUF focus on current feelings that constantly ebb and flow in both nature and degree. It is possible for an older individual to feel terribly frightened and alone after the death of a loved one in one moment, to furiously blame the departed in the next, and to be utterly mired in guilt moments later. Bewilderment and loss of control are equally important feelings to be acknowledged by the nurse. The nurse could state, for example, "It sounds as if you are feeling confused and overwhelmed by a lot of different and uncomfortable feelings. What more do you want to tell me about this?" Only by maintaining a focus on present feelings can the nurse hope to match the older adult step for step in the grieving process (Moses & Kearney, 1995).

Nurses, no less than their patients, will feel the need to make sense out of what is happening. To this end they may follow the urge to focus on content rather than feeling in order to get the story straight. If the nurse responds to this urge, both nurse and older patient will be diverted by details and circumstances and lose the focus necessary to continue the work of grieving. The pathway back to normal, purposeful grieving requires awareness on the part of the nurse that collusion has occurred in the relationship to avoid the anxiety of the grieving process. Returning to a focus on feelings is essential.

ENUF is a set of attitudes intended to guide both the nurse and the older patient on the difficult journey of grieving. Because each nurse is a unique individual, no two practitioners will engage in the process in exactly the same way. There is never a single right thing to say nor a right time to say it because each meeting between nurse and elder constitutes a unique moment between two unique individuals. ENUF is also a self-correcting process that is constantly revalidated. Nurses who try to intervene "perfectly" by rigidly following "the model" or the intellectual concepts involved in the process lose their authenticity, honesty, and ability to take risks. If the nurse isn't able to take risks, how can the older patient dare to try? The practice of ENUF is designed to create an environment that facilitates the work of grieving. The creation of safety, to which the gerontologic nurse must be committed, is the

safety *for* risk-taking, not the safety *from* risk-taking. Once elders allow themselves to struggle emotionally to redefine, reevaluate, and create new ways of perceiving the issues attached to their feelings, they will be able to cope better with the loss (Moses & Kearney, 1995).

Several of the activities listed under the NIC intervention label Grief Work Facilitation reflect partial elements of ENUF: "Assist the patient to identify the initial reaction to the loss" (Empathy); "Encourage expression of feelings about the loss" (Feeling Focus); "Communicate acceptance of discussing the loss" (Nonjudgmental); and "Support progression through personal grieving stages" (Unconditional Positive Regard). However, the ENUF intervention is not just a formula, a technique, or a set of activities. In fact, by focusing the interaction on the relationship this response places a premium on presence. When ENUF is used effectively, it decreases the telling of facts, details, ideas, or abstractions that is emphasized in the Grief Work Facilitation intervention and increases the use of personal and emotional referents. The older patient experiences rapport with the nurse and becomes more willing to take risks, to struggle with attachment, and to accept feedback (Moses & Kearney, 1995). It is concern with these more interpersonal elements of the grieving process that primarily differentiates the NIC intervention label from ENUF. It is proposed here that the key elements of ENUF be incorporated into an effective nursing intervention for facilitating grief work.

CASE STUDY 1

Forcing an older individual in denial like Mrs. Fox to experience the full force of a loss without internal and external supports in place can lead to emotional collapse (Moses, 1983). A more efficient and purposeful approach would be to offer suggestions, recommendations, and information while supporting the legitimacy of the older person's denial. Validating the older individual's value, even when he cannot cope with catastrophic loss, is even more important. The process of working through denial is highly individualized and can take a long period of time (Ersek, 1992; Manousos & Williams, 1998). Although it is not necessary to quantify (as per a rating scale) the "amount" of denial experienced by elderly patients, the nurse should use each encounter with the elder to assess the types of denial being exhibited and to evaluate readiness to alter attitudes, behaviors, values, and feelings.

Attitudes of nurses, family, and friends can strongly affect the pressure that older persons experience in the context of their loss(es). The most important function nurses and other helpers serve is to legitimize anxious feelings. Asking the anxious elder to "calm down" is both futile and counterproductive. Anxiety will continue, even if chemically or psychologically "masked," until it serves its productive purpose. Moreover, anxiety facilitates the restructuring of attitudes necessary to regain balance in the context of loss. The injunction to "calm down" devalues the elderly person's internal experience and the tremendous coping task she faces. The nurse should use one of the standardized measures of anxiety discussed in Chapter 44 to monitor the elder's level of anxiety, at baseline, on a monthly basis until normative values are achieved and every 6 months thereafter. If the elder has been given anxiolytic medications, levels of anxiety should monitored more closely to determine the efficacy of the psychotropic drugs.

Mrs. Fox's nurse engaged her in the following dialogue:

NURSE: So you've never had to worry before about finances, and it doesn't seem necessary now to start? You believe your daughter is overreacting?

MRS. FOX: Yes. She makes me so nervous when she keeps talking about it.

NURSE: If you believe there is nothing to worry about and talking about it makes you nervous, I can understand why you'd want her to stop talking about the finances. [Empathetic and nonjudgmental response]

MRS. FOX: You do? (Pauses) I don't think my daughter understands. She's always pushing me about these bills and now my insurance policy. (Starts to cry) I just hate it all. I don't want to think about it—I never had to before. (Crying, but voice sounds angry) [Denial of impact on life—breaking into feelings concerning impact]

NURSE: You're crying but your voice sounds angry. Do you feel angry when you feel your daughter is pushing you? [Empathy—checking for accuracy]

MRS. FOX: I guess I do, but I don't know why. She's a good daughter.

NURSE: You just said, "I don't want to think about it—I never had to before." Tell me about that.

MRS. FOX: Well, I didn't, I just let my husband take care of things. (Looks around and becomes more agitated) Oh, I wish she'd stop. If she just wouldn't push me. (Angry voice)

NURSE: It feels like your daughter is pushing you, and it makes you feel angry with her?

MRS. FOX: Yes, I do get angry with her but . . . I guess it isn't her fault.

NURSE: What isn't her fault?

MRS. FOX: (Long pause, then whispers) That my husband died and I don't know what to do about paying bills. (Starts crying. Nurse moves in to hold Mrs. Fox's hand while she cries)

Mrs. Fox had been in denial concerning the fact of a problem with her finances. To acknowledge that there was a problem with her finances, Mrs. Fox had to acknowledge the painful impact of her husband's death that resulted in the need for change, which took many months. Her daughter's insistence created the anxiety necessary to begin to deal with the feeling. However, Mrs. Fox felt no understanding or acceptance from her daughter concerning her pain about changing. When the nurse gently and empathetically acknowledged this pain without insisting that she change, Mrs. Fox felt supported and valued enough to begin to acknowledge the feelings: first anger at the unfairness, then an overwhelming sense of depression concerning her inadequacy to deal with the impact. Empathetic support and acceptance allowed Mrs. Fox to struggle with the issues of fairness and adequacy. She moved quickly into expressing her anger and depression and worked with the nurse and then with her daughter to find alternatives for dealing with her financial situation.

CASE STUDY 2

The best response to elders experiencing guilt during the grieving process is to listen sensitively and accept the legitimacy of the elder's feelings. With empathetic listening by a significant other, the grieving individual can answer questions regarding causality and impact on the world. Acceptance of the guilt experience as a normal, necessary, and facilitative element of grief provides the basis of a constructive relationship with the older adult. In contrast, viewing guilt as pathologic impedes the helping relationship. Guilt outlives its usefulness only after it facilitates existential restructuring.

Significant others or health care professionals who support, accept, and encourage expression of feelings can help older individuals identify competency issues and establish new evaluative criteria. Statements that reflect this facilitative attitude can be as simple as "Tell me more about your feelings." "It sounds like you feel helpless/hopeless. Do you, and if so, why?" or "It sounds as if being confined has turned your whole world upside down. Can you tell me how things have changed for you since the doctor told you about this diagnosis?" "Cheering up" or denying the older person the right to his depressed feelings devalues the importance of that individual's struggle to reevaluate essential and core-level issues and reinforces the notion that they are indeed inadequate (see Chapter 41). The nurse should evaluate the bereaved elder's level of depression using a screening tool such as the Geriatric Depression Scale at baseline and, if the elder scores 10 or greater on the scale, at biweekly intervals until resolution of depression is achieved and every 6 months thereafter.

Mrs. Lloyd's nurse engaged her in the following dialogue:

NURSE: Mrs. Lloyd, you keep saying we should be talking about your daughter. Can you tell me why that seems so important?

MRS. LLOYD: Well, she needs help, and it's my job to take care of her, so we should be talking about her.

NURSE: So, you feel responsible for her and her well-being, and talking about other things during our time doesn't feel comfortable for you? [Empathy—checking for accuracy]

MRS. LLOYD: Well, I am responsible for her. There's no one else. I suppose I should have done something a long time ago. Do you think I was wrong to keep her with me? I probably should have put her somewhere but I couldn't, and then her father took all my time (he was ill a long time before his death). I probably neglected her, and she, you know, regressed or something. . . . (Tearful at times) [Daughter graduated from high school but was never placed in any other day programs after high school and remained isolated with mother because few services were available]

NURSE: If I'm hearing you accurately, you have a lot of concerns about the way you've dealt with your daughter over the last 10 to 20 years and lots of questions about the rightness or wrongness of your decisions. Is that correct?

MRS. LLOYD: I always worry now about whether I did okay. I feel so bad sometimes. (Cries) What if I made the wrong decisions and now she has to suffer?

NURSE: (Moving closer and touching Mrs. Lloyd's arm while she's crying; sits quietly as she cries) Tell me about your sadness. [Focus on feelings—acknowledges and values them]

MRS. LLOYD: I feel like I've done all the wrong things, and if I have—well, what kind of a mother am I? That makes me sad.

NURSE: It sounds like you are questioning your adequacy as a mother.

MRS. LLOYD: Yes, I guess I am.

NURSE: What does it mean to you if you made mistakes?

MRS. LLOYD: If they were mistakes that she has to suffer for now—well, how can I live with that? Worse, how can I leave her? (Cries some more) It's my fault if her life is awful, and now I can't do anything about it!

NURSE: You're worried that she'll suffer for mistakes you made and you won't be able to help her?

MRS. LLOYD: Yes.

NURSE: It looks like those thoughts and ideas are very painful for you. How long have you been this concerned about your decisions concerning your daughter?

MRS. LLOYD: I guess I thought the decisions were okay at the time. It felt like I didn't have very many choices, but in the last few years I've been wondering. . . .

NURSE: Any idea what started you wondering?

MRS. LLOYD: Oh, talking to other people and trying to plan for when I'm gone. (Pause) People just seemed to act like I should have done something sooner.

NURSE: So you started wondering about your decisions when other people seemed to question your choices?

MRS. LLOYD: Yes.

NURSE: Were you feeling judged?

MRS. LLOYD: Yes—and no one knows how hard it was to make those decisions. But maybe they're right.

NURSE: And if they're "right," does that make it hard to feel like you were a "good enough" mother?

MRS. LLOYD: Yes and that was all I had—being her mother. What if I did a terrible job?

NURSE: Being a good mother was the job that gave you a sense of value and worth? And now you're wondering if you still are that valuable person?

MRS. LLOYD: Oh yes—if I didn't do it right, how can I look at my life and feel okay about it?

NURSE: If you believe that being a "good and valuable mother" means not making mistakes, I can understand why you feel so sad and depressed when you think about mistakes you may have made. (Pause) Maybe we can look together at the definition you have for being a good

enough mother and where it came from to help you deal with this issue.

Mrs. Lloyd was struggling with feelings of guilt and depression in an attempt to deal with the issues of significance, adequacy, and value as a mother and as a human being. Her roles as wife and mother were her major sources for a sense of significance and meaning (hence guilt) and value and adequacy (hence depression). In the face of her own impending death, she was reviewing these issues and struggling with doubts about her significance and adequacy (value). The nurse's responses allowed Mrs. Lloyd to examine the definitions and criteria she was using and to reevaluate the usefulness of those definitions. If the nurse's reply to Mrs. Lloyd had been "Don't feel guilty," the reevaluation process would not have been facilitated.

CASE STUDY 3

It is crucial that older individuals express the anger they feel in the face of loss or change. Nurses can assist elders in this process by accepting and relating to their anger. Unfortunately, anger often is directed toward nurses, threatening their sense of adequacy and value. However, nurses must encourage the elderly person's expression of feelings in order to facilitate healing interaction and promote the grieving process. Older individuals who express their feelings of anger verbally are unlikely to act them out. "Acting out" usually occurs when persons are frustrated in their efforts to express their anger (Moses, 1983). Nurses should understand the underlying dynamics of anger, examine their own motives carefully, and accept the older person's expressions of anger as a preventive measure against the potentially more destructive form of "acting out."

Mr. Smythe's nurse engaged him in the following dialogue:

NURSE: Mr. Smythe, it sounds like you feel you don't have control over your own life anymore. Is that how you feel? [Empathy—checking for accuracy]

MR. SMYTHE: Well, they'd like to think that they can tell me how to run my life, but I'll be damned if I'll let them.

NURSE: How do you feel when you think about not having control of your own life? [Beginning to focus on feeling]

MR. SMYTHE: Now that's a stupid question. I feel angry, that's how I feel. But it doesn't do any good. They just keep doing it, telling me what to do. It isn't the way I'm used to things being, I can tell you that! [Anger, assisting with issue of unfairness]

NURSE: I can understand if you believe you don't have control of your own life that you might feel angry. It does sound like feeling out of control is not a common experience for you. You're used to being in charge a lot in your business. Is that right? [Expressing attitude of acceptance and valuing even in face of devaluing messages sent to nurse by Mr. Smythe]

MR. SMYTHE: You're darn right! (Pauses—anger diffused a little)

NURSE: Were there any times in your work life when you felt this kind of anger or "out of control" feeling? [Exploring feelings]

MR. SMYTHE: (Thoughtfully) Well, sure, I guess when someone messed up a big deal and I was afraid of losing a client or a lot of money. Yeah, I guess the anger felt like I feel now.

NURSE: What would you do in the work situation to deal with your out of control feeling?

MR. SMYTHE: Well (Laughs), I guess I would yell a lot at first at the people who I thought had messed up.

NURSE: What were you most angry about then?

MR. SMYTHE: I guess at first I was mad because my plan was messed up and it was unfair, but maybe . . . maybe I was scared too. You can lose a lot of money in the deals I'm used to putting together. I never really thought about it. [Fear—dealing with issue of vulnerability]

NURSE: So maybe some of the anger was covering up the scared feeling? It wasn't okay to let anyone know about the scared feelings? [Focusing on feelings]

MR. SMYTHE: (Laughs again) Oh, yeah, you never let the other guy know you're scared in business deals.

NURSE: Could your anger now have anything to do with being scared? What might you be scared of now?

MR. SMYTHE: Well, you know that doctor can't give me any guarantees that I won't have another one of these "MIs" even if I do everything I'm supposed to. It feels like a real chancy thing. If I start doing things like exercising, I'm taking quite a chance on having another heart attack.

NURSE: So, it feels like you don't want to take any risks without those guarantees? [Checking for accuracy]

MR. SMYTHE: Yeah.

NURSE: What do you think would help you decide to take those risks? What helped you in the work situation?

MR. SMYTHE: (Thoughtfully) Well, I guess I decided what I wanted to achieve was worth the risk and there were some things I could do to minimize some of the risks.

NURSE: It sounds like when you decide that going on with your life and enjoying some of your former pleasures are worth the risk, you'll go ahead and do that. Are there any questions I can help you get answered that might help you minimize that sense of risk?

Mr. Smythe's struggle was expressed in the feeling states of anger and fear. His anger was necessary to struggle with his sense of unfairness at his illness and its impact on his life, and it also masked the more "unacceptable" feeling of fear. The fear, once acknowledged and valued, decreased the need for the anger and allowed Mr. Smythe to use the fear to deal with his sense of vulnerability. By focusing on the fear and anger, the nurse helped Mr. Smythe to identify the issues to which the feelings were attached and to generate ideas and thoughts about how to deal with the situation.

FUTURE DIRECTIONS

Future classification work and research in the area of grieving should consider how the concept of role transi-

tions (Meleis, 1975; Schumacher, Jones, & Meleis, in press) is pertinent to the care of older adults who are grieving. According to the transition framework, a transition is precipitated by a significant marker event or turning point (in grieving it might be a loss, death of a spouse, or catastrophic diagnosis) that requires new patterns of response and involves the development of new skills, relationships, and roles. Transitions can be developmental, situational, or related to health or illness. Schumacher et al. (in press) have noted that transitions span the whole period of time from the initial marker event until harmony and stability are achieved and that this time period is variable and depends on the nature of the change and the extent to which the change influences other aspects of the person's life. NIC and NOC could be strengthened through the addition of an intervention label and outcome applicable to the grieving process that are based on the concept of role transitions. The intervention label might be "Facilitation of Healthy Transitions" and the corresponding outcome could be labeled "Healthy Transitions" or "Role Transitions" or "Role Transition."

Schumacher and colleagues (in press) have identified seven healthy transition processes and seven corresponding unhealthy processes that could be used as indicators for the proposed outcome "Healthy Transitions." These include, for example, the elder's symptom experience, functional status, sense of connectedness to a meaningful interpersonal network, sense of empowerment, and sense of integrity. Schumacher et al. (in press) have identified a number of tools for measuring these process indicators, including the Fulfillment of Meaning Scale for integrity, the Desired Control Scale for empowerment, the Mutuality Scale for connectedness, and various measures of anxiety, depression, cognitive status, and pain for symptom experience. In addition, one of the many activities of daily living or multidimensional functional assessment scales can be used to capture change in functional status. Moreover, these processes could serve as the bases for intervention activities, such as redefining meanings, modifying expectations, restructuring life routines, developing new knowledge and skills, and maintaining continuity in identity, relationships, and environment, all of which are relevant to coping with grief. Schumacher and associates also have identified assessment, reminiscence, role supplementation, creation of health environments, and mobilization of resources as nursing therapeutics related to facilitation of health transition processes.

Table 49-2 compares key elements of the NANDA diagnosis "Dysfunctional Grieving" and "Grieving" diagnosis suggested here. The activities specified by the NIC intervention "Grief Work Facilitation" are contrasted with the key building blocks of ENUF. Indicators for the NOC outcomes "Grief Resolution" and "Coping" are compared with the outcomes proposed here.

Table 49-2   Comparison of Nursing Diagnoses, Outcomes, and Interventions Related to Grieving

Nursing Diagnoses		Nursing-Sensitive Outcomes		Nursing Interventions	
Dysfunctional Grieving (NANDA)	Grieving (Whiting & Buckwalter)	Grief Resolution (NOC)	Grieving/Coping Model (Whiting & Buckwalter)	Grief Work Facilitation (NIC)	ENUF (Whiting & Buckwalter)
DEFINITION					
Extended, unsuccessful use of intellectual and emotional responses by which individuals attempt to work through the process of modifying self-concept based on the perception of loss	A normal, spontaneous, unlearned, lifelong, functional process that is part of living and is uniquely defined by the person experiencing the loss	*Indicators* Expresses feelings about loss Verbalizes reality of loss Describes meaning of the loss or death Maintains current will Discusses unresolved conflict(s) Reports decreased preoccupation with loss Maintains grooming and hygiene Reports adequate nutritional intake Seeks social support Reports involvement in social activities Expresses positive expectations about the future Expresses spiritual beliefs about death Verbalizes acceptance of loss Participates in planning funeral Maintains advance directives Reports absence of somatic distress Maintains living environment Reports absence of sleep disturbance Reports normal sexual desire Shares loss with significant others Progresses through stages of grief Identifies effective coping patterns Verbalizes sense of control Verbalizes acceptance of situation Modifies lifestyle as needed Uses available social support Identifies multiple coping strategies	Reentry into preexisting developmental tasks with new skills, perspectives, insights, and attitudes • Contain the impact of the loss • Devalue "normal" standards • Enlarge signs of values • Stay away from comparative to asset values	*Activities* Identify the loss Encourage expression of feelings about the loss Encourage discussion of previous loss experiences Encourage identification of greatest fears concerning the loss Support progression through personal grieving stages Assist to identify personal coping strategies Communicate acceptance of discussing the loss Use clear words, such as dead or died, rather than euphemisms Encourage expression of feelings in ways comfortable for the child, such as writing, drawing, or playing* Identify sources of community support Reinforce progress made in the grieving process Assist the patient to identify the nature of the attachment to the lost object or person Assist the patient to identify the initial reaction to the loss Encourage the patient to verbalize memories of the loss, both past and current	Empathy Nonjudgment Unconditional positive regard Feeling focus
DEFINING CHARACTERISTICS					
Verbal expression of loss; denial of loss; expression of unresolved issues; anger; sadness; crying; difficulty in expressing loss; alterations in: eating habits, sleep patterns, dream patterns, activity level, libido; idealization of lost object; reliving of past experiences; interference with life functioning; developmental regression; labile affect; alterations in concentration and/or pursuits of tasks	Redefinition, reevaluation, and reattachment in the context of loss Depression Anger Fear Guilt Anxiety Denial Reassessment of attitudes and values Struggle with social, emotional, and philosophic structures				

*Interventions more pertinent for children than older adults.

Continued

Table 49-2 Comparison of Nursing Diagnoses, Outcomes, and Interventions Related to Grieving—cont'd

Nursing Diagnoses		Nursing-Sensitive Outcomes		Nursing Interventions	
Dysfunctional Grieving (NANDA)	Grieving (Whiting & Buckwalter)	Grief Resolution (NOC)	Grieving/Coping Model (Whiting & Buckwalter)	Grief Work Facilitation (NIC)	ENUF (Whiting & Buckwalter)
RELATED FACTORS/ETIOLOGIES					
Actual or perceived object loss; objects may include people, possessions, a job, status, home, ideals, parts, and processes of the body	Feel/think/act/believe paradigm out of sync Inability to fulfill dreams, illusions, fantasies, and projections into the future Profound impact on existential issues related to attachment, meaning, vitality, values, choice, and ownership	Avoids unduly stressful situations Seeks professional help as appropriate Reports decrease in negative feelings Identifies ineffective coping patterns Reports decrease in stress Seeks information concerning illness and treatment Adapts to developmental changes Employs behaviors to reduce stress Uses effective coping strategies Verbalizes need for assistance Reports decrease in physical symptoms of stress Reports increase in psychologic comfort		Instruct in phases of the grieving process, as appropriate Include significant others in discussions and decisions, as appropriate Encourage patient to implement cultural, religious, and social customs associated with the loss Answer children's questions associated with the loss* Encourage children to discuss feelings* Assist the child to clarify misconceptions* Support efforts to resolve previous conflict Assist in identifying modifications needed in lifestyle	

SUMMARY

Grieving is a functional rather than a dysfunctional process. It is regarded as a normal, spontaneous, unlearned, and life-long process. It is part of living and is uniquely defined by the older person who is experiencing the loss. Through the feeling states of depression, guilt, anger, fear, and denial, the elderly individual separates from a lost dream. Nurses should support, rather than block, these feelings. Using the principles of ENUF—empathy, nonjudgment, unconditional positive regard, and feeling focus—nurses can assist bereaved elders to better cope with losses or changes in their lives and environment. Successful movement through the grieving process is accomplished when the older person has achieved a sense of personal growth and can develop new and attainable dreams.

REFERENCES

Adams, J., Hershatter, M. J., & Moritz, D. (1991, May/June). Accumulated loss phenomenon among hospice caregivers. *American Journal of Hospital and Palliative Care*, 29-37.

Aspinwall, L. G., & Brunhart, S. M. (1996). Distinguishing optimism from denial: Optimistic beliefs predict attention to health threats. *Personality and Social Psychology Bulletin, 22*(10), 993-1003.

Bell, J. M. (1995). Editorial, The dysfunction of "dysfunctional." *Journal of Family Nursing, 1*(3), 235-237.

Bowlby, J. (1961). Processes of mourning. *International Journal of Psychoanalysis, 42*, 317-340.

Clayton, P., Halikas, J., & Maurice, W. (1971). The bereavement of the widowed. *Diseases of the Nervous System, 32*, 597-604.

Collins, J., Crump, S., Buckwalter, K. C., Hall, G. R., Gerdner, L., & Kudart, P. (1995). Uncovering and managing denial during the research process. *Archives of Psychiatric Nursing, IX*(2), 62-67.

Dimond, M. (1981). Bereavement and the elderly: A critical review with implications for nursing practice and research. *Journal of Advanced Nursing, 6*, 461-470.

Dimond, M., Caserta, M., & Lund, D. (1994). Understanding depression in bereaved older adults. *Clinical Nursing Research, 3*(3), 253-268.

Engel, G. L. (1960a). Is grief a disease, a challenge? *Psychosomatic Medicine, 22*, 326-327.

Engel, G. L. (1960b). Is grief a disease? *Psychosomatic Medicine, 23*, 18-22.

Ersek, M. (1992). Examining the process and dilemmas of reality negotiation. *IMAGE: The Journal of Nursing Scholarship, 24*(1), 19-25.

Faschingbauer, T. (1981). *Texas revised inventory of grief.* Minneapolis, MN: Honeycomb.

Faschingbauer, T. R., DeVaul, R. A., & Zisook, S. (1977). Development of the Texas inventory of grief. *American Journal of Psychiatry, 134*, 696-698.

Frank, A. (1991). *At the will of the body.* New York: Houghton-Mifflin.

Freud, S. (1973). Mourning and melancholia. In *Complete psychological works (1917)* (standard ed., Vol 14, pp. 239-258). London: Hogarth Press.

Glick, I., Weiss, R. S., & Parkes, C. M. (1974). *The first year of bereavement.* New York: John Wiley & Sons.

Gordon, M. (1982). *Nursing diagnosis: Process and application.* Hightstown, NJ: McGraw-Hill.

Iowa Intervention Project. J. C. McCloskey & G. M. Bulechek (Eds.). (2000). *Nursing interventions classification (NIC)* (3rd ed.). St. Louis, MO: Mosby.

Iowa Outcomes Project. M. Johnson, M. Maas, & S. Moorhead (Eds.). (2000). *Nursing outcomes classification (NOC)* (2nd ed.). St. Louis, MO: Mosby.

Kavanaugh, K. (1995). Understanding and facilitating the grieving process. *The Brown University Long Term Care Quality Letter, 7*(17), 1-3.

Kearney, R. (1986). *Intervention therapy.* Unpublished manuscript.

Kim, M. J., & Moritz, D. A. (Eds.). (1982). *Classification of nursing diagnoses: Proceedings of the third and fourth national conferences.* Hightstown, NJ: McGraw-Hill.

Kübler-Ross, E. (1969). *On death and dying.* London: Collier-Macmillan.

Lewis, M., & Rosenblum, L. A. (1974). *The effect of the infant on its caregiver.* New York: John Wiley & Sons.

Lindemann, E. (1974). Symptomatology and management of acute grief. *American Journal of Psychiatry, 101*, 141-148.

Lowenthal, M., & Haven, C. (1968). Interaction and adaptation as a critical variable. *American Sociological Review, 33*, 20-30.

Maddison, D. C., & Viola, A. (1968). The health of widows in the year following bereavement. *Journal of Psychosomatic Research, 12*, 297-306.

Manousos, I. R., & Williams, D. I. (1998). The locus of denial. *Counseling of Psychology Quarterly, 11*(1), 15-22.

McFarland, G., & Wasli, E. (1986). *Nursing diagnosis and process in psychiatric mental health nursing.* Baltimore: Lippincott Williams & Wilkins.

Meleis, A. I. (1975). Role insufficiency and role supplementation: A conceptual framework. *Nursing Research, 24*(4), 264-270.

Morley, C. (1997). The use of denial by patients with cancer. *Professional Nurse, 12*(5), 139-152.

Moses, K. L. (1977). Effects of developmental disability on parenting the handicapped child. In M. L. Reff (Ed.), *Patterns of emotional growth in the developmentally disabled child.* The Julia S. Molloy Education Center.

Moses, K. L. (1983). The impact of initial diagnosis: Mobilizing family resources. In A. Mulick & S. M. Pueschel (Eds.), *Parent-professional partnerships* (pp. 11-41). San Diego, CA: Academic Press.

Moses, K. L. (1985). Dynamic intervention with families. In E. Cherow, N. Matkin, & R. Trybus (Eds.), *Hearing-impaired children and youth with developmental disabilities* (pp. 82-98). Washington, DC: Gallaudet University Press.

Moses, K. L. (1993). *On loss, grieving, facilitating, and intervening: Notes on helping and the dynamics of change.* Evanston, IL: Resource Networks.

Moses, K. L., & Kearney, R. (1995). *Transition therapy: An existential approach to facilitating growth in the light of loss* (pp. 2-4, 128-139). Evanston, IL: Resource Networks.

Moses, K. L., & Van Heck-Wulatin, M. (1981). The socio-emotional impact of infant deafness: A counseling model. In G. Mencher & S. Gerber (Eds.), *Early management of hearing loss* (pp. 243-278). New York: Grune & Stratton.

North American Nursing Diagnosis Association. (1999). *Nursing diagnoses: Definitions & classification 1999-2000.* Philadelphia: Author.

O'Hara, P. A., Harper, D. W., Chartrand, L. D., & Johnston, S. F. (1996). Patient death in a long-term care hospital: A study of the effect on nursing staff. *Journal of Gerontological Nursing; 22*(8), 27-35.

Parkes, C. M. (1965). Bereavement and mental illness: A clinical study of the grief of bereaved patients. *British Journal of Medicine Psychology, 38,* 1-15.

Parkes, C. M. (1972). *Studies of grief in adult life.* Madison, CT: International Universities Press.

Parkes, C. M. (1997). Bereavement and mental health in the elderly. *Reviews in Clinical Gerontology, 7,* 47-53.

Patterson, I. (1996). Participation in leisure activities by older adults after a stressful life event: The loss of a spouse. *International Journal of Aging and Human Development, 42*(2), 123-142.

Prigerson, H. G., Shear, M. K., Newsom, J. T., Frank, E. Reynolds, C. F., III., Maciejewski, P. K., Houck, P. R., Biehals, A. J., & Kupfer, D. J. (1996). Anxiety among widowed elders: Is it distinct from depression and grief? *Anxiety, 2*(1), 1-12.

Rees, W., & Lufkins, S. G. (1967). Mortality of bereavement. *British Medical Journal, 4,* 13-16.

Rogers, C. (1965). *Client centered therapy.* Boston: Houghton Mifflin.

Rosenthal, V. (1994). "Einzigerlebnstherapy: Essentials of an experiential psychotherapy." In *There is no such thing as psychotherapy and other essays.* Evanston, IL: Private Printing.

Sanders, C., Mauger, P., & Strong, P., Jr. (1979). *A manual for the Grief Experience Inventory.* Tampa, FL: University of South Florida.

Schumacher, K. L., Jones, P. S., & Meleis, A. I. (in press). *The elderly in transition: Needs and issues of care.* Unpublished manuscript.

Solari-Twadell, P. A., Bunkers, S. S., Wang, C. E., & Snyder, D. (1995). The pinwheel model of bereavement. *IMAGE: Journal of Nursing Scholarship: 27*(4), 323-326.

Vachon, M. (1976). Grief and bereavement following the death of a spouse. *Canadian Psychiatric Association Journal, 21,* 35-44.

Volkan, V. (1970). Typical findings in pathological grief. *Psychiatric Q, 44,* 231-250.

Wright, B. (1960). *Physical disability: A psychological approach.* New York: Harper & Row.

Zisook, S., & DeVaul, R. A. (1983). Grief, unresolved grief and depression. *Psychosomatics, 24,* 247-271.

Zisook, S., DeVaul, R. A., & Click, M. A. (1982). Measuring symptoms of grief and bereavement. *American Journal of Psychiatry, 139,* 1590-1593.

Zisook, S., Shuchter, S., & Schuckit, M. (1985). Factors in the persistence of unresolved grief among psychiatric outpatients. *Psychosomatics, 26,* 497-503.

CHAPTER 50

SOCIAL ISOLATION

James D. Waterman, Mary Blegen, Patricia Clinton, and Janet P. Specht

Most, if not all, of us would like to grow old surrounded by friends and family enveloped in a rich network of support. Evidence that this type of network nourishes the body, mind, and spirit is well documented (Bassuk, Glass, & Berkman, 1999; Chappell, Badger, & Ware, 1989; Knox & Uvanas-Moberg, 1998). However, death of family and friends, retirement, relocation, and other life changes can reduce social contacts, placing elders at risk for social isolation. Social isolation is the quantity and quality of social contact below that required to sustain an individual's physiologic and psychologic well-being.

Loss of social contacts limits the available social support believed to be necessary for physiologic and psychologic well-being. Limited social support is associated with early cardiovascular death, higher 5-year mortality, early hospital admissions, restricted stroke recovery, cognitive decline, depression, and other psychiatric disorders (Bassuk, Glass, & Berkman, 1999; Evans, Bishop, & Haselkorn, 1991; Knox & Uvanas-Moberg, 1998; LaVeist, Sellers, Brown, & Nickerson, 1997; Lockery, Dunkle, Kart, & Coulton, 1994; Lubben, 1988; Prince, Harwood, Blizard, Thomas, & Mann, 1997). Within a social network, members exchange resources, although not necessarily on an equal basis. As elderly persons continue to age, they may become unwilling or unable to reciprocate and participate in their social network, even though family and friends continue to provide support (Morgan, 1988). When friends and family feel unduly burdened and express resentment because of increased demands on their time, older adults can feel embarrassed for not being able to return favors. These feelings may lead to voluntary withdrawal from social networks and social isolation. This decreased social contact results in diminished social support and decreased physical and psychologic well-being.

Conceptual Framework

In its simplest form, social support is defined as ". . . the resources provided by other persons" (Cohen & Syme, 1985, p. 4). In addition, contemporary thinking differentiates between received social support and perceived social support. Received support (also known as actual, enacted, or objective support) is support that is mobilized and exchanged between members. Perceived support (also known as anticipated or subjective support) is the belief that there will be someone available to provide needed assistance. Social contact with family and friends tends to increase the amount of received support, which in turn increases the anticipation of support (i.e., perceived support) in future situations. Anticipation of support moderates the effects of psychologic distress through several theoretical mechanisms. Individuals who anticipate support are more likely to perceive stressful situations as relatively benign, gain in self-confidence in problem solving, and take risks in problem solving when they believe they have access to social support resources (Hobfoll & Stokes, 1988; Krause, Liang, & Keith, 1990).

A considerable body of literature has described the association between social support and health, especially the physiologic and psychologic well-being derived from social contacts. Individuals with more social contacts tend to receive more social support and are more likely to adopt health promotion behaviors (Cohen & Syme, 1985). On the other hand, elders who find themselves with limited opportunities for social contact tend to experience decreased physical and psychologic well-being.

Diminished social contact begins the process that leads to social isolation, diminished social support, and decreased well-being (see Figure 50-1). Factors that diminish social contact are conceptualized as barriers and divided into five categories. Each category of barriers can be linked with nursing diagnoses, interventions, and outcomes. Barriers are the etiologies for the nursing diagnosis Social Isolation.

Carpenito (1997) described barriers (constraints) to social contacts that fall within five dimensions: (1) spatial separation; (2) intrapersonal separation; (3) interpersonal separation; (4) social separation; and (5) physiofunctional separation. These barriers to social contact are viewed as etiologies of social isolation and are summarized in Table 50-1.

Spatial separation is the limited ability of the elder to bridge spatial barriers. This may include relocation, location of residence, hospitalization, loss of transportation, and facility layout (Dugan & Kivett, 1994; Lien-Gieschen, 1993; North American Nursing Diagnosis Association [NANDA], 1999).

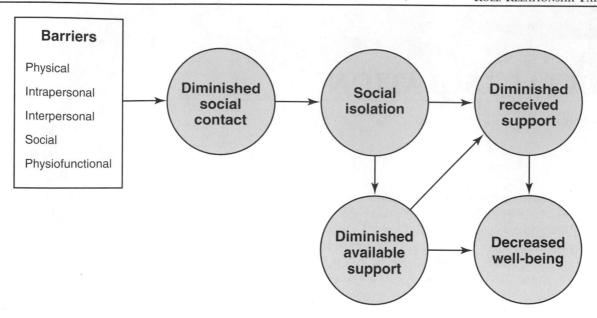

FIGURE **50-1**   Conceptual framework for social isolation. (Adapted from Krause, N., Liang, J., & Keith, V. [1990]. Personality, social support, and psychological distress in later life. *Psychology and Aging, 5,* 315-326.)

Intrapersonal separation emerges from within the elderly person and refers to limitations in personal resources or personal characteristics that restrict social contact. Potential intrapersonal barriers are poverty, caregiver burden, fear of crime, life choices, personality barriers or mental illness, and loss of spirituality (Kim, McFarland, & McLane, 1995; Lien-Gieschen, 1993; Miller & McFall, 1991; NANDA, 1999; Silverstone & Miller, 1980).

Interpersonal separation refers to a limited ability to initiate and maintain relationships. Risk factors for raising this barrier include the following: loss of attachment figures through divorce, death, retirement, or relocation of a network member; decreased communication skills; and strained relationships (Berezin, 1980; Dugan & Kivett, 1994; Elsen & Blegen, 1991; Kim, McFarland, & McLane, 1995; Lien-Gieschen, 1993; NANDA, 1999).

Social separation refers to a limited ability to interact within groups. Limited availability of social groups in the community or separation from those groups can foster social separation. Stigmatizing conditions such as obesity, disfigurement, personality traits, and/or acquired immunodeficiency syndrome (AIDS) can lead to decreased social involvement and skills (Berezin, 1980; Dugan & Kivett, 1994; Elsen & Blegen, 1991; NANDA, 1999).

Finally, physiofunctional separation refers to a limited ability to interact with the environment. These limitations can spring from loss of vision, hearing, or cognitive ability, from altered consciousness, and from physical disabilities (Dugan & Kivett, 1994; Evans, Werkhoven, & Fox, 1982; Lien-Grieschen, 1993; NANDA, 1999; Simonsick, Kasper, & Phillips, 1998).

ASSESSMENT

Diagnosis of social isolation requires assessment of the quantity and quality of social contact, loneliness, social support, physiologic and psychologic well-being, signs of separation from others, and cause of the separation. Although not all of these factors must be present, some would need to be confirmed to make a diagnosis of Social Isolation. In addition, it is important to note that individuals vary in the need for social contact and social support. Some people thrive with minimal social contact and support, while others need much higher levels.

Both objective and subjective data are useful in determining that social isolation is a problem for the client. Interviewing the client may produce the subjective data pertinent to social contacts. Objectively, the nurse could observe the number of contacts the client has within a specified time frame in hospitals or long-term care facilities. Demographic information from the client's record, such as widowhood, living alone, and recent changes in the factors leading to separation of the individual from others, are indicators of diminished social contacts (Hansson, Jones, Carpenter, & Remondet, 1986-87; Holden, 1988; Rubinstein, 1987).

Assessment of potential etiologies of social isolation (see Table 50-1 and Box 50-1) and the conditions related to social isolation (Figure 50-1) supplements the data regarding social contacts. All of these indicators could be placed in a checklist to provide reminders of these factors.

Well-being can be assessed both subjectively and objectively. The elder can be asked to rate well-being and health status on a scale. Alternatively, the nurse can observe other

	Suggested Nursing-Sensitive Outcomes and Nursing Interventions	
Table 50-1	SOCIAL ISOLATION	
Nursing Diagnosis	**Nursing-Sensitive Outcomes**	**Nursing Interventions**

SOCIAL ISOLATION
Related Factors/Etiologies
Spatial separation
 	
  • Relocation
  • Hospitalization
  • Housing location
  • Facility layout
  • Transportation difficulty
	ENVIRONMENTAL ADAPTATION
	SOCIAL SUPPORT
		ENVIRONMENTAL MANAGEMENT
		TRANSPORT
		VISITATION FACILITATION
		SECURITY ENHANCEMENT
		DISCHARGE PLANNING
		SUPPORT SYSTEM ENHANCEMENT

Intrapersonal separation
 	
  • Poverty
  • Caregiver burden
  • Fear
  • Loss of faith
  • Personality barriers
  • Mental illness
	WELL-BEING
	PSYCHOLOGIC COMFORT
	SPIRITUAL WELL-BEING
	PSYCHOSOCIAL ADJUSTMENT:
	LIFE CHANGE
	CAREGIVER WELL-BEING
	SELF-EFFICACY
	SELF-ESTEEM
	FEAR CONTROL
		ANIMAL-ASSISTED THERAPY
		CAREGIVER SUPPORT
		SELF-AWARENESS ENHANCEMENT
		SELF-ESTEEM ENHANCEMENT
		VALUES CLARIFICATION
		SECURITY ENHANCEMENT
		COPING ENHANCEMENT
		COGNITIVE RESTRUCTURING

Interpersonal separation
 	
  • Loss of attachment figure
  • Strained relationships
  • Communication barriers
	LONELINESS
	GRIEF RESOLUTION
	COMMUNICATION ABILITY
	PSYCHOSOCIAL ADJUSTMENT:
	LIFE CHANGE
		SUPPORT GROUP
		FAMILY PROCESS MAINTENANCE
		FAMILY SUPPORT
		ROLE ENHANCEMENT
		GRIEF WORK FACILITATION
		COMPLEX RELATIONSHIP BUILDING
		REMINISCENCE THERAPY

Social separation
 	
  • Social stigma
  • Ineffective social skills
  • Limited community
    resources
  • Decreased social
    involvement
	SOCIAL INTERACTION SKILLS
	SOCIAL INVOLVEMENT
	LEISURE PARTICIPATION
	RESOURCE USE
		BEHAVIOR MODIFICATIONS: SOCIAL SKILLS
		COMPUTER NETWORKING
		ACTIVITY THERAPY
		RECREATION THERAPY
		RESOURCE MOBILIZATION

Physiofunctional separation
 	
  • Physical disability
  • Mental illness
  • Limited mobility
  • Unable to drive
  • Diminished cognitive
    status
  • Diminished sensory acuity
  • Neurologic deficits
  • Altered level of
    consciousness
	MOBILITY LEVEL
	SELF-CARE: ACTIVITIES OF DAILY
	LIVING (ADL)
	SELF-CARE: INSTRUMENTAL ACTIVITIES
	OF DAILY LIVING (IADL)
	COGNITIVE ABILITY
	NEUROLOGICAL STATUS
	SENSORY PERCEPTUAL STATUS
	QUALITY OF LIFE
		EXERCISE THERAPY: AMBULATION
		EXERCISE PROMOTION
		COMMUNICATION ENHANCEMENT: HEARING
		DEFICIT
		COMMUNICATION ENHANCEMENT: VISUAL DEFICIT
		SELF-CARE ASSISTANCE
		TRANSPORT
		COGNITIVE STIMULATION

Box 50-1	Defining Characteristics SOCIAL ISOLATION

Proposed
1. Absent or decreased social contacts
2. Lack of social support
3. Diminished physiologic and psychologic well-being
4. Subjective reports of loneliness

NANDA
1. Absence of supportive significant others
2. Sad, dull affect
3. Inappropriate or immature interests/activities for developmental age/stage

4. Uncommunicative
5. Withdrawn
6. No eye contact
7. Preoccupation with own thoughts
8. Repetitive, meaningless actions
9. Projects hostility in voice, behavior
10. Seeks to be alone or exists in a subculture
11. Evidence of physical/mental handicap or altered state of wellness

indicators of health such as functional ability, stability of chronic conditions (e.g., blood pressure, diabetes), and recovery from illness or injury (e.g., stroke, fractures). Physiologic well-being is often measured using functional status indicators such as those in the Medical Outcomes Survey (Stewart, Hays, & Ware, 1988). Psychologic well-being can be measured by tools addressing life satisfaction, general quality of life, the presence of depression, or other psychologic problems.

Loneliness, a strong indicator that a person feels isolated from others, is determined subjectively by asking about feelings of aloneness, desire for more contact with people, expressions of rejection, feelings of difference from others, and inadequacy or absence of significant purpose in life (Kim, McFarland, & McLane, 1995; NANDA, 1999; Russell, Cutrona, de la Mora, & Wallace, 1997; West, Kellner, & Moore-West, 1986). Frequent social contacts with family, friends, or neighbors were found to prevent emotional and social loneliness (Bondevik & Skogstad, 1998).

Social isolation and contacts can be measured by social support scales. Describing the social network and the perception of support activities within the network (Kane & Kane, 1981; Russell et al., 1997) are frequently used measures of social support. A social network is the web of social relationships in which a person is enmeshed and can be characterized by the number of network members, the frequency of contacts, the presence of a confidant, the durability of the network, the proximity of network members to the individual, and reciprocity. Aspects of perceived support activities include acknowledging the provision of tangible support (i.e., material goods, errands, transportation), emotional support (i.e., listening, being with, empathy), and informational support (i.e., information, counseling) (Evans, Bishop, & Haselkorn, 1991; Neuling & Winfield, 1988; Norris, Stephans, & Kinney, 1990).

Well-developed and detailed measures of social support include the Older Adults Resources and Services (OARS) (Duke University, 1978), the Norbeck Social Support Questionnaire (Norbeck, Lindsey, & Carrieri, 1981), and the Personal Resource Questionnaire (Weinert,

1987). While useful for research, these tools are too long for routine clinical assessment. A shorter tool, which captures support from family and friends and which could be used for clinical assessment, is the Ulbrich and Bradsher (1993) tool. This tool uses two questions to determine support from relatives and two similar questions about friends—"Do you have close relatives (friends) living nearby?" and "If so, if you had a real problem, do you feel that you could call on any of these relatives (friends) for help?" Follow-up questions if relatives and friends were available ask "How often in the past year did you ask for help from any of them?" This scale measures the availability of friends and relatives and frequency of contact in time of need in an efficient manner that could be routinely used in clinical situations.

Another issue surrounding the measurement of social support is the reliability of responses. Reliability of responses depends on the respondent's memory, interest in the questions, and ability to understand the questions (Rossi, Wright, & Anderson, 1983). Cognitively impaired elders pose a problem in subjective measures. Moreover, if relatives or friends are used to obtain this information, there can be a bias in the responses. Nursing judgment will be needed in assessing this information.

Absent or decreased social skills can be determined by behavioral and subjective indicators, such as poor communication skills, inappropriate behavior, inept social interaction, and statements of social unease, lack of friendships, and not being understood (Kim, McFarland, & McLane, 1995).

NURSING DIAGNOSIS

NANDA includes two diagnoses relevant to social isolation in older adults. NANDA defined Social Isolation as "aloneness experienced by the individual and perceived as imposed by others as a negative or threatened state" (NANDA, 1999, pp. 49-50). The NANDA diagnosis Impaired Social Interaction has been defined as "the state in which an individual participates in an insufficient or excessive quantity or ineffective quality of social exchange"

(NANDA, 1999, p. 49). Elements from the NANDA definitions that contribute to the understanding of the concept of social isolation are "the quantity and quality of social contacts" and "a threatened state of well being." The NANDA elements "aloneness," "perception of isolation," and "imposition by others" create difficulties for the definition of Social Isolation. Social isolation can be self-imposed rather than imposed by others. Self-imposed isolation can result from fear of crime, personality disorders, alcoholism, and dislike of people (Berezin, 1980; Lien-Gieschen, 1993; Seeman & Anderson, 1983). Contributing factors leading to social isolation that are not imposed by others include fatigue, caregiver burden, decreased physical mobility, and diminished sensory acuity (Lien-Gieschen, 1993; Miller & McFall, 1991).

Social isolation can occur within a crowd. Some college students report feeling isolated despite being among hundreds to thousands of people their own age (Berezin, 1980). A similar phenomenon occurs within retirement villages and nursing homes, where some elders keep to themselves, do not interact with other residents, and report feeling isolated (Berezin, 1980). In addition, subjective appraisal of isolation by elderly people reflects a lack of quality in social relationships, not simply physical separation (West et al., 1986).

We suggest that NANDA's Social Isolation diagnosis, which focuses on the negative state of aloneness, be combined with NANDA's Impaired Social Interaction diagnosis, which focuses on the insufficient or inadequate aspects of interpersonal processes. This combination recognizes that an actual decrease in social contact and a perception of aloneness have equal importance. Subjective appraisal of isolation and feelings of loneliness constitute a real problem that should be addressed (Austin, 1989; West et al., 1986). A new, proposed definition of Social Isolation combines elements from the NANDA definitions of Impaired Social Interaction and Social Isolation. The definition proposed for this chapter would be "the quantity and quality of social contact below that are required to sustain an individual's physiologic and psychologic well being."

Infrequent and inferior social contact limits received and anticipated support, which results in diminished well-being (Krause, Liang, & Keith, 1990). Cognitive impairment and limited mobility can interfere with the elder's ability to make social contacts, which in turn can limit the quality of available support resources (Krause et al., 1990). Poor timing, inappropriate interaction, and inept interaction all contribute to inferior social contacts and result in lack of social support (Evans, Bishop, & Haselkorn, 1991; Peters-Golden, 1982). For instance, visits that upset a member of the household, visits when the elderly person is very tired, or visits that occur with the expectation that the visitors will receive a meal can impose further hardship rather than provide support for the elderly person.

Defining Characteristics

Diminished physiologic and psychologic well-being is a major consequence of social isolation (NANDA, 1999) and, when combined with signs and symptoms of absent or decreased social contact and perceived loneliness, is evidence of the presence of social isolation. Feelings of loneliness, described as the subjective appraisal of deficiencies in social relationships (Elsen & Blegen, 1991; West et al., 1986), can indicate social isolation. Social support emanates from social interaction and increases well-being. Therefore absence of social support is an indicator (defining characteristic) of social isolation. Box 50-1 contrasts the defining characteristics for Social Isolation proposed here and those listed by NANDA.

CASE STUDY 1

E. Jones is an 83-year-old white female who lives alone in her home of 50 years in a suburb of a large city in the Midwest. Mrs. Jones is a widow of 10 years and lost her only child in the Vietnam War. Her nearest relatives are two grand-nieces who live in New York and with whom Mrs. Jones exchanges Christmas cards but rarely contacts. Mrs. Jones does not drive and either walks to stores and other places to run errands or depends on neighbors to drive her. Mrs. Jones belonged to a bridge club and was close to other women in the club; however, she is now the sole survivor of the club and does not have any friends left who are her age. Mrs. Jones liked to work in her garden and would talk with neighbors. Six months ago Mrs. Jones fractured her right hip and underwent an open reduction and internal fixation. Mrs. Jones was transferred from the hospital to a skilled nursing facility to regain strength and returned home 2 weeks ago. Her nieces have called twice a week to check on her, but the phone calls were brief. Only one neighbor knew Mrs. Jones was home and has been checking on her once a week in order to run errands. Her physical status has deteriorated since returning home, she has difficulty ambulating with a walker, and routine activities have become challenging. Her personal hygiene is now poor, meals are often skipped, and there is evidence that Mrs. Jones is increasingly forgetful. The neighbor contacted Mrs. Jones' physician, who arranged a home visit by a nurse from the home health department at the local hospital.

Assessment revealed that she had talked with her nieces twice in the last week, had a neighbor visit once in the last week, but felt that she had no one to confide in, she often felt lonely, and she was somewhat unhappy about how infrequent her nieces contacted her. Additionally, she could not identify anyone who would take care of her if she were sick. Assessment data are presented in the first column of Table 50-2.

Related factors contributing to the social isolation are spatial and physical separation (geographic distance from nieces and inability to walk far), social separation (lack of involvement in social groups), interpersonal separation (loss of spouse and peers and reluctance to ask for help from

Table 50-2	Nursing Diagnoses, Outcomes, and Interventions for MRS. JONES		

Nursing Diagnoses	Nursing-Sensitive Outcomes	Nursing Interventions
SOCIAL ISOLATION ***Defining Characteristics*** Absence of close family and friends Decreased social contacts Loss of peers and spouse	**SOCIAL INVOLVEMENT** ***Indicators*** Interaction with family members Interaction with neighbors Interaction with close friends	**SOCIALIZATION ENHANCEMENT** ***Activities*** Encourage enhanced involvement in already established relationships Encourage social and community activities Give feedback about improvement in care of personal appearance or other activities Give positive feedback when patient reaches out to others
Expressions of loneliness	**LONELINESS** ***Indicators*** Expression of social isolation Expression of loss due to separation from another Difficulty in establishing contact with other people Decrease in ability to concentrate Eating disturbance	**FAMILY INVOLVEMENT PROMOTION** ***Activities*** Identify family member's capabilities for involvement in care of patient Identify family member's preferences for involvement with patient Determine level of patient dependency on family Encourage family members to keep or maintain family relationships Discuss options for type of home care **ANIMAL-ASSISTED THERAPY** ***Activities*** Determine patient's acceptance of animals as therapeutic agents Provide therapy animals for patient such as dogs, cats, horses, snakes, turtles, gerbils, guinea pigs, and birds Encourage patient to feed/groom animals
Reports there is no one to help her	**SOCIAL SUPPORT** ***Indicators*** Reports of confidant relationship Reports of persons who could help when needed Evidence of willingness to call on other for help Reports of help being offered by others Resource use Uses senior transportation service to attend senior center	**SUPPORT SYSTEM ENHANCEMENT** ***Activities*** Assess psychologic response to situation and availability of support system Determine adequacy of existing social network Determine barriers to using support systems Assess community resource adequacy to identify strengths and weaknesses Provide services in a caring and supportive manner Explain to concerned others how they can help
Impaired mobility after hip fracture	**AMBULATION: WALKING** ***Indicators*** Walks with effective gait Walks short distance Walks moderate distance	**EXERCISE THERAPY: AMBULATION** ***Activities*** Consult physical therapy about ambulation plan Assist patient to establish realistic increment in distance for ambulation Encourage independent ambulation within safe limits
Poor hygiene Poor nutritional status Increased forgetfulness	**WELL-BEING** ***Indicators*** Satisfaction with social interaction Satisfaction with physiologic functioning Satisfaction with ability to express emotions	**SELF-CARE ASSISTANCE** ***Activities*** Monitor patient's ability for independent self-care Encourage independence, but intervene when patient is unable to perform

the neighbors), and intrapersonal separation (increasing memory loss). Evidence of loss of well-being includes poor grooming, poor nutritional status, and loss of strength in ambulating. The diagnosis of Social Isolation was made on the evidence that there is a decrease in social contacts, expressions of loneliness, and diminished well-being.

To address Mrs. Jones' isolation, the nurse would need the following additional data: community resources that might be available to Mrs. Jones and how she feels about using them; whether or not she had ever been or continued to be involved with a church; what her emotional relationship is with the nieces; if there are other possible causes for the poor nutritional intake (poverty? getting groceries? eating alone? depression?); other causes for poor hygiene (unable to get in tub or shower?); and causes for increased forgetfulness (recent relocation from nursing home?). These additional data will help support the initial diagnosis and help identify possible interventions, outcomes, and other problems that need to be addressed (Table 50-2).

CASE STUDY 2

H. Smith is a 73-year-old black male who was unable to live alone after his wife died. He has arthritic contractures of his hands, making it difficult for him to cook and care for his home; otherwise he is in fairly good health. Two years ago he was admitted to a residential care facility. Mr. Smith occasionally comes to the common areas in the facility but seldom interacts with anyone and spends much time alone in his room. He has no close friends at the facility, generally seems very sad, and talks of feeling lonely and worthless. Prior to coming to the residential facility, Mr. Smith attended a senior center daily and was an avid bird watcher. He no longer pursues this interest.

The initial diagnosis for Mr. Smith is Social Isolation related to social and interpersonal separation as evidenced by the death of his wife, decreased social interactions with other residents, and the time he spends alone in his room. Other indicators of social isolation are his expressions of loneliness, worthlessness, and sadness (Table 50-3).

Additional data are needed to identify the impact of his arthritis on his comfort and mobility level and how it affects his ability to be socially involved. There is also limited information about his family and friends and their availability to provide support. Additionally, there is a need to pursue his previous interests and hobbies and how those could be promoted or rekindled.

NURSING-SENSITIVE OUTCOMES

The conceptual model presented in this chapter provides a framework for selecting nursing outcomes for elders who are socially isolated. Based on the model, enhancing social contacts increases received and available social support, which decreases social isolation and increases physiologic and psychologic well-being. Overall, the desired outcome is enhanced well-being. Nursing outcomes for socially iso-

lated elders include improved well-being, enhanced social contact, improved social skills, enhanced social support, reduced loneliness, and improved well-being. The Nursing Outcomes Classification (NOC) (Iowa Outcomes Project, 2000) has identified outcomes consistent with this framework. Table 50-1 presents outcomes related to each of the etiologies of Social Isolation.

The NOC outcome Well-Being (Iowa Outcomes Project, 2000), defined as "an individual's expressed satisfaction with health status" (p. 443), is a key outcome for all etiologies of Social Isolation. The indicators for Well-Being address satisfaction with the following aspects of physical and psychologic well-being: physiologic functioning, performance of activities of daily living, happiness, psychologic functioning, and social interaction. Well-being indicates the effectiveness of the interventions at resolving the known or suspected etiologies of isolation. In addition, outcomes can be used to address improved well-being for specific health problems. In a situation with a client who is socially isolated and has hypertension, an outcome indicating well-being would be the indicators systolic and diastolic blood pressure.

A NOC outcome for received and available social support is Social Support (Iowa Outcomes Project, 2000), defined as "perceived availability and actual provision of reliable assistance from other persons" (p. 406). The indicators for Social Support include reports of persons willing to help when needed, reports of confidant relationship(s), reports of stable social network, and reports of money, time, labor, and information provided by others. An appropriate goal for persons with social isolation is that they will participate in more social activities. The outcome Loneliness (Iowa Outcomes Project, 2000) is defined as "the extent of emotional, social, or existential isolation response" (p. 297). Indicators of Loneliness include expression of desperation, extreme hopelessness, social isolation, and difficulty in planning and establishing contact with other people. Obviously, the outcome established for a patient should be a decrease in loneliness. An indicator of reaching the desired outcome is verbal expression of satisfaction with social contacts (Cox et al., 1997).

Increasing social interaction is consistent with the NOC outcome Social Involvement (Iowa Outcomes Project, 2000), defined as the "frequency of an individual's social interactions with persons, groups, or organizations" (p. 405). Indicators of Social Involvement include interaction with close friends, neighbors, or family members and participation in organizations or leisure activities. Furthermore, increasing social interaction is consistent with the NOC outcome Social Interaction Skills (Iowa Outcomes Project, 2000), defined as "an individual's use of effective interaction behaviors" (p. 404). Indicators of Social Interaction Skills include disclosure, receptiveness, engagement, trust, and compromise. Appropriate goals include identifying strengths and limitations in current patterns of social interaction and using enhanced social skills in both

Table 50-3	Nursing Diagnoses, Outcomes, and Interventions for MR. SMITH	
Nursing Diagnoses	**Nursing-Sensitive Outcomes**	**Nursing Interventions**
SOCIAL ISOLATION *Defining Characteristics* Absence of close friends and family Decreased social contacts Loss of spouse	SOCIAL INVOLVEMENT *Indicators* Interaction with neighbors (fellow residents) Participation in leisure activities	DISCUSSION GROUP *Activities* Determine the purpose of the group Form a group of optimal size: 5-12 members Establish a time and place for group meeting Encourage members to share things they have in common with one another
	SOCIAL INTERACTION SKILLS *Indicators* Disclosure Engagement Relaxation	SOCIALIZATION ENHANCEMENT *Activities* Encourage relationships with persons who have common interests and goals Encourage sharing of common problems with others
	ENVIRONMENTAL ADAPTATION *Indicator* Attends meals and other group activities	ENVIRONMENTAL MANAGEMENT *Activities* Structure environment to promote socialization Provide individualized and consistent seating arrangement for meals Provide space for group activities
Expressions of loneliness Sad expressions	LONELINESS *Indicators* Expression of social isolation Expression of loss due to separation from another Difficulty in establishing contact with other people	ACTIVITY THERAPY *Activities* Assist to identify meaningful activities Assist person to schedule specific periods for diversional activity in daily routine Assist to explore the personal meaning of usual activity and/or favorite leisure activities
Expressions of worthlessness	SELF-ESTEEM *Indicators* Description of self Description of success in social groups Balance of participation and listening in social groups	SELF-ESTEEM ENHANCEMENT *Activities* Encourage to identify strengths Explore previous achievements of success Assist in identifying positive responses from others

familiar and new interpersonal situations in order enhance mutuality (Kim, McFarland, & McLane, 1995).

While many of the NOC outcomes provide good measures of effectiveness of interventions for social isolation, several potentially useful outcomes are missing. Environmental Adaptation, the desired effect when trying to intervene with Social Isolation related to spatial separation, is not included. Indicators of Environmental Adaptation might include the ability to find one's way around and the ability to use services and equipment. An outcome is also needed to measure progress in resource use when lack of, or poor use of, resources is the etiology, as is the case in social isolation related to social separation or spatial separation. A new outcome Resource Use could include contacting social services agencies such as transportation, attending senior center activities, and participating in community groups.

CASE STUDY 1

Five goals were developed with Mrs. Jones and confirmed with her nieces: (1) moderate interaction with neighbors and family (a "3" rating on the 5-point indicator scale for social involvement); (2) feelings of loneliness would decrease to moderate (a "3" rating on a 5-point scale); (3) use of transportation to attend senior center activities and social support would be at a substantial level (a "4" on a 5-point rating scale); (4) ability to walk up to one block independently with an assistive device; and (5) report of moderately compromised well-being (Table 50-2). Initial outcome assessments were to be completed weekly for the first month and then every 2 weeks for the next 2 months.

CASE STUDY 2

The goals developed by the nurse with Mr. Smith included the following: (1) increase in social involvement by participation in a discussion group weekly and daily visits with neighbors to a moderate level (a "3" rating on a 5-point scale); (2) increase in comfort and ease with interactions with others to a moderate level (a "3" rating on a 5-point scale); (3) decrease in feelings of loneliness to a moderate level (a "3" rating on a 5-point scale); and (4) increase in feelings of self-worth so they are often positive (a "4" rating on a 5-point scale) (Table 50-3). Mr. Smith's progress toward the established goals would be reassessed by the nurse and Mr. Smith every 2 weeks for the first month and then monthly for 3 months. If improvement were noted, assessments would be done quarterly.

NURSING INTERVENTIONS

A wide variety of nursing interventions can be appropriate for persons experiencing social isolation (Table 50-1). Interventions for Social Isolation have two functions: to overcome barriers to social contact and to support the patient until the barriers are breached. Interventions designed for the first function target specific spatial, intrapersonal, interpersonal, social, and physiofunctional barriers that lead to isolation. Interventions designed for the second function support individuals at times of crisis and stress until the social network can be mobilized or rebuilt.

Two types of support may be particularly useful: informational support and emotional support. Informational support can be provided to both patients and family members through the NIC interventions Anticipatory Guidance, Counseling, and Crisis Intervention (Bore, 1994; Evans, Bishop, & Haselkorn, 1991; Goodman & Pynoos, 1990; Iowa Intervention Project, 2000). Anticipatory Guidance alerts the patient and family to expected developmental changes and/or potential situational crises. For example, it is important to prepare the elderly patient in advance when relocation is necessary. This may be as simple as explaining why changing rooms is necessary or as complex as preparing a move from home to a long-term care facility. In addition, Counseling and Crisis Intervention enhance coping skills. Effective interaction with the patient and family can help alleviate anxiety and facilitate smooth transitions (see Chapter 48).

Emotional support is equally important. Active Listening and Touch (both NIC interventions) and a respectful and caring manner are important skills in the nurse's repertoire. However, peers in a group setting or one-on-one visitation can be even more effective in providing reassurance, acceptance, and encouragement (Harris & Bodden, 1978; Hoffmann, 1993; Meagher, Gregor, & Stewart, 1987; Vinokur-Kaplan, Cibulski, Spero, & Bergman, 1982). The NIC intervention Visitation Facilitation (Iowa Interven-

tion Project, 2000), defined as "promoting beneficial visits by family and friends" (p. 698), would also be helpful. Fick (1993) has suggested that animals can decrease loneliness in elders. The NIC intervention Animal-Assisted Therapy emphasizes the use of animals as a source of affection, attention, diversion, and relaxation.

Interventions that target spatial separation are designed to assist the patient in spanning physical barriers. The elder's ability to walk can be facilitated through Exercise Promotion and Exercise Therapy: Ambulation (Iowa Intervention Project, 2000). Environmental Management can be used to change the patient's environment in order to enhance movement and encourage interaction with other people. For example, a nursing home can rearrange furniture to remove barriers from one point to the next. Additionally, the television can be removed as the focal point of a day room, and chairs and tables can be arranged to encourage residents to gather around them. The NIC intervention Transport (Iowa Intervention Project, 2000), defined as "moving a patient from one location to another" (p. 672), can be used to prescribe arrangement or provision of transportation to outside activities.

Intrapersonal interventions are designed to enhance personal resources that facilitate interaction with others. Self-Awareness Enhancement (Iowa Intervention Project, 2000), defined as "assisting a patient to explore and understand his/her thoughts, feelings, motivations and behaviors" (p. 574), helps the patient to comprehend how his behavior affects others. Self-Esteem Enhancement (Iowa Intervention Project, 2000) is "assisting a patient to increase his personal judgment of self-worth" (p. 580) by enhancing the ability to be assertive. Exercise Therapy: Ambulation is used to increase the ability to walk and move about in one's environment to enhance self-care ability and the likelihood of desiring social interaction.

Interpersonal interventions, such as Socialization Enhancement, Communication Enhancement, and Support Group, are designed to improve social skills (Iowa Intervention Project, 2000) (Table 50-1). The COSTAR Programme in Baltimore is a mobile mental health program that takes nurses, social workers, counselors, and psychiatrists into the community for frequent contacts with the long-term mentally ill (Thornicroft & Breakey, 1991). Social functioning was shown to improve in the patients involved with COSTAR.

The NIC intervention Reminiscence Therapy is defined as "using the recall of past events, feelings, and thoughts to facilitate pleasure, quality of life, or adaptation to present circumstances" (Iowa Interventions Project, 2000, p. 554). One of the activities for the reminiscing intervention is conducting a group discussion of life history. Otherwise the reminiscing intervention is aimed at individuals rather than groups. Reminiscence groups for older persons can be conducted in a number of settings, and studies have linked reminiscence with increased self-esteem, decreased depression, decreased confusion, improved life satisfaction, and increased social interaction (Hamilton, 1992). Therapy Group, another NIC intervention that takes place in a group context, is defined as "application of psychotherapeutic techniques to a group, including the utilization of interactions between members of the group" (Iowa Interventions Project, 2000, p. 666). An advantage of therapy groups is that they promote interaction among the members of the group.

Social interventions are designed to improve social interaction. Recreation Therapy is the "purposeful use of recreation to promote relaxation and enhancement of social skills" (Iowa Intervention Project, 2000, p. 549). Groups are another useful social intervention. Group interventions offer the advantage of helping a greater number of clients, strengthening peer identification, and promoting social interaction and self-growth (Burnside, 1989; Hamilton, 1992). There are many types of groups, including discussion groups, therapy groups, support groups, reminiscence groups, and interest groups. One

program developed in Sweden used recreational groups as a way to enhance social contacts among the participants. Groups were formed in botany, art history, music, song, and outings for picnics and theater (Arnetz, Eyre, & Theorell, 1982). Thus there is a need for a NIC intervention specifying a more generic group intervention in which the primary goals are promoting socialization and sharing of interests. Outcomes for each type of group are quite similar, particularly increased social interaction and self-growth. Another potentially helpful intervention that is not part of NIC would be computer networking, which is the encouragement of elders to use the Internet as a way of making connections with others in society. For example, caregivers of elders often find it difficult to leave the home. Computer access to bulletin boards and chat rooms would give them an opportunity to interact with others, particularly other caregivers.

Physiofunctional interventions such as Exercise Promotion are designed to overcome physiologic or functional limitations to enhance social interaction (Table 50-1).

Table 50-4 Mrs. Jones's Progress With Outcomes

	Base	Week 2	Week 4	Week 8
SOCIAL INVOLVEMENT	2	2	3	3
Interaction with family members	2	3	3	3
Interaction with neighbors	2	3	3	3
LONELINESS	1	2	2	3
Expression of social isolation	1	2	2	3
Expression of loss due to separation	2	2	2	2
Difficulty in establishing contact with people	1	2	2	2
Decrease in ability to concentrate	2	2	3	3
Eating disturbance	3	3	3	4
SOCIAL SUPPORT	1	2	2	2
Reports of confidant relationship	1	1	2	2
Reports of persons who could help	2	2	2	2
Evidence of willingness to call on others for help	1	2	2	2
Reports of help being offered by others	1	2	2	2
Uses community resources to attend senior center	1	1	1	1
AMBULATION: WALKING	2	2	4	4
Walks with effective gait	2	2	4	4
Walks short distance	2	2	4	4
Walks moderate distance	2	2	4	4
WELL-BEING	1	2	2	2
Satisfaction with social interaction	1	2	2	2
Satisfaction with physiologic function	1	2	3	2
Satisfaction with willingness to express emotion	1	2	3	3

Nursing Outcomes Classification (NOC) 5-point Likert measurement scales:

Social Involvement: 1 = None; 2 = Limited; 3 = Moderate; 4 = Substantial; 5 = Extensive.
Loneliness: 1 = Extensive; 2 = Substantial; 3 = Moderate; 4 = Limited; 5 = None.
Social Support: 1 = None; 2 = Limited; 3 = Moderate; 4 = Substantial; 5 = Extensive.
Ambulation: Walking: 1 = Dependent, does not participate; 2 = Requires assistive person and device;
3 = Requires assistive person; 4 = Independent with assistive device; 5 = Completely independent.
Well-Being: 1 = Extremely compromised; 2 = Substantially compromised; 3 = Moderately compromised;
4 = Mildly compromised; 5 = Not compromised.

Correction or compensation of hearing and vision (Communication Enhancement) is important to increasing an elder's ability to interact with others. For family caregiver clients who are often overburdened by their responsibilities, Respite Care provides emotional and physical rest and enhances opportunities for social interaction.

CASE STUDY 1

The home health nurse set outcomes with Mrs. Jones to enhance self-care and mobility and increase social interactions. Interventions included Socialization Enhancement, Family Involvement Promotion, Animal-Assisted Therapy, Support System Enhancement, Exercise Therapy: Ambulation, and Self-Care Assistance (Table 50-2). The nieces were contacted to inform them of the situation, and the neighbor who visited weekly was given suggestions on how to help Mrs. Jones. It was decided that professional assistance was needed until Mrs. Jones and her nieces could decide what to do. Home health aides went to Mrs. Jones' home on a daily basis to assist with cooking and grooming. In-home physical therapy was arranged in order to increase Mrs. Jones' general muscle strength. Over a period of 2 weeks, Mrs. Jones gained 4 pounds and was able to ambulate from the bedroom to kitchen without assistance. However, after extensive discussions, Mrs. Jones and her nieces decided that she should move to New York to be near relatives who were willing to check

on her several days a week. Table 50-4 records the progress Mrs. Jones made toward the established goals using the selected outcomes.

CASE STUDY 2

Several interventions were prescribed for Mr. Smith: Discussion Group, Socialization Enhancement, Environmental Management, Activity Therapy, and Self-Esteem Enhancement (Table 50-3). The nurse noted Mr. Smith's reluctance to join in conversations and suggested that he join a weekly discussion group. The discussion group consisted of 10 residents from Mr. Smith's floor and the nurse who acted as the group facilitator. Usually the group began by one member talking about events of the past week, which led to a discussion on a topic of interest. Mr. Smith eventually discovered that others in the group had similar problems related to loss of a loved one, loss of self-esteem, and loss of physical health. The sharing of concern, experiences, and feelings brought Mr. Smith closer to the other members of the group. He began to form friendships and interacted with others in planning social activities on the weekends and evenings. He expressed less loneliness and began to gain confidence in his ability to contribute to the group and to friendships. Table 50-5 shows Mr. Smith's progress toward the desired outcomes for his interventions.

Table 50-5 Mr. Smith's Progress With Outcomes	Base	Week 2	Week 4	Week 8
SOCIAL INVOLVEMENT	2	3	3	4
Interaction with fellow residents	2	2	3	4
Participation in leisure activities	1	2	2	3
SOCIAL INTERACTION SKILLS	2	2	3	3
Disclosure	2	2	2	3
Engagement	2	2	3	4
Relaxation	2	3	3	3
ENVIRONMENTAL ADAPTATION				
Attends meals and other group activities	2	2	3	4
LONELINESS	2	2	2	3
Expression of social isolation	1	2	2	3
Expression of loss due to separation	1	2	2	2
Difficulty in establishing contact with others	1	2	2	3
SELF-ESTEEM	2	2	3	4
Description of self	2	2	3	4
Description of success in social groups	1	1	2	2
Balance of participation and listening in groups	1	2	3	4

Key: Social Involvement: 1 = None; 2 = Limited; 3 = Moderate; 4 = Substantial; 5 = Extensive.
      Social Interaction Skills: 1 = None; 2 = Limited; 3 = Moderate; 4 = Substantial; 5 = Extensive.
      Environmental Adaptation: 1 = None; 2 = Limited; 3 = Moderate; 4 = Substantial; 5 = Extensive.
      Loneliness: 1 = Extensive; 2 = Substantial; 3 = Moderate; 4 = Limited; 5 = None.
      Self-Esteem: 1 = Never positive; 2 = Rarely positive; 3 = Sometimes positive; 4 = Often positive;
                                           5 = Consistently positive.

SUMMARY

Social isolation can have a devastating effect on well-being. Nurses, however, are in a position to assess, diagnose, and intervene to improve the well-being of elders. By assisting the client to overcome the barriers to social contacts, networks can be revitalized, increasing both available and received social support.

Ultimately the client must establish and maintain social contacts. Nurses and other health professionals can continue to be a member of the elder's social network, although not the only member. Once appropriate outcomes such as social support or social involvement have been identified, the nurse can introduce interventions that permit the elderly client to fully participate in social interactions. As these outcomes are realized, both physiologic and psychosocial well-being are increased.

REFERENCES

Arnetz, B. B., Eyre, E., & Theorell, T. (1982). Social activation of the elderly: A social experiment. *Social Science in Medicine, 16*, 1685-1690.

Austin, A. G. (1989). Becoming immune to loneliness: Helping the elderly fill a void. *Journal of Gerontological Nursing, 15*(9), 25-28.

Bassuk, S. S., Glass, T. A., & Berkman, F. (1999). Social disengagement and incident cognitive decline in community-dwelling elderly persons. *Annals of Internal Medicine, 131*(3), 165-173.

Berezin, M. A. (1980). Isolation in the aged: Individual dynamics, community and family involvement. Intrapsychic isolation in the elderly. *Journal of Geriatric Psychiatry, 13*(1), 5-18.

Bondevik, M., & Skogstad, A. (1998). The oldest old, ADL, social network, and loneliness. *Western Journal of Nursing Research, 20*(3), 325-343.

Bore, J. (1994). Occupational therapy home visits: A satisfactory service? *British Journal of Occupational Therapy, 57*(3), 85-88.

Burnside, I. (1989). Group work with elder women: A model to improve the quality of life. *Journal of Women and Aging, 1*(1,2,3), 265-290.

Carpenito, L. (1997). *Nursing diagnosis: Application to clinical practice* (7th ed.). Baltimore, MD: Lippincott Williams & Wilkins.

Chappell, N. L., Badger, M., & Ware, I. (1989). Social isolation and well-being. *Journal of Gerontology, 44*, S169-S176.

Cohen, S., & Syme, S. L. (1985). Issues in the study and application of social support. In S. Cohen & S. L. Syme (Eds.), *Social support and health*. San Diego, CA: Academic Press.

Cox, H. C., Hinz, M. D., Lubno, M. A., Newfield, S. A., Ridenour, N. A., Slater, M. M., & Sridaromont, K. L. (1997). *Clinical applications of nursing diagnosis: Adult, child, women's, psychiatric, gerontic, and home health considerations* (3rd ed.). Philadelphia: F. A. Davis.

Dugan, E., & Kivett, V. R. (1994). The importance of emotional and social isolation to loneliness among very old rural adults. *The Gerontologist, 34*, 340-346.

Duke University Center for the Study of Aging and Human Development. (1978). *Multidimensional assessment: The OARS methodology*. Durham, NC: Duke University.

Elsen, J., & Blegen, M. (1991). Social isolation. In M. Maas, K. Buckwalter, & M. A. Hardy (Eds.), *Nursing diagnoses and interventions for the elderly* (pp. 519-529). Reading, MA: Addison Wesley Longman.

Evans, R. L., Bishop, D. S., & Haselkorn, J. K. (1991). Factors predicting satisfactory home care after stroke. *Archives of Physical Medicine and Rehabilitation, 72*, 144-147.

Evans, R. L., Werkhoven, W., & Fox, H. R. (1982). Treatment of social isolation and loneliness in a sample of visually impaired elderly persons. *Psychological Reports, 51*, 103-108.

Fick, K. M. (1993). The influence of an animal on social interactions of nursing home residents in a groups setting. *The American Journal of Occupational Therapy, 47*, 529-534.

Goodman, C. C., & Pynoos, J. (1990). A model telephone information and support program for caregivers of Alzheimer's patients. *The Gerontologist, 30*, 399-404.

Hamilton, D. B. (1992). Reminiscence therapy. In G. M. Bulechek & J. C. McCloskey (Eds.), *Nursing interventions: Essential nursing treatments* (2nd ed., pp. 292-302). Philadelphia: W. B. Saunders.

Hansson, R. O., Jones, M. H., Carpenter, B. N., & Remondet, J. H. (1986-87). *International Journal of Aging and Human Development, 24*(1), 41-53.

Harris, J. E., & Bodden, J. L. (1978). An activity group experience for disengaged elderly persons. *Journal of Counseling Psychology, 25*, 325-330.

Hobfoll, S. E., & Stokes, J. P. (1988). The process and mechanics of social support. In S. Duck, D. F. Hay, S. E. Hobfoll, W. Ickes, & B. M. Montgomery (Eds.), *Handbook of personal relationships: Theory, research, and interventions* (pp. 497-517). New York: John Wiley & Sons.

Hoffmann, H. (1993). The round table in a community-based outpatient service. *Acta Psychiatry Scandinavia, 87*, 153-159.

Holden, K. C. (1988). Poverty and living arrangements among older women: Are changes in economic well-being underestimated? *Journal of Gerontology, 43*, 522-527.

Iowa Intervention Project. J. C. McCloskey & G. M. Bulechek (Eds.). (2000). *Nursing interventions classification (NIC)* (3rd ed.). St. Louis, MO: Mosby.

Iowa Outcomes Project. M. Johnson, M. Maas, & S. Moorhead (Eds.). (2000). *Nursing outcomes classification (NOC)* (2nd ed.). St. Louis, MO: Mosby.

Kane, R. A., & Kane, R. L. (1981). *Assessing the elderly: A practical guide to measurement*. Lexington, MS: Lexington Books.

Kim, M. J., McFarland, G. K., & McLane, A. M. (1995). *Pocket guide to nursing diagnoses* (6th ed.). St. Louis, MO: Mosby.

Knox, S. S., & Uvanas-Moberg, K. (1998). Social isolation and cardiovascular disease: An atherosclerotic pathway? *Psychoneuroendocrinology, 23*(8), 877-890.

Krause, N., Liang, J., & Keith, V. (1990). Personality, social support, and psychological distress in later life. *Psychology and Aging, 5*, 315-326.

LaVeist, T. A., Sellers, R. M., Brown, K. A., & Nickerson, K. J. (1997). Extreme social isolation, use of community-based senior support services, and mortality among African American elderly women. *American Journal of Community Psychology, 25*(5), 721-732.

Lien-Gieschen, T. (1993). Validation of social isolation related to maturational age: Elderly. *Nursing Diagnosis, 4*(1), 37-44.

Lockery, S. A., Dunkle, R. E., Kart, C. S., & Coulton, C. J. (1994). Factors contributing to the early rehospitalization of elderly people. *Health & Social Work, 19*, 182-191.

Lubben, J. E. (1988). Gender differences in the relationship of widowhood and psychological well-being among low income elderly. *Women & Health, 14*, 161-189.

Meagher, D. M., Gregor, F., & Stewart, M. (1987). Dyadic social-support for cardiac surgery patients a Canadian approach. *Social Science in Medicine, 25,* 833-837.

Miller, B., & McFall, S. (1991). The effect of caregiver's burden on change in frail older persons' use of formal helpers. *Journal of Health and Social Behavior, 32,* 165-179.

Morgan, D. L. (1988). Age differences in social network participation. *Journal of Gerontology, 43,* S129-S137.

Neuling, S. J., & Winfield, H. R. (1988). Social support and recovery after surgery for breast cancer: Frequency and correlation of supportive behaviors by family, friends, and surgeon. *Social Science in Medicine, 27,* 385-392.

Norbeck, J. S., Lindsey, A. M., & Carrieri, V. L. (1981). The development of an instrument to measure social support. *Nursing Research, 30,* 264-269.

Norris, V. K., Stephans, M. A., & Kinney, J. M. (1990). The impact of family interactions on recovery from stroke: Help or Hindrance? *The Gerontologist, 30,* 532-542.

North American Nursing Diagnosis Association. (1999). *Nursing diagnoses: Definitions & classification 1999-2000.* Philadelphia: Author.

Peters-Golden, H. (1982). Breast cancer: Varied perceptions of social support in the illness experience. *Social Science in Medicine, 16,* 483-491.

Prince, M. J., Harwood, R. H., Blizard, R. A., Thomas, A., & Mann, A. H. (1997). Social support deficits, loneliness, and life events as risk factors for depression in old age. *Psychological Medicine, 27*(2), 323-332.

Rossi, P. H., Wright, J. D., & Anderson, A. B. (1983). *Handbook of survey research.* San Diego, CA: Academic Press.

Rubinstein, R. L. (1987). Never married elderly as a social type: Re-evaluating some images. *The Gerontologist, 27,* 108-113.

Russell, D. W., Cutrona, C. E., de la Mora, A., & Wallace, R. B. (1997). Loneliness and nursing home admissions among rural older adults. *Psychology & Aging, 12*(4), 574-589.

Seeman, M., & Anderson, C. S. (1983). Alienation and alcohol: The role of work, mastery, and community in drinking behavior. *American Sociological Review, 48,* 60-77.

Silverstone, B., & Miller, S. (1980). Isolation in the aged: Individual dynamics, community and family involvement: The isolation of the community elderly from informal social structure: Myth or reality? *Journal of Geriatric Psychiatry, 13*(1), 27-47.

Simonsick, E. M., Kasper, J. D., & Phillips, C. L. (1998). Physical disability and social interaction. Factors associated with low social contact and home confinement in disabled older women. *Journals of Gerontology. Series B, Psychology and Social Sciences, 53*(4), 5209-5217.

Stewart, A. L., Hays, R. D., & Ware, J. E. (1988). The MOS short-form general health survey: Reliability and validity in a patient population. *Medical Care, 26,* 724-735.

Thornicroft, G., & Breakey, W. R. (1991). The COSTAR programme. 1: Improving social networks of the long-term mentally ill. *British Journal of Psychiatry, 159,* 245-249.

Ulbrich, P. M., & Bradsher, J. E. (1993). Perceived support, help seeking, and adaptation to stress among older black and white women living alone. *Journal of Aging and Health, 5,* 365-386.

Vinokur-Kaplan, D., Cibulski, O., Spero, S., & Bergman, S. (1982). "Oldster to oldster": An example of mutual aid through friendly visiting among Israeli elderly. *Journal of Gerontological Social Work, 4*(1), 75-91.

Weinert, C. (1987). A social support Measure: PRQ85. *Nursing Research, 36,* 273-277.

West, D. A., Kellner, R., & Moore-West, M. (1986). The effects of loneliness: A review of literature. *Comprehensive Psychiatry, 27,* 351-363.

CHAPTER 51

IMPAIRED COMMUNICATION

Brenda Emick-Herring

Impaired communication is a clinical problem that nurses, especially gerontology nurses, frequently encounter. The causes are variable, but the diagnosis has a high preponderance in older adults. Cerebrovascular disease, Alzheimer's disease, Parkinson's disease, multi-infarct dementia, acute confusion, head trauma, alcohol abuse, and tumor are very prevalent in elders and gravely compromise communication (Damasio, 1992; Foreman & Zane, 1996; Groher, 1990; Hall & Wakefield, 1996; Rakowiez & Hodges, 1998; Roussel, 1995; Simmons-Mackie, 1995). Recent literature suggests that adults with motor neuron disease such as amyotrophic lateral sclerosis (ALS) and those with life-threatening illnesses such as cancer also develop language deficits that impair the quality of life (Rakowiez & Hodges, 1998; Salt & Robertson, 1998). In the nursing literature, communication deficits are often addressed via NANDA's (1982) nursing diagnosis Impaired Verbal Communication. This chapter, however, focuses on the broader concept of impaired communication, which subsumes this specific nursing diagnosis and additional impairments related to nonverbal communication.

Communication is a complex and intricate process. Samovar and Rintye (1979) described seven distinct components involved in communication, including (1) a sender, (2) an encoding action, (3) a message, (4) a channel (medium), (5) a decoding action, (6) a receiver, and (7) feedback. Cusack (1991) stressed that codes ". . . are the embodiment of language—the system of symbols by which messages are transmitted" (p. 530). She emphasized that language is expressed (encoded) in two major ways—speaking and writing—and is received (decoded) by listening and reading.

Communication has many components, including verbal and nonverbal modalities, the senses (especially hearing and vision), motor planning and execution, attention, memory, and various cognitive functions. Verbal communication pertains to the understanding and use of words (symbols) that have shared meaning among senders and receivers. In contrast, nonverbal communication involves transmission of messages without necessarily using words.

A person's verbal and nonverbal communication abilities contribute to reasoning, problem solving, decision making, goal attainment, independence, and emotional well-being. Though verbal and nonverbal components are both key aspects of communication, one does not preclude the other. For example, an individual may speak three or four sentences that flow smoothly, have voice inflection, and have correct sentence structure, but the message conveys no meaning. Conversely, some people who cannot speak or sign may be adept at communicating via facial expressions, body movements, posture, gaze, and gestures.

Communication has intrigued and mystified society for many years. It is the primary avenue that humans have for translating thoughts into language so they can be shared with others. The neural processes for normal and abnormal language have been studied by scientists in many fields.

Bronstein, Popovich, and Stewart-Amidei (1991) emphasized the difference between speech and language. Speech is the act of speaking. It occurs when one forces air through the vocal cords. Language, however, is wider in scope and includes speaking, writing, reading, and auditory comprehension. Boss (1991) describes language in terms of conveying and comprehending thoughts and ideas by the use of symbols (written, oral, and signing) in a sequential and grammatical manner. McFarland and Naschinski (1985) stress that communicators need to have a mutual understanding of the meanings of code symbols to enhance understanding and gratification during exchanges.

From a practical standpoint, language has three basic yet hierarchical elements: phonology, semantics, and syntax. Phonology is speech sounds and the order in which they are placed in a word or phrase. In the English language, word sounds and ordering are represented by syllables. For example, pajamas is "pa-ja-mas." Semantics involves relating a symbol to an object or concept so that a word has meaning and a phrase relays a message (e.g., the word "stop" means to quit doing a motion or activity). Syntax includes the grammar, rules, plurality, tense, and ordering of words to portray a more complex thought. For instance, "She went upstairs to get her medicine and a glass of water."

The frontal and temporal lobes of the brain contain major language and speech structures. Language formulation originates in the left frontal lobe. This is where thoughts are organized and converted to a spoken, written, or signage format to be shared with others. The left temporal lobe is responsible for hearing, interpreting auditory stimuli, and comprehending speech and written words.

The occipital lobe integrates visual impulses for sight and then stores visual images (such as symbols) in the form of visual memories. The occipital lobe and the parietal lobe have neural interconnections with the temporal lobe, thus working closely to interpret written words for reading.

Subcortically, the left thalamus and left basal ganglia have been identified as playing a role in language (Bronstein et al., 1991; Damasio, 1992). The actual motor mechanics of speech formulation involve precise integration of the frontal lobe, frontal association area, brainstem, descending motor pathways, several of the cranial nerves, and the respiratory system. Because there is close proximity of the language centers and functional overlap, damage to more than one of these cerebral areas may produce similar language impairments (Figure 51-1). Moreover, because symptoms vary depending on the cause, specific characteristics of impaired communication are described in the context of particular etiologies.

RELATED FACTORS/ETIOLOGIES

Age-related changes in the sensory system can affect communication skills. Hearing loss from aging itself, presbycusis, and cerumen accumulation can interfere with correct understanding of verbal comments. Reduced vision from homonymous hemianopsia, visual field cuts, cataracts, glaucoma, retinopathy, and macular degeneration can disrupt reading, writing, and interpretation of facial expressions, gestures, lip reading, and nonverbal feedback (Roussel, 1995; Simmons-Mackie, 1995). Many elderly persons have a history of chronic lung disease, which diminishes airflow and can decrease speech volume to the point that speech is difficult to understand (McConnell &

Murphy, 1996). However, language as a "learned" process does not seem to decline with normal aging.

Neurogenically based disorders such as Parkinson's disease, Alzheimer's disease, and stroke can produce a high incidence of communication problems. Bryan and Maxim (1998) indicated that demented or very old elders with language deficits may experience further language decline when living in long-term care facilities.

Language deterioration in the aged most commonly results from hypoxic, hemorrhagic, occlusive, hypoglycemic, metabolic, degenerative, or infectious causes (Boss, 1984a; Cusack, 1991; Loen, 1991; McConnell & Murphy, 1996). Many of these physiologic processes also interfere with cerebral circulation and thus lead to anatomic defects and respiratory distress (see Related Factors in Table 51-1).

One language deficit that is very common in elders is aphasia. Aphasia results from brain damage and, simply stated, is the impaired ability to produce language (to speak, gesture, or write) and to comprehend language (to understand gestures and spoken or written words). Individuals with aphasia frequently and repeatedly make errors sending or receiving messages. The following statements exemplify such errors:

1. "Cil-pen" instead of "pen cil" (abnormal phonology).
2. "You ought to be shrapped and basseled you rooty toot"—said to a nurse when she mistakenly left the plastic cover on an electric razor (abnormal semantics).
3. "Go . . . sit . . . toilets . . . now"—stated by a patient who needed to use a commode (abnormal syntax).

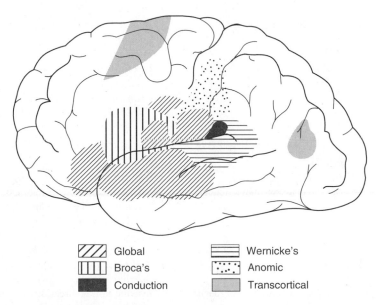

Global
Broca's
Conduction
Wernicke's
Anomic
Transcortical

FIGURE 51-1   Lesions in various types of aphasia. (From Kertesz, A., Lesk, D., & McCabe, P. [1977]. Isotope localization of infarcts in aphasia. *Archives of Neurology, 34,* 590-601.)

	Suggested Nursing-Sensitive Outcomes and Nursing Interventions	
Table 51-1	IMPAIRED VERBAL COMMUNICATION*	
Nursing Diagnosis	**Nursing-Sensitive Outcomes**	**Nursing Interventions**
IMPAIRED VERBAL COMMUNICATION* *Related Factors/Etiologies* Decrease in circulation to brain; brain tumor; physical barrier (tracheostomy, intubation); anatomic defect (cleft palate); psychologic barriers (psychosis, lack of stimuli); cultural difference, developmental or age related. *Progressive neurologic disease, e.g., Parkinson's disease, Alzheimer's disease; cortical damage; cranial nerve damage, hearing loss or deafness; glossectomy*	COMMUNICATION: EXPRESSIVE ABILITY *Indicators* Use of written language, *e.g., writes* Use of spoken language: vocal	COMMUNICATION ENHANCEMENT: SPEECH DEFICIT *Activities* *Practice signing name, writing serial symbols and habitual words. Use written flash cards or word board as a communication tool. Ask person to type letters/words.* Solicit family's assistance in understanding patient's speech. Stand in front of the patient when speaking and listen attentively. *Request timely referral for speech therapy.* Provide verbal prompts/reminders. Encourage patient to repeat words. *Reinforce prescriptive speech-language activities during informal interactions with patient. Carry on one-way conversations as appropriate.* Provide positive reinforcement and praise *for language efforts.* Use pictures/*word* board if appropriate. Refrain from shouting at patient with communication disorders. *Arrange for speech therapy after discharge if needed. See interventions for Case Study 1 for more strategies.*
	Use of spoken language: esophageal	Provide verbal prompts/reminders. Listen attentively. Provide positive reinforcement and praise.
	Use of clarity of speech, *e.g., able to articulate and organize speech; adequate vocal volume, cadence, tone, and rate*	Solicit family's assistance in understanding patient's speech. Listen attentively *and intuitively. Ask patient to say* simple words and short sentences. Refrain from shouting and dropping your voice at the end of sentences. Use picture/*word* board, if appropriate. *Reinforce* speech language *activities* during informal interactions. Encourage patient to repeat words. *Ask patient to raise voice volume, pause between words, stress the last sound of each word, and practice prescribed oral-motor exercises.*
	Use of pictures and drawings	Use picture/*word* board as appropriate. *Ask patient to draw pictures or point to pictures (or objects) that depict his/her needs.*
	Use of sign language	Use interpreter as necessary. *Learn to sign basic words. Use gestures, facial expressions, body movements, and demonstrations.*
	Use of nonverbal communication	Use of picture/*word* board. Provide positive reinforcement and praise as appropriate. *Encourage pictures, gestures, pantomime, pointing, and use of facial expressions. See additional activities at end of this table.*
	COMMUNICATION: RECEPTIVE ABILITY *Indicators* *Comprehends* written language, *e.g., reads*	COMMUNICATION ENHANCEMENT FOR RECEPTIVE DEFICITS *Activities* *Practice picture matching with written words. Practice reading aloud from enlarged print flash cards. Help patient find familiar written words in greeting cards, menu, etc. Tape word labels on functional objects and have patient read them while using objects. After reading words/phrases ask patient what he/she remembers. As reading comprehension improves, write simple messages to patient.*
	Comprehends spoken language	Give one simple direction at a time. Use short words and sentences. Refrain from shouting at patient with communication disorders. Stand in front of patient

*This author recommends using the nursing diagnosis Impaired Communication versus Impaired Verbal Communication.

Table 51-1	Suggested Nursing-Sensitive Outcomes and Nursing Interventions—cont'd IMPAIRED VERBAL COMMUNICATION*—cont'd	
Nursing Diagnosis	**Nursing-Sensitive Outcomes**	**Nursing Interventions**
		when speaking. Use picture board as appropriate. Use hand gestures, *pantomime, environmental cues, and facial expression while speaking. Use patient's name, light touch, and eye contact before speaking. Validate what you think patient said. If nurse can't understand patient (due to jargon, paraphasia, etc.), ask patient to describe it. If still unclear, ask patient to act it out or "show me." Avoid joking, teasing, and using idioms and colloquialisms. Limit patient speaking time and reduce praise given if patient is verbose. See interventions for Case Study 2 for more strategies.*
	COMMUNICATION ABILITY ***Indicators*** *Comprehends* pictures and drawings *Comprehends* sign language *Comprehends* nonverbal language	**COMMUNICATION ENHANCEMENT FOR SOCIAL ABILITIES** ***Activities*** *Use simple photos or sketches if appropriate.* Use interpreter, as necessary. *Learn to sign and do so.* *Use short and literal instructions and/or emphatic gestures, since patients often do not understand subtle body language, actions, posture, or sighs. Explain this to family, since misunderstandings can occur if family expects patient to "read" their nonverbal messages. Gently teach and role model the role of speaker.*
	Directs message appropriately	Use picture/*word board. Support patient's attempts to communicate. Cue/explain how to initiate a conversation, take turns speaking, avoid interrupting, and ask questions of others. Role model these behaviors.*
	Exchanges messages with others	*Respectfully explain and remind patient about social conversational skills, e.g., turn-taking, maintaining the topic, completing a thought/sentence, speaking with appropriate rate and voice volume, and listening to others. Allow patient to practice these skills. Gently discuss potential consequences of inappropriate conversational skills.*
	Acknowledgement of messages received	*Say "I understand" and/or nod your head in affirming way. Use simple photos or sketches if appropriate.* *Shake the patient's hand or give a thumb's up sign.*
	Demonstrates appropriate nonverbal communication	*Explain appropriate nonverbal behaviors and rationale for why they are suitable, e.g., how close to stand or sit to another, what polite eye gaze is and when to make eye contact, when to shake or raise hands, the importance of listening, proper gestures, and changing one's facial expression. Avoid assuming patient is depressed if there are limited facial expressions; rather, ask patient if depression is present or not. If present, report it. Eventually explain how others' nonverbal behaviors may represent an emotion.*

Although these simple illustrations portray language problems common to aphasics, they cannot begin to demonstrate the multiple errors that haunt persons with aphasia as they try to communicate. Language recovery becomes an exhausting struggle and can be very irritating.

Therefore health care professionals, significant others, and caretakers should be prepared to intervene for frustration and fatigue in this population (Leppink, 1991).

Aphasia arises from left hemispheric neural damage in most persons. There are many different types of aphasia, and individuals may simultaneously experience more than one kind, which makes nursing assessment and intervention challenging. Unfortunately, accompanying neurologic deficits such as muscle weakness, neglect, emotional liability, poor attention span, and memory problems often coexist with aphasia and complicate the care-planning issues faced by the health care team and family members. Aphasia should not be confused with the thought-processing disorders that are seen in schizophrenia or in major depressive disorders; rather, it is a language reception and/or expression disorder.

In addition to aphasic disorders, it is not uncommon for elderly persons to experience motor speech problems that result from cerebral insults or various disease processes. Two specific types of motor problems, apraxia and dysarthria, plus multiple types of aphasia are further explained throughout this chapter.

Nonfluent Aphasia

Nonfluent or Broca's (expressive) aphasia typically occurs from lesions in the left, posterior, frontal lobe (see Figure 51-1). Contralateral hemiplegia, apraxia of the arm to commands, and apraxia of speech are also common in this aphasic population. Speech production is severely affected and sometimes absent except for a few habituated phrases such as "yes," "okay," "damn," or serial words such as "1, 2, 3, . . ." and "Monday, Tuesday, Wednesday. . . .

An individual with nonfluent aphasia speaks short utterances that are slow, labored, and telegraphic. Content words such as nouns and verbs are expressed, but little else is said and many pauses occur. For example, a hungry person may state, "eat . . . supper . . . now." Overall, spoken language seems to be very difficult to produce and the person has problems finding or retrieving words and naming objects (anomia). Often the person with nonfluent aphasia also has at least some difficulty comprehending what is being said.

Individuals with nonfluent aphasia appear cautious, slow to respond, and frustrated; they can become depressed and emotionally distraught, since they are aware of their speech inaccuracies. Reading, a parallel function, is often impaired as well. Persons with nonfluent aphasia might be able to copy and write with fairly good penmanship, but cannot successfully translate their thoughts into written script.

CASE STUDY 1

Mr. Jones, age 70, had suffered a large left middle cerebral artery stroke. He has right-sided hemiplegia and neglect. His wife and two daughters are overly protective because they still fear for his life. Mr. Jones has nonfluent aphasia and only moderate comprehension; he follows 70% of one-step commands per the speech pathology report. He frequently says automatic obscenities, and he has poor to fair spontaneous speech ability that is dysarthric in nature. He is easily agitated and angered when he can't express himself. About half of his statements have word substitutions (paraphasic errors). He is able to write his name and city. Nurses have noted that Mr. Jones follows simple gestural commands, responds to facial expressions, and has fairly intact word repetition skills.

Fluent Aphasia

Fluent aphasia is also known as Wernicke's or receptive aphasia. It emerges following damage to the left posterior, superior, and temporal lobe. Residual deficits are more semantic in nature, since individuals have difficulty receiving and understanding language, especially when abstract content is present. It is important for nurses to note that comprehension, if partially intact, primarily will focus on "trunk or whole body" commands. In other words, the person will be more likely to understand requests to "roll over" or "sit down" than commands to "lift a foot" or "grasp the spoon" (Boss & Abney, 1996; Simmons-Mackie, 1995).

Surprisingly, a person with fluent aphasia can produce lengthy, flowing speech that contains appropriate melody, voice inflection, and a normal to rapid rate. However, the speech produced has little meaning and relevancy to listeners due to incorrect word choices, paraphasias, and neologisms (nonsense words) that are stated. Paraphasia involves substituting one word in place of another or substituting individual sounds within a word. A classic example of word substitution is a patient who wanted an appointment made at the beauty shop. She repeatedly shouted, "We've got to get to the fire department to get the girl to get a shave." In this example fire department was used in place of telephone, girl was substituted for beauty operator, and shave replaced haircut. Individual sound errors includes adding or deleting a sound, for example "cromb" for "comb." If done repeatedly in words, sentences, and conversations, speech may be unrecognizable. An example of this is, "We could faspheta or pupa, okay?" meaning, "We could have spaghetti for supper."

Patient frustration escalates in situations such as these, but for different reasons than it does for persons with nonfluent aphasia. Persons with fluent (receptive) aphasia believe they are making a request or statement clearly and do not understand why the listener does not act or respond accordingly. They commonly become angry with others for not understanding. Due to impaired comprehension abilities, the person with fluent aphasia is unable to detect or rectify personal speech errors. Reading comprehension and writing ability are also greatly affected, thus complicating their communication problems. Statements written by persons with fluent aphasia are wordy but empty of meaning.

Conduction Aphasia

Language and speech pathways involve a highly complex neural network within the brain. The pathway between Broca's area and Wernicke's area is known as the arcuate fasciculus (see Figure 51-1). Damage here creates a distinct set of characteristics in which persons are not able to verbally repeat words/phrases, especially when asked to, nor are they able to read out loud. They commonly have trouble naming and make sound substitutions while speaking and writing. Their penmanship reveals misspelled or omitted words as well as incorrect letter and word sequencing.

Global Aphasia

This type of aphasia results from gross damage to the frontal and temporoparietal regions of the brain. Language formulation and comprehension are severely impaired; thus individuals say and understand very little. The speech that is present may be jargon or have nonfluent aphasia characteristics (as discussed earlier). Words may be stated over and over, e.g., "Yes . . . Yes . . . Yes," and may or may not be reliable for what is intended. Swearing occurs frequently and is often used in correct context. The ability to hum and sing previously learned songs is commonly intact. Rote speech ability such as counting, saying the alphabet, or reciting the months of the year may still be present. Comprehension of words is reduced to just a few nouns, verbs, and expressions common to the elderly person's geographic region and cultural background.

Anomic Aphasia

Anomic aphasia is the most common type of aphasia. It involves intense problems finding and naming words. Knowing what they want to say but being unable to say the right word causes persons to try to describe an item or activity. For instance, when trying to ask where one's eyeglasses are, the person may state, "Have you seen my, ahhh, you know, my, they are brown, oh . . . and I use them to read." This description (circumlocution) is often successful and helps the listener figure out what the person wants/needs; however, when numerous words cannot be retrieved, the speech content may seem vague to the listener. Boss and Abney (1996) described four very specific types of anomias; the interested reader is referred to their article for detailed information.

Transcortical Aphasia

Less prevalent than other aphasias, transcortical aphasia is differentiated by a preserved ability to repeat sentences. Persons with this disorder have nonfluent aphasia patterns, problems initiating speech, neologisms, and anomia, and they may echo other people's comments, which is known as echolalia (Boss, 1996; Boss & Abney, 1996; Bronstein et al., 1991; Damasio, 1992). Again, these references provide more detailed information about the three specific types of transcortical aphasia.

Apraxia

Apraxia of speech is a rather difficult concept to understand. Speech and articulation are quite inconsistent. The muscles used for speaking are not paralyzed nor all that weak, yet the person is unable to voluntarily move the muscles for articulation. This motor "planning" deficit ranges from mild to severe and usually causes frustration in the person, since auditory and written comprehension abilities are intact. Automatic speech abilities are preserved. Frontal lobe damage is the most prevalent cause of apraxic speech, but it is also associated with parietal or temporal lobe lesions. Apraxia often coexists with aphasia or dysarthria.

Dysarthria

Whereas apraxia is a motor speech "planning" problem, dysarthria is a motor speech "production" problem secondary to muscle weakness. Dysarthria is caused by damage to the brainstem, basal ganglia, cerebellum, cranial or phrenic nerves, peripheral nerves, or respiratory system. It is characterized by speech so poorly articulated that it is easily misunderstood by others.

The dysarthric person's speech varies and voice quality may sound breathy, harsh, muffled, hypernasal (air escapes through the nose), or denasal (nasal stuffiness). Pitch is frequently affected, and speech rate becomes faster or slower. Consonants are mispronounced and unclear, especially at the end of words. The person tends to run words together so it is hard to tell where one sentence stops and the next begins. Overall, speech sounds "slurred." There are five distinct types of dysarthria, described in more detail by Boss and Abney (1996), Bronstein et al. (1991), and Simmons-Mackie (1995). Hypokinetic dysarthria occurs in many elderly people with Parkinson's disease. Because their voices sound monotone and because facial expression is lost, such persons have a solemn and masklike appearance. This can lead to the misperception that they are unintelligent and unemotional, yet quite the opposite is true.

Right Hemisphere Deficits

The role that the right hemisphere plays in communication is now more clearly understood. Research in this area is relatively new, yet findings suggest that nonverbal communication is the major function of the right hemisphere. It mediates the emotional, gestural, pragmatic, and facial expression components of language during human interactions and is significantly influenced by cultural factors.

The right brain also processes the music and rhythms of songs and rhymes (Boss, 1996; Boss & Abney, 1996; Bronstein et al., 1991; Levy, 1985; Loen, 1991; Simmons-Mackie, 1995; Thompkins & Mateer, 1985; Wapner, Hamby, & Garner, 1981). The right hemisphere is associated with emotional, affective, socially appropriate, and interactive parts of communication. It also allows one to "organize a narrative" (i.e., tell a story, make a joke, or write a letter) (Damasio, 1992, p. 537).

Although much of the medical literature refers to behavioral gestures as part of right brain function (Boss, 1996; Boss & Abney, 1996; Bronstein et al., 1991), research findings vary as to whether gestures are controlled by the left or right hemisphere (Heilman, Scholes, & Watson, 1975; Ross, 1981; Ross & Mesulam, 1979). Gestures are important in

Learning outcome 2

Page 671 - 672.

Prognatics

normal pragmatics include respecting others' personal space, taking turns talking, sticking to the topic, asking questions of others, listening without cutting in, using acceptable hand and facial gestures appropriate to the conversation, sensitively reacting to another person's comments, and telling jokes at the proper time (Boss, 1996; Boss & Abney, 1996; Bronstein et al., 1991; Kleppe-Yeager, 1995; Simmons-Mackie, 1995; Sohlberg & Mateer, 1989).

Prosody provides the affective and emotional components of speech. It is the ability to vary the tone of voice, melody, loudness, dialect, accent, rhythms, and pauses while conversing or reading out loud. It adds interest and zest to speech content.

Any of the preceding functions of the right hemisphere may become impaired when the right side of the brain is injured. To illustrate how abnormal pragmatics and prosody (aprosodia) can influence communication, recitation of the pledge of allegiance in a public setting is used. Characteristically the person with abnormal pragmatics would say the words correctly, but the manner in which they were expressed would likely be improper. For instance, the individual might unknowingly stay seated while reciting the words, or look away from the flag, put his hand in a coat pocket instead of across the heart, or giggle or cry while saying the lines. Concurrently, potential aprosodic errors might include shouting out the words at a faster rate than others are reciting the pledge, using a sarcastic or silly voice inflection, saying words without accenting any of the syllables, and/or ignoring pauses between the lines.

Additional communication problems that frequently result from damage to the right brain include the inability to understand abstract concepts, jokes, humor, voice intonation, and figurative speech (e.g., "fork it over" or "hold your horses"). Persons display excessive talking (verbosity) and flat affect and have difficulty recognizing faces and making inferences from spoken and written information. Other features also can emerge, including reduced concentration, disorientation, poor awareness/insight, and left neglect. All of these disturbances/behaviors can adversely impact communication/socialization. When many of them are present, the person is said to have a syndrome called right hemispheric dysfunction (RHD) (Benton & Bryan, 1996; Boss, 1990; Kleppe-Yeager, 1995; Studer & ... 1994).

As these characteristics wear heavily on them, persons with right hemispheric damage become self-centered and egocentric. They require a great deal of supervision to remain safe, and they need a lot of help to successfully complete even simple activities.

CASE STUDY 2

A 67-year-old woman, Mrs. Yoder, was in a car accident and hit her head on the windshield, sustaining diffuse brain damage with resultant traumatic brain injury (TBI). According to her husband, Mrs. Yoder was unconscious for about 20 minutes. She has fluent aphasia, speech motor problems, and speech confusion as a result of information processing impairments. Acute rehabilitation is necessary for in-depth evaluation and treatment by psychiatry, speech, neuropsychology, occupational therapy, and physical therapy. On admission to rehabilitation, Mrs. Yoder presents with several language impairments, including reduced auditory and reading comprehension, fluent but "empty" speech, confabulation, echolalia, trouble shifting topics, and poor attention, judgment, and memory.

Mrs. Yoder's speech deficits include apraxia, dysfluency, and hoarse vocal quality. Her nonverbal and pragmatic skills are also impaired. Mrs. Yoder gets too close to people as she speaks, making them uncomfortable. She has few facial expression changes. Mrs. Yoder talks too loudly, too fast, does not pause, and monopolizes conversations. Her pragmatic problems are secondary to poor self-monitoring and inattention.

Box 51-1	Specific Language Impairments and Strategies for Persons With Alzheimer's Disease

Specific Language Impairments Seen in Alzheimer's Disease	Special Strategies for Persons With Alzheimer's Disease
Word retrieval problems with compensatory circumlocution	See the items in Table 51-1 that pertain to Receptive Communication Abilities
Loss of meaningful (semantic) communication, i.e., fluent aphasia	Minimize fatigue; allow an AM and PM nap even if person wakes up during the night
Speech perseveration (getting "stuck" on a word or phrase, and repeating it over and over)	Learn about the patient's past experiences and relationships
Focus on self, past roles, interests, and family regardless of what others are talking about; they unexpectedly shift topics	Do not refute or reorient persons when they fantasize; rather, acknowledge such experiences and use them to get the patient to perform a desired task
Asking fewer and fewer questions of others	Incorporate funny stories, story telling, fun songs, or personal anecdotes if the person responds positively to this strategy (Buckwalter, Gerdner, Hall, Stolley, Kudart, & Ridgeway, 1995)
Difficulty repairing their own conversational errors (Orange, Lubinski, & Higginbotham, 1996)	
Inability to produce or respond when others ask them to clarify their comments (Orange et al., 1996)	Use validation techniques, reminiscence therapy, and conversation analysis (Bryan & Maxim, 1998; Hall & Buckwalter, 1991)
Diminished interactive conversational skills and initiation of conversation; the person seems unable to follow the rules of conversation	Distract the person or encourage an oral motor activity (offer a drink or a piece of gum) to stop speech perseveration; distraction may also work when frustration or refusal to do a task occurs
Apparent inability to follow commands; the person might not want to do the requested activity	
Inability to write except to sign their name (Hall, personal communication, December 1996)	Combine environmental cues, actions, facial expression, and pantomime with verbal communication
Decreased reading comprehension	Verbalize one simple thought/topic per statement and allow adequate processing time
Inability to follow written directions and instructions (Hall & Buckwalter, 1991)	Use polite gestures with verbal invitations rather than giving task commands
Inability to use orienting cues in the environment, such as clocks and calendars	Teach family members strategies to repair conversational errors that their loved one makes when conversing with others (Orange et al., 1996)
Misperception of sensory information, especially visual and auditory information (mirrors, pictures, and intercom/paging systems), and resulting verbal and/or behavioral outbursts	
Nonsensical speech and mumbling	

Alzheimer's Disease

Persons with Alzheimer's disease are anxious and fearful about embarrassing themselves, losing control, or being rendered helpless (Hall, 1994). Persons with Alzheimer's disease can exhibit a particular set of language impairments, which are detailed in Box 51-1.

ASSESSMENT

It is rare that someone presents with just one language problem, since the neuronal circuitry is interconnected among many cortical and subcortical areas that are in close anatomic proximity. The goals of a communication assessment are to (1) provide a foundation for understanding patients' language strengths and deficits so staff can interact with them and (2) develop therapeutic interventions and teaching plans to facilitate relearning of communication skills. Assessment Guide 51-1 details the components of a comprehensive nursing assessment.

A team approach for assessing and intervening for communication and sensory deficits is extremely valuable,

since the impairments may be quite complex. Groher (1990) illustrated how the assessment should govern the treatment approach when he wrote, "For instance if the patient responds best to gesture and short auditory input from the left visual field, then this fact should be communicated to staff and family" (p. 296). This quotation also stresses that the health care professionals and family members alike should develop and use a consistent communication approach with patients.

From a nursing care perspective, it is wise to establish yes/no reliability as soon as possible by asking questions about the patient and her surroundings, such as "Is the TV on?" "Are you sitting in a chair?" "Are you wearing shoes?" and "Is the sun shining?" Avoid asking orientation-based questions such as "Do you live in Iowa?" since they test more than just yes/no reliability. If yes/no responses are reliable, the nurse has a beginning communication tool to use with the person. If not, communication will be challenging, since the person may indicate yes but actually mean no. Any nursing assessment for an older adult should reference the person's premorbid education level, dominant language, culture, speaking/writing/reading

Similarly, the existing NIC definition is too limiting, since it focuses on "speech" deficits rather than all communication impairments that may occur. In addition, the current definition is confusing; it is as if the content is stated backward. This author suggests that clarity could be improved by expanding and reordering the definition to "Assistance in learning alternate methods of communication and in accepting and living with language impairments." This would greatly extend the patient population base for whom this nursing intervention and its activities could be applied.

The third column of Table 51-1 lists in nonitalicized text the existing NIC intervention "activities." As currently written, these "activities" tend to focus on measures for oral expressive difficulties and lack measures for comprehension, reading, writing, nonverbal communication, and motor speech deficits. Because nurses interact with and care for persons with multiple and diverse communication impairments, NIC activities need to be updated so they are more specific for various deficits and individualized patient care. Proposed intervention activities appear in *italics* in the text of the third column of Table 51-1 and are incorporated into the interventions developed for patients discussed in the two case studies.

Persons with Alzheimer's disease often require unique approaches to communication. Several strategies that are appropriate for use with this population are found in Box 51-1.

Two NIC intervention "activities" can be questioned from legal and patient advocacy standpoints. The activities "Teach esophageal speech as appropriate" and "Instruct patient and family on use of speech aids (e.g., tracheal-esophageal prosthesis and artificial larynx)" are beyond the scope of nursing practice unless nurses have had formal course work or training in this method of speech production and the corresponding mechanical aids. Esophageal speech is a very specialized, labor-intensive, and precise way of producing speech. It is difficult for trained professionals to teach and for patients to successfully learn. Therefore rather than teaching the techniques, nurses may be better advised to be sensitive to this form of vocalization, encourage patients to practice it, and consistently help and remind patients to use any recommended speaking devices. Rewording to this effect is included in Table 51-1 under the NIC activity, corresponding with the NOC indicator, "Use of spoken language: esophageal."

Boss (1984a, 1984b, 1991, 1996) developed a model that succinctly organizes nursing management principles for persons with communication impairments into four categories: (1) environmental management; (2) supportive behaviors; (3) behaviors to enhance communication; and (4) education of person, family, and significant others about content within the first three categories. Many of the NIC intervention "activities" identified during the NIC

research process may have indirectly originated from Boss's earlier model (1984b), since there is great overlap when comparing the two.

Finally, within the cognitive rehabilitation arena, researchers are developing strategies for cognitive retraining. These strategies emphasize attention and concentration, memory and retention, abstraction and concept learning, problem solving, rehearsal, decision making, organization, self-expression, forward thinking, and social competence. The areas of self-expression and social competence specifically involve listening, parsimony of speech, and grammar. Social competence also entails understanding social signals and recognizing voice inflections (Parente, 1995). Some of the team strategies for helping patients relearn these concepts are appropriate for nurses to reinforce. They would also complement the NOC outcome of Cognitive Abilities. See Chapter 34 for more specific information about cognition.

As the ability to comprehend spoken words improves, nurses must be aware that a "fatigue phenomenon" often occurs (Boss, 1984a). Neural processing abilities wane in a patient as additional verbal information is received. Consequently, important comments should be stated first, then "nice-to-know" information and pleasantries can be added subsequently. For instance, when explaining a new medication, the nurse should first state the purpose and rationale for the pill. Next, simply and briefly they should share the potential side effects. Social comments (about the weather, how one slept, etc.) should be put aside until the end of the exchange.

CASE STUDY 1

Interventions for Mr. Jones were organized around Boss's nursing management model (Boss, 1984b, p. 213-215). Following Mr. Jones's stroke, a calm, unhurried approach and a structured environment was recommended. Caregivers worked to help Mr. Jones continue to view speaking as a "pleasant experience" (Boss, 1984b, p. 213), and they allowed ample opportunity for Mr. Jones to practice speaking and for him to hear intact speech. The following specific management strategies also were included in his plan:

1. Mr. Jones was engaged in at least one or two sit-down, face-to-face conversational exchanges in the morning, afternoon, or evening. Sitting at eye level was recommended to make Mr. Jones feel less rushed and to enable him to see the speaker's mouth and facial expressions.
2. Distractions were removed, Mr. Jones was addressed by name, and eye contact was maintained.
3. The nurse reminded family and visitors that, when a group was present, they would need to speak one at a time and would need to allow Mr. Jones extra time to respond. The nurse explained that he will need more time even for yes and no questions.

4. Mr. Jones was approached from the left side (or verbally cued to turn toward the right), since he had right neglect.
5. Mr. Jones was encouraged to attend an inpatient stroke support group twice per week to promote socialization.
6. Brief, positive language experiences were structured, including listening to the morning news on TV (since he is rested then), attending hospital chapel services with his wife, and participating in conversations with nurses and other team members.

It was important for staff to develop and implement strategies to support Mr. Jones' success. Staff acknowledged the tendency for frequent angry outbursts but tried to remain calm and reassure Mr. Jones with supportive voice inflections that it was okay to feel frustration (his right brain could still understand emotions associated with other peoples' voice tones). Mr. Jones was treated as an adult and spoken to naturally, with normal volume, with a slower rate, and without exaggerating words. Mr. Jones was praised honestly for his hard efforts; even small gains were recognized by clapping and/or giving verbal praise (using gestures with words to help his comprehension). Staff pointed out Mr. Jones' capabilities to prevent him from dwelling on his mistakes (to build his confidence). He was allowed to do all the tasks he was capable of and his family was reminded of his abilities. Staff attempted to distinguish between when Mr. Jones needed help to speak and when it was appropriate to wait and let him find and say the statement he was struggling with. If he became too frustrated, staff would go ahead and model the word. This approach was reviewed with family so that they did not automatically speak for him.

Finally, strategies were developed to enhance communication. Staff talked about things that interested Mr. Jones. They also used the following specialized techniques for speech production and/or comprehension:

1. Asking simple, brief, yes/no questions to collect information from Mr. Jones.
2. Rewording to validate his response; for instance, if a nurse asked Mr. Jones if his wife visited and he indicated no, the nurse would validate by saying, "Mrs. Jones stayed home today?"
3. Asking Mr. Jones to name objects and body parts during nursing cares. (If he could not initiate the name, the nurse would do it and encourage him to verbally repeat it, since he was capable of imitation.)
4. Encouraging imitation of single words, greetings, affirmations, salutations, and thanks.
5. Restating what the nurse thought Mr. Jones intended to say and modeling correct speech production rather than correcting errors.
6. Producing the first sound of the word Mr. Jones might be attempting to say (phonetic cueing) as a cue to help him finish the word. For instance, the nurse might say, "I think you are asking about your d _____" (daughter).
7. Constructing open-ended sentences such as "You would like your _____?"

8. Encouraging Mr. Jones to state greetings, farewells, habitual phrases such as "okay," "how are you," and "thanks," and to engage in automatic speech, for example, "January, February, March. . . ."
9. Assessing whether Mr. Jones can sing and, if so, encouraging him to do so when he likes.
10. Asking key questions when Mr. Jones was highly frustrated and continuing to ask questions to target his concern or need.
11. Avoiding asking Mr. Jones to write; he would not be able to write a word that he couldn't say.
12. Offering Mr. Jones simple picture flash cards to indicate his concrete needs.

Mr. Jones and his family needed to learn and share with others how he could be assisted to communicate. His family was taught that he might need repeated reassurance, support, and answers to questions. The family also was cautioned against excluding Mr. Jones from decision making and repressing his independence. Family-centered interventions included the following:

1. Discussing with Mr. Jones' daughter the language inconsistencies that are commonly seen in aphasics, since they keep asking him to "just try harder" to speak.
2. Explaining this care plan to Mrs. Jones and letting her practice with supervision.
3. Encouraging Mrs. Jones and her daughters to participate in speech therapy sessions with the speech-language pathologist.
4. Allowing time for the family to verbalize their fears, anxiety, and questions.

Because Mr. Jones had nonfluent aphasia, dysarthria, fair comprehension, and a high frustration level, it was initially wise for nurses to ask him yes/no questions to simply meet his needs for toileting, thirst, food, and comfort. Later he was asked to gesture, to point to objects or pictures, and to "show" the nurses and his family what he needed and wanted. Mr. Jones seemed to relax a bit once such a system was in place. He attempted to say words on his own, smiled more, his appetite improved, and he had fewer episodes of profanity.

Since Mr. Jones was able to say automatic words such as "hi," "okay," "thanks," and "not now," the nurses spent more time asking him to name items during meals, dressing, and bathing. With encouragement and extra processing time, he could repeat the names of many common two-syllable words. Nurses then took the time twice a shift to sit down at eye level and encourage him to verbalize brief words and phrases to express his emotions or talk about his day. They often had to remind his family not to automatically speak for him as he struggled for words, and he sometimes shook his finger at them to be quiet.

Mr. Jones was discharged home 15 days after his stroke. He had progressed to saying two or three short sentences in a row and only needed initial phonetic cueing occasionally. He returned for speech therapy twice per week.

CASE STUDY 2

Mrs. Yoder had sustained diffuse brain injury in the motor vehicle accident and experienced numerous residual deficits, including various communication problems and symptoms of right hemisphere dysfunction (RHD). Consequently a key strategy was to reduce distractions in her environment. To improve Mrs. Yoder's attention and concentration skills, her nurse caregivers used alerting statements such as "look at me" and called Mrs. Yoder by name to get her attention before all interactions. They had her attend to simple tasks such as pushing a touch tone call light or washing her face or hands, and they always allowed extra processing time.

The team reoriented Mrs. Yoder with each contact and posted a calendar, clock, and daily schedule within her visual range. They established a structured routine and consistent daily schedule that they reviewed with her in the morning, afternoon, evening, and as needed to improve her short-term memory (use repetition). The nursing plan specified that, when appropriate, Mrs. Yoder would be taught and reminded to use more complex memory aids such as a memory book, appointment calendar, calculator, or voice-activated dialing telephone. She would be assigned by the team and her nurses to make/use lists and practice following short, written directions as her reading improves. The strategies of repetition and rehearsal help memory and can be used creatively by nurses. For example, if Mrs. Yoder were to forget when her husband visited, the nurses could have him sign and date a guest book, show it to her while reading what it says, have her "sign" it and, before leaving, open the book, point to his entry and read it aloud to remind her it is there. The book could be used later to remind her of the visit. This approach has the advantage of stimulating auditory, visual, and tactile senses.

One-step commands, accompanied by gestures, pantomime, pointing, and animated facial expressions, were used to improve Mrs. Yoder's auditory comprehension deficits. Whenever comprehension is not achieved, nurses would repeat the statement once, then rephrase it to see if comprehension could be achieved. Staff spoke concretely and avoided figurative phrases. Physical cues such as pointing were also used to improve comprehension.

Statements such as "It's morning so it is time to get dressed" were used to help Mrs. Yoder focus and shift topics or tasks more easily. Nurses tried to pause, giving her extra time before changing topics or activities.

The nurse considered limiting Mrs. Yoder's group activities, but chose instead to implement other strategies that would help her to function better in group situations. Because Mrs. Yoder was verbose and had speech comprehension difficulties, the treatment team needed to establish and teach her predetermined signals, such as making a "T" for time out to indicate it is someone else's turn to talk. When Mrs. Yoder talked too loudly, putting a finger to the lips and pursing them was used as a signal to remind her to lower her voice. Staff briefly pointed out when she was too close to others. As Mrs. Yoder gained insight and social competence, nurses asked her questions about normal personal space, for instance, "How far apart do strangers stand? How far apart do friends stand?" The plan specified that additional conversational and social graces would be discussed and practiced as Mrs. Yoder improved.

Exercises and drills for Mrs. Yoder's speech motor problems were encouraged. Interventions for her apraxia included the following: (1) promoting a calm, unhurried environment; (2) encouraging word repetition with Mrs. Yoder able to clearly see the speaker's mouth; (3) asking Mrs. Yoder to use gestures and act things out as she speaks (the treatment team consistently role modeled this technique in return); (4) having Mrs. Yoder practice speech by singing, or tapping out a rhythm as she spoke (for example, "bath"/TAP "room"/TAP) (Wood, 1986); and (5) asking Mrs. Yoder to paraphrase what had been said, since paraphrasing facilitates understanding, develops summary skills, and increases memory storage. After acute rehabilitation, Mrs. Yoder was likely to require outpatient therapy or at least structured lessons and exercises from a speech pathologist to practice at home.

Mrs. Yoder's poor attention, poor memory, and fluent aphasia required frequent verbal cues and simple demonstrations. For example, she could attend to eating a finger food for 30 seconds and then needed verbal reminders to proceed. She could say the date and day of the week after six or seven verbal reminders in which the nurse simultaneously showed her the calendar. She had just begun to visually scan her room independently to find the calendar when asked these questions.

Nurses learned to recognize some of her paraphasic statements. For example, when she said to "open the window," it meant she wanted the side rail down on the bed. By the tenth day of hospitalization, Mrs. Yoder marked off days on the calendar with an "x" and could read the day of the week aloud from the calendar. She was able to state three words while tapping her fingers, e.g., "cof"/TAP "ee"/TAP; "lip"/TAP "stick"/TAP; and "out"/TAP "side"/TAP. Mrs. Yoder became able to attend to repeating eight or nine simple words that her husband read to her from his crossword puzzle book while visiting. Mrs. Yoder remained quite verbose but recognized the hand signal to lower her voice.

Mrs. Yoder continued to have difficulty recognizing another person's personal space and she often stood right next to strangers in the elevator on her way to therapy. Because she continued to have great difficulties with language, cognition, short-term memory, and social skills, she continued her recovery program in an adult day care center near her home.

SUMMARY

The inability to communicate produces frustration and anxiety and can contribute to depression, withdrawal, and social isolation, conditions for which elders are already at risk (McConnell & Murphy, 1996; Valente, 1994; Wolanin, 1983). In direct contrast, intact communication skills convey an individual's innermost thoughts, feelings, desires, and needs. Positive communication is imperative to establishing and maintaining relationships, vocational responsibilities, leisure and social activities, and role fulfillment as a partner, confidant, grandparent, mentor, colleague, or neighbor.

In today's healthcare delivery system, nurses working in acute care, rehabilitation, sub-acute care, skilled, or intermediate care, day care and community or home health care often encounters persons with various language and communication disturbances. Nurses can play a pivotal role in assessing for communication impairments, helping to establish meaningful communication approaches for persons experiencing such difficulties, accessing appropriate referrals for specialized evaluation and treatment, reinforcing specific speech and language prescriptive strategies and exercises, and helping families and friends to understand and manage communication impairments.

REFERENCES

Benton, E., & Bryan, K. (1996). Right cerebral hemisphera damage: Incidence of language problems. *International Journal of Rehabilitation Research, 19*(1), 47-54.

Boss, B. J. (1984a). Dysphasia, dyspraxia, and dysarthria: Distinguishing features, part I. *Journal of Neurosurgical Nursing, 16*(3), 151-160.

Boss, B. J. (1984b). Dysphagia, dyspraxia, and dysarthria: Distinguishing features, part II. *Journal of Neurosurgical Nursing, 16*(4), 211-216.

Boss, B. J. (1991). Managing communication disorders in stroke. *Nursing Clinics of North America, 26*(4), 985-996.

Boss, B. J. (1996). Pragmatics: Right brain communication. *Axon, 17*(4), 81-85.

Boss, B. J., & Abney, K. L. (1996). Communication: Language and pragmatics. In S. P. Hoeman (Ed.), *Rehabilitation nursing: Process and application* (2nd ed., pp. 542-571). St. Louis, MO: Mosby.

Bronstein, K. S., Popovich, J., & Stewart-Amidei, C. (1991). *Promoting stroke recovery: A research-based approach for nurses* (pp. 200-215). St. Louis, MO: Mosby.

Bryan, K., & Maxim, J. (1998). Enabling care staff to relate to older communication disabled people. *International Journal of Language & Communication, 33*(Suppl.), 121-125.

Buckwalter, K. C., Gerdner, L. A., Hall, G. R., Stolley, J. M., Kudart, P., & Ridgeway, S. (1995). Shining through: The humor and individuality of persons with Alzheimer's disease. *Journal of Gerontological Nursing, 21*(3), 11-16.

Cusack, D. (1991). Impaired verbal communication. In M. Maas, K. Buckwalter, & M. A. Hardy (Eds.), *Nursing diagnoses and interventions for the elderly* (pp. 530-541). Reading, MA: Addison Wesley Longman.

Damasio, A. R. (1992). Medical progress: Aphasia. *The New England Journal of Medicine, 326*(8), 531-539.

Folstein, M. F., Folstein, S. M., & McHugh, P. R. (1975). Mini-mental state: A practical method for grading the cognitive state of patients for the clinician. *Journal of Psychiatric Research, 12*(3), 189-198.

Foreman, M. D., & Zane, D. (1996). Nursing strategies for acute confusion in elders. *American Journal of Nursing, 96*(4), 44-52.

Groher, M. E. (1990). Speech and language assessment. In M. Rosenthal, M. R. Bond, E. R. Griffith, & J. D. Miller (Eds.), *Re-*

habilitation of the adult and child with traumatic brain injury (pp. 294-309). Philadelphia: F. A. Davis.

Hall, G. R. (1994). Caring for people with Alzheimer's disease using the conceptual model of progressively lowered stress threshold in the clinical setting. *Nursing Clinics of North America, 29*(1), 129-140.

Hall, G. R., & Buckwalter, K. C. (1991). Clinical outlook: Whole disease care planning: Fitting the program to the client with Alzheimer's disease. *Journal of Gerontological Nursing, 17*(3), 38-41.

Hall, G. R., & Wakefield, B. (1996). Acute confusion in the elderly. *Nursing 96, 27*(7), 32-37.

Heilman, K. M., Scholes, R., & Watson, R. T. (1975). Auditory affective agnosia: Disturbed comprehension of affective speech. *Journal of Neurology, Neurosurgery, and Psychiatry, 38*(1), 69-72.

Inouye, S. K., Van Dyck, C. H., Alessi, C. A., Balkin, S., Siegal, A. P., & Horwitz, R. I. (1990). Clarifying confusion: The confusion assessment method; a new method for detection of delirium. *Annals of Internal Medicine, 113*, 941-948.

Iowa Intervention Project. J. C. McCloskey & G. M. Bulechek (Eds.). (2000). *Nursing interventions classification (NIC)* (3rd ed.). St. Louis, MO: Mosby.

Iowa Outcomes Project. M. Johnson, M. Maas, & S. Moorhead (Eds.). (2000). *Nursing outcomes classification (NOC)* (2nd ed.). St. Louis, MO: Mosby.

Kleppe-Yeager, K. (1995). *Right hemisphere syndromes: Facilitating functional independence.* (Lecture September 21), Younker Rehabilitation Center, Des Moines, Iowa.

Leppink, M. H. (1991). Tiredness after a stroke. *Stroke Connection Magazine, 13*(2), 5-6.

Levy, J. (1985). Right brain, left brain: Fact and fiction. *Psychology Today, 19*(5), 38, 42-44.

Loen, M. (1991). Impairment in verbal communication. In M. Snyder (Ed.), *A guide to neurological and neurosurgical nursing* (2nd ed., pp. 235-256). Albany, NY: Delmar Publishers, Inc.

McConnell, E. S., & Murphy, A. T. (1996). Nursing diagnoses related to physiological alterations. In M. A. Matteson, E. S. McConnell, & A. D. Linton (Eds.), *Gerontological nursing: Concepts and practice.* (2nd ed., pp. 447-455). Philadelphia: W. B. Saunders.

McFarland, G. K., & Naschinski, C. E. (1985). Impaired communication. *Nursing Clinics of North America, 20*(4), 775-785.

Neelon, V. J., Champagne, M. T., Carlson, J. R., & Funk, S. G. (1996). The NEECHAM confusion scale: Construction, validation, and clinical testing. *Nursing Research, 45*(6), 324-330.

North American Nursing Diagnosis Association. (1999). *Nursing diagnoses: Definitions & classification 1999-2000.* Philadelphia: The Association.

Orange, J. B., Lubinski, R. B., & Higginbotham, D. J. (1996). Conversational repair by individuals with dementia of the Alzheimer's type. *Journal of Speech & Hearing Research, 39*(4), 881-895.

Parente, R. (1995). *A relentless quest: Techniques for memory and learning following brain injury.* Workshop presented on April 6, 1995, Des Moines, IA.

Rakowiez, W. P., & Hodges, J. R. (1998). Dementia and aphasia in motor neuron disease: An under recognized association. *Journal of Neurology, Neurosurgery, & Psychiatry, 65*(6), 881-889.

Ross, E. D. (1981). The aprosodias: Functional-anatomic organization of the affective components of language in the right hemisphere. *Archives of Neurology, 38*(9), 561-569.

Ross, E. D., & Mesulam, M. M. (1979). Dominant language functions of the right hemisphere? Prosody and emotional gesturing. *Archives of Neurology, 36*(3), 144-148.

Roussel, L. A. (1995). The neurological system and its problems in the elderly. In M. Stanley & P. G. Beare (Eds.), *Gerontological nursing* (pp. 174-187). Philadelphia: F. A. Davis.

Salt, N., & Robertson, S. J. (1998). A hidden client group? Communication impairment in hospice patients. *International Journal of Language & Communication, 33*(Suppl.), 96-101.

Samovar, L. A., & Rintye, E. D. (1979). Group communication: Theory and practice. *Small group discussion: A reader* (3rd ed.). Dubuque, IA: Wm. C. Brown.

Simmons-Mackie, N. N. (1995). Disorders in oral, speech, and language functions. In D. A. Umphred (Ed.), *Neurological rehabilitation* (3rd ed., pp. 747-768). St. Louis, MO: Mosby.

Sohlberg, M. M., & Mateer, C. A. (1989). *Introduction to cognitive rehabilitation: Theory and practice.* New York: Guilford Press.

Studer, M., & Kleppe-Yeager, K. (1994, June). The cognitive and the motor inseparable: A transdisciplinary approach. *PT Magazine,* 52-56.

Thompkins, C., & Mateer, C. A. (1985). Right hemisphere appreciation of prosodic and linguistic indication of implicit attitude. *Brain and Language, 24,* 185-203.

Valente, S. M. (1994). Recognizing depression in elderly patients. *American Journal of Nursing, 94*(12), 19-24.

Wapner, W., Hamby, S., & Garner, H. (1981). The role of the right hemisphere in the apprehension of complex linguistic materials. *Brain and Language, 14,* 15-33.

Wolanin, M. P. (1981). Physiologic aspects of confusion. *Journal of Gerontological Nursing, 7*(4), 236-242.

Wolanin, M. P. (1983). Scope of the problem and its diagnosis. *Geriatric Nursing, 4*(4), 227-230.

Wood, P. (1986). *Apraxia.* Patient teaching material for Younker Rehabilitation Center, Des Moines, IA.

CHAPTER 52

CAREGIVER ROLE STRAIN

Barbara A. Given, Sharon L. Kozachik, Clare E. Collins, Danielle N. DeVoss, and Charles W. Given

As a result of changes in the health care system, ongoing personal, technical, and emotional care responsibilities are being undertaken increasingly by family caregivers. Family caregivers provide unpaid care for family members who become dependent or need assistance because of the physical or mental effects of a chronic health problem. In the most common family caregiving situation, a woman over 55 years of age receives support primarily from family members who may or may not reside with her. As a consequence of the longevity of women's lives, elderly females are generally cared for by adult children, while older males are generally cared for by their female spouses. Caregiving is a fluid process, shifting as needs change. Caregivers report that they assume a "stand-by" role when patients are providing for their own care needs, then step in when caregiver involvement is needed (Schumacher, 1996).

Family members are now providing the majority of care, taking primary responsibility for the management of treatment effects and symptoms, for personal and intimate care tasks, and for the supervision and monitoring of overall patient health status (Haley, 1997). This care is not without personal costs and role strain. The essence of caregiver role strain is the recognition by families that they are too overloaded to meet the care demands thrust on them.

RELATED FACTORS/ETIOLOGIES

Caregiver role strain results from subjective and objective caregiver stressors that are generated by the role. Fluctuations, uncertainties, and changes in patient status can require family members to assume new roles and reorganize long-established roles within and outside of the caregiving role. Incorporating care roles into existing daily roles can require learning new skills and cause serious disruption to the caregiver. Care role expectations, competing role demands, demands on time, and demands on financial resources that are expended contribute to role strain (Aneshensel, Pearlin, & Schuler, 1993; Ferrell, Ferrell, Rhiner, & Grant, 1991; Haley, 1997; Oberst & Scott, 1988). Role strain can be impacted by the availability of assistance with care. In addition, characteristics of the caregiver and the care-recipient, family relationships, and living arrangements can affect role strain. Care role demands can become imbalanced relative to caregivers' social, family, and financial roles and the physical, emotional, and formal and informal supportive resources they have available. These imbalances can escalate as demands increase, as available resources decrease, or as both occur.

Care Role Expectations

The inability of the patient to perform self-care activities and the amount of supervision or assistance required of the caregiver have been related to role strain (Siegel, Raveis, Houts, & Mor, 1991; Yost, McCorkle, Buhler-Wilkerson, Schulz, & Lusk, 1993). Caregiver role strain can be brought about by the performance of direct care tasks, by the administration of medication and complex medical treatments, and by assistance with daily living activities. Providing care to a dependent care-recipient can deplete the physical or emotional energy resources of the caregiver. Patient disability and care demands, especially lifting, turning, and movement, can add to physical energy depletion. Loss or interruption of sleep due to care can contribute to caregiver physical and emotional exhaustion. Troublesome, inappropriate, disruptive, or resistant patient behavior, cognitive impairment, or emotional problems can lead to loss of caregiver emotional energy and contribute to increased caregiver stress (Goode, Haley, Roth, & Ford, 1998; Scharlach, Sobel, & Roberts, 1991; Penning, 1998). Providing ongoing care to recipients who have memory problems also contributes to caregiver strain (Almberg, Grafstrom, & Winblad, 1997; Kramer, 1997; Scharlach et al., 1991).

Competing Role Demands

Care activities and demands often compete with the performance of other roles within the household, family, employment, and social network. Penning (1998) found that 92% of the caregivers ($n = 687$) had multiple roles in which they were concurrently engaged. Thirty-one percent of the sons or sons-in-law and 25% of the daughters or daughters-in-law were engaged in four major roles: spouse; parent to a home-dwelling child; caregiver to a parent; and career. Competing and multiple role demands have been shown to add to role overload and role conflict, leading to role strain. The preexisting roles of caregivers directly influence their availability, capability, and willingness to provide care. Caregivers are forced to adjust other roles each time a change in care demand or alteration in usual patient role performance occurs. Setting priorities, allocation of time to other roles, and management of financial resources add to role conflicts. The caregiver does not lessen care provided, but instead sacrifices personal, social, or leisure activities (Mui, 1992; Ory, Hoffman, Yee, Tennstedt, & Schulz, 1999; Stoller & Pugliesi, 1989). Because of the competing role demands of work, social roles, and their own family roles (e.g., child rearing), adult daughters and daughters-in-law who provide care are more likely than older spouses to experience role captivity and role conflicts (Buehler & Lee, 1992; Hooyman & Gonyea, 1995; Young & Kahana, 1989).

Intergenerational issues also add to role conflicts. Adult children often feel uncomfortable providing intimate and personal care such as bathing, toileting, or caring for incontinence. This role difficulty may arise, for example, when a son provides care for his mother or a daughter or daughter-in-law provides care for a father or father-in-law. Role captivity can ensue when the caregiver feels trapped in a position that is unwanted, either due to uneasiness in providing care, time constraints, concurrent role demands, or the previous or present relationship with the care-recipient (Aneshensel et al., 1993).

Intragenerational caregivers (generally spouses) can experience role entrenchment when they are left alone to care. As isolation reduces the opportunity for interaction, caregiver role strain can develop. Elderly spouse caregivers may have fewer social roles to perform than adult children caregivers and may become completely focused on providing care.

Employed caregivers can have difficulty maintaining their work roles and can experience increased work absences, decreased hours worked, and reduction in work productivity because of care demands. Once the caregivers' accrued paid time off (e.g., vacation) has been depleted, then the utilization of unpaid time off, a leave of absence, termination of employment, or early retirement might be necessary (Given et al., 1993; Ory et al., 1999; Perry & Roades de Meneses, 1989; Siegel et al., 1991). The Family Medical Leave Act, which became active in 1993, required employers bound by the act to provide up to 12 weeks of unpaid leave each year for eligible employees to care for a child, spouse, or parent with a serious health condition (Westerfield & Rini, 1996). However, the act mandated unpaid leave only for persons employed in their current job for at least 12 months with at least 1250 hours of accumulated work and who work 25 or more hours per week. Moreover, for the family caregiver with a low income, paid time off and an unpaid leave are not realistic. Caregivers are at risk for role conflict when forced to continue employment and balance work and demands of care. For some caregivers, however, employment provides respite and emotional support (Barusch & Spaid, 1989).

Indeed, not being employed for pay outside the home has been associated with greater levels of caregiver stress; employment, therefore, can serve as a buffer for caregivers (Penning, 1998).

Demands on Time

Lack of time can quickly lead to caregiver role strain. Illness duration and stage of illness influence the impact that time has on the care situation. The multidimensional tasks of caregiving are emotionally and physically draining and also place excessive demands on time. Caregivers have to modify usual daily schedules and roles because they spend many hours a day assisting patients. Caregivers often are required to provide prolonged assistance when patient problems are not readily resolved (McCorkle & Wilkerson, 1991; Oberst & Scott, 1988). Additionally, stand-by care (monitoring the patient's status) requires a great deal of time (Bugge, Alexander, & Hagen, 1999). Time spent providing care is time not spent in other family, social, or work-related roles, it can lead to deprived interactions and relationships with other family members, and it can result in role conflicts. Tasks of care often are boring, repetitive, and completed in isolation of individuals other than the patient. Lack of social interaction and emotional resources adds to caregiver role strain (Northouse & Wortman, 1990; Oberst et al., 1989; Ory et al., 1999; Scharlach et al., 1991). Because social roles often must be put aside, the time expended in providing care reflects a social cost of care. Role strain might not be related only to the amount of time or hours per day devoted to caring; it can also be related to an inability to control the timing of tasks and to a lack of personal or supportive resources (Carey, Oberst, McCubbin, & Hughes, 1991; Fink, 1995). Providing more care to a patient has been associated with increased caregiver stress (Bugge et al., 1999; Penning, 1998). Additionally, not having as much personal time with the care recipient has been associated with increased caregiver strain (Bugge et al., 1999).

Demands on Finances

The out-of-pocket costs of transportation, medications, equipment, and telephone, as well as the wages that are lost by both patient and caregiver, can cause strain (Siegel et al., 1991; Stommel, Given, & Given, 1993). Adequate financial resources can facilitate purchasing necessary assistive services and prevent disruption of work, family, and social roles. Individuals with low incomes, those who receive only the minimum wage, and those who are unemployed might be at greater risk for role strain. If the care-recipient does not have insurance or has insurance that does not cover costly deductibles or co-payments, financial resources may be strained. Interference with promotions or job transfers can occur (Ory et al., 1999). Having fewer financial resources results in reduced capacity to respond to the demands of care (Davis-Ali, Chesler, & Chesney, 1993).

Assistance With Care

Assistance with caregiving by either the formal or informal care system can affect role strain, especially when the caregiver experiences role overload, has outside employment, is having difficulty or discomfort completing the tasks, or finds the role undesirable. The family system usually comprises the primary caregiver (a spouse or adult child), secondary family caregivers, and non-family caregivers. The availability of informal caregivers to provide assistance to the primary caregiver depends on family network and structure, family stage, caregiver and care-recipient age, and prior family relationships (Dilworth-Anderson, Williams, & Cooper, 1999). Support initially offered by secondary carers wanes over time depending on the physical care needs of the patient (Given et al., 1992). Elderly female spouses provide care with little assistance; in contrast, middle-aged caregivers are provided assistance because others see them as having competing role demands. Perceived family assistance and community resources influence caregiver role strain and are more important than actual quality or quantity of support received (Bull, Maruplema, & Luo, 1995; Fink, 1995). The use of formal assistive services can produce contradictory effects on the caregiver. When viewed as being provided for respite (to benefit the caregiver), the formal service can reduce the burden felt by the caregiver. If, however, the caregiver views the formal service addition as an indicator that she is unable to meet the care needs of the patient, she can have increased concerns about her role (Call, Finch, Huck, & Kane, 1999).

Community agencies, though not a substitute for the care that family members give, can provide complementary services such as home health aides, transportation, and nutrition assistance (Stommel, Given, Given, & Collins, 1995). Eligibility criteria for community services prevent some families from obtaining assistance. Community services need to be legitimized to the family, as they may be either unaware of how to access them or reluctant to accept help (Collins, Given, & Given, 1994). Overall family well-being can be maintained when caregivers have the necessary resources and supports available to them (Fink, 1995).

Caregiver Characteristics

Caregiver characteristics and related factors (e.g., gender, self-concept, the illness trajectory, care requirements, patients' mental and physical status, prior family relationships, loss of role relationships) influence how role strain is experienced. When a family member takes on the role of caregiver, he brings a multiplicity of personal characteristics to the care situation. Gender, age, physical and emo-

tional health status, developmental stage, and self-concept are all personal caregiver characteristics that affect the caregiving situation (Raveis, Karus, & Siegel, 1998).

The gender-based division of family labor in care tasks is well documented; overall, women most frequently provide care. When couples share household and child care tasks and responsibilities, women typically perform more tasks that are personal, relentless, repetitive, and routine; men tend to be involved with more narrowly focused tasks, which are infrequent, irregular, and non-routine. Unlike age and socioeconomic status, gender is consistently related to caregiver role strain. Female caregivers typically are more adversely affected by their caregiving role functions than male caregivers (sons as well as husbands); this pattern holds true among caregivers of physically impaired individuals and stroke, heart disease, and cancer patients (Given et al., 1993; Haley, Levine, Brown, & Bartolucci, 1987; Schulz, 1991).

Providing care is a task generally fulfilled by late middle-age or older adults primarily for individuals with chronic physical or mental illnesses. Older female spouses are seen as "available" to care. In younger families, however, the caregiver role is often "off time" and not supported by normative expectations. Caregivers of younger patients may therefore report more role strain than those caring for older patients, due to the other multiple and competing roles they fulfill (e.g., spouse, family, career) and the competing demands of care they face (Given et al., 1993; Schumacher, Dodd, & Paul, 1993). Young and middle-aged family caregivers may have more need for assistance with care than older individuals because of these competing demands and role conflicts. Adult child caregivers become sandwiched between competing roles and care role implementation, which adds to increased role strain (Brody, 1981; Penning, 1998).

Caregivers often bring their personal chronic health problems and a compromised health status to the care situation. Caregivers often dismiss their own health care problems in light of the demands of providing patient care. As a result of role strain, healthy caregivers can experience changes in physical health status such as fatigue, irregular eating, mental and physical exhaustion, and sleep disorders (Whitlach, Feinberg, & Sebestra, 1997). Physical health alterations become evident in increased utilization of the primary health care system. If the primary caregiver becomes ill, then caregiving duties have to be reassigned to another family member or to a formal health care agency in order to ensure continuity of care. Institutionalization of the family member often occurs when the health of the caregiver is compromised.

Preexisting emotional health states can influence caregiver role strain. Frustration, anxiety, anger, guilt, and depression take their toll on the caregivers' mental health status and contribute to role strain. Emotional stressors such as lack of privacy, lack of personal time and energy, hopelessness, the pervasive nature of care, and decreased satisfaction in relationships with family members can result from care involvement and further compromise existing problems (Northouse & Peters-Golden, 1993; Whitlach et al., 1997).

Emotional distress can interfere with the caregiver's capacity to perform requisite role tasks. Self-destructive behaviors such as substance abuse can occur when the caregiver experiences distressful emotional episodes. Depression is a common consequence of family caregivers, especially in long-term caregiving and in transitions such as institutionalization or bereavement (Collins, Stommel, Wang, & Given, 1994).

The caregiving experience is directly related to the developmental and life stage of the caregiver and the care-recipient. Developmentally, the adult child caregiver is enmeshed in activities related to generativity, where the primary tasks are maintaining intimate relationships and developing a family (Cook & Fontaine, 1991). If the adult child is involved in a caregiving situation where this development is slowed, crisis occurs and stagnation results. When a caregiver has dependent children, it is important to consider the impact that the caregiving situation has on both the caregiver's intimate relationship and and family member development.

The elder spousal caregiver can be enmeshed in a struggle between integrity (attempting to accept one's life as it has proceeded and maintaining a positive self-concept) and despair (Cook & Fontaine, 1991). Caregivers, especially spouses, can become snarled in caregiving and isolated from social exchange, causing a loss of identity separate from caregiving. If the elder feels burdened, then acceptance of the care situation cannot occur and the elder becomes at risk of developing a negative self-concept.

Care-Recipient Characteristics

The status of the care-recipient, including the trajectory of the illness, the care that is required, and physical and emotional status affect role strain. In addition, the nature of the relationship between caregiver and care-recipient and their living arrangements can affect role strain.

The stability and severity of illness and the onset and pattern of the illness trajectory are central to caregiver role strain. The demands of care and the number and type of tasks depend upon the stage and trajectory of illness and treatment. Overall patient status (i.e., prognosis, recuperation, stabilization, recurrence, or terminal status) can influence caregiver reaction. Rapid onset of dependency can cause disruption and loss of equilibrium. However, gradual changes in cognition also can result in wear and tear on the caregiver (Scharlach et al., 1991).

Four types of caregiver demands exist: activities of daily living; instrumental tasks; cognitive assistance; and expressive tasks. Activities of daily living include personal care needs, such as dressing, bathing, or toileting. Instrumental care requirements encompass housekeep-

ing chores (e.g., cooking, cleaning, laundry), maintenance of the home, and transportation. Cognitive care requirements refer to linkage or brokerage services, such as appointment scheduling, medication schedules, and financial management. The expressive tasks include emotional support, personal contact, telephone check-in, offering comfort, and insuring that the care-recipient feels loved, connected, and valued by the family (Hooyman & Gonyea, 1995). These different categories of care requirements require different knowledge, skills, and caregiver behaviors and are related to caregiver role strain.

The health status of the care-recipient is at the forefront of the caregiver's mind and is related to the role strain experience. If the care-recipient improves in health status, then the caregiving tasks may be associated with a positive emotional response in the caregiver. However, if the care-recipient has an illness that is chronic, physically debilitating, or terminal or that requires complex care that the caregiver is unable to provide, increased caregiver strain can result (Call, Finch, Huck, & Kane, 1999). Care-recipients can experience negative psychosocial responses as a result of their own dependency. This negative impact may manifest itself through expressions of fatalism, powerlessness, helplessness, anxiety, grief, or depression.

Family Relationships

Family caregiving tasks must be placed within the historical context of family relationships, as the bonds of affection and reciprocity that sustain caregiving take root in past relationships. Both the care-recipient and the giver of care bring a history of family role interactions to the care process. The influence of types of family relationships and family roles and also the quality of the patient/family caregiver relationship should be considered in terms of the intensity of role strain (Zarit & Pearlin, 1993). Social restrictions, excessive demands, and a loss of attachment feelings add to feelings of being trapped. When caregivers are restricted by providing care and have to withdraw from preferred roles, they become angry, anxious, or depressed (Neufeld & Harrison, 1998).

Deterioration of a spousal relationship between caregiver and care-recipient can occur due to changes brought on by gradual declines in physical health or cognitive status. In these situations the relationship between the dyad deteriorates and becomes characterized by less mutuality and interaction, contributing to caregiver strain (Call et al., 1999; Kneeshaw, Considine, & Jennings, 1999). Grief can occur as a response to the loss of a relationship. For a spouse caregiver involved in an unsatisfying marital relationship, a spouse burdened by substance abuse, or a spouse who has been emotionally or physically abused, being tenured in a caregiving role can cause intrapersonal and interpersonal conflict (Schulz, 1991).

For the child caregiver, losing an affectionate relationship with a parent and being required to assume a pseudo parenting role can be devastating and can contribute to role strain (Almberg, Grafstrom, & Winblad, 1997). Adult child caregivers often feel "obligated" to provide care to a parent. In these situations, care is provided, in essence, on a quid pro quo basis, since the parent provided care and nurturing to the child during the formative years. The adult child who does not desire to perform caregiving services, yet feels obligated to provide care, is at risk for caregiver role strain. Nonspouse caregivers might have lower obligations and expectations and be unwilling to accept the personal cost of providing care. Patients with relatives other than a spouse or adult child as caregivers are at greater risk of institutionalization when they become physically dependent (Barusch & Spaid, 1989; Pruchno & Potashnik, 1989; Schumacher et al., 1993).

Living Arrangements

Living arrangements affect patterns of care. Co-residence enables caregivers to provide instrumental (e.g., housekeeping) assistance (Hooyman & Gonyea, 1995). The scope and intensity of care provided by co-residential caregivers is different from caregivers not residing with the care-recipient (Tennstedt, Crawford, & McKinlay, 1993). Caregivers who live with the patient may be more depressed and distressed than those who live in separate households due to the presence of constant role demands and role expectations (Oberst et al., 1989; Stommel & Kingry, 1991). Those who live in separate households have some respite from care. Caregivers who do not live with patients, however, have to schedule the time to coordinate and provide care as well as continue their own household activities. These related factors are important considerations if one is to have a comprehensive perspective of factors influencing role strain.

ASSESSMENT

Assessment is crucial to the diagnosis and monitoring of caregiver role strain and to the selection and evaluation of nursing intervention(s). Health care professionals need to assess and evaluate the needs of the caregiver based on defining characteristics, related factors, and the nature of the patient care needs. Based on the demand for care, nurses need to help identify strategies to prevent, moderate, or alleviate caregiver role strain.

A complete caregiver assessment should be conducted. Not only do the needs of caregivers differ based on defining characteristics, they also differ based on related factors. When assessing the caregiver for the presence of caregiver role strain, it is essential that a multidimensional assessment be performed, including the financial, biophysical, psychosocial, and spiritual aspects of care. A set of assessment areas and related questions appear in Table 52-1.

CASE STUDY

Jill Duran is a 41-year-old woman who is employed full-time at a state university. Her husband Dave is an accountant at a local utility company. They have three children, ages 14, 11, and 9. Jill's mother, P. Reisen, was admitted to the hospital for weakness and weight loss and was diagnosed with untreatable, end-stage lung cancer. Mrs. Reisen, widowed for 6 months, was discharged from the hospital to live with her daughter. A referral was made to the local hospice. On the initial assessment visit the hospice nurse made the following observations. All of the Duran family members expressed willingness to care for Mrs. Reisen. Mrs. Reisen stated she was concerned about becoming a burden. Jill expressed shock at her mother's diagnosis, stating that she was just beginning to recover from her father's death. She also confided to the nurse that she was concerned about how her children might have to adjust, especially since her mother tended to be demanding. Mrs. Reisen was able to manage her medications without assistance. Though frail, she could ambulate safely throughout the house and use the telephone. She felt safe to be in the house alone while the Durans were at work and school. She did not complain of specific symptoms other than fatigue. The nurse agreed to visit weekly to assess Mrs. Reisen. The nurse also arranged for the hospice social worker to set up regular weekly visits to provide support to Mrs. Reisen and her family.

On the nurse's third visit, Jill reported that her mother had grown fearful of bathing by herself. Consequently, Jill had begun assisting her with a tub bath each evening. This had worked well for a few days, but soon Mrs. Reisen began giving reasons for not bathing, such as her skin was dry, or she was cold, or she was too tired. Jill had the impression that these reasons were fabricated, though she could not prove it. But it was taking longer and longer for her to get her mother bathed, and she was exhausted by the time Mrs. Reisen got to bed. The nurse recommended that a home health aide be brought in three times per week to help with bath care. Mrs. Reisen was reluctant to have help from a stranger, but she agreed to try it. Two days later, Jill and Mrs. Reisen were introduced to Nancy, a certified home health aide. Mrs. Reisen responded well to Nancy, and bath care went well.

Over the next several days, the Durans observed that Mrs. Reisen became more demanding and less predictable. She frequently complained that the children disturbed her, that the washing machine was noisy, that the room temperature was either too hot or too cold, and that food wasn't cooked correctly. She refused to get into the bathtub, insisted on receiving sponge baths from Nancy, then complained that she was never clean. Jill suspected that she was not taking her medications correctly and decided to take over medication administration. One day, Jill returned from work to find her mother lying on the kitchen floor. She denied being hurt, but couldn't remember how she got on the floor. She thought that perhaps she "had tripped over one of the babies." The nurse received an anxious phone call from Jill, stating that she didn't know how to manage.

Table 52-1	Caregiver Assessment
Inadequate caregiver resources to ensure care	Have outside support and resources been used in the past?
	What psychologic resources (e.g., optimism, hardiness) exist?
	With what care activities does the patient require assistance?
	How long has the caregiver been providing care?
	What are the hours of care provided per week (direct and indirect)? Per day?
	What personal losses has the caregiver suffered because of the care responsibilities?
	What formal agency support is used?
	What resources exist with friends and family?
	Are financial resources adequate for the family?
Caregiver ability to perform care activities	What are the positive aspects of the caregiving role?
	Are there adequate knowledge and skills needed to provide care?
	Does the caregiver feel prepared and competent to care?
	What areas of care are difficult?
	What areas of care have been mastered?
	Does the caregiver feel overloaded?
Role conflict/interference with other competing roles	What other family, work, or social roles exist?
	What working role alternatives have been considered?
	What roles have been altered or relinquished?
	How well is the caregiver able to manage household responsibilities?
	Does the caregiver understand the nature of the caring role?
Loss of relationship with care-recipient/ history of poor relationship with the care-recipient	Is the caregiver trapped by this role?
	How has the relationship between the caregiver and the care-recipient changed since the need for caregiving arose?
	What was the relationship like prior to the recipient's need for assistance with care?
Family conflict	What family support is utilized to help with care?
	What are the family expectations about the care situation?
	What gender-specific roles need to be altered?
	How are the role tasks distributed to other family members?
	What previous conflicts are of concern?
	Which aspects of caregiving cause family disagreement?
	Where are the areas of family conflict?
Emotional status with relationships	What is most distressing about the care provision?
	Does the caregiver perceive that she is providing adequate care?
	Has the caregiver begun to question the meaning of this experience?
	What aspects of care cause the caregiver to feel depressed, anxious?
Disease status of the patient	What is the age of the patient? The gender?
	What is the date of the original diagnosis?
	What is the expected course of the disease and treatment?
	What are the goals of care: cure or palliation?
	Can the care-recipient participate in the care?
Emotional and physical health of the caregiver	Does the caregiver have any chronic health deficits?
	How often does the caregiver see his own primary care provider?
	Does the caregiver follow through on own health promotion and illness/disease screening needs?
Developmental (caregiver)	How old is the caregiver?
	In which developmental stage is the caregiver currently engaged?
	What is the relationship of the caregiver to the care-recipient?
	Does the caregiver have her own family?
	Are there children in the household?
	How does the caregiver manage stress/stressful situations?
Care-recipient and family psychosocial factors	Is the care-recipient cognitively impaired?
	What emotional support is needed by the patient?
	How does the family system communicate?
	How is the family system presently coping?
	Does the patient exhibit problematic behaviors?

Table 52-1	Caregiver Assessment—cont'd
Situational factors	Is the caregiver abusive (i.e., physically, emotionally, sexually) toward the care-recipient?
	Does the caregiver omit care tasks?
	What is the socioeconomic status of the family?
Financial/employment factors	What is the financial status of the caregiver?
	Has any new debt been incurred as a result of the caregiving situation?
	Has the caregiver's employment status been altered due to the caregiving role (exhausted paid time off, personal days, taken days off without pay)?

Data from Given, C. W., Given, B., Stommel, M., Collins, C., King, S., & Franklin, S. (1992). The caregiver reaction assessment (CRA) for persons with chronic physical and mental impairments. *Research in Nursing and Health, 15*(4), 271-283.

The hospice nurse suspected that Mrs. Reisen was experiencing confusion and had her seen by her physician, who determined that the confusion resulted from brain metastases. The nurse informed Jill that it was no longer safe to leave her mother alone. Jill took 2 weeks of vacation from her job to serve as caregiver. Initially, being home brought relief because Jill did not have to worry about how her mother was doing. But Mrs. Reisen became more inconsistent, more demanding, and more critical of Jill. Moreover, she began wandering at night, so Jill's sleep was frequently interrupted. When the nurse visited toward the end of this 2-week period, she found Jill to be frustrated, angry, and exhausted.

NURSING DIAGNOSIS

Family caregiving is part of a set of normative family responsibilities and, in many cases, is carried out for long periods of time (often years) with love, personal commitment, attachment, and a sense of obligation. The ways in which the demands of care affect the caregiver can result in multidimensional role conflicts and role overload, which lead, in turn, to role strain (Aneshensel et al., 1993; Cicirelli, 1992; Gallagher-Thompson, 1994; Given & Given, 1996; Lawton, Moss, Kleban, Glicksman, & Rovine, 1991).

Caregiver Role Strain can be defined as the "felt difficulty" in fulfilling the care role due to persistent physical, psychologic, social, work, financial, and family relationship hardships and role changes due to illness and care requirements of an ill family member (Given & Given, 1996; Oberst, Thomas, Gass, & Ward, 1989; Ory et al., 1999; Stetz, 1989; Stommel, Wang, Given, & Given, 1992). The North American Nurses Association (NANDA) has defined Caregiver Role Strain as "a caregiver's felt difficulty in performing the family caregiver role" (NANDA, 1999, p. 59).

The defining characteristics of caregiver role strain include difficulty performing required activities, inadequate resources, role conflict, and altered relationships. The caregiver role typically is a new role, one for which many caregivers are unprepared. Lack of preparation makes it difficult for caregivers to perform required activities. Families typically lack sufficient knowledge and skills required to solve problems, to manage symptoms, to understand treatment modalities, to operate complex equipment, to make decisions, to monitor disease status and emotional states, and to change or adapt as the patient's status changes (Houts, Nezu, Nezu, & Bucher, 1996; Lawton et al., 1991; Pearlin, Mullan, Semple, & Skaff, 1990). The family caregiver can be overwhelmed by a fear of role incompetence as the new role is acquired. Concern for competence is expressed by caregivers as they seek to acquire the role of caring. Furthermore, fear generated by lack of competence and lack of control over the care situation adds to caregiver role strain.

Due to the multiple tasks of care, caregivers can experience role overload—the internal experience of being overwhelmed by care tasks and responsibilities. Role overload is characterized by a relentless feeling of mental or physical exhaustion that creates a sense of difficulty in providing care (Aneshensel et al., 1993). Performance of and/or assistance with tasks of care, such as activities of daily living, symptom management, dealing with emotional responses (e.g., anger or depression), and carrying out medical care procedures can be overwhelming to the caregiver. The demands and tasks of daily care can require attention 24 hours a day and can last for years. Physical care can at times be discrete and amenable to planning and scheduling. In contrast, the inappropriate or difficult behaviors of the cognitively deteriorating patient often are not easily managed. Planning, organizing, monitoring, anticipating, and supervising the care processes requires differing dynamic intensity and complex levels of skills, knowledge, and time. Spouse caregivers appear to be at particular risk for caregiver role overload. They typically provide the most extensive, focused, and comprehensive care, they maintain their role longer, they tolerate greater levels of patient disability, and they have less assistance (Siegel et al., 1991).

NURSING-SENSITIVE OUTCOMES

Outcomes are the means through which the efficacy of nursing actions can be measured. Evaluation of outcomes must occur within a longitudinal frame, as interventions have both immediate and long-term effects. The caregiver must be afforded the opportunity to establish her own goals to be attained from the therapeutic relationship. The nurse works with the caregiver to determine the outcomes that are desired from the interventions. For nurses working with caregivers, it is important that outcome indicators be shared with the caregiver from the outset, so that both parties can monitor the caregiver's progress. If the nurse and caregiver are to be successful in abating caregiver role strain, then both must view their therapeutic alliance as a partnership with the goal of maximizing positive psychosocial outcomes for the caregiver.

If nursing interventions are successful, reduced role strain should be observed (see Table 52-2). The following *Nursing Outcomes Classification (NOC)* outcomes and definitions are specific to caregiver role strain:

Caregiver Emotional Health—"Feelings, attitudes, and emotions of a family care provider while caring for a family member or significant other over an extended period of time" (Iowa Outcomes Project, 2000, p. 140)

Caregiver Performance: Direct Care—"Provision by family care provider of appropriate personal and health care for a family member or significant other" (p. 146)

Caregiver Performance: Indirect Care—"Arrangement and oversight of appropriate care for a family member or significant other by family care provider" (p. 148)

Caregiver Physical Health—"Physical well-being of a family care provider while caring for a family member or significant other over an extended period of time" (p. 149)

Caregiver Well-Being—"Primary care provider's satisfaction with health and life circumstances" (p. 151)

Coping—"Actions to manage stressors that tax an individual's resources" (p. 192)

Decision Making—"Ability to choose between two or more alternatives" (p. 194)

Grief Resolution—"Adjustment to actual or impending loss" (p. 223)

Knowledge: Disease Process—"Extent of understanding conveyed about a specific disease process" (p. 262)

Knowledge: Health Resources—"Extent of understanding conveyed about health care resources" (p. 271)

Knowledge: Treatment Regimen—"Extent of understanding conveyed about a specific treatment regimen" (p. 294)

Leisure Participation—Use of restful or relaxing activities as needed to promote well-being" (p. 296)

Role Performance—"Congruence of an individual's role behavior with role expectations" (p. 370)

Social Involvement—"Frequency of an individual's social interactions with persons, groups, or organizations" (p. 405)

Social Support—"Perceived availability and actual provision of reliable assistance from other persons" (p. 406)

Spiritual Well-Being—"Personal expression of connectedness with self, others, higher power, all life, nature, and the universe that transcend and empower the self" (p. 407)

Box 52-1 presents NOC outcomes and selected indicators. The indicators provided are not exhaustive, and readers are encouraged to refer to the *Nursing Outcomes Classification (NOC)* (Iowa Outcomes Project, 2000) for additional outcome indicators. Table 52-2 shows how caregiver-specific indicators can be written into a plan of care (see Table 52-2).

NURSING INTERVENTIONS

Nursing interventions should be directed toward assisting the caregiver to use personal and social resources and gain competence to care. Interventions relevant to assisting family members to reduce or prevent role strain include mobilizing and maintaining resources and support system enhancement; facilitating effective coping; respite care; role acquisition, evaluation, and enhancement; competency; teaching; complex relationship building and intimate exchange; active listening; caregiver support; decision-making support; anticipatory guidance; problem-solving and counseling; family integrity; and spiritual support.

Those interventions and their definitions are:

Active Listening—"Attending closely to and attaching meaning to a caregiver's verbal and nonverbal messages" (Iowa Interventions Project, 2000, p. 127)

Anticipatory Guidance—"Preparation of caregiver for an anticipated developmental and/or situational crisis" (p. 145)

Caregiver Support—"Provision of necessary information, advocacy, and support to facilitate primary patient care by someone other than a health care professional" (p. 200)

Complex Relationship Building—"Establishing a therapeutic relationship with a patient who has difficulty interacting with others" (p. 227)

Counseling—"Use of an interactive helping process focusing on the needs, problems, or feelings of the patient and significant others to enhance or support coping, problem-solving, and interpersonal relationships" (p. 238)

Decision-Making Support—"Providing information and support for a patient or caregiver who is making a decision regarding health care" (p. 243)

Respite Care—"Provision of short-term care to provide relief for the family caregiver" (p. 560)

Role Enhancement—"Assisting a patient, significant other, and/or family to improve relationships by clarifying and supplementing specific role behaviors" (p. 569)

Spiritual Support—"Assisting the patient or caregiver to feel balance and connection with a greater power" (p. 607)

Support System Enhancement—"Facilitation of support to patient or caregiver by family, friends, and community" (p. 624)

Box 52-1   Nursing-Sensitive Outcomes for Caregiver Role Strain

Caregiver Emotional Health
Indicators

Reports satisfaction with life, sense of control, self-esteem, freedom from guilt, anger, anxiety, or depression, and use of psychotropic drugs

Caregiver Performance: Direct Care
Indicators

Provides emotional support to the care-recipient

Understands the disease process and treatment plan

Anticipates the needs of the care recipient

Monitors the health status and behavior of the care-recipient

Demonstrates unconditional positive regard for the care-recipient

Demonstrates competence in monitoring own caregiving skill level

Caregiver Performance: Indirect Care
Indicators

Expresses confidence in problem solving

Demonstrates ability to obtain needed services

Shows skill in overseeing needed services

Shows skill in pursuing care problems with direct care providers

Caregiver Physical Health
Indicators

Expresses satisfaction with use of health providers, perceived general health, physical function and comfort, energy and mobility levels, and sleep pattern

Caregiver Well-Being
Indicators

Expresses satisfaction with physical and emotional health, lifestyle, performance of usual roles, social, professional, and instrumental support, and caregiver role

Coping
Indicators

Identifies effective and ineffective coping patterns

Verbalizes a sense of control, acceptance of situation, and need for assistance

Modifies lifestyle as needed

Reports decrease in negative feelings and physical symptoms of stress

Uses available social support

Seeks professional help as appropriate

Decision Making
Indicators

Identifies relevant information, alternatives, potential consequences of each alternative, and resources necessary to support each alternative

Acknowledges social context of the situation and relevant legal implications

Recognizes contradiction with others' desires

Grief Resolution
Indicators

Expresses feelings about loss and spiritual beliefs about death

Verbalizes reality and acceptance of the loss

Has adequate sleep pattern, adequate nutritional intake, and involvement in social activities

Maintains grooming and hygiene

Knowledge: Disease Process
Indicators

Describes disease process, cause or contributing factors, risk factors, effects of disease, signs and symptoms of disease, usual disease course, measures to minimize disease progression, complications, signs and symptoms of complications, and precautions to prevent complications

Knowledge: Health Resources
Indicators

Describes resources that enhance health, when to contact a health professional, emergency measures, resources for emergency care, need for follow-up care, community resources available for assistance, and how to connect with needed services

Knowledge: Treatment Regimen
Indicators

Describes the rationale for a treatment regimen, prescribed medications, procedures, exercise, activity, diet, performance of treatment procedures, and the expected effects of treatment

Leisure Participation (Respite)
Indicators

Participates in activities other than work

Expresses satisfaction with leisure activities

Uses appropriate social and interactional skills

Demonstrates creativity through leisure activities

Identifies recreational options

Reports restfulness of leisure activities

Role Performance
Indicators

Meets role expectations

Navigates role transition periods

Performs family, community, work, friendship, and intimate role behaviors

Describes behavioral changes with illness, disability, or elderly dependents

Reports strategies for role changes and comfort with role experiences

Social Involvement
Indicators

Interacts with close friends, neighbors, family members, and members of work groups

Participates as a member of church, club member, volunteer group member, or in leisure activities

Social Support
Indicators

Reports time, money, labor, information, or emotional assistance provided by others

Reports confidant relationships

Spiritual Well-Being
Indicators

Expresses faith, hope, meaning and purpose in life, spiritual world view, serenity, love, forgiveness, connectedness with inner self and others

Engages in prayer, worship, meditation, and/or spiritual reading

Participates in spiritual rites and passages

Table 52-2	Nursing Care Plan for Caregivers	
Nursing Diagnosis	**Nursing-Sensitive Outcomes**	**Nursing Interventions**
CAREGIVER ROLE STRAIN *Defining Characteristics* Reports feeling overwhelmed Reports needing help with completing care tasks Reports not feeling competent to manage some of the care tasks Reports feeling anxious and depressed from performing care tasks Reports decreased sense of mastery	**CAREGIVER EMOTIONAL HEALTH** *Indicators* Satisfaction with life Sense of control Self-esteem Free of anger Free of depression Perceived adequacy of resources	**ACTIVE LISTENING** *Activities* Encourage expression of feelings Listen for the unexpressed message and feeling, as well as content of the conversation Verify understanding of message **COUNSELING** *Activities* Demonstrate empathy, warmth, and genuineness Encourage expression of feelings Assist caregiver to identify the problem or situation that is causing the distress Assist caregiver to identify strengths, and reinforce these **CAREGIVER SUPPORT** *Activities* Determine caregiver's acceptance of role Teach caregiver stress management techniques Educate caregiver about the grieving process Support caregiver through the grieving process Identify sources of respite care Inform caregiver of health care and community resources
	CAREGIVER PERFORMANCE: DIRECT CARE *Indicators* Knowledge of disease process Performance of treatments Assists with activities of daily living Assists with instrumental activities of daily living Confidence in performing the needed tasks	**CAREGIVER SUPPORT** *Activities* Determine caregiver's level of knowledge Determine caregiver's acceptance of role Explore with the caregiver strengths and weaknesses Provide information about the patient's condition in accordance with patient preferences Teach caregiver the patient's therapy in accordance with patient preferences **ROLE ENHANCEMENT** *Activities* Assist caregiver to identify behaviors needed for new or changed roles Assist caregiver to identify specific role changes required due to illness or disability Serve as role model for learning new behaviors Facilitate opportunity for caregiver to role play new behaviors Teach new behaviors needed by caregiver to fulfill new role
	DECISION MAKING *Indicators* Identifies alternatives Identifies potential consequences of each alternative Identifies resources necessary to support each alternative Weighs alternatives Chooses among alternatives	**DECISION-MAKING SUPPORT** *Activities* Determine whether there are differences between the caregiver's view of the patient's condition and the view of the health care providers Inform caregiver of alternative views or solutions Help caregiver identify the advantages and disadvantages of each alternative Provide information requested by the caregiver Serve as liaison between caregiver and family Serve as liaison between caregiver and other health care providers Facilitate collaborative decision making

Table 52-2	Nursing Care Plan for Caregivers—cont'd	
Nursing Diagnosis	**Nursing-Sensitive Outcomes**	**Nursing Interventions**
	COPING	COUNSELING
	Indicators	*Activities*
	Identifies effective coping patterns	Establish a therapeutic relationship based on trust and respect
	Verbalizes sense of control	Demonstrate empathy, warmth, and genuineness
	Reports decreased stress	Assist the caregiver to identify the problem or situation that is causing distress
	Uses available social support	Use techniques of reflection and clarification to facilitate expression of concerns
	Verbalizes need for assistance	Ask caregiver to identify what he can or cannot do about what is happening
	Seeks professional help as appropriate	Verbalize the discrepancy between the caregiver's feelings and behaviors
		Assist caregiver to identify strengths, and reinforce these
		Discourage decision making when the caregiver is under severe stress

Mobilize and Maintain Resources and Support System Enhancement

Interventions that build resources or help family caregivers mobilize existing resources can moderate role strain. Nurses can help caregivers by enlisting the services of community agencies. Families with high levels of strain and weak social skills might need to be assisted to mobilize resources, while those with lower levels and strong social skills might be able to take a more active role in developing the resources themselves (Fink, 1995). By monitoring the current family situation, the nurse is capable of assessing family dynamics and communication patterns and eliciting alliances within the family system. For the family caregiver who has not been able to successfully adjust to the role acquisition, mobilizing psychosocial resources can afford opportunities for the caregiver to become empowered to care. Reasonable expectations and goals should be encouraged, so that caregivers feel as if they can succeed. Caregivers need assistance to reevaluate their personal commitment and capacity to care.

When anticipating the fluctuating demands of care on caregivers, available social resources should be determined, as they may enhance family caregiver well-being. It is important that the health care professional does not impose unwanted assistance onto the caregiver. Therefore it is imperative that the nurse seeks permission from the caregiver to acquire additional assistance when the caregiver identifies the existence of a need. If the care-recipient is cognitively impaired, the caregiver may experience feelings of isolation. Assessing the adequacy of existing social networks and subsequently encouraging the caregiver to establish social contact with a friend or family member on a regular basis can help reduce caregiver feelings of isolation. Increased social support can facilitate decreased levels of role strain for caregivers (Fink, 1995).

Social support to family caregivers can be supplied formally through professional services or informally through tangible or intangible assistance from other family members or friends. Formal health care system support can be provided by health care professionals, home care aides, and chore service providers. Formal agencies do not substitute for family care, but families need to be taught how to work with health care professionals to maximize appropriate use of community services. Assessment of any barriers, perceived or actual, to successful utilization of support systems can facilitate increased usage by the caregiver. Different patient-caregiver relationships (e.g., adult child–parent) and different phases of illness require different types and amounts of assistance from the formal system.

Plans for assisting caregivers should link the clinical course of the disease and treatment with a set of outcome goals. Caregivers' methods of organizing care should be accepted to assist caregivers to mobilize family support. Involving other family members, friends, or significant others in the planning and implementation of care can free up caregivers to afford them opportunities for self-rejuvenation. Home health aides and volunteers and other resources such as mobile meals should be considered. Effective discharge planning and referral to home health care or case management can assist family members to deal with caregiver role strain (Bull et al., 1995; McCorkle et al., 1989).

Dispositional traits (such as optimism or hardiness) are resources of the family caregiver that can buffer caregiver role strain. Assessing optimism and other enduring traits can help to specify which family members may be successful in handling caregiver role strain.

Facilitate Effective Coping. When effectively mobilized, coping skills can facilitate resolution of crises (e.g., intrapersonal and/or interpersonal conflicts) and control internal and environmental stressors. Caregivers experiencing role strain due to increased role tasks and demands may deal with coping in ways that either facilitate adaptation (e.g., seek assistance with role tasks, vent feelings, take time out from role demands) or augment the role strain (e.g., project blame, consume alcohol, use drugs, deny that a problematic situation exists). Successful resolution of a crisis leads to growth in coping abilities and skills. Only with continuity can the family become prepared, develop problem-solving skills, enhance family communication, and explore alternative strategies that will facilitate coping as the care situation changes.

Cognitive behavioral therapy can facilitate the integration of coping strategies within the caregiver, altering thought patterns, feelings, and behaviors (Hartman & Lazarus, 1992; Thase & Beck, 1993). Cognitive therapy is used when an individual feels overwhelmed or inadequate and involves establishing a therapeutic alliance with the caregiver based on mutual trust and the identification and evaluation of problems. The caregiver's strengths and resources are identified through a collaborative effort (of nurse and caregiver), and a plan of action is formulated.

To effectively cope, families must make interpersonal adjustments, including grieving the previously held relationship with the ill family member, adjusting existing family relationships, maintaining social networks, and establishing collaborative relations with health care providers. Families deal with day-to-day challenges, coordinate formal and informal support services, rearrange preexisting personal and family schedules, and divide labor among family members. Finally, the caregiver integrates individual developmental trajectories with tasks of care and adjusts career and work commitments (Smyer & Birkel, 1991).

Enhance Problem Solving and Counseling.   When engaged in a caregiving situation, family caregivers can become so isolated or so overwhelmed that they temporarily lose the capacity to solve problems. The overwhelming nature of role tasks and demands seemingly overrides this function. Caregivers need assistance to assess problem areas and to identify services or support that can help them accomplish role tasks and demands (Houts, Nezu, Nezu, & Bucher, 1996).

Caregivers need assistance in evaluating all competing role demands in order to identify where conflicts are likely to occur, what the sources of these conflicts are, who can help to alleviate them, and where role realignment is needed. Through establishing rapport with the family system and engaging in interactions based on genuine concern and empathy, the nurse can support both the family caregiver and the larger family system through tumultuous periods. Family conferences can be a useful strategy to help caregivers examine and deal with role changes, family conflicts, and the setting of priorities; con-

ferences also can be a nonthreatening arena for expressing concerns and identifying family strengths.

Role reduction can occur as care demands increase and other concurrent role demands either increase or remain stable. The nurse must assist the caregiver to establish and set priorities. Urgent care tasks (e.g., toileting, medication administration) and care tasks that can be deferred (e.g., laundry, grocery shopping) should be distinguished. Family involvement in care, family mobilization of resources, and support system enhancement can facilitate role reduction and relieve role overload.

Respite Care.   As caregivers become overwhelmed by providing care and maintaining other family, employment, and social roles, the utilization of respite services can be made an integral part of care. Respite can include relief from direct care and relief from the provision of instrumental activities. A few hours of respite each week allows the caregiver some personal time, reduces burden, and subsequently enables the caregiver to continue providing care (Call et al., 1999). The nurse must monitor the endurance of the family caregiver. If the family caregiver is unable to continue within that role, then the nurse will need to enlist the assistance of family, friends, volunteers, or formal care assistance. The nurse might be called upon to provide emergency care to the care-recipient in the event that the caregiver is unable to continue fulfilling his role functions.

Facilitate Role Acquisition, Evaluation, and Role Enhancement.   Successfully acquiring a new role requires an investment of time, personal involvement, commitment to the role, and learning the requisite role tasks. The first strategy in this process is role-making, which entails taking the characteristics of the role, synthesizing them, and integrating them into role functioning. Role-making involves "trying the new role on for size" under the supervision of a mentor or professional, tailoring the role to be congruent with one's personal values. The nurse can facilitate this role transition by being a role model and teaching the caregiver those behaviors that will be required in order to successfully become enculturated into the caregiver role.

The nurse might need to sit with the caregiver to assess current family, work, and social/civic roles in which she is currently engaged. The degree to which these competing roles will need to be altered or sacrificed will impact not only the caregiver, but also the care-recipient. Other family members should also be called upon to assess how their competing roles might need to be altered or sacrificed.

A clear, explicit explanation of the caregiver role and role components should be offered. Knowledge of the illness, treatment, and anticipated care challenges creates feelings of caregiver competency. The caregiver should be advised of the role transitions that will occur (1) as care demands change, (2) when the care-recipient requires institutional care, and (3), in the case of terminal illness, following the death of the care-recipient (Schumacher, 1996). The nurse must explore with the caregiver what capacities exist that will facilitate caregiver role acquisition. Role enhancement can clarify and supplement specific role behaviors and allow for greater ease in role acquisition. Assistance to caregivers enables them to master the techniques of care and role components. Becoming accomplished and successful caregivers can produce a sense of personal pride and can contribute to caregiver well-being (Archbold, Stewart, Greenlick, & Harvath, 1990; Lawton et al., 1991; Miller, Campbell, Farran, Kaufman, & Davis, 1995; Younger, 1991). Family members' positive responses to providing care result from the knowledge that one is successfully fulfilling a responsibility and personal challenge while meeting the care needs of a family member (Picot, Youngblut, & Zeller, 1997).

Part of attaining a sense of competence includes having adequate skills to provide the requisite care tasks and information regarding the disease process and illness trajectory. Medication administration (e.g., times, doses, side effects), treatments (e.g., sterile versus aseptic technique with dressing changes), special nutritional needs, and/or management of disruptive behaviors (e.g., wandering at night) are crucial areas of emphasis for caregiver education (Houts et al., 1996). The nurse will need to ensure that role tasks and skills are being performed and that role acquisition has successfully taken place. Booster sessions and positive feedback might need to be provided periodically to the caregiver.

Nurses need to be sensitive to the "care-problems" of families. Family caregivers need to be assessed for capacity, ability, and desire to provide and continue care. Caregivers most at risk for needing assistance from the formal care system are those who are emotionally challenged, who experience role captivity, who have limited social, family, and financial resources, and who are themselves experiencing chronic illnesses. Nurses need either to assist these families to cope with care and achieve care competency or to provide the forum and support for the family caregiver to choose to relinquish the caregiving role, devoid of guilt.

Teach Required Skills and Provide Information. Written information and guidelines can assist family members to understand and recall useful strategies, but should never take the place of open, ongoing verbal instruction. Family members might not be ready to hear or comprehend information until the need actually exists. Reiteration and reinforcement need to take place as the patient moves to an altered level of care demands (i.e., improvement or deterioration). Information obtained from the health care team is better than that from lay sources. Providing a knowledge base can help to create a sense of control, competence, confidence, and security.

Provide Counseling, Guidance, Decision-Making Support, and Caregiver Support. Confusion about care can actually disrupt the channels of communication between nurses and family caregivers and between the patient-caregiver dyad. Caregivers often have difficulty in adequately communicating fear, confusion, and problems. Patients and caregivers also can have different expectations about the provision and reception of care. Without thorough knowledge of the illness situation and open discussion of the role of caregiver and needs of the care-recipient, conflict likely will arise. If this conflict is not mediated, caregiver role strain will be greatly heightened. If open communication is encouraged and supported, this openness will resurface in family conversations. Tension between the patient and caregiver is almost unavoidable. Caregivers are often overwhelmed and frustrated, which leads to feelings of resentment and guilt. While caregivers often state that they enjoy the caregiving role and experience feelings of gratification and love, they also express discontent and an inability to properly cope. Open channels of communication between nurse, patient, and caregiver should be encouraged and can help to mediate destructive feelings and resolve family conflict. It is important that the nurse ascertains whether or not there are differences among the perceptions of the caregiver, other family members, and the health care professional.

The emotional needs of the caregiver should be monitored, and plans must be made to facilitate coping with frustration, anger, anxiety, grief, depression, and overall caregiver burden. The difficulties, stresses, and strains experienced must be analyzed, and the value and contribution of caregiver efforts should be acknowledged. Caregivers should also be encouraged to express feelings and difficulties, especially guilt, grief, anger, and resentment. Interventions to deal with emotions can include teaching caregivers to identify the feelings, perceptions, and interpretations that contribute to their distress and assisting them to use coping strategies to manage these responses. Encouraging caregivers to attend to their own personal needs, to take time for self-care, or to participate in support groups can be essential.

Facilitate Intimate Exchange and Complex Relationship Building. For the caregiver who is caring for a spouse afflicted by a cognitive impairment or physically debilitating illness, physical touching can occur only during tasks of care. The nurse needs to be sensitive to the needs of the caregiver and to feelings that arise due to the loss of previously held relationships. Reminiscence therapy can bring comfort by allowing the caregiver to focus on the past positive aspects of the relationship. Browsing through old photo albums or reading birthday, anniversary, or other greeting cards previously received from the care-recipient can comfort the caregiver. The promotion of family cohesion can foster feelings of love and belonging for the caregiver toward the care-recipient, despite the lack of current intimate interaction.

Sexuality for the spousal caregiver and care-recipient often remains unaddressed. The mental or physical status and/or the complexity of health care needs of the care-recipient or the mental or physical status of the spousal caregiver can interrupt and/or halt the previously established sexual relationship. Nursing can facilitate the expression of sexual needs or desires between the spousal caregiver and care-recipient and negotiate how to meet both the caregiver's and the care-recipient's needs without compromising either's well-being. For the adult child caregiver, discussing sexual needs with a parent (or parent-in-law) may be an uncomfortable experience, as many children do not view their parents as sexual beings. In this case the nurse can function in the role of a mediator and facilitator by broaching the subject with both the child caregiver and the parent care-recipient.

If the care-recipient is afflicted with a cognitive impairment that negatively impacts verbal communication, then the nurse will need to assist the caregiver in assigning meanings to both verbal and nonverbal forms of communication. Unfortunately, this often is accomplished through trial and error. If the care-recipient is engaging in problematic behaviors, then the nurse will need to assist the caregiver in setting firm limits on these behaviors. Providing positive feedback to the care-recipient for acceptable behaviors can reinforce these behaviors. However, as the cognitive impairment progresses, the effectiveness of this intervention diminishes.

Active Listening. Active listening, a deliberate and active behavior, requires the nurse to be attentive to both the verbal and nonverbal cues provided by the caregiver (Koshy, 1989). Components include eye contact, relaxed body posture, absence of distractions, and the utilization of therapeutic communication. Active listening conveys empathy, caring, and concern to the caregiver, the care-recipient, and the family system. The nurse must be attentive to both the content of conversations and to the affective presentation. If the expressed affective range is incongruent with either the content or the mood of the caregiver, then the nurse must assess for psychosocial manifestations of role strain. Being aware of the caregiver's body language (posture, eye contact, presentation of trunk) can also clue the nurse that the caregiver might be experiencing psychosocial difficulties. Caregivers also can benefit from having the opportunity to express their feelings of guilt and anger over the loss of the previous level of intimacy with the care-recipient. Guilt work facilitation (helping another to cope with painful feelings of responsibility) can foster such expression.

Anticipatory Guidance. Nurses need to note the changes and transitions that occur within the caregiving situation, determine who is at risk, and anticipate potential problems and needs for those deemed at risk. There may be times when work, family, or other issues outside of (but in addition to) the caregiving role require management. Hastily made decisions can have serious implications for patient and caregiver. If role strain is anticipated, plans can be formed and strategies can be designed to prevent, moderate, or reduce role strain.

Some of the strain that arises can be mediated or avoided by information and preparedness: describing the intricacies of the caregiving role, providing gentle warnings about possible complications or situational crises that may arise, identifying the stressors the patient and caregiver may face (e.g., financial), locating informal and formal sources of assistance, making referrals, and teaching the caregiver how to seek social support (Houts et al., 1996).

The nurse might need to schedule additional visits during phases of the illness trajectory where care demands are high. It also is helpful to provide the caregiver with an emergency phone number to call for assistance, if needed.

Spiritual Support. It is important that spiritual needs be addressed, as caregivers experience and express anger, frustration, guilt, and loss (Koenig, 1994). Being thrust into a caregiving situation brings disruption and chaos to a life that may have, heretofore, been predictable and comfortable. Nurses can assist caregivers through encouraging the use of biblical passages, existential philosophical readings, or inspirational readings. The inner peace and feelings of unconditional love that result from prayer, meditation, or readings can relieve some caregiver psychologic burden. Spiritual needs cannot be ignored by nurses because they are intimately related to both the physical and psychologic health of the caregiver (Koenig, 1994).

CASE STUDY

The nurse assisted Jill to identify her goals and options and to choose from those options. Jill stated that her main goals were to have her mother's needs met, to regain a sense of her own coping, and to have her family regain a sense of normality. Jill agreed to have home health aide assistance 4 hours each morning, 5 days per week, for both bath care and respite. The hospice would also try to schedule volunteer respite for the afternoons. Jill and Dave would alternate taking time off work when volunteers could not be scheduled. The hospice also scheduled 3 hours of respite each weekend by a nurse volunteer so that the entire Duran family could get away. In addition, since Mrs. Reisen seemed less amenable to interacting with the social worker, the social worker agreed to focus on the Durans.

Within a week, Jill reported a decrease in her anxiety and frustration, which she attributed to home health aide assistance and respite and being able to go to work most days. The entire Duran family looked forward to their weekend time together. Jill was able to express feelings of grief to the social worker. She realized that her grief over her father had not resolved and that, due to mental status changes, it seemed as though her mother had already died.

Mrs. Reisen's mental and physical status continued to deteriorate. She became more demanding, more critical, and eventually combative. Jill continued to find the various hospice services helpful and supportive, but acknowledged that caring for her mother was very disruptive. The nurse again helped Jill to review her options. This time Jill selected nursing home placement as the top option. Within a week Mrs. Reisen was transferred to a nearby nursing facility. The hospice nurse continued to supervise her care there, and the social worker continued to counsel the Durans in their home. Although Jill admitted to having some feelings of guilt about her decision, she also saw her family's relief. Moreover, she realized that she felt much less angry and frustrated with her mother. When Mrs. Reisen died 2 months later, Jill felt supported by her family and expressed confidence that she would cope well.

SUMMARY

Care for a family member creates physical, mental, and emotional demands not previously experienced by most family members. The pattern of care demands varies in magnitude and type and changes depending on the stage or phase of illness. Interventions directed toward the family need to be dynamic and responsive as the family moves through care transitions characterized by uncertainty and role change. Interventions that help families anticipate illness demands and gain a sense of self-competence and self-esteem can facilitate their ability to continue care and influence the level of caregiver role strain. Families need assistance in reframing the caregiving experience so that they focus on the strengths they bring to the care situation.

Today and in the foreseeable future, family members will be engaged in more and more care responsibilities. In this time of cost containment and dramatic shifts in care from the formal to the informal system, role strain exhibited by caregivers can have profound impact on patient care outcomes. It is critical that family caregivers be supported and their levels of role strain monitored.

Interventions for family caregivers will be successful if they are tailored to patient and caregiver needs, that is, developed considering the defining characteristics, influencing characteristics, and related factors that contribute to caregiver role strain experience. The goal of care is to meet the needs of both the patient and the family caregiver, thereby enhancing the quality of life of the family unit and limiting the role strain of family members caring for their loved ones.

REFERENCES

Almberg, B., Grafstrom, M., & Winblad, B. (1997). Major strain and coping strategies as reported by family caregivers who care for aged demented relatives. *Journal of Advanced Nursing, 26*(4), 683-691.

Aneshensel, C. S., Pearlin, L. I., & Schuler, R. H. (1993). Stress, role captivity, and the cessation of caregiving. *Journal of Health and Social Behavior, 34,* 54-70.

Archbold, P. G., Stewart, B. J., Greenlick, M. R., & Harvath, T. (1990). Mutuality and preparedness as predictors of caregiver role strain. *Research in Nursing and Health, 13*(6), 375-384.

Barusch, A. S., & Spaid, W. M. (1989). Gender differences in caregiving: Why do wives report greater burden? *The Gerontologist, 29*(5), 667-676.

Brody, E. M. (1981). "Women in the middle" and family help to older people. *The Gerontologist, 21*(5), 471-480.

Buehler, J., & Lee, H. (1992). Exploration of home care resources for rural families. *Cancer Nursing, 15*(4), 299-308.

Bugge, C., Alexander, H., & Hagen, S. (1999). Stroke patients' informal caregivers: Patient, caregiver, and service factors that affect caregiver strain. *Stroke, 30*(8), 1517-1523.

Bull, M., Maruplema, G., & Luo, D. (1995). Testing of a model for post hospital transitions of family caregivers for elderly persons. *Nursing Research, 44*(3), 132-138.

Call, K. T., Finch, M. A., Huck, S. M., & Kane, R. A. (1999). Caregiver burden from a social exchange perspective: Caring for older people after hospital discharge. *Journal of Marriage and the Family, 61,* 688-699.

Carey, P. J., Oberst, M. T., McCubbin, M. A., & Hughes, S. (1991). Appraisal and caregiving burden in family members caring for patients receiving chemotherapy. *Oncology Nursing Forum, 18*(8), 1341-1348.

Cicirelli, V. (1992). *Family caregiving: Autonomous and paternalistic decision making* (vol. 186). Thousand Oaks, CA: Sage Publications.

Collins, C. E., Given, B. A., & Given, C. W. (1994). Interventions with family caregivers of persons with Alzheimer's disease. *Nursing Clinics of North America, 29*(1), 195-207.

Collins, C. E., Stommel, M., Wang, S., & Given, C. W. (1994). Caregiving transitions: Changes in depression among family caregivers of relatives with dementia. *Nursing Research, 43*(4), 220-225.

Cook, J. S., & Fontaine, K. L. (1991). *Essentials of mental health nursing* (2nd ed.). Reading, MA: Addison Wesley Longman.

Davis-Ali, S., Chesler, M., & Chesney, B. (1993). Recognizing cancer as a family disease: Worries and support reported by patients and spouses. *Social Work in Health Care, 19*(2), 45-65.

Dilworth-Anderson, P., Williams, S. W., & Cooper, T. (1999). Family caregiving to elderly African Americans: Caregiver types and structures. *Journal of Gerontology, 54B*(4), S237-S241.

Ferrell, B., Ferrell, B., Rhiner, M., & Grant, M. (1991). Family factors influencing cancer pain management. *Postgrad Medical Journal, 67*(Suppl 2), S64-S69.

Fink, S. (1995). The influence of resources and family demands on the strains and well-being of family caregivers. *Nursing Research, 44*(3), 139-146.

Gallagher-Thompson, D. (1994). Clinical intervention strategies for distressed caregivers: Rationale and development of psychoeducational approaches. In F. Light, G. Niederehe, & B. D. Lebowitz (Eds.), *Stress effects on family caregivers of Alzheimer's patients: Research and interventions* (pp. 260-277). New York: Springer.

Given, B., & Given, C. W. (1996). Family caregiver burden from cancer care. In S. B. Baird, R. McCorkle, & M. Grant (Eds.), *Cancer nursing: A comprehensive textbook* (2nd ed., pp. 93-109). Philadelphia: W. B. Saunders.

Given, C. W., Given, B., Stommel, M., Collins, C., King, S., & Franklin, S. (1992). The caregiver reaction assessment (CRA) for persons with chronic physical and mental impairments. *Research in Nursing and Health, 15*(4), 271-283.

Given, C. W., Stommel, M., Given, B., Osuch, J., Kurtz, M., & Kurtz, J. C. (1993). The influence of cancer patients' symptoms and functional states on patients' depression and family caregivers' reaction and depression. *Health Psychology, 12*(4), 277-285.

Goode, K. T., Haley, W., Roth, D. L., & Ford, G. R. (1998). Predicting longitudinal changes in caregiver physical and mental health: A stress process model. *Health Psychology, 17*(2), 190-198.

Haley, W. E. (1997). The family caregiver's role in Alzheimer's disease. *Neurology, 48*(5, Suppl. 6), S25-S29.

Haley, W. E., Levine, E. G., Brown, S. L., & Bartolucci, A. A. (1987). Stress, appraisal, coping, and social support as predictors of adaptational outcome among dementia caregivers. *Psychology and Aging, 2*(4), 323-330.

Hartman, C., & Lazarus, L. (1992). Psychotherapy with elderly depressed patients. *Clinics in Geriatric Medicine, 8*(2), 355-362.

Hooyman, N. R., & Gonyea, J. (1995). *Feminist perspectives on family care: Policies for gender justice.* Thousand Oaks, CA: Sage.

Houts, P. S., Nezu, A. M., Nezu, C. M., & Bucher, J. A. (1996). The prepared family caregiver: A problem-solving approach to family caregiver education. *Patient Education and Counseling, 27*(1), 63-73.

Iowa Intervention Project. J. C. McCloskey & G. M. Bulechek (Eds.). (2000). *Nursing interventions classification (NIC)* (3rd ed.). St. Louis, MO: Mosby.

Iowa Outcomes Project. M. Johnson, M. Maas, & S. Moorhead (Eds.). (2000). *Nursing outcomes classification (NOC)* (2nd ed.). St. Louis, MO: Mosby.

Kneeshaw, M. F., Considine, R. M., & Jennings, J. (1999). Mutuality and preparedness of family caregivers for elderly women after bypass surgery. *Applied Nursing Research, 12*(3), 128-135.

Koenig, H. G. (1994). *Aging and God: Spiritual pathways to mental health in midlife and later years.* Birmingham, NY: NYL Hayworth Pastoral Press.

Koshy, K. T. (1989). I only have ears for you. *Nursing Times, 85*(30), 26-29.

Kramer, B. J. (1997). Differential predictors of strain and gain among husbands caring for wives with dementia. *The Gerontologist, 37*(2), 239-249.

Lawton, M. P., Moss, M., Kleban, M. H., Glicksman, A., & Rovine, M. (1991). A two-year factor model of caregiving appraisal and psychological well-being. *Journal of Gerontology, 46*(4), 181-189.

McCorkle, R., Benoliel, J. Q., Donaldson, G., Georgiadou, F., Moinpour, C., & Goodell, B. (1989). A randomized clinical trial of home nursing care for lung cancer patients. *Cancer, 64*(6), 1375-1382.

McCorkle, R., & Wilkerson, K. (1991). *Home care needs of cancer patients and their caregivers.* (Final Report No. NR01914). Philadelphia: University of Pennsylvania School of Nursing.

Miller, B., Campbell, R., Farran, C., Kaufman, J. E., & Davis, L. (1995). Mastery and caregiving distress. *Journal of Gerontology: Psychological Sciences, 50B*(6), S374-S382.

Mui, A. C. (1992). Caregiver strain among black and white daughter caregivers: A role theory perspective. *The Gerontologist, 32*(2), 203-212.

Neufeld, A., & Harrison, M. J. (1998). Men as caregivers: Reciprocal relationships or obligation? *Journal of Advanced Nursing, 28*(5), 959-968.

North American Nursing Diagnosis Association. (1999). *Nursing diagnoses: Definitions & classification 1999-2000.* Philadelphia: Author.

Northouse, L. L., & Peters-Golden, H. (1993). Cancer and the family: Strategies to assist spouses. *Seminars in Oncology Nursing, 9*(2), 74-82.

Northouse, L. L., & Wortman, C. B. (1990). Models of helping and coping in cancer care. *Patient Education and Counseling, 15,* 49-64.

Oberst, M. T., & Scott, D. W. (1988). Post discharge distress in surgically treated cancer patients and their spouses. *Research in Nursing and Health, 11*(4), 223-233.

Oberst, M. T., Thomas, S. E., Gass, K. A., & Ward, S. E. (1989). Caregiving demands and appraisal of stress. *Cancer Nursing, 12*(4), 209-215.

Ory, M., Hoffman, R. R., Yee, Y. L., Tennstedt, S., & Schulz, R. (1999). Prevalence and impact of caregiving: A detailed comparison between dementia and nondementia caregivers. *The Gerontologist, 39*(2), 177-185.

Pearlin, L. I., Mullan, J. T., Semple, S. J., & Skaff, M. M. (1990). Caregiving and the stress process: An overview of concepts and their measures. *Gerontologist, 30*(5), 583-594.

Penning, M. J. (1998). In the middle: Parental caregiving in the context of other roles. *Journal of Gerontology: Psychological Sciences, 53B*(4), S188-S197.

Perry, G. R., & Roades de Meneses, M. (1989). Cancer patients at home: Needs and coping styles of primary caregivers. *Home Healthcare Nurse, 7*(6), 27-30.

Picot, S. J., Youngblut, J., & Zeller, R. (1997). Development and testing of a measure of perceived caregiver rewards in adults. *Journal of Nursing Measurement, 5*(1), 33-52.

Pruchno, R. A., & Potashnik, S. L. (1989). Caregiving spouses: Physical and mental health in perspective. *Journal of the American Geriatrics Society, 37*(8), 697-705.

Raveis, V. H., Karus, D. G., & Siegel, K. (1998). Correlates of depressive symptomatology among adult daughter caregivers of a parent with cancer. *Cancer, 83*(8), 1652-1663.

Scharlach, A. E., Sobel, E. L., & Roberts, R. E. L. (1991). Employment and caregiver strain: An integrative model. *The Gerontologist, 31*(6), 778-787.

Schulz, R. (1991). Theoretical perspectives on caregiving: Concepts, variables, and methods. In D. E. Biegel & A. Blum (Eds.), *Aging and caregiving: Theory, research, and policy* (pp. 27-52). Thousand Oaks, CA: Sage.

Schumacher, K. L. (1996). Reconceptualizing family caregiving: Family-based illness are during chemotherapy. *Research in Nursing & Health, 19*(4), 261-271.

Schumacher, K. L., Dodd, M. J., & Paul, S. M. (1993). The stress process in family caregivers of persons receiving chemotherapy. *Research in Nursing and Health, 16*(6), 395-404.

Siegel, K., Raveis, V., Houts, P., & Mor, V. (1991). The relationship of spousal caregiver burden to patient disease and treatment-related conditions. *Annals of Oncology, 2,* 511-516.

Smyer, M. A., & Birkel, R. C. (1991). Research focused on interventions with families of the chronically mentally ill elderly. In E. Light & B. D. Lebowitz (Eds.), *The elderly with chronic mental illness* (pp. 111-130). New York: Springer.

Stetz, K. M. (1989). The relationship among background, characteristics, purpose of life, and caregiving demands on perceived health of spouse caregivers. *Scholarly Inquiry for Nursing Practice: An International Journal, 3*(2), 133-153.

Stoller, E. P., & Pugliesi, K. L. (1989). Other roles of caregivers: Competing responsibilities or supportive resources. *Journal of Gerontology, 44*(6), S231-238.

Stommel, M., Given, B., Given, C. W., & Collins, C. (1995). The impact of the frequency of care activities on the division of labor between primary caregivers and other care providers. *Research on Aging, 17*(4), 412-433.

Stommel, M., Given, C. W., & Given, B. (1993). The cost of cancer home care to families. *Cancer, 71*(5), 1867-1874.

Stommel, M., & Kingry, M. (1991). Support patterns for spouse-caregivers of cancer patients: The effect of the presence of minor children. *Cancer Nursing, 14*(4), 200-205.

Stommel, M., Wang, S., Given, C. W., & Given, B. (1992). Confirmatory factor analysis (CFA) as a method to assess measurement equivalence. *Research in Nursing and Health, 15,* 399-405.

Tennstedt, S. L., Crawford, S. L., & McKinlay, J. B. (1993). Is family care on the decline? A longitudinal investigation of the substitution of formal long-term care services for informal care. *Milbank Quarterly, 71*(4), 601-624.

Thase, M. E., & Beck, A. T. (1993). An overview of cognitive behavioral therapy. In J. H. Wright, M. E. Thase, A. T. Beck, & J. W. Ludgate (Eds.), *Cognitive therapy with inpatients* (pp. 3-34). New York: Guilford Press.

Westerfield, J., & Rini, A. G. (1996). Family Medical Leave Act: Ready or Not! *Nursing Management, 27*(4), 25, 29.

Whitlach, C. J., Feinberg, L. F., & Sebestra, D. S. (1997). Depression and health in family caregivers: Adaption over time. *Journal of Aging and Health, 9*(2), 222-243.

Yost, L. S., McCorkle, R., Buhler-Wilkerson, K., Schulz, D., & Lusk, E. (1993). Determinants of subsequent home health care nursing service use by hospitalized patients with cancer. *Cancer, 72*(11), 3304-3312.

Young, R. F., & Kahana, E. (1989). Specify caregiver outcomes: Gender and relationship aspects of caregiving strain. *The Gerontologist, 29*(5), 660-666.

Younger, J. B. (1991). A theory of mastery. *Advanced Nursing Science, 14*(1), 76-89.

Zarit, S. H., & Pearlin, L. I. (1993). Family caregiving: Integrating informal and formal care systems for care. In S. H. Zarit, L. I. Pearlin, & K. Schaie (Eds.), *Caregiving systems: Formal and informal helpers* (pp. 303-316). Hillsdale, NJ: Lawrence Erlbaum Associates.

CHAPTER 53

RISK FOR VIOLENCE: SELF-DIRECTED OR DIRECTED AT OTHERS

Todd N. Ingram

Violence has become an increasingly high-profile concern for government officials and representatives, as well as for the general public. Federal and state legislatures have responded to this concern by passing new laws that attempt to increase protection for society from violent crime and to maximize penalties for those who commit such crimes.

On a smaller scale, violence continues to be a concern for nursing caregivers in a variety of settings. Acute, long-term, and home care settings each can be an environment of occasional violence by clients toward themselves or others. The significance of the problem for clients, nurses, and other caregivers cannot be minimized.

RISK FACTORS

The foundation for preventing violence is prediction of violent behavior. Prediction of violent behavior, in turn, requires understanding the factors that can lead to violent behavior. Stokman (1984), in a study of aggression among hospitalized mentally ill offenders, specified three spheres of influence that predict violent behavior: long-term vulnerabilities, short-term stressors, and contextual triggers. These categories provide a useful framework to discuss the various theories and research findings related to both other-directed and self-directed violence. It is important to note that long-term, short-term, and triggering factors are not mutually exclusive of one another. Factors from all categories usually are present when violence occurs, and it is not unusual to find multiple stressors from the first two categories present and interacting when a violent episode is triggered.

Violence Directed at Others

Long-term vulnerabilities are individual client traits or life situations that have been present for many years—perhaps since childhood. Some investigators have suggested that violence directed at others is instinctual and was used for self-preservation (Lorenz, 1966). Other studies illustrating long-term vulnerabilities have described biologic phenomena such as abnormal electroencephalograms (Bach-y-Rita, Lion, Climent, & Ervin, 1971; Moyer, 1976; Williams, 1976), testosterone elevation (Sheard, 1979), monoamine metabolite levels in spinal fluid (Roy &

Pollack, 1994), and low cholesterol levels (Golier, Marzuk, Leon, Weiner, & Tardiff, 1995). Social learning theory (Bandura, 1973) focuses on behavior patterns acquired from experience or observation. An individual learns to be aggressive or nonaggressive by a complex system of perceived rewards obtained by witnessing the emotional and behavioral responses of others. More recent research support for this theory comes from Davis and Boster (1988) and Morrison (1992a), who described a coercive interactional style as characteristic of potentially violent individuals. Further support for social learning theory comes from documented childhood traits and behaviors, including enuresis, fire setting, cruelty to animals, and deviant, abusive family environments (Convit, Jaeger, Lin, Meisner, & Volavka, 1988; Justice, Justice, & Kraft, 1974).

In a prospective study of patient assaults on nursing staff in three geriatric psychiatric units, Cooper and Mendonca (1989) found that the most common diagnoses associated with violent behavior were mental retardation and dementia. These individuals were prone to misinterpret reality or perceive helping gestures as threats. Consequently, they were about twice as likely to commit violent acts. Still other investigators have noted the role of substance abuse mixed with chronic psychiatric illness as a precursor to violent behavior directed at others (Mulvey, 1994; Torrey, 1994). Finally, additional research has pointed to a variety of long-term factors influencing violence directed at others, including sensory impairments (Kolanowski, Hurwitz, Taylor, Evans, & Strumpf, 1994), a coercive interactional style (Kolanowski et al., 1994; Morrison, 1992a), and changing social support networks (Estroff, Zimmer, Lachicotte, & Benoit, 1994). These conditions can lead individuals to interpret helping gestures as threats or can produce situations where there is chronic distrust of others. Individuals with these attributes often use argument rather than mediation when attempting to resolve conflict.

Short-term or current stressors are recent situations or changes in a client's life that add to emotional load. One early psychologic theory suggested that violence was a response to frustration (Dollard, Dobb, Miller, Mowerer, & Sears, 1939). Berkowitz (1974, 1982) saw this as goal directed and labeled it instrumental violence. He also distinguished this from random violence. Recent research related to frustration as a short-term stressor has been conducted on short- and long-term care units with a variety of age-groups. These studies looked at unit milieu, structure, rules, and rule enforcement (Davis, 1991; Katz & Kirkland, 1990; Lanza, 1988; Morrison, 1987, 1989; Roper & Anderson, 1991). The consensus is that patients often feel powerless and confused regarding unit rules and their stress threshold decreases while frustration increases. The following additional stressors apply more specifically to elderly clients in various care settings: sudden illnesses that can create a delirium episode (Foreman, 1990; Lawlor & Sunderland, 1988); prescription drug reactions (Allen, Yanchick, Cook, & Foss, 1990); sleep disturbance, which can lead to agitation and aggression (Cohen-Mansfield & Marx, 1990); and delusional thinking in clients with Alzheimer's dementia (Gilley, Wilson, Beckett, & Evans, 1997; Gormley, Rizwan, & Lovestone, 1998).

Contextual triggers are the immediate events that spark a violent episode. These can occur during seemingly routine interactions between a client and a caregiver or the environment. Examples of triggering events described by researchers include rule enforcement (Lanza, 1988; Morrison, 1987, 1989), impulsive events within unit milieus (Gallop, McCay, & Esplen, 1992), seclusion and restraint procedures, and activities of daily living assistance situations (Cooper & Mendonca, 1989; Sheridan, Henrion, Robinson, & Baxter, 1990). Enforcement of therapeutic and social rules in hospital care settings is frequently cited as a precursor to violence (Lanza, 1988; Morrison, 1987, 1989). Violence has been reported to occur often when requests were denied or when social or therapeutic rules (e.g., taking medication) were enforced by the staff. Other studies have mentioned seclusion and restraint procedures (Sheridan, Henrion, Robinson, & Baxter, 1990) and situations involving staff assistance in feeding, lifting, bathing, and ambulation as trigger events for violence (Cooper & Mendonca, 1989; Winger, Schirm, & Stewart, 1987). In these situations individuals can feel threatened by invasion of personal space and interpret helping routines as sexual assault.

Self-Directed Violence

Research on long-term vulnerabilities related to self-directed violence has focused on personality characteristics and chronic depression, both of which can lead to neglect and suicide. Rickelman and Houfek (1995) described an interactional model that includes cognitive rigidity, attributional style, stress, hopelessness, and depression. Individuals who fit into this model tend to be inflexible and have difficulty solving problems. This leads to increased stress and hopelessness and greater vulnerability to suicide. Another investigator correlated depression with hardiness and attitudes about death (Cataldo, 1994). She found that healthy death attitudes are related to low depression scores, and that nonhardiness and fearful or escape-oriented death attitudes predicted depression. In

an extensive review article, Lum (1988) listed the following long-term factors that are influential in depression and suicide: chronic pain, other chronic illnesses, learned helplessness, chronic substance abuse, and a family history of mood disturbance.

However, Conwell, Raby, and Caine (1995), reflecting the increasing body of research on older individuals, suggested the possibility that certain biologic aspects of aging might influence self-directed violence. It is important for clinicians to note, though, that current research shows that the single most significant factor in assessing self- or other-directed violence in elders is a history of violent behavior. Numerous researchers have documented the importance of a previous history of other-directed violence (Asnis, Kaplan, van Praag, & Sanderson, 1994; Hwang & Segal, 1996; Monahan, 1981).

Several studies have supported the importance of past suicide attempts as a top risk factor for self-directed violence (Malone, Haas, Sweeney, & Mann, 1995; Nordstrom, Asberg, Aberg-Wistedt, & Nordin, 1995; Roy & Draper, 1995). The Depression Guideline Panel of the Agency for Health Care Policy and Research (AHCPR) (1993) listed the following top five suicide risk factors: white race, male gender, advanced age, living alone, and previous suicide attempt. *The Handbook of Mental Illness*, published by the Iowa Alliance for the Mentally Ill (1995), reported that the highest rates of suicide nationally are found in individuals over 65 years of age. Psychiatric illnesses, especially long-term mood disorders, place the elderly person at greater risk for self-directed violence (Ahrens, Berghofer, Wolf, & Muller-Oerlinghausen, 1995; Beautrais et al., 1996) (see Chapter 41). Other psychiatric illnesses related to increased suicide rates in elders are posttraumatic stress disorder (Lehmann, McCormick, & McCracken, 1995), schizophrenia (Roy & Draper, 1995), and substance abuse (Anderson, Howard, Walker, & Suchinsky, 1995). Social and environmental factors related to suicide include chronic sensory impairments (Johnston & Walker, 1996) and affective and cognitive constriction (Duberstein, 1995; Rickelman & Houfek, 1995; Schmid, Manjee, & Shah, 1994). Individuals with these conditions can appear so blunted that self-harm intent is not obviously evident.

Current stressors affecting self-directed violence include involuntary hospitalization (Cardell & Horton-Deutsch, 1994; Roy & Draper, 1995), change in marital status, alcohol abuse (Stack & Wasserman, 1995), hopelessness that persists after remission of a major depressive episode (Rifai, George, Stack, Mann, & Reynolds, 1994; Zweig & Hinrichsen, 1993), a history of cancer (Grabbe, Demi, Camann, & Potter, 1997), and an impaired ability to communicate and feelings of helplessness (Johnston & Walker, 1996). When short-term stressors lead to a risk for self-directed violence, psychiatric illness frequently is present. Andreasen and Black (1995) reported that more than 90% of persons who successfully committed suicide had a major psychiatric illness. A second leading factor listed by the authors is alcohol abuse or dependence. There is additional evidence that depression and suicide might be biologically mediated by a decrease in norepinephrine and serotonin levels in the brain (Andreasen & Black, 1995; Kurlowicz, 1994; Lum, 1988). Other short-term factors that might lead to depression and increased risk for suicide include effects of medications such as antihypertensives and narcotic analgesics, physical illnesses such as metabolic disturbances, cardiovascular illnesses, neurologic problems, and bereavement (Kurlowicz, 1994).

Triggers for self-directed violence are often less clear than those for other-directed violence. Suicide can be a person's final act after a long downward spiral of depression (Andreasen & Black, 1995), or it can occur as a reaction to a sudden event such as medical or psychiatric hospitalization (Cardell & Horton-Deutsch, 1994; Kurlowicz, 1994). Another significant factor is the presence of a lethal means such as a firearm (Fawcett, Clark, & Busch, 1993). Close monitoring of a client's reaction to changes in health or to loss becomes critical.

ASSESSMENT

The various predictors for violence in elders (summarized in Table 53-1) span all categories of the Stokman model. More importantly, violent individuals typically have several liabilities: a chronic psychiatric illness mixed with substance abuse or a dementia combined with placement in a new environment. This strengthens the argument that caregivers must assess the elderly client for all possible liabilities to make an accurate diagnosis of risk for violence. Further research will clarify and expand the risk factors that are significant in the elderly population. Indeed, a new diagnosis of risk for violence specific to elders may be very useful for caregivers in the future.

Selected Assessment Scales

Since much of the risk for suicide in elderly persons is related to depression and hopelessness, whether from a

Table 53-1   Risk Factors for Prediction of Violence: Adapted for the Elderly Client

Long-Term Vulnerabilities	Self- or Other-Directed
(Individual client traits or conditions that are present for many years)	
History of violence	Both
Neurologic conditions (e.g., seizure disorder, mental retardation)	Other
Chronic sensory impairments	Both
Progressive dementia	Other
Advanced age	Self
Lives alone	Self
Chronic mood disorder (major depression)	Self
Schizophrenia	Both
Posttraumatic stress disorder	Self
History of substance abuse	Both
Coercive interactional style	Other
Changes in social support system	Other
Affective and cognitive blunting	Self

Short-Term Stressors	Self- or Other-Directed
(Recent situations or changes that add to the client's emotional load)	
Hospitalization	Self
Involuntary hospitalization	Both
Care setting rules	Other
Delirium	Other
Prescription medication reactions	Other
Sleep disturbance	Other
Acute alcohol intoxication	Both
Persistent hopelessness after remission of a major depressive episode	Self
Divorce/loss of spouse	Self

Contextual Triggers	Self- or Other-Directed
(Immediate events that spark a violent episode)	
Care setting rule enforcement	Both
Seclusion and restraint procedures	Other
ADL care assistance	Other

psychiatric illness or from a reaction to loss, a scale that measures depression in elderly persons is particularly helpful. The Geriatric Depression Scale (Yesavage et al., 1983) offers a reliable scale to measure depression in elders (see Chapter 41). The scale has 30 questions that can be self or clinician administered; a yes/no answer format simplifies the decision-making process. Of special note is the scale's avoidance of measuring somatic symptoms, many of which are found in nondepressed elders.

A variety of instruments assess agitation and threatening behaviors that indicate a risk for other-directed violence in the elderly population (Gerdner & Buckwalter, 1994). All deal with client behaviors that define the diagnosis Risk for Violence: Directed at Others as developed for the North American Nursing Diagnosis Association (NANDA) (1999). A newer instrument called the Violence Scale (Morrison, 1993) is intriguing for several reasons. It is brief, containing only five judgmental statements. It uses a Likert response scale. It is based on clinician observation and knowledge of a client's history of aggression or violence, and it is behaviorally based, making use of Morrison's hierarchy of escalating aggressive to violent behavior (Table 53-2). This scale is under continuing study and needs to be validated with elderly populations. Yet its simplicity and use of actual behavioral observation make it potentially useful for tracking escalation or reduction of risk for violence directed at others during a client's duration of care.

Table 53-2	Violence Scale
Violence Toward Others*	**Level of Violence (Morrison, 1992b)**
1. This person has physically harmed another person.	1. Violence
2. This person has touched another person in a threatening manner.	2. Violence
3. This person has verbally threatened another person and had a plan of action to carry it out.	3. Aggression
4. This person has verbally threatened to harm another person, but did not have a plan of action to carry out the threat.	4. Aggression
5. This person has engaged in arguments with others including bragging of previous violence.	5. Aggression

Adapted from Morrison, E. (1993). The measurement of aggression and violence in hospitalized psychiatric patients. *International Journal of Nursing Studies, 30*(1), 51-64.

*Items are randomized to decrease rater bias.

CASE STUDY 1

K. Dodd is a 78-year-old man who has been admitted to a locked, acute care psychiatric unit from home because his wife can no longer manage his combative behavior. Mr. Dodd was diagnosed 6 months ago with an unspecified but rapidly progressing dementia. He responds to his name but is disoriented in all other spheres. At home he was beginning to wander and, when his wife attempted to stop him, he would become enraged and strike her with his fists. He has accused her of "sneaking out with another man" and feels she is intentionally keeping him in so he will not discover this. His wife reports that Mr. Dodd drank heavily 3 to 4 times a week for about 25 years but has not consumed alcohol for about the last 5 years. After admission, Mr. Dodd began trying the locked doors and was difficult to redirect. At times he became combative when confronted by the staff and had to be secluded and restrained. One time he entered the dayroom, spontaneously punched another elderly man, and accused him of trying to "steal" his wife. The staff noted that Mr. Dodd responded positively to diversions such as shuffling cards, playing catch with a foam ball, and occasionally reminiscing.

CASE STUDY 2

D. Bailey is an 82-year-old female who is being seen weekly at the psychiatric outpatient clinic following hospitalization for an episode of major depression. Mrs. Bailey's husband died about 6 months ago after over 50 years of marriage. Mrs. Bailey did well for a while and was able to continue to care for herself and her own home. However, a neighbor noticed that Mrs. Bailey was not getting out as much as usual a month ago. When she checked on her, she discovered that Mrs. Bailey had lost weight, looked disheveled, seemed confused, and was slow to respond. A daughter living about 300 miles away was notified, and Mrs. Bailey was admitted to the hospital. After several weeks of medication, she was well enough to return home. During several weekly follow-up visits in the clinic, the advanced practice nurse in the clinic determined that Mrs. Bailey was remaining at home most days, continued to feel lost and hopeless without her husband around, and still was not sleeping well. The nurse practitioner discovered that Mrs. Bailey had experienced some "spells" when she was younger that were similar to this, but her husband always had taken care of things until she got back on her feet. Mrs. Bailey had three daughters, but none within a 300-mile radius. She reported that they stay in touch but cannot visit much. Mrs. Bailey denied current suicide ideation, but her affect continued to look very flat.

NURSING DIAGNOSIS

Aggression and violence are often found to be synonymous in early writings on the subject. More recent investigators have separated the two terms so that *aggression* refers to threatening behavior toward others, whereas *violence* refers to physical behavior that results in harm to self or others (Monahan, 1981; Morrison, 1992b). The NANDA handbook (1999) combined both aggressive and violent behaviors to define two nursing diagnoses, Risk for Violence: Directed at Others and Risk for Violence: Self-Directed. Box 53-1 presents the risk factors for both of these diagnoses that have been listed by NANDA.

- Risk for Violence: Directed at Others—"Behaviors in which an individual demonstrates that he/she can be physically, emotionally, and/or sexually harmful to others" (p. 127).
- Risk for Violence: Self-Directed—"Behaviors in which an individual demonstrates that he/she can be physically, emotionally, and/or sexually harmful to self" (p. 129).

NURSING-SENSITIVE OUTCOMES

The *Nursing Outcomes Classification (NOC)* (Iowa Outcomes Project, 2000) includes several outcomes that are relevant to persons at risk for violence directed at others: Aggression Control; Impulse Control; Distorted Thought Control; Risk Control: Alcohol Use; and Risk Control: Drug Use (Box 53-2). Indicators that an individual is successful in meeting the outcome Aggression Control might include refraining from striking at others, harming others, violating others' personal space, and destroying property, as well as maintaining self-control without supervision (Box 53-3). The NOC outcomes most relevant to persons at risk for violence directed at self include Suicide Self-Restraint and Impulse Control. Important indicators that an individual is successful in meeting the outcome Suicide Self-Restraint include expression of feelings, maintaining connectedness in relationships, and refraining from formulating a plan for committing suicide or gathering tools

Box 53-1	Risk for Violence—Factors Significant for the Elderly
Self-Directed	**Directed at Others**
Multiple attempts	History of violence: against self or others
Over 45	Neurologic impairment
Marital status: single, widowed, divorced	Cognitive impairment
Recent job loss or failure	History of family violence
Family history of conflict and/or suicide	History of cruelty to animals
Mental illness: depression, psychosis, personality disorder, substance abuse	History of fire setting
Hopelessness, despair	History of drug and/or alcohol abuse
Suicidal ideation: frequent	Pathologic intoxication
Suicide plan: special, lethal	Psychotic symptomology
Social isolation	Antisocial character
	Organic brain syndrome
	Toxic reactions to medication

Data from Depression Guideline Panel. (1993). *Depression in primary care: Detection and diagnosis: Volume 1* (AHCPR Pub. 93-0551). Washington, DC: Agency for Health Care Policy and Research; Justice, B., Justice, R., & Kraft, I. (1974). Early warning signs of violence: Is triad enough? *American Journal of Psychiatry, 131,* 457-459.

Box 53-2	Selected Outcomes and Interventions for Elderly Clients **RISK FOR VIOLENCE: SELF-DIRECTED OR DIRECTED AT OTHERS**
Outcomes	**Interventions**
Aggression Control	Anger Control Assistance
Impulse Control	Environmental Management: Violence Prevention
Suicide Self-Restraint	Anxiety Reduction
Distorted Thought Control	Behavior Management
Quality of Life	Crisis Intervention
Risk Control: Alcohol Use	Delusion Management
Risk Control: Drug Use	Dementia Management
Risk Detection	Substance Use Prevention
	Suicide Prevention
	Support System Enhancement
	Surveillance: Safety

Box 53-3	Suggested Nursing-Sensitive Outcomes and Nursing Interventions **RISK FOR VIOLENCE: DIRECTED AT OTHERS**

Nursing Diagnosis
Risk for Violence: Directed at Others
Risk factors
Antisocial character
Organic brain syndrome
Seizure disorder
Toxic medication reactions
Increased anxiety
Repetition of verbalizations
Body language: clenched fists, tense facial expression, rigid
    posture
Hostile, threatening verbalizations
Environmental destruction
Suspicion of others
Delusions
Hallucinations
Substance abuse

Nursing-Sensitive Outcomes
Aggression Control
Indicators
Refrains from verbal outbursts
Refrains from violating others' personal space
Refrains from striking others
Refrains from destroying property
Identifies when frustrated

Impulse Control
Indicators
Identifies social support systems
Accepts referrals for treatment
Maintains self-control without supervision

Distorted Thought Control
Risk Control: Alcohol Use
Risk Control: Drug Use

Nursing Interventions
Anger Control Assistance
Activities
Establish basic trust and rapport with patient
Limit access to frustrating situations until patient is able to
    express anger in an adaptive manner
Monitor potential for inappropriate aggression and intervene
    before its expression
Prevent physical harm if anger is directed at self or others
    (e.g., restrain and remove potential weapons)
Instruct in use of calming measures
Provide physical outlets for expression of anger or tension
Reinforce appropriate expression of anger

Environmental Management: Violence Prevention
Activities
Monitor patient during use of potential weapons
Remove other individuals from the vicinity of a violent or
    potentially violent patient
Provide ongoing surveillance for clients at risk

to commit suicide (Box 53-4). Other related outcomes include Quality of Life and Risk Detection.

NURSING INTERVENTIONS

Nursing interventions to prevent violence directed at others must vary depending on individual client characteristics. Persons with dementias, for example, might require interventions that are not needed with persons who do not have dementia. Gerdner and Buckwalter (1994) identified the following as significant areas of intervention for this population: provision of physical safety, a sense of control, and physical comfort; compensation for sensory and cognitive deficits; communication; and environmental modification. Other researchers have suggested individualizing communication and fostering greater awareness of the individual and the environment during feeding and hygiene activities (Allen, 1999; Brannan, 1988; Kayser-Jones & Schell, 1997; Namazi & Johnson, 1996; Williams, 1989; Winger et al., 1987). Reducing stress and preventing fatigue through environmental control have been advocated for the same population (Hall, Kirschling, & Todd, 1986; Janelli & Kanski, 1997).

For clients with chronic mental illnesses who live in the community, intensive case management offers an alterna-

tive to hospitalization as symptoms increase (Buckwalter & Stolley, 1991; Dvoskin & Steadman, 1994). It can be helpful to individualize care by providing consistent caregivers, frequent availability, and stronger linkages to community services for the chronically mentally ill. Dvosken and Steadman also advocate strong ties to substance abuse treatment since this is an all-too-frequent problem among chronically mentally ill clients of all ages.

Older individuals at risk for self-directed violence require increased supervision for safety (Green & Grindel, 1996; Moore, Berman, Knight, & Devine, 1995). For those where the risk is not so great, cognitive-based therapies (Boettcher, 1983), spiritual well-being models (Morris, 1996), and support groups (Devons, 1996) are recommended to assist them in coping with illnesses, losses, and low self-esteem. The use of humor (Richman, 1995) and reminiscence (Lewis & Butler, 1974) can decrease depressive symptoms and increase social cohesion.

The *Nursing Interventions Classification (NIC)* (Iowa Intervention Project, 2000) includes several relevant interventions (see Box 53-2). Anger Control Assistance and Environmental Management: Violence Prevention are fundamental to decreasing the risk for violence directed at others (see Box 53-3). Suicide Prevention is the key intervention for decreasing the risk for self-directed vio-

Box 53-4	Suggested Nursing-Sensitive Outcomes and Nursing Interventions RISK FOR VIOLENCE: SELF-DIRECTED

Nursing Diagnosis
Risk for Violence: Self-Directed
Risk factors
Age: over 45
Marital status: single, widowed, divorced
Recent job loss/failure
Family background: conflictual
History of suicide in family
Chronic illness
Severe depression
Psychosis
Severe personality disorder
Chronic substance abuse
Hopelessness
Multiple past attempts
Suicide plan: clear and specific
Socially isolated: unresponsive family

Nursing-Sensitive Outcomes
Suicide Self-Restraint
Indicators
Maintains connectedness in relationships
Seeks help when feeling self-destructive
Verbalizes control of impulses
Refrains from gathering means for suicide

Refrains from using mood-altering substance(s)
Upholds suicide contract
Maintains self-control without supervision

Impulse Control
Indicators
Recognizes risks in environment
Seeks help when experiencing impulses
Identifies social support systems

Nursing Interventions
Suicide Prevention
Activities
Determine whether patient has specific suicide plan identified
Determine history of suicide attempts
Facilitate support of patient by family and friends
Observe closely during suicidal crisis
Protect patient from harming self

Substance Use Treatment
Support System Enhancement
Activities
Determine adequacy of existing social networks
Determine barriers to using support systems
Encourage the patient to participate in social and community activities

Data from Depression Guideline Panel. (1993). *Depression in primary care: Detection and diagnosis: Volume 1* (AHCPR Pub. 93-0551). Washington, DC: Agency for Health Care Policy and Research.

lence. Support System Enhancement and Substance Use Treatment are also important (see Box 53-4).

CASE STUDY 1

The nursing staff recognized that Mr. Dodd had several significant risk factors for the diagnosis Risk for Violence: Directed at Others related to neurologic and cognitive deficits secondary to the progressive dementia. Risk factors included the following:

- Recent history of violence
- Current spontaneous combative behavior
- Paranoid delusions regarding his wife
- Frequent anger and rage reactions
- History of alcohol abuse

Mr. Dodd's primary nurse and his wife agreed that the desired goals were decreased aggression and decreased abusive behavior. The nurse chose Environmental Management: Violence Prevention; Delusion Management; Dementia Management; and Distraction as the key nursing interventions. Mr. Dodd was moved to a room close to the nurses' station. The staff closely supervised Mr. Dodd's interactions with other residents and intervened when he became agitated. When he became angry, other residents were removed from the area. The staff then tried to engage him in playing catch or gave him a deck of cards to distract him. The staff also attempted to provide Mr. Dodd with more consistency in caregivers. Finally, the staff instructed Mrs. Dodd to speak in a calm voice, to refuse to argue with her husband, and to call for assistance if he became agitated. Greater consistency in caregivers and a calmer approach by his wife and staff seemed to decrease his agitation. When he did become agitated, distraction was usually successful. Table 53-3 summarizes Mr. Dodd's progress in meeting the specified outcomes.

CASE STUDY 2

The clinic nurse decided that although Mrs. Bailey was not suicidal, she was persistently hopeless enough for the nurse to make a diagnosis of Risk for Violence: Self-Directed related to ongoing situational stressors. Significant risk factors for Mrs. Bailey included the following:

- History of depression/mood disturbance
- Persistent hopelessness after a depressive episode
- Recent loss of spouse
- Decreased social activity
- Inconsistent family support

The nurse worked with Mrs. Bailey to identify desired outcomes. Mrs. Bailey was able to state that she wanted to feel closer to others. The nurse suggested that Mrs. Bailey also consider learning how to identify and express her

Table 53-3	Mr. Dodd's Progress With Identified Outcomes		
	Ratings		
	Week 1	Week 2	Week 3
SELECTED LABELS AND INDICATORS			
AGGRESSION CONTROL			
Refrains from striking others	2	3	4
Refrains from harming others	2	3	4
Refrains from violating others' personal space	2	3	3
Refrains from destroying property	3	3	5
Maintains self-control without supervision	1	2	3
ABUSIVE BEHAVIOR SELF-CONTROL			
Avoids physically abusive behavior	3	3	4
Avoids emotionally abusive behavior	2	2	3
Demonstrates impulse control	2	3	4
Participates in treatment as needed	2	2	3

Nursing Outcomes Classification (NOC) 5-point Likert measurement scale:

Aggression Control and Abusive Behavior Self-Control: 1 = Never demonstrated; 2 = Rarely demonstrated; 3 = Sometimes demonstrated;
4 = Often demonstrated; 5 = Consistently demonstrated.

Table 53-4	Mrs. Bailey's Progress With Identified Outcomes			
	Week 1	Week 2	Week 3	Week 4
SELECTED LABELS AND INDICATORS				
SUICIDE SELF-RESTRAINT				
Expresses feelings	3	4	4	5
Maintains connectedness in relationships	2	3	4	5
Refrains from gathering means for suicide	5	5	5	5
Maintains self-control without supervision	5	5	5	5
IMPULSE CONTROL				
Identifies feelings that lead to impulsive actions	3	4	4	5
Verbalizes control of impulses	4	4	5	5
Identifies social support systems	3	4	5	5
Accepts referrals for treatment	3	4	4	5

Nursing Outcomes Classification (NOC) 5-point Likert measurement scale:

Suicide Self-Restraint and Impulse Control: 1 = Never demonstrated; 2 = Rarely demonstrated; 3 = Sometimes demonstrated;
4 = Often demonstrated; 5 = Consistently demonstrated.

feelings so that they would not overwhelm her. Mrs. Bailey agreed to do this. Key nursing interventions included Coping Enhancement, Distraction, Mood Management, and Support System Enhancement. The clinic nurse encouraged Mrs. Bailey to get involved in church activities again and to play cards with her club once a week. She also got in touch with the daughter who lives closest across the state to explain the situation and encourage more frequent contact. At weekly appointments the nurse assisted Mrs. Bailey to identify her feelings and encouraged her to express those feelings. The nurse also administered the Geriatric Depression Scale to measure improvement. Within a month Mrs. Bailey looked brighter and seemed to have more energy. She was able to state that she enjoyed playing cards and felt supported by people at her church.

Table 53-4 summarizes Mrs. Bailey's progress with the identified outcomes.

SUMMARY

The keys to preventing violence are accurate assessment of risk and diligent, careful intervention. Because violence is less predictable in elderly clients with progressive organic disorders, caregivers must be ready to intervene quickly. Nurses also need to be prepared to intervene to decrease the risk of suicide in older adults. Adequate training can help nurses manage most potentially violent situations so that both clients and staff remain safe.

REFERENCES

Ahrens, B., Berghofer, A., Wolf, T., Muller-Oerlinghausen, B. (1995). Suicide attempts, age and duration of illness in recurrent affective disorders. *Journal of Affective Disorders, 36*(1-2), 43-49.

Allen, L. (1999). Treating agitation without drugs. *American Journal of Nursing, 99*(4), 36-41.

Allen, M., Yanchick, V., Cook, J., & Foss, S. (1990). Do drugs affect social behavior in the confused elderly? *Journal of Gerontological Nursing, 16*(12), 34-39.

Anderson, B., Howard, M., Walker, R., & Suchinsky, R. (1995). Characteristics of substance-abusing veterans attempting suicide: A national study. *Psychological Reports, 77*(3), 1231-1242.

Andreasen, N., & Black, D. (1995). *Introductory textbook of psychiatry.* Washington, DC: American Psychiatric Press.

Asnis, G., Kaplan, M., van Praag, H., & Sanderson, W. (1994). Homicidal behaviors among psychiatric outpatients. *Hospital and Community Psychiatry, 45*(2), 127-132.

Bach-y-Rita, G., Lion, J., Climent, C., & Ervin, F. (1971). Episodic dyscontrol: A study of 130 violent patients. *American Journal of Psychiatry, 127,* 1473-1478.

Bandura, A. (1973). *Aggression: A social learning analysis.* Upper Saddle River, NJ: Prentice-Hall.

Beautrais, A., Joyce, P., Mulder, R., Fergusson, D., Deavoll, B., & Nightingale, S. (1996). Prevalence and comorbidity of mental disorders in persons making serious suicide attempts: A case-control study. *American Journal of Psychiatry, 153*(8), 1009-1014.

Berkowitz, L. (1974). Some determinates of impulsive aggression: Role mediated associations with reinforcements for aggression. *Psychological Review, 81,* 165-176.

Berkowitz, L. (1982). Violence and rule following behavior. In L. Marsh & A. Campbell (Eds.), *Aggression and violence* (pp. 91-101). Oxford: Basil Blackwell.

Boettcher, E. (1983). Preventing violent behavior: An integrated theoretical model for nursing. *Perspectives in Psychiatric Care, 21*(2), 54-58.

Brannan, P. (1988). Using nursing skills instead of restraints. *Geriatric Nursing, 9*(2), 114-115.

Buckwalter, K., & Stolley, J. (1991). Managing mentally ill elders at home. *Geriatric Nursing, 12*(3), 135-139.

Cardell, R., & Horton-Deutsch, S. (1994). A model for assessment of inpatient suicide potential. *Archives of Psychiatric Nursing, 8*(6), 366-372.

Cataldo, J. (1994). Hardiness and death attitudes: Predictors of depression in the institutionalized elderly. *Archives of Psychiatric Nursing, 8*(5), 326-332.

Cohen-Mansfield, J., & Marx, M. (1990). The relationship between sleep disturbances and agitation in a nursing home. *Journal of Aging and Health, 2*(1), 42-57.

Convit, A., Jaeger, J., Lin, S., Meisner, M., & Volavka, J. (1988). Predicting assaultiveness in psychiatric inpatients: A pilot study. *Hospital and Community Psychiatry, 38*(4), 429-434.

Conwell, Y., Raby, W., & Caine, E. (1995). Suicide and aging II: The psychobiological interface. *International Psychogeriatrics, 7*(2), 165-181.

Cooper, A., & Mendonca, J. (1989). A prospective study of patient assaults on nursing staff in a psychogeriatrics unit. *Canadian Journal of Psychiatry, 34,* 399-403.

Davis, D., & Boster, L. (1988). Multifaceted therapeutic interventions with the violent psychiatric inpatient. *Hospital and Community Psychiatry, 39*(8), 867-869.

Davis, S. (1991). Violence by psychiatric inpatients: A review. *Hospital and Community Psychiatry, 42*(6), 585-590.

Depression Guideline Panel. (1993). *Depression in primary care: Detection and diagnosis: Volume 1* (AHCPR Pub. 93-0551). Washington, DC: Agency for Health Care Policy and Research.

Devons, C. (1996). Suicide in the elderly: How to identify and treat patients at risk. *Geriatrics, 51*(3), 67-68, 70-73.

Dollard, J., Dobb, L., Miller, B., Mowerer, O., & Sears, R. (1939). *Frustration and aggression.* New Haven, CT: Yale University Press.

Duberstein, R. (1995). Openness to experience and completed suicide across the second half of life. *International Psychogeriatrics, 7*(2), 183-198.

Dvoskin, J., & Steadman, H. (1994). Using intensive case management to reduce violence by mentally ill persons in the community. *Hospital and Community Psychiatry, 45*(7), 679-684.

Estroff, S., Zimmer, C., Lachicotte, W., & Benoit, J. (1994). The influence of social networks and social support on violence by persons with serious mental illness. *Hospital and Community Psychiatry, 45*(7), 669-678.

Fawcett, J., Clark, D., & Busch, K. (1993). Assessing and treating the patient at risk for suicide. *Psychiatric Annals, 23*(5), 244-255.

Foreman, M. (1990). Complexities of acute confusion. *Geriatric Nursing, 11*(3), 136-139.

Gallop, R., McCay, E., & Esplen, M. (1992). The conceptualization of impulsivity for psychiatric nursing practice. *Archives of Psychiatric Nursing, 6*(6), 366-373.

Gerdner, L., & Buckwalter, K. (1994). A nursing challenge: Assessment and management of agitation in Alzheimer's patients. *Journal of Gerontological Nursing, 20*(4), 11-20.

Gilley, D., Wilson, R., Beckett, L., & Evans, D. (1997). Psychotic symptoms and physically aggressive behavior in Alzheimer's disease. *Journal of the American Geriatrics Society, 45*(9), 1074-1079.

Golier, J., Marzuk, P., Leon, A., Weiner, C., & Tardiff, K. (1995). Low serum cholesterol level and attempted suicide. *American Journal of Psychiatry, 152*(3), 419-423.

Gormley, N., Rizwan, M., & Lovestone, S. (1998). Clinical predictors of aggressive behavior in Alzheimer's disease. *International Journal of Geriatric Psychiatry, 13*(2), 109-115.

Grabbe, L., Demi, A., Camann, M., & Potter, L. (1997). The health status of elderly persons in the last year of life: A comparison of deaths by suicide, injury, and natural causes. *American Journal of Public Health, 87*(3), 434-437.

Green, J., & Grindel, C. (1996). Supervision of suicidal patients in adult inpatient psychiatric units in general hospitals. *Psychiatric Services, 47*(8), 859-863.

Hall, G., Kirschling, M., & Todd, S. (1986). Sheltered freedom: An Alzheimer's unit in an IFC. *Geriatric Nursing, 7*(3), 132-137.

Hwang, S., & Segal, S. (1996). Criminality of the mentally ill in sheltered care: Are they more dangerous? *International Journal of Law and Psychiatry, 19*(1), 93-105.

Iowa Alliance for the Mentally Ill. (1995). *The handbook of mental illness.* Des Moines: Author.

Iowa Intervention Project. J. C. McCloskey & G. M. Bulechek (Eds.). (2000). *Nursing interventions classification (NIC)* (3rd ed.). St. Louis, MO: Mosby.

Iowa Outcomes Project. M. Johnson, M. Maas, & S. Moorhead (Eds.). (2000). *Nursing outcomes classification (NOC)* (2nd ed.). St. Louis, MO: Mosby.

Janelli, L., & Kanski, G. (1997). Music intervention with physically restrained patients. *Rehabilitation Nursing, 22*(1), 14-19.

Johnston, M., & Walker, M. (1996). Suicide in the elderly: Recognizing the signs. *General Hospital Psychiatry, 18*(4), 257-260.

Justice, B., Justice, R., & Kraft, I. (1974). Early warning signs of violence: Is triad enough? *American Journal of Psychiatry, 131*, 457-459.

Katz, P., & Kirkland, F. (1990). Violence and social structure on mental hospital wards. *Psychiatry, 53*, 262-277.

Kayser-Jones, J., & Schell, E. (1997). The mealtime experience of a cognitively impaired elder: Ineffective and effective strategies. *Journal of Gerontological Nursing, 23*(7), 33-39.

Kolanowski, A., Hurwitz, S., Taylor, L., Evans, L., & Strumpf, N. (1994). Contextual factors associated with disturbing behaviors in institutionalized elders. *Nursing Research, 43*(7), 73-78.

Kurlowicz, L. (1994). Depression in hospitalized medically ill elders: Evolution of the concept. *Archives of Psychiatric Nursing, 8*(2), 124-136.

Lanza, M. (1988). Factors relevant to patient assault. *Issues in Mental Health Nursing, 9*, 239-257.

Lawlor, B., & Sunderland, T. (1988). Causes and treatment of behavioral change. *Consultant, 28*(1), 43-48.

Lehmann, L., McCormick, R., & McCracken, L. (1995). Suicidal behavior among patients in the VA health care system. *Psychiatric Services, 46*(10), 1069-1071.

Lewis, M., & Butler, R. (1974). Life review therapy: Putting memories to work in individual and group psychotherapy. *Geriatrics, 29*, 165-173.

Lorenz, K. (1966). *On aggression*. Philadelphia: Harcourt Brace.

Lum, T. (1988). An integrated approach to aging and depression. *Archives of Psychiatric Nursing, 2*(4), 211-217.

Malone, K., Haas, G., Sweeney, J., & Mann, J. (1995). Major depression and the risk of attempted suicide. *Journal of Affective Disorders, 34*(3), 173-185.

Monahan, J. (1981). *The clinical prediction of violent behavior*. Rockville, MD: NIMH.

Moore, P., Berman, K., Knight, M., & Devine, J. (1995). Constant observation: Implications for nursing practice. *Journal of Psychosocial Nursing and Mental Health Services, 33*(3), 46-50.

Morris, L. (1996). A spiritual well-being model: Use with older women who experience depression. *Issues in Mental Health Nursing, 17*, 439-455.

Morrison, E. (1987). Determining social and therapeutic rules for psychiatric inpatients. *Hospital and Community Psychiatry, 38*(9), 994-995.

Morrison, E. (1989). Theoretical modeling to predict violence in hospitalized psychiatric patients. *Research in Nursing and Health, 12*, 31-40.

Morrison, E. (1992a). A coercive interactional style as an antecedent to aggression in psychiatric patients. *Research in Nursing and Health, 15*, 421-431.

Morrison, E. (1992b). A hierarchy of aggressive behaviors among psychiatric inpatients. *Hospital and Community Psychiatry, 43*(5), 505-506.

Morrison, E. (1993). The measurement of aggression and violence in hospitalized psychiatric patients. *International Journal of Nursing Studies, 30*(1), 51-64.

Moyer, K. (1976). *The psychobiology of aggression*. New York: Harper and Row.

Mulvey, E. (1994). Assessing the evidence of a link between mental illness and violence. *Hospital and Community Psychiatry, 45*(7), 663-668.

Namazi, K., & Johnson, D. (1996). Issues related to behavior and the physical environment: Bathing cognitively impaired patients. *Geriatric Nursing, 17*(5), 234-239.

Nordstrom, P., Asberg, M., Aberg-Wistedt, A., & Nordin, C. (1995). Attempted suicide predicts suicide risk in mood disorders. *Acta Psychiatrica Scandinavica, 92*(5), 345-350.

North American Nursing Diagnosis Association. (1999). *Nursing diagnoses: Definitions & classification 1999-2000*. Philadelphia: Author.

Richman, J. (1995). The lifesaving function of humor with depressed and suicidal elderly. *Gerontologist, 35*(2), 271-273.

Rickelman, B., & Houfek, J. (1995). Toward an interactional model of suicidal behaviors: Cognitive rigidity, attributional style, stress, hopelessness, and depression. *Archives of Psychiatric Nursing, 9*(3), 158-168.

Rifai, A., George, C., Stack, J., Mann, J., & Reynolds, C. (1994). Hopelessness in suicide attempters after acute treatment of major depression in late life. *American Journal of Psychiatry, 151*(11), 1687-1690.

Roper, J., & Anderson, N. (1991). The interactional dynamics of violence, part 1: An acute psychiatric ward. *Archives of Psychiatric Nursing, 5*(4), 209-215.

Roy, A., & Draper, R. (1995). Suicide among psychiatric hospital in-patients. *Psychological Medicine, 25*(1), 199-202.

Roy, A., & Pollack, S. (1994). Are cerebrospinal fluid or urinary monoamine metabolite measures stronger correlates of suicidal behavior in depression? *Neuropsychobiology, 29*(4), 164-167.

Schmid, H., Manjee, K., & Shah, T. (1994). On the distinction of suicide ideation versus attempt in elderly psychiatric inpatients. *The Gerontologist, 34*(3), 332-339.

Sheard, M. (1979). Testosterone and aggression. In M. Sandler (Ed.), *Psychopharmacology of aggression* (pp. 111-121). New York: Raven Press.

Sheridan, M., Henrion, R., Robinson, L., & Baxter, V. (1990). Precipitants of violence in a psychiatric inpatient setting. *Hospital and Community Psychiatry, 41*(7), 776-780.

Stack, S., & Wasserman, I. (1995). Marital status, alcohol abuse and attempted suicide: A logit model. *Journal of Addictive Diseases, 14*(2), 43-51.

Stokman, C. (1984). Dangerousness and violence in hospitalized mentally ill offenders. *Psychiatric Quarterly, 56*(2), 138-143.

Torrey, E. (1994). Violent behavior by individuals with serious mental illness. *Hospital and Community Psychiatry, 45*(7), 653-662.

Williams, C. (1989). Liberation: Alternative to physical restraints. *The Gerontologist, 29*(5), 585-586.

Williams, D. (1976). Neural factors related to habitual aggression. In K. Moyer (Ed.), *Physiology of aggression* (pp. 169-186). New York: Raven Press.

Winger, J., Schirm, V., & Stewart, D. (1987). Aggressive behavior in long-term care. *Journal of Psychosocial Nursing, 25*(4), 28-33.

Yesavage, J., Brink, T., Rose, T., Lum, O., Huang, V., Adey, M., & Otto Leirer, V. (1983). Development and validation of a geriatric depression screening scale: A preliminary report. *Journal of Psychiatric Research, 17*, 37-49.

Zweig, R., & Hinrichsen, G. (1993). Factors associated with suicide attempts by depressed older adults: A prospective study. *American Journal of Psychiatry, 150*(11), 1687-1692.

CHAPTER 54

SELF-DETERMINATION

Kay Weiler and Sue A. Moorhead

Interest in the concept of self-determination has increased greatly since the passage of the Patient Self-Determination Act (PSDA) in 1990 (Pub. L. N. 101-508). A growing number of articles address a variety of topics related to advance directives, such as the prevalence of use of advance directives (Berrio & Levesque, 1996; Rein et al., 1996; Schonwetter, Walker, & Robinson, 1995), their use in home health (Davitt & Kaye, 1996; Gates, Schins, & Smith, 1996), their use in long-term care (Cohen-Mansfield et al., 1991; Walker & Blechner, 1995-6), and their use in hospital medical/surgical units and critical care (Collins & Mozdzierz, 1996; Kolcaba & Fisher, 1996; Rein et al., 1996). In addition, the literature contains articles focusing on the use of advance directives by patients with cancer (Collins & Mozdierz, 1996; Schonwetter, Walker, Solomon, Indurkhya, & Robinson, 1996), Alzheimer's disease (Mezey, Kluger, Maislin, & Mittelman, 1996), acquired immunodeficiency syndrome (AIDS) (Klaus, 1995), and renal failure (Perry, Nicholas, Molzahn, & Dossetor, 1995) and by elders (High, 1991; Pearlman & Uhlmann, 1988). Issues such as ambiguous advance directives (Campbell, 1995), lack of patient knowledge about advance directives (Gamble, McDonald, & Lichstein, 1991; Ott & Hardie, 1997; Sabino, 1996; Schonwetter, Walker, & Robinson, 1995), recognition of advance directives across care settings (Meier et al., 1996), life values assessment (Schirm & Stachel, 1996; Schonwetter et al., 1996), and ethical concerns (Ferdinand, 1996; Hepburn & Reed, 1995; Mouton, Johnson, & Cole, 1995) are frequently the focus of discussions on advance directives. Finally, some of this literature addresses the knowledge base of nurses (Weiler, Eland, & Buckwalter, 1996) and the role of the nurse (American Nurses' Association, 1991; Huth, 1995; Johns, 1996).

The right of a competent older person in the United States to accept or to reject medical care is based on the common law right to self-determination and the constitutional right to privacy: "No right is held more sacred, or is more carefully guarded by the common law, than the right of every individual to the possession and control of his own person, free from all restraint or interference of others, unless by clear and unquestionable authority of law" (*Matter of Conroy*, 1985, p. 1221, *Union Pacific Railroad Co. v. Botsford*, 1891, p. 251).

The origin of this right has been described in the following terms: "Every human being of adult years and sound mind has a right to determine what shall be done with his own body . . ." (*Schloendorff v. Society of New York Hospital*, 1914, p. 92). Simply stated, it is the right of the person "to be let alone" (Cooley, 1930, p. 29). The right of an elderly person to make health care decisions is protected by the Constitutional right to privacy. While not explicitly stated in the Constitution, this right has been found within the penumbra or zone of rights in the ninth (*Griswold v. Connecticut*, 1965) and fourteenth amendments (*Roe v. Wade*, 1973). Although the Constitution does not explicitly state the right to privacy, the Supreme Court has determined that this right is implied in the intent and wording of the Constitution (*Griswold v. Connecticut*, 1965). This right recognizes the individual's interest in preserving ". . . the inviolability of his person . . ." (*Superintendent of Belchertown v. Saikewicz*, 1977, p. 424; *quoting Pratt v. Davis*, 1905, p. 166). The New Jersey Supreme Court has found that the constitutional right to privacy is "broad enough to encompass a patient's decision to decline medical treatment under certain circumstances" even if that personal decision would foreseeably result in death (*Matter of Quinlan*, 1976, p. 663).

Although the common law right to self-determination and the Constitutional right to privacy have been established, these rights are not absolute. These personal rights are balanced against societal interests in (1) preservation of human life, (2) prevention of suicide, (3) protection of the interests of innocent third parties, and (4) preservation of the integrity of the medical profession (*Brophy v. New England Sinai Hospital, Inc.*, 1986).

The preservation of life is generally considered the most significant of the four societal interests. It expresses the societal belief in the sanctity of all human life and is predicated on the belief that the existence of all human life should be protected (*Matter of Conroy*, 1985; *Matter of Spring*, 1980; President's Commission for the Study of Ethical Problems in Medicine and Biomedical and Behavioral Research, Deciding to Forego Life-Sustaining Treatment [hereafter President's Commission], 1983; *Superintendent of Belchertown v. Saikewicz*, 1977). However, this abstract interest in preserving life has often yielded to the personal interest that the individual has in directing his own life (Somers, 1986).

Prevention of suicide, the second societal interest, is an important consideration when attempting to determine whether the elderly individual who is refusing medical care wants to exert the right to self-determination or wants to implement self-destruction (*Matter of Conroy,* 1985). Two critical differences distinguish the refusal of health care from suicide (1) in refusing treatment, the person does not wish to die, and (2), even if death is desired, the cause of death is natural and is not from self-inflicted injuries (*Matter of Quinlan,* 1976; President's Commission, 1983; *Superintendent of Belchertown v. Saikewicz,* 1977).

The protection of innocent third parties is recognized when the needs and interests of dependent children are balanced against an adult's right to self-determination in a health care decision (*Application of President & Directors of Georgetown College, Inc.,* 1964; *Norwood Hospital v. Munoz,* 1991). This interest is also considered when a patient with a communicable disease makes a health care decision considered to create a harmful risk to the community (*Jacobson v. Massachusetts,* 1905).

Preservation of the integrity of the medical profession is a significant issue when patients assert their right to self-determination in a direction contrary to the physician's or health care provider's professional judgment. Questions regarding this issue arise when patients seek to compel health care providers and institutions to take specific health care treatment measures. Concerns also arise from health care institutions seeking to clarify their position, specifically when there is a question about the capacity of the individual to forego treatment (*President's Commission,* 1983).

This interest in the preservation of the integrity of the medical profession has been countered with the following two responses: (1) "medical ethics do not require medical intervention in disease at all costs" (*Matter of Conroy,* 1985, p. 1224), and (2) the right to make an individual health care decision is only valid when there is a right to refuse health care treatment (*Matter of Conroy,* 1985, p. 1225). The concept of self-determination raises difficult and complex ethical and legal questions for the general public and for legal and health care professions.

An individual's ability to exert self-determination in health care treatment rests on three related concepts: mental capacity, the presence of an advance directive, and the availability of a substitute decision maker. As a competent adult, each person has the right to make decisions regarding personal health care treatment. However, that right, as identified earlier, is not an absolute right and is balanced against four societal interests. In the balancing process, the potential conflicts among the individual's preferences; the individual's capacity to express treatment preferences; and the presence of an advance directive, family preferences, health care providers' preferences, and the societal interests discussed previously may require judicial analysis.

Individuals who anticipate the need for future health care decisions may communicate their treatment prefer-ences through a variety of means. Verbal comments, a living will, and a durable power of attorney have been recognized as valid advance directives for future health care treatment decisions. One method of communication of treatment preferences is the use of oral statements made by the elderly person in relation to potential health care problems and possible treatment decisions. Verbal comments indicating a thoughtful and consistent approach have been recognized by the courts as valid indicators of the person's preferred approach to potential treatment alternatives (*In re Storar,* 1981).

The Patient Self-Determination Act (PSDA), which became effective on December 1, 1991, is a legislative attempt to enhance the patient's role in health care treatment decisions (Pub. L. N. 101-508). The PSDA requires that all adults admitted to inpatient, nursing home, home health, and hospice care must receive information about the legal options available in that state for documenting present or future health care treatment decisions. The legislation was enacted (Pub. L. N. 101-508):

(A) to provide written information to each such individual concerning
   (i) an individual's rights under State law (whether statutory or as recognized by the courts of the State) to make decisions concerning such medical care, including the right to accept or refuse medical or surgical treatment and the right to formulate advance directives . . .
   (ii) the written policies of the provider or organization respecting the implementation of such rights;
(B) to document in the individual's medical record whether or not the individual has executed an advance directive. If the health care provider fails to provide the patient with the identified information, the facility may lose Medicare and Medicaid payments.

The writing of an advance directive gives some assurance to the individual that undesired care will be avoided and increases the chance that the type of care the individual wishes will be provided. The purpose of the Patient Self-Determination Act is not to require patients to have such a document but to make people aware of the alternatives available to them. With increased patient knowledge and awareness, it is expected that the number of patients with advance directives will increase. It is also expected that nurses will have increased encounters with these documents (Weiler, Eland, & Buckwalter, 1996).

Two forms of formal written advance directives have recently become important in health care decision-making situations: the living will and the durable power of attorney. Both provide future guidelines in the event that the person is incapable of participating in the decision-making process.

Living Will

A living will authorizes an adult to control decisions regarding the administration of life-sustaining treatment.

By declaring instructions that indicate to the primary health care provider the individual's wishes to have life-sustaining treatment withheld or withdrawn, the individual provides directions to be followed in the event that the person is both in a terminal condition and is unable to participate in medical treatment decisions.

Living will legislation is limited to situations in which life-sustaining treatment is being considered for an adult who both has a terminal condition and who is unable to participate in the treatment decision (Uniform Rights of the Terminally Ill Act [U.L.A.], 1985, prefatory note). It does not apply to life-sustaining measures for minors, adults who have not written a living will, or treatment decisions made by a proxy decision maker (Uniform Rights of the Terminally Ill Act [U.L.A.], 1985, prefatory note). States have varied definitions of specific terms such as *life-sustaining treatment* or *terminal illness* based on the perceived needs or best interests of the residents within that state.

The living will declaration becomes effective when (1) the declaration has been communicated to the attending physician, (2) the declaring adult is determined by the attending physician to be in a terminal condition, and (3) the declaring adult is incapable of making a health care treatment decision (Uniform Rights of the Terminally Ill Act [U.L.A.], 1985, § 3). The living will may be revoked at any time by the declarant, and the revocation is effective when the attending physician is notified of the revocation decision (Uniform Rights of the Terminally Ill Act [U.L.A.], 1985, § 4).

Living will legislation is particularly appropriate in view of the multiple health care needs and concerns of elders. It does not rely on another person to form the substituted judgment of that decision. It does depend on health care personnel, especially physicians and nurses, to carry out the decision (Cohn, 1983).

Durable Power of Attorney for Health Care

The traditional power of attorney is a private agreement between parties that authorizes one person (the agent) to act in the place of or on behalf of another person (the principal) (Restatement, Second, Agency, 1958, § 1). The traditional power of attorney explicitly becomes ineffective if the principal becomes mentally incapacitated (Restatement, Second, Agency, 1958, § 133). This specific characteristic of the traditional power of attorney renders this relationship inappropriate for health care decisions. The situation of diminished capacity or lack of capacity occurs precisely when an agent for decision making is needed. Therefore, some states have enacted legislation that provides for the creation of a relationship that remains in effect even if the principal becomes mentally incapacitated and unable to make decisions. This *durable* power of attorney, the second form of written advance directive, is especially important in health care decisions related to elders.

The following characteristics are required for a durable power of attorney for health care: (1) the principal must be mentally competent at the time that the relationship is created; (2) it is a private written agreement between two persons in a principal-agent relationship; and (3) the document creating the relationship must contain words showing the principal intended that the authority conferred would be exercisable even if the principal became incapacitated or disabled (Uniform Durable Power of Attorney Act [U.L.A.], 1979 § 1 and comments). Words that may be used to indicate this durability include "This power of attorney shall not be affected by subsequent disability or incapacity of the principal or lapse of time" (Uniform Durable Power of Attorney Act [U.L.A.], 1984 §§ 1, 2).

As identified in the description of the durable power of attorney relationship, there must be a person who writes the document and another person who is willing to serve as the agent or substitute decision maker. A clear limitation of this legal advance directive is the availability of someone who is willing to serve as a substitute decision maker. This legal advance directive offers greater flexibility for the person who writes the document because it is not limited to life-sustaining measures; it may apply to nursing home placement or the administration of antibiotics or other forms of non-emergency treatment. However, the major limitation of the durable power of attorney for health care is the requirement of having someone who is willing to serve in the role of substitute decision maker. Unfortunately, many elderly adults have outlived their spouses, siblings, and friends. Therefore, unless they have another relative (e.g., adult child, grandchild, niece, nephew) or close friend, they are not able to benefit from the assistance of a personal substitute decision maker or the flexibility offered by the durable power of attorney for health care.

Substitute Decision Making

If a person has not anticipated the need for health care treatment decisions and has become mentally incapacitated, then the individual is no longer capable of understanding or executing an advance directive. However, that does not mean that she has lost all control concerning pertinent health care treatment decisions. The law recognizes that a substitute or surrogate decision maker may be appointed after the person becomes incapacitated. This does not fall under the umbrella of advance planning but does provide a spokesperson to participate in the health care treatment decision making process.

All states have legislation authorizing the court to appoint a substitute decision maker, usually referred to as a *guardian,* for a minor or a cognitively incapacitated adult (Hurme, 1995-6). This legal authority, developed from the states' *parens patriae* power, identifies the states' power to protect individuals who are not able to protect themselves.

The purpose of appointing a guardian is to provide a legal mechanism for the transfer of an individual's authority for personal decisions to a responsible adult (Weiler, Helms, & Buckwalter, 1993).

NURSING DIAGNOSIS

Nursing diagnosis content related to the concept of self-determination was originally labeled as Altered Role Performance: Right of Self-Determination. In the first edition of this book, the relevant chapter attempted to identify the interrelationship between a person's legal right to make health care treatment decisions and nursing practice (Weiler, 1991). The relevance and significance of the content to the theoretical and practical aspects of the nursing profession were unquestioned. However, the question "Where does this fit within the nursing diagnosis framework?" arose several times.

The current chapter was originally conceptualized under that same classification. However, in writing the chapter, it became evident that interventions such as Patient Rights Protection and Decision-Making Support were relevant to the case studies. Questions then arose regarding the level of congruity between identified interventions and the previously developed diagnosis based on Altered Role Performance (Weiler, 1991). In addition to the disparity between the interventions and the previous diagnosis, desired outcomes such as Participation: Health Care Decisions, Decision Making, and Dignified Dying were not consistent with the literature review or the previous diagnosis. These inconsistencies led the authors to

conceptualize creation of a new diagnosis. Specifically, this chapter proposes that the old diagnosis Altered Role Performance: Right to Self-Determination should be revised to Risk for Loss of Self-Determination. Box 54-1 presents the defining characteristics and related factors for the new nursing diagnosis.

The remainder of this chapter is structured around four case studies that illustrate situations in which the right of self-determination might be challenged. The case studies are used to demonstrate how nursing interventions from the *Nursing Interventions Classification (NIC)* (Iowa Intervention Project, 2000) and patient outcomes from the *Nursing Outcomes Classification (NOC)* (Iowa Outcomes Project, 2000) can be linked to the new diagnosis. Legal case studies have been selected because they depict actual events that have created great controversy within the health care setting and have led to judicial resolution. These actual cases vividly depict (1) the potential situations that might require an individual to exercise self-determination in his or her own care, (2) the advantages of having executed an advance directive, and (3) the personal anguish that can arise for family members and health care professionals when an individual does not have the cognitive capacity to make essential decisions and has not written an advance directive.

Norwood Hospital v. Munoz (1991)

Yolanda Munoz, a thirty-eight year old woman who lives . . . with her husband, Ernesto Munoz, and their minor son. Ernesto's father, who is over seventy-five years old, also lives in the same household.

Box 54-1 Comparison of the Previous and Suggested Diagnoses for Self-Determination

Previous Nursing Diagnosis (Weiler, 1991)
Altered Role Performance: Right to Self-Determination
Defining characteristics
Negative attitude/knowledge of caregivers regarding right of self-determination
Change in others' perception of role
Change in usual patterns of responsibility
Lack of knowledge regarding right of self-determination
Lack of advocates, social support
Lack of social contacts/interactions
Incongruence of patient's stated/documented wishes regarding treatment prescribed/provided by health care professionals/caregivers
Family members'/caregivers' uncertainty regarding client's competence
Loss of autonomy/decision-making authority

Related factors/etiologies
Change in physical/mental capacity
Institutionalization
Lack of advance directive

Suggested Nursing Diagnosis
Risk for Loss of Self-Determination
Defining characteristics
Risk for or actual loss of decision-making capacity
Change in physical capacity
Change in mental capacity
Change in health status
Change in caregiver's usual pattern of responsibility regarding patient
Family members'/caregivers' uncertainty regarding patient's wishes concerning treatment
Incongruence between one's stated wishes regarding treatment and the treatment provided by caregivers

Related factors/etiologies
Change in level of personal independence
Institutionalization
Lack of advocate
Change in others' perception of patient's decision-making capacity
Lack of knowledge of advance directive
Lack of advance directive

Ms. Munoz has a history of stomach ulcers. Approximately ten years ago she underwent surgery for a bleeding ulcer. On April 11, 1989, Ms. Munoz vomited blood and collapsed in her home. During the week that she collapsed, Ms. Munoz had taken two aspirin every four hours to alleviate a pain in her arm. The aspirin apparently made her ulcer bleed. Ernesto took his wife to the Norwood Hospital emergency room. Physicians at Norwood Hospital gave Ms. Munoz medication which stopped the bleeding. Ms. Munoz was then admitted to the hospital . . . her hematocrit . . . was 17%. It was (her physician's) medical opinion that the patient had a 50% probability of hemorrhaging again. If Ms. Munoz started to bleed, (her physician) believed that she would in all probability die unless she received a blood transfusion. Ms. Munoz, however, refused to consent to a blood transfusion in the event of a new hemorrhage.

Ms. Munoz and her husband were baptized as Jehovah's Witnesses over sixteen years ago. . . . A principal tenet of the Jehovah's Witnesses religion is a belief, based on interpretations of the Bible, that the act of receiving blood or blood products precludes an individual resurrection and everlasting life after death.

Norwood Hospital sought a judicial opinion regarding Ms. Munoz's rights to refuse the transfusion and the hospital's obligations to provide indicated treatment. Ms. Munoz recovered and left the hospital without having another episode of bleeding; therefore, the judicial determination regarding her specific case became moot. However, the court agreed to review the case regarding a competent adult's refusal of life-saving medical treatment because the issue was one of public importance and capable of repeating itself while evading judicial review.

In examining a patient's right to refuse medical treatment that is considered necessary to save the patient's life, the court recognized that competent individuals have a common law right to determine for themselves whether to allow a physical invasion of their bodies (*Brophy v. New England Sinai Hospital Inc.*, 1986, p. 633; *Norwood Hospital v. Munoz*, 1991, p. 122). In addition to the common law right to refuse treatment, individuals also have a constitutional right (*Brophy v. New England Sinai Hospital Inc.*, 1986, p. 633; *Griswold v. Connecticut*, 1965; *Norwood Hospital v. Munoz*, 1991, p. 122; *Roe v. Wade*, 1973; *Superintendent of Belchertown v. Saikewicz*, 1977). All parties agreed that Ms. Munoz was a competent adult; therefore, there was no controversy regarding her capacity to make the health care treatment decision for herself (*Norwood Hospital v. Munoz*, 1991, p. 117). However, the court identified that the right to refuse medical treatment in life-threatening situations is not absolute and that four countervailing interests must be considered: (1) the prevention of suicide, (2) the preservation of life, (3) the maintenance of the ethical integrity of the medical profession, and (4) the protection of innocent third parties.

The court used the testimony to quickly decide that Ms. Munoz had no intention of committing suicide and did not want to die. In reviewing the interest in preservation of life, the court identified two relevant but distinct interests: the preservation of a specific individual's life and the sanctity of all life. In this case the issue was the preservation of one specific life—Ms. Munoz. The court concluded that, even though the State has an interest in preserving a specific life, that interest is weakened when the decision maker (the individual who refuses the treatment) is also the person whom the State is seeking to protect. In situations in which the decision maker is competent and has chosen to refuse medical treatment, the State's interest in preserving the life does not override the individual's decision. In examining the more abstract concept of protecting the sanctity of life, the court quoted a prior decision, "The duty of the State to preserve life must encompass a recognition of an individual's right to avoid circumstances in which the individual (herself) would feel that efforts to sustain life demean or degrade (her) humanity" (*Brophy v. New England Sinai Hospital Inc.*, 1986, p. 635). Because Ms. Munoz clearly believed that a blood transfusion would violate a sacred religious belief, receiving a transfusion would have diminished the quality and integrity of her life. The court determined that the State's interest in preserving life was secondary to Ms. Munoz's decision to refuse treatment.

In reviewing the preservation of the ethical integrity of the medical profession, the court recognized that medical ethics do not require that a patient's life be preserved in all circumstances (*Brophy v. New England Sinai Hospital Inc.*, 1986, p. 639). Also the court noted that, "If the doctrines of informed consent and right of privacy have as their foundations the right to bodily integrity . . . and control of one's own fate, then those rights are superior to the institutional considerations" (*Superintendent of Belchertown v Saikewicz*, 1977, p. 427). Therefore Ms. Munoz's rights to refuse the treatment outweighed the interest in preserving the ethical integrity of the medical profession.

Finally, the court examined the most difficult aspect of the case, the protection of innocent third parties. The controversy presented to the court was the potential conflict between Ms. Munoz's right to determine for herself which health care treatment she would accept or reject and her responsibilities, both to her family and to society, to provide care for her young son. The State's interest in protecting Ms. Munoz's minor son was discussed at length by the court. The testimony indicated that Ms. Munoz was the primary caregiver for her son. Mr. Munoz worked long hours driving his own commercial truck. Mr. Munoz' father, who lived with the family, was an elderly individual and did not contribute to the care or upbringing of the child. Therefore an argument was made that if Ms. Munoz died as a result of having a bleeding ulcer she would effectively be abandoning her child. However, that argument was countered when it was identified that, if Ms. Munoz were to die, Mr. Munoz had the financial resources to provide for daily care and the material needs of his son. Additionally, Mr. Munoz's sister and brother-in-law had supported Ms. Munoz's decision to refuse the blood transfusion and had volunteered to assist in caring for and raising her son. In examining Ms. Munoz's right, as a competent adult, to determine which health care she would accept and which she would reject, the court identified that none of the State's interests outweighed her right to make her own decisions.

In this case it is clear that Ms. Munoz had the mental capacity to make this decision. It is also clear that her decision was based on a religious belief that was supported by her family. In this case the nursing diagnosis Risk for Loss of Self-Determination would be appropriate. It is important that nurses support a patient's decision and serve as an advocate for the patient and family. Box 54-2 identifies the primary outcome and intervention that would be appropriate for this case study. The major goal in Ms. Munoz' situation would be her participation in health care decision making. The NOC outcome Participation: Health Care Decisions focuses on involving patients in health care treatment options. It is defined as "personal involvement in selecting and evaluating health care options" (Iowa Outcomes Project, 2000, p. 335). Several key indicators for this outcome that relate to this case study are included in Box 54-2. Other NOC outcomes to consider for this case include Decision Making, Will to Live, Acceptance: Health Status, and Health Beliefs: Perceived Threat (Iowa Outcomes Project, 2000).

The focus of the nurse's intervention should be on protecting Ms. Munoz's right to decide what health care treatment she receives. The NIC intervention Patient Rights Protection is defined as the "protection of the health care rights of a patient, especially a minor, incapacitated, or incompetent patient unable to make decisions" (Iowa Intervention Project, 2000, p. 497). However, Ms. Munoz's ability to decide her care, although mentally competent, was challenged in the courts because of her incapacitated condition. Several key nursing activities for this intervention are included under this intervention in Box 54-2.

Other nursing interventions appropriate for this case include the NIC interventions Decision-Making Support, defined as "providing information and support for a patient who is making a decision regarding health care" (Iowa Intervention Project, 2000, p. 243) and Values Clarification, defined as "assisting another to clarify her/his own values in order to facilitate effective decision-making" (Iowa Intervention Project, 2000, p. 693). These interventions would be particularly helpful if the nurse were involved during the time the patient was in the process of deciding between the possible treatment options.

Lane v. Candura (1978)

This case concerns a 77-year-old widow, Mrs. Rosaria Candura, of Arlington, . . . a patient at the Symmes Hospital in Arlington suffering from gangrene in the right foot and lower leg. . . . Her daughter, . . . filed a petition in Probate Court for Middlesex County seeking appointment of herself as temporary guardian with authority to consent to the operation on behalf of her mother. An order and a judgment were entered in the Probate Court to that effect, from which the guardian *ad litem* appointed to represent Mrs. Candura has appealed. . . .

The principal question arising on the record before us, therefore, is whether Mrs. Candura has the legally requisite competence of mind and will to make the choice for herself. The (trial court) decision does not include a clear-cut finding that Mrs. Candura lacks the requisite legal competence. . . .

We hold that Mrs. Candura has the right under the law to refuse to submit either to medical treatment or a surgical operation, that on the evidence and findings in this case the decision is one that she may determine for herself, and that therefore her leg may not be amputated unless she consents to that course of action. . . .

Mrs. Candura was a 77-year-old widow who had a history of an infected toe on the right foot in 1974, which had became gangrenous and was amputated. Mrs. Candura reinjured her right foot in 1977, gangrene

---

Box 54-2	Nursing Diagnosis, Outcome, and Intervention for *Norwood Hospital v. Munoz*

Nursing Diagnosis
Risk for Loss of Self-Determination
Defining characteristics
Incongruence between one's stated wishes regarding treatment and the treatment provided by caregivers

Related factors/etiologies
Change in health status
Change in level of personal independence
Institutionalization

Nursing-Sensitive Outcome
Participation: Health Care Decisions
Indicators
Claims decision-making responsibility
Specifies health outcome preferences

Identifies health outcome priorities
Negotiates for care preferences
Evaluates satisfaction with health care outcomes

Nursing Intervention
Patient Rights Protection
Activities
Determine whether patient's wishes about health care are known
Provide patient with *Patient's Bill of Rights*
Work with the physician and administration to honor patient and family wishes
Refrain from forcing treatment
Note religious preference

resulted, and a portion of the right foot was amputated. In 1978, after a difficult recovery, Mrs. Candura injured the right leg again and the surgical decision was to amputate the remainder of the right foot. Mrs. Candura originally consented to and then refused the surgical procedure.

The trial court found that Mrs. Candura was disappointed in the failure of the earlier operations to arrest the gangrene. The court determined that she did not believe that the operation would cure her and that she did not want to live as an invalid in a nursing home. Furthermore, the court stated that she did not fear death but welcomed it. She was described as stubborn, somewhat irascible, hostile to certain doctors, and occasionally combative in response to questions. Although her conception of time was distorted, overall she demonstrated a high degree of awareness and acuity in response to the question of her possible surgery. She was clear in her decision to refuse surgery, even though the decision could lead to her death.

Each adult is presumed competent to make personal health care decisions unless evidence demonstrates that the person is incompetent. The burden is not on the patient to establish competence but on the petitioners to establish incompetence. The court in Mrs. Candura's case decided that there was not sufficient evidence to defeat the presumption of competence. Although the choice of refusing surgery may have been medically irrational, it did not justify a conclusion of incompetence.

Mrs. Candura suffered a change in her physical capacity, refused surgery, and contradicted her daughter's wishes for her to have surgery. Therefore, her daughter questioned Mrs. Candura's decision-making ability and petitioned the court for the right to make personal care decisions for her mother. The court found, however, that Mrs. Candura demonstrated the requisite mental capacity to appreciate the nature and consequences of her act, and, therefore, she retained her self-determination and the freedom of individual choice.

Cases, such as Mrs. Candura's arise when a person has such extreme physical disability that the refusal of care would result in the individual's imminent death. However, in this case, Mrs. Candura still had mental capacity and, therefore, retained the right of self-determination in health care treatment decisions. Her ability to decide her own care was established by the courts. Box 54-3 identifies the key outcome and intervention that would be appropriate for this case study. The NOC outcome Decision Making is defined as the "ability to choose between two or more alternatives" (Iowa Outcomes Project, 2000, p. 194). Mrs. Candura was able to demonstrate her ability to accomplish the indicators that support this outcome. Other relevant NOC outcomes for this case study are Cognitive Ability, defined as the "ability to execute complex mental processes" (Iowa Outcomes Project, 2000, p. 170) and Health Beliefs: Perceived Control, defined as "personal conviction that one can influence a health outcome" (Iowa Outcomes Project, 2000, p. 228).

The primary nursing intervention in this case would be to support Mrs. Candura's decision-making process. The relevant nursing activities for the NIC intervention Decision-Making Support (Iowa Intervention Project, 2000) are highlighted in Box 54-3. Additional interventions that could be helpful are Family Process Maintenance, defined as "minimization of family process disruption effects" (Iowa Intervention Project, 2000, p. 336) and Coping Enhancement, defined as "assisting a patient to adapt to perceived stressors, changes, or threats that interfere with meeting life demands and threats" (Iowa Intervention Project, 2000, p. 234).

Box 54-3   Nursing Diagnosis, Outcome, and Intervention for *Lane v. Candura*

Nursing Diagnosis
Risk for Loss of Self-Determination
Defining characteristics
Change in physical capacity
Change in health status
Incongruence between stated wishes for treatment and the treatment provided by caregivers

Related factors/etiologies
Change in level of personal independence
Institutionalization
Change in others' perception of patient's decision-making capacity
Lack of knowledge of advance directives

Nursing-Sensitive Outcome
Decision Making
Indicators
Identifies relevant information
Identifies alternatives

Identifies potential consequences of each alternative
Recognizes contradictions with others' desires
Acknowledges relevant legal implications
Acknowledges social context of the situation
Chooses among alternatives

Nursing Intervention
Decision-Making Support
Activities
Determine whether there are differences between the patient's view of own condition and the view of health care providers
Inform patient of alternative views or solutions
Facilitate collaborative decision making
Help patient explain decision to others as needed
Serve as a liaison between patient and family
Refer to legal aid, as appropriate
Serve as a liaison between patient and other health care providers

Bartling v. Superior Court (1984)

. . . Mr. Bartling was 70 years old and suffered from emphysema, chronic respiratory failure, arteriosclerosis, an abdominal aneurysm . . . and a malignant tumor of the lung. Mr. Bartling also had a history of . . . 'chronic acute anxiety/depression' and alcoholism.

(Mr. Bartling) was placed on a ventilator . . . remained on the ventilator until the time of his death, and efforts to "wean" him from the machine were unsuccessful. A living will, signed by Mr. Bartling with an "X" and properly witnessed . . . stated in part: "If at such time the situation should arise in which there is no reasonable expectation of my recovery from extreme physical or mental disability, I direct that I be allowed to die and not be kept alive by medications, artificial means, or heroic measures."

A "Durable Power of Attorney for Health Care," executed by Mr. Bartling . . . stated in part: "I do not wish to continue to live under these conditions. It is therefore my intent to refuse to continue on ventilator support and thereby to permit the natural process of dying to occur—peacefully, privately, and with dignity" . . .

The trial court . . . findings, include(ed): (1) Mr. Bartling's illnesses were serious but not terminal . . .; (2) although Mr. Bartling was attached to a respirator to facilitate breathing, he was not in a vegetative state and was not comatose; and (3) Mr. Bartling was competent in the legal sense . . .

There is no question in our minds that Mr. Bartling was, as the trial court determined, competent in the legal sense to decide whether he wanted to have the ventilator disconnected . . .

Having resolved the threshold issue of whether or not Mr. Bartling was legally competent, we turn to the major issue in this case: whether the right of Mr. Bartling, as a competent adult, to refuse unwanted medical treatment, is outweighed by the various state and personal interests . . .

In California, "a person of adult years and in sound mind has the right, in the exercise of control over his own body, to determine whether or not to submit to lawful medical treatment."

Mr. William Bartling was a 70-year-old man with an extensive medical history, who was admitted to a private religious hospital for treatment of his depression. On admission, a routine chest x-ray identified the presence of a lung tumor. The tumor was examined by a needle biopsy, which resulted in a collapsed lung. The lung did not reinflate, a tracheostomy tube was placed, and respiratory support with a ventilator was provided. Mr. Bartling's physicians identified that he was seriously ill. However, he was not terminally ill, and death was not imminent.

There was no disagreement between Mr. Bartling, his wife, the physician, the hospital, or the court that Mr. Bartling was competent to make his health care decisions. Mr. Bartling wanted to live but preferred death to life on a ventilator. In the event that Mr. Bartling became incompetent to make health care treatment decisions, he executed a written living will, which stated his desire to cease his daily struggle with life. He also made and signed a durable power of attorney for health care, naming his wife as the attorney-in-fact.

Mr. Bartling tried to detach the ventilator from the tracheostomy tube himself. He was subsequently restrained with soft restraints so that he could not accidentally or intentionally disconnect the ventilator. The hospital sought an injunction to prevent Mr. Bartling or his representative from disconnecting the ventilator. The hospital argued that as a religious hospital it could not ethically participate in this patient's suicide. The hospital also expressed concern about potential civil and criminal liability if they disconnected the respirator.

The question before the court was whether a competent adult's right to refuse unwanted medical treatment is outweighed by various state and personal interests. The court decided an adult has the right to determine whether or not to accept medical treatment. The Bartling decision is viewed as extending the right to self-determination to situations in which there is a serious but not a terminal illness.

The factors that were relevant in evaluating Mr. Bartling's right of self-determination included his change in physical capacity, his questionable change in mental capacity, the hospital's refusal to follow his verbal or written directives, and the hospital's application for a court injunction. All of these were important in evaluating Mr. Bartling's right of self-determination.

Mr. Bartling communicated his decision regarding his health care treatment and provided two written advance directives that were to be followed in the event that he was no longer able to personally communicate those wishes. He did not need to rely on the ability of another person to make his decision. However, he did provide written advance directives in the event that they were needed. These written directives had been communicated to his wife, the physicians, the hospital, and the court. These directives served as verification that he wished to have his wife serve as his substitute decision maker if he became incapable of making his own decisions.

This case study varies from the two discussed previously in that Mr. Bartling had taken steps to control the types of treatments he could receive by writing a living will and appointing a surrogate decision maker. It is clear that there were treatments that were unacceptable to him (such as life on a ventilator). Mr. Bartling appointed his wife as his decision maker should he become incapacitated and unable to make his own decisions. Box 54-4 highlights the outcome and interventions that are appropriate for this case study.

Mr. Bartling's desire to control his destiny in terms of medical treatment focused on his desire to control his own death based on his values of life and his personal view of quality. The NOC outcome Health Beliefs: Perceived Threat, defined as "personal conviction that a health problem is serious and has potential negative consequences for lifestyle" (Iowa Outcomes Project, 2000, p.

| Box 54-4 | Nursing Diagnosis, Outcome, and Intervention for *Bartling v. Superior Court* |

Nursing Diagnosis
Risk for Loss of Self-Determination
Defining characteristics
Risk for or actual loss of decision-making capacity
Change in physical capacity
Incongruence between one's stated wishes regarding treatment and the treatment provided by caregivers
Change in mental capacity

Related factors/etiologies
Institutionalization
Change in level of personal independence
Change in others' perception of patient's decision-making capacity

Nursing-Sensitive Outcome
Health Beliefs: Perceived Control
Indicators
Perceived responsibility for health decisions
Requested involvement in health decisions

Maintains sense of control of remaining time
Belief that own decisions control health outcomes
Belief that own actions control health outcomes
Willingness to designate surrogate decision maker
Willingness to have current living will

Nursing Intervention
Patient Rights Protection
Activities
Work with physicians and hospital administration to honor patient and family wishes
Honor a patient's wishes expressed in a living will or durable power of attorney for health care
Know the legal status of living wills in the state
Determine whether patient's wishes about health care are known
Work with the physician and administration to honor patient and family wishes
Refrain from forcing treatment

---

230), is relevant to this case study. Other NOC outcomes that could be used are Dignified Dying, defined as "maintaining personal control and comfort with the approaching end of life" (Iowa Outcomes Project, 2000, p. 198), Decision Making, and Participation: Health Care Decisions.

Once again the role of the nurse is to work with the patient and his family. The nursing intervention Patient Rights Protection focuses on protecting his right to control decisions (Iowa Intervention Project, 2000). Additional interventions that would be useful in this case are Decision-Making Support and Dying Care (Iowa Intervention Project, 2000).

Cruzan v. Director, Missouri Department of Health (1990)

On the night of January 11, 1983, Nancy Cruzan lost control of her car. The vehicle overturned, and Cruzan was discovered lying face down in a ditch without detectable respiratory or cardiac function. Paramedics were able to restore her breathing and heartbeat at the accident site, and she was transported to a hospital in an unconscious state. An attending neurosurgeon diagnosed her as having sustained probable cerebral contusions compounded by significant anoxia (lack of oxygen). She now lies in a Missouri state hospital in what is commonly referred to as a persistent vegetative state: generally, a condition in which a person exhibits motor reflexes, but evinces no indications of significant cognitive function. . . .

After it had become apparent that Nancy Cruzan had virtually no chance of regaining her mental faculties, her parents asked hospital employees to terminate the artificial nutrition and hydration procedures. All agreed that such removal would cause her death. The employees refused to honor the request without court approval. The parents then sought and received authorization from the state trial court for termina-

tion. The Court found that a person in Nancy's condition had a fundamental right under the State and Federal Constitutions to refuse or direct the withdrawal of "death prolonging procedures." . . . The court also found that Nancy's "expressed thoughts at age twenty-five in a somewhat serious conversation with a house-mate friend that if sick or injured she would not wish to continue her life unless she could live at least halfway normally, suggests that given her present condition she would not wish to continue on with her nutrition and hydration." . . .

The Supreme Court of Missouri reversed on a divided vote. The court recognized a right to refuse treatment embodied in the common-law doctrine of informed consent, but expressed skepticism about the application of that doctrine in the circumstances of this case. . . .

We granted *certiorari* to consider the question whether Cruzan has a right under the United States Constitution which would require the hospital to withdraw life-sustaining treatment from her under these circumstances. . . .

The logical corollary of the doctrine of informed consent is that the patient generally possesses the right not to consent, that is, to refuse treatment . . . most courts have based a right to refuse treatment either solely on the common-law right to informed consent or on both the common-law right and a constitutional privacy right . . . Distilling certain state interests from prior case law—the preservation of life, the protection of the interests of innocent third parties, the prevention of suicide, and the maintenance of the ethical integrity of the medical profession— . . . the issue is not whether, but when, for how long, and at what cost to the individual [a] life may be briefly extended. . . .

But in the context presented here, a State has more particular interests at stake. The choice between life and death is a deeply personal decision of obvious and overwhelming finality. We believe Missouri may legitimately seek to safeguard the personal element of this choice through the imposition of heightened evidentiary requirements. It cannot be disputed that the Due Process Clause protects an interest in life as well as an interest in refusing life-sustaining medical treatment. . . . (w)e think a State may properly decline to make judgments about the "quality" of life that a particular individual may enjoy, and simply assert an unqualified interest in the preservation of human life to be weighed against the constitutionally protected interests of the individual.

In our view, Missouri has permissibly sought to advance these interests through the adoption of a "clear and convincing" standard of proof to govern such proceedings. "The function of a standard of proof, as that concept is embodied in the Due Process Clause and in the realm of fact finding, is to "instruct the fact finder concerning the degree of confidence our society thinks he should have in the correctness of factual conclusions for a particular type of adjudication'" (citations omitted). "This Court has mandated an intermediate standard of proof—'clear and convincing evidence'—when the individual interests at stake in a state proceeding are both 'particularly important' and 'more substantial than mere loss of money'" (citations omitted). . . .

In sum, we conclude that a State may apply a clear and convincing evidence standard in proceedings where a guardian seeks to discontinue nutrition and hydration of a person diagnosed to be in a persistent vegetative state. . . .

The Supreme Court of Missouri held that in this case the testimony adduced at trial did not amount to clear and convincing proof of the patient's desire to have hydration and nutrition withdrawn. The judgment of the Supreme Court of Missouri is Affirmed.

Nancy Cruzan was injured in an automobile accident on January 11, 1983, and the next month a gastrostomy feeding tube was placed. At the time of her accident, Nancy Cruzan was 25 years old, had been in good health, and had never written any advance directive regarding her potential health care treatment. Nancy had, however, had serious discussions with a housemate about her beliefs regarding the quality of life that she would find intolerable and not worth living. In October of 1987, her parents, as her guardians, petitioned the county court judge to remove the feeding tube and he approved their request. The Missouri Attorney General appealed the case to the Missouri Supreme Court, which overturned the lower court ruling and held that there was no clear and convincing evidence of what Nancy would have wanted to have done if she could have chosen her own course of treatment (*Cruzan v. Harmon*, 1988).

The Missouri Supreme Court decision was appealed to the United States Supreme Court and the State court decision was upheld. Therefore, under the United States Supreme Court ruling, the gastrostomy feeding tube could not be removed from Nancy's body (*Cruzan v. Director, Missouri Department of Health*, 1990).

As identified earlier, a person has a Constitutional and common law right to accept or reject health care treatment. However, this is not an absolute right but is balanced against several societal interests. The critical question in the United States Supreme Court Cruzan decision was whether the state of Missouri, in a attempt to protect society's interest in all human life, could require clear and convincing evidence of the individual's previously stated or written preferences for health care treatment before authorizing the withdrawal of treatment. This question was particularly important because it seemed clear that the removal of the gastrostomy tube would hasten Nancy's death.

The United States Supreme Court held that Missouri could require clear and convincing evidence of the individual's preferences before removing care that could end her life. For Nancy and her parents this seemed to indicate either that more information was needed to clearly and convincingly establish Nancy's verbal expressions of her preferences before her accident or that Nancy would have to continue to live with a gastrostomy tube. In August, 1990, Nancy's parents brought a second petition to the original county court judge with additional testimony regarding comments which Nancy had made before her accident about living in an impaired condition. Her parents, as her guardians, asserted that they were acting in a substitute decision making capacity for Nancy, based upon additional testimony, and were requesting the removal of the gastrostomy tube. The State of Missouri did not challenge the second petition, so the Cruzan's second request for removal of the feeding tube was granted by the county court on December 14, 1990. Nancy Cruzan died on December 26, 1990.

This case study illustrates a situation where a patient is unable to make her own decisions about health care because of loss of cognitive ability. As her substitute decision makers, her parents' desired outcome was that she have a dignified death. The NOC outcome Dignified Dying, defined as "maintaining personal control and comfort with the approaching end of life" (Iowa Outcomes Project, 2000, p. 198) is an appropriate outcome for this case study. As Box 54-5 illustrates, there are only two indicators for this outcome that work in this situation. The outcome focuses on patient behaviors that imply the patient is cognitively intact. Additional indicators need to be added to this outcome to include living wills, durable power of attorney for health care, and surrogate decision makers for individuals who were cognitively impaired at birth or those who have become cognitively impaired. This case illustrates that a broader view of dignified dying is needed for this outcome to include the patient's ability to plan and control health care by using surrogate decision makers. Once again the NIC intervention Patient Rights Protection (Iowa Intervention Project, 2000) would be appropriate for this case.

The four case studies presented in this chapter provide examples of actual patient situations that have challenged the right to self-determination. Box 54-6 provides a summary of the NIC interventions and NOC outcomes that were useful in these case studies. It is clear that outcomes and interventions linked to the nursing diagnosis Risk for Loss of Self-Determination are useful and important in today's health care environment.

Box 54-5   Nursing Diagnosis, Outcome, and Intervention for *Cruzan v. Director, Missouri Department of Health*

Nursing Diagnosis
Risk for Loss of Self-Determination
Defining characteristics
Change in mental capacity
Change in health status
Change in physical capacity
Change in caregivers' usual patterns of responsibility regarding the patient
Actual loss of decision-making capacity
Family members/caregivers uncertainty regarding patient's wishes concerning treatment
Incongruence between one's stated wishes regarding treatment and the treatment provided by caregivers
Change in others' perception of patient's decision-making capacity
Institutionalization

Related factors/etiologies
Change in level of personal independence
Lack of advance directive

Nursing-Sensitive Outcome
Dignified Dying
Indicators
Shares feelings about dying
Controls treatment choices

Nursing Intervention
Patient Rights Protection
Activities
Determine whether patient's wishes about health care are known
Determine who is legally empowered to give consent for treatment or research
Work with physician and hospital administration to honor patient and family wishes

---

Box 54-6   Summary of Outcomes and Interventions
RISK FOR LOSS OF SELF-DETERMINATION

Outcomes
Participation: Health Decisions
Decision Making
Will to Live
Acceptance: Health Status
Health Beliefs: Perceived Threat
Cognitive Ability
Health Belief: Perceived Control
Dignified Dying

Interventions
Patient Rights Protection
Decision-Making Support
Values Clarification
Family Process Maintenance
Coping Enhancement
Dying Care

SUMMARY

The relevance of the concept of self-determination to nursing practice is in the early stages of development. During the last two decades, health care treatments based on technology have become very common. As the complexity of health care increases, patients' desire to control the treatments they receive will continue and the potential for conflict may increase for patients, family members, and care providers.

The American Nurses' Association Code for Nurses explicitly identifies the nurse's role with regard to patient autonomy: "The nurse provides services with respect for human dignity and the uniqueness of the client unrestricted by considerations of social or economic status, personal attributes, or the nature of health problems" (American Nurses' Association, 1985). The accompanying interpretive statements clarify that clients have a moral right to determine what will be done to their own person and that "truth-telling and the process of reaching informed choice underlie the exercise of self-determination . . ." (American Nurses' Association, 1985). Ideally, families would discuss these serious issues before needing legal documents, and patients would understand the options available to them before admission to a hospital or clinic setting. In lieu of this ideal, nurses must teach patients how to protect their ability to control their health care treatments. To assist patients, nurses will have to have knowledge of state laws regarding advance directives and understand the strengths and weaknesses of the various documents. Providing public and professional education are critical roles for the nurse in the implementation of the Patient Self-Determination Act (American Nurses' Association, 1991).

Hospitals are now required to ask patients on admission if they have an advance directive (Pub. L. N. 101-508); however, the ability to create such a document while hospitalized is not easy. Although an example of an advance directive protocol for nurses was recently published (Mezey, Bottrell, Ramsey & NICHE faculty, 1996), it will continue to be difficult to accomplish the writing of these legal documents in the hospital setting. Hospital employees usually are not allowed to witness such documents. Patients facing major surgeries and life-threatening illnesses are not in the optimum physical or mental health and need to have support for their decision making. Nurses need to continue efforts to assist patients with advance directives. Nurses also must facilitate the completion of advance directives by patients who wish to write living wills and durable powers of attorney.

It is imperative that nursing knowledge and practice advance in the area of self-determination. It has been proposed that a new diagnosis Risk for Loss of Self-Determination be developed. Assessment parameters need to include questions pertaining to living wills, durable powers of attorney for health care, and the presence of a guardian (Mezey, Bottrell, Ramsey, & NICHE faculty, 1996). It would also be helpful to develop a nursing diagnosis that addresses the knowledge component of self-determination. For example, a nursing diagnosis entitled Knowledge Deficit: Advance Directives would be useful, and nursing interventions focused on teaching could be developed to address this problem (e.g., Teaching: Advance Directive). Box 54-6 provides a summary of the NIC interventions and NOC outcomes that are currently available to address Risk for Loss of Self-Determination. An outcome such as Self-Determination needs to be developed to address the behaviors an individual must complete to ensure protection of the right of self-determination. An intervention such as Self-Determination Enhancement could be developed to assist patients and families to address these issues. As nursing moves into more community and home settings, the opportunities to use such an intervention will be greatly increased.

REFERENCES

American Nurses' Association. (1991). *Position statement on nursing and the patient self-determination act.* Kansas City, MO: Author.

American Nurses' Association. (1985). *Code for nurses with interpretive statements.* Kansas City, MO: Author.

Application of President & Directors of Georgetown College, Inc. (1964). 331 F.2d 1000, 1008 (D.C.Cir), cert. denied, 377 U.S. 978, 84 S.Ct. 1883, 12 L.Ed.2d 746.

Bartling v. Superior Court. (1984). 209 Cal. Rptr. 220.

Berrio, M. W., & Levesque, M. E. (1996). Advance directives: Most patients don't have one. Do yours? *American Journal of Nursing, 96*(8), 24-29.

Brophy v. New England Sinai Hospital Inc. (1986). 497 N.E.2d 626.

Campbell, M. L. (1995). Interpretation of an ambiguous advance directive. *Dimensions of Critical Care Nursing, 14*(5), 226-233.

Cohen-Mansfield, J., Rabinovich, B., Lipson, S., Fein, A., Gerber, B., Weisman, S., & Pawlson, G. (1991). The decision to execute a durable power of attorney for health care and preferences regarding the utilization of life-sustaining treatments in nursing home residents. *Archives of Internal Medicine, 151,* 289-294.

Cohn, S. D. (1983). The living will from the nurse's perspective. *Law, Medicine & Health Care, 11*(3), 121-124, 136.

Collins, E., & Mozdzierz, G. (1996). Ethical considerations in treating oncology patients in the intensive care unit. *Critical Care Nursing Quarterly, 18*(4), 44-53.

Cooley, T. M. (1930). *A treatise on the law of torts.* (National Textbook Series) 29.

Cruzan v. Director, Missouri Department of Health. (1990). 110 S. Ct. 2841.

Cruzan v. Harmon. (1988). 760 SW 2d. 408.

Davitt, J. K., & Kaye, L. W. (1996). Supporting patient autonomy: Decision making in home health care. *Social Work: Journal of the National Association of Social Workers, 41*(1), 41-50.

Ferdinand, R. (1996). Ethical dilemmas. Jehovah's Witnesses and advance directives. *American Journal of Nursing, 96*(3), 64.

Gamble, E., McDonald, P., & Lichstein, P. (1991). Knowledge, attitudes, and behavior of elderly persons regarding living wills. *Archives of Internal Medicine, 151,* 277-280.

Gates, M. F., Schins, I., & Smith, A. S. (1996). Applying advanced directive regulations in home health agencies. *Home Health Care Nurse, 14*(2), 127-133.

Griswold v. Connecticut. (1965). 381 U.S. 479.

Hepburn, K., & Reed, R. (1995). Ethical and clinical issues with Native-American elders: End-of-life decision making. *Clinics in Geriatric Medicine, 11*(1), 97-111.

High, D. (1991). A new myth about families of older people. *The Gerontologist, 31*(5), 611-618.

Hurme, S. B. (1995-6). Current trends in guardianship reform. *Maryland Journal of Contemporary Legal Issues, 7*(1), 143-189.

Huth, J. (1995). Practical points. Advanced directives and the Patient Self-Determination Act: What is a nurse to do? *Journal of Post-Anesthesia Nursing, 10*(6), 336-339.

In re Storar. (1981). 420 N.E.2d 64.

Iowa Intervention Project. J. C. McCloskey & G. M. Bulechek (Eds.). (2000). *Nursing intervention classification* (3rd ed.). St. Louis, MO: Mosby.

Iowa Outcomes Project. M. Johnson, M. Maas, & S. Moorhead (Eds.). (2000). *Nursing outcomes classification (NOC)* (2nd ed.). St. Louis, MO: Mosby.

Jacobson v. Massachusetts. (1905). 197 U.S. 11.

Johns, J. L. (1996). Advance directives and opportunities for nurses. *Image: The Journal of Nursing Scholarship, 28*(2), 149-153.

Klaus, B. D. (1995). Advance directives: Matters of life and death. *Nurse Practitioner: American Journal of Primary Health Care, 20*(10), 88, 90.

Kolcaba, K. Y., & Fisher, E. M. (1996). A holistic perspective on comfort care as an advance directive. *Critical Care Nursing Quarterly, 18*(4), 66-76.

Lane v. Candura. (1978). 376 N.E.2d 1232.

Matter of Conroy. (1985). 486 A.2d 1209.

Matter of Quinlan. (1976). 355 A.2d 647.

Matter of Spring. (1980). 405 N.E.2d 115.

Meier, D. E., Fuss, B. R., O'Rourke, D., Baskin, S. A., Lewis, M., & Morrison, R. S. (1996). Marked improvement in recognition and completion of health care proxies. A randomized controlled trial of counseling by hospital patient representatives. *Archives of Internal Medicine, 156*(11), 1227-1232.

Mezey, M., Bottrell, M. M., Ramsey, G., & The NICHE Faculty. (1996). Advance directives protocol: Nurses helping to protect patient's rights. *Geriatric Nursing, 17,* 204-210.

Mezey, M., Kluger, M., Maislin, G., & Mittelman, M. (1996). Life-sustaining treatment decisions by spouses of patients with Alzheimer's disease. *Journal of the American Geriatrics Society, 44*(2), 144-150.

Mouton, C. P., Johnson, M. S., & Cole, D. R. (1995). Ethical considerations with African-American elders. *Clinics in Geriatric Medicine, 11*(1), 113-129.

Norwood Hospital v. Munoz. (1991). 409 Mass. 116.

Ott, B. B., & Hardie, T. L. (1997). Readability of advance directive documents. *Image: The Journal of Nursing Scholarship, 29*(1), 53-57.

Patient Self-Determination Act. (1990). Pub. L. N. 101-508.

Pearlman, R. A., & Uhlmann, R. F. (1988). Quality of life in chronic diseases: Perceptions of elderly patients. *Journal of Gerontology, 43*(2), M25-M30.

Perry, L. D., Nicholas, D., Molzahn, A. E., & Dossetor, J. B. (1995). Attitudes of dialysis patients and caregivers regarding advance directives. *ANNA Journal, 22*(5), 457-463, 481.

Pratt v. Davis. (1906). 118 Ill. App. 161, 166 (1905), aff'd 224 Ill. 300, 79 N.E.562.

President's Commission for the Study of Ethical Problems in Medicine and Biomedical and Behavioral Research. (1983). Deciding to Forego Life-Sustaining Treatment, 32.

Rein, A. J., Harshman, D. L., Frick, T., Phillips, J. M., Lewis, S., & Nolan, M. T. (1996). Advance directive decision making among medical patients. *Journal of Professional Nursing, 12*(1), 39-46.

Restatement, Second, Agency. (1958). St. Paul, MN: American Law Institute.

Roe v. Wade. (1973). 410 U.S. 113.

Sabino, C. P. (1996). Ten legal myths about advance directives. *Journal of Nursing Law, 3*(1), 35-41.

Schirm, V., & Stachel, L. (1996). The values history as a nursing intervention to encourage use of advance directives among older adults. *Applied Nursing Research, 9*(2), 93-96.

Schloendorff v. Society of New York Hospital. (1914). 105 N.E. 92.

Schonwetter, R. S., Walker, R. M., & Robinson, B. E. (1995). The lack of advanced directives among hospice patients. *Hospice Journal: Physical, Psychological, & Pastoral Care of the Dying, 10*(3), 1-11.

Schonwetter, R. S., Walker, R. M., Solomon, M., Indurkhya, A., & Robinson, B. E. (1996). Life values, resuscitation preferences, and the applicability of living wills in an older population. *Journal of the American Geriatrics Society, 44*(8), 954-958.

Somers, T. H. (1986). *In re* Conroy: Self-determination: Extending the right to die. *Journal of Contemporary Health Law and Policy, 2,* 351-363.

Superintendent of Belchertown v. Saikewicz. (1977). 370 N.E.2d 417.

Uniform Durable Power of Attorney Act (U.L.A.). (1979). § 1 and comments.

Uniform Durable Power of Attorney Act (U.L.A.). (1984). §§ 1, 2.

Uniform Rights of the Terminally Ill Act (U.L.A.). (1985).

Union Pacific Railroad Co. v. Botsford, 141 U.S. 250, (1891).

Walker, L., & Blechner, B. (1995-6). Continuing implementation of the Patient Self-Determination Act in nursing homes: Challenges, opportunities, and expectations. *Generations, 19*(4), 73-77.

Weiler, K. (1991). Altered role performance: Potential loss of right of self-determination. In M. Maas, K. Buckwalter, & M. Hardy (Eds.), *Nursing diagnoses and interventions in the elderly* (pp. 561-570). Reading, MA: Addison-Wesley Longman.

Weiler, K., Eland, J., & Buckwalter, K. C. (1996). Iowa nurses' knowledge of living wills and perceptions of patient autonomy. *Journal of Professional Nursing, 12*(4), 245-252.

Weiler, K., Helms, L. B., & Buckwalter, K. C. (1993). A comparative study of guardianship petitions for adults and elder adults. *Journal of Gerontological Nursing, 19*(9), 15-25.

CHAPTER 55

ALTERED FAMILY PROCESSES

Linda Lindsey Davis

By 2030 as much as one third of the population in the United States will be 65 or older (U.S. Senate, 1990). Recent estimates of the numbers of community-dwelling elders who need help with activities of daily living range from 1.8 to 5.1 million elders (American Association of Retired Persons [AARP] and the Travelers Foundation, 1988; Select Committee on Aging, 1987; Stone, Cafferata, & Sangl, 1987). As more individuals live longer, more families will have the experience of caring for an aged member with some degree of functional dependence. Families are considered to be the foundation of community-based care, and the significant contributions that families make to the care of elders are well-known. However, the effects of elder care on families and the implications for nursing practice with these caregiving families are less well explored. The purpose of this chapter is to present a theoretical and empirical justification for the nursing diagnosis Altered Family Processes (Carroll-Johnson, 1989, p. 535). This diagnosis is concerned with "a change in family relationships and/or functioning" (North American Nursing Diagnosis Association [NANDA], 1999, p. 58). The intent of the chapter is to provide a knowledge base for family-focused nursing interventions and expected outcomes when there is family dysfunction around caring for a dependent elder.

Several factors make elder caregiving more likely for families in the future. First, with increasing longevity, more middle-age adults will find themselves with living parents who need some form of assistance. Second, as more women enter the workforce, there will be fewer women in the home to function as primary caregivers for family elders. Third, the trend toward smaller families means there will be fewer family members to call on for elder care. Finally, because of the combination of greater longevity and smaller families, families will be multigenerational collectives in which grandchildren and great grandchildren must assist with elder caregiving (Lieberman & Fisher, 1999).

The majority of published studies of caregiving for a frail, dependent elder have focused on home care in stroke or dementia. Each of these illnesses presents chal-

lenges for families because of the functional losses and dependencies that result. Families first take over instrumental activities of daily living (IADL), such as managing finances and providing transportation for their aging elders. When stroke is the causative factor for caregiving, families also begin to assist with basic activities of daily living (ADL), such as eating, dressing, and bathing. For the 20% to 50% of elders over age 85 with some degree of dementia (Cross & Gurland, 1986), memory loss, confusion, agitation, depression, repetitive behaviors, paranoia, and hallucinations can create a compendium of elder behaviors that distress their families and require family members to develop skills in managing behavioral problems.

Negative family caregiver outcomes associated with long-term home care for a physically and/or cognitively impaired elder are well documented in the literature. As a result of caring for a dependent elder, family members can experience a decline in their own health and well-being (Haley & Pardo, 1989), increased life stress (Davis, 1992), increased depressive symptoms (Shields, 1992; Vitaliano, Russo, Young, Teri, & Maiuro, 1991), family or marital conflicts (Semple, 1992), and feelings of burden and social isolation (Draper, Poulos, Cole, Poulos, & Ehrlich, 1992; Zarit, Orr, & Zarit, 1985). Every family system has values, traditions, and a history of experiences that influence the way the family responds. Family caregiving for a dependent elder also is affected by the following factors:

- The extent of the elder's functional dependence and the existence of specific elder behaviors that distress or disrupt family life (Gold, Reis, Feldman, Markiewicz, & Andres, 1995)
- The history and quality of relationships between the dependent elder and other family members (Rose & DelMaestro, 1990)
- The living arrangements (shared versus separate) of the elder and family caregivers (Tennstedt, Crawford, & McKinlay, 1993)
- The nature and scope of family caregiving activities (Davis & Grant, 1994)
- The consequences of caregiving on the work, family roles, and relationships of other family members (Lieberman & Fisher, 1995; Semple, 1992; Szabo & Strang, 1999; Winslow & Carter, 1999)

The author wishes to acknowledge funding support for preparation of this chapter from the School of Nursing and the Alzheimer's Disease Center at the University of Alabama at Birmingham.

- The availability and acceptability of formal and informal caregiving assistance (Mittelman et al., 1993; 1996)

ASSESSMENT

Family assessment provides the database on which family nursing diagnoses and interventions are based. It is important to assess the context of family caregiving for the elder. What are the living arrangements of the elder and other family members? Are formal and informal support services used to assist with caregiving? What has been the impact of caregiving on the work and family roles of the elder and other family members? Which family members are involved in direct caregiving (assisting with ADL) and indirect caregiving services (assisting with IADL)? A caregiving genogram can be helpful in providing a comprehensive picture of who is involved in elder caregiving. Figure 55-1 shows a caregiving genogram for a 72-year-old stroke patient who receives assistance with IADL from his three children and direct care (ADL) assistance from his spouse and a part-time sitter.

It is important to identify coexisting family life changes and crises. Are there other dependent family members such as young children or other elders receiving care? Has the family recently experienced the illness or death of another family member? Has the family recently had to cope with job loss, divorce, or moving into or out of a home? The situational and developmental stresses associated with caring for a dependent elder can place significant demands on a family already challenged by other life changes.

It is also important to have the family's perspective of the elder caregiving situation. Do other family members believe that elder caregiving is the sole responsibility of a single family member? If not, how are decisions made about the division of caregiving responsibilities? Is there a plan for respite for the primary caregiver? Answers to these questions can provide information on how the family is managing an elder caregiving situation.

Family Assessment Measures

Because of the profound impact of elder caregiving on families, a thorough and systematic family assessment of family functioning is important. A number of published measures can be used for family assessment. In general, most family assessment measures are either self-report or observational in nature (Grotevant & Carlson, 1989); both types of measures have strengths and limitations.

Self-report measures are useful for assessing the structure, functioning, and responses of the caregiving family through the eyes of one or more family members. These self-report measures can be used to explore the insider perspective of family caregiving for a dependent elder, a critical and much-needed factor in planning family care. The majority of family caregiving studies have used self-report measures to gain a family-oriented perspective of family functioning. However, the choice of family member to complete the self-report measure can influence the results of the family assessment. Some investigators have noted that family caregivers' ratings of a dependent elder's health status and behaviors generally are lower than the ratings by the elder or other family members and can be influenced by the caregiver's feelings about caregiving (Kiyak, Teri, & Borson, 1994; Knapp & Hewison, 1999).

Observation measures are used for family assessment because of their potential for offering an outsider perspective of family coping and adaptation. However, observational measures are greatly dependent on the ability of raters not to let their personal reactions affect their ratings of family situations they observe. In addition, observa-

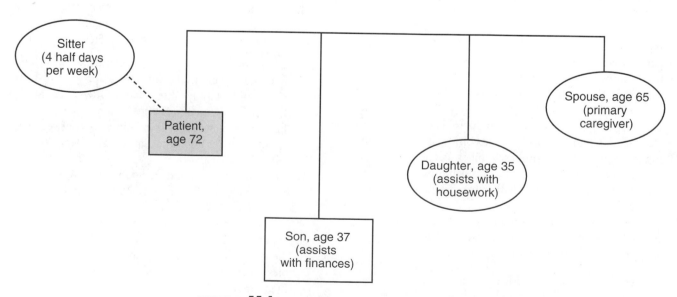

FIGURE **55-1**   A caregiving genogram for a frail elder.

tional measures require extensive training and ongoing monitoring of raters to ensure consistency in the use of the measure. Perhaps the most comprehensive approach to family assessment around elder caregiving is to combine self-report by two or more family members with observational assessment by the nurse. Table 55-1 lists descriptive characteristics of five family assessment measures

frequently cited in the elder caregiving literature over the past decade.

NURSING DIAGNOSIS

NANDA (1999, p. 58) has defined Altered Family Processes as "a change in family relationship and/or functioning."

Table 55-1	Characteristics of Five Commonly Used Family Assessment Measures			
Measures	**Type and Theoretical Focus**	**Family Constructs**	**Documented Psychometric Properties/ Administration**	**Uses**
McMaster Clinical Rating Scale (CRS)	Observational measure (7 items) Family systems theory	Rates family as functional or dysfunctional in problem solving, roles, communication, involvement, responsiveness, behavior control, overall functioning	Reliability (interrater) Validity (criterion) Raters must be trained to make clinical inferences about family functioning	Useful in determining need for clinical intervention with a family
Family Adaptability and Cohesion Scale (FACES)	Self-report (20 items) Circumplex model of family systems	Measures perceived family adaptability and cohesion	Reliability (internal consistency and test-retest) Validity (construct) Easy to administer and score	Classifies families according to 16 types of functioning
Family Environment Scale (FES)	Self-report (90 items) Social-ecologic-psychologic theory, family systems theory	Three dimensions: interpersonal relationships, basic organizational structure, personal growth	Reliability (internal consistency) Validity (construct and criterion) Three forms: measures real (Form R), ideal (Form I), and expected (E) family environment	Can be used with family members as young as age 11 to assess family functioning
Family Assessment Device (FAD)	Self-report (60 items) Structure/organization of family system	Seven scales: problem solving, roles, communication, affective responsiveness, affective involvement, behavior control, general functioning	Reliability (internal consistency and test-retest) Validity (predictive, concurrent, and construct) Easy to administer, simple to score	Useful in differentiating healthy from unhealthy families
Family Inventory of Life Events and Changes (FILE)	Self-report (71 items) Sum of normative and non-normative successors and intrafamilial strains experienced in past year Family stress theory	Nine scales: intrafamily strain, marital strain, pregnancy and childbearing strain, finance and business strain, work and family transition strains, illness and family events for a family losses, transition in or out of family, legal	Reliability (internal consistency and test-retest) Validity (concurrent) Easy to administer, simple to score	Estimates stressful life events for a family

Signs and symptoms of Altered Family Processes include changes in family roles and responsibilities, disruption in family routines, loss of privacy/autonomy of family members, isolation from others in the social network, and frequent, unresolved intrafamilial conflicts.

CASE STUDY

S. Dicklin was 71 years old when she went to live with her son Paul, his wife Janice, and their three children. A retired high school teacher, Mrs. Dicklin had always been independent and active in numerous school and church projects. After the death of her husband from a massive coronary 5 years ago, Mrs. Dicklin had managed quite well, putting her energies into a favorite civic project: teaching nonliterate adults to read. However, increasing problems with forgetfulness and impaired judgment over the past 6 months had caused her son and daughter-in-law to fear for her safety. Paul and Janice became concerned because of repeated phone calls from neighbors who reported seeing her arguing with neighbors and wandering in the street in her nightgown. Such behavior was most unusual for the elderly woman, who was well respected in her community for her friendly relations with others. Their family physician diagnosed her situation as "probable Alzheimer's disease." Moving Mrs. Dicklin into her son and daughter-in-law's home would mean that their 13- and 15-year-old daughters had to share a room, but Paul and Janice concluded that this move was preferable to constant trips across town to check on the safety of this increasingly impaired elder.

When Mrs. Dicklin first moved in, things went well. Her daughter-in-law included the elder Mrs. Dicklin in many of her own daily activities, and her granddaughters accepted the need to share a room reasonably well. The whole family participated in helping Mrs. Dicklin settle into household routines, and the children spent extra time with their grandmother in the afternoon when they came home from school. However, over the past 3 months Mrs. Dicklin's increasing memory loss, her tendency to get up and wander in the house during the night, and her declining interest in her personal hygiene began to cause numerous family problems. Janice reported that arguments ensued with her mother-in-law when she tried to get her to take a bath and change clothes. An embarrassing episode with her mother-in-law at a club luncheon caused Janice to give up many of her own social activities in an effort to spend more time at home.

Both girls began to complain that their grandmother often came into their shared bedroom and went through their things. They reported that they no longer felt comfortable inviting friends into the house because of their lack of privacy and their uncertainty about how their grandmother might respond. The noisy play of 6-year-old Jamie agitated the elderly woman and caused her to lose her temper, pace the floor, and scold everyone. Once an outgoing and conscientious child, Jamie had become sullen and began to argue with his sisters about doing household chores. As a result of the tensions around Mrs.

Dicklin's behavior and the children's reactions, Paul and Janice had numerous disagreements around what should be done. Paul began to stay late at the office every evening to avoid the worsening family situation.

Janice asked the family physician to prescribe medication to reduce her mother-in-law's agitation and to make a referral for a visiting nurse. The family decided to have a nurse from the home health agency come 3 days a week to help with hygiene care for Mrs. Dicklin. Janice remarked to the nurse with some anger, "I guess it's up to me to decide when we put Mom Dicklin in a nursing home."

The Dicklin family's altered family functioning is easily seen in the loss of personal privacy for family members and the isolation from friends and neighbors. The cumulative effects of these stressors are manifested in conflicts between family members and Mrs. Dicklin, and with each other. Paul's avoidance behavior contributes to family stress and to Janice's sense of abandonment to manage this situation alone. The confusion, growing dependence, and behavioral problems of Mrs. Dicklin, previously a highly valued, senior family member and respected community leader, have resulted in role reversal in the family. Faced with the need to become full-time caregivers, Paul, Janice, and the children now must develop new role skills and abilities.

Because of the emotionally charged and highly stressful situation around elder caregiving for the Dicklin family, the nurse elected to conduct two additional assessment visits in the home. In the first home visit the nurse met with the entire family to observe general family functioning. Using the McMaster Clinical Rating Scale (Epstein, Baldwin, & Bishop, 1982) as an observational guide, the nurse assessed family problem solving, roles, communication, mutual involvement, social responsiveness, behavior control in the stressful interview situation, and overall family functioning. During this interview Mrs. Dicklin was by turns silent and withdrawn or she interrupted and disagreed with comments made by other family members. The three children did not speak unless asked direct questions. Marital conflict between Janice and Paul was evidenced by Janice's frequent observation that she was responsible "for everything that happened in the home" and by Paul's unwillingness to look at Janice when she spoke directly to him. The nurse concluded from this interview that the family was experiencing significant functional disruption.

In the second interview the nurse met with the younger Dicklin family and had them complete the F-COPES measure (Olson et al., 1982). On the F-COPES, the family scored themselves as rating high on life stressors, as having difficulty mobilizing their personal and social resources, and as struggling with appraising their problems as capable of solution. Janice and Paul agreed that these findings were not typical of their family and were the result of family distress related to Mrs. Dicklin's memory problems, confusion, depression, and agitation. However, all of them were in agreement that they wanted to provide home care for their elder.

The nurse's next step was to consult with the physician, who reported that Mrs. Dicklin had a depressive reaction. This reaction likely developed in response to a moderate decline of cognitive function, as evidenced by her score of 22 on the Mini-Mental State Examination. The MMSE score can range from 30 to 0, with lower scores indicating greater impairment (Folstein, Folstein, & McHugh, 1975). The physician treated Mrs. Dicklin with a low-dosage antidepressant, a cerebral vasodilator, and a memory-enhancing drug.

As a result of these three assessments, the nurse concluded that the younger Dicklin family could benefit from nursing interventions designed to increase both their caregiving knowledge and skills and their ability to use simple behavioral management techniques to alleviate Mrs. Dicklin's depressive symptoms and troubling behaviors.

NURSING-SENSITIVE OUTCOMES

The nursing outcomes specific to the diagnosis Altered Family Processes are oriented toward reducing family caregiving stressors, enhancing the family's decision-making abilities around elder caregiving, and reducing family life disruption (Table 55-2) (Iowa Interventions Project, 2000; Iowa Outcomes Project, 2000). Specific indicators that caregiver stress has been reduced might include improvements in role performance, social interactions, work performance, and the caregiver-patient relationship, as well as an increase in perceived social support. Specific indicators for the outcome Decision Making might include family identification of relevant information, alternatives, and consequences of each alternative and increased ability to weigh and choose among alternatives. Finally, indicators related to disruption in the caregivers' lifestyle might include increased satisfaction with life circumstances, increased opportunities for privacy and diversional activities, and improvements in relationships, social interactions, and work productivity.

NURSING INTERVENTIONS

A major consideration in intervening with families is to focus care on the entire family system. Family-focused care may be delivered either to an individual within the context of her family or to the family as a unit. For example, although the home health nurse who implements a continence retraining program for an elderly stroke patient would be mindful of how this activity might affect family functioning, the focus for nursing care remains on the individual patient. However, should the family become conflicted around assisting with continence care for the elder, nursing interventions then might consist of convening family discussion groups for conjoint problem solving and conflict resolution. In this situation the family has become the unit for nursing intervention. Nursing activities must include a focus on assessment and intervention with the family as a caregiving unit. Intergen-

erational caregiving for a frail elder involves development of family cooperation and management of caregiving resistance of selected family members, as well as attendance to the needs of multiple generational family members. Balancing the individual needs of family members while promoting interdependence of the family as a caregiving unit is a challenge for community-based nursing practitioners.

As shown in Table 55-2, specific nursing interventions with families experiencing altered functioning as a result of caring for an impaired elder can be grouped into the following three categories: family support interventions to reduce caregiving stress, skill training interventions to enhance family problem solving and decision making around home care issues, and interventions that promote family cohesion and unity in caregiving. Numerous studies document the benefits of these three types of interventions with family caregivers of dependent elders. Interventions from all three categories typically are combined when intervening with a family.

Family Support Interventions

Many families experience anger, depression, avoidance behaviors, and a growing sense of burden as a result of caring for a physically and cognitively impaired elder. Numerous studies document the value of family counseling in helping caregiving families manage their negative reactions to elder caregiving. Based on their work with dementia patients and their families, Schmidt and Keyes (1985) found that supportive counseling sessions could reduce negative affect in caregivers. Zarit, Anthony, and Boutselis (1987) reported that family counseling was more effective than individual counseling of the primary caregiver in reducing burden around home care for a frail elder. Ferris, Steinberg, Shulman, Kahn, and Reisberg (1987) found that a combined supportive intervention for families that included home visits for family counseling, support group activities for the primary caregiver, and ad hoc telephone counseling in times of crisis could reduce depression, anger, and anxiety in family caregivers. Mittelman and colleagues (1993) noted that family involvement in counseling sessions increased the likelihood that families would provide assistance and respite for the primary family caregiver. Furthermore, when caregivers received that support, institutionalization of the dependent elder member was significantly delayed. Although these and similar studies document that families of dependent elders benefit from supportive interventions, affective support has limitations when used in isolation.

Skill Training Interventions

Families with dependent elders benefit from caregiving skill training. Pinkston, Linsk, and Young (1988) successfully

Table 55-2 Suggested Nursing-Sensitive Outcomes and Nursing Interventions
ALTERED FAMILY PROCESSES

Nursing Diagnosis	Nursing-Sensitive Outcomes	Nursing Interventions
ALTERED FAMILY PROCESSES: CARING FOR THE DEPENDENT ELDERLY FAMILY MEMBER ***Defining Characteristics*** Changes in family roles and responsibilities Disruption in daily family routines Loss of privacy/autonomy of family members Isolation from others in the social network Frequent, unresolved intrafamilial conflicts	**CAREGIVER STRESSORS** ***Indicators*** Impairment of usual role performance Impairment of social interactions Perceived lack of social support Impairment of usual work performance Amount of care or oversight required Impairment of caregiver-patient relationship	**FAMILY SUPPORT** ***Activities*** Conduct family discussion sessions to define caregiving problems and to facilitate consensus around desired caregiving outcomes Provide necessary knowledge of options to family that will assist them to make decisions about patient care Assist family in developing a list of family caregiving strengths and skills Assist family to acquire necessary knowledge, skills, and equipment to sustain their decision about patient care
	DECISION MAKING ***Indicators*** Identifies relevant information Identifies alternatives Identifies potential consequences of each alternative Recognizes contradiction with others' desires Acknowledges social context of the situation Weighing alternatives Chooses among alternatives	**FAMILY INVOLVEMENT PROMOTION** ***Activities*** Conduct family education session around the etiology, prognosis, and progressive nature of elder's health problem(s) Conduct family problem-solving and skill training sessions around managing the elder's behavioral deficits (in IADL and ADL) and behavioral excesses (e.g., agitation, anger, wandering, argumentativeness) Conduct family sessions on managing affective reactions to elder care (management of family caregiver stress, feelings of anger, hopelessness, depression) Facilitate family understanding of the medical aspects of illness Facilitate family management of the medical aspects of illness Identify other situational stressors for the family
	CAREGIVER LIFESTYLE DISRUPTION ***Indicators*** Dissatisfaction with life circumstances Role performance impaired Opportunities for privacy compromised Relationships with other family members disrupted Social interactions disrupted Diversional activities compromised Work productivity compromised Role responsibilities compromised Relationship with friends impaired	**FAMILY INTEGRITY PROMOTION** ***Activities*** Collaborate with family in increasing opportunities for daily pleasant family life events that include the dependent elder, as well as other family members Consult with family on community-based resources for respite services (for adult day care, family night out, and family vacations) Facilitate a tone of togetherness within/among the family Assist family to maintain positive relationship

taught family caregivers operand conditioning principles for improving the troubling behaviors of their dementia-impaired relatives. Teri and Uomoto (1991) reported success in teaching caregivers to monitor their agitated or depressed elder's mood and to improve the elder's affect through behavioral shaping techniques. Pynoos and Ohta (1991) individualized family caregiver skill training programs according to the specific problems that 25 families reported and enabled those caregivers to provide long-term home care for their frail elders. Quayhagen, Quayhagen, Corbeil, Roth, and Rodgers (1995) successfully trained family caregivers in the use of cognitive stimulation skills for reducing or improving their impaired elder's memory and behavior problems.

Numerous studies have documented the positive benefits of teaching stress management techniques to family caregivers. Greene and Monahan (1989) reported that family caregivers ($n = 244$) who participated in stress reduction training experienced an improvement in negative affect and a reduction in caregiving distress. Gallagher-Thompson and Steffen (1994) were successful in helping family caregivers improve their own mood and affect by teaching them how to increase the number of pleasant events in their daily lives. These and similar studies document the benefits of family caregiver skill training for behavioral management, stress management, and mood improvement. These findings also demonstrate the abilities of family caregivers to master highly complex cognitive and behavioral management skills.

Interventions That Promote Family Cohesion and Unity

Whenever possible, it is important to help families maintain or regain their sense of unity and perceived competency in managing their own problems around caregiving for an elder. Montgomery and Borgatta (1989) reported that families of frail elders ($n = 541$) seek services that enable them to solve their own caregiving problems. When offered a choice among educational seminars, support group activities, respite care, and in-home family consultation on home care skills, families chose in-home consultation services over all other types of services more than 90% of the time.

Seltzer, Ivry, and Litchfield (1987) taught caregivers and their families ($n = 157$) to function as their own case managers in securing and coordinating services for a frail, elderly family member. Families who received training successfully performed twice as many case management functions for their impaired family member as did families who did not receive such training. These investigators concluded that families of impaired elders could manage many of their own home care problems if they first received support in finding and negotiating with community-based health care systems.

CASE STUDY

Based on the results of these and similar caregiving studies, the home health nurse used the results of the family assessment to develop a program of supportive counseling and family skill training. The nurse focused on interventions that supported the Dicklin family's cohesion and unity in becoming managers of their own caregiving situation. The following five focal areas were used to organize nursing interventions and activities for this highly stressed family with a dependent elder:

Family Problem Solving. Participate with the Dicklin family in scheduling and conducting weekly family problem-solving meetings. Teach family members how to identify the ABCs (antecedents-behaviors-consequences) of a behavior problem situation. Help each member to identify ways of reducing stressful antecedent stimuli that result in the problem situation. Encourage each family member to collaborate in identifying the three priority problems for that week. Use those three priority problems to construct a caregiving diary for tracking problems. Assist the family in exploring alternative solutions for each problem and each member's contribution in solving the problem. Review weekly progress with family members.

Family Skill Training. Teach the family techniques for cueing Mrs. Dicklin's failing memory. For example, help the family to construct a refrigerator-mounted calendar of her daily schedule, showing the times of Mrs. Dicklin's favorite TV shows, plans for a trip to the store, and anticipated visits from children and grandchildren. Refer her to the schedule frequently so she can anticipate upcoming events each day. Encourage the family to sit down with Mrs. Dicklin each day and discuss the calendar of events. Help the family in developing a list of pleasurable, easily accomplished activities that Mrs. Dicklin enjoys, such as listening to music, playing simple games, and taking a favorite walk or a short car trip. Be sure to include some of these pleasurable events on the family's daily schedule. Suggest that these pleasant events be included in discussions at family meetings.

Family Health Maintenance. Remind the younger Dicklins that their own family health and well-being is a caregiving resource; thus it is important to schedule some personal time-outs and pleasant life events exclusively for themselves. Provide resources on sitter services and information on adult day care centers so they can schedule family night out on a regular basis.

Family Stress Management. Teach the family cognitive reframing skills and stress management techniques for reducing their own caregiving stress. Review those skills and techniques weekly as needed.

Family Support. Reassure the Dicklin family that behavioral management takes time and that their realistic goal should be to stabilize the frequency of problem occurrences. Once each month review family progress and management successes.

Over the course of several months, the home health nurse used weekly family meetings with the younger Dicklins to work with them on these desired outcomes. First, the nurse helped the family to put together a resource notebook of printed educational materials on the problems of dementing illness and a list of contact information on family caregiver assistance programs in their community. Then, to reduce caregiving stressors and facilitate family problem solving, the nurse worked with the Dicklin family to identify the priority caregiving problems they wanted to solve. The family identified Mrs. Dicklin's memory loss and nighttime wandering and their own loss of family privacy as priority problems they wanted to manage better. The nurse then worked with the family to outline simple behavioral management strategies that could be used to enhance Mrs. Dicklin's remaining memory function and to redirect her attention when she became confused. Through a daily family life event diary, the nurse also helped the family to identify and reduce environmental stimuli that triggered Mrs. Dicklin's nocturnal wandering behaviors. Finally, to reduce family life disruption, the nurse worked with the family to develop community-based resources that would allow them to have 1 evening each week and 1 weekend every 6 to 8 weeks away from caregiving responsibilities.

As a result of these nursing interventions, Janice enrolled Mrs. Dicklin in their church's weekly evening elder social and, through her contacts with the local Alzheimer's family support group, found a long-term care facility in the community that offered a monthly family caregiver respite program consisting of Friday-to-Sunday elder lodging at a reasonable cost.

After 4 months of nursing interventions through family meetings, the Dicklin family reported a reduction in stress levels. The nurse agreed, rating them overall much improved in the area of caregiver stressors, with the greatest improvements in the nursing outcomes of family role performance, social interactions, and caregiver-patient relationships. The Dicklins also reported reductions in family lifestyle disruptions, which they attributed to their regular weekly and monthly family respite activities. The nurse agreed with their conclusions and attributed this improvement to increased family opportunities for privacy and diversional activities. On a 5-point Family Lifestyle Disruption scale (Iowa Outcomes Project, 2000), the nurse rated overall family lifestyle disruption as improved from a preintervention score of "2" (substantial disruption) to a "3" (moderate disruption).

The nurse also rated this family's overall decision making to be improved, giving them a score of 4 (often demonstrated) on the 5-point Decision-Making scale (Iowa Outcomes Project, 2000). However, Decision Making proved to be a difficult nursing-sensitive outcome to achieve with this young family struggling to care for a progressively impaired elder. Over a period of 6 months, the nurse focused on family skill training for managing a growing number of dementia-related behavioral deficits and excesses associated with the erratic but progressive decline in Mrs. Dicklin's condition. Choosing among alternatives proved to be difficult for this family. As Janice commented sadly in a family problem-solving meeting, "Sometimes there really aren't good alternatives to choose from in making decisions about my mother-in-law." Family problem solving and decision making around a constantly changing home care situation remained the long-term focus for nursing interventions with this family.

SUMMARY

Many community-based nursing practitioners work with families attempting to cope with the stressors of elder caregiving. A family assessment that enables the practitioner to determine both the family's current functional patterns and its caregiving problems is the crucial first step in developing nursing-sensitive outcomes and data-based nursing interventions. Families benefit most from nursing interventions that combine family support and counseling, family skill training in providing home care, and strategies to promote family integrity in solving their own caregiving problems.

REFERENCES

American Association of Retired Persons and the Travelers Foundation. (1988). *A national survey of caregivers: A final report.* Washington, DC: American Association of Retired Persons.

Carroll-Johnson, R. (Ed.). (1989). *Classification of nursing diagnosis: Proceedings of the eighth conference.* Baltimore: Lippincott Williams & Wilkins.

Cross, P., & Gurland, B. (1986). *The epidemiology of dementing disorders* (Report to the Office of Technology Assessment, US Congress). Washington, DC: U.S. Government Printing Office.

Davis, L. (1992). Building a science of caring for family caregivers. *Family & Community Health, 15,* 1-9.

Davis, L., & Grant, J. (1994). Constructing the reality of recovery: Family home care management strategies. *Advances in Nursing Science, 17*(2), 66-76.

Draper, B., Poulos, C., Cole, A., Poulos, R., & Ehrlich, F. (1992). A comparison of caregivers for elderly stroke and dementia victims. *Journal of the American Geriatrics Society, 40*(9), 896-901.

Epstein, N. B., Baldwin, L. M., & Bishop, D. S. (1982). *McMaster clinical rating scale.* Unpublished manuscript. Providence, RI: Brown/Butler Family Research Program.

Ferris, S., Steinberg, G., Shulman, E., Kahn, R., & Reisberg, B. (1987). Institutionalization of Alzheimer's disease patients: Reducing precipitating factors through family counseling. *Home Health Care Services Quarterly, 8*(1), 23-51.

Folstein, M., Folstein, S., & McHugh, P. (1975). Mini-mental state: A practical method for grading the cognitive state of patients for the clinician. *Journal of Psychiatric Research, 12*(3), 189-198.

Gallagher-Thompson, D., & Steffen, A. (1994). Comparative effects of cognitive-behavioral and brief psychodynamic psychotherapies for depressed family caregivers. *Journal of Consulting and Clinical Psychology, 62*(3), 543-549.

Gold, D., Reis, M. F., Feldman, M., Markiewicz, D., & Andres, D. (1995). When home caregiving ends: A longitudinal study of outcomes for caregivers of relatives with dementia. *Journal of the American Geriatrics Society, 43*(1), 10-16.

Greene, V., & Monahan, D. (1989). The effect of a support and education program on stress and burden among family caregivers of frail elderly persons. *The Gerontologist, 29*(4), 472-477.

Grotevant, H., & Carlson, C. (1989). *Family assessment: A guide to methods and measures.* New York: Guilford Press.

Haley, W. E., & Pardo, K. M. (1989). Relationship of severity of dementia to caregiving stressors. *Psychology and Aging, 4*(4), 389-392.

Iowa Intervention Project. J. C. McCloskey & G. M. Bulechek (Eds.). (2000). *Nursing interventions classification (NIC)* (3rd ed.). St. Louis, MO: Mosby.

Iowa Outcomes Project. M. Johnson, M. Maas, & S. Moorhead (Eds.). (2000). *Nursing outcomes classification (NOC)* (2nd ed.). St. Louis, MO: Mosby.

Kiyak, H. A., Teri, L., & Borson, S. (1994). Physical and functional health assessment in normal aging and in Alzheimer's disease: Self-reports vs. family reports. *The Gerontologist, 34*(3), 324-330.

Knapp, P., & Hewison, J. (1999). Disagreement in patient and carer assessment of functional abilities after stroke. *Stroke, 30,* 934-938.

Lieberman, M., & Fisher, L. (1995). The impact of chronic illness on the health and well-being of family members. *The Gerontologist, 35*(1), 94-102.

Lieberman, M., & Fisher, L. (1999). The effects of family conflict resolution and decision-making on the provision of help for an elder with Alzheimer's disease. *The Gerontologist, 39,* 156-166.

Mittelman, M., Ferris, S., Shulman, E., Steinberg, M., & Levin, B. (1996). A family intervention to delay nursing home placement of patients with Alzheimer's disease: A randomized, controlled study. *Journal of the American Medical Association, 276*(21), 1725-1731.

Mittelman, M., Ferris, S., Steinberg, M., Shulman, E., Mackell, J., Ambinder, A., & Cohen, J. (1993). An intervention that delays institutionalization of Alzheimer's Disease patients: Treatment of spouse-caregivers. *The Gerontologist, 33*(6), 730-740.

Montgomery, R., & Borgatta, E. (1989). The effect of alternative support strategies on family caregiving. *The Gerontologist, 29*(4), 457-464.

North American Nursing Diagnosis Association. (1999). *Nursing diagnoses: Definitions & classification 1999-2000.* Philadelphia: Author.

Olson, D. H., McCubbin, H. I., Barnes, H., Larsen, A., Muxen, M., & Wilson, M. (1982). *Family inventories: Inventories used in a national survey of families across the family life cycle.* Minneapolis: University of Minnesota.

Pinkston, E., Linsk, N., & Young, R. (1988). Home-based behavioral family treatment of the impaired elderly. *Behavior Therapy, 19*(3), 331-344.

Pynoos, J., & Ohta, R. (1991). In-home interventions for persons with Alzheimer's disease and their caregivers. *Physical & Occupational Therapy in Geriatrics, 9,* 83-92.

Quayhagen, M. P., Quayhagen, M., Corbeil, R. R., Roth, P. A., & Rodgers, J. A. (1995, May/June). A dyadic remediation program for care recipients with dementia. *Nursing Research, 44*(3), 153-159.

Rose, J., & DelMaestro, S. (1990). Separation-individuation conflict as a model for understanding distressed caregivers: Psychodynamic and cognitive case studies. *The Gerontologist, 30*(5), 693-697.

Schmidt, G., & Keyes, B. (1985). Group psychotherapy with family caregivers of demented patients. *The Gerontologist, 25*(4), 347-350.

Select Committee on Aging, U.S. House of Representatives. (1987). *Exploding the myths: Caregiving in America* (Committee Publication No. 99-611). Washington, DC: U.S. Government Printing Office.

Seltzer, M., Ivry, J., & Litchfield, L. (1987). Family members as case manager's: Partnership between the formal and informal support networks. *The Gerontologist, 27*(6), 722-728.

Semple, S. (1992). Conflict in Alzheimer's caregiving families: Its dimensions and consequences. *The Gerontologist, 32*(5), 648-655.

Shields, C. (1992). Family interaction and caregivers of Alzheimer's disease patients: Correlates of depression. *Family Process, 31,* 19-33.

Stone, R., Cafferata, G. L., & Sangl, J. (1987). Caregivers of the frail elderly: A national profile. *The Gerontologist, 27*(5), 616-626.

Szabo, V., & Strang, V. (1999). Experiencing control in caregiving. *IMAGE: Journal of Nursing Scholarship, 31,* 71-75.

Tennstedt, S., Crawford, S., & McKinlay, J. (1993). Determining the pattern of community care: Is co-residence more important than caregiver relationship? *Journal of Gerontology: Social Sciences, 48*(2), S74-S83.

Teri, L., & Uomoto, J. (1991). Reducing excess disability in dementia patients: Training caregivers to manage patient depression. *Clinical Gerontologist, 10*(2), 49-63.

U.S. Senate. (1990). *Aging America: Trends and projections* (Serial 101-J). Washington, DC: U.S. Government Printing Office.

Vitaliano, P., Russo, J., Young, H., Teri, L., & Maiuro, R. (1991). Predictors of burden in spouse caregivers of individuals with Alzheimer's disease. *Psychology and Aging, 6*(3), 392-402.

Winslow, B., & Carter, P. (1999). Patterns of burden in wives who care for husbands with dementia. *Nursing Clinics of North America, 34,* 275-287.

Zarit, S., Anthony, C., & Boutselis, M. (1987). Intervention with caregivers of dementia patients: Comparison of two approaches. *Psychology and Aging, 2*(3), 225-234.

Zarit, S., Orr, N., & Zarit, J. (1985). *The hidden victims of Alzheimer's disease: Families under stress.* New York: New York University Press.

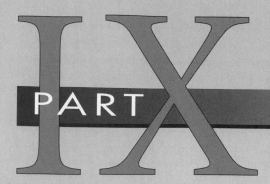

PART IX

Sexuality-Reproductive Pattern

OVERVIEW

Sexual intimacy contributes to positive body and self-image for older adults. In Chapter 56, Normal Changes With Aging, Wright reviews the usual patterns and practices of older adults, emphasizing that many elders are sexually active.

In Chapter 57 Wright analyzes the often ignored diagnosis Sexual Dysfunction among elders. The author describes the relationship between dysfunction and several common physical and functional problems, including dementia. She also details sexual difficulties following surgery, chemotherapy, and radiation treatment, as well as

difficulties related to knowledge deficit and misinformation. She discusses nursing interventions and nursing-sensitive outcomes for each type of sexual dysfunction.

Chapter 58, Altered Sexuality Patterns, focuses on etiologies inherent in the normal aging process that alter patterns of sexuality. From the perspective of the aging individual, Wright explores altered body function or structure, knowledge or skill deficit and misinformation, impaired relationships or lack of partner, and other common causes of sexual pattern change. She identifies nursing-sensitive outcomes and recommends interventions based on the described etiologies.

CHAPTER 56

NORMAL CHANGES WITH AGING

Lore K. Wright

From the Middle Ages into the twentieth century, Western cultural beliefs have held that old age is the life stage of decay, that sexual activity even between older married couples is unnatural, inappropriate, and perverse, and that sexual intimacy is appropriate only for procreation (Covey, 1989). The landmark studies by Masters and Johnson in 1966 documented that sexual activity among older people is much more common than thought, but even this evidence did not erase negative cultural stereotypes and prejudice about sexuality in older people.

However, sexuality is no longer viewed solely as the prerogative of the young. In the 1990s several factors have contributed to changing societal attitudes toward sexuality in older persons. Probably the most important factors are an increased life expectancy and better overall health of older people. Since the turn of the century, life expectancy has steadily increased. Between 1900 and 1902 the median age at death was 58 years; it rose to 74 years by the 1960s and to 79 years by the 1990s (National Center for Health Statistics, 1994). The majority of today's elders remain in fairly good physical health well into their 70s and even into their 80s (United States Bureau of the Census, 1998).

Increased attention has been given to the special needs of older people, including issues surrounding sexuality (Maas, Buckwalter, & Hardy, 1991). Seeking to gain insight into elders' own perspectives, Steinke (1994) surveyed knowledge and attitudes about sexuality in community-residing adults (total $n = 303$) ranging in age from 60 to 85. Based on open-ended questions and the Aging Sexual Knowledge and Attitude Scale (ASKAT) developed by White (1982), Steinke documented that older adults have moderate amount of knowledge and permissive attitudes, that most are sexually active and, importantly, that males and females do not differ significantly on these indicators.

OLDER PERSONS AND THEIR SEXUAL PARTNERS

For most mature men and women, intimate relationships still occur within the context of marriage. But this fact gives a clear advantage to older men, who are two to three times more likely to be married than older women. Remarriage statistics after widowhood or divorce underscore the gender differences. Widowed men age 65 and older are nearly twice as likely to remarry than are women the same age. In addition, widowed men often remarry within a year or less, whereas widowed women tend to live alone for 2 to 10 years before remarriage (Travis, 1987). Similarly, divorced men age 65 and older are about two times more likely to remarry than women age 65 and older, and these men often marry women considerably younger than themselves (United States Bureau of the Census, 1998). Overall, these statistics translate into fewer sexual partners for older women.

However, remarriage rates might not tell the full story. Some older men and women choose to live together without getting married for financial, personal, and family reasons. For example, previously married older women may not wish to lose pension or alimony payments or, if financial security permits it, both partners might wish to maintain their own residence, even though they predominantly live in one.

Remarriage plans also can lead to discord between older persons and their grown children. In the past, issues surrounding an aging parent's sexuality and issues surrounding inheritance contributed to feelings of dismay in grown children. Today, inheritance issues are still of concern, although elders are quite adept at making appropriate legal and financial arrangements.

However, dismay over sexuality in aging parents seems less of an issue in the 1990s. It is not uncommon to hear a grown daughter advise her mother to "have all the fun you want" but to be weary of remarriage. Often, the long-term illness and subsequent nursing home care costs of the previous spouse (the grown child's parent) are remembered. The awareness that caregiving responsibilities could again be required might contribute to the elder person's decisions to opt for a "companion" relationship without remarriage. National statistics support these interpretations. The number of unmarried couples 65 years old and over living together in the same household has increased by 35% in the last 9 years, i.e., from 127,000 to 195,000 (United States Bureau of the Census, 1998).

It is also of interest to note that older adults living in age-segregated, leisure-type retirement communities report significantly more sexual interest, sexual activity, and liberal attitudes than middle-income older adults who live in mainstream, age-integrated communities (Weinstein & Rosen, 1988). Obviously, age-segregated housing increases the availability of suitable partners, and it may indirectly contribute to more liberal sexual attitudes.

PATTERNS OF SEXUALITY IN OLDER PERSONS

It is generally agreed on that sexuality refers to more than physical intercourse and the achievement of orgasm. Walz and Blum (1987), in their practical guide *Sexual Health in Later Life,* provide several elegant, as well as humorous, definitions of sexuality. Sexuality, they state, is being a man or a woman and being sensual. Sexuality is the expression of feelings and self in an intimate way. And "sexuality is something that takes place more often between the ears than between the legs" (Walz & Blum, 1987, p. 4).

Sexuality, then, involves the total person and is part of a love relationship. In an earlier study Reedy, Birren, and Schaie (1982) compared young, middle-age, and older adults on five "components of love," which included communication, respect, loyalty, emotional security, as well as help and play behaviors and sexual intimacy. Adults in all three groups ranked emotional security as most characteristic of their relationship, that is, considerably higher than sexual intimacy. However, the ranking of sexual intimacy itself showed interesting patterns. Compared with young and middle-age adults, older adults ranked it as much less characteristic of their relationships (Reedy, Birren, & Schaie, 1982).

The finding of decreased sexual intimacy is consistent with the declines in sexual activity reported in a number of cross-sectional studies (Jacoby, 1999; Mulligan & Moss, 1991; Rowland, Greenleaf, Dorfman, & Davidson, 1993; Weizman & Hart, 1987). For example, Mulligan and Moss (1991) documented that sexual interest of both partners showed a gradual decline with increasing age; on average, touching or caressing occurs weekly up to age 59 and monthly for elders age 60 to 99. Sexual intercourse occurs weekly up to age 49, monthly between ages 50 and 69, and yearly at ages 70 to 99. Another study found that intercourse of 4 times a month was reported by 64% of 60 to 65 year olds, but by only 47% of those age 66 to 71 (Weizman & Hart, 1987). Interestingly, however, masturbation appears to increase with age. Whereas 9% of the 60- to 65-year-old men reported masturbation of more than 4 times per month, 26% of those age 66 to 71 reported such frequency (Weizman & Hart, 1987).

In 1984 Consumer Reports conducted a survey of sexual behavior of approximately 4200 men and women age 50 to 93 (Brecher, 1984). With increasing age, a decline in all sexual behavior was reported by both men and women. Between the ages 50 and 59, 98% of married men and 95% of married women reported being sexually active. The percentages were 93 for men and 89 for women between the ages 60 and 69. At age 70 and above, 81% of men and women were sexually active. In the 50-to-59 age-group, 90% of males and 73% of females reported to have sex at least once per week. A survey conducted by the American Association of Retired People (AARP)/Modern Maturity with 1384 adults age 45 and older found similar

trends, but slightly lower percentages for each age-group when a regular partner was present (Jacoby, 1999). However, without a regular partner, only 6% of males and less than half a percent of females over the age of 60 reported having intercourse once per week. In both the 1984 Consumer Report Survey and the 1999 AARP survey, masturbation was reported more often by males than females. Homosexual experiences after age 50 were reported by only 3.6% of men and 1.4% of women (Brecher, 1984).

A more recent national study of older married persons also documented decreased sexual frequency with increasing age, but there were no differences between males and females or between white and black respondents (Marsiglio & Donnelly, 1991). In the same study, length of marriage was found to be negatively related to frequency of sexual activity.

However, decreased sexual activity with aging is not a universal finding, and some investigators contribute decline not to the aging process itself, but to chronic illness, to psychologic factors such as boredom, and to social factors such as isolation (Mooradian & Greiff, 1990). One of the few longitudinal studies on sexual activity found that only a small subgroup of 278 married men and women age 46 to 71 reported decreased sexual activity (George & Weiler, 1981). The majority (58.3%) reported stable, i.e., exactly the same, level of sexual activity over a period of 6 years. Younger subjects (under 56 years of age at start of the study) reported a decrease in sexual activity over 6 years more often than older subjects, and women reported significantly lower levels of sexual interest and activity than their male peers. Cessation of sexual activity was highest for the over-65 age-group.

Another important finding in the longitudinal study was that "both men and women overwhelmingly attributed cessation of sexual relations to the attitudes or physical condition of the male partner" (George & Weiler, 1981, p. 922). These findings corroborate previously discussed claims that for women, a decrease in sexual activities is mainly linked to the availability of a (potent) partner.

Only recently has some attention been paid to the issues faced by older homosexuals, gays, and lesbians (Butler, Lewis, Hoffman, & Whitehead, 1994). According to a population-based study, homosexual behavior in the United States occurs in 6.2% of men and 3.6% of women (Sell & Wells, 1995). Unfortunately, the study was limited to ages 16 to 50. However, a national survey of lesbians has documented that females 55 years of age and older represent 3.1% of the total lesbian population (Bradford, Ryan, & Rothblum, 1994).

Increased acknowledgment of sexual activity has less to do with more accepting societal attitudes toward homosexuality than with fear because of the known increased risk of HIV infections and other transmittable diseases in this population (Forrester & Murphy, 1992; Taylor & Robertson, 1994). Although homosexuals continue to experience discrimination, Quam and Whitford (1992) documented that, overall, older gays and lesbians report high life satisfaction. However, loneliness and not being active in lesbian or gay social organizations hinders adjustment to aging.

PHYSIOLOGIC CHANGES WITH AGING RELATED TO SEXUALITY

Men and women experience a number of physiologic changes as part of the aging process that affect general appearance, the sex organs, and possibly psychologic and cognitive well-being. The more visual signs of aging, e.g., wrinkled skin and brown spots, a less firm body and varicose veins, do not seem to be important for sexual intimacy in established relationships, although they may become important for forming new relationships. Physiologic changes affecting the sex organs can contribute to decreasing sexual intimacy. In turn, these changes become intertwined with psychologic functioning.

The female hormone estrogen plays an important role in maintaining the structural integrity of female genitalia, and there is some evidence that other hormones, i.e., androgens and gonadotropins, have a facilitory role (Mooradian & Greiff, 1990). During menopause, ovarian function declines, leading to markedly reduced estradiol and progesterone production. The structural integrity of the vagina becomes affected. Blood flow is reduced, a thinning of tissue walls takes place, and vaginal pH becomes more alkaline; the length, width, and flexibility of the vagina decrease, and vaginal secretions (lubrication) also decrease. In addition, there is loss of fat in the mons veneris, thinning of pubic hair, shrinkage of the labia majora, and thinning of the labia minora, leading to exposure of the clitoris.

Changes related to sexual responsiveness in the older female include decreased breast engorgement during arousal and a change in orgasmic response. During orgasm, the vagina will become less responsive, and the number of contractions are decreased to about half that of younger women (Mooradian & Greiff, 1990). These changes do not tend to interfere with sexual enjoyment.

Testosterone is produced in the interstitial cells of Leydig of the testes. After age 50 testosterone production shows a small but reliable age-related decline, with the lowest serum androgen levels observed in men over the age of 70 (Matsumoto, 1993). This phenomenon, which has been observed in numerous studies, is sometimes called "andropause" in an attempt to equate it with the female hormonal changes during menopause (Vermeulen, 1991). However, the importance of lower testosterone levels to male sexual functioning, i.e., arousal, is not clear. Some studies support a correlation between male sexual functioning and serum or bioavailable testosterone, whereas others do not (Rowland et al., 1993).

It is not surprising that there has been so much emphasis on discovering a possible link between testosterone levels and male functioning, because most men, as well as health care professionals, equate male sexuality with potency, the ability to achieve an erection, and the sexual capacity for intercourse (Butler et al., 1994). However, Korenman (1995) points out that the principal sex organ is the brain. Erotic stimuli are recognized through one or more of the five senses or through fantasy. Sensory experiences are then processed and integrated in the sexual response centers of the hypothalamus. Subsequently, autonomic responses and neurotransmitters are involved in causing male erections. Korenman (1995) states that even with severe testosterone deficiency, normal erectile function can be achieved in response to erotic stimuli; however, testosterone deficiency does inhibit nocturnal penile tumescence.

Because serum testosterone levels affect a number of androgen-dependent body tissues, aging males experience several physiologic changes, including the loss of penile muscle tone and weight. It requires several minutes of sexual stimulation to achieve an erection versus the few seconds required by younger males (Rowland et al., 1993). Erection tends to be less firm, and the angle of the erect penis tends to point at 90 degrees in older men, whereas in younger men it points up at 40 degrees (Thienhaus, 1988). Secretory activity from Cowper's gland before ejaculation is also reduced. Urgency for ejaculation decreases, ejaculation may take longer, and sometimes there is orgasm without ejaculation. Semen may seep out or is ejected retrograde into the bladder. This does lessen sexual pleasure to some extent.

During orgasm, the frequency of penile contractions lessens, and the force with which semen is expelled is reduced as is the quantity of semen. Sperm production generally ends in the mid-70s, but it is important to note that fertility (sperm production) "has no connection with potency (erectile capacity)" (Butler & Lewis, 1993, p. 44).

Following orgasm, erection is lost more quickly for older men, and there is a longer refractory period; it may take days before another erection can be achieved (Thienhaus, 1988). Overall, however, an older man's sexual functioning tends to reflect those of his earlier years.

SUMMARY

Sexual intimacy is more than intercourse; it includes caressing, stroking, and kissing and being an emotional companion to the partner. Sexual pleasure, although it is not absolutely essential for a fulfilled later life, can add greatly to older persons' quality of life. Intercourse not only provides physical pleasure, but it can also be considered an exercise. It is equivalent to walking three blocks or climbing two and a half flights of stairs. Moreover, sexual intimacy of any form contributes to a positive body and self-image. To be touched and embraced offers physical evidence that one is loved and desired and that wrinkles, brown spots, varicose veins, and gray hair do not really matter (Walz & Blum, 1987).

REFERENCES

Bradford, J., Ryan, C., & Rothblum, E. D. (1994). National lesbian health care survey: Implications for mental health care. *Journal of Consulting & Clinical Psychology, 62*(2), 228-242.

Brecher, E. M. (1984). *Love, sex, and aging.* Boston: Little, Brown and Company.

Butler, R. N., & Lewis, M. I. (1993). *Love and sex after 60.* New York: Ballentine Books.

Butler, R. N., Lewis, M. I., Hoffman, E., & Whitehead, E. D. (1994). Love and sex after 60: How physical changes affect intimate expression. *Geriatrics, 49*(29), 21-27.

Covey, H. C. (1989). Perceptions and attitudes toward sexuality of the elderly during the middle ages. *The Gerontologist, 29*(1), 93-100.

Forrester, D. A., & Murphy, P. A. (1992). Nurses' attitudes toward patients with AIDS and AIDS-related risk factors. *Journal of Advanced Nursing, 17*(1), 1260-1266.

George, L. K., & Weiler, S. J. (1981). Sexuality in middle and late life: The effects of age, cohort, and gender. *Archives of General Psychiatry, 38,* 919-923.

Jacoby, S. (1999). Great sex. What's age got to do with it. *Modern Maturity, 42R*(5), 43-45, 74.

Korenman, S. G. (1995). Advances in the understanding and management of erectile dysfunction. *Journal of Clinical Endocrinology and Metabolism, 80*(7), 1985-1988.

Maas, M., Buckwalter, K., & Hardy, M. A. (1991). *Nursing diagnosis and interventions for the elderly.* Reading, MA: Addison Wesley Longman.

Marsiglio, W., & Donnelly, D. (1991). Sexual relations in later life: A national study of married persons. *Journal of Gerontology, 46*(6), S338-S344.

Masters, W. H., & Johnson, V. E. (1966). *Human sexual response.* Boston: Little, Brown, and Company.

Matsumoto, A. M. (1993). "Andropause"—Are reduced androgen levels in aging men physiologically important? *Western Journal of Medicine, 159*(5), 618-620.

Mooradian, A. D., & Greiff, V. (1990). Sexuality in older women. *Archives of Internal Medicine, 150,* 1033-1038.

Mulligan, T., & Moss, C. R. (1991). Sexuality and aging in male veterans: A cross-sectional study of interest, ability, and activity. *Archives of Sexual Behavior, 20*(1), 17-25.

National Center for Health Statistics. (1994). *Vital statistics of the United States, 1990* (DHHS Publication No. [PHS] 95-1101). Washington, DC: Public Health Service.

Quam, J. K., & Whitford, G. S. (1992). Adaptation and age-related expectations of older gay and lesbian adults. *The Gerontologist, 32*(3), 367-374.

Reedy, M. N., Birren, J. E., & Schaie, W. K. (1982). Age and sex differences in satisfying love relationships across the adult life span. In K. Warner, W. K. Schaie, & J. Geweitz (Eds.), *Readings in adult development and aging* (pp. 154-165). Boston: Little, Brown, and Company.

Rowland, D. L., Greenleaf, W. J., Dorfman, L. J., & Davidson, J. M. (1993). Aging and sexual function in men. *Archives of Sexual Behavior, 22*(6), 545-557.

Sell, R. L., & Wells, J. A. (1995). The prevalence of homosexual behavior and attraction in the United States, the United Kingdom and France: Results of national population-based samples. *Archives of Sexual Behavior, 24*(3), 235-248.

Steinke, E. E. (1994). Knowledge and attitudes of older adults about sexuality in aging: A comparison of two studies. *Journal of Advanced Nursing, 19,* 477-485.

Taylor, I., & Robertson, A. (1994). The health needs of gay men: A discussion of the literature and implications for nursing. *Journal of Advanced Nursing, 20*(3), 560-566.

Thienhaus, O. J. (1988). Practical overview of sexual function and advancing age. *Geriatrics, 43*(8), 63-67.

Travis, S. S. (1987). Older adults' sexuality and remarriage. *Journal of Gerontological Nursing, 13*(6), 8-14.

United States Bureau of the Census. (1998). *Statistical abstract of the United States* (118th ed.). Washington, DC: Author.

Vermeulen, A. (1991). Androgens in the aging male. *Journal of Clinical Endocrinology & Metabolism, 73,* 221-224.

Walz, T. H., & Blum, N. S. (1987). *Sexual health in later life.* St. Charles, IL: Heath, D. C. and Company.

Weinstein, S., & Rosen, E. (1988). Senior adult sexuality in age segregated and age integrated communities. *International Journal of Aging & Human Development, 27*(4), 261-270.

Weizman, R., & Hart, J. (1987). Sexual behavior in healthy married elderly men. *Archives of Sexual Behavior, 16*(1), 39-44.

White, C. (1982). A scale for the assessment of attitudes and knowledge regarding sexuality in the aged. *Archives of Sexual Behavior, 11,* 491-502.

CHAPTER *57*

SEXUAL DYSFUNCTION

Lore K. Wright

The prefix *dys*, derived from Greek, indicates an impaired, abnormal, or difficult state. Sexual Dysfunction, therefore, refers to sexual difficulties that can be linked to disease, pathology, or surgery. This conceptualization is congruent with diagnostic criteria established by the American Psychiatric Association (1994), which recognizes sexual dysfunction caused by a general medical condition. Difficulties that can be attributed to normal changes with aging were the focus of Chapter 58, entitled *Altered Sexuality Patterns.*

Sexual dysfunction can result from several different etiologies: altered body function or structure related to disease, surgery, chemotherapy, radiation therapy, or medication or knowledge deficit or misinformation related to disease, surgery, chemotherapy, radiation therapy, or medication. Nursing interventions and nursing-sensitive outcomes are closely linked to these varying etiologies. To make these links clear, specific characteristics of Sexual Dysfunction and available nursing interventions are discussed in the context of specific etiologies.

NURSING DIAGNOSIS

The North American Nursing Diagnosis Association (NANDA) has defined Sexual Dysfunction as "a state in which an individual experiences a change in sexual function that is viewed as unsatisfying, unrewarding, inadequate (NANDA, 1999, pp. 57-58). Defining characteristics are based on the patient's verbalization of problems about actual or perceived limitations imposed by disease and/or therapy.

Many elders are indeed confronted with adjusting to disease, surgery, or medications that impact sexual functioning. The criterion that the patient has to verbalize problems can hinder diagnosis unless health care professionals take an active role in addressing sexual issues during acute and chronic illnesses and in pre- and post-surgical situations. Generally, illness and surgery are viewed as acceptable causes of problems. Patients and health care professionals should, therefore, be ready to discuss relevant sexual issues. Nevertheless, initiating and facilitating teaching about actual or potential sexual dysfunction remains a major nursing obligation. If at all possible, the patient's sex partner needs to be included in these discussions.

RELATED FACTORS/ETIOLOGIES

The most common related factors or etiologies pertaining to sexual dysfunction in older persons include (1) altered body structure or function resulting from disease, surgery, other treatments and (2) medications. Intertwined with almost every dysfunction is lack of knowledge or misinformation. Disturbances in body image are frequent accompanying problems. In Table 57-1 etiologies and related factors pertaining to sexual dysfunction in older people are summarized and their adverse impact on sexual function for males and females are indicated.

Altered Body Structure or Function: Diseases

Cardiovascular Disease. Cardiovascular disease is the most common cause of death in the United States (National Center for Health Statistics, 1994). Before age 70, the overall male/female ratio is 4:1; after age 70 it is 1:1. Women with severe arteriosclerosis are likely to experience reduced intensity of excitement and shorter orgasms, although precise studies examining reduced vulvovaginal blood flow and response impairment are lacking (Mooradian & Greiff, 1990). After a heart attack, women might anticipate pain or have fears about precipitating another incident. Such fears decrease the frequency of intercourse in over 40% of cases, and 27% of women tend not to resume sexual activity (Papadopoulos, Beaumont, Shelly, & Larrimore, 1983). However, some studies show that these fears are less common in females than in males (Baggs & Karch, 1987).

In men, arterial disease contributes to impotence, or vascular erectile dysfunction (ED). Following a heart attack, physiologic as well as psychologic reasons contribute to impotence, and frequency of sexual intercourse is reduced in 43% to 76% of cases. Too much food and drink before sexual intercourse taxes the heart and can lead to chest pain; chest pain, in turn, causes fear and can prevent an erection (Butler & Lewis, 1993).

More recently, vascular changes in the penis itself have also been linked to impotence. Tissue examination of the penis in patients with vascular disease show profound ischemic changes of the corpora cavernosa. These changes include incompressible veins, as seen in Peyronie's disease (Korenman, 1995). In this rare condition, fibrous thicken-

Sexual Dysfunction Related to Altered Body Structure or Function: Diseases, Surgery, Treatments, and/or Medications†	Related Factors/Etiologies	
	Male	**Female**
Cardiovascular disease	Intercourse frequency reduced • Fear of pain and precipitating heart attack: impotence Ischemic changes in penis: problems with intercourse (Peyronie's disease)	Excitement reduced Same fears: intercourse reduced or abstained from
Stroke	Erectile and ejaculation difficulties Motor and cognitive impairments Deny problems or the illness	Decreased vaginal lubrication Motor and cognitive impairments Deny problems or the illness
Cancer	Diagnosis itself causes anxiety, depression, and reduced desire for sexual relations. Prostate or metastatic prostate cancer: reduced sexual desire or frequency of intercourse once treatment with antihormonal therapy and medical or surgical castration is started	Diagnosis itself causes anxiety and depression Partners report no desire for sexual relations with diagnosis of cervical cancer
COPD	Avoidance of sexual intimacy Lower serum testosterone level and impotence	Avoidance of sexual intimacy
Diabetes	Impotence attributed to neurologic and circulatory interference to the penis Erectile difficulties in older men can be diagnostic	Late onset type II: vaginal dryness and significant sexual difficulties Less physiologic arousal to erotic stimuli Vaginal infections and dyspareunia
Urinary disorders	Overflow incontinence associated with prostatic hyperplasia Experience incontinence as embarrassing and distasteful	Vaginal dryness and sexual difficulties Incontinence during deep vaginal penetration and during orgasm Experience, more than males, incontinence as embarrassing and distasteful
Arthritis	Pain and stiffness Hip discomforts interfere with intercourse Reduce activity to avoid pain and fatigue Sjögren's syndrome and scleroderma Painful erections and difficulties with intercourse	Pain and stiffness Hip discomforts interfere with intercourse Reduced activity to avoid pain and fatigue Lack of lubrication
Low back pain	Weak back muscles, slipped disk limit sexual activity	Low back pain limits sexual activity
Dementia	Memory loss profoundly affects a couple's relationship No longer each other's confidant Husband caregivers abstain from sexual intercourse out of fear of guilt, exploitation, or rape Over 70% lose sexual desire 14% develop hypersexuality, causing emotional and physical distress to the spouse caregiver Sexual overtures made to relatives or strangers	Memory loss profoundly affects a couple's relationship No longer each other's confidant Consent to sex becomes a question Nursing home female patients climbing into bed with male patients Sexual abuse of demented elderly women living in the community Sexual overtures made to relatives or strangers
Nutritional deficits	Anemia, depression, decreased sexual functioning Low levels of zinc associated with taking antihypertensive medications	Anemia, depression, decreased sexual functioning

*NANDA etiologies for Sexual Dysfunction applicable to disease, surgery, or treatments; etiologies attributable to normal aging are excluded.

†Closely related factors are lack of knowledge and disturbance in self-image.

Table 57-1	Sexual Dysfunction in the Elderly: Related Factors/Etiologies*—cont'd	
Sexual Dysfunction Related to Altered Body Structure or Function: Diseases, Surgery, Treatments, and/or Medications†	**Related Factors/Etiologies**	
	Male	**Female**
Coronary artery bypass	Fear of sudden death during intercourse Fear and performance anxiety contribute to impotence	Lower sexual desire in women Less fear of sudden death
Genital and pelvic surgery (chemotherapy and radiation)		Pelvic floor surgery for nonmalignant conditions: decreased libido and lubrication Decreased genital sensations Dyspareunia may either be eliminated or become a new symptom Deterioration of sexual function with poor or ambivalent partner relationship Vulvectomy experiences: dyspareunia, decreased libido and arousal, too small vaginal orifice, reduced frequency of intercourse Sexually inactive Psychologic problems: depression, low self-confidence, poor body image Increased sexual dysfunction with chemotherapy and radiation for gynecologic cancer Sexual activity lowest at completion of radiation therapy: complaints: vaginal shortening, dyspareunia, and bleeding
Neuroleptics	Erectile difficulties, dry ejaculation, and priapism	Decreased vaginal lubrication
Tricyclic antidepressants	Loss of libido, impotence, delayed and painful ejaculation and orgasm	Decreased libido, absent orgasm
Trazodone and MAO inhibitors	Priapism	
SSRIs	Higher incidence of side effects than with tricyclics	Sexual dysfunction, including anorgasmia
Antiparkinsonian medications	Increased libido, hypersexuality	Depression: decreased libido
Antihypertensives	Decreased libido, ejaculatory difficulties, impotence	Depression: decreased libido
Beta blockers	Decreased libido, ejaculatory difficulties, impotence	Migraine headaches interfere with intimacy
Digoxin	Decreased libido, ejaculatory difficulties, impotence	Fatigue: decreased libido
Morphine	Decreased libido, ejaculatory difficulties, impotence	Decreased libido
Diuretics	Exacerbated sexual dysfunction	Not known
Mastectomy and chemotherapy		No significant difference regardless of which procedure was used Chemotherapy contributes to sexual dysfunction, poorer body image, more psychologic distress, marital problems
Prostatectomy, chemotherapy and radiation treatment	Surgical intervention leads to impotence TURP procedure: sexual functioning declines in 10% of patients; 15% of patients experience incontinence	

Continued

Table 57-1	Sexual Dysfunction in the Elderly: Related Factors/Etiologies*—cont'd	
Sexual Dysfunction Related to Altered Body Structure or Function: Diseases, Surgery, Treatments, and/or Medications†	**Related Factors/Etiologies**	
	Male	**Female**
	Nerve-sparing retropubic prostatectomy preserves potency on 70%	
	Perineal surgery causes impotence in 100% of patients	
	Radiation therapy causes erectile dysfunction in 25% of the cases	
	Hormone treatment results in dysfunction in 80% of the cases	
Colon resection, colostomy, and ileostomy	Stoma patients have higher levels of psychologic distress and sexual dysfunction	Stoma patients have higher levels of psychologic distress and sexual dysfunction
	Sexual difficulties: adjustment to diarrhea, leakage, embarrassing bowel sounds	Sexual difficulties: adjustment to diarrhea, leakage, embarrassing bowel sounds
	Resection of the rectum and anus leaves males impotent	

ing of the walls of blood vessels produces an upward bowing of the penis, and the shaft tends to be angled to the right or left (Butler & Lewis, 1993). The angle causes intercourse to be painful and sometimes makes it impossible.

Stroke. Stroke is the third leading cause of death in the United States. With advancing age, the incidence of stroke increases dramatically, doubling with every decade after the age of 55 (United States Department of Health and Human Services [USDHHS], 1995). Currently, about 3 million people in the United States endure varying degrees of disability from strokes. Men have a 30% higher incidence of strokes than women, and African-American men have a 50% higher incidence than white men (USDHHS, 1995). Following a stroke, women can experience decreased vaginal lubrication. Men are likely to experience erectile and ejaculation difficulties (Ebersole & Hess, 1998). Although sexual activity is not contraindicated following a stroke, associated functional (motor) and cognitive impairments can contribute to sexual difficulties. Body positioning can compensate for problems caused by paralysis. However, cognitive impairment can severely affect intimate relationships. With nondominant (usually right) hemisphere strokes, patients may not recognize sensory stimuli in their left visual field and, more importantly, may deny problems or the illness; male patients may deny that they have erection problems. Emotional disturbances, such as delusions, apathy, or personality changes, can further complicate intimate relationships.

Cancer. Cancer is the second leading cause of death in the United States. Cancer of the genital organs shows the highest death rates for ages 55 to 84, with rates five to

ten times higher for whites than African Americans (National Center for Health Statistics, 1994). A similar pattern is observed for (female) breast cancer and for prostate cancer, with rates at least five times higher for whites than blacks above age 55.

A diagnosis of genital or breast cancer affects sexual functioning in approximately 90% of women (Mooradian & Greiff, 1990). One year after a diagnosis of breast cancer, 50% of women continue to report sexual dysfunction (Schag et al., 1993). The diagnosis itself causes anxiety and depression, which can become compounded by body disfiguration and a poor self-image resulting from treatment (Hamilton, 1999). Interestingly, however, body image disturbances seem to occur more often in women with gynecologic cancer than in women with breast cancer (Andersen & Jochimsen, 1985). Cervical cancer has an especially negative impact on sexual behavior, with 74% of affected older women and 42% of their partners reporting no desire for sexual relations (Thranov & Klee, 1994).

For men, the diagnosis of cancer of the prostate gland can cause anxiety and depression, which in turn can affect sexual performance. However, in a sample of patients with stage C or D carcinoma (limited to prostate or metastatic prostate cancer), reduced sexual desire or frequency of intercourse was not present at the time of diagnosis. Desire and frequency were negatively affected in over 50% of patients once treatment with antihormonal therapy combined with medical or surgical castration was started (Rousseau, Dupont, Labrie, & Couture, 1988).

Chronic Obstructive Pulmonary Disease. Chronic obstructive pulmonary disease (COPD) is the fifth leading cause of death, with the highest rates occurring between the ages of 50 to 89 (USDHHS, 1995). Over 10 million people in the United States suffer from this condition, which is characterized by shortness of breath, dyspnea, and fatigue. All of these symptoms can lead to avoidance of sexual intimacy. In women, a direct link between chronic stress associated with COPD and sexual dysfunction has not been demonstrated. In men, however, hypoxia is associated with a lower serum testosterone level and impotence; in addition, side effects from medications to treat COPD can exacerbate impotence (Semple et al., 1983; Thompson, 1986).

Diabetes.   Over 7 million people in the United States have diabetes, and 90% of the adult diabetic population has type II or non–insulin-dependent diabetes mellitus. Early studies failed to identify sexual dysfunction in older women with diabetes. In subsequent research, women with late onset type II diabetes reported vaginal dryness and significant sexual difficulties, whereas women with type I diabetes did not (Schreiner-Engel, Schiavi, Vietorisz, & Smith, 1987; Staab & Hodges, 1996). Objective measures (vaginal capillary engorgement) demonstrated that although there was less physiologic arousal to erotic stimuli in women with diabetes, their subjective responses to stimuli were similar to those of healthy controls (Wincze, Albert, & Bansal, 1993). Complicating factors include recurrent vaginal infections and dyspareunia because of lack of lubrication (Mooradian & Greiff, 1990).

Men who have had diabetes most of their lives are two to five times more likely to become impotent than men in the general population (Ebersole & Hess, 1998). This problem cannot be attributed to psychologic distress or psychotic disorders; rather neurologic and circulatory interference to the penis causes the problem (Schiavi, Stimmel, Mandeli, Schreiner-Engel, & Ghizzani, 1995). In older men, erectile difficulties and impotence can be a diagnostic clue for diabetes, particularly if sexual desire is unchanged.

Urinary Disorders.   Among community-residing adults aged 60 and older, the prevalence of urinary incontinence ranges from 15% to 30%. Women are twice as likely to be afflicted with this ailment than men, and, among nursing home residents, the prevalence of urinary incontinence is ≥50% (USDHHS, 1992). Close to half of all women with urinary incontinence experience vaginal dryness and sexual difficulties. Incontinence is often experienced during deep vaginal penetration and during orgasm (Vierhout & Gianotten, 1993). In addition, urinary tract infections and dysuria are common. The fragile urethral wall and the urethra become irritated during intercourse, especially when the male partner has delayed ejaculation. (Mooradian & Greiff, 1990). In men, overflow incontinence is associated most often with prostatic hyperplasia, less frequently with prostatic carcinoma or urethral stricture. Incontinence can be embarrassing and distasteful, and it contributes to abstaining from intercourse. However, women experience incontinence as

more distasteful than men (Debus-Thiede & Dimpfl, 1993; Staab & Hodges, 1996).

Arthritis.   Over 40 million people in the United States are afflicted with arthritis; women suffer from this ailment twice as often as men (Butler & Lewis, 1993). Osteoarthritis causes pain and stiffness that results from wear and tear on the aging bone structure. Rheumatoid arthritis, a systemic disease, affects joints, muscles, and tendons, resulting in pain on movement. Hip discomfort related to arthritis is common and can interfere with intercourse. In an effort to avoid pain and fatigue, many patients reduce activity and movement (Ebersole & Hess, 1998). Inactivity tends to "freeze up" joints and further limit motion. Intercourse becomes even more difficult.

Two other rheumatic diseases, Sjögren's syndrome and scleroderma, both affect mobility of the joints and muscles and interfere with sexual functioning. Women afflicted with either disorder often have a marked lack of vaginal lubrication (Walz & Blum, 1987). Men afflicted with scleroderma can experience painful erections and difficulties with intercourse.

Low Back Pain.   Low back pain, a common complaint in older persons, can severely limit sexual enjoyment. In women, the most likely cause of low back pain is osteoporosis, resulting from post-menopausal estrogen deficiency (Scharbo-Dehaan, 1994). Brittle vertebrae and intervertebral disk atrophy (spondylosis) cause the pain. In men, weak back muscles and a slipped disk can cause severe discomforts and limit sexual activity.

Dementia.   With every decade after age 65, the incidence of dementia increases. Spurred by an aging baby boomer generation, 14 million people in the United States are expected to have dementia by the year 2030 (National Institutes of Health, 1994; Wright, 1997). The incidence is higher in women; a likely contributing factor is higher female longevity. The most common causes of dementia are Alzheimer's disease, comprising approximately 66% of all cases, and vascular dementias (formerly referred to as *multi-infarct dementia* or *MID*), comprising approximately 15% of all cases. Over 70 other conditions can cause or simulate dementia (National Institutes of Health, 1993). All dementias are characterized by memory impairment, other cognitive deficits, and impaired social functioning (American Psychiatric Association, 1994).

A diagnosis of dementia does not rule out the presence of other diseases, which could also negatively impact sexual functioning. However, memory loss alone profoundly affects a couple's relationship. Partners can no longer be each other's confidants, and it becomes questionable whether a demented partner can consent to sex. Husbands in the caregiver role may abstain from sexual intercourse out of fear and guilt, thinking that intimacy with the memory-impaired spouse is exploitation or rape (Litz, Zeiss, & Davies, 1990; Wright, 1993a).

Over 70% of patients in the middle phases of Alzheimer's disease lose sexual desire, but approximately 14% of male-afflicted spouses develop hypersexuality (or 50% of those who remain sexually active) (Wright, 1993a). They demand daily intercourse, sometimes even several times a day because they forget the previous encounter. This behavior causes emotional and physical distress to the spouse caregiver, including frequent bouts of cystitis. Male hypersexuality is likely to disappear in the late phases of dementia (Wright, 1993b, 1994).

Sexual overtures also can be made toward relatives or strangers; this causes embarrassment regardless of whether the demented elder is male or female. There are anecdotal reports of female demented nursing home patients climbing into bed with male patients and engaging in sexual touching. In the community, a different concern is the possibility of demented elderly women being sexually abused (Wright, 1997). Signs of abuse include difficulty with walking or sitting; torn, stained, or bloody underclothing; complaints of pain or itching in the genital area; and bruises or bleeding in the external genital, vaginal, or anal areas (Fulmer & Edelman, 1991).

Nutritional Deficits. Nutritional deficits can cause anemia, which negatively affects general well-being. Depression and decreased sexual functioning, including impotence, are part of the symptom sequel. Low levels of zinc associated with taking antihypertensive medications can also contribute to impotence (Khedun, Naicker, & Maharaj, 1995). There is no scientific evidence, however, that vitamin E deficiency causes impotence or that treatment with megadoses of vitamin E improves erectile function (Butler & Lewis, 1993).

Altered Body Structure or Function: Surgery, Chemotherapy, and Radiation Treatment

Coronary Artery Bypass. Following cardiac surgery, sexual desire in women tends to decrease, but sexual arousal remains intact. Women have less fear than men of sudden death during intercourse (Mooradian & Greiff, 1990). In men, fear and performance anxiety, rather than limitations imposed by the surgery, contribute to impotence (Butler & Lewis, 1993).

Genital and Pelvic Surgery, Chemotherapy, and Radiation. Nonmalignant conditions require surgery only, whereas cancer of the genital organs and pelvic floor may be treated surgically or in combination with chemotherapy or radiation. Following pelvic floor surgery for nonmalignant conditions, 29% of women experience decreased libido, 38% experience reduced lubrication, and 18% experience decreased genital sensations. Dyspareunia that was present before surgery can resolve with surgery. Conversely, dyspareunia can become a new symptom following surgery (Poad & Arnold, 1994). Following subtotal

hysterectomy, preoperative dyspareunia is relieved in the majority of cases. The frequency of intercourse tends to increase, and desire and frequency of orgasm remain unchanged (Helstrom, Lundberg, Sorbom, & Backstrom, 1993). Deterioration of sexual function after subtotal hysterectomy is more common in women who have poor or ambivalent partner relationships before surgery (Helstrom, Sorbom, & Backstrom, 1995).

More than half of women undergoing a vulvectomy experience some type of sexual dysfunction. Common complaints are dyspareunia, decreased libido and arousal, a vaginal orifice that is too small, and reduced frequency of intercourse; close to one third of women become sexually inactive (Andersen, Turnquist, LaPolla, & Turner, 1988; Andreasson, Moth, Jensen, & Bock, 1986). More than half of all women undergoing vulvectomy experience psychologic problems ranging from depression to low self-confidence and poor body image (Andreasson et al., 1986). Significantly less sexual dysfunction and less misdirection of the urine stream is reported by women who undergo radical vulvar surgery with the added technique of a skin flap reconstruction of the perineal defect (Landoni et al., 1995).

Most studies indicate that when surgery is combined with chemotherapy and radiation therapy for gynecologic cancer, increased sexual dysfunction results. Level of sexual activity is lowest at the completion of radiation therapy, and complaints of vaginal shortening, dyspareunia, and bleeding are common (Cartwright-Alcarese, 1995; Flay & Matthews, 1995). Patients treated with chemotherapy or radiation without surgery also experience a high incidence of dyspareunia and decreased sexual desire, but over half of these patients stay sexually active (Thranov & Klee, 1994).

Mastectomy and Chemotherapy. Surgical procedures in the treatment of cancer of the breast include radical mastectomy, partial mastectomy with and without reconstruction, and lumpectomy. No significant difference in postsurgical sexual function and self-image have been found regardless of which procedure was used (Schover et al., 1995; Wilmoth & Townsend, 1995). Furthermore, no significant differences in long-term adjustment have been found between women who have breast reconstruction and those who wear external breast prostheses (Reaby & Hort, 1995). Hormonal and radiation therapy does not measurably affect quality of life; however, the addition of chemotherapy contributes to long-term sexual dysfunction, poorer body image, more psychologic distress, and marital problems (Schover et al., 1995).

Prostatectomy, Chemotherapy, and Radiation Treatment. Enlargement of the prostate gland is almost universal in men over the age of 50. The enlargement causes urinary urgency and difficulty with voiding or urinary retention. It is not known what triggers an enlarged prostate gland to turn cancerous. Over half of all cases require some type of surgical intervention, and many of these lead to impotence (Butler & Lewis, 1993).

A relatively new procedure for benign prostatic hyperplasia (BPH), called *transurethral ultrasound-guided laser-induced prostatectomy (TULIP),* has been shown to cause no sexual dysfunction (Takahashi, Homma, Minowada, & Aso, 1994). Disadvantages of this procedure are delayed recovery (prolonged catheterization and irritative symptoms) and missing incidental prostate cancer because no tissue for histology examination is obtained (Schulze, 1995).

Transurethral resection of the prostate (TURP) is a common procedure. In 90% of the cases, sexual functioning is either regained or increased, but 15% of men after TURP experience some urinary incontinence (Butler & Lewis, 1993). When the prostate gland is very large, suprapubic or retropubic, surgery will be performed. The modified nerve-sparing retropubic prostatectomy preserves potency in 70% of patients. Perineal surgery is used when there is substantial enlargement and the patient is in poor physical condition; it causes impotence in 100% of patients (Butler & Lewis, 1993).

Nonsurgical treatments also have side effects. Radiation therapy for cancer of the prostate gland causes erectile dysfunction in approximately 25% of cases, whereas hormone treatment results in dysfunction in 80% of cases (Schover, 1993). However, the drug sildenafil citrate (Viagra) shows promise for patients with erectile dysfunction after radiation treatment for localized prostate cancer. In one study, 15 out of 21 patients (71%) had a positive response to sildenafil (Kedia, Zippe, Agarwal, Nelson, & Lakin, 1999).

Colon Resection, Colostomy, and Ileostomy.   Resection of colorectal cancer can be sphincter-saving or, depending on the site of the cancer, result in a colostomy or ileostomy. Stoma patients report higher levels of psychologic distress and sexual dysfunction than those with intact sphincters (Strangers, Taal, Aaronson, & te Velde, 1995). Stomas require considerable adjustment to bouts of diarrhea, embarrassing bowel sounds, and leakage. For men and women, these changes in body function translate into sexual difficulties even if surgery did not involve the lower part of the rectum or alter the physiology of sexual functions.

Surgery for cancer, which requires resection of the rectum and anus, can cause damage to nerve fibers in males and leave them impotent; women, however, retain capacity for sexual arousal and orgasm. For patients requiring total resection of the lower third of the rectum and anorectal junction, a restorative procedure known as a colic J-shaped pouch and a hand sewn pouch-endoanal anastomosis has been used with reasonable success (Leo et al., 1993). Patients who had this procedure reported less than two bowel movements a day, and none complained of severe sexual dysfunction.

Altered Body Structure or Function: Medications

Over 100 medications are known to affect sexual function, with estimates of incidence ranging from 4% to 96% (Seagraves, 1992). While effects on males are well documented, there is considerably less information about the effects of medications on female sexual function (Duncan & Bateman, 1993; Prisant, Carr, Bottini, Solursh, & Solursh, 1994). The most commonly cited medications of concern to older people are psychotropics, antihypertensives, beta blockers, and diuretics.

Dopamine increases sexual behavior, serotonin inhibits it, and norepinephrine cause conflicting effects (Gitlin, 1994). Neuroleptics are often associated with erectile difficulties, dry ejaculation, and priapism (painful, persistent erections) in men and with decreased vaginal lubrication in women. Tricyclic antidepressants can improve sexual function because of a general increase in well-being and activity, but negative side effects include loss of libido, impotence, or delayed and painful ejaculation and orgasm in men and decreased libido and retarded or absent orgasm in women. Trazodone and MAO inhibitors have the added problem of causing priapism (Clayton, Owens, & McGarvey, 1995). The newer selective serotonin reuptake inhibitors (SSRIs) are reported to have a higher incidence of side effects than the tricyclics, with women reporting more sexual dysfunction, including anorgasmia, than men (Balon, Yeragani, Pohl, & Ramesh, 1993; Gitlin, 1994). Anxiolytics cause mild, nonspecific sexual side effects. Antiparkinsonian medication (including dopamine) tends to increase libido, and in a small number of patients has resulted in hypersexuality (Uitti et al., 1989).

Additional medications commonly associated with sexual dysfunction include antihypertensives, beta blockers, digoxin, and morphine. These drugs cause decreased libido, ejaculatory difficulties, and impotence. Zinc deficiencies associated with diuretics to treat hypertension and alcoholism can exacerbate sexual dysfunction (Ebersole & Hess, 1998; Khedun et al., 1995).

Knowledge Deficit or Misinformation: Diseases

Lack of knowledge or misinformation about diseases can aggravate sexual dysfunction. For cardiovascular disease, typical examples include fear of precipitating a heart attack and heavy food and alcohol intake before intercourse. In stroke situations, inappropriate body positioning, lack of lubrication, and a male's denial or misperception of impotence exacerbates problems. A diagnosis of cancer can lead to anxiety and depression and requires specific knowledge about anticipated body changes and how both partners might be affected by these changes. Inappropriate body positioning during intercourse can aggravate COPD. Women with type II diabetes might use inadequate or inappropriate lubrication, and older men with erectile difficulties might not question whether diabetes could be the underlying cause of their dysfunction. Lack of knowledge about managing incontinence increases sexual dysfunction, including dyspareunia, vaginal infections, and abstaining from intimacy. Patients with arthritis and those suffering from low back pain might not use adequate pain control, exercise, and appropriate body positioning during intimacy. When the disease is dementia, unresolved psychologic conflicts can limit a caregiver husband's sexuality; inappropriate sexual behavior by demented elders can escalate if caregivers do not know how to structure the environment and set limits. All diseases can be complicated by knowledge deficits regarding adequate nutritional intake.

Knowledge Deficit or Misinformation: Surgery, Chemotherapy, and Radiation Treatment

Patients may lack knowledge or be misinformed about a proposed surgery and how it will affect their sexual function. They may not know when to resume sexual intercourse following bypass surgery or understand the special problems following vulvectomy surgery. The time at the end of radiation treatment is particularly difficult for both partners. Mastectomy patients may not know that the addition of chemotherapy requires greater adjustment and psychologic support than is required for surgery alone. For male patients, knowledge about the different types of prostatectomies and potentials for sexual dysfunction are important. Lack of knowledge about stoma management can greatly contribute to sexual dysfunction in both men and women.

Lack of Knowledge or Misinformation: Medications

Patients taking prescribed medications may not be aware of common side effects; symptoms such as loss of libido, erectile difficulties, impotence, and decreased or retarded orgasm can be incorrectly attributed to relationship problems. Male patients may not know that priapism, a possible side effect of neuroleptics, trazodone and MAO inhibitors, is considered a urologic emergency.

NURSING-SENSITIVE OUTCOMES

Important outcomes for patients experiencing sexual dysfunction during acute and chronic illnesses include the following: Knowledge: Disease Process; Knowledge: Treatment Regimen; Knowledge: Medication; Symptom Control through behaviors or management strategies; Safety Behavior: Personal; Health Seeking Behavior; Caregiver Well-Being; and Acceptance of the new Health Status. Knowledge, symptom control, safety, health-seeking behaviors, and

caregiver well-being can minimize negative effects of disease, surgery, other treatments, and medication. Acceptance can strengthen the emotional bond between sex partners, regardless of whether intercourse is resumed or not. Nursing-sensitive outcomes are listed in Table 57-2 and related to the two major related factors ("Altered Body Structure or Function" and "Knowledge Deficit or Misinformation") and to suggested nursing interventions.

Knowledge: Disease Process, Treatment Procedure(s), or Treatment Regimen

The outcomes "Knowledge: Disease Process, Treatment Procedure(s), or Treatment Regimen" (Iowa Outcomes Project, 2000) pertains to patients' verbalized understanding of sexual dysfunction associated with a specific disease, surgery, or treatment regimen. The patient's partner, if available, also needs to have this understanding. When choices about treatment regimens or types of surgery are possible, patients and their partners should be able to compare the differential impact of these treatments/surgical procedures. For example, women need to understand that different types of mastectomy surgeries are not related to more or less sexual dysfunction, that the addition of chemotherapy can contribute to long-term problems, and that relationship issues with a partner require particular attention (Schover et al., 1995).

Similarly, patients undergoing vulvectomies need to be able to compare surgical procedure options. They should know that there is a lower rate of sexual dysfunction with a skinflap reconstruction and that the addition of chemotherapy and radiation therapy increases the risk of sexual dysfunction (Cartwright-Alcarese, 1995; Landoni et al., 1995). An excellent example of patients demonstrating appropriate knowledge and decision making is the interactive videodisc-based shared decision-making program about treatment options for benign prostatic hyperplasia reported by Barry, Fowler, Mulley, Henderson, and Wennberg (1995). Additional outcome indicators of adequate knowledge are decreased anxiety and verbalized emotional support from the patient's sex partner.

Knowledge: Medication

The outcome Knowledge: Medication refers to the patient's "extent of understanding conveyed about the safe use of medication" (Iowa Outcomes Project, 2000, p. 279). This is important because medications are often part of the overall treatment regimen. Outcome indicators include the following: ability to refer to a list of potential side effects and feel comfortable reporting sexual dysfunction that might be attributable to medications, ability to make informed decisions about changing to a different medication, knowledge about serious interaction effects with drugs enhancing sexual performance, and conveying understanding of the necessity to adapt to side effects.

Table **57-2**	Suggested Nursing-Sensitive Outcomes and Nursing Interventions **SEXUAL DYSFUNCTION**	
Nursing Diagnosis	**Nursing-Sensitive Outcomes**	**Nursing Interventions**
SEXUAL DYSFUNCTION *Related Factors/Etiologies** Altered body structure or function	**KNOWLEDGE: DISEASE PROCESS** **TREATMENT PROCEDURE(S)** **TREATMENT REGIMEN** *Indicators* Patient verbalizes understanding of impact of disease, surgery, radiation, medication side effects; makes informed choices	**SEXUAL COUNSELING** **LEARNING FACILITATION** **TEACHING: PROCEDURE/TREATMENT** **ANXIETY REDUCTION** **DECISION-MAKING SUPPORT**
	KNOWLEDGE: MEDICATION *Indicators* Patient knows side effects and when/how to report them; can discuss medication options; description of side effects of medications	**SEXUAL COUNSELING** **TEACHING: PRESCRIBED MEDICATION** (caution regarding concomitant use of sildenafil and organic nitrates) **DECISION-MAKING SUPPORT**
	SYMPTOM CONTROL *Indicators* Patient and partner report management strategies that minimize sexual dysfunction; able to give return demonstration of devices; report use of strategies to overcome/reduce impotence and vaginal problems; patient/partner can choose appropriate body positions from schematic drawings; reports controlling symptoms; uses available resources	**SEXUAL COUNSELING** **TEACHING: PSYCHOMOTOR SKILL** **COPING ENHANCEMENT** **EMOTIONAL SUPPORT** **PELVIC MUSCLE EXERCISE** **REFERRAL**
Knowledge deficit or misinformation	**SAFETY BEHAVIOR: PERSONAL** *Indicators* Patient verbalizes correct time frames for safe resumption of intercourse after illness/surgery; able to recognize emergency situations and knows how to respond	**SEXUAL COUNSELING** **CARDIAC PRECAUTIONS** **CARDIAC CARE: REHABILITATIVE** **ANTICIPATORY GUIDANCE**
	HEALTH SEEKING BEHAVIOR *Indicators* Patient reports exercise program; provides record of dietary intake; body weight is within normal limits; potency in male diabetic patient restored; adheres to self-development strategies to eliminate unhealthy behavior; describes strategies to maximize health	**HEALTH EDUCATION** **HOPE INSTILLATION** **HUMOR** **EXERCISE PROMOTION**
	CAREGIVER WELL-BEING *Indicators* Report of reduced or eliminated inappropriate sexual behavior or demands from cognitively impaired spouse/family member; caregiver reports environmental restructuring, limit setting	**CAREGIVER SUPPORT** **DEMENTIA MANAGEMENT** **ENVIRONMENTAL MANAGEMENT: SAFETY** **LIMIT SETTING** **EMOTIONAL SUPPORT**

*Based on NANDA's related factors for Sexual Dysfunction if applicable to disease, surgery, other treatments, or medications common to older persons. Normal changes with aging excluded.

Continued

Table 57-2	Suggested Nursing-Sensitive Outcomes and Nursing Interventions—cont'd SEXUAL DYSFUNCTION—cont'd	
Nursing Diagnosis	**Nursing-Sensitive Outcomes**	**Nursing Interventions**
	ACCEPTANCE: HEALTH STATUS *Indicators* Willingness of both partners to discuss problems and make adaptations; partner voices support; patients with urinary incontinence or stomas able to verbalize appropriate management strategies to prevent leakage, injury; patients know how to reach nurse specialist; reduction of anxiety and/or depression; scores on standardized measures of emotional health and sexual functioning; peacefulness; expressed feelings about health status; pursuit of information	SEXUAL COUNSELING SELF-ESTEEM ENHANCEMENT EMOTIONAL SUPPORT ANXIETY REDUCTION BODY IMAGE ENHANCEMENT CULTURAL BROKERAGE TEACHING: SAFE SEX

Symptom Control Behavior

The outcome Symptom Control refers to "personal actions to minimize perceived adverse changes in physical and emotional functioning" (Iowa Outcomes Project, 2000, p. 419). An important outcome indicator is the reporting of the use of strategies by their sexual partners to minimize sexual dysfunction caused by disease, surgery, and other treatments. However, some strategies or techniques may need to be evaluated through return demonstrations. Successful outcomes overlap with the patient and partner's sense of well-being. Important examples are the management of impotence and vaginal problems and the use of appropriate body positions.

Impotence. Impotence management strategies can help patients with COPD, diabetes, stroke, and nutritional deficits, as well as those on medication regimens that include cardiac drugs, vasodilators, antihypertensives, and tricyclic antidepressants. Postsurgically, patients who have had a prostatectomy, resection of the rectum, or bypass surgery and patients who have had chemotherapy for prostate cancer also require knowledge of impotence management. Management strategies to alleviate or compensate for male impotence should be verbalized by both partners. If a vacuum tumescence device or injections are to be used, a successful return demonstration can provide evidence of adequate knowledge. Reports of resumption of sexual intimacy are another outcome criterion. Reduction of accompanying anxiety and depression is another indicator that impotence is being managed successfully.

Vaginal Problems. Strategies to compensate for vaginal problems are especially important when a dysfunction is caused by diabetes, urinary incontinence, low back pain, vulvectomy or other pelvic surgery, radiation therapy, chemotherapy, medication, the male partner's ejaculatory difficulties, or hypersexuality. Women need to report using appropriate and adequate vaginal lubrication and management strategies that prevent discomfort, as well as reporting a decrease of dyspareunia, vaginal infections, and cystitis.

Body Positioning. Body positioning is especially important for patients with COPD, arthritis, low back pain and after stroke and cardiac and pelvic surgery. Both partners need to indicate an understanding of different body positions that can be used during sexual intercourse to compensate for sexual dysfunction caused by illness. The partners should be able to identify appropriate positions from a range of schematic drawings (Cartwright-Alcarese, 1995; Lueckenotte, 1996; McCormick, Riffer, & Thompson, 1986; Thompson, 1986; Walz & Blum, 1987). Successful symptom control behavior overlaps with the patient's safety status.

Safety Behavior: Personal

The outcome Safety Behavior: Personal refers to "individual or caregiver efforts to control behaviors that might cause physical injury" (Iowa Outcomes Project, 2000, p. 375). Indicators of successful outcomes occur when patients verbalize time frames about safe resumption of intercourse after a heart attack, bypass surgery, or pelvic surgery, use symptom control behaviors described previously, and verbalize how to recognize and deal with emergency situations. The safety status of the patient is closely linked to health seeking behaviors.

Health Seeking Behavior: Adherence

The outcome Health Seeking Behavior: Adherence refers to "actions to promote optimal wellness, recovery, and rehabilitation" (Iowa Outcomes Project, 2000, p. 233). Evidence of health seeking behaviors are reports of exercise programs, adequate dietary intake and supplements if necessary, body weight that is age and height appropriate, blood counts within normal limits, and reports from male patients with late-onset diabetes that potency has returned.

Caregiver Well-Being

The outcome Caregiver Well-Being refers to "primary care providers satisfaction with health and life circumstances" (Iowa Outcomes Project, 2000, p. 151). This outcome is especially important when the patient's sexual dysfunction is caused by cognitive impairment. Successful outcome in such situations are the caregivers' report of reduced or eliminated inappropriate sexual behaviors or demands made by the ill person. Caregivers need to feel supported in handling this difficult problem and report trying environmental restructuring, limit setting, and possibly prescription medication. For caregivers who mourn the loss of intimacy because of the partner's cognitive impairment, outcomes can be acceptance of abstinence or forming a new relationship. The outcome Caregiver Well-Being, therefore, overlaps with acceptance of the patient's health status.

Acceptance: Health Status

The outcome Acceptance: Health Status refers to "reconciliation to health circumstances" (Iowa Outcomes Project, 2000, p. 108). Some outcome indicators apply to all patients with sexual dysfunction. An example would be a partner's willingness to discuss problems and be supportive in making necessary adaptations; this may or may not include resumption of intercourse. Partnership issues are important for all patients, but acceptance of health status is difficult when sexual dysfunction is related to urinary incontinence or stomas. Patients and their partners need to be able to verbalize appropriate management strategies to prevent leakage and odors, and they need to know how to contact a nurse specializing in urinary incontinence or stoma care if additional assistance is required. Related outcome indicators are for the couple to evidence reduced anxiety and depressive symptoms and to report that their sexual relationship has improved.

Evidence of reduction in anxiety and depression can be made by observing the patient's (and partner's) affect and behavior or can be based on scores obtained with standardized scales. Depression can be evaluated with the Short Zung Depression Scale (Tucker, Ogle, Davinson, & Eilenberg, 1987) or the Geriatric Depression Scale (Yesavage & Brink, 1983). In addition, depression and anxiety can be assessed with subscales of the Symptom Check List (SCL-90-R) (Derogatis & Cleary, 1977). Each scale takes about 10 to 15 minutes to administer. Standardized scales should be viewed as a guide to judging improvement or making a mental health referral.

Several standardized measures are also available to obtain an overall evaluation of the patient's sexual function/dysfunction. Examples are the Changes in Sexual Function Questionnaire (Clayton et al., 1995) or the Derogatis Sexual Function Inventory (DSFI) (Derogatis, 1980). Both scales cover a wide range of sexual behaviors but because of their length are more suited for research purposes than routine clinical evaluations. In clinical settings, the 10-item sexual satisfaction subscale of the DSFI can be helpful, with a higher score providing an indication of improved partner relationships. Another useful outcome measure is the Global Sexual Satisfaction Index (GSSI), which is part of the DSFI. Patients completing this index rate sexual quality/activities of their relationship on a simple nine point scale ranging from 8 = "could not be better" to 0 = "could not be worse" (Derogatis, 1980). Two other short scales can be helpful for evaluating outcomes in clinical settings. Prisant et al. (1994) have used a 5-item sexual function/dysfunction scale for men and another similar 5-item scale for women. A lower score on any item would indicate improvement.

Another outcome measure specific to women after mastectomy surgery is the Mastectomy Attitude Scale (MAS) developed by Heyl (1977) and reported by Feather and Wainstock (1989). This 33-item scale addresses emotional concerns, sexuality, appearance, life outlook, concealment, openness, and necessity (of surgery). Subscales pertinent to the patient's symptoms could be used for outcome evaluations.

NURSING INTERVENTIONS

In Chapter 58 it is argued that interventions by a skilled nurse begin during the assessment phase and that outcome targets are adjusted as new information is obtained. The same process applies to sexual dysfunction that is caused by disease or surgery. A helpful approach in addressing sexual dysfunction in older people is to "give permission" to talk about sexual issues: "People who are faced with your condition (e.g., surgery, treatment) often want to know how it will affect their sex life. Do you have a question about sexual issues?" Although this approach contributes to the assessment, it is at the same time an intervention strategy aimed at reducing anxiety.

The PLISSIT heuristic developed by Annon (1976) can be used as a guide to identify levels of interventions: P = permission giving; LI = limited information; SS = specific suggestions; IT = intensive therapy. Nurses are likely to use the first three levels of interventions but not intensive sex therapy unless specially trained to meet qualifications identified by the American Association of Sex Educators, Counselors, and Therapists (ASSECT).

The most frequently used nursing interventions to obtain desired outcomes for sexual dysfunction are the following: Learning Facilitation defined as "promoting the ability to process and comprehend information" (Iowa Intervention Project, 2000, p. 423), Teaching: Procedure/Treatment, or "preparing a patient to understand and mentally prepare for a prescribed procedure or treatment"

(p. 652), Teaching: Prescribed Medication, or "preparing a patient to safely take prescribed medications and monitor for their effects" (p. 650), Sexual Counseling, or the "use of an interactive helping process focusing on the need to make adjustments in sexual practice or to enhance coping with a sexual event/disorder" (p. 584), Anxiety Reduction, or "minimizing apprehension, dread, foreboding, or uneasiness related to an unidentified source of anticipated danger" (p. 146), Emotional Support, or the "provision of reassurance, acceptance, and encouragement during times of stress" (p. 300), Referral, or the "arrangement for services by another care provider or agency" (p. 551), Limit Setting, or "establishing the parameters of desirable and acceptable patient behavior" (p. 428), and Caregiver Support, or the "provision of the necessary information, advocacy, and support to facilitate primary patient care by someone other than a health care professional" (p. 200). Interventions listed in Table 57-2 are based on the Nursing Intervention Classification (NIC) criteria (Iowa Intervention Project, 2000). These interventions are described in the context of specific etiologies for Sexual Dysfunction.

Nursing Interventions for Sexual Dysfunction Related to Altered Body Structure and Function

To ensure that patients have adequate knowledge of the cause(s) of their sexual dysfunction, teaching interventions typically focus on several issues: the disease process, preparing the patient during the preoperative period for surgery and the postoperative period, preparing the patient for other treatments or procedures, and discussing medication effects. This teaching cannot be ignored because the patient is an elderly individual, because the number of minutes allocated per clinic visit are too few, or because the length of hospital stay has been drastically reduced. Nurses must insist on adequate time to address sexual issues. Illness-specific information has been presented at the beginning of this chapter; the nurse facilitates learning by presenting this information at the patient's level of comprehension; the nurse then assists patients with making informed choices. Sexual Counseling should involve the patient's partner if at all possible, and referrals to specialists are made as appropriate.

Many medications cause sexual dysfunction. Teaching about prescribed medications includes preparing patients to take their medicine safely and to monitor side effects. Patients receiving medications are usually given a list of potential side effects; it is important that the list mentions potential sexual dysfunction. Psychotropic medications, antihypertensives, beta blockers, digoxin, and diuretics are known to contribute to impotence in men and to decreased libido and orgasmic difficulties in women (see Table 57-1). Reduced libido and orgasmic difficulties attributable to antidepressant medications can be managed by waiting if the therapy is short-term (6 weeks), by giving

a brief drug holiday, or by lowering the dose. Another strategy is to switch to a different agent (e.g., from SSRI antidepressants, which are associated with the highest rate of sexual dysfunction, to bupropion [Gitlin, 1994; Rothschild, 1995]). Specific antidotes such as cyproheptadine and yohimbine may also reverse side effects.

Priapism caused by neuroleptics requires immediate intervention. Patients should be told to come for treatment within the first 4 to 6 hours of occurrence in order to prevent the possibility of permanent impotence and the need for invasive procedures. Treatment, usually performed by a urologist, consists of irrigating the corpora cavernosa with saline or metaraminol to promote venous constriction and detumescence (Gitlin, 1994).

Antihypertensive and diuretic medications often cause impotence in men and decreased vaginal lubrication in women. Switching from high-dose thiazide diuretics to other classes of antihypertensive agents can alleviate impotence in men (Prisant et al., 1994). Zinc supplements can alleviate diuretic induced impotence in men, and, interestingly, weight reduction seems to ameliorate sexual problems in both men and women (Duncan & Batemen, 1993; Khedun et al., 1995; Prisant et al., 1994). Patients requesting sildenafil (Viagra) need to be questioned about all other medications; the concomitant use of organic nitrates and Viagra can cause fatal hypotension (Billner, 1998; Goldstein et al., 1998).

Hypersexuality, which on rare occasions is associated with antiparkinsonian therapy, can be treated by reducing the dosage. A neuroleptic may be added in selected cases (Uitti et al., 1989).

To facilitate symptom control, special nursing interventions are required for impotence, vaginal problems, and conditions where special body positions during intercourse need to be advocated. Sexual counseling for impotence is the most important intervention for male patients because many different ailments cause this problem. Importantly, the nurse should address this issue at check-up visits following successful (and sometimes life-saving) surgery. Although before surgery patients often consider the complication of impotence as unimportant, at 9 months it tends to become central to their lives (Black, 1994). Teaching will focus on the use of a vacuum pump, injection, medication, or the type of surgery that may be recommended. Manufacturers of mechanical devices often provide helpful brochures; video tapes explaining the use of the devices might also be available. Examples of devices are surgical implants with an inflatable reservoir that activates a "squeeze" pump in the scrotum to obtain an erection. Vacuum tumescent devices consist of a plastic cylinder that is placed over the penis; a pumping device creates negative pressure thus drawing blood into the penis. A rubber band is placed at the base of the penis to restrict venous return of the blood; this maintains an erection for 15 to 30 minutes (Staab & Hodges, 1996). Return demonstration in the presence of the partner may be necessary. The nurse should alert the patient about possible trauma from the rubber band that can lead to self-limiting hematomas (Korenman & Viosca, 1992).

Teaching of injection techniques can be a nursing intervention when pharmacologic erection programs (PEP) have been prescribed. Papaverine hydrochloride or papaverine combined with phentolamine mesylate injection leads to an erection in 65% to 100% of cases, lasting for 30 to 40 minutes. Solutions containing prostaglandin E_1 (PGE_1) may be preferred over papaverine because of lower incidence of priapism and penile scarring (Korenman, 1995; Staab & Hodges, 1996). Androgen therapy in the form of weekly intramuscular injections of testosterone enanthate has become more widespread. The patient must be told about potential adverse effects, including stimulation of benign or malignant prostate growth and reduction of HDL-cholesterol; the latter can increase the risk of coronary artery disease (Korenman, 1995; Matsumoto, 1993).

If the patient has retained some erectile function, the patient or partner can be taught to massage the penis and push it down, not up toward the abdomen where it will lose blood. Pressure should be applied to the base of the penis, enabling it to hold blood (Shell & Smith, 1994). This technique can be helpful for male patients with late-onset diabetes. These patients should be told that potency can return once the diabetic condition is controlled with medication or diet.

Impotence can be especially difficult to accommodate in stroke patients who deny erectile problems. Teaching should focus on helping the female partner to understand what causes the male's perceptual problems. Strategies to compensate for impotence can be explained, but the partner's willingness to use such strategies needs to be respected, and emotional support needs to be given.

Nursing interventions for vaginal problems are commonly needed by women with diabetes, urinary incontinence, low back pain, vulvectomy and other pelvic surgery, and radiation and chemotherapy. In addition, a male partner's ejaculatory difficulties or hypersexuality, resulting from medication side effects, can require women to develop coping strategies. Sexual counseling can include teaching the following techniques. Before intercourse, both partners need to wash their genitalia. Adequate amounts of a water-soluble lubrication should be used. Women should void before and immediately after intercourse. The vaginal orifice can be wiped with a premoistened feminine towelette (e.g., sold by Massengill) to prevent irritation and odors. To reduce risk of cystitis, different body positions should be tried to avoid prolonged pressure on the urethra. After intercourse, a large glass of water or cranberry juice should be taken. For women who have had radiation therapy, the following additional special techniques are required. Positions that provide the woman with control over depth of penetration and angle of movement can be used to compensate for shortening of the vaginal canal. Vaginal stenosis can be prevented or minimized if women stay sexually active throughout the course of the radiation treatment. As an alternative, using a vaginal dilator with a water-soluble lubricant for 10 minutes 3 times per week can be helpful. Painful vaginal penetration results from decreased elasticity, scarring, and thinning of the vaginal epithelium; anticipation of discomfort can result in tensing the perineal muscles and can cause vaginismus. Women can practice different Kegel perineal exercises to relax muscles and decrease pain (Cartwright-Alcarese, 1995). Hormone replacement therapy (HRT) also might be appropriate for women with no contraindications.

Sexual Counseling to teach different body positions can be especially helpful to patients with COPD, arthritis, low back pain, and after stroke and cardiac and pelvic surgery. Instead of the traditional male superior position, the female superior position is less energy-demanding for men. When the patient is the woman, different positions can make breathing more comfortable. For example, the female can lie on the edge of the bed with her back supported by pillows and her feet touching the floor; her partner can then face her kneeling on the floor. Another position is for the female to kneel on the floor while supporting her chest on the bed; the male then penetrates from behind (Thompson, 1986).

Male stroke patients can find a comfortable position in a wheelchair with removable arms, with the female allowing entry from in front or behind (McCormick et al., 1986). Patients with arthritis are advised to use pain medications and a hot bath before intercourse and to use pillows and positions to avoid abduction of the hips. Male patients with a protruding abdomen may find the following "triangle" superior position comfortable: the male places his hips under the female's sharply bent knees and the female lies on her back (Shell & Smith, 1994). Schematic drawings of different body positions can be found in textbooks by Walz and Blum (1987) and Lueckenotte (1996) and in the article by McCormick et al. (1986).

Nursing Interventions for Sexual Dysfunction Related to Knowledge Deficit/Misinformation

Patients need knowledge to adapt to sexual dysfunction caused by disease, surgery, other therapies, or medications. Ignorance and being unprepared for treatment and its consequences is still reported by researchers as "the most striking finding" (Lancaster, 1993). Sexual Counseling, together with the partner if possible, must be initiated to teach strategies that can compensate for Sexual Dysfunction. A number of previously identified key issues are likely to be the focus of the counseling, but the nurse with expert knowledge guides patients to adapt strategies to their specific illness and social circumstances.

The patient's safety status after a heart attack, bypass surgery, stroke, or abdominal surgery requires special nursing interventions. Patients are counseled that sexual intercourse can usually be resumed after 4 to 6 weeks, although a longer recuperation might be required. In addition, Health Education, Cardiac Precautions, and Anticipatory Guidance are provided. The medication sildenafil (Viagra) must not be taken with organic nitrates such as nitroglycerin (Billner, 1998). Heavy meals and drinking should be avoided before intercourse. Masturbation is less taxing and can be practiced as an alternative. Patients can evaluate their own cardiopulmonary readiness and energy level required for intercourse by taking a brisk walk around a block or by rapidly walking up two flights of stairs (Ebersole & Hess, 1998). If no discomfort is noted, taking one to two tablets of nitroglycerin sublingually 5 to 10 minutes before intercourse provides additional safety. If discomfort occurs, the tablets can be repeated in 5 minutes but no more than 3 tablets should be taken within 15 minutes (Spratto & Woods, 1996). If pain persists, the physician/primary health care provider needs to be contacted.

Another nursing intervention is Health Education. Patients are advised to stop smoking and begin a regular exercise program. Level of exertion is tailored to the patient's condition, and dietary changes or supplements are recommended to treat anemia or medication-induced deficiencies. Writing down the instructions in form of a "care plan" can motivate patients to adhere to health seeking behaviors.

Nursing interventions for sexual dysfunction associated with cognitive impairment are especially challenging. Interventions for hypersexuality associated with Alzheimer's disease or inability to recognize sexual dysfunction following a stroke must include Emotional Support for the spouse or other family caregiver. To decrease inappropriate sexual behaviors by the patient, prescription tranquilizers may be tried, but, more importantly, Environmental Management needs to be taught, including use of separate bedrooms or use of clothing that cannot be easily removed. Caregiver spouses must be supported in their decision to set limits on unwanted sexual intercourse. Community nurses might need to intervene if sexual abuse is suspected (Wright, 1996).

Nursing interventions that focus on helping patients and their partners to accept the new health status include the following: Sexual Counseling, Emotional Support, Self-Esteem Enhancement, Anxiety Reduction, Cultural Brokerage, Body Image Enhancement, and Referral.

If at all possible, both partners need to be included in Sexual Counseling; this is the most important strategy for improving the couple's relationship. The nurse provides Emotional Support and Self-Esteem Enhancement by acknowledging to the patient and partner that illness requires adaptation and that some aspects of sexual dysfunction can be compensated for through specific management strategies. This not only provides the necessary information but also helps to increase communication between patient and partners and helps to reduce anxiety.

In this respect, homosexual patients and their partners are in need of special counseling. After abdominoperineal resection, for example, anal intercourse is no longer possible. These patients and their sex partners need to be counseled that the stoma must not be abused and that AIDS and other sexually transmitted diseases can be transmitted via the stoma (Black, 1994). Alternative methods for expressing affection need to be discussed, and the patient's psychological state, including suicidal ideation, needs to be monitored.

Another important nursing intervention in this context is Cultural Brokerage (i.e., linking patients from different cultures or religions to the orthodox health care system). For example, non–English speaking Asian patients are very private individuals, and it is not appropriate to ask a housekeeping staff member to function as a translator; rather, a health care professional who can act as translator needs to be found (Black, 1994). Moreover, the nurse needs to be alert to the possibility that a patient might be told what the translator thinks the patient wants to hear instead of the information the nurse wants to give.

Helping patients and their partners adjust to a new health status is also important when the diagnosis is breast cancer. This necessitates that the nurse provide different emotional support to wives and husbands and that the support be specific to the diagnostic phase, the treatment phase, and the recovery periods (Northouse, 1992). Emotional Support and Body Image Enhancement are provided during the most difficult time after completion of radiation treatment for vulvectomy surgery (Flay & Matthews, 1995; Northouse, 1992). Symptoms of depression need to be monitored in both partners; if clinical depression or suicidal ideation are noted, referral to a mental health professional needs to be made.

CASE STUDY

L. Daniel, a 72-year-old, white male, was admitted to a psychiatric unit for evaluation of paranoid ideation, aggressive and abusive behavior toward his wife, and sexual preoccupation. He had suffered a right hemisphere stroke 2 years ago; his speech was intact, but he had left-sided hemiplegia and was wheelchair dependent. He had been cared for at home by his wife with daily assistance from a nurse's aide.

Mr. Daniel insisted that his wife had a lover in her bedroom because she refused to have sex with him. He thought that "three times a week should not be too much to ask." He threatened he would find himself another woman if his wife would not cooperate. When asked how he would find another women, he stated he would just drive to the local bar. He did not seem to recognize his physical limitations.

Mrs. Daniel was a slightly built woman aged 66. During a counseling session with the nurse, Mrs. Daniel described her husband's abusive behavior. He had grabbed her several times when she provided physical assistance, pulled her into bed, and tried to have intercourse. "But he just can't do it, even when he tries for 2 hours," she stated tearfully; she sounded very distressed. Mrs. Daniel was asked whether the use of mechanical devices to compensate for impotence had ever been discussed. She looked shocked and stated: "I just couldn't do those kind of things."

When the nurse suggested a counseling session together with her husband, Mrs. Daniel became very anxious and wanted to know if this was to force her to agree to have sex again. The nurse assured her that the goal for the meeting was to have open communication about the problem. Perhaps an agreement about how to show affection for each other could be reached, and that affection did not have to mean intercourse. The nurse also explained the reason for Mr. Daniel's inability to recognize physical limitations and dysfunctions after his stroke, and the nurse mentioned that Mr. Daniel had shown no inappropriate behavior toward the nurses on the unit during bathing and other personal care.

During the couple's counseling session, Mrs. Daniel told her husband that she loved him, that she would always care for him, that they could hug and lie in bed together, but that there just could not be any sex. Mr. Daniel sat quietly for a while. He then said that he was very relieved to hear she would not leave him, he had thought she was planning to get out of the marriage. Mrs. Daniel again said she would stay, but there just could not be any sex. Mr. Daniel looked sad. "That will be difficult to accept," he said. The session continued by discussing different ways of expressing affection, or "how to be nice to each other." The counseling session seemed to end peacefully, and some agreement seemed to have been reached.

Subsequently, while Mrs. Daniel attended to discharge arrangements, the nurse stayed with Mr. Daniel. He suddenly turned to the nurse and said: "Now, does my wife understand that we will have sex at least three times a week?" Before the (surprised) nurse could formulate a response, Mrs. Daniel returned reporting that discharge procedures were completed, and the couple left.

The concerned nurse had subsequent telephone contacts with Mrs. Daniel, who reported that things were a lot better. Her husband no longer accused her of having another man, and they hugged a lot. "You told me something very important," Mrs. Daniel said. "You said he did not grab the nurses in the hospital, so that means he can control himself. So now, when he starts to talk about sex, I just tell him no, and get out of the way. I do show him affection, but there just can't be any sex."

Was Mrs. Daniel's limit setting the best possible intervention? Perhaps. There was expression of affection between the couple, and Mrs. Daniel remained committed to caring for her husband. It appears that the outcome Caregiver Well-Being had been achieved.

SUMMARY

Teaching elderly patients and their partners the effects of disease, surgeries, and treatments on sexuality and management strategies to compensate for sexual dysfunction are crucial nursing interventions. Nurses must have expert knowledge, sensitivity, and excellent communication skills to help patients and their partners achieve desired outcomes. Even when patients report that targeted outcomes have been reached, the nurse

might never fully know which intervention was the most meaningful to a couple's emotional and physical well-being.

REFERENCES

American Psychiatric Association. (1994). *Diagnostic and statistical manual of mental disorders* (4th ed.). Washington, DC: Author.

Andersen, B. L., & Jochimsen, P. R. (1985). Sexual functioning among breast cancer, gynecologic cancer, and healthy women. *Journal of Consulting & Clinical Psychology, 53*(1), 25-32.

Andersen, B. L., Turnquist, D., LaPolla, J., & Turner, D. (1988). Sexual functioning after treatment of in situ vulvar cancer: Preliminary report. *Obstetrics & Gynecology, 71*(1), 15-19.

Andreasson, B., Moth, I., Jensen, S. B., & Bock, J. E. (1986). Sexual function and somatopsychic reactions in vulvectomy operated women and their partners. *Acta Obstetricia et Gynecologica Scandinavica, 65,* 7-10.

Annon, J. (1976). The PLISSIT model: A proposed conceptual scheme for the behavioral treatment of sexual problems. *Journal of Sex Education & Therapy, 2*(1), 1-15.

Baggs, J. G., & Karch, A. M. (1987). Sexual counseling of women with coronary heart disease. *Heart & Lung, 16*(2), 154-159.

Balon, R., Yeragani, V., Pohl, R., & Ramesh, C. (1993). Sexual dysfunction during antidepressant treatment. *Journal of Clinical Psychiatry, 54*(6), 209-212.

Barry, M. J., Fowler, F. J. Jr., Mulley, A. G. Jr., Henderson, J. V. Jr., & Wennberg, J. E. (1995). Patient reactions to a program designed to facilitate patient participation in treatment decisions for benign prostatic hyperplasia. *Medical Care, 33*(8), 771-782.

Billner, K. L. (1998). Erectile dysfunction and sildenafil. *Nurse Practitioner, 23*(1), 111.

Black, P. K. (1994). Hidden problems of stoma care. *British Journal of Nursing, 3*(14), 707-711.

Butler, R. N., & Lewis, M. I. (1993). *Love and sex after 60.* New York: Ballantine Books.

Cartwright-Alcarese, F. (1995). Addressing sexual dysfunction following radiation therapy for gynecologic malignancy. *Oncology Nursing Forum, 22*(8), 1227-1232.

Clayton, A. H., Owens, J. E., & McGarvey, E. L. (1995). Assessment of paroxetine-induced sexual dysfunction using the changes in sexual functioning questionnaire. *Psychopharmacology Bulletin, 31*(2), 397-413.

Debus-Thiede, G., & Dimpfl, T. (1993). The psychological status of the female with urinary incontinence. (German). *Zentralblatt fur Gynakologie, 115*(7), 332-335.

Derogatis, L. R. (1980). Psychological assessment of psychosexual functioning. *Psychiatric Clinics of North America, 3*(1), 113-131.

Derogatis, L. R., & Cleary, P. A. (1977). Confirmation of the dimensional structure of the SCL-90: A study in construct validation. *Journal of Clinical Psychology, 33*(4), 981-989.

Duncan, L., & Bateman, D. N. (1993). Sexual function in women. *Drug Safety, 8*(3), 225-234.

Ebersole, P., & Hess, P. (1998). *Toward healthy aging: Human needs and nursing response* (5th ed.). St. Louis, MO: Mosby.

Feather, B. L., & Wainstock, J. M. (1989). Perceptions of postmastectomy patients. Part II. *Cancer Nursing, 12*(5), 301-309.

Flay, L. D., & Matthews, J. H. (1995). The effects of radiotherapy and surgery on the sexual function of women treated for cervical cancer. *International Journal of Radiation Oncology, Biology, Physics, 31*(2), 399-404.

Fulmer, T. T., & Edelman, C. L. (1991). Adult day care. In M. S. Harper (Ed.), *Management and care of the elderly* (pp. 269-289). Thousand Oaks, CA: Sage.

Gitlin, M. J. (1994). Psychotropic medications and their effects on sexual function: Diagnosis, biology, and treatment approaches. *Journal of Clinical Psychiatry, 55*(9), 406-413.

Goldstein, I., Lue, T. F., Padma-Nathan, H., Rosen, R., Steers, W., & Wicker, P. (1998). Oral sildenafil in the treatment of erectile dysfunction. *New England Journal of Medicine, 20*(338), 1397-1404.

Hamilton, A. B. (1999). Psychological aspects of ovarian cancer. *Cancer Investigation, 17*(5), 335-341.

Helstrom, L., Lundberg, P. O., Sorbom, D., & Backstrom, T. (1993). Sexuality after hysterectomy: A factor analysis of women's sexual lives before and after subtotal hysterectomy. *Obstetrics and Gynecology, 81*(3), 357-362.

Helstrom, L., Sorbom, D., & Backstrom, T. (1995). Influence of partner relationship on sexuality after subtotal hysterectomy. *Acta Obstetricia et Gynecologica Scandinavica, 74*(2), 142-146.

Heyl, M. (1977). *Attitudes toward a mastectomy: The development of a measurement scale.* Dissertation. Greensboro, NC: University of North Carolina-Greensboro.

Iowa Intervention Project. J. C. McCloskey & G. M. Bulechek (Eds.). (2000). *Nursing interventions classification (NIC)* (3rd ed.). St. Louis, MO: Mosby.

Iowa Outcomes Project. M. Johnson, M. Maas, & S. Moorhead (Eds.). (2000). *Nursing outcomes classification (NOC)* (2nd ed.). St. Louis, MO: Mosby.

Kedia, S., Zippe, C. D., Agarwal, A., Nelson, D. R., & Lakin, M. M. (1999). Treatment of erectile dysfunction with sildenafil citrate (Viagra) after radiation therapy for prostate cancer. *Urology, 54*(2), 308-312.

Khedun, S. M., Naicker, T., & Maharaj, B. (1995). Zinc hydrochlorothiazide and sexual dysfunction. *Central African Journal of Medicine, 41*(10), 312-315.

Korenman, S. G. (1995). Advances in the understanding and management of erectile dysfunction. *Journal of Clinical Endocrinology and Metabolism, 80*(7), 1985-1988.

Korenman, S. G., & Viosca, S. P. (1992). Use of a vacuum tumescence device in the management of impotence in men with a history of penile implant or severe pelvic disease. *Journal of the American Geriatrics Society, 40*(1), 61-64.

Lancaster, J. (1993). Women's experiences of gynaecological cancer treated with radiation. *Curationis, 16*(1), 37-42.

Landoni, F., Proserpio, M., Maneo, A., Cormio, G., Zanetta, G., & Milani, R. (1995). Repair of the perineal defect after radical vulvar surgery: Direct closure versus skin flaps reconstruction. A retrospective comparative study. *Australian and New Zealand Journal of Obstetrics & Gynaecology, 35*(3), 300-304.

Leo, E., Belli, F., Baldini, M. T., Vitellaro, M., Santoro, N., Mascheroni, L., Andreola, S., Bellomi, M., Rebuffoni, G., & Zucali, R. (1993). Total rectal resection, colo-endoanal anastomosis and colic reservoir for cancer of the lower third of the rectum. *European Journal of Surgical Oncology, 19*(3), 283-293.

Litz, B. T., Zeiss, A. M., & Davies, H. D. (1990). Sexual concerns of male spouses of female Alzheimer's disease patients. *The Gerontologist, 30*(1), 113-116.

Lueckenotte, A. G. (1996). *Gerontologic Nursing.* St. Louis, MO: Mosby.

Matsumoto, A. M. (1993). "Andropause"—Are reduced androgen levels in aging men physiologically important? *Western Journal of Medicine, 159*(5), 618-620.

McCormick, G. P., Riffer, D. J., & Thompson, M. M. (1986). Coital positioning for stroke afflicted couples. *Rehabilitation Nursing, 11*(2), 17-19.

Mooradian, A. D., & Greiff, V. (1990). Sexuality in older women. *Archives of Internal Medicine, 150,* 1033-1038.

National Center for Health Statistics. (1994). *Vital statistics of the United States.* DHHS Publication No. (PHS) 95-1101. Washington, DC: Public Health Service.

National Institutes of Health. (1993). *Advisory panel on Alzheimer's disease.* Washington, DC: U.S. Government Printing Office.

National Institutes of Health. (1994). *Alzheimer's disease.* NIH Publication No. 94-3676. Washington, DC: National Institute of Mental Health.

North American Nursing Diagnosis Association. (1999). *Nursing diagnoses: Definitions & classification 1999-2000.* Philadelphia: Author.

Northouse, L. L. (1992). Psychological impact of the diagnosis of breast cancer on the patient and her family. *Journal of the American Medical Women's Association, 47*(5), 161-164.

Papadopoulos, C., Beaumont, C., Shelly, S. I., & Larrimore, P. (1983). Myocardial infarction and sexual activity of the female patient. *Archives of Internal Medicine, 143,* 1528-1530.

Poad, D., & Arnold, E. P. (1994). Sexual function after pelvic surgery in women. *Australian and New Zealand Journal of Obstetrics and Gynaecology, 34*(4), 471-474.

Prisant, L. M., Carr, A. A., Bottini, P. B., Solursh, D. S., & Solursh, L. P. (1994). *Archives of Internal Medicine, 154*(7), 730-736.

Reaby, L. L., & Hort, L. K. (1995). Postmastectomy attitudes in women who wear external breast prostheses compared to those who have undergone breast reconstructions. *Journal of Behavioral Medicine, 18*(1), 55-67.

Rothschild, A. J. (1995). Selective serotonin reuptake inhibitor–induced sexual dysfunction: Efficacy of a drug holiday. *American Journal of Psychiatry, 152*(10), 1514-1516.

Rousseau, L., Dupont, A., Labrie, F., & Couture, M. (1988). Sexuality changes in prostate cancer patients receiving antihormonal therapy combining the antiandrogen flutamide with medical (LHRH agonist) or surgical castration. *Archives of Sexual Behavior, 17*(1), 87-98.

Schag, C. A., Ganz, P. A., Polinsky, M. L., Fred, C., Hirji, K., & Peterson, L. (1993). Characteristics of women at risk for psychosocial distress in the year after breast cancer. *Journal of Clinical Oncology, 11*(4), 783-793.

Scharbo-Dehaan, M. (1994). Management strategies for hormonal replacement therapy. *Nurse Practitioner, 19*(12), 47-57.

Schiavi, R. C., Stimmel, B. B., Mandeli, J., Schreiner-Engel, P., & Ghizzani, A. (1995). Diabetes, psychological function and male sexuality. *Journal of Psychosomatic Research, 39*(3), 305-314.

Schover, L. R. (1993). Sexual rehabilitation after treatment for prostate cancer. *Cancer, 71*(3 Suppl), 1024-1030.

Schover, L. R., Yetman, R. J., Tuason, L. J., Meisler, E., Esselstyn, C. B., Hermann, R. E., Grundfest-Broniatowski, S., & Dowden, R. V. (1995). Partial mastectomy and breast reconstruction. A comparison of their effects on psychosocial adjustment, body image, and sexuality. *Cancer, 75*(1), 54-64.

Schreiner-Engel, P., Schiavi, R. C., Vietorisz, D., & Smith, H. (1987). The differential impact of diabetes type on female sexuality. *Journal of Psychosomatic Research, 31*(1), 23-33.

Schulze, H. (1995). TULIP: Transurethral ultrasound-guided laser-induced prostatectomy. *World Journal of Urology, 13*(2), 94-97.

Seagraves, R. T. (1992). Overview of sexual dysfunction complicating the treatment of depression. *Journal of Clinical Psychiatry, Monograph, 10*(2), 4-10.

Semple, P. D. A., Beastall, G. H., Brown, T. M., Stirling, K. W., Mills, R. J., & Watson, W. S. (1983). Sex hormone suppression and sexual impotence in hypoxic pulmonary fibrosis. *Thorax, 39,* 46-51.

Shell, J. A., & Smith, C. K. (1994). Sexuality and the older person with cancer. *Oncology Nursing Forum, 21*(3), 553-558.

Spratto, G. R., & Woods, A. L. (1996). *Nurse's drug reference.* Albany, NY: Delmar.

Staab, A. S., & Hodges, L. C. (1996). Problems with sexuality. In A. S. Staab & L. C. Hodges (Eds.), *Gerontological nursing* (pp. 370-390). Baltimore: Lippincott Williams & Wilkins.

Strangers, M. A., Taal, B. G., Aaronson, N. K., & te Velde, A. (1995). Quality of life in colorectal cancer: Stoma vs. non-stoma patients. *Diseases of the Colon & Rectum, 38*(4), 361-369.

Takahashi, S., Homma, Y., Minowada, S., & Aso, Y. (1994). Transurethral ultrasound-guided laser-induced prostatectomy (TULIP) for benign prostatic hyperplasia: Clinical utility at one-year follow-up and imaging analysis. *Urology, 43*(6), 802-807.

Thompson, W. L. (1986). Sexual problems in chronic respiratory disease. *Sexual Dysfunction 79*(7), 41-52.

Thranov, I., & Klee, M. (1994). Sexuality among gynecologic cancer patients—a cross-sectional study. *Gynecologic Oncology, 52*(1), 14-19.

Tucker, M. A., Ogle, S. J., Davinson, J. G., & Eilenberg, M. D. (1987). Validation of a brief screening test for depression in the elderly. *Age and Aging, 16,* 139-144.

Uitti, R. J., Tanner, C. M., Rajput, A. H., Goetz, C. G., Klawans, H. L., & Thiessen, B. (1989). Hypersexuality with antiparkinsonian therapy. *Clinical Neuropharmacology, 12*(5), 375-383.

United States Department of Health and Human Services. (1992). *Urinary incontinence in adults: Clinical practice guideline.* AHCPR Pub. No. 92-0038. Rockville, MD: Agency for Health Care Policy and Research.

United States Department of Health and Human Services. (1995). *Post-stroke rehabilitation: Clinical practice guideline.* AHCPR Pub. No. 95-0662. Rockville, MD: Agency for Health Care Policy and Research.

Vierhout, M. E., & Gianotten, W. L. (1993). Unintended urine loss in women during sexual activities. (Dutch). *Nederlands Tijdschrift voor Geneeskunde, 137*(18), 913-916.

Walz, T. H., & Blum, N. S. (1987). *Sexual health in later life.* Lexington, MA: Lexington Books.

Wilmoth, M. C., & Townsend, J. (1995). A comparison of the effects of lumpectomy versus mastectomy on sexual behaviors. *Cancer Practice, 3*(5), 279-285.

Wincze, J. P., Albert, A., & Bansal, S. (1993). Sexual arousal in diabetic females: Physiological and self-report measures. *Archives of Sexual Behavior, 22*(6), 587-601.

Wright, L. K. (1993a). *Alzheimer's disease and marriage.* Thousand Oaks, CA: Sage.

Wright, L. K. (1993b). The impact of Alzheimer's disease on marriage and sexuality. *The Gerontologist, 33,* Special Issue, 46.

Wright, L. K. (1994). Alzheimer's disease–afflicted spouses who remain at home: Can human dialectics explain the findings? *Social Science and Medicine, 38*(8), 1037-1046.

Wright, L. K. (1997). Elderly persons with mental illness. In N. K. Worley (Ed.), *Mental health nursing in the community* (pp. 385-402). St. Louis, MO: Mosby.

Yesavage, J. A., & Brink, T. L. (1983). Development and validation of a geriatric depression screening scale: A preliminary report. *Journal of Psychiatric Research, 17*(1), 37-49.

CHAPTER 58

ALTERED SEXUALITY PATTERNS

Lore K. Wright

In Chapter 56 normal changes with aging and their impact on sexuality were discussed. Changes in sexuality patterns that result from disease, pathology, or surgery were discussed in Chapter 57. This chapter focuses on changes in sexuality patterns that result from normal aging processes.

NURSING DIAGNOSIS

The North American Nursing Diagnosis Association (NANDA) has defined Altered Sexuality Patterns as "the state in which an individual expresses concern regarding his/her sexuality" (NANDA, 1999, p. 65). Sexual behavior is highly individual and variable. Some older people are sexually active, others are not, and neither situation may be of concern to the individual. It is only when the client expresses concern over sexual issues that a nursing diagnosis can be used. Only when the client voices concern can etiologies be explored, goals for outcomes be established, and interventions be implemented.

This diagnostic formulation also presents difficulties. Although societal attitudes toward sexually active older persons are changing, there is still great reluctance on the part of both older persons and health care professionals to discuss sexual concerns (Butler, Lewis, Hoffman, & Whitehead, 1994). Thus many elders may have concerns and think and worry about sexual issues but not express (verbalize) these concerns to health care professionals. The number of elders who could potentially meet the nursing diagnosis Altered Sexuality Patterns is probably much larger than is known.

Yet it is not difficult to facilitate verbalization of problems or concerns. Any assessment, whether physical or psychosocial, needs to include a simple, matter-of-fact question delivered in an unhurried and attentive manner: "Do you have any questions or concerns about sexual intimacy?" The word *intimacy* rather than *intercourse* conveys a more inclusive definition of sexuality and may also be perceived as less confrontive or embarrassing by elders.

RELATED FACTORS/ETIOLOGIES

Change in sexuality patterns can result from several different etiologies: altered body function or structure, knowledge or skill deficits, impaired relationships, lack of

a sexual partner, lack of privacy, conflicts surrounding sexual orientation or variant preferences, values conflicts, and fear of acquiring a sexually transmitted disease. An older client's verbalized concerns are likely to be related to more than one etiology. Some of these are specific to women, some to men, and many are experienced by both men and women. In Table 58-1 only those etiologies encountered in elderly people and only those attributable to normal aging are listed; thus the list draws from criteria for "altered patterns" as well as for "sexual dysfunction." Accompanying symptoms have been categorized for females versus males. Nursing interventions and nursing-sensitive outcomes are closely linked to these varying etiologies. To make these links clear, specific characteristics of changes in sexuality patterns and available nursing interventions are discussed in the context of specific etiologies.

Altered Body Function or Structure

Altered Sexuality Pattern Related to Body Image Disturbance or Structure is one of the most common diagnoses associated with normal aging. Both men and women experience symptoms that warrant the diagnosis.

Function and Structure Changes in Older Women. For older women, typically around age 50, symptoms of vaginal dryness, dyspareunia, dysuria, and cystitis following intercourse are indicative of estrogen deficiency associated with the cessation of ovarian function, or menopause. In addition, about 85% of menopausal women experience vasomotor instability (hot flushes/flashes), and anxiety or nervousness and irritability typically accompany the symptoms (McKeon, 1994; Sheehy, 1992). However, there is insufficient epidemiologic evidence of increased depression during menopause (American Psychiatric Association, 1994). For older women engaged in sexual relations, menopausal physical changes can lead to dyspareunia and vaginitis. There is also increased risk for greater shock and abrasion to the urethra and bladder, which often results in cystitis (Mooradian & Greiff, 1990). When a woman verbalizes menopausal discomforts to a health care professional, the use of appropriate lubrication and a change in body positions during intimacy may be discussed, but in all likeli-

Table 58-1	Related Factors/Etiologies ALTERED SEXUALITY PATTERNS	
NANDA Criteria Applicable to Older Clients	**Symptoms**	
	Female	Male
Altered body function or structure	Vaginal dryness Dyspareunia Dysuria, cystitis	Slower sexual response Less firm erections Changes in ejaculation Anxiety, depression
Knowledge/skill deficit about alternative responses to health transitions; misinformation	Use of inappropriate substances, techniques Misinterpretation of normal aging changes Reluctance to discuss problems with health care professional Anxiety	Use of inappropriate substances, techniques Misinterpretation of normal aging changes Reluctance to discuss problems with health care professional Anxiety Depression
Impaired relationship with a significant other	Diminished or absent sexual intimacy Communication problems	Diminished or absent sexual intimacy Communication problems
Lack of significant other	Grief over disabled or deceased partner Isolation, low self-esteem	Grief over disabled or deceased partner Depression
Lack of privacy	Complaints over changed living arrangements (moving in with children, group home, or institutionalization) Low self-esteem	Complaints over changed living arrangements (moving in with children, group home, or institutionalization) Anger, hostility
Conflicts with sexual orientation	Perceived societal intolerance of variant preferences Lesbian relationship Anxiety, isolation	Perceived societal intolerance of variant preferences Gay relationship Anxiety, isolation
Values conflict	Adherence to religious principles Monetary considerations Anxiety, isolation	Less likely Monetary considerations Anxiety, isolation
Fear of acquiring a sexually transmitted disease	Reluctance to form new relationship; Anxiety, doubts	Reluctance to form new relationship Anxiety, doubts

hood, hormone replacement therapy (HRT) will at least be considered (McKeon, 1994). A blood test typically will reveal a level of more than 40 mIU/mL of the follicle-stimulating hormone (FSH) versus the less than 30 mIU/mL found in nonmenopausal women (Kee, 1995; Lemcke, Marshall, & Pattison, 1995). Decreased production of ovarian estrogen and the loss of negative feedback from the ovaries stimulates the pituitary gland to secrete more FSH (Lemcke et al., 1995).

Estrogen replacement has been used since the 1930s. In the late 1970s, unopposed estrogen was linked to a dramatic rise in endometrial cancer (Sharbo-Dehaan, 1994). Subsequently, combined regimens of estrogen and progesterone were adopted for women who had not undergone a hysterectomy. Currently, approximately 40 million women in the United States are over the age of 50, and every year for the next 10 years another 2 to 3 million women will be faced with deciding whether to use or reject hormone replacement (United States Bureau of the Census, 1998). At present, only 15% to 25% of menopausal women receive hormone replacement therapy (Andrews, 1995).

There is considerable debate whether a normal aging process should be "medicalized" and whether the advantages of hormone replacement therapy outweigh the disadvantages (Herrick, Douglas, & Carlson, 1995). Much of the medical literature continues to portray menopause as a deficiency disease requiring a cure; in contrast, most women would reject a disease label. Nevertheless, lack of estrogen, in addition to causing the menopausal symptoms already described, has adverse effects on the body. Estrogen deficiency leads to rapid bone demineralization, increased risk of heart disease, and, possibly, memory problems. Rapid demineralization of bone tissue (osteoporosis) is an especially serious problem, affecting 60 million postmenopausal women. In 40% of women over the age 70, osteoporosis causes bone fractures, and some of these fractures result in permanent disability or death (Butler & Lewis, 1993). In addition, lack of estrogen decreases high density lipoprotein (HDL or the "good" cholesterol) and increases low density lipoprotein (LDL or the "bad" cholesterol), which can lead to heart disease. Lack of estrogen may also contribute to the formation of fatty deposits in the arteries, thus contributing to heart attacks and strokes (McKeon, 1994). There is weak and contradictory evidence that estrogen deficiency increases the risk of developing Alzheimer's disease (Brenner et al., 1994; Henderson, Paganini-Hill, Emanuel, Dunn, & Buckwalter, 1994; Hogervorst, Boshuisen, Riedel, Willeken, & Jolles, 1999; Paganini-Hill & Henderson, 1994).

Clearly, estrogen replacement therapy (ERT) provides several benefits to the older woman. But there are also some risks, the most important being endometrial adenocarcinoma and breast cancer. Unopposed estrogen is invariably related to adenomatous endometrial hyperplasia, which is a precursor of endometrial cancer (McKeon, 1994). The addition of progesterone reduces the occurrence of endometrial hyperplasia and, at high doses, causes preexisting hyperplasia to regress. (The combination of estrogen and progesterone therapy is often referred to as HRT to distinguish it from ERT, estrogen replacement alone). Unfortunately, the addition of progesterone may negate the beneficial effects of unopposed estrogen on the lipid profile already described; however, these effects may be only temporary and may reverse with time (Miller et al., 1991; Whitehead, Hillard, & Crook, 1990).

The second major risk, breast cancer, has received considerable attention. Findings from the Nurses' Health Study reported a relative risk of 1.36 of breast cancer among those women who used ERT (Colditz et al., 1990). However, other studies did not support these findings nor did several meta-analyses of the conflicting reports (McKeon, 1994). To date, there is a growing consensus that with long-term use of ERT (more than 15 years), there is a modest increase in risk for developing breast cancer, but short-term use (5 years or less) is not associated with increased risk. As yet, it is not known whether the combination of estrogen and progesterone increases or decreases the risk of developing breast cancer (McKeon, 1994).

More recently, the medication raloxifene hydrochloride (Evista), a synthetic "designer" estrogen, has been shown effective in reducing the risk of osteoporosis (Ettinger et al., 1999). Unlike estrogen, raloxifene does not stimulate breast or uterine tissue; it lowers LDL cholesterol and appears to lower the risk of breast cancer (Ettinger et al., 1999). However, raloxifene does not increase vaginal lubrication.

Function and Structure Changes in Older Men.
Older men, beginning around age 40, begin to experience several changes: a slower erectile response, less firm erections, erections that are lost quickly, different sensations during ejaculations, and a lengthened refrac-

tory period (time between ejaculations) (Butler, Finkel, Lewis, Sherman, & Sunderland, 1992). Men are even less likely to talk about these changes than women talk about their menopausal symptoms. Men tend to worry that the changes they are experiencing are the first signs of impotence. This "performance anxiety," as it is sometimes referred to, can lead to avoidance of intimacy and even depression (Butler & Lewis, 1993; Thienhaus, 1988). Thus the etiology of "altered body function or structure," which is attributable to normal changes with aging, becomes intertwined with "knowledge/skill deficit," "misinformation," and "impaired relationship with a significant other."

While the changes occurring with menopause in women can be linked to estrogen deficiency, a corresponding male hormone deficit that could be linked to changes in sexual functioning in older men has not been clearly established. Testosterone levels decrease very slowly with increasing age, and some men in their eighties have levels similar to those of young men (Rowland, Greenleaf, Dorfman, & Davidson, 1993). However, the absence of a meaningful age-related decrease in testosterone observed in several studies might be due to age-related differences when testosterone levels peak. Testosterone levels peak in younger men in the morning. Testosterone levels peak in older men in the afternoon. Consequently, if blood samples in these studies had been collected in the afternoon, age differences would not have been found (Matsumoto, 1993).

A few studies have shown that administering oral testosterone to healthy elderly males who had serum testosterone levels of less than 350 ng/dl had no adverse effects and did increase libido and feelings of well-being (Matsumoto, 1993). But there are concerns that the use of testosterone replacement therapy in elderly men with mild androgen deficiency might stimulate benign or malignant prostate growth or reduce HDL cholesterol levels, thereby increasing the risk for coronary artery disease (Swerdloff & Wang, 1993).

Knowledge or Skill Deficit and Misinformation

Because menopause is a defined physiologic event, women tend to receive more information about anticipated body changes related to aging than do older men. But even women are not fully informed; only 44% of perimenopausal women reported that they were very satisfied with the information they received from their physician (Utian & Schiff, 1994), and the majority were not aware of long-term health concerns associated with menopause (Andrews, 1995).

Women may also be misinformed about appropriate lubricants to compensate for vaginal dryness and may use an oil-based lubricant such as Vaseline instead of a water-based lubricant such as K-Y jelly. Oil-based lubricants are inappropriate, insoluble substances that provide a medium for microorganisms and subsequent vaginal infection. Women who experience dyspareunia and cystitis might not be aware that irritation to the vaginal wall, urethra, and bladder contributes to the problem. Also, they might not know that different body positions for intercourse can alleviate the problems (such as the "on top" position and requesting the partner to thrust his penis downward toward the back of the vagina, toward the rectum, instead toward the upper part of the vagina) (Butler & Lewis, 1993; Heiman, 1995). Increased fluid intake and urination before and after intercourse also might not be practiced.

Although knowledge and skill deficits can lead to anxiety, many women remain reluctant to discuss these problems with a health professional (Heiman, 1995). Women also might shy away from openly discussing concerns with their sex partner. In such situations, lack of knowledge and/or skills can lead to refusing continued intimacy, which in turn can lead to "impaired relationship with a significant other."

Men who lack knowledge about normal changes with aging are not likely to request increased penile stimulation from their sex partner; they misinterpret less firm erections and diminished sensations during ejaculation as signs of impotence (Thienhaus, 1988). "This misconception literally scares men into impotence" (Butler et al., 1992, p. 63). Thus anxiety over "performance" can lead to a vicious cycle of discouragement, avoidance of sexuality, depression, and further difficulties during the next attempt (National Institutes of Health, 1992). Men, even more so than women, are reluctant to discuss these issues with a health professional. Even though the drug sildenafil citrate (Viagra) has received extensive media coverage, reluctance to discuss sexual dysfunction is reflected in recent statistics: Only one in 10 older men try sex-enhancing treatments (Jacoby, 1999), and only 5% receive adequate treatment from a geriatrician, even though 67% of men aged 70 have erectile dysfunctions (Godschalk, Sison, & Mulligan, 1997). Anxiety, depression, and relationship problems can result.

The presence of emotional problems in an older male should alert the health professional to question changes in sexual functioning. The Adult Sexuality Knowledge and Attitude Test (ASKAT), developed by Walz and Blum in 1987, still provides a good assessment of the client's insight and can be used as a starting point for more focused assessment questions. Severity of anxiety and depression can be assessed with standardized scales such as the Short Zung Depression Scale (Tucker, Ogle, Davinson, & Eilenberg, 1987), the Geriatric Depression Scale (Yesavage & Brink, 1983), or the subscales for depression, anxiety, and interpersonal sensitivity of the Symptom Check List (SCL-90-R) (Derogatis & Cleary, 1977). Referral to a mental health professional should be considered.

Impaired Relationship With a Significant Other

In long-term relationships, complaints of diminished or absent intimacy are, in all likelihood, indications of communication problems. Despite years of marriage, partners might not be open with each other about their changing sexual experiences. Long-term relationships also can experience boredom caused by monotony of repetitious sexual relations, and one partner's desire might not match that of the other (Byers, 1983; Heiman, 1995). In addition, interpersonal problems such as one partner's preoccupation with a hobby or business can cause impaired sexual intimacy (Byers, 1983).

Altered Sexuality Patterns Related to Lack of Significant Other

Widowhood and divorce are the most common reasons for lack of a significant partner. Women are three times more likely to experience isolation than men (United States Bureau of the Census, 1998). Low self-esteem results if an older women perceives herself as physically unattractive (Kuhlman, 1996). Older men who do not remarry within a relatively short time after the death of a spouse are vulnerable to depression, and the risk of suicide is highest among elder widowed or divorced white males (Ebersole & Hess, 1998).

Lack of Privacy

Moving in with grown children, moving into a group home, or being placed into a nursing home all carry with them loss of independence. Elders might not complain directly that changed living arrangements interfere with privacy needs; rather, lack of privacy can be manifest in expressions of low self-esteem, anger, and hostility.

Sexual Orientation or Variant Preferences

In addition to experiencing the same problems as other sexually active elders, aging homosexuals face intolerant societal attitudes. Approximately one third of lesbians come out after the age of 50, undoubtedly accompanied by conflict. Most older lesbians continue to prefer monogamous relationships more so than gay men. Gay older men rarely have long-term relationships, possibly due to a lifelong pattern of multiple partners and death of a loved one (Ebersole & Hess, 1998). Those who are active in the gay and lesbian community tend to experience less anxiety and isolation (Quam & Whitford, 1992).

Values Conflict

Cultural or religious principles can create values conflicts, especially for older women who consider entering a sexual relationship without marriage. These conflicts can be compounded by monetary considerations, such as loss of a pension in case of remarriage, or by disapproval from grown children (Butler & Lewis, 1993). The conflict is likely to cause anxiety and, if not resolved, isolation. It appears, however, that an increasing number of elders choose to live together without remarriage (United States Bureau of the Census, 1998).

Fear of Acquiring a Sexually Transmitted Disease

Ten percent of persons over the age of 50 have human immunodeficiency virus (HIV) infection; the rate is 4% for persons over age 70 (Butler & Lewis, 1993). Most of these HIV cases have resulted from blood transfusions. Elders entering a new relationship have to be concerned about acquiring HIV or other sexually transmitted diseases. Increased public education has raised anxiety levels and doubts about the wisdom of entering into a new intimate relationship, but increased awareness can also contribute to appropriate preventive practices.

NURSING-SENSITIVE OUTCOMES

Successful outcomes for a diagnosis of Altered Sexuality Patterns are those that meet the patients' expressed needs. Thus whether sexual intimacy is resumed, continues, declines, or ceases is less important than is helping patients to become comfortable with age-related changes. Also, many symptoms attributable to normal changes with aging can be alleviated. The key to need satisfaction is adequate knowledge about normal changes in sexual functioning with aging. Once patients have this knowledge, other outcomes can build on this foundation. Because the diagnosis of Altered Sexuality Patterns often has several etiologies, typically more than one outcome is formulated.

Nursing outcomes most frequently targeted include the following: increased knowledge about sexual functioning; adjustment to normal changes with aging and obtaining desired levels of sexual intimacy; increased communication skills about sexuality; control of menopausal symptoms; knowledge about hormone replacement medication; acceptance of aging body image; grief resolution associated with loss of sexual partner; social restructuring to facilitate sexual behaviors; conflict resolution over sexual preferences or divergent values; and risk control for sexually transmitted diseases (Iowa Outcomes Project, 2000). Outcomes pertaining to various etiologies and suggested nursing interventions are summarized in Table 58-2.

Knowledge: Sexual Functioning

The outcome Knowledge: Sexual Functioning pertains to the patient's "extent of understanding conveyed about sexual development and responsible sexual practices"

(Iowa Outcomes Project, 2000, p. 291). Women and men should have knowledge both about their own functioning and about their partner's functioning. This knowledge should facilitate decisions about alternative practices or alleviation of symptoms.

Crucial areas of knowledge about women are changes associated with menopause and accompanying symptoms such as vaginal dryness, dyspareunia, dysuria, and cystitis. Essential areas of knowledge pertaining to males are the slower sexual response with aging, less firm erections, and changes in sensations during and frequency of ejaculation. Correct answers on the Adult Sexuality Knowledge and Attitude Test (ASKAT) (Walz & Blum, 1987) can provide evidence of the client's insight and knowledge; incorrect answers can be targeted for interventions.

Adjustment to Aging: Sexual Functioning

The outcome Adjustment to Aging: Sexual Functioning pertains to an individual's skills in adapting to age-associated physiologic changes in sexual functioning. Outcome indicators for women include the use of adequate and water-soluble vaginal lubricants and experimentation with different body positions during intimacy. Outcome indicators for men include correct interpretation and acceptance of physiologic changes and the use of increased penile stimulation during intimacy.

Men and women need to obtain their own desired level of sexual intimacy, a level that is agreeable to both partners. Such outcomes are intertwined with achieving improved communication skills between sexual partners. Successful adjustments will decrease anxiety and depressive symptoms. If deemed necessary, pre and post-intervention anxiety and depressive symptom scores on standardized tests can be evaluated.

Communication: Sexual Functioning

The outcome Communication: Sexual Functioning pertains to an individual's ability to communicate concerns about sexual functioning to a significant other and/or health professional. Health professionals who routinely address these issues can overcome barriers to communication. Patients who have improved their communication skills are likely to report enhanced or resumed sexual intimacy.

Symptom Control: Menopausal Symptoms

The outcome Symptom Control: Menopausal Symptoms pertains to the alleviation of physical and emotional discomforts associated with loss of ovarian function. The patient needs to become knowledgeable about oral HRT and vaginally administered HRT. Women also need to understand the following alternatives to hormone replacement: vaginal moisturizers, vitamin E and B complex

Table 58-2	Suggested Nursing-Sensitive Outcomes and Nursing Interventions ALTERED SEXUALITY PATTERNS		

Nursing Diagnoses	Nursing-Sensitive Outcomes	Nursing Interventions
ALTERED SEXUALITY PATTERNS *Related Factors/Etiologies* Altered body function or structure, illness or medical	KNOWLEDGE: SEXUAL FUNCTIONING ANXIETY CONTROL COMFORT LEVEL	LEARNING FACILITATION HUMOR SEXUAL COUNSELING ANXIETY REDUCTION REFERRAL
Knowledge/skill deficit about responses to health-related transitions	KNOWLEDGE: SEXUAL FUNCTIONING PSYCHOSOCIAL ADJUSTMENT: LIFE CHANGE COMMUNICATION: SEXUAL FUNCTIONING KNOWLEDGE: MEDICATION (ERT/HRT) ANXIETY CONTROL COMFORT LEVEL	LEARNING FACILITATION TEACHING: PRESCRIBED MEDICATION HUMOR SEXUAL COUNSELING REFERRAL COPING ENHANCEMENT TEACHING: SEXUALITY TEACHING: PRESCRIBED MEDICATION MEDICATION MANAGEMENT ANXIETY REDUCTION REFERRAL
Impaired relationship with a significant other	COMMUNICATION: SEXUAL FUNCTIONING KNOWLEDGE: SEXUAL FUNCTIONING PSYCHOSOCIAL ADJUSTMENT: SEXUAL FUNCTIONING	COPING ENHANCEMENT SEXUAL COUNSELING LEARNING FACILITATION HUMOR REFERRAL
Lack of significant other	GRIEF RESOLUTION SELF-ESTEEM COMFORT LEVEL SOCIAL INTERACTION SKILLS BODY IMAGE: SEXUALLY ATTRACTIVE	GRIEF WORK FACILITATION EMOTIONAL SUPPORT SELF-ESTEEM ENHANCEMENT REFERRAL SOCIALIZATION ENHANCEMENT BODY IMAGE ENHANCEMENT
Lack of privacy	SOCIAL INTERACTION SKILLS ANXIETY CONTROL SELF-ESTEEM	ENVIRONMENTAL MANAGEMENT VISITATION FACILITATION LEARNING FACILITATION EMOTIONAL SUPPORT SELF-ESTEEM ENHANCEMENT
Conflict with sexual orientation or variant preferences	COMFORT LEVEL ANXIETY CONTROL SOCIAL INTERACTION SKILLS KNOWLEDGE: SEXUAL FUNCTIONING ACCEPTANCE: HEALTH STATUS	COUNSELING EMOTIONAL SUPPORT ANXIETY REDUCTION REFERRAL SOCIALIZATION ENHANCEMENT LEARNING FACILITATION RISK IDENTIFICATION REFERRAL

Continued

Table 58-2	Suggested Nursing-Sensitive Outcomes and Nursing Interventions—cont'd ALTERED SEXUALITY PATTERNS—cont'd		
Nursing Diagnoses	**Nursing-Sensitive Outcomes**	**Nursing Interventions**
Values conflict	PSYCHOSOCIAL ADJUSTMENT: LIFE CHANGE ANXIETY CONTROL KNOWLEDGE: SEXUAL FUNCTIONING SOCIAL INTERACTION SKILLS	SELF-AWARENESS ENCHANCEMENT VALUES CLARIFICATION FAMILY INVOLVEMENT PROMOTION EMOTIONAL SUPPORT SUPPORT SYSTEM ENHANCEMENT CULTURAL BROKERAGE ANXIETY REDUCTION LEARNING FACILITATION—HUMOR SOCIALIZATION ENHANCEMENT
Fear of acquiring a sexually transmitted disease	RISK CONTROL COMMUNICATION: SEXUAL FUNCTIONING ANXIETY CONTROL	RISK IDENTIFICATION TEACHING: SAFE SEX ANTICIPATORY GUIDANCE EMOTIONAL SUPPORT ANXIETY REDUCTION

supplements, and homeopathic remedies such as ginseng tea, dong quai, and bee pollen (Scharbo-Dehaan, 1994). Relief or control of menopausal symptoms overlaps with adjustment to aging and, for HRT, with knowledge about medication.

Knowledge: Medication (ERT/HRT)

The outcome Knowledge: Medication is defined as the "extent of understanding conveyed about the safe use of medication" (Iowa Outcomes Project, 2000, p. 279). Knowledge: Medication pertains to a women's understanding of hormone replacement therapy. Women should be able to verbalize advantages, disadvantages, and contraindications of ERT or HRT. It is also important that women do not replace one set of symptoms (e.g., hot flushes, vaginal dryness, cystitis) with another set of discomforts (e.g., abdominal distension, weight gain, breast tenderness). Rather, the level of hormone replacement medications should be adjusted to the individual woman's body responses (McKeon, 1994; Scharbo-Dehaan, 1994).

Body Image: Sexual Attractiveness

The outcome Body Image: Sexual Attractiveness pertains to the older person's psychologic adjustment to an aging body, typically characterized by wrinkled skin, brown spots, varicose veins, and a less firm body. Because American society still equates sexual attractiveness with a youthful, slim appearance, this outcome is especially important for older women who seek a new partner (Butler et al., 1994; Travis, 1987). It is desired that older persons view themselves and their partner as sexually attractive and value the emotional security in established relationships.

Grief Resolution: Sexual Partner

The outcome Grief Resolution: Sexual Partner pertains to an older person's psychologic adjustment to an impaired or lost sexual relationship. Indicators that this outcome has been met include statements regarding resolution of grief, increased self-esteem, decreased depressive symptoms, and increased social participation. Accomplishing this outcome does not necessarily lead to a new sexual relationship.

Social Restructuring: Facilitation of Sexual Behaviors

The outcome Social Restructuring: Facilitation of Sexual Behaviors pertains to older persons' ability to request and accomplish adequate privacy in living arrangements. Outcome indicators include acknowledgement by family members or staff in institutional settings of older persons' sexual desires and efforts by family and staff to accommodate elders' need and right for privacy (Ebersole & Hess, 1998). Successful social restructuring will increase an older person's self-esteem and decrease anger and hostility.

Conflict Resolution: Sexual Preferences/Variants and Values

The outcome Conflict Resolution: Sexual Preferences/ Variants and Values pertains to an older person expressing acceptance of and comfort with personal preferences and values despite family members' or societal disapproval. Decreased anxiety and increased social participation can indicate that this outcome has been met (Deevey, 1990; Ebersole & Hess, 1998).

Risk Control: Sexually Transmitted Diseases

The outcome Risk Control: Sexually Transmitted Diseases pertains to knowledge and practice of safe sex. Patients should be able to verbalize safe sex techniques and to assess safety ranging from absolute safe, to very safe, probably safe, and risky (Staab & Hodges, 1996). This is especially important for homosexual relationships.

NURSING INTERVENTIONS

Interventions typically are conceptualized as occurring subsequent to the formulation of desired outcomes, which occurs following assessment. In reality, however, interventions begin during the assessment phase. When the nurse questions a patient in a friendly, respectful manner about intimate (sexual) issues, assessment is only one aspect of this interaction. Another component is the nurse's role modeling, the conveyed message that it is all right to talk about sexual concerns. This practice decreases barriers to communication, and, thus, the exchange serves as an intervention. Indeed, every exchange between the nurse and the patient holds an opportunity for intervention, be it increasing the patient's knowledge, decreasing anxiety, or providing emotional support.

The most frequently used nursing interventions for Altered Sexual Patterns include the following: Learning Facilitation, Humor, Sexual Counseling, Referral, Anxiety Reduction, Emotional Support, and Socialization Enhancement. Additional interventions are listed in Table 58-2. All interventions are based on Nursing Intervention Classification (NIC) criteria (Iowa Intervention Project, 2000). These interventions are discussed below in the context of specific etiologies.

Altered Body Function and Structure

Increasing the patient's knowledge of normal changes with aging that affect sexual functioning is facilitated in an environment conducive to learning (i.e., a private and unhurried exchange) and by adjusting the information to the client's level of knowledge and understanding. Humor can be used in moderate levels to decrease embarrassment; the patient's attempts at humor should be responded to positively.

Sexual Counseling is defined as the "use of an interactive helping process focusing on the need to make adjustments in sexual practice or to enhance coping with a sexual event/disorder" (Iowa Intervention Project, 2000, p. 584). Sexual Counseling differs from Sex Therapy. If in-

depth treatment for serious sexual problems is necessary, the nurse must either have specialized training and meet qualifications identified by the American Association of Sex Educators, Counselors, and Therapists (AASECT) or the patient must be referred to a qualified sex therapist. Sexual Counseling is a less intense level of intervention. During counseling, specific aspects of sexual functioning can be discussed, alternative methods can be explained, and popular books can be recommended, including "Love and Sex after 60" (Butler & Lewis, 1993), "The New Our Bodies, Ourselves" (Boston Women's Health Book Collective, 1992), and the older but still accurate "Sexual Health in Later Life" (Walz & Blum, 1987), which contains the ASKET questionnaire.

Anxiety reduction is achieved by listening attentively and encouraging verbalization of feelings, perceptions, and fears. If high levels of anxiety and/or depression are noted (possibly confirmed by a standardized assessment scale), the patient should be referred to a mental health professional. It is important to remember that older clients might deny feelings of depression and focus instead on somatic complaints (Wright, 1996).

Knowledge or Skill Deficit and Misinformation

Knowledge deficits and misinformation require Learning Facilitation, defined as "promoting the ability to process and comprehend information" (Iowa Intervention Project, 2000, p. 423) and Humor, which is "facilitating the patient to perceive, appreciate, and express what is funny, amusing, or ludicrous in order to establish relationships, relieve tension, release anger, facilitate learning, or cope with painful feelings" (Iowa Intervention Project, 2000, p. 380). Teaching provided during Sexual Counseling should be consistent with the patient's values.

Coping is enhanced by appraising and discussing alternatives, such as the use of adequate amounts or different types of water-soluble lubricants (e.g., K-Y jelly, Slippery Stuff, Astroglide). Alternative body positions during intimacy can be explained using drawings provided in the book by Walz and Blum (1987). Lueckenotte (1996) also provides this information. The need for increased penile stimulation for older men can be explained to both partners. Older men should be given information about the role of testosterone, testosterone levels, and the risks associated with testosterone medication. Information about the new drug sildenafil citrate (Viagra) can be provided (Goldstein et al., 1998). The mechanism of this drug's action can be summarized as follows: an erection is maintained in the presence of cyclic guanosine monophosphate (cGMP), but is lost when cGMP is removed by the enzyme cGMP phosphodiesterase. Sildenafil citrate inhibits the phosphodiesterase and minimizes the breakdown of cGMP, thereby sustaining the erection. Contraindications for the use of sildenafil (i.e., the concomitant use of organic nitrates) must be added to the information provided.

For women, adequate fluid intake to prevent cystitis should be stressed. If a woman has a lifelong habit of douching, occasional vinegar or saline douches (not alkaline substances such as soda) are recommended (Carnevali, 1993). Women who experience menopausal symptoms need to be given information not only about ERT or HRT, but also about alternative remedies. For example, there are anecdotal reports that hot flashes can be reduced or relieved through relaxation and guided imagery, through daily supplementation of vitamin B complex and 400 to 800 international units of vitamin E, and with ginseng tea, dong quai, and bee pollen (Scharbo-DeHaan, 1994).

When ERT or HRT is considered, the risks and benefits need to be explained. Contraindications have to be ruled out, such as current breast or endometrial cancer, undiagnosed vaginal bleeding, acute liver disease, or thrombophlebitis. Other contraindications to be considered include, but are not limited to, past history of breast or endometrial cancer, recent myocardial infarction, or chronic liver disease (McKeon, 1994). Clearly, before ERT/HRT can be recommended, a thorough physical examination should be performed either by a nurse practitioner or by a physician. If a woman is already receiving hormone therapy, teaching should focus on the prescribed medication, especially side effects such as breast tenderness, weight gain, bloating, and headaches. About 10% of women receiving HRT experience such effects. Lowering the dosage of progesterone and switching to a combined regimen of estrogen and progesterone (at lower dosages) can alleviate these side effects (McKeon, 1994; Scharbo-Dehaan, 1994). Emotional responses such as anxiety and depression must always be monitored and addressed. If indicated, patients need to be referred to a mental health professional.

Impaired Relationship With Significant Other

At the root of an impaired relationship with a sexual partner is impaired communication. Teaching new communication and coping skills is essential, for example, the ability to tell a partner what is pleasing and what is not. Sexual Counseling might need to include the spouse or sexual partner. Referral to a sex therapist might be necessary.

Lack of Significant Other

Grief Work Facilitation, which is the "assistance with the resolution of a significant loss" (Iowa Intervention Project, 2000, p. 358), can be used with patients who have lost their sexual partner. Feelings about the loss, including anger or relief, should be explored, and patients can be encouraged to describe memories of the relationship, good or bad,

past or recent. The nurse should permit ambivalent feelings to surface and not automatically assume that the loss pertains to someone who was truly loved (Staab & Hodges, 1996). Emotional Support is the "provision of reassurance, acceptance, and encouragement during times of stress" (Iowa Intervention Project, 2000, p. 300) and is crucial throughout. Self-esteem Enhancement is "assisting a patient to increase his/her personal judgment of self-worth" (p. 580) and is undertaken by monitoring the patient's statements of self-worth and providing encouragement for pursuing new challenges.

When interacting with older widowed and divorced men who live alone, monitoring of depression and suicidal ideation is especially important. Older white males have the highest suicide rate in the United States. Opportunities for intervention with these persons exist, since many of them visit a health professional within 6 months prior to committing suicide. Direct questioning, such as "Are you having thoughts of wanting to end your life?" is important (Wright, 1996).

To counteract isolation, Socialization Enhancement, which is the "facilitation of another person's ability to interact with others" (Iowa Intervention Project, 2000, p. 604), is used, i.e., encouraging relationships with persons who have common interests. Arranging attendance at a support group can play a vital role in grief resolution. In addition, Support Group is the "use of a group environment to provide emotional support and health-related information for members" (p. 623) and offers opportunities to meet a potential new partner. This is especially important for older women who, in addition to grief, might need to deal with a change in body image. The nurse helps the patient to separate physical appearance from feelings of personal worth. Humor is again an appropriate strategy, such as helping a woman to say, "I think I earned my wrinkles."

Lack of Privacy

Interventions that address lack of privacy are different for institutional versus live-in family situations. Federal nursing home regulations for intermediate care facilities (ICFs) and for skilled nursing facilities (SNFs) now include provisions to ensure privacy during spousal visits, unless medically contraindicated. "Do-not-disturb" signs can be placed on closed doors to ensure privacy (Richardson & Lazur, 1995). However, nursing home staff may not feel comfortable with such arrangements (Ebersole & Hess, 1998). Knowledge Facilitation, i.e., helping staff members to understand, accept, and support older persons' sexuality, might be needed.

If an older person lives with grown children, interventions will have to include the family. Stress levels of all concerned are likely to be high, but a home visit by the nurse to assess and recommend a solution can be of value. Churches can play an important role by requesting a nurse to speak about this topic at the congregation's educational meetings.

Conflicts With Sexual Orientation/Variant

Conflict resolution regarding sexual identity is especially important for older lesbians. Approximately one third come out after the age of 50, and 40% were previously married (Deevey, 1990; Ebersole & Hess, 1998). Assessment techniques such as asking, "Who is most important to you" (instead of "Are you married?") and "Do you consider yourself primarily heterosexual, homosexual, or bisexual?" (to convey recognition of sexual variety) are important to build trust and to facilitate self-acceptance (Ebersole & Hess, 1998).

Given the high incidence of suicidal ideation and suicidal attempts among lesbians, Emotional Support, Anxiety Reduction, and Referral for depression with suicidal ideation are important interventions. Older gay men might need Counseling due to loss of a partner and lesser opportunities for new relationships. Recommending involvement in the gay and lesbian community (Socialization Enhancement) can decrease isolation.

Both gays and lesbians are faced with the same changes in sexual functioning with aging as heterosexual elders. Thus Knowledge Facilitation is used in addition to risk identification for sexually transmitted diseases.

Values Conflict

Values conflicts are likely to focus on whether to remarry, just "live together," or remain alone. Conflict resolution is facilitated through Values Clarification. For example, the patient can be helped to define advantages and disadvantages of changing living arrangements or remarriage. Anticipating the consequences of decisions will contribute to self-awareness and to the identification of positive as well as ambivalent (angry or depressed) feelings. The nurse helps the patient to evaluate life priorities with respect to economic impact, family wishes, and societal acceptance. Family discussions might need to be facilitated, and legal council should be advised.

Interventions that focus on values conflicts must also address changes in sexual functioning associated with aging. The nurse can provide structured learning opportunities as well as encouraging elders to join groups whose members are of similar age and have similar concerns. However, group discussions might not be acceptable for some patients. Many traditional Asian patients, for example, are very private and will discuss sexual issues with a health professional only (Black, 1994). Should a translator be required for a non-English-speaking person, the nurse might have to become a cultural broker; for example, traditional Asian patients would likely choose another health professional rather than a family member or a member of the housekeeping staff as translator (Black, 1994).

Fear of Acquiring a Sexually Transmitted Disease

When patients verbalize fear of acquiring a sexually transmitted disease, Risk Identification and Teaching: Safe Sex are as important for older as for younger partners. Mutually monogamous sex between noninfected partners and any sexual activity between noninfected partners, including solo or mutual masturbation, can be considered absolutely safe. Very safe are noninsertive sexual practices, manual stimulation of the partner, and dry kissing, providing that skin is intact and free of lesions. Probably safe are insertive sexual practices with the use of condoms and spermicide. Everything else should be considered risky (Staab & Hodges, 1996).

As risk factors and safe techniques are discussed, anxiety surrounding this issue and fears in anticipation of a new relationship need to be recognized and dealt with. Patients can be assisted with reaching a decision and can be encouraged to rehearse communicating with their partner about sexual issues.

CASE STUDY

C. Newman, a 58-year-old widow for 7 years, had gone through menopause when her husband was dying of cancer. She had been placed on a combination regimen of estrogen and progesterone because of hot flushes. She had stopped the medication after about 1 year "because too much was going on at the time."

Mrs. Newman requested to talk with the clinical nurse specialist because she needed "to talk things over." Mrs. Newman had recently become reacquainted with a former high school friend who lost his wife about a year ago. She thought their relationship was heading toward intimacy. She wanted to discuss whether or not to resume HRT.

The nurse recognized the importance of the new relationship in Mrs. Newman's life, but began with the patient's stated need to discuss HRT, a less sensitive issue. Advantages, disadvantages, and contraindications were explained; at the same time, the nurse listened attentively to Mrs. Newman's verbal and nonverbal responses. It became clear that Mrs. Newman had done considerable reading on the subject and she had seemed to reach the conclusion that for her advantages outweighed any risks, particularly since her mother had suffered from osteoporosis. Her real concerns were the following: how to ask her family physician, who had also been her late husband's physician, for a prescription ("it's a bit embarrassing"), and whether she should discuss HIV risks with her male friend ("How do you ask about something like this when you haven't even done it?").

The nurse recognized Mrs. Newman's anxiety. She acknowledged Mrs. Newman's sensitivity about sexual issues and supported her concern over sexually transmitted diseases by sharing statistical information pertaining to HIV in older adults. She asked Mrs. Newman whether she wanted to find a new health care provider; the answer was no. The nurse then helped Mrs. Newman to process how the physician could be approached and how Mrs. Newman could phrase questions to her friend. This exchange reduced Mrs. Newman's anxiety; her voice and demeanor became calmer as she verbalized options and phrases she would use. The nurse also provided Mrs. Newman with information on normal changes in sexual functioning in older men and how Mrs. Newman could adapt to these changes. Helpful readings on the topic were suggested. Mrs. Newman declined making a follow-up appointment with the nurse, but stated that she would call if she needed additional help. She did call the nurse about 3 weeks later, sounding upbeat. She reported that she told her friend "what the nurse had said." They both thought it highly unlikely that either of them carried HIV. Nevertheless, before becoming intimate, they had decided to have a blood test and give each other the report. "It's a really good relationship," Mrs. Newman said.

SUMMARY

Interventions related to altered sexuality patterns require that the nurse possesses expert knowledge, sensitive assessment skills, and the ability to target realistic outcomes. Maturity, tact, and good timing when implementing interventions are also crucial. Older people tend to trust nurses with sensitive issues. Nurses who are uncomfortable with discussing sexual issues support that trust by making appropriate referrals.

REFERENCES

American Psychiatric Association. (1994). *Diagnostic and statistical manual of mental disorders* (4th ed.). Washington, DC: Author.

Andrews, W. C. (1995). The transitional years and beyond. *Obstetrics and Gynecology, 85*(1), 1-5.

Black, P. K. (1994). Hidden problems of stoma care. *British Journal of Nursing, 3*(14), 707-711.

Boston Women's Health Book Collective. (1992). *The new our bodies, ourselves: A book by & for women. Updated and expanded for the 1990's.* New York: Simon & Schuster.

Brenner, D. E., Kukull, W. A., Stergachis, A., van Belle, G., Bowen, J. D., McCormick, W. C., Teri, L., & Larson, E. B. (1994). Postmenopausal estrogen replacement therapy and the risk of Alzheimer's disease: A population-based case-control study. *American Journal of Epidemiology, 140*(3), 262-267.

Butler, R. N., Finkel, S. I., Lewis, M. I., Sherman, F. T., & Sunderland, T. (1992). Aging and mental health: Primary care of the healthy older adult. *Geriatrics, 47*(5), 54-65.

Butler, R. N., & Lewis, M. I. (1993). *Love and sex after 60.* New York: Ballantine Books.

Butler, R. N., Lewis, M. I., Hoffman, E., & Whitehead, E. D. (1994). Love and sex after 60: How physical changes affect intimate expression. *Geriatrics, 49*(29), 21-27.

Byers, J. P. (1983). Sexuality and the elderly. *Geriatric Nursing, 4*(4), 293-297.

Carnevali, D. (1993). Genital problems. In D. L. Carnevali & M. Patrick (Eds.), *Nursing management for the elderly* (3rd ed., pp. 504-509). Baltimore: Lippincott Williams & Wilkins.

Colditz, G. A., Stampfer, M. J., Willett, W. C., Hennekens, C. H., Rosner, B., & Speizer, F. E. (1990). Prospective study of estrogen replacement therapy and risk of breast cancer in postmenopausal women. *Journal of the American Medical Association, 264*(20), 2648-2653.

Deevey, S. (1990). Older lesbian women. An invisible minority. *Journal of Gerontological Nursing, 16*(5), 35-39.

Derogatis, L. R., & Cleary, P. A. (1977). Confirmation of the dimensional structure of the SCL-90: A study in construct validation. *Journal of Clinical Psychology, 33*(4), 981-989.

Ebersole, P., & Hess, P. (1998). *Toward healthy aging: Human needs and nursing response* (5th ed.). St. Louis, MO: Mosby.

Ettinger, B., Black, D. M., Mitlak, B. H., Knickerbocker, R. K., Nickelsen, T., Genant, H. K., Christiansen, C., Delmas, P. D., Zanchetta, J. R., Stakkestad, J., Gluer, C. C., Krueger, K., Cohen, F. J., Eckert, S., Ensrud, K. E., Avioli, L. V., Lips, P., & Cummings, S. R. (1999). Reduction of vertebral fracture risk in postmenopausal women with osteoporosis treated with raloxifene. Results from a 3-year random clinical trial. *Journal of the American Medical Association, 282*(7), 637-645.

Godschalk, M. F., Sison, A., & Mulligan, T. (1997). Management of erectile dysfunction by the geriatrician. *Journal of the American Geriatrics Society, 45*(10), 1240-1246.

Goldstein, I., Lue, T. F., Padma-Natham, H., Rosen, R., Steers, W., & Wicker, P. (1998). Oral sildenafil in the treatment of erectile dysfunction. *New England Journal of Medicine, 20*(338), 1397-1404.

Henderson, V. W., Paganini-Hill, A., Emanuel, C. K., Dunn, M. E., & Buckwalter, J. G. (1994). Estrogen replacement therapy in older women. *Archives of Neurology, 51*(9), 896-900.

Heiman, J. R. (1995). Evaluating sexual dysfunctions. In D. P. Lemcke, J. Pattison, L. A. Marshall, & D. S. Cowley (Eds.), *Primary care of women* (pp. 124-130). Norwalk, CT: Appleton & Lange.

Herrick, C. A., Douglas, V., & Carlson, J. H. (1995). Menopause and hormone replacement therapy from holistic and medical perspectives. *Issues in Mental Health Nursing, 17*, 153-168.

Hogervorst, E., Boshuisen, M., Riedel, W., Willeken, C., & Jolles, J. (1999). The effect of hormone replacement therapy on cognitive function in elderly women. *Psychoneuroendocrinology, 24*(1), 43-68.

Iowa Intervention Project. J. C. McCloskey & G. M. Bulechek (Eds.). (2000). *Nursing interventions classification (NIC)* (3rd ed.). St. Louis, MO: Mosby.

Iowa Outcomes Project. M. Johnson & M. Maas (Eds.). (2000). *Nursing outcomes classification (NOC)* (2nd ed.). St. Louis, MO: Mosby.

Jacoby, S. (1999). Great sex. What's age got to do with it. *Modern Maturity, 42R*(5), 43-45, 74.

Kee, L. J. (1995). *Laboratory and diagnostic tests with nursing implications.* Norwalk, CT: Appleton & Lange.

Kuhlman, G. (1996). Applying the nursing process with the elderly. In S. H. Wilson & C. R. Kneisl (Eds.), *Psychiatric nursing* (pp. 902-920). Reading, MA: Addison Wesley Longman.

Lemcke, D. P., Marshall, L. A., & Pattison, J. (1995). Menopause and hormone replacement therapy. In D. P. Lemcke, J. Pattison, L. A. Marshall, & D. S. Cowley (Eds.), *Primary care of women* (pp. 161-172). Norwalk, CT: Appleton & Lange.

Lueckenotte, A. G. (1996). *Gerontological Nursing.* St. Louis, MO: Mosby.

Matsumoto, A. M. (1993). "Andropause"—Are reduced androgen levels in aging men physiologically important? *Western Journal of Medicine, 159*(5), 618-620.

McKeon, V. A. (1994). Hormone replacement therapy: Evaluating the risks and benefits. *Journal of Obstetric, Gynecologic, & Neonatal Nursing, 23*(8), 647-657.

Miller, V. T., Muesing, R. A., LaRosa, J. C., Stoy, D. B., Phillips, E. A., & Stillman, R. J. (1991). Effects of conjugated equine estrogen with and without three different progestogens on lipoproteins, high-density lipoprotein subfractions, and apolipoprotein A-I. *Obstetrics & Gynecology, 77*(2), 235-240.

Mooradian, A. D., & Greiff, V. (1990). Sexuality in older women. *Archives of Internal Medicine, 150*(5), 1033-1038.

National Institutes of Health. (1992). Impotence. *NIH Consensus Statement, 10*(4), 1-29.

North American Nursing Diagnosis Association (1999). *Nursing diagnoses: Definitions & classification 1999-2000.* Philadelphia: Author.

Paganini-Hill, A., & Henderson, V. W. (1994). Estrogen deficiency and risk of Alzheimer's disease in women. *American Journal of Epidemiology, 140*(3), 256-261.

Quam, J. K., & Whitford, G. S. (1992). Adaptation and age-related expectations of older gay and lesbian adults. *The Gerontologist, 32*(3), 367-374.

Richardson, J. P., & Lazur, A. (1995). Sexuality in the nursing home patient. *American Family Physician, 51*(1), 121-124.

Rowland, D. L., Greenleaf, W. J., Dorfman, L. J., & Davidson, J. M. (1993). Aging and sexual function in men. *Archives of Sexual Behavior, 22*(6), 545-557.

Scharbo-Dehaan, M. (1994). Management strategies for hormonal replacement therapy. *Nurse Practitioner, 19*(12), 47-48, 50-52, 55-57.

Sheehy, G. (1992). *The silent passage.* New York: Random House.

Staab, A. S., & Hodges, C. L. (1996). Problems with sexuality. In A. S. Staab & L. C. Hodges (Eds.), *Gerontological nursing* (pp. 370-390). Baltimore: Lippincott Williams & Wilkins.

Swerdloff, R. S., & Wang, C. (1993). Androgen deficiency and aging in men. *Western Journal of Medicine, 159*(5), 579-585.

Thienhaus, O. J. (1988). Practical overview of sexual function and advancing age. *Geriatrics, 43*(8), 63-67.

Travis, S. S. (1987). Older adults' sexuality and remarriage. *Journal of Gerontological Nursing, 13*(6), 8-14.

Tucker, M. A., Ogle, S. J., Davinson, J. G., & Eilenberg, M. D. (1987). Validation of a brief screening test for depression in the elderly. *Age & Ageing, 16*(3), 139-144.

United States Bureau of the Census. (1998). *Statistical abstracts of the United States* (118th ed.). Washington, DC: United States Bureau of the Census.

Utian, W. H., & Schiff, I. (1994). North American Menopause Society—Gallup survey on women's knowledge, information sources and attitudes to menopause and hormone replacement therapy. *Menopause. Journal of North American Menopause Society, 1,* 39-48.

Walz, T. H., & Blum, N. S. (1987). *Sexual health in later life.* Lexington, MA: Heath, D. C.

Whitehead, M. I., Hillard, T. C., & Crook, D. (1990). The role and use of progestogens. *Obstetrics & Gynecology, 75*(suppl.), S59-S76.

Wright, L. K. (1996). The elderly with mental illness. In N. Worley (Ed.), *Mental health nursing in the community* (pp. 385-402). St. Louis, MO: Mosby.

Yesavage, J. A., & Brink, T. L. (1983). Development and validation of a geriatric depression screening scale: A preliminary report. *Journal of Psychiatric Research, 17*(1), 37-49.

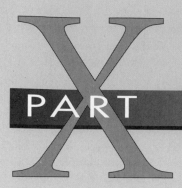

PART X

Coping–Stress Tolerance Pattern

OVERVIEW

Old age, along with other stages of life, involves adaptation to many changes. For elders, successful coping with losses of functional abilities can often avoid further losses such as forced removal from one's own home. In Chapter 59 Bunten discusses coping–stress tolerance patterns among elders and suggests that elders are more vulnerable than younger adults to stress associated with threats of loss. The author suggests that although older adults may be more vulnerable to psychologic and physiologic stress and may have reduced adaptive capacity, life coping patterns influence coping ability. She advises that nursing interventions to reduce stress can enhance an older person's adaptation.

Ineffective Individual Coping, the topic of Chapter 60, is presented in the context of Lazarus and Folkman's model, a holistic framework that includes personal, environmental, social, and spiritual aspects of coping. Stolley explains how the use of mediators during stressful events (coping activities, social support, and religiosity or spirituality) determines the outcome results of effective or ineffective coping. Outcomes of the coping process are briefly identified, and further development of the nursing diagnosis is suggested. Nursing interventions are identified and illustrated using a case study.

CHAPTER 59

NORMAL CHANGES WITH AGING

Donna Bunten

STRESS IN THE ELDER

Illness and infirmity, life-threatening disease, loss of loved ones, loss of material resources, loss of autonomy, loss of roles, loneliness, isolation, boredom, and concern with dying can occur at any stage of life. However, older persons are more likely than younger persons to experience these stressful circumstances. Moreover, these stressors can have a different significance when they occur in late life (Lazarus, 1987). The timing of stressful events is also important to consider, as the elderly person may find multiple personal and/or environmental stresses occurring concurrently.

The ability to handle stressful events and the coping mechanisms used will vary from elder to elder, just as in any other age group (Lachman, 1996). Some older adults develop a tremendous tolerance to stress through a lifetime of coping with stress (Aldwin, Sutton, Chiara, & Spiro, 1996). Others find that even small changes in their lives precipitate inordinate stress. The personality characteristics of an individual are reported to remain fairly stable throughout the life span; accordingly, the ways that elderly individuals deal with new events and new situations related to old age are a function of personality and reflect long-standing lifestyles (Brody, 1985; Dohrenwend, 1985). Researchers who have studied the effects of stress on the lives of older people have identified other mediating variables: cognitive style, coping strategies, personal efficacy, social skills, the availability of support systems, a sense of control or power, sense of humor, and personality traits (Clarke, 1984; Folkman, Lazarus, Pimley, & Novacck, 1987; Wooten, 1996). The manner in which one perceives an event as affecting one's life is thought to be another critical factor in the production of stress (McCrae, 1989). Thus coping with stress can be viewed as a lifelong process one learns in order to adjust needs to the demands of the environment.

The term *stress* refers to either external events or circumstances that tax the ability to adapt. Stress is also used to describe the emotional distress and physiologic arousal that the events produce (McCrae, 1989). As Lazarus and Folkman (1984) point out, the individual's perception of the situation as a challenge, threat, or loss makes it stressful. McCrae (1984) elaborates on this theme by suggesting that if events are classified as challenges, threats, and losses, some clear age differences are seen. Most challenges

(e.g., marriage, starting a family, job hunting) are associated with young adulthood. Threats or losses (e.g., loss of independence, serious illnesses) are more likely to occur in old age. Nurses are, for example, familiar with the stress and anxiety that frequently accompany relocation of the elder to a health care setting (Thomasma, Yeaworth, & McCabe, 1990). Haight, Michel, and Hendrix (1998) describe frail elders who are relocated to nursing homes as being at risk for developing depression and suicide ideation.

Holmes and Rahe (1962) proposed that any event that significantly changes a person's routine pattern of life should be considered stressful. They prepared a list of life events (normative events such as marriage or retirement and events that occur all too commonly such as divorce and bereavement) and assigned values to each to reflect how much adaptive effort is needed to adjust to them. Items on the Holmes and Rahe Scale reflect situations that are most commonly linked to lives of young to middle-aged adults. Variations on this theme have been produced that better reflect events in later life. The Geriatric Social Readjustment Rating Scale (GSRRS) was developed by Amster and Krauss in 1974. The loss of a spouse was considered to be the most stressful event for persons on the Holmes and Rahe Scale. On the GSRRS, loss of a spouse is among the top four most stressful events, along with institutionalization, death of a close family member, and major personal injury or illness. Neugarten (1970) suggested that loss of a spouse might be less traumatic for older persons than for younger men and women. Subsequent research has found that stress is less intense when it is expected or predicted for both the young and the old (Binstock & George, 1990; Moneyham & Scott, 1995).

COPING MECHANISMS

Elders are frequently stereotyped as worrying excessively about the threats and losses associated with aging; they also have been described as having diminishing and less effective coping skills. However, the majority of research challenges such a perspective (Powers, Winsocki, & Whitbourne, 1992). Moneyham and Scott (1995) studied a small group of elderly people and found that they shared a rather dim view about the future and an acceptance that loss was inevitably coming into their lives. These researchers described the participants' behaviors as being in a proactive mode of coping, which they called "anticipatory coping." The elderly subjects were focusing on preventing or minimizing their losses as much as possible while holding the belief that loss was inevitable in their future. Other studies also indicate that elderly individuals adapt to coping demands; if coping strategies in elders change from those used as younger adults, it is a matter of facing different types of stress (McCrae, 1984; Lazarus & Folkman, 1984).

McCrae (1984) describes some of the mechanisms elderly persons reported using when facing different demands:

> Faith, fatalism, and expression of feelings were used especially when subjects had experienced a loss; wishful thinking, faith and fatalism were used by subjects facing a threat. A number of mechanisms were used more under conditions of challenge, including rational action, perseverance, positive thinking, intellectual denial, restraint, self-adaptation, drawing strength from adversity, and humor (p. 919).

McCrae also found older persons to be more forgiving and less likely to vent emotions on others.

Folkman et al. (1987) described older respondents as less likely than younger persons to seek social support or to use confrontational coping mechanisms, hostile reactions, or escapist fantasy when coping with stressful events. The older persons in their cross-sectional study were more likely to report using distancing and positive reappraisal of stressful events when coping. The availability of social support for these subjects was not addressed. Moneyham and Scott (1995) reported that social support was consistently found to moderate the effects of stress on subsequent physical and psychologic stress.

Coyne and DeLongis (1986) suggest that relatively healthy aged individuals can and do successfully cope with the most stressful situations that occur in life. Although some experience low morale and depression following a major life change, most eventually find a solution to problems. When an individual by virtue of early developmental processes and other life experiences is able to cope with the demands of life events, especially life changes, stress can function to increase learning and the ability to cope and, thus, be associated with growth. In fact, the experience of successfully coping with stress may be a precondition to the development of a mature personality and, hence, good mental health.

Some elders never experience long-term or chronic stress; some never experience a crisis situation that their repertoire of coping skills doesn't enable them to manage. However, the elderly person whose inner resources and support systems have diminished may find coping strategies inadequate. Anxiety, helplessness, hopelessness, and loss of a sense of control over their lives can result. Advanced age alone is not believed to influence either the frequency or the intensity of these affective states. Neverthe-

less, elders are particularly vulnerable to illnesses associated with stress. Thomas (1988) points out that elderly individuals are found to have diminishing adaptive capacity, which hinders their ability to maintain homeostasis. "It doesn't make a difference whether stress is physical or emotional, the elder requires more time to recover and return to prestress levels than when they were younger" (Thomas, 1988, p. 26). High levels of stress also can exacerbate mental, emotional, or organic illness at any age.

It is not the purpose of this chapter to describe the physiologic effects of stress (see Ebersole & Hess, 1998 for an excellent review), but to emphasize that elderly persons who are experiencing physiologic or psychologic symptoms of stress can be assisted in reducing stress. Various methods are suggested in the literature for teaching the elder stress reduction: problem-solving approaches, progressive muscle relaxation, guided imagery, nutrition, proper rest and sleep, exercise and fitness training, education to remove uncertainty, and using humor (Clarke, 1984; Weinberger, 1991; Wooten, 1996). Nurses also can assist those elders who are found in various health care settings to restore a sense of control, which is ". . . basic to moving beyond the helplessness experienced during crises, illness, and stress" (Ebersole & Hess, 1998).

SUMMARY

Elderly individuals can be faced with a multiplicity of personal and environmental stressors. Definite conclusions about whether or not coping abilities and strategies for responding to stress change with age are premature. Nevertheless, nurses are encouraged to view the elder as being responsibly and actively involved in dealing with stress and capable of employing various methods of coping. Nurses are in a primary position to facilitate each individual elderly client's efforts to deal with problems and to respond appropriately and realistically to the demands of the environment, situation, or condition.

REFERENCES

Aldwin, C. M., Sutton, K. J., Chiara, G., & Spiro, A., III. (1996). Age differences in stress, coping, and appraisal: Findings from the Normative Aging Study. *Journals of Gerontology. Series B, Psychological Sciences & Social Sciences, 51*(14), P179-P188.

Amster, L. E., & Krauss, H. H. (1974). The relationship between life crisis and mental deterioration in old age. *International Journal of Aging and Human Development, 5*(1), 51-55.

Binstock, R. H., & George, L. K. (1990). *Handbook of aging and the social sciences* (3rd ed.). San Diego, CA: Academic Press.

Brody, E. M. (1985). *Mental and physical health practices of older people.* New York: Springer.

Clarke, M. (1984). Stress and coping: Constructs for nursing. *Journal of Advanced Nursing, 9,* 3-13.

Coyne, J. C., & DeLongis, A. (1986). Going beyond social support: The role of social relationships in adaptation. *Journal of Counseling and Clinical Psychology, 54,* 454-460.

Dohrenwend, B. P. (1985). "Hassels" in the conceptualization and measurement of life stress variables. *American Psychologist, 40,* 780-785.

Ebersole, P., & Hess, P. (1998). *Toward healthy aging: Human needs and nursing response* (5th ed.). St. Louis, MO: Mosby.

Folkman, S., Lazarus, R. S., Pimley, S., & Novacck, J. (1987). Age differences in stress and coping processes. *Psychology and Aging, 2,* 171-184.

Haight, B. K., Michel, Y., & Hendrix, S. (1998). Life review: Preventing despair in newly relocated nursing home residents short- and long-term effects. *International Journal of Aging & Human Development, 47*(2), 119-142.

Holmes, T. H., & Rahe, R. H. (1962). The social readjustment rating scale. *Journal of Psychosomatic Research, 11,* 213-218.

Lachman, V. D. (1996). Stress and self-care revisited: A literature review. *Holistic Nursing Practice, 10*(2), 1-12.

Lazarus, R. S. (1987). Stress and coping. In G. L. Maddox (Ed.), *The encyclopedia of aging* (pp. 647-649). New York: Springer.

Lazarus, R. S., & Folkman, S. (1984). *Stress, appraisal and coping.* New York: Springer.

McCrae, R. R. (1984). Situational determinants of coping response: Loss, threat and challenge. *Journal of Personality and Social Psychology, 46,* 919-928.

McCrae, R. R. (1989). Age differences and changes in the use of coping mechanisms. *Journal of Gerontology, 44*(6), 161-169.

Moneyham, L., & Scott, C. B. (1995). Anticipatory coping in the elderly. *Journal of Gerontological Nursing, 21*(7), 23-28.

Neugarten, B. L. (1970). Adaptation and the life cycle. *Journal of Geriatric Psychology, 4,* 71-87.

Powers, C. B., Winsocki, P. A., & Whitbourne, S. K. (1992). Age difference and correlates of worrying in young and elderly adults. *The Gerontologist, 32,* 82-88.

Thomas, B. L. (1988). Self-esteem and life satisfaction. *Journal of Gerontological Nursing, 14*(12), 25-30.

Thomasma, M., Yeaworth, R. C., & McCabe, B. W. (1990). Moving day: Relocation and anxiety in institutionalized elderly. *Journal of Gerontological Nursing, 16*(7), 18-24.

Weinberger, R. (1991). Teaching the elderly stress reduction. *Journal of Gerontological Nursing, 17*(10), 23-27.

Wooten, P. (1996). Humor: An antidote for stress. *Holistic Nursing Practice, 10*(2), 49-56.

CHAPTER 60

INEFFECTIVE INDIVIDUAL COPING

Jacqueline M. Stolley

The North American Nursing Diagnosis Association (NANDA) has defined Ineffective Individual Coping as the "inability to form a valid appraisal of the stressors, inadequate choices of practiced responses, and/or inability to use available resources" (Ackley & Ladwig, 1993, p. 154; NANDA, 1999, p. 70). Several NANDA diagnoses are related to coping: Ineffective Individual Coping, developed in 1978; Impaired Adjustment, developed in 1986; and Defensive Coping, developed in 1988. Another diagnosis, Potential for Enhanced Spiritual Well-Being, developed in 1994, could be related to coping in view of the theoretical framework presented later in this chapter. Coping often occurs in the context of a family or community setting. However, this chapter will focus on the nursing diagnosis Ineffective Individual Coping and the outcomes and interventions that can be implemented by nurses to assist elders to cope (Box 60-1).

It is important for the gerontologic nurse to differentiate between the reactions to stressful situations that represent a normal part of life and those that represent ineffective coping. For example, using defense mechanisms can be a healthy way to deal with stress on a short-term basis. It is the nurse's role to explore the use of defense mechanisms with the older client to mutually determine if they are deleterious (McFarland & McFarlane, 1997), and to examine with the client outcomes to short- and long-term events that are appraised as stressful. The key to understanding any particular individual's responses lies in understanding his cognitive appraisal and exploring its specific dimensions. To judge the effectiveness of specific coping strategies or responses requires a clear understanding of the purposes they serve for the individual (McFarland & McFarlane, 1997).

Several scholars have conceptualized coping paradigms (Pargament et al., 1990; Pearlin & Schooler, 1978; Valliant, 1967), but for purposes of this chapter, the primary theoretical framework for stress and coping is a modification of the paradigm set forth by Lazarus and Folkman (1984). This theoretical framework is especially useful for gerontologic nurses because it not only considers the major concepts of stress, appraisal, and coping, but also presents a holistic view of the coping process that incorporates personal, environmental, social, and spiritual aspects of the person.

Coping is a complex phenomenon that is used by humans to mediate stress. The coping process is initiated in response to an event or situation (or stress) that the individual must appraise, using cognitive processes, to determine if the event or situation poses a threat, is harmful, or provides a challenge. Following the appraisal, the individual uses mediators to cope with the stress. These mediators include coping activities, social support, and religiosity or spirituality. By using these mediators the outcomes of effective or ineffective coping result.

Scholars have postulated that coping paradigms are shaped by specific stressful situations, building on or modifying general coping structures (Lazarus & Folkman, 1984; Pearlin, Turner, & Semple, 1989). In fact, coping functions will be more effective if they are fluid and varied (Pearlin & Schooler, 1978). It is therefore important for the gerontologic nurse to understand that a person might react differently to various life events and situations that have the potential to produce stress and that these varied reactions can be healthy.

Lazarus and Folkman (1984) emphasized stress that concerns the relationship between the person and the environment. Different consequences of stress result from miscellaneous antecedent conditions that arise out of the environment and within the individual. What influences the interpretation is the appraisal of the situation or event (Lazarus & Folkman, 1984). Through the process of cognitive appraisal the individual determines the potential for threat (primary appraisal) and his capability for coping with the threat (secondary appraisal). Appraisal also enables the individual to assess the degree of stress and evaluate the strength of emotional outcomes (Lazarus & Folkman, 1984).

Reappraisal (positive or negative) can occur as a result of new information from the environment and/or insight into the individual's reactions (Lazarus & Folkman, 1984). For example, individuals can change their original feelings about an event or situation after evaluating coping activities or gaining new knowledge. It can be difficult to separate the reappraisal process and outcomes of the coping process because outcomes, good and bad, impact reappraisal (Lazarus & Folkman, 1984).

The process of cognitive appraisal does not stand alone. Personal and situational factors influence the appraisal process and resulting coping activities. Personal factors

| Box 60-1 | Suggested Nursing-Sensitive Outcome and Nursing Intervention INEFFECTIVE INDIVIDUAL COPING |

Nursing Diagnosis
Ineffective Individual Coping
Related to the caregiving role

Verbalization of inability to cope or inability to ask for help (must be present for this nursing diagnosis) (Becket, 1991; Collard, Jones, Murphy, & Fitzmaurice, 1987; Tack & Gillis, 1990; Vincent, 1986)*

Inability to meet role expectations (Becket, 1991; Collard et al., 1987; Tack & Gillis, 1990; Vincent, 1986)

Inability to meet basic needs (Becket, 1991; Collard et al., 1987; Tack & Gillis, 1990; Vincent, 1986)

Inadequate problem solving (must be present for this nursing diagnosis) (Collard et al., 1987; Vincent, 1986)*

Decreased use of social support (Collard et al., 1987; Vincent, 1986)*

Destructive behavior toward self or others (Collard et al., 1987; Vincent, 1986)

Inappropriate use of defense mechanisms (Vincent, 1986)*

Change in usual communication patterns (Collard et al., 1987)

Verbal manipulation

High illness rate (Collard et al., 1987; Vincent, 1986)

Non-NANDA defining characteristics
Verbalization of appearance of (Becket, 1991; Collard et al., 1987)

Anxiety (Collard et al., 1987; Vincent, 1986)

Expression of Depression (Vincent, 1986; Tack & Gillis, 1990)

Expression of Impatience (Tack & Gillis, 1990)

Expression of Irritability (Tack & Gillis, 1990)

Expression of discouragement of (Tack & Gillis, 1990)*

Reported life stress (Vincent, 1986)*

Nursing-Sensitive Outcome
Coping
Identifies effective coping patterns*

Identifies ineffective coping patterns*

Verbalizes sense of control*

Reports decrease in stress*

Verbalizes acceptance of situation*

Seeks information concerning illness and treatment*

Modifies lifestyle as needed*

Adapts to developmental changes*

Uses available social support*

Employs behaviors to reduce stress

Identifies multiple coping strategies

Uses effective coping strategies*

Avoids unduly stressful situations

Verbalizes need for assistance*

Seeks professional help as appropriate

Reports decrease in physical symptoms of stress*

Reports decrease in negative feelings

Reports increase in psychologic comfort

Nursing Intervention
Coping Enhancement
Appraise a patient's adjustment to change in body image, as indicated*

Appraise the impact of the patient's life situation on roles and relationships*

Encourage patient to identify a realistic description of change in role*

Appraise the patient's understanding of the disease process of the disease*

Appraise and discuss alternative responses to situation*

Use a calm, reassuring approach*

Provide an atmosphere of acceptance*

Assist the patient in developing an objective appraisal of the event*

Help patient to identify the information she is most interested in obtaining

Provide factual information concerning diagnosis, treatment, and prognosis*

Provide the patient with realistic choices about certain aspects of care

Encourage an attitude of realistic hope as a way of dealing with feelings of helplessness*

Evaluate the patient's decision-making ability

Seek to understand the patient's perspective of a stressful situation

Discourage decision making when the patient is under severe stress

Encourage gradual mastery of the situation*

Encourage patience in developing relationships

Encourage relationships with persons who have common interests and goals*

Encourage social and community activities*

Encourage the acceptance of limitations of others*

Acknowledge the patient's spiritual and cultural background*

Encourage the use of spiritual resources, if desired*

Explore patient's previous achievements of success*

Explore patient's reasons for self-criticism*

Confront patient's ambivalent (angry or depressed) feelings*

Foster constructive outlets for anger and hostility

Arrange situations that encourage patient's autonomy*

Assist patient in identifying positive responses from others

Encourage the identification of specific life values

Explore with the patient previous methods of dealing with life problems*

Introduce patient to persons (or groups) who have successfully undergone the same experience*

Support the use of appropriate defense mechanisms

Encourage verbalization of feelings, perceptions, and fears*

Discuss consequences of not dealing with guilt and shame

Encourage the patient to identify own strengths and abilities*

*Indicates suggested signs and symptoms, NOC indicators, and NIC activities for Mrs. Foster.

Continued

Box 60-1 Suggested Nursing-Sensitive Outcome and Nursing Intervention—cont'd
INEFFECTIVE INDIVIDUAL COPING—cont'd

Assist the patient in breaking down complex goals into small, manageable steps	Provide appropriate social skills training
Reduce stimuli in the environment that could be misinterpreted as threatening	Assist the patient to identify positive strategies to deal with limitations and manage needed lifestyle or role changes*
Appraise patient's needs and desires for social support*	Assist the patient to solve problems in constructive manner
Assist the patient to identify available support systems*	Instruct the patient on the use of relaxation techniques, as needed*
Determine the risk of the patient's inflicting self-harm	Assist the patient to clarify misconceptions
Encourage family involvement, as appropriate*	Encourage the patient to evaluate own behavior*

Nursing Outcomes Classification (NOC) 5-point Likert measurement scale:

Coping =   1 = Never demonstrated; 2 = Rarely demonstrated; 3 = Sometimes demonstrated; 4 = often demonstrated;
        5 = Consistently demonstrated.

that affect appraisal are commitments and beliefs. Deep commitment can increase the potential for threat and challenge or drive a person to act effectively and help maintain hope (Lazarus & Folkman, 1984). Beliefs affect expectations for personal control in response to the stress and can empower the individual to find meaning and sustain hope at difficult times (Lazarus & Folkman, 1984). Situational factors that affect appraisal are the novelty, uncertainty, duration, imminence, and timing of the situation or the event that may be appraised as stress.

Coping mediators include coping activities, social support, and individual characteristics and resources, and constraints on coping. Fig. 60-1 depicts the Stress, Appraisal, and Coping paradigm as described by Lazarus and Folkman (1984). For purposes of this chapter the paradigm of coping is modified to incorporate the following mediators of coping: coping activities, social support, and religiosity or spirituality. Caregiver characteristics and resources as well as personal and environmental constraints are considered factors that affect the mediators of coping. This modified paradigm is described in the following pages and is depicted in Fig. 60-2.

Coping activities can be broadly categorized into problem-focused coping (the management of the source of stress) and emotion-focused coping (the regulation of stressful emotions). While most stressors elicit both types of coping, problem-focused coping seems to be most prominent when people believe that something productive can be done. Emotion-focused coping is used when people feel that the stressor is something that must be withstood (Lazarus & Folkman, 1984). Most scholars have further refined coping activities to include multifaceted coping activities (Jalowiec, 1979, 1987; Smyth & Yarandi, 1996; Vitaliano, Russo, Carr, Maiuro, & Becker, 1985; Wineman, Durand, & Steiner, 1994).

Social networks are the entirety of an individual's relationships, but social support involves only the help a person receives from a segment of that network. Support

can be further delineated into formal support (by professionals) and informal support (by family and friends). The availability of social support is an important factor for both physical and mental health in elders (Ryan & Austin, 1989). Lack of social support has been implicated in negative physical and emotional response (Haley, Ellen, Levine, Brown, & Bartolucci, 1987; Pruchno & Resch, 1989). The most significant positive components of social support and the coping process in elderly persons have been found to be reassurance of worth and tangible assistance (Russell & Cutrona, 1991).

The role of religiosity and spirituality in coping has been studied in the form of organized religious activity, nonorganized religious activity, and intrinsic religious activity. Religion and religiosity have been found to be spontaneously mentioned as a coping resource by older individuals (Ferraro & Koch, 1994; Koenig, George, & Siegler, 1988; Rosen, 1982; Stolley, Buckwalter, & Koenig, 1999; Swanson & Harter, 1971). Scholars have found that self-esteem and self-worth are highest among those with the greatest, as well as the least, amount of religious commitment, and lowest among elderly people with only modest levels of religiosity (Beckman & Houser, 1982; Blazer & Palmore, 1976; Hunsberger, 1985; Koenig et al., 1988; Krause, 1995). Religious coping has been used even in the presence of severe physical illness, helping elders deal with the illness and reduce the incidence of depression (Koenig et al., 1992).

Interestingly, Reed (1991) found that self-transcendence is one significant correlate of mental health among the oldest-old as well as among younger groups of elders. Intrinsic religiosity may be a reflection of self-transcendence. Nelson (1990) found that those who are more intrinsically oriented to religion experience less depression. Furthermore, prayer has been identified as a coping activity employed by elders (Conway, 1985; Kaye & Robinson, 1994; Manfredi & Pickett, 1987; Pargament et al., 1990; Pearlin et al., 1989; Stolley et al., 1999; Whitlach, Meddaugh, & Langhout, 1992; Wilson, 1989). Thus religiosity and spirituality

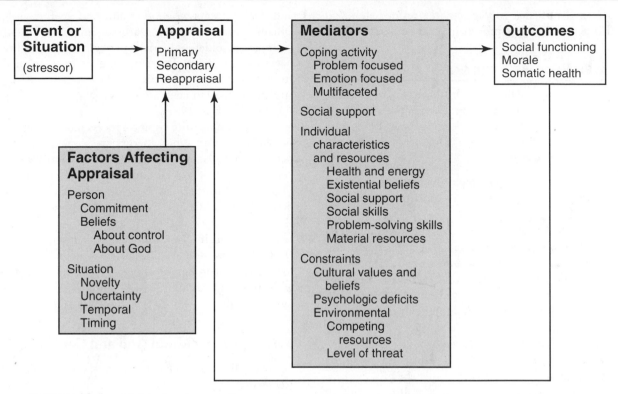

FIGURE **60-1**   Model of coping paradigm. (Data from Lazarus, R., & Folkman, S. [1984]. *Stress, appraisal, and coping.* New York: Springer.)

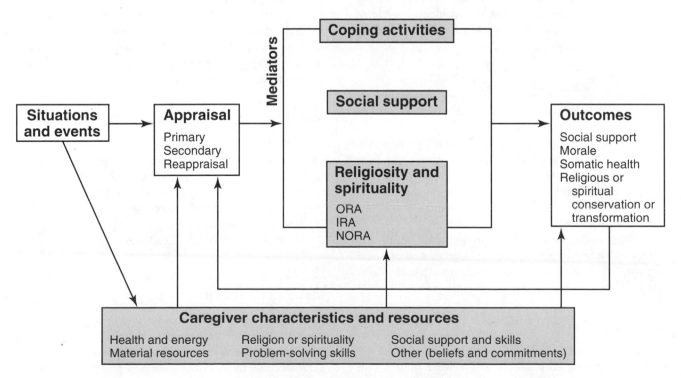

FIGURE **60-2**   Modified coping model.

have been identified as coping activities or mediators that contribute to the coping process in older adults.

RELATED FACTORS/ETIOLOGIES

Ineffective coping can be caused by three categories of etiologies: situational crises, maturational crises, and personal vulnerability (McFarland & McFarlane, 1997). McFarland and McFarlane (1997) further describe the following related factors:

1. Physical or psychologic impairment, such as memory loss, disease processes, or previous psychiatric treatment
2. Impaired self-efficacy or self-concept, including feelings of powerlessness, lowered self-competency, and lack of perceived control, hardiness, or social support
3. Stress event or illness, including events or situations that result in the loss of a loved one, pain, overload, conflict, poor psychosocial development, and threats to security
4. Situation or context, including a lack of resources, instability in the social or cultural realm, and lack of or exhaustion of treatments
5. Inaccurate appraisal of stress, event, or illness, resulting in denial or lack of realistic goals
6. Inaccurate response repertoire, including guilt, destructive behavior, or avoidance
7. Inappropriate deployment of coping resources

These related factors are well grounded in the conceptual framework set forth by Lazarus and Folkman (1984). When considering whether the older client is experiencing ineffective coping, it is imperative to consider these related factors in order to develop individualized interventions and facilitate positive outcomes.

RISK FACTORS

Lazarus and Folkman (1984) have identified individual characteristics and resources and personal and environmental constraints as risk factors for coping. However, these concepts are threaded through the coping paradigm and acknowledged to affect all aspects of the coping process. Thus factors that affect the coping process are considered underlying strengths and weaknesses that contribute to the stress and coping paradigm.

Coping resources include an individual's health and energy, existential beliefs or general beliefs about personal control, commitments, social support, social skills, problem-solving skills, and material resources.

Health and Energy

Although research suggests that people of all ages are capable of coping surprisingly well despite poor health and depleted energy, good health and energy certainly enhance coping efforts (Lazarus & Folkman, 1984). For example, an older individual in poor health might not have the physical and/or emotional reserves to manage stress. Conversely, good physical health can provide the strength needed to facilitate stress evaluation and mediation (McGoldrick, 1989).

Age can impact the coping process and coping activities when health and energy are considered. Older persons use less confrontive coping styles and are less inclined to solicit social support (Folkman, Lazarus, Pimley, & Novacek, 1987). Elders are more likely to become withdrawn and use positive reappraisal to cope. Furthermore, they tend to use less emotional expression, self-blame, and information seeking than younger adults (Felton & Revenson, 1987). Furthermore, increasing age may enhance coping, depending on previous experience with stress and coping (Aldwin, Sutton, Chiara, & Spiro, 1996).

Positive Beliefs About God and Control

Positive beliefs about God and control can contribute to a feeling of hope and a sense that outcomes are controllable (Lazarus & Folkman, 1984). Positive beliefs about God might contribute more to successful coping than do actual feelings of control (Schaefer & Gorsuch, 1991).

Commitments and Social Support

The role of commitments affects both the appraisal of stress and other aspects of the coping process. Similarly, while social support is an individual resource that contributes to the coping process, it is also seen as a major mediating variable that impacts the coping process. Ongoing use of social support resources will have an effect on outcomes of the coping process.

Social Skills and Problem-Solving Skills

Social skills help the individual better manage the problems of daily living and maintain levels of social support (Gilovich, 1990; Griffin, Dunning, & Ross, 1990). Additionally, they enable the person to better use problem-solving skills, a coping resource that enhances the ability to search for information, analyze situations, and generate courses of action (Lazarus & Folkman, 1984; Rosenbaum, 1980).

Material Resources

Material resources include money and the capacity to buy goods and services. Strong relationships have been found among economic status, stress, and adaptation. Those individuals who have money and who possess the skills to use it effectively generally fare much better than those without material resources (Lazarus & Folkman, 1984). Monetary resources expand coping options in nearly all stressful situations, providing easier and probably more effective access to legal, medical, financial, and other professional assistance (Lazarus & Folkman, 1984). Even when money is not spent directly on managing the stressor, financial security can reduce the impact of the stressor, facilitating effective coping.

Personal Constraints

Personal constraints include cultural values and beliefs that inhibit particular ways of conduct and the individual's unique psychologic development. For example, cultural values and/or psychologic makeup may determine whether or not the individual uses pertinent resources (Lazarus & Folkman, 1984).

Environmental Constraints

Environmental constraints include requirements that compete for the same resources. Decisions may need to be made on how to spend scarce resources or time. The level of threat also affects appraisal and coping activities. The perceived level of threat can affect the degree to which resources on hand are used for coping (Lazarus & Folkman, 1984).

ASSESSMENT

Lazarus and Folkman (1984) developed the Ways of Coping Checklist (WCCL), which has been used extensively with all adult age groups and which captures problem- and emotion-focused coping. Later research on the WCCL conducted by Aldwin, Folkman, Schaefer, Coyne, and Lazarus (1980) used factor analysis to elicit seven factors or types of coping behavior. Using the Lazarus and Folkman (1984) framework, Jalowiec (1979) developed the Jalowiec Coping Scale (JCS). A revised version of the JCS taps a larger domain of coping behavior and identifies the following eight coping styles: confrontive, evasive, optimistic, fatalistic, emotive, palliative, supportive, and self-reliant (Jaloweic, 1987). The revised JCS also contains an effectiveness scale for each coping style. While the effectiveness rating of the JCS does not provide an objective view of coping effectiveness, it does give the gerontologic nurse and the client insight into the subjective effectiveness of these coping styles.

Even though these and other assessment tools are available, the assessment of coping in older adults remains a complicated process. The WCCL and JCS were designed for research purposes and could be cumbersome and time consuming to use in the clinical arena. Vincent (1986) recommends that a tool be developed that can be incorpo-

rated into nursing assessments. However, nurses can determine if ineffective coping is a concern by reviewing the defining characteristics specified for the related nursing diagnosis and following up with an assessment of other components of the stress and coping paradigm such as appraisal, morale, health problems, social functioning, and religiosity or spirituality. Tools exist that can assess components of the stress and coping process in general and specific situations. Selected examples include the Philadelphia Geriatric Center Caregiving Appraisal Scale (Lawton, Kleban, Moss, Rovine, & Glicksman, 1989), the Geriatric Depression Rating Scale (Yesavage et al., 1983), the Social Provisions Scale (Cutrona & Russell, 1987), and the Profile of Mood States (McNair, Lorr, & Droppleman, 1971). Used in conjunction with an in-depth nursing assessment that contains many of the characteristics, resources, and constraints of coping, the gerontologic nurse can develop a nursing care plan that effectively deals with ineffective individual coping. Table 60-1 identifies meaningful domains for data collection, using the modified version of the coping paradigm. The gerontologic nurse can use these domains to learn if the older individual's resources relate to the requirements of the event and if acceptable goals are likely to be met.

When assessing coping methods in the elderly client, it is important to keep in mind that coping does not differ significantly from other age groups. Older persons can have diminished resources and be subject to multiple stressors that must be considered. Further, older persons tend to use less confrontive coping styles, to solicit less social support than their younger counterparts (Folkman et al., 1987), and to report lower use of emotional expression, self-blame, and information seeking (Felton & Revenson, 1987).

NURSING DIAGNOSIS

The nursing diagnosis Ineffective Individual Coping was approved at the Fourth National Conference of NANDA (Ferrera & Fitzpatrick, 1982) after being refined through clinical research studies (Guzzetta & Forsyth, 1979). At that time, 11 defining characteristics were chosen based on the belief that they represented the client experiencing coping difficulties. As of the Eleventh National Conference (Matthewman et al., 1995), nine published studies and two unpublished studies were found that included the diagnosis of Ineffective Individual Coping.

Defining characteristics accepted by NANDA are presented in Table 60-1, with citations of the studies that support each defining characteristic. It is interesting to note that none of the studies support the defining characteristic of verbal manipulation. Nevertheless, the recommendation of the Eleventh Conference was that the 11 original NANDA defining characteristics be maintained. This recommendation was made despite the fact that none of the studies validated verbal manipulation as a defining characteristic, and characteristics validated through research were ignored. These include verbalization or appearance of ineffective coping (Becket, 1991; Collard, Jones, Murphy, & Fitzmaurice, 1987), anxiety (Collard et al., 1987; Vincent, 1986), depression—expression of (Tack & Gillis, 1990; Vincent, 1986), fear (Collard et al., 1987), frustration—expression of (Tack & Gillis, 1990), discouragement—expression of (Tack & Gillis, 1990), and reported life stress (Vincent, 1986). While these defining characteristics have not yet been accepted by NANDA, it is important for the gerontologic nurse to keep them in mind when assessing ineffective individual coping and to consider their relationship to other defining characteristics that may be present in the older adult. In fact, recommendations at the Eleventh Conference (Matthewman et al., 1995) included continued study of the 11 current defining characteristics as well as of the additional nine defining characteristics supported by research.

Another consideration when assessing coping effectiveness is to determine whether the preferred nursing diagnosis is Ineffective Individual Coping, Impaired Adjustment, or both (Matthewman et al., 1995, pp. 50-51). Ineffective Individual Coping is defined by NANDA as the "inability to form a valid appraisal of the stressors, inadequate choices of practiced responses, and/or inability to use available resources" (NANDA, 1999, p. 70). For Impaired Adjustment, the NANDA definition is "inability to modify lifestyle/behavior in a manner consistent with a change in health status" (p. 71).

CASE STUDY

The Fosters were referred to a gerontologic nurse consultant through the local chapter of the Alzheimer's Association. Mrs. Foster is a 79-year-old female whose husband was diagnosed with Alzheimer's disease (AD) 1 year ago. They have been married for 55 years. Mr. Foster is in the early stages of AD, exhibiting losses in short-term memory, impairment in judgment and impulse control, and loss of personality "spark." Mrs. Foster has difficulty dealing with her husband's diagnosis and vacillates between believing that her husband's memory is "OK" because he remembers things sometimes and a feeling of hopelessness about his diagnosis. Even though Mr. Foster has periods of poor judgment using the car, Mrs. Foster refuses to deny him driving privileges. Throughout the marriage, Mrs. Foster always deferred to Mr. Foster, and while he has never been abusive, their marriage has been very traditional with Mr. Foster acting as the "head of the house." Thus Mrs. Foster remains reluctant to challenge her husband.

Although the post-retirement period was supposed to be a time of increased freedom, Mrs. Foster now finds herself more tied down than ever. Mrs. Foster states that she is unable to cope with the changing roles in her marriage and the problematic behavior arising from Mr. Foster's disease process. She admits that it is difficult for her to find solutions to problems. At times she experiences headaches and loss of appetite, which she attributes to stress. She has frequent periods of crying, "When I'm alone and no one can see."

Mrs. Foster enjoys good physical health, as does Mr. Foster, excluding his diagnosis of AD. They live on an adequate retirement income and have savings that were to be used to enjoy their retirement, to travel, to buy gifts for their children and grandchildren, and to leave to their heirs. They have two children (one son and one daughter) who live over 1000 miles away. Mrs. Foster is reluctant to burden them with her problems because "they have their own lives to live." Both of the Fosters have been active members of their church and describe their friends as those they know from church. However, since Mr. Foster has behavior problems, they no longer go to organized religious activities. Additionally, Mrs. Foster has not confided the diagnosis of AD to anyone at church, even the minister, because she is afraid of being rejected or pitied and is somewhat embarrassed by Mr. Foster's behavior. Thus the Fosters have gone from a very active religious life to one that consists of nonorganized religious activities such as watching religious TV programs and intrinsic religious activities, such as prayer. Both of the Fosters express faith in God and believe that God will help them with their problems. Mrs. Foster firmly believes AD happens for a reason and that "God never gives us a burden we cannot carry ourselves. God will provide help, but I must be independent and help myself." Nevertheless, they miss the socialization and camaraderie of organized religious activities.

Mrs. Foster is beginning to show the strains of the caregiving role. She complains of fatigue, states she does not know how long she can go on, and feels very much alone with her burden. She is visibly depressed, appears pale, and shows some restlessness during the interview. She does not know much about AD because her physician did not provide information or referral to community support services. She only called the Alzheimer's Association out of desperation and loneliness, and her knowledge deficit about the disease and its management is very apparent.

The nurse consultant assesses the information gleaned about Mrs. Foster's situation and makes the initial nursing diagnosis of Ineffective Individual Coping based on the following defining characteristics: (1) verbalization of inability to cope (at times) and the inability to ask for help; (2) inability to problem solve; (3) alteration in societal participation; and (4) inappropriate use of defense mechanisms (denial). Mrs. Foster also meets the "unofficial" defining characteristics for depression, discouragement, and reported life stress. Later administration of the JCS supported the nursing diagnosis of Ineffective Individual Coping. Table 60-1 shows assessment data that lead to this diagnosis based on the conceptual framework set forth in this chapter.

Table 60-1 Assessment for Coping	
Assessment Criteria	**Assessment for Mrs. Foster**
The event or situation that contributes to or causes stress *Appraisal:* primary, secondary, reappraisal	Caregiving for her beloved husband who has behavioral problems caused by Alzheimer's disease Mrs. Foster's primary appraisal includes realistic and unrealistic interpretations of the event, such as her vacillation between recognizing the disease and denying that anything is wrong. Therefore her appraisal is faulty, causing confusion for Mrs. Foster and making it difficult to mobilize coping activities consistently. As a result, secondary appraisal is also faulty because Mrs. Foster is unable to evaluate options and prospects she has to manage the situation. Reappraisal is done inconsistently depending on Mrs. Foster's accurate or inaccurate primary appraisal of the caregiving situation.
Factors affecting appraisal: personal factors: commitment and beliefs about God and personal control; situational factors: novelty, uncertainty, and timing; and temporal factors	Mrs. Foster is deeply committed to her husband of 55 years, which is why she has difficulty realistically appraising the magnitude of the caregiving situation and accepting the diagnosis of AD. She has the sincere desire to do what is best for him, a strength that may lead to more realistic appraisal and subsequent interventions. Her religious and spiritual beliefs are also strengths, although religiosity is not fully utilized, since Mrs. Foster has "dropped out" of organized religious activities. Her beliefs about personal control are reflected in her statement, "God never gives us a burden we cannot handle ourselves. God will provide help, but I must be independent and help myself." The situation of caregiving for a person with AD is difficult: it is novel—something that Mrs. Foster has never experienced; there is uncertainty about the course of the disease, especially since Mrs. Foster has not sought further knowledge; the timing of the event in the life course is not "out of sync" because AD frequently occurs in older persons (vs. younger persons), but it has interfered with the "golden years." Thus Mrs. Foster has responsibilities she did not expect. Temporal factors, particularly the duration of AD (2 to 20 years), are necessary to consider in order to appropriately appraise the situation. Mrs. Foster tends to deny that some changes need to be made now in her caregiving strategies and that the caregiving process will be of long duration. The duration of caregiving must be considered for accurate ongoing assessment and planning.
Mediators of coping: coping activities (problem focused, emotion focused, multifaceted), social support, religiosity, and spirituality	Mrs. Foster's primary method of coping is denial of the existence of the problem of AD and refusal to accept her husband's disease. Problem-focused coping is not well developed for Mrs. Foster because she tends to deny the situation and does not implement strategies that are productive. She tends to use more emotion-focused activities, such as her tendency to believe that God gave her a burden she can handle alone, causing anxiety and depression. Using Jalowiec's descriptions, Mrs. Foster's activities are avoidance, evasive, fatalistic, and emotive. Elderly person tend to use fewer confrontive coping strategies than younger counterparts, and this is true of Mrs. Foster. Even though Mrs. Foster had a strong support system in the past through church activities, friends, and children, she does not use these resources, a factor also more typical of older clients. She totally believes that others will not understand, and she does not want to be a burden. Her religiosity and spirituality are strong coping activities for Mrs. Foster, although she has given up organized religious activities. She uses nonorganized religious activities such as watching religious programs on television and prayer as her primary coping activities. While these provide her with a sense of meaning and purpose, her lack of involvement in previous organized religious activities is inhibited. She does not want her pastor and church friends to know about the situation.

Continued

Table 60-1	Assessment for Coping—cont'd
Assessment Criteria	**Assessment for Mrs. Foster**
Factors affecting the coping process: individual characteristics and resources—health and energy, existential beliefs, social support, social skills, problem-solving skills, material resources; constraints—cultural values and beliefs, psychologic deficits, environmental constraints	Fortunately, Mrs. Foster is in good physical health for her age, although her older age may inhibit physical resources needed for coping; her existential beliefs are strong and she believes that God had a purpose in giving Mr. Foster this disease (at times she is willing to accept it), and that God will provide her with strength to follow through. She has many potential sources of social support through her church, her children, and the Alzheimer's Association, but she does not use those because of embarrassment and her belief that she and God can handle it. Normally, her social skills are good because she had lots of experience in the past, but she has not used these skills to obtain needed help or gain information. Problem-solving skills are compromised because of her tendency to deny the problem and subsequent inability to ask for help or learn more about the disease. Material resources are adequate for the Fosters, even if in-home care or institutionalization becomes necessary. Constraints that impact the coping process include Mrs. Foster's cultural values and beliefs that prohibit her from asking for help and those that continue to contribute to Mrs. Foster's submissiveness. Psychologic deficits are manifested in her denial of the disease and the impact of the caregiving situation as well as her wish to keep the situation "secret." Environmental constraints can also be seen with the lack of organizational religious activity—Mr. Foster behaves embarrassingly in church so they don't go, but they have always gone in the past and enjoyed it. Finally, the level of threat and the fact that at times Mrs. Foster realizes the impact of the disease and its subsequent course immobilize her from truly facing the disease realistically and seeking the help that would contribute to effective coping.
Outcomes: somatic health, social functioning, morale, religiosity and spirituality	Mrs. Foster has no major health problems, but does complain of frequent headaches and fatigue, probably related to the caregiving situation and her inability to deal with it. Social functioning is greatly impaired, with the Fosters becoming relative recluses—something that is a major change from their previous habits. Even their children have not been informed of Mr. Foster's illness, nor have they been given the opportunity to provide support in this situation. Mrs. Foster exhibits symptoms of depression and anxiety. She clearly is not comfortable with her emotional response. Finally, organized religious activity, which had once been so important in the Fosters' lives, is now nonexistent. Similarly, she does not use friends associated with church to provide support. Her main religious and spiritual strength is nonorganized religious activity and intrinsic religious activity. In some ways her religiosity and spirituality impede effective coping because she believes that she must carry this burden alone.

NURSING-SENSITIVE OUTCOMES

Adaptational outcomes include social functioning, morale, and somatic health (Lazarus & Folkman, 1984). Social functioning includes role fulfillment and satisfaction with interpersonal relationships and life conditions. Morale is linked to happiness, satisfaction, and subjective well-being. Somatic health refers to physical health, such as illness, and physical symptoms, such as headaches (Lazarus & Folkman, 1984).

Religiosity and/or spirituality may be impacted by the stress and coping process, thus becoming an outcome along with somatic health, social functioning, and morale. A situation or event can stimulate an examination of religious and spiritual beliefs, with the result being conservation or transformation of significance of these beliefs

(Pargament, 1995). Thus outcomes of the coping process impact negatively or positively on somatic health, social functioning, morale, and religious or spiritual conservation or transformation.

The following expected outcomes can be derived both from the original Lazarus and Folkman (1984) framework and from the modified framework: good somatic health; appropriate morale; satisfying social functioning; and healthy religiosity and spirituality, whether it is conserved or transformed. Obviously, effective coping includes positive outcomes in these areas and ineffective coping includes more negative outcomes.

The Nursing Outcome Classification (NOC) system measures actual rather than expected outcomes. The NOC label Coping is relevant to the diagnosis presented and is defined as "actions to manage stressors that tax an individual's resources" (Iowa Outcomes Project, 2000, p. 192). Other outcomes that could be appropriate for a caregiver like Mrs. Foster include the following: Psychosocial Adjustment: Life Change, Caregiver Emotional Health, Caregiver Physical Health, Caregiver Stressors, Caregiver Well-Being, Mood Equilibrium, and Social Involvement. Outcomes need to be individualized for each client, depending on assessment and interventions. Outcomes guide the gerontologic nurse in revising interventions and associated nursing activities.

NURSING INTERVENTIONS

The Nursing Interventions Classification (NIC) Coping Enhancement incorporates nursing activities that assist the client in dealing with the situation or event that contributes to stress. Coping Enhancement is defined as "assisting a patient to adapt to perceived stressors, changes, or threats which interfere with meeting life demands and roles" (Iowa Intervention Project, 2000, p. 234). The NIC label of Coping Enhancement and associated activities are listed in Box 60-1.

Other NIC labels potentially appropriate for the nursing diagnosis Ineffective Individual Coping include Anger Control Assistance, Anxiety Reduction, Decision-Making Support, Support System Enhancement, Presence, Spiritual Support, Emotional Support, Teaching: Individual, and Learning Facilitation. This list is not exhaustive, and the reader is referred to the *Nursing Interventions Classification (NIC)* (Iowa Intervention Project, 2000).

CASE STUDY

The NIC intervention label of Coping Enhancement was incorporated into Mrs. Foster's plan of care (see Box 60-1). These activities correspond to McFarland and McFarlane's (1997) strategies for nursing management of the client with a diagnosis of Ineffective Individual Coping in various ways. The assessment data obtained using the conceptual framework presented in this chapter (Table 60-1) guided the gerontologic nurse in determining appropriate nursing activities.

The gerontologic nurse consultant began the intervention of Coping Enhancement by educating Mrs. Foster about AD and about management strategies to deal with Mr. Foster's progressive loss of cognitive abilities. Through this educational process, Mrs. Foster learned how to appraise the situation more accurately and to rely on her past experience to implement successful problem solving. It also served to reduce her anxiety and depression by providing her with problem-solving skills necessary to deal with her husband's AD and understand the disease.

The importance of family, church, and community support was stressed by the nurse, who assured Mrs. Foster that she could better cope with the situation and care for her husband by increasing the support that would enable her to take care of both him and herself. With Mrs. Foster the nurse provided information to her children about AD. The children were concerned, expressed a need to be involved with their father's care, and made arrangements to assist with his care in whatever way possible. For example, they offered decision-making support to Mrs. Foster, and each of their children arranged to spend considerable time with their parents.

With Mrs. Foster's consent the minister of the church was also informed and educated about the disease process. He was open and accepting and encouraged Mrs. Foster to attend services and participate in church-related activities. He offered to make home visits on a regular basis and to assist Mrs. Foster in informing close friends and members of the congregation about AD and its effects, as well as identifying ways these friends could provide assistance. The nurse encouraged Mrs. Foster to continue with nonorganized religious activities and intrinsic religious activities because they provided her with a sense of hope, meaning, and connection. Thus the coping mediators of social support and religiosity were enhanced through family and church resources.

Finally, the nurse contacted the Alzheimer's Association to arrange for continued consultation and to obtain information about support groups for families of persons with AD. Mrs. Foster found it helpful to attend support groups, where she learned of strategies that other family members used successfully. She also was able to enroll her husband in a support group for victims of AD. The Alzheimer's Association provided information on respite and day care, services that enabled Mrs. Foster to complete tasks and participate in social activities.

Throughout her interactions with Mrs. Foster, the gerontologic nurse consultant was accepting and nonjudgmental. Further positive reinforcement was provided by praising Mrs. Foster for her achievements and by listening as she described perceived deficits in her caregiving. In this way, Mrs. Foster was able to learn in a nonthreatening environment to ventilate the feelings she was experiencing. Because of this atmosphere, Mrs. Foster was better able to work through her feelings of hopelessness and depression. She was further able to identify coping styles that were beneficial for her and those that were not. With this information, Mrs. Foster and the gerontologic nurse consultant were able to reevaluate strategies and maximize the use of coping mediators.

As of result of nursing interventions, Mrs. Foster was better able to identify and use effective coping patterns and to avoid those that were ineffective. She used a variety of coping styles to balance emotion-focused and problem-focused activities. She verbalized a greater sense of control over the caregiving situation most of the time, with a subsequent decline in her reported levels of stress. Importantly, Mrs. Foster was able to ask for and to accept help when needed. With acceptance of the situation and enhanced knowledge of AD, Mrs. Foster was able to obtain information, modify her lifestyle, and adapt to changes that were made necessary by her husband's progressively deteriorating cognitive condition. She learned that her participation in organized religious activities was still possible, and being with those of similar beliefs enhanced her feelings of being connected. She continued with nonorganized religious activities and intrinsic religious activities, realizing that these resources contributed to her feelings of well-being. She continued to believe that a higher power was helping her in her caregiving role. Because of increased knowledge of AD, Mrs. Foster was able to appropriately challenge her husband and to be less submissive and more self-sufficient. Finally, Mrs. Foster was able to ask for the help she needed from her family, clergyman, and friends in addition to the services provided by community organizations such as the Alzheimer's Association. As a result, Mrs. Foster expressed a greater sense of mastery and satisfaction in her caregiving role and experienced less burden and better emotional responses. Physically, Mrs. Foster reported fewer headaches and higher energy levels.

These actual outcomes led to the achievement of expected outcomes as described by Lazarus and Folkman (1984) and the modified paradigm. Mrs. Foster experienced better social functioning because she was able to share her situation with family and friends. She was no longer embarrassed and ashamed of her husband's behavior, recognizing that others were there to assist. In addition, she was able to participate in formal support systems effectively through day care, respite, and AD support groups. Because she no longer felt alone in her situation and was skilled in problem solving and caregiving mastery as a result of her involvement with the gerontologic nurse, Mrs. Foster experienced less depression and anxiety. Her headaches were much less frequent because of the reduction in anxiety. Finally, her religiosity became healthier, particularly her participation in organized activities, which she had previously abandoned.

SUMMARY

The diagnosis of Ineffective Individual Coping requires an assessment of many domains of the patient's person and environment. When using the diagnosis, it is important for gerontologic nurses to recognize the individual, incorporate that person's strengths, and minimize weaknesses. It is also important to differentiate between normal adjustment and ineffective coping, recognizing that negative emotions may initially be normal responses to particular life events. Using the framework set forth by Lazarus and Folkman (1984) and modified in this chapter, the gerontologic nurse uses an in-depth assessment of the client to determine not only the appropriate nursing diagnosis and related factors, but also sound individualized nursing activities and realistic outcomes. Gerontologic nurses are in a position to view the elderly holistically, to mobilize resources that are available to the elderly, and to intervene to facilitate their effective coping.

REFERENCES

Ackley, B. J., & Ladwig, G. B. (1993). *Nursing diagnosis handbook.* St. Louis, MO: Mosby.

Aldwin, C., Folkman, S., Schaefer, S. C., Coyne, C., & Lazarus, J. C. (1980). *Ways of coping: A process measure.* Presented at the Eighth Annual Meeting of the American Psychological Association, Montreal, Quebec, Canada.

Aldwin, C. M., Sutton, K. J., Chiara, G., & Spiro, A., III. (1996). Age differences in stress, coping, and appraisal: Findings from the Normative Aging Study. *Journals of Gerontology. Series B, Psychological Sciences & Social Sciences, 51*(4), P179-P188.

Becket, N. (1991). Clinical nurses' characterizations of patient coping problems. *Nursing Diagnosis, 2*(2), 72-78.

Beckman, L. J., & Houser, B. B. (1982). The consequences of childlessness on the social-psychological well-being of older women. *Journal of Gerontology, 37*(2), 243-250.

Blazer, D., & Palmore, E. (1976). Religion and aging in a longitudinal panel. *The Gerontologist, 16*(1), 82-85.

Collard, A. F., Jones, D. A., Murphy, M. A., & Fitzmaurice, J. B. (1987). The occurrence of nursing diagnoses in ambulatory care. In A. M. McLane (Ed.), *Classification of nursing diagnoses: Proceedings of the seventh conference* (pp. 283-289). St. Louis, MO: Mosby.

Conway, K. (1985). Coping with the stress of medical problems among black and white elderly. *International Journal of Aging and Human Development, 21*(1), 39-56.

Cutrona, C. E., & Russell, D. W. (1987). The provisions of social relationships and adaptation to stress. *Advances in Personal Relationships, 1,* 37-67.

Felton, B. J., & Revenson, T. A. (1987). Age differences in coping with chronic illness. *Psychology and Aging, 2,* 164-170.

Ferrera, A. R., & Fitzpatrick, J. J. (1982). *Classification of nursing diagnoses: Proceedings of the third and fourth national conferences.* Hightstown, NJ: McGraw-Hill.

Ferraro, K. F., & Koch, J. R. (1994). Religion and health among black and white adults: Examining social support and consultation. *Journal for the Scientific Study of Religion, 33*(4), 362-375.

Folkman, S., Lazarus, R. S., Pimley, S., & Novacek, J. (1987). Age differences in stress and coping processes. *Psychology and Aging, 2*(4), 171-184.

Gilovich, T. (1990). Differential construal and the false consensus effect. *Journal of Personality and Social Psychology, 59*(4), 623-634.

Griffin, D. W., Dunning, D. V., & Ross, L. (1990). The role of construal processes in overconfident predictions about the self and others. *Journal of Personality and Social Psychology, 59*(6), 1128-1139.

Guzzetta, C. E., & Forsyth, G. L. (1979). Nursing diagnosis pilot study: Psychophysiological stress. *Advances in Nursing Science, 2,* 27-44.

Haley, W. E., Ellen, G., Levine, S., Brown, L., & Bartolucci, A. A. (1987). Stress, appraisal, coping and social supports as predictors of adaptational outcome among dementia caregivers. *Psychology and Aging, 2*(4), 323-330.

Hunsberger, B. (1985). Religion, age, life satisfaction, and perceived sources of religiousness: A study of older persons. *Journal of Gerontology, 40*(5), 615-620.

Iowa Intervention Project. J. C. McCloskey & G. M. Bulechek (Eds.). (2000). *Nursing interventions classification (NIC)* (3rd ed.). St. Louis, MO: Mosby.

Iowa Outcomes Project. M. Johnson, M. Maas, & S. Moorhead (Eds.). (2000). *Nursing outcomes classification (NOC)* (2nd ed.). St. Louis, MO: Mosby.

Jalowiec, A. (1979). Stress and coping in hypertensive and emergency room patients. Master's thesis. University of Illinois, Chicago.

Jalowiec, A. (1987). *Jaloweic Coping Scale (revised).* Unpublished manuscript. University of Illinois, Chicago.

Kaye, J., & Robinson, K. (1994). Spirituality among caregivers. *IMAGE: Journal of Nursing Scholarship, 26*(3), 218-221.

Koenig, H. G., Cohen, H. J., Blazer, D. G., Pieper, C., Meador, K. G., Shelp, F., Goli, V., & DiPasquale, B. (1992). Religious coping and depression among elderly, hospitalized medically ill men. *American Journal of Psychiatry, 149,* 1693-1700.

Koenig, H. G., George, L. K., & Siegler, I. C. (1988). The use of religion and other emotion-regulating coping strategies among older adults. *The Gerontologist, 28,* 303-310.

Krause, N. (1995). Religiosity and self-esteem among older adults. *Journal of Gerontology, 50B*(5), P236-P246.

Lawton, M. P., Kleben, M. H., Moss, M., Rovine, M., & Glicksman, A. (1989). Measuring caregiving appraisal. *Journal of Gerontology: Psychological Sciences, 44,* 61-71.

Lazarus, R., & Folkman, S. (1984). *Stress, appraisal, and coping.* New York: Springer.

Manfredi, C., & Pickett, M. (1987). Perceived stressful situations and coping strategies utilized by the elderly. *Journal of Community Health Nursing, 4*(2), 99-110.

Matthewman, J., Fosse, E., Miller, B. K., Pesut, D. J., Doenges, M. E., Gordon, M., Jakob, D., Vincent, K. G., Kelley, J., Coenen, C., & Frisch, N. (1995). Ineffective individual/family coping. In M. J. Rantz & P. LeMone (Eds.), *Classification of nursing diagnoses: Proceedings of the eleventh conference* (pp. 413-419). Glendale, CA: Cinahl Information Systems.

McFarland, G. K., & McFarlane, E. A. (1997). Coping-stress tolerance pattern, ineffective individual coping. In G. K. McFarland & E. A. McFarlane (Eds.), *Nursing diagnosis and intervention, planning for patient care* (3rd ed.). St. Louis, MO: Mosby.

McGoldrick, A. E. (1989). Stress, early retirement and health. In K. S. Markides & C. L. Cooper (Eds.), *Aging, stress and health* (pp. 91-118). New York: John Wiley & Sons.

McNair, D. M., Lorr, M., & Droppleman L. F. (1971). *Profile of mood states manual.* San Diego, CA: Educational and Industrial Testing Service.

Nelson, P. B. (1990). Intrinsic/extrinsic religious orientation of the elderly: Relationship to depression and self-esteem. *Journal of Gerontological Nursing, 16*(2), 29-35.

North American Nursing Diagnosis Association. (1999). *Nursing diagnoses: Definitions & classification 1999-2000.* Philadelphia: Author.

Pargament, K. I., Ensing, D. S., Falgout, K., Olsen, H., Reilly, B., Van Haitsma, K., & Warren, R. (1990). God help me (I): Religious coping efforts as predictors of the outcomes to significant negative life events. *American Journal of Community Psychology, 18,* 793-824.

Pargament, K. I. (1995). Religious methods of coping: Resources for the conservation and transformation of significance. In E. Shafranske (Ed.), *Religion and the clinical practice of psychology,* Washington, DC: APA Books.

Pearlin, L. I., & Schooler, C. (1978). The structure of coping. *Journal of Health and Social Behavior, 19,* 2-21.

Pearlin, L. I., Turner, H., & Semple, S. (1989). Coping and the mediation of caregiver stress. In E. Light & B. Lebowitz (Eds.), *Alzheimer's disease: Mental treatment and family stress. Directions for research* (pp. 198-217). Washington, DC: National Institute of Mental Health.

Pruchno, R. A., & Resch, N. L. (1989). Aberrant behaviors and Alzheimer's disease: Mental health effects of spouse caregivers. *Journal of Gerontology, 44,* S177-S182.

Reed, P. G. (1991). Self-transcendence and mental health in oldest-old adults. *Nursing Research, 40*(1), 5-11.

Rosen, C. C. (1982). Ethnic differences among impoverished rural elderly in use of religion as a coping mechanism. *Journal of Rural Community Psychology, 3,* 27-34.

Rosenbaum, M. (1980). A schedule for assessing self-control behaviors: Preliminary findings. *Behavior Therapy, 11,* 109-112.

Russell, D. W., & Cutrona, C. E. (1991). Social support, stress, and depressive symptoms among the elderly: Test of a process model. *Psychology and Aging, 6*(2), 190-201.

Ryan, M., & Austin, A. (1989). Social supports and social networks in the aged. *Image: Journal of Nursing Scholarship, 21*(3), 176-180.

Schaefer, C. A., & Gorsuch, R. L. (1991). Psychological adjustment and religiousness: The multivariate belief-motivation theory of religiousness. *Journal for the Scientific Study of Religion, 20,* 448-467.

Smyth, K., & Yarandi, H. N. (1996). Factor analysis of the ways of coping questionnaire for African American women. *Nursing Research, 45*(1), 25-29.

Stolley, J. M., Buckwalter, K. C., & Koeniz, H. G. (1999). Prayer and religious coping for caregivers of persons with Alzheimer's disease and related disorders. *American Journal of Alzheimer's Disease, 14*(3), 181-191.

Swanson, W. C., & Harter, C. L. (1971). How do elderly blacks cope in New Orleans. *International Journal on Aging and Human Development, 2,* 210-216.

Tack, B. B., & Gillis, C. L. (1990). Nurse-monitored cardiac recovery: A description of the first eight weeks. *Heart & Lung: Journal of Critical Care, 19*(5 part 1), 491-499.

Valliant, G. E. (1967). *Adaptation to life.* Boston: Little, Brown.

Vincent, K. G. (1986). The validation of a nursing diagnosis: A nurse-consensus survey. In M. E. Hurley (Ed.), *Classification of nursing diagnoses: Proceedings of the sixth conference* (pp. 207-214). St. Louis, MO: Mosby.

Vitaliano, P. P., Russo, J., Carr, J. R., Maiuro, R. D., & Becker, J. (1985). The ways of coping checklist: Revision and psychometric properties. *Multivariate Behavioral Research, 20,* 3-26.

Whitlach, A. M., Meddaugh, D. I., & Langhout, K. J. (1992). Religiosity among Alzheimer's disease caregivers. *The American Journal of Alzheimer's Disease and Related Disorders & Research, 7*(6), 11-20.

Wilson, H. S. (1989). Family caregiving for a relative with Alzheimer's dementia: Coping with negative choices. *Nursing Research, 38,* 94-98.

Wineman, N. M., Durand, E. J., & Steiner, R. P. (1994). A comparative analysis of coping behaviors in individuals with multiple sclerosis or a spinal cord injury. *Research in Nursing and Health, 17,* 184-194.

Yesavage, J. A., Brink, R. A., Rose, T. L., Lum, O., Huang, V., Adey, M., & Leirer, V. (1983). Development and validation of a geriatric depression screening scale: A preliminary report. *Journal of Psychiatric Research, 17,* 37-49.

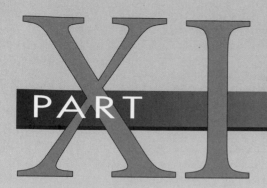

PART XI

Value-Belief Pattern

OVERVIEW

Because of loss of control, the relative imminence of death, and loss of traditional support systems, elders are believed to be particularly susceptible to spiritual distress. However, as Bunten points out in Chapter 61, success with spiritual developmental tasks and challenges associated with growing older may be satisfying and enriching. The author discusses research and other resources that may assist the nurse to understand and promote spiritual growth for elderly patients.

In Chapter 62, Spiritual Distress, LeMone argues that the outcome of this experience can be positive or negative and that a holistic view on the part of the nurse will enable better diagnosis, intervention, and positive outcomes. She discusses quantitative and qualitative assessment of spiritual distress, suggests interventions based on related factors, and discusses nursing's impact on the diagnosis in terms of well-being related to spiritual wellness of elders.

CHAPTER 61

NORMAL CHANGES WITH AGING

Donna Bunten

The belief or value system that each individual holds provides strength, hope, and meaning to his or her life (Carpenito, 1993). Beliefs and values provide a framework for understanding life and one's purpose and place here on earth (Eliopoulis, 1987; Oldnall, 1996). They guide the choices we make throughout our life span, whether we are consciously aware of them or not. Our perception of whether events are stressful is affected by our beliefs and values. This holds true and may become even more important as elderly individuals address developmental tasks associated with later adulthood.

The neo-Freudian work of Erik Erikson (1963) described the challenges of old age. Erikson believed that in the last stage of life, before satisfaction can be experienced, individuals must put their lives into perspective. They must accept the good and bad about their lives and find that their lives had meaning and usefulness. If this task, called "ego integrity," cannot be successfully accomplished, the aging person will experience despair. Erikson's final stage of development, "ego-integrity vs. despair" is a "spiritual task" of aging (Blazer, 1991). Elders need to seek satisfaction not only from the life they have lived, but also from the tasks they face during aging itself, including learning to live with illness and infirmity and the ultimate task of preparing for death (Butler & Lewis, 1982).

In old age there is an ever-present awareness of the finiteness of time. Rosowsky (1996) describes a psycho-spiritual mission calling the elder to ". . . review, reflect, resolve, repair and prepare" (p. 196), which helps elders to ameliorate pain and fear as they approach the end of life. Along with the knowledge that one's life is finite and nearing its end comes a heightened spiritual need (Koenig, Larson, and Matthews, 1996). These tasks not only challenge elders, but also provide an opportunity for spiritual growth during the aging process (Berggren-Thomas & Griggs, 1995; Price, Stevens, & LaBarre, 1995).

SPIRITUALITY

The concept of holistic nursing directs nurses to be attentive to the biologic, psychologic, sociologic, and spiritual needs of their clients (Ellis, 1992; Espeland, 1999). Nurturing of the elder's spiritual life is important in a healthy balancing of mind, body, and spirit (Hungelmann, Kenkel-Rossi, Klassen, & Stollenwerk, 1996). Spirituality encompasses, but is not limited to, religiosity (O'Conner, 1988). Although spirituality has traditionally been associated with religion, a person who is experiencing spiritual needs might not necessarily be religious or participate in religious rituals and practices (Burnard, 1993). Goddard (1995) suggests that spirituality be thought of as energy capable of producing internal harmony of body, mind, and spirit. Spirituality may be dependent on any aspect of the human experience that stimulates meaning of life for an individual and is, thus, unique to each human being (Blazer, 1991). Nurses can learn more about the spiritual needs of their clients by asking what nourishes their spirits than by asking them about their religious orientation (O'Connor, 1988). "Spirituality has to do with intangibles of vital importance to all human beings: values, relationships, and the discovery of meaning and purpose in life" (Jewell, 1999, p. 10).

Elders are faced with many spiritual challenges: loss of roles, loss of identity, incapacities, loss of loved ones, and the approach of death (Berggren-Thomas & Griggs, 1995; Blazer, 1991). These losses challenge the elder to achieve greater self-transcendence, to feel a greater sense of connection to others, and to come to an understanding and acceptance of what their life has held (Blazer, 1991). Nurses can consider spiritual growth to be a life-long journey and spiritual nurturing to be a need of many elderly.

RELIGIOSITY

Although religiosity is but one aspect of spirituality, it has been the topic of considerable research. Religion has been found to provide many people with a baseline and framework from which to establish values and beliefs and assists them to come to some understanding of their inner being or spirituality. Elderly persons who have not been religious in earlier life are not likely to become religious in late life. Those who are religious seem to have a greater sense of meaning or purpose in later life (Forbis, 1988). Tobin (1991) found that religion is a mechanism by which elderly persons can cope with the changes in their lives.

Nelson (1990) observed a positive relationship between the degree of intrinsic religious orientation (defined as living one's faith) and self-esteem in elderly persons: as the level of intrinsic faith increased, depression decreased.

Koenig, Kavale, and Ferrel (1988) reported that a strong religious commitment in the elder reduces the level of perceived stress by providing life with meaning and purpose and a means to cope with physical illness and other stressors. Koenig (1995) reported that elders who frequently attend church, pray, or read religious books are healthier, happier, and more satisfied with their lives. In addition, these elders were less depressed, anxious, lonely, or likely to abuse alcohol than less religiously committed elders. Elders have cited the following benefits of church attendance: interacting with other people, finding emotional support, giving meaning to life, and enhancing spiritual growth (Pieper, 1981). Other researchers have discussed the effects of religious practice on both mental and physical health. Kennedy, Kelman, Thomas, and Chen (1996) found that failure to attend religious services was associated with both the emergence and the persistence of depressive symptoms in older adults of various denominations. Ai, Dunkle, Peterson, and Bolling (1998) reported greater psychologic well-being in aged coronary bypass surgery patients who practiced private prayer. McBride, Arthur, Brooks, and Pilkington (1998) also found that spiritual commitment can enhance prevention, coping, and recovery from illness and surgery. Some individuals who are hospitalized or relocated to a nursing home experience a lack of privacy and separation from religious ritual (McCavery, 1984), including limited availability of services, chapel areas, and religious literature. Elderly persons who are homebound can experience these barriers as well.

SUMMARY

Nursing education often has failed to address adequately the fulfillment of clients' spiritual needs (Oldnall, 1996). Nurses may consider spiritual needs to be the domain of chaplains or other clergy who, in fact, may have lacked seminary course work in gerontology-related ... 1988). Lack of ...

leaves
s that
often
sure-
ding
der-
rily

ials
sh   are
to   rt-
abl   o-
tio   d
phi   is
insi
resp
othe
tual
pers

... professional life.

REFERENCES

Ai, A. L., Dunkle, R. E., Peterson, C., & Bolling, S. F. (1998). The role of private prayer in psychological recovery among midlife and aged patients following cardiac surgery. *The Gerontologist, 38*(5), 591-601.

Berggren-Thomas, P., & Griggs, M. J. (1995). Spirituality in aging: Spiritual need or spiritual journey. *Journal of Gerontological Nursing, 21*(30), 5-10.

Blazer, D. (1991). Spirituality and aging well. *Generations, 15*(1), 61-65.

Burnard, P. (1993). Giving spiritual care. *Journal of Community Nursing, 6*(10), 16-18.

Butler, R. N., & Lewis, M. I. (1982). *Aging and mental health: Positive psychosocial and biomedical approaches* (3rd ed.). St. Louis, MO: Mosby.

Carpenito, L. J. (1993). *Nursing diagnosis: Application to clinical practice* (5th ed.). Baltimore: Lippincott Williams & Wilkins.

Eliopoulis, C. (1987). *Gerontological nursing* (2nd ed.). Baltimore: Lippincott Williams & Wilkins.

Ellis, R. (1992). Characteristics of significant theories. In L. H. Nicoll (Ed.), *Perspectives on nursing theory* (pp. 317-324) (2nd ed.). Baltimore: Lippincott Williams & Wilkins.

Erikson, E. (1963). *Childhood and society* (2nd ed.). New York: Horton.

Espeland, K. (1999). Achieving spiritual wellness: Using reflective questions. *Journal of Psychosocial Nursing, 37*(7), 36-40.

Forbis, P. A. (1988). Meeting patients' spiritual needs. *Geriatric Nursing, 9*, 158-159.

Goddard, N. C. (1995). Spirituality vs. integrative energy: A philosophical analysis as requisite precursor to holistic nursing practice. *Journal of Advanced Nursing, 22*, 808-815.

Hungelmann, J., Kenkel-Rossi, E., Klassen, L., & Stollenwerk, R. (1996). Focus on spiritual well-being: Harmonious interconnectedness of mind-body-spirit—Use of the JAREL spiritual well-being scale. *Geriatric Nursing, 17*(6), 262-266.

Jewell, A. (1999). *Spirituality and ageing.* Philadelphia: Jessica Kinglsey.

Kennedy, G. J., Kelman, H. R., Thomas, C., & Chen, J. (1996). The relation of religious preference and practice to depressive symptoms among 1,855 older adults. *Journal of Gerontology: Series B, Psychological Sciences & Social Sciences, 51*(6), P301-P308.

Koenig, H. (1995). *Research on religion and aging.* New York: Greenwood Press.

Koenig, H., Kavale, J., & Ferrel, C. (1988). Religion and well-being in later life. *The Gerontologist, 28*, 18-27.

Koenig, H., Larson, D. B., & Matthews, D. A. (1996). Religion and psychotherapy with older adults. *Journal of Geriatric Psychiatry, 29*(2), 155-184.

McBride, J. L., Arthur, G., Brooks, R., & Pilkington, L. (1998). The relationship between a patient's spirituality and health experiences. *Family Medicine, 30*, 122-126.

McCavery, R. (1984). Spiritual care in acute illness. In O. McGillowat (Ed.), *Nursing and spiritual care* (pp. 129-143). London: Harper & Row.

Nelson, P. B. (1990). Intrinsic/extrinsic religious orientation of the elderly: Relationship to depression and self-esteem. *Journal of Gerontological Nursing, 16*(2), 29-35.

O'Connor, P. (1988). Spiritual elements of hospice care. *American Journal of Hospice Care, 2*(2), 99-108.

Oldnall, A. (1996). A critical analysis of nursing: Meeting the spiritual needs of patients. *Journal of Advanced Nursing, 23,* 139-144.

Peterson, E. A., & Nelson, K. (1987). How to meet your clients' spiritual needs. *Journal of Psychosocial and Mental Health Services, 25*(5), 34-39.

Pieper, H. C. (1981). Church membership and participation in church activities among the elderly. *Activities, Adaptation and Aging, 1*(3), 23-29.

Price, J. L., Stevens, H. O., & LaBarre, M. C. (1995). Spiritual caregiving in nursing practice. *Journal of Psychosocial Nursing, 33*(22), 5-9.

Rosowsky, E. (1996). Wisdom and spirituality: Their special importance in clinical work with older adults. *Journal of Geriatric Psychiatry, 29*(2), 123-128.

Stiles, M. K. (1990). The shining stranger, nurse-family spiritual relationship. *Cancer Nursing, 13,* 235-245.

Tobin, S. S. (1991). *Personhood in advanced old age: Implications to practice.* New York: Springer.

Wilderquest, J., & Davidhizar, R. (1994). The ministry of nursing. *Journal of Advanced Nursing, 19,* 647-652.

CHAPTER 62

SPIRITUAL DISTRESS

Priscilla LeMone

Spiritual distress, or distress of the human spirit, is a subjective human response to a "disruption in the life principle which pervades a person's entire being and which integrates and transcends one's biological and psychosocial nature" (North American Nursing Diagnosis Association [NANDA], 1999, p. 67). Although the experience of spiritual distress is not unique to elders, they are a population at risk for its development as a result of multiple interrelated factors. These factors include a lack of meaning or purpose in daily activities, loneliness, regret for unaccomplished life goals, fear of an uncertain future, and the loss of physical health, support systems, human contact, and hope (Dugan, 1987, 1988; Kierkegaard, 1962).

The human spirit is an intangible dimension of the whole person, expressed in the term *spirituality.* Although the terms *spirituality* and *religiosity* are often used interchangeably, they are not identical. Spirituality includes but is not limited to religious beliefs. Yet difficulty can arise both in separating spirituality from religiosity and in separating problems in the spiritual dimension from those in the psychosocial dimension (Mansen, 1993). Spirituality, a basic or inherent quality of all humans, is a broad multidimensional concept encompassing an individual's purpose and meaning of life (Dossey, Guzzetta, & Kenner, 1992; Haase, Britt, Coward, Leidy, & Penn, 1992). Stoll (1989) provided a framework for spirituality that includes both a vertical and a horizontal dimension. The vertical dimension is concerned with consciously or unconsciously chosen values that organize one's life and serve as motivators for fulfilling goals, needs, and aspirations. The horizontal strand reflects the experiences of one's relationships with a higher being, as well as one's beliefs and values, lifestyle, quality of life, and interactions with self, others, and nature. These strands interrelate through forgiveness, love, and trust to give meaning, purpose, and hope to life.

Reed (1992) defined spirituality as "an expression of the developmental capacity for self-transcendence . . . the propensity to make meaning through a sense of relatedness to dimensions that transcend the self in such a way that empowers and does not devalue the individual" (p. 350). Self-transcendence is a characteristic of later life in which personal boundaries are expanded toward others and the environment, toward greater awareness of beliefs and values, and toward integration of the past and future in the present (Reed, 1991a, 1996). Thus spirituality, through transcendence, serves as a resource and source of strength when faced with inevitable change and loss. As described by Walton (1996), "spirituality can arise at any time and out of any situation, whether it involves pain, sorrow, or joy" (p. 242).

If spirituality is a life force and an affirmation of life, what then is spiritual distress? It can be a sense of not having purpose and meaning, of not being in harmony with a life force, and/or of not being bonded to others. It can include experiencing a moral crisis and questioning a belief in a deity, in self, or in others. Having spiritual distress, however, does not mean giving up on life. It can mean that the person is struggling with the meaning and mystery of life. This struggle can be a positive experience if it brings the person to a deeper sense of peace, meaning, and purpose. Conversely, if the distress leads to feelings of abandonment, isolation, or hopelessness, it can be a negative experience.

RELATED FACTORS/ETIOLOGIES

A variety of factors can precipitate the experience of spiritual distress in elders. These factors, related to a challenge to a person's belief system or to separation from spiritual ties, include loss of a body part or body function, terminal illness, chronic illness, intense or chronic pain, disability, or trauma. Therapeutic regimens, such as surgery, radiation and chemotherapy, blood transfusions, dietary restrictions, and medications, can cause a conflict between personal values and beliefs and the prescribed therapy. Personal factors that can result in spiritual distress are death or illness of a loved one and separation from family and friends. Environmental factors include barriers to spiritual practices and rituals, such as lack of privacy, lack of transportation, moving to a different living environment, immobility, and inability to access special foods. The elderly person also can experience spiritual distress resulting from a feeling of embarrassment about practicing spiritual activities or perceiving that others do not have the same beliefs.

To incorporate spirituality into care, nurses must identify the social, cultural, and environmental factors that precipitate spiritual distress (Smucker, 1995). A variety of frameworks have been suggested, including personal spirituality and universality (Stoll, 1989) and spiritual needs (Fish & Shelley, 1983; Highfield & Cason, 1983; Stallwood & Stoll, 1975).

ASSESSMENT

As one ages, inevitable changes and multiple losses occur. Along with declining physical resources comes loss of fulfilling work and income, loss of relationships, and possible relocation. Affirming life in the face of change and loss and finding a sense of purpose and meaning in life are difficult for some elders. Developmental stages and tasks, common to all persons as they age, can alter usual methods of coping. According to Erikson (1963), old age provides a time for a reminiscence of life events to attain purpose and fulfillment. However, if the aging adult looks back and sees a life filled with failures or missed achievements, a sense of despair can occur. The aging process, with related losses and stressors, can negatively affect an individual's sense of meaning and purpose, means of forgiveness, and/or sources of love and relatedness (Peterson, 1990).

An initial nursing assessment should be conducted to serve as a basis for making a diagnosis related to spiritual distress and for providing spiritual support. Ongoing, regular assessments should be planned to evaluate the effectiveness of the interventions. Questions that can provide cues to spiritual needs include the following (Carpenito, 1995):

- What is your source of spiritual strength or meaning?
- How do you practice your spiritual beliefs?
- Are there any practices that are important for your spiritual well-being?
- Do you have a spiritual advisor?

- Has being (sick, hurt, moved, etc.) affected your spiritual beliefs?
- How can I help you maintain your spiritual strength? (e.g., contact your pastor, priest, or rabbi; provide reading materials or music important to you; provide privacy at certain times; arrange for transportation to religious services; pray with you)

The nurse assesses the patient's behavioral response to questions about spiritual needs, noting altered responses (anger, crying, or withdrawal). It is important to assess for physical or treatment-related factors that interfere with the patient's usual spiritual practices, such as an inability to kneel during prayer or dietary conflicts. The nurse should also determine patients' knowledge of their illness, reason for moving (as from own home to a long-term care facility), and medical regimen. Other areas of assessment include the patient's level of cognitive functioning, ability to read, relationships with family and significant others, communications, affect and attitude, self-concept, and body image (Peterson, 1990). Further cues to spiritual needs are the presence of articles significant to the patient (Bible, rosary, prayer book, religious medals, church papers), the amount and type of visitors, and requests for spiritual assistance.

Several assessment tools are available for assessing spiritual needs or spiritual well-being. These tools with related information are outlined in Table 62-1. These tools provide indications of spiritual concerns and indicate cues to support making the diagnosis.

Stoll (1979) proposed guidelines for a spiritual assessment that is based on (1) concept of God or deity, (2) sources of strength and hope, (3) religious practices, and (4) relationship between spiritual beliefs and health. Within these four areas, 13 questions are asked to identify the person's concept of a transcendent being or life force,

Table 62-1	Tools to Assess Spirituality
Name/Author(s)	**Description**
Spiritual Distress Index/ Flesner (1981)	22-item Likert scale based on areas in which a person can experience spiritual distress: (1) forgiveness, (2) love, (3) hope, (4) trust, and (5) meaning and purpose. Has high test-retest reliability and high positive correlation with the Spiritual Well-Being Scale.
The Spiritual Well-Being Scale/ Paloutzian & Ellison (1982)	20-item measure gives three scores: (1) spiritual well-being, (2) existential well-being, and (3) religious well-being. Uses Likert scale, has established validity and reliability.
Spiritual pilgrimage or timeline/ Tubesing & Tubesing (1983)	Draws a timeline of one's spiritual pilgrimage from birth to the present, and then extends it into the future; provides information about perceptions of spiritual growth.
Personal reflection guide/ Tubesing & Tubesing (1983)	Encourages reflection about values, beliefs, and commitments; spiritual truths and beliefs; meaningful spiritual rituals; aspects of spirituality that are missing and how rituals can help; and advice for younger persons on developing a richer spiritual life.
Indexes of Spiritual Well-Being/ Moberg (1984)	82-item questionnaire, used to identify factors that may influence spiritual well-being: social attitudes, self-perceptions, activities serving others, and religious orientation and experiences. Is specific to Christianity.
The Serenity Scale/ Roberts & Aspy (1993)	40-item self-report summated scale to evaluate serenity status. Alpha coefficient = 0.92, item-to-total correlation ranges from 0.25 to 0.67.

persons and practices that provide strength and hope, important religious practices and symbols, use of prayer or meditation, and alteration of religious practices by illness. The assessment interview should always be open-ended and nonthreatening, allowing the individual sufficient time for self-expression.

O'Brien (1982) developed a spiritual assessment guide based on data collected from hemodialysis patients. The guide has questions about six areas of spirituality: (1) general spiritual beliefs; (2) personal spiritual beliefs; (3) identification with institutionalized religion; (4) spiritual or religious support systems; (5) spiritual or religious rituals; and (6) spiritual deficit or distress. The spiritual deficit or distress section contains questions to assess spiritual pain, alienation, anxiety, guilt, anger, loss, and despair. A shorter tool, the Spiritual Needs Survey developed by Hess (Fish & Shelley, 1983), asks five questions that focus on the patient's spiritual needs and personal efforts to address them. This tool was designed for use in hospitals and extended-care facilities. A spiritual well-being scale, illustrated in Table 62-2, was developed as part of the Nursing Outcomes Classification (NOC) by the College of Nursing at the University of Iowa (Iowa Outcomes Project, 2000) and provides a means of measuring indicators of spiritual well-being for patients in a variety of settings. The choice

of instrument used in the clinical setting is individualized by nursing expertise in the use of quantitative measures and the patient's cognitive and physical status.

NURSING DIAGNOSIS

Nursing has long recognized the importance of including the spiritual dimension as an inseparable component of holistic care. However, as with other subjective human experiences, the assessment and diagnosis of an altered spiritual response are often difficult. Spiritual Distress, as a nursing diagnosis, was first introduced as Alterations in Spiritual Comfort Level by NANDA in 1973 at the First National Classification Conference (Gebbie & Lavin, 1975) and later changed to Alterations in Faith, with subcategories of alterations in faith of self, faith in others, and faith in God. The single diagnosis of Spiritual Distress (Distress of the Human Spirit) and refinements of the definition, etiologies, related factors, and defining characteristics were adopted at the Fourth National Classification Conference in 1978 (Kim & Moritz, 1982) and remain in current use (Carroll-Johnson, 1989).

Other diagnostic labels for alterations in spirituality have been suggested. Although NANDA did not change the diagnosis, participants at the Fifth National Confer-

Table 62-2	Measuring Spiritual Well-Being				
	Extremely Compromised 1	Substantially Compromised 2	Moderately Compromised 3	Mildly Compromised 4	Not Compromised 5
SPIRITUAL WELL-BEING					
Indicators	1	2	3	4	5
Expresses faith	1	2	3	4	5
Expresses hope	1	2	3	4	5
Expression of meaning and purpose in life	1	2	3	4	5
Expression of spiritual world view	1	2	3	4	5
Expression of serenity	1	2	3	4	5
Expression of love	1	2	3	4	5
Expression of forgiveness	1	2	3	4	5
Mystical experiences	1	2	3	4	5
Prayer	1	2	3	4	5
Worship	1	2	3	4	5
Participation in spiritual rites and passages	1	2	3	4	5
Interaction with spiritual leaders	1	2	3	4	5
Meditation	1	2	3	4	5
Expression through song	1	2	3	4	5
Spiritual reading	1	2	3	4	5
Other (Specify)	1	2	3	4	5

Data from Iowa Outcomes Project. M. Johnson, M. Maas, & S. Moorhead (Eds.). (2000). *Nursing outcomes classification (NOC)* (2nd ed.). St. Louis, MO: Mosby.

ence suggested the labels of Spiritual Distress related to forgiveness, love, hope, trust, meaning, and purpose as separate diagnoses. O'Brien (1982) developed several diagnoses based on data collected for developing a spiritual assessment guide: Spiritual Pain, Spiritual Alienation, Spiritual Anxiety, Spiritual Guilt, Spiritual Anger, Spiritual Loss, and Spiritual Despair.

Defining characteristics of the NANDA diagnosis Spiritual Distress are listed in Box 62-1. Validation studies of these defining characteristics have reported conflicting findings. Weatherall and Creason (1987) analyzed both literature on the topic and assessment data from hospitalized patients and found support for verbal cues of the meaning of suffering, concern about relationship with deity, and inner conflict about beliefs. Two other characteristics, hopelessness and cues having to do with relationships with others, were identified and found to be gender and age related. McHolm (1991) surveyed members of the Oncology Nursing Society and found diagnostic validity for all but two of the NANDA characteristics (anger toward God and apathy). McHolm also identified other nonspecific indicators of distress, including somatic complaints, feelings of guilt, fear, depression, anorexia, silence, and bitterness. Hensley (1994) surveyed American Nurses Association certified nurses to determine the diagnostic content validity of the NANDA characteristics and found support for all but description of nightmares/sleep disturbances and gallows humor. All researchers recommended continued validation and refinement of the list of defining characteristics.

Examples of diagnostic statements for Spiritual Distress in elders include the following:

• Spiritual Distress related to inability to reconcile spiritual beliefs with loss of spouse and diagnosis of cancer as manifested by withdrawal from social activities and expressions of anger toward God.
• Spiritual Distress related to inability to forgive self and others for perceived failures in life as manifested by negative statements and bitterness.

• Spiritual Distress related to inability to practice spiritual rituals in nursing home as manifested by expressions of loneliness and isolation.

Spirituality is an important dimension of well-being for elders. For the elderly person, spirituality can reduce stress and anxiety and help maintain a sense of self and purpose in life (Reed, 1991b). Spiritual wellness can also facilitate living with chronic illness and preparing for death (Miller, 1985). It is essential, therefore, that nurses integrate spiritual assessments and interventions to enhance spirituality in elders in acute-care, long-term care, community-based, and home settings.

CASE STUDY

R. Porter is a frail 88-year-old woman of Irish descent. Her husband died 14 years ago of a cerebral vascular accident. Mrs. Porter lived in her own home until 1 year ago. At that time she was diagnosed with metastatic breast cancer and moved to a nursing home following surgery, radiation, and chemotherapy. She has been told that her life expectancy is less than a year. Although she has little pain at the present, she needs assistance with activities of daily life and mobility. Mrs. Porter has no living relatives.

Mrs. Porter has been quiet and withdrawn since moving to the nursing home. She cries often, refuses to take part in activities, and often spends an entire day lying on her bed in the dark. She eats very little and has lost 10 pounds since admission. She tells the staff that she misses her husband, her house, and her garden. She also says that she is angry because she has suffered so much. Mrs. Porter holds her rosary constantly and only cheers briefly after visits from her priest. The assessment scale in Table 62-2 was administered to Mrs. Porter; her low scores on the instrument indicated low spiritual well-being and further supported a diagnosis of Spiritual Distress.

Box 62-1	**Defining Characteristics** **SPIRITUAL DISTRESS**

Expresses concern with meaning of life/death and/or belief systems*
Anger toward God
Questions meaning of suffering
Verbalizes inner conflict about beliefs
Verbalizes concern about relationship with deity
Questions meaning of own existence
Unable to participate in usual religious practices

Seeks spiritual assistance
Questions moral/ethical implications of therapeutic regimen
Gallows humor
Displacement of anger toward religious representatives
Description of nightmares/sleep disturbances
Alteration in behavior/mood (evidenced by anger, crying, withdrawal, preoccupation, anxiety, hostility, apathy, etc.)

Data from North American Nursing Diagnosis Association. (1999). *Nursing diagnoses: Definitions & classification 1999-2000* (p. 67). Philadelphia: Author.
*Critical defining characteristic.

NURSING-SENSITIVE OUTCOMES

The spiritual dimension of individuals is a legitimate focus for nursing interventions. The outcome concept appropriate in designing and implementing care for patients with spiritual distress is Spiritual Well-Being (Iowa Outcomes Project, 2000), defined as the "personal expression of connectedness with self, others, higher power, all life, nature, and the universe that transcend and empower the self" (p. 407). This outcome concept is especially significant to elders who are at risk for or have Spiritual Distress. The 1971 White House Conference on Aging presented a classic description of age-related changes that affect spirituality, encompassing losses of physical faculties, societal roles, loved ones, home and freedom, and an everlasting future. Aging stresses those components most central to spirituality: having meaning and purpose in life, experiencing forgiveness, and having love and relatedness.

Alternate labels and definitions of spiritual well-being as a positive expression of spirituality are found in the literature. Hawks, Hull, Thalman, and Richins (1995) defined spiritual health as follows:

A high level of faith, hope, and commitment in relation to a well-defined world view or belief system that provides a sense of meaning and purpose to existence in general, and that offers an ethical path to personal fulfillment which includes connectedness with self, others, and a higher power or larger reality (p. 373).

Haase et al. (1992) suggested that it is spiritual perspective, rather than spirituality, that is responsive to nursing interventions. Spiritual perspective is defined as "a highly individualized awareness of one's spirituality and its qualities" (p. 143). The awareness of one's spirituality through spiritual perspective facilitates the expression of one's purpose in life. Using the diagnostic label Potential for Enhanced Spiritual Well-Being, NANDA (1999) defined spiritual well-being as the "process of an individual's developing/unfolding of mystery through harmonious interconnectedness that springs from inner strengths" (p. 68). Miller (1985) described spiritual well-being as manifested by expressions of satisfaction with the relationship with a higher power, the perception of life as having meaning, and satisfaction with one's life.

Although spiritual well-being is recognized as a critical element in maintaining wellness and quality of life, research into this phenomenon has been minimal. NANDA diagnoses and defining characteristics have been approved for clinical testing. Studies have validated some of the defining characteristics of Spiritual Distress through research (Hensley, 1994; McHolm, 1991; Weatherall & Creason, 1987), but continued research to validate and refine the list is recommended. Both Nursing Outcomes Classification (NOC) and Nursing Interventions Classification (NIC) for Spiritual Distress are being classified by the University of Iowa College of Nursing. However, because spirituality is subjective and multidimensional, further clarification and knowledge development through research of the outcomes and intervention activities is also necessary.

Table 62-3 lists the nursing diagnosis, signs and symptoms, nursing outcome and indicators, and nursing interventions and activities synthesized from the literature on Spiritual Distress and Spiritual Well-Being (Brooke, 1987; Carpenito, 1995; Conco, 1995; Gustafson, 1992; Haase et al., 1992; Hawks et al., 1995; Iowa Intervention Project, 2000; Iowa Outcomes Project, 2000; Lane, 1987; NANDA, 1999; Peterson, 1990; Thompson, McFarland, Hirsch, & Tucker, 1998). The signs and symptoms, outcome indicators, and nursing intervention activities have been divided into categories of intrapersonal "connectedness" (as a "connectedness" with self), interpersonal connectedness (in the context of others and the natural environment), and transpersonal connectedness (referring to a sense of relatedness to the unseen, God, or a power greater than the self and ordinary resources), which were developed by Reed (1992) in her work with spirituality and transcendence. The table integrates and expands NANDA defining characteristics, NOC indicators, and NIC interventions for the clinical care of elders diagnosed with Spiritual Distress.

Research on spirituality in elders suggests that, while formal participation in religious activities may decrease, spiritual involvement and personal spiritual development often increase (Blazer & Palmore, 1976; Hungelmann, Kenkel-Rossi, Klassen, & Stollenwerk, 1985). The elderly person might find it more difficult to participate in formal religious groups as a result of varying factors, including lack of transportation, physical impairments or disabilities, or illness. However, spirituality as a resource is evidenced by the use of prayer to facilitate coping and decrease anxiety (Ai, Dunkle, Peterson, & Bolling, 1998; Carson, 1989) and by transcending, or looking beyond, who and what one is (Lane, 1987). Research by Koenig and colleagues (Koenig, George, & Siegler, 1988; Koenig, Kvale, & Ferrel, 1988) identified that community-dwelling elders who are actively involved in religious activities are more likely to have higher morale and that religion (especially prayer) is often used as a coping behavior to assist with the stresses and uncertainties of life.

Cognitively intact elders use abstract reasoning to solve problems based on personal experiences and lifelong ways of knowing. As a result, spirituality is enhanced as a result of "freedom from constricted thinking, enhanced skill in making meaning, philosophical stance, and holistic view of life" (Reed, 1991c, pp. 15-16). As personal spirituality may be integrated into the perspective of and approach to life in elders, it is essential for the nurse to regard each older person as a spiritual being and to design care to enhance this essential area of personhood.

Table 62-3	Suggested Nursing-Sensitive Outcome and Nursing Intervention SPIRITUAL DISTRESS		
Nursing Diagnosis	**Nursing-Sensitive Outcome**	**Nursing Intervention**
SPIRITUAL DISTRESS *Defining Characteristics* Questions meaning of suffering	**SPIRITUAL WELL-BEING** *Indicators* Expression of meaning and purpose in life	**SPIRITUAL SUPPORT** *Activities* Use therapeutic communications to establish trust and empathic caring Be available to listen to patient's feelings Be open to patient's feelings about illness and death Express empathy with patient's feelings Assure patient that nurse will be available to support patient in time of suffering
Questions meaning of own existence	Makes positive statements about purpose in and satisfaction with life Connectedness with others to share thoughts, feelings, and belief	Use values clarification techniques to help patient clarify beliefs and values Encourage patient to review past life and focus on events and relationships that provided spiritual strength and support
Expresses feelings of loneliness, powerlessness, and/or worthlessness	Verbalizes self-worth and satisfaction with life events Connectedness with inner self	Treat patient with dignity and respect Be open to patient's expressions of loneliness and powerlessness Encourage life review through reminiscence Encourage participation in interactions with family members, friends, and others
Limits usual religious rituals or practices as a result of living environment, disease process, or treatment regimen	Participates in usual religious rituals or practices, adapting as necessary to restrictions imposed by living environment, disease process, or treatment regimen	Encourage the use of and participation in usual religious rituals or practices that are not detrimental to health Encourage chapel service attendance, if desired Encourage the use of spiritual resources, if desired Provide desired spiritual articles according to patient's preferences Provide privacy and quiet times for spiritual activities Consult with other members of the health care team about alternate methods of therapy
Questions moral/ethical implications of therapeutic regimen	Discusses moral/ethical conflicts openly and states that conflict has been reduced or eliminated	Assist with values clarification as appropriate Support patient's decisions about therapeutic regimen
Alteration in behavior/mood evidenced by anger, crying, withdrawal, preoccupation, anxiety, hostility, apathy, etc. Gallows humor	Verbalizes inner sense of peace and connectedness with self, others, and a higher power Verbalizes reduced anxiety, peace, comfort, inner strength, hopefulness, calmness, and a positive outlook on life Expression of serenity	Encourage participation in support groups Teach methods of relaxation, meditation, and guided imagery

Continued

Table 62-3	Suggested Nursing-Sensitive Outcome and Nursing Intervention—cont'd SPIRITUAL DISTRESS—cont'd		
Nursing Diagnosis	**Nursing-Sensitive Outcome**	**Nursing Intervention**	
Expresses concern with meaning of life/death and/or belief systems	Expression of meaning and purpose in life Expression of serenity	Share own beliefs about meaning and purpose Share, as appropriate, own spiritual perspective	
Verbalizes inner conflict about beliefs	Connectedness with others to share thoughts, feelings, and belief Freely expresses beliefs and values Expression of spiritual world view Expresses conflict resolution	Provide opportunities for discussion of various belief systems and world views	
Expresses anger toward God	Expression of forgiveness Expression of love Verbalizes acceptance of God, self, and/or others	Assist patient to properly express and relieve anger in appropriate ways	
Verbalizes concern about relationship with higher power and/or of having failed God Verbalizes concern about relationship with deity	Expression of faith Verbalizes acceptance of forgiveness by a higher power	Be open to patient's expressions of concern Arrange visits by patient's spiritual advisor Refer to spiritual advisor of patient's choice	
Seeks spiritual assistance	Participation in spiritual rites and passages Prayer Worship Meditation Expression through song Spiritual reading	Facilitate patient's use of meditations, prayer, and religious traditions and rituals Pray with the patient Listen carefully to patient's communication, and develop a sense of timing for prayer or spiritual rituals Provide videotapes from religious services Provide music, literature, or radio or TV programs significant to the patient in providing spiritual support Encourage the use of spiritual resources, if desired Refer to spiritual advisor of patient's choice	

A variety of individualized goals may be established to meet the outcome. Three possible goals are listed below and linked to the indicators listed in Table 62-2.

Identifying spiritual beliefs and values that meet needs for meaning and purpose, love and relatedness, and forgiveness
   Expresses faith/belief
   Expresses hope
   Expresses spiritual world view
   Expresses peace/serenity
   Expresses love
   Expresses forgiveness
Developing and using spiritual practices that nurture communication with self, others, a higher power, all life, nature, and the universe

   Reports mystical experiences
   Prays
   Worships
   Participates in religious/spiritual rites and passages
   Requests interaction with spiritual leaders
   Meditates
   Sings
   Reads spiritual materials
Expressing satisfaction with life
   Expresses meaning and purpose in life

Although not used often in the clinical setting, there are quantitative measures of spirituality. The instruments outlined in Table 62-1 are useful in providing indicators, but should be used with caution with elders. Measures such as these can prove upsetting and are only approximate indications of the elderly person's spiritual state. However, they can provide valuable information. Before using any quantitative measure, the nurse should have knowledge of tests and measures, be sensitive to the administration of the instrument, and be knowledgeable of the limitations of pencil and paper measurements.

Qualitative indicators of spirituality are probably used most often to assess both concerns with spirituality and individualized activities that support spirituality as an outcome. Qualitative indicators include verbal expressions, nonverbal cues, mood, environment, and relationships with others. A patient's verbalizations of having or experiencing satisfaction in prayer and having a deeper relationship with God are some indicators of increased spirituality. Other indicators include decreased anger and bitterness and increased socialization with family, friends, and other patients or residents.

NURSING INTERVENTIONS

The nursing intervention concept used to treat Spiritual Distress is Spiritual Support. Spiritual Support is defined as "assisting the patient to feel balance and connection with a greater power (Iowa Intervention Project, 2000, p. 607). The activities are individualized to each patient's needs, remembering that "what may be therapeutic to one person may not necessarily be therapeutic to another" (Oldnall, 1966, p. 139). The spiritual dimension is a vital component of a patient's overall well-being that integrates the physical, mental, social, and psychologic dimensions. Because it is integral to the whole person, the totality of human needs cannot be met without also providing spiritual support.

Nurses are often reluctant to include spiritual assessments or interventions in care. Although the exact reasons are unknown, it is postulated that this avoidance of the spiritual dimension is the result of factors such as its subjective nature, discomfort with discussion of a topic considered private, limited time and knowledge, interference by own beliefs, and disregard for the importance of spiritual care. One survey of 817 practicing nurses found that nurses most frequently assess for fears, sources of strength, and feelings of hope (Boutell & Bozett, 1990). Less frequently assessed areas were integration, giving love to God, and transcendence. Yet Peterson (1990) found that, of 100 hospitalized older adults, 71% indicated they would appreciate a nurse asking about religious beliefs and 75% said they would appreciate a nurse helping them integrate their religious beliefs with their attitudes toward their illness.

The nurse who is treating a patient for spiritual distress must choose activities that will not offend the patient's cultural or belief system (Leetun, 1996). This might seem an impossible task given the great variety of cultural, religious, and spiritual expressions in the United States. But intervention activities can be implemented that are devoid of any religious context and that are culture sensitive. For example, the use of prayer and healing of memories can simply use meditation, imagery, and reminiscence. However, some authorities believe that cognitive and behavioral interventions are more effective when they do include the individual's faith system (Benson, 1985; Propst, 1980). When practicing meditation or relaxation the person might focus on a word or phrase, such as "shalom" or "the Lord is my shepherd" from his or her own faith system to make the technique more personally relevant and meaningful (Benson, 1985).

Many different activities provide spiritual support, including therapeutic use of self, prayer, healing of memories, and reminiscence therapy. Regardless of how spiritual support is provided, nursing interventions should include mutually determining the best method or resource to meet spiritual needs, providing a safe and private environment for expression to enhance spirituality, coordinating the patient's schedule to provide opportunity and privacy for spiritual practices, and assisting the patient with requested spiritual activities as needed (Wesorick, 1995). When carrying out interventions to promote Spiritual Well-Being, the nurse must be aware of cultural influences on both the nurse's values and beliefs and those of the patient (Engebretson, 1996).

Therapeutic Use of Self

Perhaps the most effective intervention for providing spiritual support and enhancing spirituality is the nurse's own presence and development of a therapeutic relationship. This relationship allows the nurse to learn about the patient as a unique individual, to communicate personal spiritual strength, and to indicate an availability to listen (Carson, 1989). Being present to touch another's spirit requires five essential elements: listening, empathy, vulnerability, humility, and commitment (Fish & Shelley, 1983). The therapeutic use of self allows the nurse to facilitate the patient's personal exploration of the following aspects of spirituality:

- Source of strength, hope, and peace (e.g., significant other, higher power/God, nature, "centeredness," universe)
- Usual patterns of dealing with crisis, emotional expression, and skills of choice making
- Concept of spirituality
- Special practices or rituals that enhance spirituality (e.g., positive affirmations, prayer, music, reading, nature, meditation, imagery, books, symbols, articles, food)
- Purpose and meaning of present events or illness and connection with greatest accomplishments, purposes, and meaning of life
- Relationships among spiritual beliefs, present event or illness, healing force, and recovery rate
- Relationships with significant others (Wesorick, 1995, p. 119)

In all interactions the nurse treats the patient with dignity and respect and is open to expressions of anger, loss, grief, loneliness, powerlessness, and worthlessness. Being present, listening, being empathic, providing support during decision making, sharing feelings and experiences, and allowing time for change are all critical nursing activities in providing spiritual support. The nurse also can help resolve value conflicts and altered behavioral responses through value clarification techniques, inclusion in family or support group discussions, and counseling.

Prayer

If prayer is meaningful to an individual, it can be an important intervention in providing spiritual support. Prayer, one of the oldest forms of healing therapy, is "an intimate conversation between an individual and God or a higher being" (Gustafson, 1992, p. 281). Prayer is common to all faiths and societies and may be conversational, spontaneous, silent, spoken, or written. Prayer can be implemented with the patient alone, with a group of patients of similar faith, or (in the case of the patient receiving home care) with all family members.

Prior to praying with or for a patient, the nurse must assess both the patient's need for prayer and the nurse's own beliefs and comfort in using this intervention. A question like "Has (being sick, having to move, etc.) made any difference in your practice of praying?" (Stoll, 1979) elicits data to support prayer as an intervention activity. Carson (1989, p. 169) provides the following guidelines about prayer:

1. Prayer or any spiritual intervention is *never* used out of intuition, but follows a careful assessment that reveals the presence of a spiritual need.
2. Prayer is *never* to be used as an activity or substitute for the nurse's time and presence with the patient.
3. Prayer is *never* used to meet the nurse's needs but only to facilitate the patient's relationship with God.
4. Prayer is not used to communicate a magical view of God that conveys a false sense of hope and expectation.

Nurses may pray for or with the patient, may use a book of prayers to read a favorite scripture or prayer, or may sit quietly with the patient while listening to music that provides spiritual support (Fish & Shelley, 1983; Peterson, 1990). Whatever the choice, it is important to consider the religious background of the patient as well as the types of prayer that have been meaningful in the past. If the nurse does not feel comfortable with prayer, consultation with or referral to another member of the health care team or to the patient's spiritual advisor should be scheduled.

Alternate methods of providing spiritual support through prayer include encouraging chapel or church service attendance, playing audio tapes and/or videotapes of religious services, and providing times and stations of radio and television programs of the patient's preference (e.g., church services, gospel music, symphony music, religious movies) (Lowis & Hughes, 1997). The patient may also read materials that are spiritually strengthening or, if a visual deficit exists, may listen to books or materials on tape.

Healing of Memories

The use and method of healing of memories through prayer is a process based on the use of imagery and the healing power of prayer for persons known to pray (Linn & Linn, 1978). The process is very similar to reminiscence therapy, discussed later. Linn and Linn (1978) viewed inner healing of memories as a twofold process: (1) seeking forgiveness of self and (2) forgiving others. This process also entails going through five stages of healing life's hurts: denial, anger, bargaining, depression, and acceptance of life's hurts. As the person works through these stages, feelings of anxiety, anger, fear, and guilt are relieved. The healing of past hurts allows those hurts to become strengths and is especially important for the elderly person. This integration helps the elderly person find meaning in the past life and a sense of harmony with the past, present, and future.

The use of healing of memories has had limited investigation. Schlientz (1981) studied the use of healing of memories on the emotion of anger, finding that subjects who used this process had less anger than a control group. Propst (1980) compared the effectiveness of religious and nonreligious imagery on treating mild depression in religious individuals. She found religious imagery to be significantly more effective in decreasing depression than nonreligious imagery. This may be especially true for the elderly person, who often has a strong personal sense of faith.

Reminiscence Therapy

Reminiscence Therapy is defined as "using the recall of past events, feelings, and thoughts to facilitate pleasure, quality of life, or adaptation to present circumstances" (Iowa Intervention Project, 2000, p. 554). Reminiscence, or reviewing one's past life, is a method of providing spiritual support for elders. Reminiscence may be verbal or silent and, depending on the type and depth of the review, provides the elderly person with different benefits. Simple or informative life review helps in the review and informs others of history. Therapeutic or integrative life review facilitates resolution of conflicts. More intense review, called obsessional or ruminative, may be elicited from the elder who is depressed, is in pain, is in despair, or has had an ungratifying past (Hamilton, 1992; Klausner et al., 1998). Reminiscence can be used in any setting to facilitate psychologic comfort and a sense of purpose in elders (Haight,

Box 62-2	Activities REMINISCENCE THERAPY	
Choose a comfortable setting	Comment on the affective quality accompanying the memories in an empathic manner	
Set aside adequate time		
Encourage verbal expression of both positive and negative feelings of past events	Use direct questions to refocus back to life events, if patient digresses	
Ask open-ended questions about past events	Encourage writing of past events	
Encourage writing of past events	Inform family members about the benefits of reminiscence	
Tape the reminiscence and play it back to the client, as appropriate	Gauge the length of the session to the patient's attention span	
Use the patient's photo albums or scrapbook to stimulate memories	Avoid using with persons who are in a state of generativity or with those who are avoiding reality	
Help the patient to begin a family tree or to write his or her oral history	Acknowledge previous coping skills	
Encourage the patient to write to old friends or relatives	Monitor for defensiveness about the past	
Use communication skills such as focusing, reflecting, and restating to develop the relationship	Repeat session weekly or more often over prolonged period	

1988; Sherman, 1987; Taft & Nehrke, 1990). Box 62-2 outlines the definition and activities for reminiscence therapy (Iowa Intervention Project, 2000).

CASE STUDY

Mrs. Porter was diagnosed with Spiritual Distress related to the crisis of illness/suffering/death. Spiritual support interventions were implemented to facilitate spiritual well-being. The primary nurse was responsible for Mrs. Porter's care and first had to gain her trust and confidence through caring presence, empathic listening, and patience. The nurse began by sitting quietly beside Mrs. Porter for 15 minutes each day. At first the 15 minutes were spent in silence, but slowly Mrs. Porter began to talk about her past life, her feelings of anger and loneliness, and her feelings of guilt for having alienated herself from her religious practices and prayer. The nurse asked Mrs. Porter to tell her about her past life and her spiritual practices. Mrs. Porter and the nurse began to talk about some of the past hurts in her life and especially her feelings about the death of her husband and her present illness. The nurse asked Mrs. Porter to tell her some prayers and religious practices that had been especially important in both the good and bad times of her life and encouraged Mrs. Porter to use them each day. The nurse also told Mrs. Porter that it was all right to be angry with God and to express those angry feelings in her prayers. A special time was set aside each day for Mrs. Porter and the nurse to have private time together for reminiscence and prayer. The prayers were often silent, but sometimes the nurse read aloud from the Bible or played music selected by Mrs. Porter. The nurse asked the priest to visit Mrs. Porter on a regular basis and made sure that Mrs. Porter was wheeled to the television room each Sunday to watch a local church service.

Mrs. Porter began to look forward to the daily sessions with the nurse and stated that she felt comforted by them. As she became more comfortable with herself, she began to participate in the activities of the home, even joining a group of women who quilted each day. She shared with these new friends that she now believed her life to have had meaning and purpose, that she was no longer afraid of death, and that she knew she would see her husband and God in heaven. Through her conversations and interactions, as well as by having a higher spiritual well-being score (Table 62-2), Mrs. Porter demonstrated that she felt connected with herself, others, and a higher power and had reached a higher level of spiritual well-being. Shortly after finishing a quilt that she especially enjoyed working on with other residents, Mrs. Porter died peacefully in her sleep.

SUMMARY

The human spirit, expressed as one's spirituality, is an inseparable dimension of the whole person. Although spiritual distress can occur at any age, elders are at particular risk for this human response. As a person ages, transcendence facilitates spirituality through an expansion toward others, greater awareness of beliefs and values, and integration of the past and future in the present. Spiritual distress can serve as either a negative experience with feelings of abandonment, isolation, or hopelessness or as a positive experience that brings one closer to a deeper sense of peace, meaning, and purpose.

As a person grows older, spiritual growth increases. If the elderly person's spiritual self is blocked by a past or present hurt, the nurse is in an ideal situation to establish a therapeutic, trusting relationship in which spiritual well-being and growth can be enhanced. Through presence, listening, and empathy with the patient's spiritual needs, the nurse assesses defining characteristics and related factors and implements individualized activities to provide spiritual support for spiritual distress. By providing spiritual support, the nurse not only provides holistic care, but also facilitates a sense of spirituality as a source of strength and continued development in elders.

REFERENCES

Ai, A. L., Dunkle, R. E., Peterson, C., & Bolling, S. E. (1998). The role of private prayer in psychological recovery among midlife and aged patients following cardiac surgery. *The Gerontologist, 38*(5), 591-601.

Benson, H. (1985). *Beyond the relaxation response.* Berkley, CA: Berkley Books.

Blazer, D., & Palmore, E. (1976). Religion and aging in a longitudinal panel. *The Gerontologist, 1*(1), 82-85.

Boutell, K. A., & Bozett, F. W. (1990). Nurses' assessment of patients' spirituality: Continuing education implications. *The Journal of Continuing Education in Nursing, 21*(4), 172-176.

Brooke, V. (1987). The spiritual well-being of the elderly. *Geriatric Nursing, 8*(4), 194-195.

Carpenito, L. J. (1995). *Nursing diagnosis: Application to clinical practice* (6th ed.). Baltimore: Lippincott Williams & Wilkins.

Carroll-Johnson, R. (Ed.). (1989). *Classification of nursing diagnoses: Proceedings of the eighth conference.* Baltimore: Lippincott Williams & Wilkins.

Carson, V. B. (1989). *Spiritual dimensions of nursing practice.* Philadelphia: W. B. Saunders.

Conco, D. (1995). Christian patients' views of spiritual care. *Western Journal of Nursing Research, 17*(3), 266-276.

Dossey, B., Guzzetta, C., & Kenner, C. (1992). *Critical care nursing: Body-mind-spirit.* Philadelphia: Lippincott.

Dugan, D. O. (1987, 1988). Essays on the art of caring in nursing: The human spirit in stress management. *Nursing Forum, 23*(3), 108-117.

Engebretson, J. (1996). Considerations in diagnosing in the spiritual domain. *Nursing Diagnosis, 7*(3), 100-107.

Erikson, E. (1963). *Childhood and society.* New York: W. W. Norton.

Fish, S., & Shelley, J. (1983). *Spiritual care: The nurse's role.* Downers Grove, IL: Intervarsity Press.

Flesner, R. (1981). *Development of a measure to assess spiritual distress in the responsive adult.* Unpublished manuscript. Marquette University at Milwaukee, WI.

Gebbie, K., & Lavin, M. (1975). *Proceedings of the first national conference: Classification of nursing diagnoses.* St. Louis, MO: Mosby.

Gustafson, M. (1992). Prayer. In M. Snyder (Ed.), *Independent nursing interventions* (2nd ed., pp. 280-286). Albany, NY: Delmar.

Haase, J., Britt, T., Coward, D., Leidy, N., & Penn, P. (1992). Simultaneous concept analysis of spiritual perspective, hope, acceptance and self-transcendence. *IMAGE: Journal of Nursing Scholarship, 24*(2), 141-147.

Haight, B. (1988). The therapeutic role of a structured life review process in homebound elderly subjects. *Journal of Gerontology, 43*(2), 40-44.

Hamilton, D. B. (1992). Reminiscence therapy. In G. M. Bulechek & J. C. McCloskey (Eds.), *Nursing interventions: Essential nursing treatments* (2nd ed., pp. 292-303). Philadelphia: W. B. Saunders.

Hawks, S., Hull, M., Thalman, R., & Richins, P. (1995). Review of spiritual health: Definition, role, and intervention strategies in health promotion. *American Journal of Health Promotion, 9*(5), 371-378.

Hensley, L. D. (1994). Spiritual distress: A validation study. In R. M. Carroll-Johnson & M. Paquette (Eds.), *Classification of nursing diagnoses: Proceedings of the tenth conference* (pp. 200-202). Baltimore: Lippincott Williams & Wilkins.

Highfield, M., & Cason, C. (1983). Spiritual needs of patients: Are they recognized? *Cancer Nursing, 6,* 187-191.

Hungelmann, J., Kenkel-Rossi, E., Klassen, L., & Stollenwerk, R. (1985). Spiritual well-being in older adults: Harmonious interconnectedness. *Journal of Religious Health, 24*(2), 147-154.

Iowa Intervention Project. J. C. McCloskey & G. M. Bulechek (Eds.). (2000). *Nursing interventions classification (NIC)* (3rd ed.). St. Louis, MO: Mosby.

Iowa Outcomes Project. M. Johnson, M. Maas, & S. Moorhead (Eds.). (2000). *Nursing outcomes classification (NOC)* (2nd ed.). St. Louis, MO: Mosby.

Kierkegaard, S. (1962). *Works of love.* New York: Harper & Row.

Kim, M. J., & Moritz, D. A. (Eds.). (1982). *Classification of nursing diagnosis: Proceedings of the third and fourth national conferences.* St. Louis, MO: Mosby.

Klausner, E. J., Clarkin, J. F., Spielman, L., Pupo, C., Abrams, R., & Alexopoulos, G. S. (1998). Late-life depression and functional ability: The role of goal-focused group psychotherapy. *International Journal of Geriatric Psychiatry, 13*(10), 707-716.

Koenig, H., George, L., & Siegler, I. (1988). The use of religion and other emotion-regulating coping strategies among older adults. *The Gerontologist, 28*(3), 303-310.

Koenig, H., Kvale, J., & Ferrel, C. (1988). Religion and well-being in later life. *The Gerontologist, 28*(1), 18-28.

Lane, J. A. (1987). The care of the human spirit. *Journal of Professional Nursing, 3,* 332-337.

Leetun, M. (1996). Wellness spirituality in the older adult: Assessment and intervention protocol. *Nurse Practitioner, 21*(8), 60, 65-70.

Linn, D., & Linn, M. (1978). *Healing life hurts: Healing memories through five stages of forgiveness.* New York: Paulist Press.

Lowis, J. J., & Hughes, J. (1997). A comparison of the effects of sacred and secular music on elderly people. *Journal of Psychology, 131*(1), 45-55.

Mansen, T. (1993). The spiritual dimension of individuals: Conceptual development. *Nursing Diagnosis, 4*(4), 140-147.

McHolm, F. A. (1991). A nursing diagnosis validation study: Defining characteristics of spiritual distress. In R. M. Carroll-Johnson (Ed.), *Classification of nursing diagnoses: Proceedings of the ninth conference* (pp. 112-119). Baltimore: Lippincott Williams & Wilkins.

Miller, J. F. (1985). Assessment of loneliness and spiritual well-being in chronically ill and healthy adults. *Journal of Professional Nursing, 1,* 79-85.

Moberg, D. O. (1984). Subjective measures of spiritual well-being. *Review of Religious Research, 25*(4), 351-364.

North American Nursing Diagnosis Association. (1999). *Nursing diagnoses: Definitions & classification 1999-2000.* Philadelphia: Author.

O'Brien, M. E. (1982). The need for spiritual integrity. In H. Yura & M. B. Walsh (Eds.), *Humans' needs and the nursing process* (pp. 85-116). Norwalk, CT: Appleton & Lange.

Oldnall, A. (1996). A critical analysis of nursing: Meeting the spiritual needs of patients. *Journal of Advanced Nursing, 23,* 138-144.

Paloutzian, R., & Ellison, C. (1982). Loneliness, spiritual well-being and quality of life. In L. Peplau & D. Perlmann (Eds.), *Loneliness: A sourcebook of current theory, research, and therapy* (pp. 227-237). New York: John Wiley & Sons.

Peterson, E. (1990). The physical . . . the spiritual . . . can you meet all of your patient's needs? *Journal of Gerontological Nursing, 11*(10), 23-27.

Propst, L. R. (1980). The comparative efficacy of religious and non-religious imagery for the treatment of mild depression in religious individuals. *Cognitive Therapy Research, 4,* 167-178.

Reed, P. G. (1991a). Toward a nursing theory of self-transcendence: Deductive reformulation using developmental theories. *Advances in Nursing Science, 13*(4), 64-77.

Reed, P. G. (1991b). Self-transcendence and mental health in oldest-old adults. *Nursing Research, 40*(1), 5-11.

Reed, P. G. (1991c). Spirituality and mental health in older adults: Extant knowledge for nursing. *Family Community Health, 14*(2), 14-25.

Reed, P. G. (1992). An emerging paradigm for the investigation of spirituality in nursing. *Research in Nursing & Health, 15,* 349-357.

Reed, P. G. (1996). Transcendence: Formulating nursing perspectives. *Nursing Science Quarterly, 9*(1), 2-4.

Roberts, K. T., & Aspy, C. B. (1993). Development of the serenity scale. *Journal of Nursing Measurement, 1*(2), 145-164.

Schlientz, M. A. (1981). *A study of the decrease of unresolved anger through a teaching protocol and healing prayer as a nursing intervention in spiritual care.* Unpublished doctoral dissertation. University of Pittsburgh.

Sherman, E. (1987). A phenomenological approach to reminiscence and life review. *Clinical Gerontologist, 3*(4), 3-16.

Smucker, C. (1995). A phenomenological description of the experience of spiritual distress. In M. Rantz & P. LeMone. (Eds.), *Classification of nursing diagnoses: Proceedings of the eleventh conference* (pp. 136-149). Glendale, CA: Cinahl Information Systems.

Stallwood, J., & Stoll, R. (1975). Spiritual dimension of nursing practice. In L. Beland & J. Passos (Eds.), *Clinical nursing* (3rd ed., pp. 1086-1098). New York: Macmillan.

Stoll, R. I. (1979). Guidelines for spiritual assessment. *American Journal of Nursing, 79,* 1574-1577.

Stoll, R. I. (1989). The essence of spirituality. In V. B. Carson (Ed.), *Spiritual dimensions of nursing practice* (pp. 4-23). Philadelphia: W. B. Saunders.

Taft, L., & Nehrke, M. (1990). Reminiscence: Life review ego integrity in nursing home residents. *International Journal of Aging and Human Development, 30*(3), 189-196.

Thompson, J., McFarland, G., Hirsch, J., & Tucker, S. (1998). *Mosby's clinical nursing* (4th ed.). St. Louis, MO: Mosby.

Tubesing, D., & Tubesing, N. (1983). *The caring question.* Augsburg.

Walton, J. (1996). Spiritual relationships: A concept analysis. *Journal of Holistic Nursing, 14*(3), 237-250.

Weatherall, J., & Creason, N. S. (1987). Validation of the nursing diagnosis, spiritual distress. In A. M. McLane (Ed.), *Classification of nursing diagnoses: Proceedings of the seventh conference* (pp. 182-185). St. Louis, MO: Mosby.

Wesorick, B. (1995). Consensual validation of interventions categorized by nursing diagnosis. In M. R. Rantz & P. LeMone (Eds.), *Classification of nursing diagnoses: Proceedings of the eleventh conference* (pp. 115-124). Glendale, CA: Cinahl Information Systems.

FUTURE DIRECTIONS FOR RESEARCH, EDUCATION, AND PRACTICE

Much work remains to be done in the conceptual development and testing of nursing diagnoses, interventions, and outcomes that are responsive to nursing interventions. Some of the issues that arose during the writing of this book include the lack of the following: (1) complete explications of the standardized languages; (2) clinical validation of the languages; (3) funding and administrative support for clinical validation of the concepts and their linkages; and (4) knowledge regarding the use of the standardized nomenclatures among administrators, educators, and clinicians for education, practice, research, and the development of health policy.

The problem of incomplete development and standardization of nomenclatures is noted by several nurse scholars and clinicians (Aydelotte & Peterson, 1987; Bulechek & McCloskey, 1990; Gordon, 1994; Maas, 1986; Warren, 1985). We regard this as a natural part of taxonomic development in a discipline. Some NANDA diagnoses, NOC outcomes, and NIC interventions (e.g., those in the psychosocial and health promotion or wellness domains) are less well developed than others and need input from scholars and practitioners, as well as more qualitative and quantitative research to develop and validate relevant concepts. Some diagnostic, intervention, and outcome concepts are vague or ambiguous and lack sufficient specificity for optimum clinical usefulness. Diagnoses, interventions, and outcomes in each of the classifications are at various levels of abstraction. However, we encourage nurses to resist the temptation for premature closure and undue criticisms of the taxonomies. This book is intended to be heuristic in that it will help clarify some concepts for taxonomic development and revision. The aim is to stimulate clinical testing and research to identify, define, and validate additional diagnostic, intervention, and outcome concepts; to compare diagnoses, interventions, and outcomes across a variety of client populations and settings; and to encourage research to examine and validate linkages among the diagnoses, interventions, and outcomes in different populations of elders. Clearly, nursing needs to continue the development and testing of taxonomies, both inductively from practice and deductively from theories, using qualitative and quantitative research strategies.

The rapid development of computerized clinical information systems to support nursing assessment, diagnosis,

outcome, and intervention evaluation makes it imperative that standardized nursing nomenclatures be used in these systems. Although much remains to be done to clinically validate the taxonomies, efforts to develop and maintain standardized nursing languages will continue to make strides for the profession. The leadership of the American Nurses Association (ANA) Committee on Uniform Nursing Databases is encouraging. Use of the standardized languages to enable the collection, storage, and retrieval of Nursing Minimum Data (Werley & Lang, 1988) will improve the documentation and research efforts of nurses in a variety of practice and educational settings, as well as the overall quality of care of clients, including elders. While the standardized nursing languages are evolving, they may appear to be incompatible. However, the editors believe that in time, and with refinement, the taxonomies will coalesce to more validly and completely capture nursing phenomena.

There is need for resources to support the development and validation of standardized nursing languages and taxonomies and to enable clinical research on the relationships among diagnoses, outcomes, and interventions. Support of studies of the outcomes effectiveness and efficacy of nursing interventions to treat specific nursing diagnoses also is needed. This is an especially important need for elderly persons because of their increasing numbers, the preponderance of problems that nurses treat for elders, and the proportion of health care dollars that is spent to care for elderly clients. Nursing organizations are shortsighted if they ignore these fundamentally important agendas in their funding priorities.

Opportunities to report and disseminate the results of nursing classification research in peer reviewed journals should be expanded, but the quantity and quality of research in the area also must increase. Nurses need to gain skill in classification research and related research strategies to continue the development and validation of standardized languages and investigation of the relationships among diagnoses, outcomes, and interventions. Many nurses continue to have minimal exposure to standardized nursing languages and nursing classification research. Many also have attitudinal barriers and regard standardized language and taxonomies as irrelevant to clinical practice. Thus there is a need for nurses to gain knowledge about the classifications to overcome these barriers. Edu-

NURSING PRACTICE DATA: THREE LEVELS

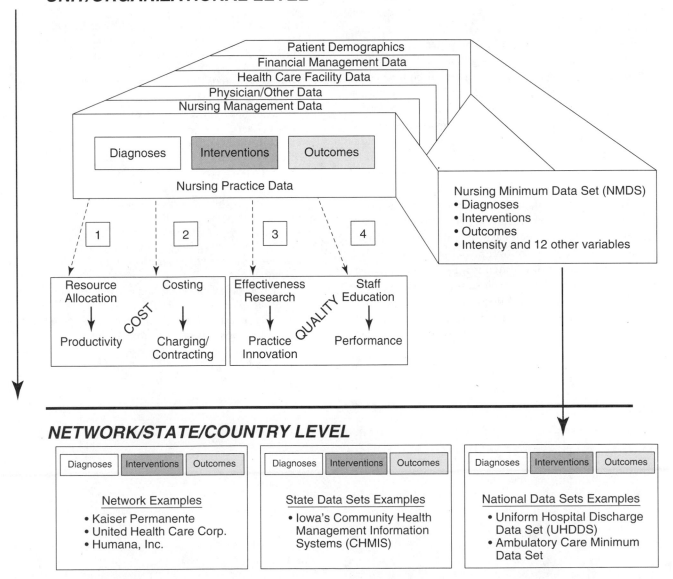

FIGURE **1** Nursing practice data: Three levels. (Copyright © 1997 Iowa Intervention Project.)

cational programming (generic, graduate, and continuing education) is required so that nurses are prepared to use standardized languages in their practice and conduct or participate in research to validate the concepts and test the linkages among nursing diagnoses, outcomes, and interventions. To this end, nursing textbooks in general and nursing research texts in particular should include more information about classification research and a variety of methods for conducting research on these phenomena. For example, most research texts currently used in graduate nursing programs do not emphasize content on how to conduct rigorous qualitative and quantitative validation studies or on the many difficult methodological dilemma encountered in doing nursing language classification or effectiveness research.

Nursing diagnoses, outcomes, and interventions for elders are particular challenges because of the complex interplay among physical, mental, social, spiritual, and environmental factors in the population. At present, many nursing settings and practitioners do not use standardized nursing languages. Yet nursing documentation using standardized languages, especially if computerized, enhances communication among clinical nurses, administrators, clients, and members of other health care disciplines. Standardized nursing data also enable nursing administrators to identify more clearly the clinical foci for programming, such as staff education and outcomes effectiveness evaluation. Figure 1 illustrates the multiple uses of local and larger standardized nursing data sets. These data sets need to be developed in all settings where nursing is practiced.

In the final analysis, whatever nursing hopes to accomplish is predicated on its ability to demonstrate and document its outcomes, interventions, and associated costs. This requires a greater emphasis on data-based decisions in clinical practice. We are optimistic that the future will bring a proliferation of research to validate nursing diagnoses, outcomes, and interventions that are responsive to nursing and to analyze the effectiveness of nursing interventions. This will require that more nurses become involved in the work to validate, use, and refine the NANDA,

NOC, and NIC classifications (Iowa Intervention Project, 2000; Iowa Outcomes Project, 2000; NANDA, 1999). To encourage this involvement, we include a NANDA enrollment form (Appendix B) and information about how to contact the Iowa Nursing Classification Center (Appendix E). Procedures for submission of new or revised diagnoses, outcomes, and interventions to NANDA, NOC, and NIC (Appendix C and Appendix D) also are included. We hope this book will stimulate readers who work with elders to be part of these important efforts by participating actively in increasing the knowledge, research, and literature base for nursing practice with elders.

REFERENCES

Aydelotte, M., & Peterson, K. H. (1987). Keynote address: Nursing taxonomies state of the art. In A. McLane (Ed.), *Proceedings of the seventh conference* (pp. 1-16). St. Louis, MO: Mosby.

Bulechek, G. M., & McCloskey, J. C. (1990). Nursing intervention taxonomy development. In J. C. McCloskey & H. K. Grace (Eds.), *Current issues in nursing* (3rd ed., pp. 23-28). St. Louis, MO: Mosby.

Gordon, M. (1994). *Nursing diagnosis: Process and application* (3rd ed.). St. Louis, MO: Mosby.

Iowa Intervention Project. J. C. McCloskey & G. M. Bulechek (Eds.). (2000). *Nursing interventions classification (NIC)* (3rd ed.). St. Louis, MO: Mosby.

Iowa Outcomes Project. M. Johnson, M. Maas, & S. Moorhead (Eds.). (2000). *Nursing outcomes classification (NOC)* (2nd ed.). St. Louis, MO: Mosby.

Maas, M. (1986). Nursing diagnoses in a professional model of nursing: Keystone for effective nursing administration. *Journal of Nursing Administration, 16*(12), 39-42.

North American Nursing Diagnosis Association. (1999). *Nursing diagnoses: Definitions & classification 1999-2000.* Philadelphia: Author.

Warren, J. (1985). Accountability and nursing diagnosis. *Journal of Nursing Administration, 13*(10), 34-37.

Werley, H. H., & Lang, N. M. (Eds.). (1988). *Identification of the nursing minimum data set.* New York: Springer.

THE PROGRESSION OF KNOWLEDGE AND THE NURSING PROFESSION

Ada Jacox

The evolution of nursing diagnosis has chronicled the problems and progress of nursing since 1950 (Jacox, 1991). This publication shows just how quickly nursing has moved to link nursing diagnoses, first to interventions and now to nursing-sensitive patient outcomes. Most classifications of nursing phenomena focused on diagnosis of problems and interventions. There was acknowledgment of a need for identification of patient outcomes that are sensitive to nursing care, but little work had been published. It is remarkable that in this short time the editors and authors of this book were able to undertake the major task of linking nursing diagnoses, nursing interventions, and nursing-sensitive patient outcomes in elders. The work shows the great value of an extended program of research grounded in practice.

Some of the book's contributing authors have an association with the Iowa Veterans' Home, an institution that has a history of 30 years of progress in developing an enlightened and autonomous organizational model for professional practice (Maas & Jacox, 1977). Nurses working at that facility acknowledged in the late 1960s that if nursing was, indeed, the major service delivered to their clients, then nurses had an obligation to develop a better knowledge base. A few dozen nurses at this long-term care setting established, among other things, a set of bylaws for the nursing department that specified authority for nursing care, a peer review system, and a committee to do research in gerontologic nursing at a time when these ideas were just beginning to take root in nursing. Their clearly stated policy was that nursing was the most essential service provided to institutionalized elders, and they have continued over time to improve that service.

Some of those who began this work at the Iowa Veterans' Home later moved to the University of Iowa and joined others in the development of the Iowa nursing classification systems. During the 1990s they established a center for nursing classification, recruited others to expand their productive team of experienced researchers and clinicians, and developed research programs within research programs with some extending nationally and even internationally. The intellectual work on classification being done at Iowa is having, and will continue to have, a major positive impact on the nursing profession.

The editors and authors take a clear-headed, critical look at what we know and do not know. They correctly assume that it is the business of every profession to organize its knowledge in the clearest and most useful ways to enable clinicians to use it in practice and test it through research. The authors show the value of nursing classification systems without proselytizing about them. They take a balanced and reasoned tone of criticism of existing work and use professional judgment and new research findings to suggest what nursing knowledge should be.

As the editors noted, the percentage of older people in the United States has increased, and the older population is getting older. Selection of this population for illustration of the nursing classifications provided a rich resource for clarifying the nature of nursing knowledge and for extending its theoretical and research boundaries. Elders and chronically ill account for a significant percentage of health care expenditures and will increasingly consume even a higher percentage. The editors make a cogent argument for focusing serious efforts on learning how best to prevent problems and how to treat developing problems quickly to promote maximum independence of elders for as long as possible. Making the problem of knowing how to care for elders even more difficult is the fact that the percentage of older people who are members of minority populations is increasing. The scarcity of research findings dealing with problems of prevention and treatment is even more serious for elderly minorities.

The book has two major foci: (1) care of elders; and (2) nursing classification systems. Developing either theme well would represent a serious undertaking; tackling them simultaneously was a gargantuan task successfully accomplished. The two themes strengthen each other. The use of classification systems enables a broader conceptualization of the problems of elders, interventions to address them, and nursing-sensitive patient outcomes relevant to this population. In turn, using care of elders as a means to demonstrate linkages among diagnoses, interventions, and outcomes results in a richer discussion than would have been possible had nursing practice been addressed more generally and abstractly. The book illustrates well how theory (classification of nursing phenomena) informs practice (care of elders) and vice versa. The emphasis on using research to describe problems, interventions, and outcomes in the care of elders completes the circle and provides a clear example of the interrelationships among theory, research, and practice. Much of the theory, research, and practice has implications for other disciplines, as well as for nursing.

Although nurses have always operated in interdisciplinary settings, care is becoming increasingly interdisciplinary and interdependent. Some classifications of nursing interventions distinguish between *independent* and *dependent interventions*. These are terms that are relative and dynamic, in large part politically defined through licensing laws, reimbursement policies, and common practice. Some nurses have tried to avoid overlap with other disciplines by defining mutually exclusive diagnoses and interventions. Such an undertaking is impossible in a health care system that requires overlap across health care professionals. Many of the problems that nurses diagnose and manage are the same as those dealt with by other health care professionals. Nurses, however, often focus on a different subset of problems and choose interventions and combinations of interventions or aspects of interventions that differ from those used by other professionals. Patient outcomes that are sensitive to nursing care also are influenced by care given by others, though many outcomes are more specifically identified with nursing care. It is the complex of problems, interventions, and outcomes in their totality that differentiates nursing from other disciplines. The differences and similarities are reflected in the three classifications of nursing language—diagnoses, interventions, and outcomes—treated in this book.

Consider the overlap among health care professionals in a few of the phenomena discussed by the authors. Nurses and psychologists deal with many of the same phenomena, such as anxiety, confusion, coping, and depression. There is overlap with physicians in the focus on pain, fluid volume deficits, and pressure ulcers; with physical therapists in the concern for physical mobility; with respiratory therapists in the concern for effective breathing patterns; with nutritionists in their interest in nutritional deficiencies; and with pharmacists in the care of drug toxicity. What distinguishes nursing from other disciplines is the comprehensive focus on all of these problems and how each affects and is affected by the others. Furthermore, nurses often are concerned with aspects of care that are of more peripheral interest to other disciplines. With regard to drugs, for example, the diagnosis of Risk for Poisoning: Drug Toxicity reflects a common problem in elders and other patients who use medications. Patient knowledge of medication and control of drug risks reflect nursing-sensitive outcomes in elders, particularly those who are noninstitutionalized. Thus nurses must understand not only the drugs and their pharmacodynamics and pharmacokinetics in elderly persons, but also how to teach patients and families about effective and safe drug use to prevent and manage drug-related problems. The point is not that other professionals are totally unaware of these problems and the need to prevent them. It is that dealing with these kinds of problems represents a major focus for nurses who work closely with patients in both institutional and noninstitutional settings. Moreover, it illustrates how nursing is differentiated from other disciplines in its knowledge and practice. The approach used in this book should serve as a blueprint for the development of evidence-based nursing practice.

Estimates of the extent to which practice is based on research range from 1% (IOM) to approximately 20% (Medical Alert, 1989). There is a preponderance of research showing variability in practice across geographic regions, treatment settings, clinical populations, and practitioners, often with little understanding of what works best to produce desirable patient outcomes. The remainder of this epilogue addresses evidence-based practice and the need for the nursing profession to take stronger action to promote nursing's agenda in the health care system. The discussion draws heavily on the nursing classification systems and the care of elders, which are the themes of this book.

EVIDENCE-BASED PRACTICE

Nursing has long promoted the need for using research to guide practice. A federally funded project in the late 1970s, "The Conduct and Utilization of Research in Nursing" (Horsley & Crane, 1983), joined nursing faculty and nursing staff in the search for areas with sufficient research to guide practice. They identified several areas as having an adequate research base but were disappointed in the amount of research generally available to serve as a basis for practice.

Now, 2 decades later, there is widespread acknowledgement of the need for all in health care to make a concerted effort to use scientific evidence as a basis for practice, and the term *evidence-based practice* is pervasive in the literature. Evidence-based practice is the conscientious and judicious use of the best research evidence in the management of patients (Sackett, 1997). There are many issues involved in evidence-based practice. Two of them are (1) what counts as scientific evidence, and (2) how can evidence and professional judgment best be combined in practice? The issue of what constitutes scientific evidence is one that has been widely debated in nursing and other disciplines. Postpositivists have a different view of scientific evidence than do humanists, for example, with some of the former still believing that something is not scientific unless it can be reduced to biochemical or physiologic measures, and that the only scientifically acceptable research designs are experiments. The issue has been prominent in the development of evidence-based clinical practice guidelines, with some arguing strongly that only randomized controlled trials (experimental studies) are appropriate for making recommendations for practice. Others, recognizing the dearth of research in many areas, argue for a "best evidence" synthesis, in which the best available research is used as a basis for guidelines. That is, if there are sufficient experimental studies to do a meta-analysis, and if the meta-analysis is clear in what works or does not work, that constitutes the evidence base and studies with weaker designs such as cohort analysis are not needed. In areas in which the research is limited to descriptive studies, the evidence from those studies must suffice to make a recommendation for practice until better evidence from stronger designs becomes available.

There is a fast-growing industry developing in the synthesis of scientific evidence. The U.S. Agency for Health Care Policy and Research (AHCPR), now the Agency for Healthcare Research and Quality (AHRQ), for example, largely for political reasons, has abandoned the development of practice guidelines and instead identified 12 agencies as evidence-based practice centers (EPCs) (AHCPR, 1998). The EPCs develop evidence reports and technology assessments based on rigorous and comprehensive reviews of scientific literature. The expectation is that professional associations, health plans, providers, and others will use the evidence reports to develop practice guidelines or other tools for improving the quality of care.

Another fast-growing enterprise to promote evidence-based practice is the Cochrane Collaboration. This organization, which was developed in England in the early 1990s, involves multiple researchers throughout the world Cochrane Centers (Cochrane Collaboration, 1998). Their function is to review scientific evidence, limited primarily to experimental studies, in specific practice areas. Neither the AHRQ nor the Cochrane Collaboration develops guidelines, but both make their reviews available for use in making practice decisions and recommendations.

The realization that more than 80% of practice does not rest on a strong science base makes it clear that something in addition to research must be used as a basis for practice decisions. This is professional judgment, based on clinicians' expertise gained through experience. There is a whole set of interrelated issues regarding how professional judgment can be combined with scientific evidence to make practice decisions. One issue is which professionals are consulted for their expertise—that is, who are considered to have professional expertise in the field of health care? This is not a new issue to nursing, which has long tried to articulate its professional expertise and how it differs from other disciplines, particularly medicine. The problem is that if it is only physicians whose professional expertise is combined with the scientific evidence, then problems and expertise outside the physician's area of knowledge will be overlooked. This is where the value of the present book on nursing classification systems and care of elders becomes clear.

Until fairly recently, much nursing practice has been invisible to others because nursing had not described clearly and comprehensively the problems with which nurses deal, the interventions they use, and the patient outcomes that are affected by nursing care. In the last decade enormous strides have been made by the profes-

sion in understanding the need for well established and well understood classifications of nursing terms. This was begun by the North American Nursing Diagnosis Association (NANDA) movement in the early 1970s and gradually evolved into the development of a number of classifications of interventions. Most recently, the focus has extended to nursing-sensitive patient outcomes. Work done from 1989 to the present by the ANA Steering Committee on Databases to Support Clinical Nursing Practice has been instrumental in promoting acceptance of the need for classification systems (American Nurses Association Steering Committee, 1995). The committee worked with staff in the National Library of Medicine (NLM) to incorporate several nursing classification languages into the NLM databases. These include, among others, NANDA, the *Nursing Interventions Classification (NIC)*, and the *Nursing Outcomes Classification (NOC)*, all used in the present book. The need to classify nursing terms also has been recognized by the International Council of Nurses, which has combined segments from many of the nursing classification systems developed around the world, particularly in the United States, into an overarching system to describe nursing care throughout the world.

The value of the work reflected in this book cannot be overestimated. The comprehensive approach taken in viewing the body and mind from the spiritual to the psychosocial and physiologic illustrates the richness and complexity of nursing. The authors of individual chapters express considerable breadth and variation in their conceptual focus. Frantz, for example, deals with the description of the anatomic and physiologic basis for pressure ulcers, and Reese presents a sophisticated discussion of fluid volume deficit. In contrast, LeMone writes about spiritual distress and Bunten discusses spiritual challenges associated with growing older. Chapters on other phenomena, such as confusion and pain, deal more explicitly with mind-body connections. Most authors discuss both prevention of problems, as well as their management once developed. All of the authors identify specific nursing diagnoses or problems along with interventions that may be useful with the problems and patient outcomes that may be affected by the interventions. In doing this, the authors generally selected diagnoses from NANDA, interventions from the *Nursing Interventions Classification (NIC)*, and outcomes from the Iowa *Nursing Outcomes Classification (NOC)*, without being confined only to terms now in those classification systems. As the authors attempt to identify and link diagnoses, interventions, and outcomes, they discover and describe ways in which the classifications work and when they do not. Reese, for example, clarifies distinctions between *potential for* fluid volume deficit and actual fluid volume deficit in ways that make both more understandable. Frantz clarifies nursing diagnoses that had been confusing because the terms adopted had not reflected generally accepted knowledge and terminology and were not technically correct. This kind of work will help to make the concept of nursing diagnosis more accepted by both nurses and other health care professionals, will make it easier to relate what nurses do to what others do, and will make nursing practice more understandable to nurses and others alike.

In some cases authors propose revisions in NANDA diagnoses suggested by trying to make links with nursing interventions and nursing-sensitive outcomes. They identify diagnoses that could be combined, modified, or expanded and add new diagnoses. As they discuss potential interventions, they suggest ways in which these in turn change the understanding of the problems described. Both problems and interventions are modified in the search for relevant nursing-sensitive patient outcomes. The approach illustrates the wisdom of thinking about and synthesizing the work of diagnoses, interventions, and outcomes simultaneously. The book in its totality shows that nursing diagnoses, interventions, and patient outcomes are dynamic and interrelated and that understanding the phenomena and how they are related constitutes evidence-based practice.

ADVANCING THE PROFESSION OF NURSING

This book illustrates the kind of focused effort necessary to articulate clearly nursing's knowledge base and to ground nursing practice in research. Although such individual efforts are necessary, they are not sufficient to enable a whole profession to advance. It also is necessary for numerous other researchers to undertake the many other areas of nursing, for nurses collectively to critique and debate each others' ideas, and for organized nursing to support and promote this intellectual work.

Attempts to classify nursing phenomena have produced a fair amount of criticism by nurses and others. The criticism has varied from a concern that the largely inductive approach was atheoretical and not deduced from nursing theories to assertions that nursing was being too circumscribed and partisan in defining its knowledge.

The classification of nursing phenomena is a substantial departure from development of the conceptual frameworks and theories that characterized attempts by nurses in the 1960s and 1970s to describe nursing knowledge. The classifications reflected in this book are, in fact, based on very broad conceptual frameworks that provide structure within and among the characterization of problems, interventions, and outcomes. By not embracing a particular theory, the classifications deal with nursing's core concepts in such a way that they can be used across multiple theories. Additionally, the varying levels of abstraction in the classifications present greater opportunity for empirical testing of the conceptual components and the relationships among them. The criticism that classification systems are atheoretical ignores the value of the broad conceptual frameworks reflected in the classifications. The

frameworks are both more abstract than many nursing theories and at the same time less abstract in the lower-level concepts that are directly related to practice. They provide the basis for the development and testing of multiple middle-range theories, which are much needed in nursing. The work reflected in this book could just as well have been done with neonates, children, women's or men's health, critical care, primary care, or the innumerable other ways in which nursing practice conceivably can be conceptualized.

The criticism that development of nursing classification systems is too partisan and unrelated to contemporary interdisciplinary practice ignores the important fact that interdisciplinary does not mean single discipline. It means that multiple disciplines combine their knowledge and practice in ways that complement the contributions of each other and ultimately result in better patient care. To be truly interdisciplinary, each discipline must understand what it has to offer. Otherwise, there may as well be one large discipline of health care with everyone doing essentially the same things. There is an extensive literature on how health care often has been and is viewed as synonymous with medical care. Although not so prominent in discussions today, the sociologic and professional literature of the 1960s and 1970s was replete with discussions regarding the nature of professionalism, including what comprises professions and how they differ from one another. To say that contemporary practice is interdisciplinary is not to say that there no longer is need for individual disciplines to define clearly what they know, what they do, and how this overlaps with what others know and do. This book, which applies nursing classification to care of elders, illustrates well what nursing is and how it overlaps and at the same time is distinguished from other disciplines.

It is even more important today than yesterday that nursing provide the scientific evidence for its practice as roles in the health care system become more blurred and as demands for evidence-based practice escalate, as they will. The Pew Taskforce Report (1995) in the early 1990s showed dramatic oversupply of physicians, approximately 25%. It also showed an oversupply of nurses at that time, which was substantially less than that of physicians and others. The physician oversupply, combined with continuing emphasis on reducing health care costs, is the basis for increased competitiveness. There is competition between primary care physicians and specialist physicians and between physicians and advanced practice nurses. Both kinds of conflict will increase rather than decrease in the foreseeable future. Thus it is important that nurses not only make clear what it is that they do, but also that they document the outcomes on patients and costs, showing when nurses outperform physicians or are more cost-effective, or when nurse-physician care produces better patient outcomes than care by either discipline alone.

The clarification of a profession and its contributions cannot be done by individual nurse researchers and clinicians working in isolation of each other or separately addressing different components of nursing. There is need for research and researchers to be supported by nursing collectively and for nursing to use the results of research as the basis for its political actions. The issue of how organized nursing can best represent the interests of all nurses is an old and continuing one. Recent years have seen a proliferation of specialty groups within nursing that parallels the multiple specialties in other disciplines. This is to be expected in a pluralistic society and in a profession as large and diverse as nursing. At the same time there is a need for the separate components of a profession to come together, either in coalitions for specific purposes or to establish more stable ways to coordinate and capitalize on the strength of the individual components. At an earlier time, this unity among diverse parts was represented by the American Nurses Association (ANA), when that association was one of only a few nursing organizations. During the 1960s and even into the 1980s, many researchers and clinicians identified with ANA collectively, as well as with special interest groups organized within ANA. During the 1990s, special interest groups within ANA have been eliminated or greatly weakened as the organization changed its structure, functions, and priorities. This has resulted in lack of a highly visible national forum in which interested nurse researchers and clinicians can combine their efforts to politically advance nursing at the national level. It was, for example, nurse researchers and others within organized nursing who in the early 1980s combined their efforts under the leadership of the American Nurses Association and in collaboration with the American Association of Colleges of Nursing and the National League of Nursing to articulate research needs for nursing. They were successful in moving nursing research out of the Health Resources and Services Administration and into the National Institutes of Health, which is the mainstream of health care.

The separation of nurse researchers and research from ANA's national political agenda inevitably must result in a weaker presentation of nursing. For example, at a time when nurse researchers were making enormous strides in defining the phenomena of nursing and in establishing nursing's research base, their work was essentially ignored by ANA in its articulation of patient outcomes relevant to nurses. Rather than capitalizing on the richness of nursing research, ANA contracted with an organization outside of nursing to identify measures of nursing process and nursing-sensitive patient outcomes. The resulting product, or "report card," is an overly narrow and unnecessarily restricted view of nursing that reflects the lowest common denominator of nursing practice (ANA, 1995). The report did not make visible the valuable contributions of nurses demonstrated in this book and other publications. Instead, the outcomes selected included only patient satisfaction, nosocomial infection rate, patient injury rate, and maintenance of skin integrity. We have the unusual situation in which a major nursing organization attempted to make nursing visible by depending solely on the very health care record that admittedly underrepresents and underestimates nursing! Major resources are being spent in trying to document the presence of these few bits of nursing in present systems. Thus an effort presumably intended to make nursing visible has the exact opposite effect of minimizing its contributions.

The implication of this is the imperative that the work of nurse scholars and clinicians be adequately represented in organized nursing's political efforts. The individuals and groups of scholars who develop the knowledge base for nursing cannot be expected to take sole responsibility for using that knowledge to advance nursing politically. Many clinicians and researchers, of course, will be involved in the political process, but it is critical that organized nursing go beyond what these individuals can do on their own. There is a clear and present need for some component of organized nursing or some coalition of nursing organizations to give serious attention to using research to make nursing more visible in health care. It is difficult at this juncture in nursing's history to know how nursing's researchers and its political agenda can best be joined, but it is clear that such unification must occur if nursing is to advance. Furthermore, organized nursing must be aggressive in ensuring an adequate funding base for nursing research and vigilant in seeing that the funding is used to promote research on significant nursing problems.

The intellectual and clinical work presented in this book is an excellent example of what individual researchers and clinicians can do to advance the field. It is up to nurses collectively to decide if and how organized nursing can mobilize its resources to advance nursings' agenda in the political arena.

REFERENCES

Agency for Health Care Policy and Research. (1998). *AHCPR's evidence-based practice centers. AHCPR fact sheet.* Rockville, MD: Author.

American Nurses Association. (1995). *Nursing care report card for acute care.* Washington, DC: Author.

American Nurses Association Steering Committee. (1995). *Nursing data systems: The emerging framework.* Washington, DC: American Nurses Association.

Cochrane Collaboration. (1998). Second Edition. Oxford, England: Update software.

Horsley, J. A., & Crane, J. (1983). *Using research to improve nursing practice: A guide.* New York: Grune and Stratton.

Jacox, A. (1991). Epilogue: Implications for policy, theory, research, and practice. In M. Maas, K. Buckwalter, & M. Hardy (Eds.), *Nursing diagnoses and interventions for the elderly* (pp. 615-620). New York: Addison Wesley Longman.

Maas, M., & Jacox, A. (1977, December). Guidelines for nurse autonomy: Reality not rhetoric. *American Journal of Nursing,* 2201-2208.

Medical Alert. (1989). A staff report summarizing the hearings in "The future of health care in America." *Subcommittee on Education and Health, Joint Economic Committee, Congress of the United States* (pp. 101-151). Washington, DC: U.S. Government Printing Office.

Pew Taskforce Report. (1995). *Critical challenges: Revitalizing the health professions for the twenty-first century.* San Francisco, CA: Pew Center for Health Professionals.

Sackett, D. (1997). *Evidence-based medicine: How to practice and teach EBM.* New York: Churchill Livingstone.

WEBSITE RESOURCES

http://arborcom.com

Arbor Nutrition Guide. A roadmap to quality nutrition links. This site offers in-depth information on nutrition based on current information from academic research and government sources.

http://chid.nih.gov

The Combined Health Information Database. Contains considerable health information and health education resources. Many of the materials are not indexed any other place. There is a special section on health promotion and health promotion education.

http://home.cybergrrl.com/dv/stats.html

Healthgrrl: Violence Resources for Women. Statistical resources on domestic violence and its relationship to issues such as those related to pregnancy, children, teen relationships, and elder abuse.

http://www.aafp.org/nsi

The American Academy of Family Physicians' Nutrition Screening Initiative site. Overview of the Nutrition Screening Initiatives and links to Nutrition Screening Initiative materials.

http://www.acjnet.org/

ACJNet Elder Abuse. The Access to Justice Network (ACJNet) is an electronic community that brings together people, information, and educational resources on Canadian justice and legal issues.

http://www.ahcpr.gov

Agency for Healthcare Research and Quality (AHRQ) has published many clinical practice guidelines about urinary incontinence.

http://www.alzheimers.org

The Alzheimer's Disease Education and Referral Center website. Here you will find information about Alzheimer's disease and related disorders.

http://www.alz.org

The Alzheimer's Association home page.

http://www.aoa.dhhs.gov/abuse/report/default.htm

The National Elder Abuse Incidence Study from the Administration on Aging.

http://www.apic.org

The Association for Professionals in Infection Control and Epidemiology website.

http://www.asaging.org/networks/forsa/forsa.html

American Society on Aging site. Constitutes a large national, multidisciplinary, and nondenominational community of professionals committed to examining and fostering the expression of the spiritual dimension of human existence and its role in the aging process.

http://www.bsos.umd.edu/socy/rosenberg.htm

University of Maryland Department of Sociology site. Provides access to the Rosenberg Self-Esteem Scale.

http://www.cdc.gov

The Centers for Disease Control and Prevention website.

http://www.crha-health.ab.ca/hlthconn/items/elder-ab.htm

Calgary Regional Health Authority. Abuse of the Elderly. Elder abuse definitions and prevention.

http://www.depression.com

Depression.com site. Sponsored by Squibb and provides helpful information about living with a depressed person and depression in special groups (elderly).

http://www.elderabuselaw.com/links/eabuse.html

Michael Schwartz's Compendium of Elder Abuse Law. The site claims to be the Internet's comprehensive resource for elder abuse and related law. The library and archives contain source materials, compilations, and articles concerning elder abuse, nursing homes, fiduciaries, consumer protection, and related topics.

http://www.hs.ttu.edu/sexuality&aging

Texas Tech University site. Addresses sexual issues for aging adults.

http://www.iog.wayne.edu

Wayne State University Institute of Gerontology. Contains information for those interested in gerontology, geriatrics, the process of aging, services for the elderly, or concerns of senior citizens in general.

http://www.library.utoronto.ca/www/aging/onpea.htm

Ontario Network for the Prevention of Elder Abuse. Institute for Human Development, Life Course and Aging, University of Toronto.

http://www.lungusa.org

The American Lung Association website.

http://www.mentalhealth.com

Internet Mental Health site. Has information on 54 of the most common mental disorders, including practice guidelines, and on the 72 most common psychiatric drugs.

http://www.muhealth.org/~son/scdnt/scdnt.html

University of Missouri–Columbia Sinclair School of Nursing. This site is for the discussion and dissemination of information related to Orem's Self-Care Deficit Nursing Theory.

http://www.nafc.org

The National Association for Continence (NAFC) website includes sections on "Facts About Urinary Incontinence," "How to Get Help," and "Frequently Asked Questions (FAQ)," as well as the organizational newsletter and links to related websites.

http://www.ncoa.org

The National Council on the Aging. National Interfaith Coalition on Aging. Includes representatives from all faiths, as well as others concerned with religion and aging. The coalition supports individual religious groups that serve older people.

http://www.niddk.nih.gov

National Institute of Diabetes and Digestive and Kidney Diseases (NIDDK) of the National Institutes of Health (NIH). National Kidney & Urologic Disease Information Clearinghouse.

http://www.npuap.org

The National Pressure Ulcer Advisory Panel website.

http://www.nursing.uiowa.edu/research/index.htm

The University of Iowa College of Nursing Research page containing research information regarding the elderly.

http://www.nursing.uiowa.edu/sites/chronicwound

University of Iowa College of Nursing Chronic Wound Healing site. The site is a brief tutorial on various aspects of chronic wound care. It is part of a larger CD-I (Compact Disc Interaction) created to teach chronic wound care to health care professionals.

http://www.nvc.org

National Center for Victims of Crime. Victim's advocacy organization that helps all types of victims such as victims of stalking, rape, sexual assault, and elder abuse.

http://www.senioract.com

Senior Act site. This site is for activity directors working in long-term care facilities and adult day care, retirement, assisted living, subacute, and skilled care centers. It is an area where activity directors can come to obtain instant activity program ideas, resources, and information on activity conferences in the nation.

http://www.walkers.org

Walkers web. One of the top 10 mental health websites of 1999 by Newguide. Has extensive information on mood disorder, treatment, resources, news, live chat, and bookstore.

MEMBERSHIP APPLICATION

Last Name: _____ First: _____ MI: ___

Home Address: _____

_____

City/State/Zip/Country: _____

Home telephone number: _____

FAX number: _____

E-mail: _____

Place of Employment: _____

Position or Title: _____

Business address: _____

City/State/Zip/Country: _____

Business telephone number: _____

FAX number: _____

E-mail: _____

Current RN license number: _____

State/province: _____

Demographic data (circle one in each category):

Initial nursing education:

      Diploma, Associate degree, Baccalaureate
      degree, Other

Highest degree held: BS, BSN, MS, MSN, PhD,
      DNSc, EdD, Other _____

Primary function:

      Administrator, Manager, Clinician, Staff
      Nurse, Consultant, Educator, Researcher
      Clinical Nurse Specialist, Nurse Practitioner,
      Other (Specify) _____

Area of specialization:

      Community Health, Maternal/Newborn,
      Parent/Child, Medical/Surgical, Nursing of
      Children, Critical Care, Psychiatry/Mental
      Health, Gerontology, Long-Term Care, Health
      Promotion, Nursing Administration,
      Rehabilitation, Perioperative Nursing,
      Ambulatory Care, Nursing Informatics

Are you a member of the ANA? Yes _____ No _____

Membership Fee

Regular Membership: $85.00*

Student or Retired RN Membership: $65.00*

Associate Membership: $85.00*

     *$29.00 is for a subscription to Nursing Diagnosis:
     The Journal of Nursing Language & Classification.*

Indicate Method of Payment: Checks* or money
orders should be made payable to NANDA.

     NANDA cannot accept checks in foreign currencies.

_____ Check   _____ Money Order

_____ MasterCard   _____ VISA

If using credit card complete:

Card No:

Exp. Date:

Copy this application form and send it to:

NANDA

1211 Locust St.

Philadelphia, PA 19107

FAX 215.545.8107

E-mail: NANDA@NURSECOMINC.COM

NURSING-SENSITIVE OUTCOMES CLASSIFICATION REVIEW FORM

The Nursing-Sensitive Outcomes Classification (NOC) research team is interested in feedback and submission of outcomes for review and potential addition to the NOC. Suggestions and submissions may be sent by letter or e-mail to the following address:

Lori Penaluna
Project Director
Nursing-Sensitive Outcomes Classification
462 NB, College of Nursing
The University of Iowa
Iowa City, Iowa 52242
E-mail: lori-penaluna@uiowa.edu
Phone: (319) 353-5414
FAX: (319) 335-6820

A. General Comments About the Classification

Comments about the classification in general are welcome, as are suggestions for outcomes that need to be developed.

B. Feedback on a Particular Outcome

If the submission is a revision of an existing NOC outcome, provide a paragraph clearly describing the rationale for changes, and note the changes on a copy of the existing outcome. Suggestions can include changes in the definition, indicators, or scale. Additional indicators also can be suggested.

C. Guidelines for Outcome Submission

All submissions should be typed. Three copies of all materials should be submitted. Background readings/references should be typed in American Psychological Association format. Each submission of a proposed outcome must include a label, a definition, indicators, and a short list of references that support the outcome and indicators. You also may suggest a scale to use with the outcomes. A brief paragraph describing the rationale for adding the outcome to the NOC should be included. The rationale should note how the proposed outcome is different from outcomes already included in the NOC.

General Principles for Developing Outcomes

1. Define the outcome as a variable patient or client state, behavior, or perception that is responsive to nursing intervention(s).
2. Labels should be concise, stated in five words or fewer.
3. Colons can be used to make broader concepts more specific.
4. Labels should describe concepts that can be measured along a continuum.
5. Labels should be neutral and *not* stated as goals.
6. A group of indicators that are more specific than the outcome must be listed for use in determining the status of the outcome.
7. The definition should be a brief phrase that defines the concept and encompasses the indicators.

GUIDELINES FOR SUBMISSION OF A NEW OR REVISED INTERVENTION

This appendix contains materials to assist you in preparing an intervention to submit for review or to suggest a change for an existing intervention. It is important that a submitter be familiar with NIC and with the Principles for Intervention Development and Refinement (included in this Appendix) before developing or revising an intervention.

The Materials Needed

All submissions should be typed and formatted in the same style as appears in NIC. *Three copies* of all materials should be submitted. Background readings/references should be typed in APA format. Materials that are too difficult to read or incomplete will be sent back to the submitter without being reviewed.

Each submission of a **proposed new intervention** should include a label, a definition, activities listed in logical order, and a short list of background readings that support the intervention. In addition, a *rationale for inclusion* should also be attached and the submitter *should note how the proposed new intervention differs from existing interventions.* If a new intervention would call for changes in existing interventions, these changes should also be submitted. The Demographic Information Form should be filled out and included.

Each submission for a **revised intervention** should indicate how the proposed changes relate to the existing intervention. In most instances a copy of the intervention from the NIC book with additions, deletions, and modifications made on the copy will be the best way to clearly indicate changes. If changes are substantial, however, the revised intervention should be retyped with the current intervention attached. A rationale must also be included. The Demographic Information Form should be filled out and included.

The Review Process

1. Submitted materials for proposed new or revised interventions are assigned to two or three reviewers who have expertise in the content area and who are familiar with NIC.
2. The reviewers receive a copy of what has been submitted and a review form.
3. The reviewers are asked to return their comments and their recommendations within 1 month. The initial submission and the reviewers' comments are then reviewed by the research team and a decision is made.
4. Approximately 2 to 6 months after submission, the submitter will receive a letter stating the outcome of the process and will receive a copy of the reviewers' comments. If the decision is for inclusion in NIC, the submitter will be acknowledged in the next edition.

Principles for Intervention Development and Refinement

A set of guiding principles is necessary in forming intervention labels, definitions, and activities. Such principles, used to maintain consistency and cohesion within the Classification, can help the user to understand the Classification's language and form.

General Principles for Intervention Labels. Intervention labels are concepts. The following principles should be used when selecting names for concepts.

1. They should be noun statements; no verbs.
2. They should, preferably, be three words or less; no more than five words.
3. When a two-part label is required, use a colon to separate the words (e.g., Bleeding Reduction: Nasal). Guidelines for use of the colon are: (1) avoid unless it is indicated and desired by clinical practice and (2) use to indicate a more specialized area of practice only when there are different activities that require a new intervention.
4. Capitalize each word.
5. Labels will include modifiers to represent the nurse's actions. Choose modifiers to represent the nurse's actions (e.g., Administration, Assistance, Management, Promotion). The modifier should be selected based on its meaning, how it sounds in relationship to the other words in the label, and its acceptability in general practice. Some of the possible modifiers are listed here:
   Administration—directing the movement or behavior of, having charge of; see also Management

Assistance—helping

Care—paying close attention, giving protection, being concerned about

Enhancement—making greater, augmenting, increasing; see also Promotion

Maintenance—continuing or carrying on, supporting

Management—directing the movement or behavior of, having charge of; see also Administration

Monitoring—watching and checking

Precaution—taking care beforehand against a possible danger; see also Protection

Promotion—advancing; see also Enhancement

Protection—shielding from injury; see also Precaution

Reduction—lessening, diminishing

Restoration—reinstating, bringing back to normal or unimpaired state

Therapy—having a therapeutic nature, healing

NOTE: Some of these terms mean the same thing; a choice of which one to use will depend upon which sounds better in context and whether one is already more familiar and more accepted in practice.

General Principles for Definitions of Interventions.
A definition for an intervention label is a phrase that defines the concept. It is a summary of the most distinguishing characteristics. The definition, together with the defining activities, delineates the boundaries of nurse behavior circumscribed by the label.

1. Use phrases (not complete sentences) that describe the behavior of the nurse and can stand alone without examples.
2. Avoid using terms for the patient and nurse, but when a term must be used, *patient* or *person* is preferred rather than *client*.
3. For those phrases that begin with a verb form, consider the situation and choose either the -ion form (e.g., limitation) or the -ing form (e.g., limiting).

General Principles for Activities.
Activities are actions that a nurse does to implement the intervention. The following principles relate to activities:

1. Begin each activity with a verb. Possible verbs include *assist, administer, explain, avoid, inspect, facilitate, monitor,* and *use*. Use the most active verb that is appropriate for the situation. Use the term *monitor* rather than *assess*. Monitoring is a type of assessment but is done postdiagnosis as part of an intervention rather than as preparation for making a diagnosis. Avoid the terms *observe* and *evaluate*.
2. Keep the activities as generic as possible (e.g., instead of saying, "Place on Kinair bed" or "Place on circlelectric bed," say, "Place on therapeutic bed"). Eliminate brand names.
3. Avoid combining two different ideas in one activity unless they illustrate the same point.
4. Avoid repeating an idea; when two activities are saying the same thing, even in different words, eliminate one.
5. Focus on the critical activities; do not worry about including all supporting activities. The number of activities depends on the intervention, but, on average, use a one-page list.
6. Word similar activities modifying different interventions the same for each intervention.
7. Word activities so they are clear without referring to the patient or the nurse. If the patient must be referred to, use the term *patient* or *person* in preference to *client* or other terms. Use the terms *family member(s)* or *significant other(s)* rather than *spouse*.
8. Add the phrase "as appropriate," "as necessary," or "as needed" to the end of those activities that are important but used only on some occasions.
9. Check for consistency between the activities and the label's definition.
10. Arrange the activities in the order in which they are usually carried out, when appropriate.

DEMOGRAPHIC INFORMATION FORM

(Please complete and submit with new/revised intervention[s].)

Please complete the following:

1. Are you currently employed as an RN?
   ___ (1) Yes ___ (2) No, am an RN but not currently employed as an RN
   ___ (3) No, am studying to be an RN ___ (4) No, am not an RN

2. How long have you practiced as an RN?
   ___ (0) Not practiced as an RN
   ___ (1) One Year or Less
   ___ (2) 1 to 3 Years
   ___ (3) 3 to 5 Years
   ___ (4) 5 to 10 Years
   ___ (5) Over 10 Years

3. Which of the following *best* describes the setting in which you are employed? (Check only one area.)
   ___ (1) Hospital
   ___ (2) Long-Term Care
   ___ (3) Public/Community Health
   ___ (4) Occupational Health
   ___ (5) Office Nursing
   ___ (6) School Nursing
   ___ (7) Outpatient Setting
   ___ (8) Nursing Education
   ___ (9) Other (specify) _____

4. Which of the following *best* describes the type of unit/specialty area in which you practice? (Check only *ONE* area)
   ___ (1) General Medicine
   ___ (2) General Surgery
   ___ (3) Intensive Care
   ___ (4) OB/GYN/Pediatrics
   ___ (5) Specialty Medicine
   ___ (6) Specialty Surgery
   ___ (7) Psychiatric (adult or child)
   ___ (8) Ambulatory Care/Outpatient
   ___ (9) General Long-term Care/Rehabilitation
   ___ (10) Other

5. What is your *highest* level of educational preparation?
   ___ (1) Associate Degree
   ___ (2) Diploma
   ___ (3) Baccalaureate
   ___ (4) Master's
   ___ (5) Doctorate

6. Are you currently certified by any professional organizations?
   ___ (1) Yes ___ (2) No

7. How have you used the Classification?
   ___ Clinical Practice
   ___ Teaching
   ___ Research
   ___ Administration
   ___ Other (please specify) _____

   _____

Please elaborate on how you have used the Classification:

General comments about the Classification:

If your suggestions are included in NIC, we would like to acknowledge your help in the next edition. Please sign here if you will permit us to include your name as a contributor.

   Print your name _____
   Employment title _____
   Place of employment _____
   Street _____
   City, State, and ZIP Code _____
   Telephone _____
   E-mail address _____

Please mail or fax this form along with your proposed new or revised intervention(s) to:

> **Center for Nursing Classification**
> **NIC Review**
> **The University of Iowa College of Nursing**
> **Iowa City, Iowa 52242-1121**
>
> **Fax: (319) 335-6820 or (319) 335-9990**

INDEX

Page references followed by "f" indicate
figures, "t" indicate tables, and "b" indicate
boxes.

Nursing interventions—cont'd
diversional activity
deficits—cont'd
client advocacy, 42-43
description of, 40, 41b-43b
drug holidays, 43-44
interdisciplinary approach, 40
medication administration goals
clearly defined, 40
monitoring, 40, 42
dry skin
bathing, 139t, 141-142
description of, 141
emollients, 142
humidity, 142
soap, 141
falls, 27-30, 28b-29b
fear, 585-586
fever, 213
financial abuse, 108t-109t
fluid volume deficit
description of, 186
fluid and electrolyte
monitoring, 187t
intravenous therapy, 188b
grief and grieving
description of, 639-640,
647t-648t
empathy, 640-642
feelings, 643
nonjudgmental approach, 640,
642
unconditional positive regard,
640, 642-643
guidelines for submission of, 807-
808
gustatory sensory impairment,
485-486
health promotion, 79-82
hearing loss, 485-486
heatstroke, 213
hemianopsia, 500-501
home maintenance management,
impaired, 70-71
hopelessness, 525b, 532t, 604t-
605t, 608-609
hypernatremia, 196, 197b-198b
hyperthermia, 213
knowledge deficit
counseling, 512
description of, 506-507
learning
impediments to
cognitive impairments,
509-510
lack of confidence, 510

Nursing interventions—cont'd
knowledge deficit—cont'd
literacy level, 511
memory difficulties, 510
motivation, 510
sensory impairments,
508-509
principles of, 507-508
strategies for, 511
transfer of, 508
video materials for
enhancing, 511
support groups, 512
teaching
cultural effects, 509
principles of, 507-508
repetition, 508
written materials for, 511-512
pain
analgesics
adjuvant agents, 468
administration routes, 468
description of, 466-467
dosing of, 468
nonopioid, 467-468
opioid, 467
cognitive-behavioral, 470
cutaneous stimulation, 469
description of, 465-466
massage, 470
nonpharmacologic, 468-469
nonsteroidal anti-inflammatory
drugs, 467-468
thermal agents, 469
transcutaneous electrical nerve
stimulation, 469-470
perception alterations
counseling, 485-486
environmental, 483-485
referral, 486
powerlessness, 532t, 566-568, 567b
pressure ulcers
bacterial control, 131
debridement and cleansing, 130
description of, 129-130
dressings, 130-131
moist wound environment,
130-131
overview of, 129t
preventing further injury,
131-132
substrates, 131
reflex incontinence, 255t
relocation stress syndrome, 623-
626, 627b
self-care deficits, 376-379

Nursing interventions—cont'd
self-esteem disturbances, 598-599
sensory impairment and
alterations
counseling, 485-486
environmental, 483-485
referral, 486
sexual dysfunction, 743-746
sleep, 406-408
social isolation, 653t, 659-661
spiritual distress, 787t-788t,
789-791
stress incontinence, 254t-255t
submission of, 807-808
suicide, 533
thermoregulation, 213
unilateral neglect
deficit-specific types of, 499-500
denial, 500
description of, 496-497
family intervention, 499
psychosocial support, 499
safety support, 499
sensory input, 497-499
urinary incontinence
bladder training, 271-272
catheterization, 273-274
description of, 254t-257t,
269-270
fluid increases, 272-273
habit training, 271-272
nonpharmacologic, 269t
pelvic floor exercises, 270-271
pharmacologic, 269t
urinary tract infections, 52
violence, 701-702
vision impairments, 483-486
Nursing languages, 794
Nursing phenomena, 800
Nutrition. see also Malnutrition
alcoholism effects, 119
altered (less than body
requirements)
assessment of
anthropometric
measurements, 149
biochemical tests, 149-150
clinical measures for, 147
description of, 147
laboratory tests, 149-150
nutrient intake, 148-149
tools for, 150
case study example of, 152, 155
description of, 145
indicators of, 148t
NANDA diagnosis, 150, 152b